ICD-10-PCS Code Book

Professional Edition

2022

Anne B. Casto, RHIA, CCS
Consulting Editor

AHIMA
American Health Information Management Association®

ISBN: 978-1-58426-848-2
AHIMA Product No.: AC222221

AHIMA Staff:
Rachel Schratz, MA, Assistant Editor
Christine Scheid, Content Development Manager
Megan Grennan, Director, Content Production and AHIMA Press
James Pinnick, Vice President, Content and Product Development

Cover image: © knikola, Shutterstock

The Centers for Medicare and Medicaid Services (CMS) and the National Center for Health Statistics (NCHS), two departments within the US Federal Government's Department of Health and Human Services (HHS) provide the *International Classification of Diseases, Tenth Revision, Clinical Modification* (ICD-10-CM) for coding and reporting. ICD-10-CM is the US modification to the World Health Organization's (WHO) International Classification of Diseases, Tenth Revision (ICD-10).

Coding Clinic for ICD-10-CM and ICD-10-PCS is a publication of the American Hospital Association (AHA).

For more information about AHIMA Press publications, including updates, visit https://www.ahima.org/education-events/education-by-product/books/

American Health Information Management Association
233 North Michigan Avenue, 21st Floor
Chicago, Illinois 60601-5809
ahima.org

Contents

About the Consulting Editor

Anne B. Casto, RHIA, CCS, is the president of Casto Consulting, LLC. Casto Consulting, LLC is a consulting firm that provides services to hospitals and other healthcare stakeholders primarily in the areas of reimbursement and coding. Casto Consulting, LLC specializes in linking coding and billing practices to positive revenue cycle outcomes. Additionally, the firm provides guidance to consulting firms, healthcare organizations and healthcare insurers regarding reimbursement methodologies and Medicare regulations.

Additionally, Ms. Casto is a lecturer in the HIMS department at The Ohio State University, School of Health and Rehabilitation Sciences. Over the past 20 years, Ms. Casto has taught numerous courses in the areas of healthcare reimbursement, coding, healthcare data trending, and coding analytics.

Prior to her current roles, Ms. Casto was the vice president of clinical information for Cleverley & Associates where she worked very closely with APC regulations and guidelines, preparing hospitals for the implementation of the Medicare OPPS. Ms. Casto was also the clinical information product manager for CHIPS/Ingenix. She joined CHIPS/Ingenix in 1998 and spent the majority of her time developing coding compliance products for the inpatient and outpatient settings.

Ms. Casto has been responsible for inpatient and outpatient coding activities in several large hospitals including Mt. Sinai Medical Center (NYC), Beth Israel Medical Center (NYC), and The Ohio State University. She worked extensively with CMI, quality measures, physician documentation, and coding accuracy efforts at these facilities.

Ms. Casto received her degree in Health Information Management at The Ohio State University in 1995. She received her Certified Coding Specialist credential in 1998 from the American Health Information Management Association. In 2009 Ms. Casto received her ICD-10-CM/PCS Trainer certificate from AHIMA. Ms. Casto is the author of an AHIMA-published textbook entitled *Principles of Healthcare Reimbursement*. Additionally, Ms. Casto was a contributing author to the published AHIMA books: *Severity DRGs and Reimbursement; A MS-DRG Primer* and *Effective Management of Coding Services.*

Ms. Casto received the AHIMA Legacy Award, part of the FORE Triumph Awards, in 2007 which honors a significant contribution to the knowledge base of the HIM field through an insightful publication. Additionally, Ms. Casto was honored with the Ohio Health Information Management Association's Distinguished Member Award in 2008 and the Ohio Health Information Management Association's Professional Achievement Award in 2011.

Acknowledgments

Many thanks to my family for their support during this project. Thanks to Dr. Susan White, The Ohio State University; your data manipulation skills are second to none. I thank the reviewers for their thoughtful comments and suggestions. Many thanks to Linda Hyde, RHIA, and Rachael D'Andrea, MS, RHIA, CHTS-TR, CPHQ for their very thorough technical review of the book.

ICD-10-PCS Overview

The *International Classification of Diseases, Tenth Revision, Procedure Coding System* (ICD-10-PCS) was created to accompany the World Health Organization's (WHO) ICD-10 diagnosis classification. This coding system was developed to replace ICD-9-CM procedure codes for reporting inpatient procedures. ICD-10-PCS was designed to enable each code to have a standard structure and be very descriptive, and yet flexible enough to accommodate future needs.

History of ICD-10-PCS

The WHO has maintained the International Classification of Diseases (ICD) for recording cause of death since 1893. It has updated the ICD periodically to reflect new discoveries in epidemiology and changes in medical understanding of disease. The International Classification of Diseases Tenth Revision (ICD-10), published in 1992, is the latest revision of the ICD. The WHO authorized the National Center for Health Statistics (NCHS) to develop a clinical modification of ICD-10 for use in the United States. This version of ICD-10 is called ICD-10-CM, and is intended to replace the previous US clinical modification, ICD-9-CM, that had been in use since 1979. ICD-9-CM contains a procedure classification; ICD-10-CM does not.

The Centers for Medicare and Medicaid Services (CMS), the agency responsible for maintaining the inpatient procedure code set in the United States, contracted with 3M Health Information Systems in 1993 to design and then develop a procedure classification system to replace Volume 3 of ICD-9-CM. ICD-10-PCS is the result. ICD-10-PCS was initially released in 1998. It has been updated annually since that time.

ICD-10-PCS Design

ICD-10-PCS is fundamentally different from previous procedure classification systems in its structure, organization, and capabilities. It was designed and developed to adhere to recommendations made by the National Committee on Vital and Health Statistics (NCVHS). It also incorporates input from a wide range of organizations, individual physicians, healthcare professionals, and researchers. Several structural attributes were recommended for a new procedure coding system. These attributes include a multiaxial structure, completeness, and expandability.

Multiaxial Structure

The key attribute that provides the framework for all other structural attributes is multiaxial code structure. *Multiaxial code structure* makes it possible for the ICD-10-PCS to be complete, expandable, and provide a high degree of flexibility and functionality.

ICD-10-PCS codes are composed of seven characters. Each character represents a category of information that can be specified about the procedure performed. A character defines both the category of information and its physical position in the code. A character's position can be understood as a semi-independent axis of classification that allows different specific values to be inserted into that space, and whose physical position remains stable. Within a defined code range, a character retains the general meaning that it confers on any value in that position.

Completeness

Completeness is considered a key structural attribute for a new procedure coding system. The specific recommendation for completeness included that a unique code be available for each significant procedure, that each code retain its unique definition, and that codes that have been deleted are not reused.

In ICD-10-PCS, a unique code is constructed for every significantly different procedure. Within each section, a character defines a consistent component of a code, and contains all applicable values for that character. The values define individual expressions (Open, Percutaneous) of the character's general meaning (approach) that are then used to construct unique procedure codes. Because all approaches by which a procedure is performed are assigned a separate approach value, every procedure which uses a different approach will have its own unique code. This is true of the other characters as well. The same procedure performed on a different body part has its own unique code; the same procedure performed using a different device has its own unique code, and so on.

Because ICD-10-PCS codes are constructed of individual values rather than lists of fixed codes and text descriptions, the unique, stable definition of a code in the system is retained. New values may be added to the system to represent a specific new approach or device or qualifier, but whole codes by design cannot be given new meanings and reused.

Expandability

Expandability was also recommended as a key structural attribute. The specific recommendation for expandability included that the system be capable of accommodating new procedures and technology and that these new codes could be added to the system without disrupting the existing structure.

ICD-10-PCS is designed to be easily updated as new codes are required for new procedures and new techniques. Changes to ICD-10-PCS can all be made within the existing structure because whole codes are not added. Instead, a new value for a character can be added to the system as needed. Likewise, an existing value for a character can be added to a table(s) in the system.

ICD-10-PCS Additional Characteristics

ICD-10-PCS possesses several additional characteristics in response to government and industry recommendations. These characteristics are

- Standardized terminology within the coding system
- Standardized level of specificity
- No diagnostic information
- No explicit "not otherwise specified" (NOS) code options
- Limited use of "not elsewhere classified" (NEC) code options

Standardized Terminology

Words commonly used in clinical vocabularies may have multiple meanings. This can cause confusion and result in inaccurate data. ICD-10-PCS is standardized and self-contained. Characters and values used in the system are defined in the system. For example, the word *excision* is used to describe a wide variety of surgical procedures. In ICD-10-PCS, the word *excision* describes a single, precise surgical objective, defined as "cutting out or off, without replacement, a portion of a body part."

No Eponyms or Common Procedure Names

The terminology used in ICD-10-PCS is standardized to provide precise and stable definitions of all procedures performed. This standardized terminology is used in all ICD-10-PCS code descriptions. As a result, ICD-10-PCS code descriptions do not include eponyms or common procedure names.

In ICD-10-PCS, physicians' names are not included in a code description, nor are procedures identified by common terms or acronyms such as appendectomy or CABG. Instead, such procedures are coded to the root operation that accurately identifies the objective of the procedure.

ICD-10-PCS assigns procedure codes according to the root operation that matches the objective of the procedure. By relying on the universal objectives defined in root operations rather than eponyms or specific procedure titles that change or become obsolete, ICD-10-PCS preserves the capacity to define past, present, and future procedures accurately using stable terminology in the form of characters and values.

No Combination Codes

With rare exceptions, ICD-10-PCS does not define multiple procedures with one code. This is to preserve standardized terminology and consistency across the system. A procedure that meets the reporting criteria for a separate procedure is coded separately in ICD-10-PCS. This allows the system to respond to changes in technology and medical practice with the maximum degree of stability and flexibility.

Standardized Level of Specificity

ICD-10-PCS provides a standardized level of specificity for each code, so each code represents a single procedure variation. In general, ICD-10-PCS code descriptions are much more specific than previous procedure classification systems but sometimes an ICD-10-PCS code description is actually less specific. ICD-10-PCS provides a standardized level of specificity that can be predicted across the system.

Diagnosis Information Excluded

Another key feature of ICD-10-PCS is that information pertaining to a diagnosis is excluded from the code descriptions. Adding diagnosis information limits the flexibility and functionality of a procedure coding system. It has the effect of placing a code "off limits" because the diagnosis in the medical record does not match the diagnosis in the procedure code description. The code cannot be used even though the procedural part of the code description precisely matches the procedure performed. Diagnosis information is not contained in any ICD-10-PCS code. The diagnosis codes, not the procedure codes, will specify the reason the procedure is performed.

Not Otherwise Specified (NOS) Code Options Restricted

The standardized level of specificity designed into ICD-10-PCS restricts the use of broadly applicable NOS or unspecified code options in the system. A minimal level of specificity is required to construct a valid code.

Limited Not Elsewhere Classified (NEC) Code Options

NEC options are provided in ICD-10-PCS, but only for specific, limited use. In the Medical and Surgical section, two significant NEC options are the root operation value Q, Repair, and the device value Y, Other Device. The root operation Repair is a true NEC value. It is used only when the procedure performed is not one of the other root operations in the Medical and Surgical section. Other Device, on the other hand, is intended to be used to temporarily define new devices that do not have a specific value assigned, until one can be added to the system. No categories of medical or surgical devices are permanently classified to Other Device.

ICD-10-PCS Code Structure

Undergirding ICD-10-PCS is a logical, consistent structure that informs the system as a whole, down to the level of a single code. This means the process of constructing codes in ICD-10-PCS is also logical and consistent: the spaces of the code, called *characters* are filled with individual letters and numbers, called *values*.

Characters

All codes in ICD-10-PCS are seven characters long. Each character in the seven-character code represents an aspect of the procedure. The following are two examples of the code structure: one from the Medical and Surgical section and one from the Ancillary section.

Medical and Surgical Code Structure

Character 1	Character 2	Character 3	Character 4	Character 5	Character 6	Character 7
Section	Body System	Operation	Body Part	Approach	Device	Qualifier

Imaging Section Code Structure

Character 1	Character 2	Character 3	Character 4	Character 5	Character 6	Character 7
Section	Body System	Type	Body Part	Contrast	Qualifier	Qualifier

An ICD-10-PCS code is best understood as the result of a process rather than as an isolated, fixed quantity. The process consists of assigning values from among the valid choices for that part of the system, according to the rules governing the construction of codes.

Values

One of 34 possible values can be assigned to each character in a code: the numbers 0 through 9 and the alphabet (except the letters I and O, because they are easily confused with the numbers 1 and 0). A finished code looks like this: 02103D4.

This code is derived by choosing a specific value for each of the seven characters. Based on details about the procedure performed, values for each character specifying the section, body system, root operation, body part, approach, device, and qualifier are assigned. Because the definition of each character is a function of its physical position in the code, the same value placed in a different position in the code means something different. The value 0 in the first character means something different than 0 in the second character, or 0 in the third character, and so on.

Code Structure Example

The following example defines each character using the code 0LB50ZZ, Excision of right lower arm and wrist tendon, Open approach. This example comes from the Medical and Surgical section of ICD-10-PCS.

Character 1: Section

The first character in the code determines the broad procedure category, or section, where the code is found. In this example, the section is Medical and Surgical. 0 is the value that represents Medical and Surgical in the first character.

Character 1	Character 2	Character 3	Character 4	Character 5	Character 6	Character 7
Section	Body System	Root Operation	Body Part	Approach	Device	Qualifier
0						

Character 2: Body System

The second character defines the body system—the general physiological system or anatomical region involved. Examples of body systems include Lower Arteries, Central Nervous System, and Respiratory System. In this example, the body system is Tendons, represented by the value L.

Character 1	Character 2	Character 3	Character 4	Character 5	Character 6	Character 7
Section	Body System	Root Operation	Body Part	Approach	Device	Qualifier
0	L					

Character 3: Root Operation

The third character defines the root operation, or the objective of the procedure. Some examples of root operations are Bypass, Drainage, and Reattachment. In this example code, the root operation is Excision. When used in the third character of the code, the value B represents Excision.

Character 1	Character 2	Character 3	Character 4	Character 5	Character 6	Character 7
Section	Body System	Root Operation	Body Part	Approach	Device	Qualifier
0	L	B				

Character 4: Body Part

The fourth character defines the body part or specific anatomical site where the procedure was performed. The body system (second character) provides only a general indication of the procedure site. The body part and body system values together provide a precise description of the procedure site. Examples of body parts are Kidney, Tonsils, and Thymus. In this example, the body part value is 5, Lower Arm and Wrist, Right. When the second character is L, the value 5 when used in the fourth character of the code represents the right lower arm and wrist tendon.

Character 1	Character 2	Character 3	Character 4	Character 5	Character 6	Character 7
Section	Body System	Root Operation	Body Part	Approach	Device	Qualifier
0	L	B	5			

Character 5: Approach

The fifth character defines the approach, or the technique used to reach the procedure site. Seven different approach values are used in the Medical and Surgical section to define the approach. Examples of approaches include Open and Percutaneous Endoscopic. In this example code, the approach is Open and is represented by the value 0.

Character 1	Character 2	Character 3	Character 4	Character 5	Character 6	Character 7
Section	Body System	Root Operation	Body Part	Approach	Device	Qualifier
0	L	B	5	0		

Character 6: Device

Depending on the procedure performed, there may be a device left in place at the end of the procedure. The sixth character defines the device. Device values fall into four basic categories:

- Grafts and Prostheses
- Implants
- Simple or Mechanical Appliances
- Electronic Appliances

In this example, there is no device used in the procedure. The value Z is used to represent No Device, as shown here:

Character 1	Character 2	Character 3	Character 4	Character 5	Character 6	Character 7
Section	Body System	Operation	Body Part	Approach	Device	Qualifier
0	L	B	5	0	Z	

Character 7: Qualifier

The seventh character defines a qualifier for the code. A qualifier specifies an additional attribute of the procedure, if applicable. Examples of qualifiers include Diagnostic and Stereotactic. Qualifier choices vary depending on the previous values selected. In this example, there is no specific qualifier applicable to this procedure, so the value is No Qualifier, represented by the letter Z.

Character 1	Character 2	Character 3	Character 4	Character 5	Character 6	Character 7
Section	Body System	Operation	Body Part	Approach	Device	Qualifier
0	L	B	5	0	Z	Z

0LB50ZZ is the complete specification of the procedure "Excision of right lower arm and wrist tendon, open approach."

ICD-10-PCS Organization and Official Conventions

The *ICD-10-PCS Code Book, Professional Edition,* 2022 is based on the official *International Classification of Diseases, Tenth Revision, Procedure Coding System,* issued by the US Department of Health and Human Services (HHS) and CMS. This book is consistent with the content of the government's version of ICD-10-PCS and follows the official conventions.

Index

The Alphabetic Index is provided to assist the user with locating the appropriate table to construct procedure codes. Each table contains all the information required to construct valid procedure codes. Coders should not code from the PCS Index alone; the PCS code tables should always be consulted before assigning a PCS procedure code.

Main Terms

Main terms in the Alphabetic Index reflect the root operations, third character, of procedures. The Index includes not only root operation terms, but also other common procedural terms, anatomical sites, and device terms. The main terms are listed alphabetically. After the coder has located the correct main term and subterm in the Alphabetic Index, he or she is provided with the first three to four digits of the procedure code. The coder should then move to the Tables section of the code book and locate the appropriate table to complete the code construction. Even if the entire seven-digit code is provided in the Index, the coder should still reference the Tables to ensure the correct PCS code has been constructed.

See Reference

Common procedure terms are often listed with the *see* reference. The coder is instructed to follow the reference provided in order to locate the appropriate table to construct the code. For example, the *see* reference is present for the main term Colectomy. The Index excerpt is as follows:

Colectomy

see Excision, Gastrointestinal System 0DB

see Resection, Gastrointestinal System 0DT

In this example, the coder should review the definition of the root operations Excision and Resection to determine which is consistent with the medical record documentation. The coder should then proceed to the corresponding table as suggested by the *see* reference.

Use Reference

Anatomical site terms and device terms are often listed with the *use* reference. The coder is instructed to follow the reference provided in order to locate the appropriate main term for the procedure in question. For example, the *use* reference is present for the main term Inferior rectus muscle. The Index excerpt is as follows:

Inferior rectus muscle
use Muscle, Extraocular, Left
use Muscle, Extraocular, Right

In this example, the coder should identify the root operation for the procedure, and then look for the subterm that identifies the body part indicated in the *use* reference. For example, the procedure is excision of the inferior rectus muscle. The coder would locate the main term Excision. The Index excerpt is as follows:

Excision
Muscle
Extraocular
Left 08BM
Right 08BL

In this example, the coder knows that the Code Table 08B is the correct table because the previous review of the *use* reference identified that the inferior rectus muscle is an extraocular muscle. The coder can now proceed to the 08B Table to finish constructing the PCS code.

In addition to the *use* reference, the coder may also consult appendix D for Body Part Table or appendix E for the Device Table.

Code Tables

ICD-10-PCS contains 17 sections of Code Tables, represented by the numbers 0 through 9 and the letters B through D, F through H, and X. The Tables are organized by general type of procedure. The three main sections of tables include:

1. **Medical and Surgical section**
   - Medical and Surgical (first character 0)
2. **Medical and Surgical Related sections**
   - Obstetrics (first character 1)
   - Placement (first character 2)
   - Administration (first character 3)
   - Measurement and Monitoring (first character 4)
   - Extracorporeal or Systemic Assistance and Performance (first character 5)
   - Extracorporeal or Systemic Therapies (first character 6)
   - Osteopathic (first character 7)
   - Other Procedures (first character 8)
   - Chiropractic (first character 9)
3. **Ancillary sections**
   - Imaging (first character B)
   - Nuclear Medicine (first character C)
   - Radiation Therapy (first character D)
   - Physical Rehabilitation and Diagnostic Audiology (first character F)
   - Mental Health (first character G)
   - Substance Abuse (first character H)
   - New Technology (first character X)

Each code table is defined by the first three characters of the PCS code. Each of these characters is displayed above the table. The table consists of all the options for characters 4 through 7. The root operation or root type, character 3, is present along with its official definition. Table 097 is provided here as an example of the table structure.

0 Medical and Surgical

9 Ear, Nose, Sinus

7 Dilation: Expanding an orifice or the lumen of a tubular body part

Body Part Character 4	Approach Character 5	Device Character 6	Qualifier Character 7
F Eustachian Tube, Right **G** Eustachian Tube, Left	**0** Open **7** Via Natural or Artificial Opening **8** Via Natural or Artificial Opening Endoscopic	**D** Intraluminal Device **Z** No Device	**Z** No Qualifier
F Eustachian Tube, Right **G** Eustachian Tube, Left	**3** Percutaneous **4** Percutaneous Endoscopic	**Z** No Device	**Z** No Qualifier

There can be multiple rows within the table for the first three characters, so the coder must carefully review all the applicable rows. Additionally, a table may cover multiple pages. Therefore, the coder must continue to review the code table options until the end of the table is reached to ensure the correct PCS code has been constructed.

AHA *Coding Clinic* for ICD-10-CM and ICD-10-PCS

The American Hospital Association began publishing coding guidance for ICD-10-CM and ICD-10-PCS in the fourth quarter of 2012. In this code book we identify procedure codes that are discussed in the *Coding Clinic* guidance fourth quarter 2012 through second quarter 2021. In the Medical and Surgical section, after each body system table section, there is an AHA *Coding Clinic* section that lists the references. For all other sections of the code book, the AHA *Coding Clinic* section follows the Tables section. In the AHA *Coding Clinic* section, the PCS codes included in AHA *Coding Clinic* guidance are listed with a sky blue note that alerts the coder to review the AHA *Coding Clinic* prior to assignment of the code to ensure appropriate and accurate reporting. The quarter of publication, year and page number(s) are provided in the note.

AHA CC: 4Q; 2012; pg#-pg#

AHA Coding Clinic Crosswalk for Deleted Codes

Deleted Code	Coding Clinic Reference	Replacement Code
047K3Z6	4Q, 2016, 88-89	047K3ZZ
04CK3Z6	4Q, 2016, 88-89	04CK3ZZ
04V03E6	4Q, 2016, 91-92	04V03EZ
04V03F6	4Q, 2016, 92-94	04V03FZ
0B5S0ZZ	2Q, 2016, 17-18	See 0B5T0ZZ
0BQR0ZZ	2Q, 2016, 22-23	See 0BQT0ZZ
0BQR4ZZ	3Q, 2014, 28	See 0BQT4ZZ
0BQS0ZZ	2Q, 2016, 22-23	See 0BQT0ZZ
0BQS4ZZ	3Q, 2014, 28	See 0BQT4ZZ
0NQS0ZZ	3Q, 2016, 29-30	See 0NQR0ZZ
0NSS04Z	3Q, 2014, 23-24	See 0NSR04Z
0NSS0ZZ	1Q, 2017, 20-21	See 0NSR0ZZ
0NR80JZ	3Q, 2017, 17	See 0NR70JZ

ICD-10-PCS Coding Guidelines

The ICD-10-PCS Coding Guidelines are presented here in the introduction and throughout this manual. Within the manual, the Medical and Surgical Section Guidelines are presented after the Introduction of the Medical and Surgical section. The Obstetric Section Guidelines are presented after the Introduction of the Obstetrics section. Lastly, the New Technology Guidelines are presented after the Introduction of the New Technology section.

ICD-10-PCS Official Guidelines for Coding and Reporting, 2022

The Centers for Medicare and Medicaid Services (CMS) and the National Center for Health Statistics (NCHS), two departments within the US federal government's Department of Health and Human Services (DHHS) provide the following guidelines for coding and reporting using the International Classification of Diseases, 10th Revision, Procedure Coding System (ICD-10-PCS). These guidelines should be used as a companion document to the official version of the ICD-10-PCS as published on the CMS website. The ICD-10-PCS is a procedure classification published by the United States for classifying procedures performed in hospital inpatient health care settings.

These guidelines have been approved by the four organizations that make up the Cooperating Parties for the ICD-10-PCS: the American Hospital Association (AHA), the American Health Information Management Association (AHIMA), CMS, and NCHS.

These guidelines are a set of rules that have been developed to accompany and complement the official conventions and instructions provided within the ICD-10-PCS itself. They are intended to provide direction that is applicable in most circumstances. However, there may be unique circumstances where exceptions are applied. The instructions and conventions of the classification take precedence over guidelines. These guidelines are based on the coding and sequencing instructions in the Tables, Index, and Definitions of ICD-10-PCS, but provide additional instruction. Adherence to these guidelines when assigning ICD-10-PCS procedure codes is required under the Health Insurance Portability and Accountability Act (HIPAA). The procedure codes have been adopted under HIPAA for hospital inpatient healthcare settings. A joint effort between the healthcare provider and the coder is essential to achieve complete and accurate documentation, code assignment, and reporting of diagnoses and procedures. These guidelines have been developed to assist both the healthcare provider and the coder in identifying those procedures that are to be reported. The importance of consistent, complete documentation in the medical record cannot be overemphasized. Without such documentation, accurate coding cannot be achieved.

Conventions

A1. ICD-10-PCS codes are composed of seven characters. Each character is an axis of classification that specifies information about the procedure performed. Within a defined code range, a character specifies the same type of information in that axis of classification.

Example: The fifth axis of classification specifies the approach in sections 0 through 4 and 7 through 9 of the system.

A2. One of 34 possible values can be assigned to each axis of classification in the seven-character code: they are the numbers 0 through 9 and the alphabet (except the letters I and O because they are easily confused with the numbers 1 and 0). The number of unique values used in an axis of classification differs as needed.

Example: Where the fifth axis of classification specifies the approach, seven different approach values are currently used to specify the approach.

A3. The valid values for an axis of classification can be added to as needed.

Example: If a significantly distinct type of device is used in a new procedure, a new device value can be added to the system.

A4. As with words in their context, the meaning of any single value is a combination of its axis of classification and any preceding values on which it may be dependent.

Example: The meaning of a body part value in the Medical and Surgical section is always dependent on the body system value. The body part value 0 in the Central Nervous body system specifies Brain and the body part value 0 in the Peripheral Nervous body system specifies Cervical Plexus.

A5. As the system is expanded to become increasingly detailed, over time more values will depend on preceding values for their meaning.

Example: In the Lower Joints body system, the device value 3 in the root operation Insertion specifies Infusion Device and the device value 3 in the root operation Replacement specifies Ceramic Synthetic Substitute.

A6. The purpose of the Alphabetic Index is to locate the appropriate table that contains all information necessary to construct a procedure code. The PCS Tables should always be consulted to find the most appropriate valid code.

A7. It is not required to consult the Index first before proceeding to the Tables to complete the code. A valid code may be chosen directly from the Tables.

A8. All seven characters must be specified to be a valid code. If the documentation is incomplete for coding purposes, the physician should be queried for the necessary information.

A9. Within a PCS Table, valid codes include all combinations of choices in characters 4 through 7 contained in the same row of the table. In the example below, 0JHT3VZ is a valid code, and 0JHW3VZ is *not* a valid code.

Section: **0** **Medical and Surgical**
Body System: **J** **Subcutaneous Tissue and Fascia**
Operation: **H** **Insertion:** Putting in a nonbiological appliance that monitors, assists, performs, or prevents a physiological function but does not physically take the place of a body part

Body Part (4th)	Approach (5th)	Device (6th)	Qualifier (7th)
S Subcutaneous Tissue and Fascia, Head and Neck **V** Subcutaneous Tissue and Fascia, Upper Extremity **W** Subcutaneous Tissue and Fascia, Lower Extremity	**0** Open **3** Percutaneous	**1** Radioactive Element **3** Infusion Device **Y** Other Device	**Z** No Qualifier
T Subcutaneous Tissue and Fascia, Trunk	**0** Open **3** Percutaneous	**1** Radioactive Element **3** Infusion Device **V** Infusion Pump **Y** Other Device	**Z** No Qualifier

A10. "And," when used in a code description, means "and/or," except when used to describe a combination of multiple body parts for which separate values exist for each body part (e.g., Skin and Subcutaneous Tissue used as a qualifier, where there are separate body part values for "Skin" and "Subcutaneous Tissue").

Example: Lower Arm and Wrist Muscle means lower arm and/or wrist muscle.

A11. Many of the terms used to construct PCS codes are defined within the system. It is the coder's responsibility to determine what the documentation in the medical record equates to in the PCS definitions. The physician is not expected to use the terms used in PCS code descriptions, nor is the coder required to query the physician when the correlation between the documentation and the defined PCS terms is clear.

Example: When the physician documents "partial resection" the coder can independently correlate "partial resection" to the root operation Excision without querying the physician for clarification.

Medical and Surgical Section Guidelines (section 0)

B2. Body System

General guidelines

B2.1a

The procedure codes in Anatomical Regions, General, Anatomical Regions, Upper Extremities and Anatomical Regions, Lower Extremities can be used when the procedure is performed on an anatomical region rather than a specific body part, or on the rare occasion when no information is available to support assignment of a code to a specific body part.

Examples: Chest tube drainage of the pleural cavity is coded to the root operation Drainage found in the body system Anatomical Regions, General. Suture repair of the abdominal wall is coded to the root operation Repair in the body system Anatomical Regions, General. Amputation of the foot is coded to the root operation Detachment in the body system Anatomical Regions, Lower Extremities.

B2.1b

Where the general body part values "upper" and "lower" are provided as an option in the Upper Arteries, Lower Arteries, Upper Veins, Lower Veins, Muscles and Tendons body systems, "upper" or "lower "specifies body parts located above or below the diaphragm respectively.

Example: Vein body parts above the diaphragm are found in the Upper Veins body system; vein body parts below the diaphragm are found in the Lower Veins body system.

B3. Root Operation

General guidelines

B3.1a

In order to determine the appropriate root operation, the full definition of the root operation as contained in the PCS Tables must be applied.

Official Coding Guidelines

B3.1b

Components of a procedure specified in the root operation definition or explanation as integral to that root operation are not coded separately. Procedural steps necessary to reach the operative site and close the operative site, including anastomosis of a tubular body part, are also not coded separately.

Example: Resection of a joint as part of a joint replacement procedure is included in the root operation definition of Replacement and is not coded separately. Laparotomy performed to reach the site of an open liver biopsy is not coded separately. In a resection of sigmoid colon with anastomosis of descending colon to rectum, the anastomosis is not coded separately.

Multiple procedures

B3.2

During the same operative episode, multiple procedures are coded if:

a. The same root operation is performed on different body parts as defined by distinct values of the body part character.

   Examples: Diagnostic excision of liver and pancreas are coded separately. Excision of lesion in the ascending colon and excision of lesion in the transverse colon are coded separately.

b. The same root operation is repeated in multiple body parts, and those body parts are separate and distinct body parts classified to a single ICD-10-PCS body part value.

   Examples: Excision of the sartorius muscle and excision of the gracilis muscle are both included in the upper leg muscle body part value, and multiple procedures are coded. Extraction of multiple toenails are coded separately.

c. Multiple root operations with distinct objectives are performed on the same body part.

   Example: Destruction of sigmoid lesion and bypass of sigmoid colon are coded separately.

d. The intended root operation is attempted using one approach but is converted to a different approach.

   Example: Laparoscopic cholecystectomy converted to an open cholecystectomy is coded as percutaneous endoscopic Inspection and open Resection.

Discontinued or incomplete procedures

B3.3

If the intended procedure is discontinued or otherwise not completed, code the procedure to the root operation performed. If a procedure is discontinued before any other root operation is performed, code the root operation Inspection of the body part or anatomical region inspected.

Example: A planned aortic valve replacement procedure is discontinued after the initial thoracotomy and before any incision is made in the heart muscle, when the patient becomes hemodynamically unstable. This procedure is coded as an open Inspection of the mediastinum.

Biopsy procedures

B3.4a

Biopsy procedures are coded using the root operations Excision, Extraction, or Drainage and the qualifier Diagnostic. *Examples:* Fine needle aspiration biopsy of fluid in the lung is coded to the root operation Drainage with the qualifier Diagnostic. Biopsy of bone marrow is coded to the root operation Extraction with the qualifier Diagnostic. Lymph node sampling for biopsy is coded to the root operation Excision with the qualifier Diagnostic.

Biopsy followed by more definitive treatment

B3.4b

If a diagnostic Excision, Extraction, or Drainage procedure (biopsy) is followed by a more definitive procedure, such as Destruction, Excision or Resection at the same procedure site, both the biopsy and the more definitive treatment are coded.

Example: Biopsy of breast followed by partial mastectomy at the same procedure site, both the biopsy and the partial mastectomy procedure are coded.

Overlapping body layers
B3.5

If root operations Excision, Extraction, Repair or Inspection are performed on overlapping layers of the musculoskeletal system, the body part specifying the deepest layer is coded.

Example: Excisional debridement that includes skin and subcutaneous tissue and muscle is coded to the muscle body part.

Bypass procedures
B3.6a

Bypass procedures are coded by identifying the body part bypassed "from" and the body part bypassed "to." The fourth character body part specifies the body part bypassed from, and the qualifier specifies the body part bypassed to.

Example: Bypass from stomach to jejunum, stomach is the body part and jejunum is the qualifier.

B3.6b

Coronary artery bypass procedures are coded differently than other bypass procedures as described in the previous guideline. Rather than identifying the body part bypassed from, the body part identifies the number of coronary artery sites bypassed to, and the qualifier specifies the vessel bypassed from.

Example: Aortocoronary artery bypass of the left anterior descending coronary artery and the obtuse marginal coronary artery is classified in the body part axis of classification as two coronary arteries and the qualifier specifies the aorta as the body part bypassed from.

B3.6c

If multiple coronary arteries are bypassed, a separate procedure is coded for each coronary artery that uses a different device and/or qualifier.

Example: Aortocoronary artery bypass and internal mammary coronary artery bypass are coded separately.

Control vs. more definitive root operations
B3.7

The root operation Control is defined as, "Stopping, or attempting to stop, postprocedural or other acute bleeding." Control is the root operation coded when the procedure performed to achieve hemostasis, beyond what would be considered integral to a procedure, utilizes techniques (e.g. cautery, application of substances or pressure, suturing or ligation or clipping of bleeding points at the site) that are not described by a more specific root operation definition, such as Bypass, Detachment, Excision, Extraction, Reposition, Replacement, or Resection. If a more specific root operation definition applies to the procedure performed, then the more specific root operation is coded instead of Control.

Examples: Silver nitrate cautery to treat acute nasal bleeding is coded to the root operation Control. Liquid embolization of the right internal iliac artery to treat acute hematoma by stopping blood flow is coded to the root operation Occlusion. Suctioning of residual blood to achieve hemostasis during a transbronchial cryobiopsy is considered integral to the cryobiopsy procedure and is not coded separately.

Excision vs. Resection
B3.8

PCS contains specific body parts for anatomical subdivisions of a body part, such as lobes of the lungs or liver and regions of the intestine. Resection of the specific body part is coded whenever all of the body part is cut out or off, rather than coding Excision of a less specific body part.

Example: Left upper lung lobectomy is coded to Resection of Upper Lung Lobe, Left rather than Excision of Lung, Left.

Excision for graft
B3.9

If an autograft is obtained from a different procedure site in order to complete the objective of the procedure, a separate procedure is coded, except when the seventh character qualifier value in the ICD-10-PCS table fully specifies the site from which the autograft was obtained.

Examples: Coronary bypass with excision of saphenous vein graft, excision of saphenous vein is coded separately. Replacement of breast with autologous deep inferior epigastric artery perforator (DIEP) flap, excision of the DIEP flap is not coded separately. The seventh character qualifier value Deep Inferior Epigastric Artery Perforator Flap in the Replacement table fully specifies the site of the autograft harvest.

Fusion procedures of the spine

B3.10a

The body part coded for a spinal vertebral joint(s) rendered immobile by a spinal fusion procedure is classified by the level of the spine (e.g. thoracic). There are distinct body part values for a single vertebral joint and for multiple vertebral joints at each spinal level.

Example: Body part values specify Lumbar Vertebral Joint, Lumbar Vertebral Joints, 2 or More and Lumbosacral Vertebral Joint.

B3.10b

If multiple vertebral joints are fused, a separate procedure is coded for each vertebral joint that uses a different device and/or qualifier.

Example: Fusion of lumbar vertebral joint, posterior approach, anterior column and fusion of lumbar vertebral joint, posterior approach, posterior column are coded separately.

B3.10c

Combinations of devices and materials are often used on a vertebral joint to render the joint immobile. When combinations of devices are used on the same vertebral joint, the device value coded for the procedure is as follows:

- If an interbody fusion device is used to render the joint immobile (containing bone graft or bone graft substitute), the procedure is coded with the device value Interbody Fusion Device
- If bone graft is the *only* device used to render the joint immobile, the procedure is coded with the device value Nonautologous Tissue Substitute or Autologous Tissue Substitute
- If a mixture of autologous and nonautologous bone graft (with or without biological or synthetic extenders or binders) is used to render the joint immobile, code the procedure with the device value Autologous Tissue Substitute

Examples: Fusion of a vertebral joint using a cage style interbody fusion device containing morsellized bone graft is coded to the device Interbody Fusion Device. Fusion of a vertebral joint using a bone dowel interbody fusion device made of cadaver bone and packed with a mixture of local morsellized bone and demineralized bone matrix is coded to the device Interbody Fusion Device. Fusion of a vertebral joint using both autologous bone graft and bone bank bone graft is coded to the device Autologous Tissue Substitute.

Inspection procedures

B3.11a

Inspection of a body part(s) performed in order to achieve the objective of a procedure is not coded separately.

Example: Fiberoptic bronchoscopy performed for irrigation of bronchus, only the irrigation procedure is coded.

B3.11b

If multiple tubular body parts are inspected, the most distal body part (the body part furthest from the starting point of the inspection) is coded. If multiple non-tubular body parts in a region are inspected, the body part that specifies the entire area inspected is coded.

Examples: Cystoureteroscopy with inspection of bladder and ureters is coded to the ureter body part value. Exploratory laparotomy with general inspection of abdominal contents is coded to the peritoneal cavity body part value.

B3.11c

When both an Inspection procedure and another procedure are performed on the same body part during the same episode, if the Inspection procedure is performed using a different approach than the other procedure, the Inspection procedure is coded separately.

Example: Endoscopic Inspection of the duodenum is coded separately when open Excision of the duodenum is performed during the same procedural episode.

Occlusion vs. Restriction for vessel embolization procedures

B3.12

If the objective of an embolization procedure is to completely close a vessel, the root operation Occlusion is coded. If the objective of an embolization procedure is to narrow the lumen of a vessel, the root operation Restriction is coded.

Examples: Tumor embolization is coded to the root operation Occlusion, because the objective of the procedure is to cut off the blood supply to the vessel. Embolization of a cerebral aneurysm is coded to the root operation Restriction, because the objective of the procedure is not to close off the vessel entirely, but to narrow the lumen of the vessel at the site of the aneurysm where it is abnormally wide.

Release procedures
B3.13

In the root operation Release, the body part value coded is the body part being freed and not the tissue being manipulated or cut to free the body part.

Example: Lysis of intestinal adhesions is coded to the specific intestine body part value.

Release vs. Division
B3.14

If the sole objective of the procedure is freeing a body part without cutting the body part, the root operation is Release. If the sole objective of the procedure is separating or transecting a body part, the root operation is Division.

Examples: Freeing a nerve root from surrounding scar tissue to relieve pain is coded to the root operation Release. Severing a nerve root to relieve pain is coded to the root operation Division.

Reposition for fracture treatment
B3.15

Reduction of a displaced fracture is coded to the root operation Reposition and the application of a cast or splint in conjunction with the Reposition procedure is not coded separately. Treatment of a nondisplaced fracture is coded to the procedure performed.

Examples: Casting of a nondisplaced fracture is coded to the root operation Immobilization in the Placement section.

Putting a pin in a nondisplaced fracture is coded to the root operation Insertion.

Transplantation vs. Administration
B3.16

Putting in a mature and functioning living body part taken from another individual or animal is coded to the root operation Transplantation. Putting in autologous or nonautologous cells is coded to the Administration section.

Example: Putting in autologous or nonautologous bone marrow, pancreatic islet cells or stem cells is coded to the Administration section.

Transfer procedures using multiple tissue layers
B3.17

The root operation Transfer contains qualifiers that can be used to specify when a transfer flap is composed of more than one tissue layer, such as a musculocutaneous flap. For procedures involving transfer of multiple tissue layers including skin, subcutaneous tissue, fascia or muscle, the procedure is coded to the body part value that describes the deepest tissue layer in the flap, and the qualifier can be used to describe the other tissue layer(s) in the transfer flap.

Example: A musculocutaneous flap transfer is coded to the appropriate body part value in the body system Muscles, and the qualifier is used to describe the additional tissue layer(s) in the transfer flap.

Excision/Resection followed by replacement
B3.18

If an Excision or Resection of a body part is followed by a Replacement procedure, code both procedures to identify each distinct objective, except when the Excision or Resection is considered integral and preparatory for the Replacement procedure.

Examples: Mastectomy followed by reconstruction, both Resection and Replacement of the breast are coded to fully capture the distinct objectives of the procedures performed. Maxillectomy with obturator reconstruction, both Excision and Replacement of the maxilla are coded to fully capture the distinct objectives of the procedures performed. Excisional debridement of tendon with skin graft, both the Excision of the tendon and the Replacement of the skin with a graft are coded to fully capture the distinct objectives of the procedures performed. Esophagectomy followed by reconstruction with colonic interposition, both the Resection and the Transfer of the large intestine to function as the esophagus are coded to fully capture the distinct objectives of the procedures performed.

Examples: Resection of a joint as part of a joint replacement procedure is considered integral and preparatory for the Replacement of the joint and the Resection is not coded separately. Resection of a valve as part of a valve replacement procedure is considered integral and preparatory for the valve Replacement and the Resection is not coded separately.

B4. Body Part

General guidelines

B4.1a

If a procedure is performed on a portion of a body part that does not have a separate body part value, code the body part value corresponding to the whole body part.

Example: A procedure performed on the alveolar process of the mandible is coded to the mandible body part.

B4.1b

If the prefix "peri" is combined with a body part to identify the site of the procedure, and the site of the procedure is not further specified, then the procedure is coded to the body part named. This guideline applies only when a more specific body part value is not available.

Examples: A procedure site identified as perirenal is coded to the kidney body part when the site of the procedure is not further specified. A procedure site described in the documentation as peri-urethral, and the documentation also indicates that it is the vulvar tissue and not the urethral tissue that is the site of the procedure, then the procedure is coded to the vulva body part. A procedure site documented as involving the periosteum is coded to the corresponding bone body part.

B4.1c

If a procedure is performed on a continuous section of a tubular body part, code the body part value corresponding to the anatomically most proximal (closest to the heart) portion of the tubular body part.

Examples: A procedure performed on a continuous section of artery from the femoral artery to the external iliac artery with the point of entry at the femoral artery is coded to the external iliac body part. A procedure performed on a continuous section of artery from the femoral artery to the external iliac artery with the point of entry at the external iliac artery is also coded to the external iliac artery body part.

Branches of body parts

B4.2

Where a specific branch of a body part does not have its own body part value in PCS, the body part is typically coded to the closest proximal branch that has a specific body part value. In the cardiovascular body systems, if a general body part is available in the correct root operation table, and coding to a proximal branch would require assigning a code in a different body system, the procedure is coded using the general body part value.

Examples: A procedure performed on the mandibular branch of the trigeminal nerve is coded to the trigeminal nerve body part value. Occlusion of the bronchial artery is coded to the body part value Upper Artery in the body system Upper Arteries, and not to the body part value Thoracic Aorta, Descending in the body system Heart and Great Vessels.

Bilateral body part values

B4.3

Bilateral body part values are available for a limited number of body parts. If the identical procedure is performed on contralateral body parts, and a bilateral body part value exists for that body part, a single procedure is coded using the bilateral body part value. If no bilateral body part value exists, each procedure is coded separately using the appropriate body part value.

Example: The identical procedure performed on both fallopian tubes is coded once using the body part value Fallopian Tube, Bilateral. The identical procedure performed on both knee joints is coded twice using the body part values Knee Joint, Right and Knee Joint, Left.

Coronary arteries

B4.4

The coronary arteries are classified as a single body part that is further specified by number of arteries treated. One procedure code specifying multiple arteries is used when the same procedure is performed, including the same device and qualifier values.

Examples: Angioplasty of two distinct coronary arteries with placement of two stents is coded as Dilation of Coronary Artery, Two Arteries, with Two Intraluminal Devices. Angioplasty of two distinct coronary arteries, one with stent placed and one without, is coded separately as Dilation of Coronary Artery, One Artery with Intraluminal Device, and Dilation of Coronary Artery, One Artery with no device.

Tendons, ligaments, bursae and fascia near a joint

B4.5

Procedures performed on tendons, ligaments, bursae and fascia supporting a joint are coded to the body part in the respective body system that is the focus of the procedure. Procedures performed on joint structures themselves are coded to the body part in the joint body systems.

Example: Repair of the anterior cruciate ligament of the knee is coded to the knee bursa and ligament body part in the Bursae and Ligaments body system. Knee arthroscopy with shaving of articular cartilage is coded to the knee joint body part in the Lower Joints body system.

Skin, subcutaneous tissue and fascia overlying a joint

B4.6

If a procedure is performed on the skin, subcutaneous tissue or fascia overlying a joint, the procedure is coded to the following body part:

- Shoulder is coded to Upper Arm
- Elbow is coded to Lower Arm
- Wrist is coded to Lower Arm
- Hip is coded to Upper Leg
- Knee is coded to Lower Leg
- Ankle is coded to Foot

Fingers and toes

B4.7

If a body system does not contain a separate body part value for fingers, procedures performed on the fingers are coded to the body part value for the hand. If a body system does not contain a separate body part value for toes, procedures performed on the toes are coded to the body part value for the foot.

Example: Excision of finger muscle is coded to one of the hand muscle body part values in the Muscles body system.

Upper and lower intestinal tract

B4.8

In the Gastrointestinal body system, the general body part values Upper Intestinal Tract and Lower Intestinal Tract are provided as an option for the root operations such as Change, Insertion, Inspection, Removal and Revision. Upper Intestinal Tract includes the portion of the gastrointestinal tract from the esophagus down to and including the duodenum, and Lower Intestinal Tract includes the portion of the gastrointestinal tract from the jejunum down to and including the rectum and anus.

Example: In the root operation Change table, change of a device in the jejunum is coded using the body part Lower Intestinal Tract.

B5. Approach

Open approach with percutaneous endoscopic assistance

B5.2a

Procedures performed using the open approach with percutaneous endoscopic assistance are coded to the approach Open.

Example: Laparoscopic-assisted sigmoidectomy is coded to the approach Open.

Percutaneous endoscopic approach with extension of incision

B5.2b

Procedures performed using the percutaneous endoscopic approach, with incision or extension of an incision to assist in the removal of all or a portion of a body part or to anastomose a tubular body part to complete the procedure, are coded to the approach value Percutaneous Endoscopic.

Examples: Laparoscopic sigmoid colectomy with extension of stapling port for removal of specimen and direct anastomosis is coded to the approach value Percutaneous Endoscopic. Laparoscopic nephrectomy with midline incision for removing the resected kidney is coded to the approach value Percutaneous Endoscopic. Robotic-assisted laparoscopic prostatectomy with extension of incision for removal of the resected prostate is coded to the approach value Percutaneous Endoscopic.

External approach

B5.3a

Procedures performed within an orifice on structures that are visible without the aid of any instrumentation are coded to the approach External.

Example: Resection of tonsils is coded to the approach External.

B5.3b

Procedures performed indirectly by the application of external force through the intervening body layers are coded to the approach External.

Example: Closed reduction of fracture is coded to the approach External.

Percutaneous procedure via device

B5.4

Procedures performed percutaneously via a device placed for the procedure are coded to the approach Percutaneous.

Example: Fragmentation of kidney stone performed via percutaneous nephrostomy is coded to the approach Percutaneous.

B6. Device

General guidelines

B6.1a

A device is coded only if a device remains after the procedure is completed. If no device remains, the device value No Device is coded. In limited root operations, the classification provides the qualifier values Temporary and Intraoperative, for specific procedures involving clinically significant devices, where the purpose of the device is to be utilized for a brief duration during the procedure or current inpatient stay. If a device that is intended to remain after the procedure is completed requires removal before the end of the operative episode in which it was inserted (for example, the device size is inadequate or a complication occurs), both the insertion and removal of the device should be coded.

B6.1b

Materials such as sutures, ligatures, radiological markers and temporary post-operative wound drains are considered integral to the performance of a procedure and are not coded as devices.

B6.1c

Procedures performed on a device only and not on a body part are specified in the root operations Change, Irrigation, Removal and Revision, and are coded to the procedure performed.

Example: Irrigation of percutaneous nephrostomy tube is coded to the root operation Irrigation of indwelling device in the Administration section.

Drainage device

B6.2

A separate procedure to put in a drainage device is coded to the root operation Drainage with the device value Drainage Device.

Obstetric Section Guidelines (section 1)

C. Obstetrics Section

Products of conception

C1

Procedures performed on the products of conception are coded to the Obstetrics section. Procedures performed on the pregnant female other than the products of conception are coded to the appropriate root operation in the Medical and Surgical section.

Example: Amniocentesis is coded to the products of conception body part in the Obstetrics section. Repair of obstetric urethral laceration is coded to the urethra body part in the Medical and Surgical section.

Procedures following delivery or abortion

C2

Procedures performed following a delivery or abortion for curettage of the endometrium or evacuation of retained products of conception are all coded in the Obstetrics section, to the root operation Extraction and the body part Products of Conception, Retained. Diagnostic or therapeutic dilation and curettage performed during times other than the postpartum or post-abortion period are all coded in the Medical and Surgical section, to the root operation Extraction and the body part Endometrium.

Radiation Therapy Section Guidelines (section D)

D. Radiation Therapy Section

Brachytherapy

D1.a

Brachytherapy is coded to the modality Brachytherapy in the Radiation Therapy section. When a radioactive brachytherapy source is left in the body at the end of the procedure, it is coded separately to the root operation Insertion with the device value Radioactive Element.

Example: Brachytherapy with implantation of a low dose rate brachytherapy source left in the body at the end of the procedure is coded to the applicable treatment site in section D, Radiation Therapy, with the modality Brachytherapy, the modality qualifier value, Low Dose Rate, and the applicable isotope value and qualifier value. The implantation of the brachytherapy source is coded separately to the device value Radioactive Element in the appropriate Insertion table of the Medical and Surgical section. The Radiation Therapy section code identifies the specific modality and isotope of the brachytherapy, and the root operation Insertion code identifies the implantation of the brachytherapy source that remain in the body at the end of the procedure.

Exception: Implantation of Cesium-131 brachytherapy seeds embedded in a collagen matrix to the treatment site after resection of brain tumor is coded to the root operation Insertion with the device value Radioactive Element, Cesium-131 Collagen Implant. The procedure is coded to the root operation Insertion only, because the device value identifies both the implantation of the radioactive element and a specific brachytherapy isotope that is not included in the Radiation Therapy section tables.

D1.b

A separate procedure to place a temporary applicator for delivering the brachytherapy is coded to the root operation Insertion and the device value Other Device.

Examples: Intrauterine brachytherapy applicator placed as a separate procedure from the brachytherapy procedure is coded to Insertion of Other Device, and the brachytherapy is coded separately using the modality Brachytherapy in the Radiation Therapy section. Intrauterine brachytherapy applicator placed concomitantly with delivery of the brachytherapy dose is coded with a single code using the modality Brachytherapy in the Radiation Therapy section.

New Technology Section Guidelines (section X)

E. New Technology Section

General guidelines

E1.a

Section X codes fully represent the specific procedure described in the code title, and do not require any additional codes from other sections of ICD-10-PCS. When section X contains a code title which describes a specific new technology procedure, and it is the only procedure performed, only the section X code is reported for the procedure. There is no need to report an additional code in another section of ICD-10-PCS.

Example: XW043A6 Introduction of Cefiderocol Anti-infective into Central Vein, Percutaneous Approach, New Technology Group 6, can be coded to indicate that Cefiderocol Anti-infective was administered via a central vein. A separate code from table 3E0 in the Administration section of ICD-10-PCS is not coded in addition to this code.

E1.b

When multiple procedures are performed, New Technology section X codes are coded following the multiple procedures guideline.

Examples: Dual filter cerebral embolic filtration used during transcatheter aortic valve replacement (TAVR), X2A5312 Cerebral Embolic Filtration, Dual Filter in Innominate Artery and Left Common Carotid Artery, Percutaneous Approach, New Technology Group 2, is coded for the cerebral embolic filtration, along with an ICD-10-PCS code for the TAVR procedure. An extracorporeal flow reversal circuit for embolic neuroprotection placed during a transcarotid arterial revascularization procedure, a code from table X2A, Assistance of the Cardiovascular System is coded for the use of the extracoporeal flow reversal circuit, along with an ICD-10-PCS code for the transcarotid arterial revascularization procedure.

F. Selection of Principal Procedure

The following instructions should be applied in the selection of principal procedure and clarification on the importance of the relation to the principal diagnosis when more than one procedure is performed:

1. Procedure performed for definitive treatment of both principal diagnosis and secondary diagnosis

a. Sequence procedure performed for definitive treatment most related to principal diagnosis as principal procedure.

2. Procedure performed for definitive treatment and diagnostic procedures performed for both principal diagnosis and secondary diagnosis

a. Sequence procedure performed for definitive treatment most related to principal diagnosis as principal procedure

3. A diagnostic procedure was performed for the principal diagnosis and a procedure is performed for definitive treatment of a secondary diagnosis.

a. Sequence diagnostic procedure as principal procedure, since the procedure most related to the principal diagnosis takes precedence.

4. No procedures performed that are related to principal diagnosis; procedures performed for definitive treatment and diagnostic procedures were performed for secondary diagnosis

a. Sequence procedure performed for definitive treatment of secondary diagnosis as principal procedure, since there are no procedures (definitive or nondefinitive treatment) related to principal diagnosis.

3

A

Amniocentesis
see Drainage, Products of Conception 1090
Amnioinfusion
see Introduction of substance in or on, Products of Conception 3E0E
Amnioscopy 10J08ZZ
Amniotomy
see Drainage, Products of Conception 1090
AMPLATZER® Muscular VSD Occluder
use Synthetic Substitute
Amputation
see Detachment
AMS 800® Urinary Control System
use Artificial Sphincter in Urinary System
Anal orifice
use Anus
Analog radiography
see Plain Radiography
Anastomosis
see Bypass
Anatomical snuffbox
use Muscle, Lower Arm and Wrist, Left
use Muscle, Lower Arm and Wrist, Right
Andexanet Alfa, Factor Xa Inhibitor Reversal Agent
use Coagulation Factor Xa, Inactivated
Andexxa
use Coagulation Factor Xa, Inactivated
AneuRx® AAA Advantage®
use Intraluminal Device
Angiectomy
see Excision, Heart and Great Vessels 02B
see Excision, Upper Arteries 03B
see Excision, Lower Arteries 04B
see Excision, Upper Veins 05B
see Excision, Lower Veins 06B
Angiocardiography
Combined right and left heart
see Fluoroscopy, Heart, Right and Left B216
Left Heart
see Fluoroscopy, Heart, Left B215
Right Heart
see Fluoroscopy, Heart, Right B214
SPY system intravascular fluorescence
see Monitoring, Physiological Systems 4A1
Angiography
see Computerized Tomography (CT Scan), Artery
see Fluoroscopy, Artery
see Magnetic Resonance Imaging (MRI), Artery
see Plain Radiography, Artery
Angioplasty
see Dilation, Heart and Great Vessels 027
see Repair, Heart and Great Vessels 02Q
see Replacement, Heart and Great Vessels 02R
see Dilation, Upper Arteries 037
see Repair, Upper Arteries 03Q
see Replacement, Upper Arteries 03R
see Dilation, Lower Arteries 047
see Repair, Lower Arteries 04Q
see Replacement, Lower Arteries 04R
see Supplement, Heart and Great Vessels 02U
Angioplasty *(continued)*
see Supplement, Upper Arteries 03U
see Supplement, Lower Arteries 04U
Angiorrhaphy
see Repair, Heart and Great Vessels 02Q
see Repair, Upper Arteries 03Q
see Repair, Lower Arteries 04Q
Angioscopy
02JY4ZZ
03JY4ZZ
04JY4ZZ
Angiotensin II
use Synthetic Human Angiotensin II
Angiotripsy
see Occlusion, Upper Arteries 03L
see Occlusion, Lower Arteries 04L
Angular artery
use Artery, Face
Angular vein
use Vein, Face, Left
use Vein, Face, Right
Annular ligament
use Bursa and Ligament, Elbow, Left
use Bursa and Ligament, Elbow, Right
Annuloplasty
see Repair, Heart and Great Vessels 02Q
see Supplement, Heart and Great Vessels 02U
Annuloplasty ring
use Synthetic Substitute
Anoplasty
see Repair, Anus 0DQQ
see Supplement, Anus 0DUQ
Anorectal junction
use Rectum
Anoscopy 0DJD8ZZ
Ansa cervicalis
use Nerve, Cervical Plexus
Antabuse therapy HZ93ZZZ
Antebrachial fascia
use Subcutaneous Tissue and Fascia, Lower Arm, Left
use Subcutaneous Tissue and Fascia, Lower Arm, Right
Anterior (pectoral) lymph node
use Lymphatic, Axillary, Left
use Lymphatic, Axillary, Right
Anterior cerebral artery
use Artery, Intracranial
Anterior cerebral vein
use Vein, Intracranial
Anterior choroidal artery
use Artery, Intracranial
Anterior circumflex humeral artery
use Artery, Axillary, Left
use Artery, Axillary, Right
Anterior communicating artery
use Artery, Intracranial
Anterior cruciate ligament (ACL)
use Bursa and Ligament, Knee, Left
use Bursa and Ligament, Knee, Right
Anterior crural nerve
use Nerve, Femoral
Anterior facial vein
use Vein, Face, Left
use Vein, Face, Right
Anterior intercostal artery
use Artery, Internal Mammary, Left
use Artery, Internal Mammary, Right
Anterior interosseous nerve
use Nerve, Median
Anterior lateral malleolar artery
use Artery, Anterior Tibial, Left
use Artery, Anterior Tibial, Right
Anterior lingual gland
use Gland, Minor Salivary
Anterior medial malleolar artery
use Artery, Anterior Tibial, Left
use Artery, Anterior Tibial, Right
Anterior spinal artery
use Artery, Vertebral, Left
use Artery, Vertebral, Right
Anterior tibial recurrent artery
use Artery, Anterior Tibial, Left
use Artery, Anterior Tibial, Right
Anterior ulnar recurrent artery
use Artery, Ulnar, Left
use Artery, Ulnar, Right
Anterior vagal trunk
use Nerve, Vagus
Anterior vertebral muscle
use Muscle, Neck, Left
use Muscle, Neck, Right
Anti-SARS-CoV-2 hyperimmune globulin
use Hyperimmune Globulin
Antibacterial Envelope (TYRX) (AIGISRx)
use Anti-Infective Envelope
Antibiotic-eluting Bone Void Filler
XW0V0P7
Antigen-free air conditioning
see Atmospheric Control, Physiological Systems 6A0
Antihelix
use Ear, External, Bilateral
use Ear, External, Left
use Ear, External, Right
Antimicrobial envelope
use Anti-Infective Envelope
Antitragus
use Ear, External, Bilateral
use Ear, External, Left
use Ear, External, Right
Antrostomy
see Drainage, Ear, Nose, Sinus 099
Antrotomy
see Drainage, Ear, Nose, Sinus 099
Antrum of Highmore
use Sinus, Maxillary, Left
use Sinus, Maxillary, Right
Aortic annulus
use Valve, Aortic
Aortic arch
use Thoracic Aorta, Ascending/Arch
Aortic intercostal artery
use Upper Artery
Aortography
see Plain Radiography, Upper Arteries B30
see Fluoroscopy, Upper Arteries B31
see Plain Radiography, Lower Arteries B40
see Fluoroscopy, Lower Arteries B41
Aortoplasty
see Repair, Aorta, Thoracic, Descending 02QW
see Repair, Aorta, Thoracic, Ascending/Arch 02QX
see Replacement, Aorta, Thoracic, Descending 02RW
see Replacement, Aorta, Thoracic, Ascending/Arch 02RX
see Supplement, Aorta, Thoracic, Descending 02UW
see Supplement, Aorta, Thoracic, Ascending/Arch 02UX
see Repair, Aorta, Abdominal 04Q0
see Replacement, Aorta, Abdominal 04R0
see Supplement, Aorta, Abdominal 04U0
Apalutamide Antineoplastic
XW0DXJ5
Apical (subclavicular) lymph node
use Lymphatic, Axillary, Left
use Lymphatic, Axillary, Right
ApiFix® Minimally Invasive Deformity Correction (MID-C) System
use Posterior (Dynamic) Distraction Device in New Technology
Apneustic center use Pons
Appendectomy
see Excision, Appendix 0DBJ
see Resection, Appendix 0DTJ
Appendicolysis
see Release, Appendix 0DNJ
Appendicotomy
see Drainage, Appendix 0D9J
Application
see Introduction of substance in or on
aprevo™
use Interbody Fusion Device, Customizable in New Technology
Aquablation therapy, prostate
XV508A4
Aquapheresis 6A550Z3
Aqueduct of Sylvius
use Cerebral Ventricle
Aqueous humour
use Anterior Chamber, Left
use Anterior Chamber, Right
Arachnoid mater, intracranial
use Cerebral Meninges
Arachnoid mater, spinal
use Spinal Meninges
Arcuate artery
use Artery, Foot, Left
use Artery, Foot, Right
Areola
use Nipple, Left
use Nipple, Right
AROM (artificial rupture of membranes) 10907ZC
Arterial canal (duct)
use Artery, Pulmonary, Left
Arterial pulse tracing
see Measurement, Arterial 4A03
Arteriectomy
see Excision, Heart and Great Vessels 02B
see Excision, Upper Arteries 03B
see Excision, Lower Arteries 04B
Arteriography
see Plain Radiography, Heart B20
see Fluoroscopy, Heart B21
see Plain Radiography, Upper Arteries B30
see Fluoroscopy, Upper Arteries B31
see Plain Radiography, Lower Arteries B40
see Fluoroscopy, Lower Arteries B41
Arterioplasty
see Repair, Heart and Great Vessels 02Q
see Replacement, Heart and Great Vessels 02R
see Repair, Upper Arteries 03Q
see Replacement, Upper Arteries 03R
see Repair, Lower Arteries 04Q
see Replacement, Lower Arteries 04R
see Supplement, Upper Arteries 03U
see Supplement, Lower Arteries 04U
see Supplement, Heart and Great Vessels 02U
Arteriorrhaphy
see Repair, Heart and Great Vessels 02Q
see Repair, Upper Arteries 03Q
see Repair, Lower Arteries 04Q

Arterioscopy
see Inspection, Artery, Lower 04JY
see Inspection, Artery, Upper 03JY
see Inspection, Great Vessel 02JY
Arthrectomy
see Excision, Upper Joints 0RB
see Resection, Upper Joints 0RT
see Excision, Lower Joints 0SB
see Resection, Lower Joints 0ST
Arthrocentesis
see Drainage, Upper Joints 0R9
see Drainage, Lower Joints 0S9
Arthrodesis
see Fusion, Upper Joints 0RG
see Fusion, Lower Joints 0SG
Arthrography
see Plain Radiography, Skull and Facial Bones BN0
see Plain Radiography, Non-Axial Upper Bones BP0
see Plain Radiography, Non-Axial Lower Bones BQ0
Arthrolysis
see Release, Upper Joints 0RN
see Release, Lower Joints 0SN
Arthropexy
see Repair, Upper Joints 0RQ
see Reposition, Upper Joints 0RS
see Repair, Lower Joints 0SQ
see Reposition, Lower Joints 0SS
Arthroplasty
see Repair, Upper Joints 0RQ
see Replacement, Upper Joints 0RR
see Repair, Lower Joints 0SQ
see Replacement, Lower Joints 0SR
see Supplement, Lower Joints 0SU
see Supplement, Upper Joints 0RU
Arthroplasty, radial head
see Replacement, Radius, Left 0PRJ
see Replacement, Radius, Right 0PRH
Arthroscopy
see Inspection, Upper Joints 0RJ
see Inspection, Lower Joints 0SJ
Arthrotomy
see Drainage, Upper Joints 0R9
see Drainage, Lower Joints 0S9
Articulating Spacer (Antibiotic)
use Articulating Spacer in Lower Joints
Artificial anal sphincter (AAS)
use Artificial Sphincter in Gastrointestinal System
Artificial bowel sphincter (neosphincter)
use Artificial Sphincter in Gastrointestinal System
Artificial Sphincter
Insertion of device in
Anus 0DHQ
Bladder 0THB
Bladder Neck 0THC
Urethra 0THD
Removal of device from
Anus 0DPQ
Bladder 0TPB
Urethra 0TPD
Revision of device in
Anus 0DWQ
Bladder 0TWB
Urethra 0TWD
Artificial urinary sphincter (AUS)
use Artificial Sphincter in Urinary System
Aryepiglottic fold
use Larynx
Arytenoid cartilage
use Larynx
Arytenoid muscle
use Muscle, Neck, Left
use Muscle, Neck, Right
Arytenoidectomy
see Excision, Larynx 0CBS
Arytenoidopexy
see Repair, Larynx 0CQS
Ascenda Intrathecal Catheter
use Infusion Device
Ascending aorta
use Thoracic Aorta, Ascending/Arch
Ascending palatine artery
use Artery, Face
Ascending pharyngeal artery
use Artery, External Carotid, Left
use Artery, External Carotid, Right
aScope™ Duodeno
see New Technology, Hepatobiliary System and Pancreas XFJ
Aspiration, fine needle
Fluid or gas
see Drainage
Tissue biopsy
see Excision
see Extraction
Assessment
Activities of daily living
see Activities of Daily Living Assessment, Rehabilitation F02
Hearing
see Hearing Assessment, Diagnostic Audiology F13
Hearing aid
see Hearing Aid Assessment, Diagnostic Audiology F14
Intravascular perfusion, using indocyanine green (ICG) dye
see Monitoring, Physiological Systems 4A1
Motor function
see Motor Function Assessment, Rehabilitation F01
Nerve function
see Motor Function Assessment, Rehabilitation F01
Speech
see Speech Assessment, Rehabilitation F00
Vestibular
see Vestibular Assessment, Diagnostic Audiology F15
Vocational
see Activities of Daily Living Treatment, Rehabilitation F08
Assistance
Cardiac
Continuous
Balloon Pump 5A02210
Impeller Pump 5A0221D
Other Pump 5A02216
Pulsatile Compression 5A02215
Intermittent
Balloon Pump 5A02110
Impeller Pump 5A0211D
Other Pump 5A02116
Pulsatile Compression 5A02115
Circulatory
Continuous
Hyperbaric 5A05221
Supersaturated 5A0522C
Intermittent
Hyperbaric 5A05121
Supersaturated 5A0512C
Respiratory
24-96 Consecutive Hours
Continuous Negative Airway Pressure 5A09459
Continuous Positive Airway Pressure 5A09457
Assistance *(continued)*
Respiratory *(continued)*
24-96 Consecutive Hours *(continued)*
High Nasal Flow/Velocity 5A0945A
Intermittent Negative Airway Pressure 5A0945B
Intermittent Positive Airway Pressure 5A09458
No Qualifier 5A0945Z
Continuous, Filtration 5A0920Z
Greater than 96 Consecutive Hours
Continuous Negative Airway Pressure 5A09559
Continuous Positive Airway Pressure 5A09557
High Nasal Flow/Velocity 5A0955A
Intermittent Negative Airway Pressure 5A0955B
Intermittent Positive Airway Pressure 5A09558
No Qualifier 5A0955Z
Less than 24 Consecutive Hours
Continuous Negative Airway Pressure 5A09359
Continuous Positive Airway Pressure 5A09357
High Nasal Flow/Velocity 5A0935A
Intermittent Negative Airway Pressure 5A0935B
Intermittent Positive Airway Pressure 5A09358
No Qualifier 5A0935Z
Associating liver partition and portal vein ligation (ALPPS)
see Division, Hepatobiliary System and Pancreas 0F8
see Resection, Hepatobiliary System and Pancreas 0FT
Assurant (Cobalt) stent
use Intraluminal Device
Atezolizumab Antineoplastic XW0
Atherectomy
see Extirpation, Heart and Great Vessels 02C
see Extirpation, Upper Arteries 03C
see Extirpation, Lower Arteries 04C
Atlantoaxial joint
use Joint, Cervical Vertebral
Atmospheric Control 6A0Z
AtriClip LAA Exclusion System
use Extraluminal Device
Atrioseptoplasty
see Repair, Heart and Great Vessels 02Q
see Replacement, Heart and Great Vessels 02R
see Supplement, Heart and Great Vessels 02U
Atrioventricular node
use Conduction Mechanism
Atrium dextrum cordis
use Atrium, Right
Atrium pulmonale
use Atrium, Left
Attain Ability® lead
use Cardiac Lead, Pacemaker in 02H
use Cardiac Lead, Defibrillator in 02H
Attain StarFix® (OTW) lead
use Cardiac Lead, Defibrillator in 02H
use Cardiac Lead, Pacemaker in 02H
Audiology, diagnostic
see Hearing Assessment, Diagnostic Audiology F13
see Hearing Aid Assessment, Diagnostic Audiology F14
see Vestibular Assessment, Diagnostic Audiology F15
Audiometry
see Hearing Assessment, Diagnostic Audiology F13
Auditory tube
use Eustachian Tube, Left
use Eustachian Tube, Right
Auerbach's (myenteric) plexus
use Nerve, Abdominal Sympathetic
Auricle
use Ear, External, Bilateral
use Ear, External, Left
use Ear, External, Right
Auricularis muscle
use Muscle, Head
Autograft
use Autologous Tissue Substitute
Autologous artery graft
use Autologous Arterial Tissue in Heart and Great Vessels
use Autologous Arterial Tissue in Lower Arteries
use Autologous Arterial Tissue in Lower Veins
use Autologous Arterial Tissue in Upper Arteries
use Autologous Arterial Tissue in Upper Veins
Autologous vein graft
use Autologous Venous Tissue in Heart and Great Vessels
use Autologous Venous Tissue in Lower Arteries
use Autologous Venous Tissue in Lower Veins
use Autologous Venous Tissue in Upper Arteries
use Autologous Venous Tissue in Upper Veins
Automated Chest Compression (ACC) 5A1221J
AutoPulse® Resuscitation System 5A1221J
Autotransfusion
see Transfusion
Autotransplant
Adrenal tissue
see Reposition, Endocrine System 0GS
Kidney
see Reposition, Urinary System 0TS
Pancreatic tissue
see Reposition, Pancreas 0FSG
Parathyroid tissue
see Reposition, Endocrine System 0GS
Thyroid tissue
see Reposition, Endocrine System 0GS
Tooth
see Reattachment, Mouth and Throat 0CM
Avulsion
see Extraction
AVYCAZ® (ceftazidime-avibactam)
use Other Anti-infective
Axial Lumbar Interbody Fusion System
use Interbody Fusion Device in Lower Joints
AxiaLIF® System
use Interbody Fusion Device in Lower Joints

Axicabtagene Ciloeucel
  use Axicabtagene Ciloleucel Immunotherapy
Axicabtagene Ciloleucel Immunotherapy XW0
Axillary fascia
  use Subcutaneous Tissue and Fascia, Upper Arm, Left
  use Subcutaneous Tissue and Fascia, Upper Arm, Right
Axillary nerve
  use Nerve, Brachial Plexus
AZEDRA®
  use Iobenguane I-131 Antineoplastic

B

BAK/C® Interbody Cervical Fusion System
  use Interbody Fusion Device in Upper Joints
BAL (bronchial alveolar lavage), diagnostic
  see Drainage, Respiratory System 0B9
Balanoplasty
  see Repair, Penis 0VQS
  see Supplement, Penis 0VUS
Balloon atrial septostomy (BAS) 02163Z7
Balloon Pump
  Continuous, Output 5A02210
  Intermittent, Output 5A02110
Bandage, Elastic
  see Compression
Banding
  see Occlusion
  see Restriction
Banding, esophageal varices
  see Occlusion, Vein, Esophageal 06L3
Banding, laparoscopic (adjustable) gastric
  Initial procedure 0DV64CZ
  Surgical correction
    see Revision of device in, Stomach 0DW6
Bard® Composix® (E/X)(LP) mesh
  use Synthetic Substitute
Bard® Composix® Kugel® patch
  use Synthetic Substitute
Bard® Dulex™ mesh
  use Synthetic Substitute
Bard® Ventralex™ hernia patch
  use Synthetic Substitute
Barium swallow
  see Fluoroscopy, Gastrointestinal System BD1
Baroreflex Activation Therapy® (BAT®)
  Stimulator Generator in Subcutaneous Tissue and Fascia
  use Stimulator Lead in Upper Arteries
Barricaid® Annular Closure Device (ACD)
  use Synthetic Substitute
Bartholin's (greater vestibular) gland
  use Gland, Vestibular
Basal (internal) cerebral vein
  use Vein, Intracranial
Basal metabolic rate (BMR)
  see Measurement, Physiological Systems 4A0Z
Basal nuclei
  use Basal Ganglia
Base of Tongue
  use Pharynx
Basilar artery
  use Artery, Intracranial
Basis pontis
  use Pons
Beam Radiation
  Abdomen DW03
    Intraoperative DW033Z0
  Adrenal Gland DG02
    Intraoperative DG023Z0
  Bile Ducts DF02
    Intraoperative DF023Z0
  Bladder DT02
    Intraoperative DT023Z0
  Bone
    Intraoperative DP0C3Z0
    Other DP0C
  Bone Marrow D700
    Intraoperative D7003Z0
  Brain D000
    Intraoperative D0003Z0
  Brain Stem D001
    Intraoperative D0013Z0
  Breast
    Left DM00
      Intraoperative DM003Z0
    Right DM01
      Intraoperative DM013Z0
  Bronchus DB01
    Intraoperative DB013Z0
  Cervix DU01
    Intraoperative DU013Z0
  Chest DW02
    Intraoperative DW023Z0
  Chest Wall DB07
    Intraoperative DB073Z0
  Colon DD05
    Intraoperative DD053Z0
  Diaphragm DB08
    Intraoperative DB083Z0
  Duodenum DD02
    Intraoperative DD023Z0
  Ear D900
    Intraoperative D9003Z0
  Esophagus DD00
    Intraoperative DD003Z0
  Eye D800
    Intraoperative D8003Z0
  Femur DP09
    Intraoperative DP093Z0
  Fibula DP0B
    Intraoperative DP0B3Z0
  Gallbladder DF01
    Intraoperative DF013Z0
  Gland
    Adrenal DG02
      Intraoperative DG023Z0
    Parathyroid DG04
      Intraoperative DG043Z0
    Pituitary DG00
      Intraoperative DG003Z0
    Thyroid DG05
      Intraoperative DG053Z0
  Glands
    Intraoperative D9063Z0
    Salivary D906
  Head and Neck DW01
    Intraoperative DW013Z0
  Hemibody DW04
    Intraoperative DW043Z0
  Humerus DP06
    Intraoperative DP063Z0
  Hypopharynx D903
    Intraoperative D9033Z0
  Ileum DD04
    Intraoperative DD043Z0
  Jejunum DD03
    Intraoperative DD033Z0
  Kidney DT00
    Intraoperative DT003Z0
  Larynx D90B
    Intraoperative D90B3Z0
  Liver DF00
    Intraoperative DF003Z0
Beam Radiation *(continued)*
  Lung DB02
    Intraoperative DB023Z0
  Lymphatics
    Abdomen D706
      Intraoperative D7063Z0
    Axillary D704
      Intraoperative D7043Z0
    Inguinal D708
      Intraoperative D7083Z0
    Neck D703
      Intraoperative D7033Z0
    Pelvis D707
      Intraoperative D7073Z0
    Thorax D705
      Intraoperative D7053Z0
  Mandible DP03
    Intraoperative DP033Z0
  Maxilla DP02
    Intraoperative DP023Z0
  Mediastinum DB06
    Intraoperative DB063Z0
  Mouth D904
    Intraoperative D9043Z0
  Nasopharynx D90D
    Intraoperative D90D3Z0
  Neck and Head DW01
    Intraoperative DW013Z0
  Nerve
    Intraoperative D0073Z0
    Peripheral D007
  Nose D901
    Intraoperative D9013Z0
  Oropharynx D90F
    Intraoperative D90F3Z0
  Ovary DU00
    Intraoperative DU003Z0
  Palate
    Hard D908
      Intraoperative D9083Z0
    Soft D909
      Intraoperative D9093Z0
  Pancreas DF03
    Intraoperative DF033Z0
  Parathyroid Gland DG04
    Intraoperative DG043Z0
  Pelvic Bones DP08
    Intraoperative DP083Z0
  Pelvic Region DW06
    Intraoperative DW063Z0
  Pineal Body DG01
    Intraoperative DG013Z0
  Pituitary Gland DG00
    Intraoperative DG003Z0
  Pleura DB05
    Intraoperative DB053Z0
  Prostate DV00
    Intraoperative DV003Z0
  Radius DP07
    Intraoperative DP073Z0
  Rectum DD07
    Intraoperative DD073Z0
  Rib DP05
    Intraoperative DP053Z0
  Sinuses D907
    Intraoperative D9073Z0
  Skin
    Abdomen DH08
      Intraoperative DH083Z0
    Arm DH04
      Intraoperative DH043Z0
    Back DH07
      Intraoperative DH073Z0
    Buttock DH09
      Intraoperative DH093Z0
    Chest DH06
      Intraoperative DH063Z0
    Face DH02
      Intraoperative DH023Z0
    Leg DH0B
      Intraoperative DH0B3Z0
Beam Radiation *(continued)*
  Skin *(continued)*
    Neck DH03
      Intraoperative DH033Z0
  Skull DP00
    Intraoperative DP003Z0
  Spinal Cord D006
    Intraoperative D0063Z0
  Spleen D702
    Intraoperative D7023Z0
  Sternum DP04
    Intraoperative DP043Z0
  Stomach DD01
    Intraoperative DD013Z0
  Testis DV01
    Intraoperative DV013Z0
  Thymus D701
    Intraoperative D7013Z0
  Thyroid Gland DG05
    Intraoperative DG053Z0
  Tibia DP0B
    Intraoperative DP0B3Z0
  Tongue D905
    Intraoperative D9053Z0
  Trachea DB00
    Intraoperative DB003Z0
  Ulna DP07
    Intraoperative DP073Z0
  Ureter DT01
    Intraoperative DT013Z0
  Urethra DT03
    Intraoperative DT033Z0
  Uterus DU02
    Intraoperative DU023Z0
  Whole Body DW05
    Intraoperative DW053Z0
Bedside swallow F00ZJWZ
Berlin Heart Ventricular Assist Device
  use Implantable Heart Assist System in Heart and Great Vessels
Bezlotoxumab Monoclonal Antibody XW0
Biceps brachii muscle
  use Muscle, Upper Arm, Left
  use Muscle, Upper Arm, Right
Biceps femoris muscle
  use Muscle, Upper Leg, Left
  use Muscle, Upper Leg, Right
Bicipital aponeurosis
  use Subcutaneous Tissue and Fascia, Lower Arm, Left
  use Subcutaneous Tissue and Fascia, Lower Arm, Right
Bicuspid valve
  use Valve, Mitral
Bili light therapy
  see Phototherapy, Skin 6A60
Bioactive embolization coil(s)
  use Intraluminal Device, Bioactive in Upper Arteries
Bioengineered Allogeneic Construct, Skin XHRPXF7
Biofeedback GZC9ZZZ
BioFire® FilmArray® Pneumonia Panel XXEBXQ6
Biopsy
  see Drainage with qualifier Diagnostic
  see Excision with qualifier Diagnostic
  see Extraction with qualifier Diagnostic
BiPAP
  see Assistance, Respiratory v5A09
Bisection
  see Division
Biventricular external heart assist system
  use Short-term External Heart Assist System in Heart and Great Vessels

Blepharectomy
see Excision, Eye 08B
see Resection, Eye 08T
Blepharoplasty
see Repair, Eye 08Q
see Replacement, Eye 08R
see Reposition, Eye 08S
see Supplement, Eye 08U
Blepharorrhaphy
see Repair, Eye 08Q
Blepharotomy
see Drainage, Eye 089
Blinatumomab
use Other Antineoplastic
BLINCYTO® (blinatumomab)
use Other Antineoplastic
Block, Nerve, anesthetic injection
3E0T3BZ
Blood glucose monitoring system
use Monitoring Device
Blood pressure
see Measurement, Arterial 4A03
BMR (basal metabolic rate)
see Measurement, Physiological Systems 4A0Z
Body of femur
use Femoral Shaft, Left
use Femoral Shaft, Right
Body of fibula
use Fibula, Left
use Fibula, Right
Bone anchored hearing device
use Hearing Device, Bone Conduction in 09H
use Hearing Device in Head and Facial Bones
Bone bank bone graft
use Nonautologous Tissue Substitute
Bone Growth Stimulator
Insertion of device in
Bone
Facial 0NHW
Lower 0QHY
Nasal 0NHB
Upper 0PHY
Skull 0NH0
Removal of device from
Bone
Facial 0NPW
Lower 0QPY
Nasal 0NPB
Upper 0PPY
Skull 0NP0
Revision of device in
Bone
Facial 0NWW
Lower 0QWY
Nasal 0NWB
Upper 0PWY
Skull 0NW0
Bone marrow transplant
see Transfusion, Circulatory 302
Bone morphogenetic protein 2 (BMP 2)
use Recombinant Bone Morphogenetic Protein
Bone screw (interlocking)(lag) (pedicle)(recessed)
use Internal Fixation Device in Head and Facial Bones
use Internal Fixation Device in Lower Bones
use Internal Fixation Device in Upper Bones
Bony labyrinth
use Ear, Inner, Left
use Ear, Inner, Right
Bony orbit
use Orbit, Left
use Orbit, Right
Bony vestibule
use Ear, Inner, Left
use Ear, Inner, Right
Botallo's duct
use Artery, Pulmonary, Left
Bovine pericardial valve
use Zooplastic Tissue in Heart and Great Vessels
Bovine pericardium graft
use Zooplastic Tissue in Heart and Great Vessels
BP (blood pressure)
see Measurement, Arterial 4A03
Brachial (lateral) lymph node
use Lymphatic, Axillary, Left
use Lymphatic, Axillary, Right
Brachialis muscle
use Muscle, Upper Arm, Left
use Muscle, Upper Arm, Right
Brachiocephalic artery
use Artery, Innominate
Brachiocephalic trunk
use Artery, Innominate
Brachiocephalic vein
use Vein, Innominate, Left
use Vein, Innominate, Right
Brachioradialis muscle
use Muscle, Lower Arm and Wrist, Left
use Muscle, Lower Arm and Wrist, Right
Brachytherapy
Abdomen DW13
Adrenal Gland DG12
Back
Lower DW1L
Upper DW1K
Bile Ducts DF12
Bladder DT12
Bone Marrow D710
Brain D010
Brain Stem D011
Breast
Left DM10
Right DM11
Bronchus DB11
Cervix DU11
Chest DW12
Chest Wall DB17
Colon DD15
Cranial Cavity DW10
Diaphragm DB18
Duodenum DD12
Ear D910
Esophagus DD10
Extremity
Lower DW1Y
Upper DW1X
Eye D810
Gastrointestinal Tract DW1P
Gallbladder DF11
Genitourinary Tract DW1R
Gland
Adrenal DG12
Parathyroid DG14
Pituitary DG10
Thyroid DG15
Glands, Salivary D916
Head and Neck DW11
Hypopharynx D913
Ileum DD14
Jejunum DD13
Kidney DT10
Larynx D91B
Liver DF10
Lung DB12
Lymphatics
Abdomen D716
Axillary D714
Inguinal D718
Brachytherapy *(continued)*
Lymphatics *(continued)*
Neck D713
Pelvis D717
Thorax D715
Mediastinum DB16
Mouth D914
Nasopharynx D91D
Neck and Head DW11
Nerve, Peripheral D017
Nose D911
Oropharynx D91F
Ovary DU10
Palate
Hard D918
Soft D919
Pancreas DF13
Parathyroid Gland DG14
Pelvic Region DW16
Pineal Body DG11
Pituitary Gland DG10
Pleura DB15
Prostate DV10
Rectum DD17
Respiratory Tract DW1Q
Sinuses D917
Spinal Cord D016
Spleen D712
Stomach DD11
Testis DV11
Thymus D711
Thyroid Gland DG15
Tongue D915
Trachea DB10
Ureter DT11
Urethra DT13
Uterus DU12
Brachytherapy, CivaSheet®
see Brachytherapy with qualifier Unidirectional Source
see Insertion with device Radioactive Element
Brachytherapy seeds
use Radioactive Element
Breast procedures, skin only
use Skin, Chest
Brexanolone XW0
Brexucabtagene Autoleucel
use Brexucabtagene Autoleucel Immunotherapy
Brexucabtagene Autoleucel Immunotherapy XW0
Broad ligament
use Uterine Supporting Structure
Bromelain-enriched Proteolytic Enzyme XW0
Bronchial artery
use Upper Artery
Bronchography
see Fluoroscopy, Respiratory System BB1
see Plain Radiography, Respiratory System BB0
Bronchoplasty
see Repair, Respiratory System 0BQ
see Supplement, Respiratory System 0BU
Bronchorrhaphy
see Repair, Respiratory System 0BQ
Bronchoscopy 0BJ08ZZ
Bronchotomy
see Drainage, Respiratory System 0B9
Bronchus Intermedius
use Main Bronchus, Right
BRYAN® Cervical Disc System
use Synthetic Substitute
Buccal gland
use Buccal Mucosa
Buccinator lymph node
use Lymphatic, Head
Buccinator muscle
use Muscle, Facial
Buckling, scleral with implant
see Supplement, Eye 08U
Bulbospongiosus muscle
use Muscle, Perineum
Bulbourethral (Cowper's) gland
use Urethra
Bundle of His
use Conduction Mechanism
Bundle of Kent
use Conduction Mechanism
Bunionectomy
see Excision, Lower Bones 0QB
Bursectomy
see Excision, Bursae and Ligaments 0MB
see Resection, Bursae and Ligaments 0MT
Bursocentesis
see Drainage, Bursae and Ligaments 0M9
Bursography
see Plain Radiography, Non-Axial Upper Bones BP0
see Plain Radiography, Non-Axial Lower Bones BQ0
Bursotomy
see Division, Bursae and Ligaments 0M8
see Drainage, Bursae and Ligaments 0M9
BVS 5000 Ventricular Assist Device
use Short-term External Heart Assist System in Heart and Great Vessels
Bypass
Anterior Chamber
Left 08133
Right 08123
Aorta
Abdominal 0410
Thoracic
Ascending/Arch 021X
Descending 021W
Artery
Anterior Tibial
Left 041Q
Right 041P
Axillary
Left 03160
Right 03150
Brachial
Left 0318
Right 0317
Common Carotid
Left 031J0
Right 031H0
Common Iliac
Left 041D
Right 041C
Coronary
Four or More Arteries 0213
One Artery 0210
Three Arteries 0212
Two Arteries 0211
External Carotid
Left 031N0
Right 031M0
External Iliac
Left 041J
Right 041H
Femoral
Left 041L
Right 041K
Foot
Left 041W
Right 041V
Hepatic 0413
Innominate 03120

- **Bypass** *(continued)*
  - Artery *(continued)*
    - Internal Carotid
      - Left 031L0
      - Right 031K0
    - Internal Iliac
      - Left 041F
      - Right 041E
    - Intracranial 031G0
    - Peroneal
      - Left 041U
      - Right 041T
    - Popliteal
      - Left 041N
      - Right 041M
    - Posterior Tibial
      - Left 041S
      - Right 041R
    - Pulmonary
      - Left 021R
      - Right 021Q
    - Pulmonary Trunk 021P
    - Radial
      - Left 031C
      - Right 031B
    - Splenic 0414
    - Subclavian
      - Left 03140
      - Right 03130
    - Temporal
      - Left 031T0
      - Right 031S0
    - Ulnar
      - Left 031A
      - Right 0319
  - Atrium
    - Left 0217
    - Right 0216
  - Bladder 0T1B
  - Cavity, Cranial 0W110J
  - Cecum 0D1H
  - Cerebral Ventricle 0016
  - Colon
    - Ascending 0D1K
    - Descending 0D1M
    - Sigmoid 0D1N
    - Transverse 0D1L
  - Duct
    - Common Bile 0F19
    - Cystic 0F18
    - Hepatic
      - Common 0F17
      - Left 0F16
      - Right 0F15
    - Lacrimal
      - Left 081Y
      - Right 081X
    - Pancreatic 0F1D
      - Accessory 0F1F
  - Duodenum 0D19
  - Ear
    - Left 091E0
    - Right 091D0
  - Esophagus 0D15
    - Lower 0D13
    - Middle 0D12
    - Upper 0D11
  - Fallopian Tube
    - Left 0U16
    - Right 0U15
  - Gallbladder 0F14
  - Ileum 0D1B
  - Intestine
    - Large 0D1E
    - Small 0D18
  - Jejunum 0D1A
  - Kidney Pelvis
    - Left 0T14
    - Right 0T13
  - Pancreas 0F1G

- **Bypass** *(continued)*
  - Pelvic Cavity 0W1J
  - Peritoneal Cavity 0W1G
  - Pleural Cavity
    - Left 0W1B
    - Right 0W19
  - Spinal Canal 001U
  - Stomach 0D16
  - Trachea 0B11
  - Ureter
    - Left 0T17
    - Right 0T16
  - Ureters, Bilateral 0T18
  - Vas Deferens
    - Bilateral 0V1Q
    - Left 0V1P
    - Right 0V1N
  - Vein
    - Axillary
      - Left 0518
      - Right 0517
    - Azygos 0510
    - Basilic
      - Left 051C
      - Right 051B
    - Brachial
      - Left 051A
      - Right 0519
    - Cephalic
      - Left 051F
      - Right 051D
    - Colic 0617
    - Common Iliac
      - Left 061D
      - Right 061C
    - Esophageal 0613
    - External Iliac
      - Left 061G
      - Right 061F
    - External Jugular
      - Left 051Q
      - Right 051P
    - Face
      - Left 051V
      - Right 051T
    - Femoral
      - Left 061N
      - Right 061M
    - Foot
      - Left 061V
      - Right 061T
    - Gastric 0612
    - Hand
      - Left 051H
      - Right 051G
    - Hemiazygos 0511
    - Hepatic 0614
    - Hypogastric
      - Left 061J
      - Right 061H
    - Inferior Mesenteric 0616
    - Innominate
      - Left 0514
      - Right 0513
    - Internal Jugular
      - Left 051N
      - Right 051M
    - Intracranial 051L
    - Portal 0618
    - Renal
      - Left 061B
      - Right 0619
    - Saphenous
      - Left 061Q
      - Right 061P
    - Splenic 0611
    - Subclavian
      - Left 0516
      - Right 0515
    - Superior Mesenteric 0615

- **Bypass** *(continued)*
  - Vein *(continued)*
    - Vertebral
      - Left 051S
      - Right 051R
  - Vena Cava
    - Inferior 0610
    - Superior 021V
  - Ventricle
    - Left 021L
    - Right 021K
- **Bypass, cardiopulmonary** 5A1221Z

C

- **Caesarean section**
  - *see* Extraction, Products of Conception 10D0
- **Calcaneocuboid joint**
  - *use* Joint, Tarsal, Left
  - *use* Joint, Tarsal, Right
- **Calcaneocuboid ligament**
  - *use* Bursa and Ligament, Foot, Left
  - *use* Bursa and Ligament, Foot, Right
- **Calcaneofibular ligament**
  - *use* Bursa and Ligament, Ankle, Left
  - *use* Bursa and Ligament, Ankle, Right
- **Calcaneus**
  - *use* Tarsal, Left
  - *use* Tarsal, Right
- **Cannulation**
  - *see* Bypass
  - *see* Dilation
  - *see* Drainage
  - *see* Irrigation
- **Canthorrhaphy**
  - *see* Repair, Eye 08Q
- **Canthotomy**
  - *see* Release, Eye 08N
- **Capitate bone**
  - *use* Carpal, Left
  - *use* Carpal, Right
- **Caplacizumab** XW0
- **Capsulectomy, lens**
  - *see* Excision, Eye 08B
- **Capsulorrhaphy, joint**
  - *see* Repair, Lower Joints 0SQ
  - *see* Repair, Upper Joints 0RQ
- **Caption Guidance system** X2JAX47
- **Cardia**
  - *use* Esophagogastric Junction
- **Cardiac contractility modulation lead**
  - *use* Cardiac Lead in Heart and Great Vessels
- **Cardiac event recorder**
  - *use* Monitoring Device
- **Cardiac Lead**
  - Defibrillator
    - Atrium
      - Left 02H7
      - Right 02H6
    - Pericardium 02HN
    - Vein, Coronary 02H4
    - Ventricle
      - Left 02HL
      - Right 02HK
  - Insertion of device in
    - Atrium
      - Left 02H7Z
      - Right 02H6
    - Pericardium 02HN
    - Vein, Coronary 02H4
    - Ventricle
      - Left 02HL
      - Right 02HK

- **Cardiac Lead** *(continued)*
  - Pacemaker
    - Atrium
      - Left 02H7
      - Right 02H6
    - Pericardium 02HN
    - Vein, Coronary 02H4
    - Ventricle
      - Left 02HL
      - Right 02HK
  - Removal of device from, Heart 02PA
  - Revision of device in, Heart 02WA
- **Cardiac plexus**
  - *use* Nerve, Thoracic Sympathetic
- **Cardiac Resynchronization Defibrillator Pulse Generator**
  - Abdomen 0JH8
  - Chest 0JH6
- **Cardiac Resynchronization Pacemaker Pulse Generator**
  - Abdomen 0JH8
  - Chest 0JH6
- **Cardiac resynchronization therapy (CRT) lead**
  - *use* Cardiac Lead, Defibrillator in 02H
  - *use* Cardiac Lead, Pacemaker in 02H
- **Cardiac Rhythm Related Device**
  - Insertion of device in
    - Abdomen 0JH8
    - Chest 0JH6
  - Removal of device from, Subcutaneous Tissue and Fascia, Trunk 0JPT
  - Revision of device in, Subcutaneous Tissue and Fascia, Trunk 0JWT
- **Cardiocentesis**
  - *see* Drainage, Pericardial Cavity 0W9D
- **Cardioesophageal junction**
  - *use* Esophagogastric Junction
- **Cardiolysis**
  - *see* Release, Heart and Great Vessels 02N
- **CardioMEMS® pressure sensor**
  - *use* Monitoring Device, Pressure Sensor in 02H
- **Cardiomyotomy**
  - *see* Division, Esophagogastric Junction 0D84
- **Cardioplegia**
  - *see* Introduction of substance in or on, Heart 3E08
- **Cardiorrhaphy**
  - *see* Repair, Heart and Great Vessels 02Q
- **Cardioversion** 5A2204Z
- **Caregiver training** F0FZ
- **Carmat total artificial heart** (TAH)
  - *use* Biologic with Synthetic Substitute, Autoregulated Electrohydraulic in 02R
- **Caroticotympanic artery**
  - *use* Artery, Internal Carotid, Left
  - *use* Artery, Internal Carotid, Right
- **Carotid (artery) sinus (baroreceptor) lead**
  - *use* Stimulator Lead in Upper Arteries
- **Carotid glomus**
  - *use* Carotid Bodies, Bilateral
  - *use* Carotid Body, Left
  - *use* Carotid Body, Right
- **Carotid sinus**
  - *use* Artery, Internal Carotid, Left
  - *use* Artery, Internal Carotid, Right

Carotid sinus nerve
use Nerve, Glossopharyngeal
Carotid WALLSTENT® Monorail® Endoprosthesis
use Intraluminal Device
Carpectomy
see Excision, Upper Bones 0PB
see Resection, Upper Bones 0PT
Carpometacarpal ligament
use Bursa and Ligament, Hand, Left
use Bursa and Ligament, Hand, Right
Casirivimab (REGN10933) and Imdevimab (REGN10987)
use REGN-COV2 Monoclonal Antibody
Casting
see Immobilization
CAT scan
see Computerized Tomography (CT Scan)
Catheterization
see Dilation
see Drainage
Heart
see Measurement, Cardiac 4A02
see Irrigation
see Insertion of device in
Umbilical vein, for infusion 06H033T
Cauda equina
use Spinal Cord, Lumbar
Cauterization
see Destruction
see Repair
Cavernous plexus
use Nerve, Head and Neck Sympathetic
CBMA (Concentrated Bone Marrow Aspirate)
use Concentrated Bone Marrow Aspirate
CBMA (Concentrated Bone Marrow Aspirate) injection, intramuscular XK02303
Cecectomy
see Excision, Cecum 0DBH
see Resection, Cecum 0DTH
Cecocolostomy
see Bypass, Gastrointestinal System 0D1
see Drainage, Gastrointestinal System 0D9
Cecopexy
see Repair, Cecum 0DQH
see Reposition, Cecum 0DSH
Cecoplication
see Restriction, Cecum 0DVH
Cecorrhaphy
see Repair, Cecum 0DQH
Cecostomy
see Bypass, Cecum 0D1H
see Drainage, Cecum 0D9H
Cecotomy
see Drainage, Cecum 0D9H
Cefiderocol Anti-Infective XW0
Ceftazidime-avibactam
use Other Anti-infective
Ceftolozane/Tazobactam Anti-Infective XW0
Celiac (solar) plexus
use Nerve, Abdominal Sympathetic
Celiac ganglion
use Nerve, Abdominal Sympathetic
Celiac lymph node
use Lymphatic, Aortic
Celiac trunk
use Artery, Celiac
Central axillary lymph node
use Lymphatic, Axillary, Left
use Lymphatic, Axillary, Right
Central venous pressure
see Measurement, Venous 4A04
Centrimag® Blood Pump
use Short-term External Heart Assist System in Heart and Great Vessels
Cephalogram BN00ZZZ
CERAMENT® G
use Antibiotic-eluting Bone Void Filler
Ceramic on ceramic bearing surface
use Synthetic Substitute, Ceramic in 0SR
Cerclage
see Restriction
Cerebral aqueduct (Sylvius)
use Cerebral Ventricle
Cerebral Embolic Filtration
Dual Filter X2A5312
Extracorporeal Flow Reversal Circuit X2A
Single Deflection Filter X2A6325
Cerebrum
use Brain
Cervical esophagus
use Esophagus, Upper
Cervical facet joint
use Joint, Cervical Vertebral
use Joint, Cervical Vertebral, 2 or more
Cervical ganglion
use Nerve, Head and Neck Sympathetic
Cervical interspinous ligament
use Bursa and Ligament, Head and Neck
Cervical intertransverse ligament
use Bursa and Ligament, Head and Neck
Cervical ligamentum flavum
use Bursa and Ligament, Head and Neck
Cervical lymph node
use Lymphatic, Neck, Left
use Lymphatic, Neck, Right
Cervicectomy
see Excision, Cervix 0UBC
see Resection, Cervix 0UTC
Cervicothoracic facet joint
use Joint, Cervicothoracic Vertebral
Cesarean section
see Extraction, Products of Conception 10D0
Cesium-131 Collagen Implant
use Radioactive Element, Cesium-131 Collagen Implant in 00H
Change device in
Abdominal Wall 0W2FX
Back
Lower 0W2LX
Upper 0W2KX
Bladder 0T2BX
Bone
Facial 0N2WX
Lower 0Q2YX
Nasal 0N2BX
Upper 0P2YX
Bone Marrow 072TX
Brain 0020X
Breast
Left 0H2UX
Right 0H2TX
Bursa and Ligament
Lower 0M2YX
Upper 0M2XX
Cavity, Cranial 0W21X
Chest Wall 0W28X
Cisterna Chyli 072LX
Diaphragm 0B2TX
Duct
Hepatobiliary 0F2BX
Pancreatic 0F2DX
Change device in *(continued)*
Ear
Left 092JX
Right 092HX
Epididymis and Spermatic Cord 0V2MX
Extremity
Lower
Left 0Y2BX
Right 0Y29X
Upper
Left 0X27X
Right 0X26X
Eye
Left 0821X
Right 0820X
Face 0W22X
Fallopian Tube 0U28X
Gallbladder 0F24X
Gland
Adrenal 0G25X
Endocrine 0G2SX
Pituitary 0G20X
Salivary 0C2AX
Head 0W20X
Intestinal Tract
Lower 0D2DXUZ
Upper 0D20XUZ
Jaw
Lower 0W25X
Upper 0W24X
Joint
Lower 0S2YX
Upper 0R2YX
Kidney 0T25X
Larynx 0C2SX
Liver 0F20X
Lung
Left 0B2LX
Right 0B2KX
Lymphatic 072NX
Thoracic Duct 072KX
Mediastinum 0W2CX
Mesentery 0D2VX
Mouth and Throat 0C2YX
Muscle
Lower 0K2YX
Upper 0K2XX
Nasal Mucosa and Soft Tissue 092KX
Neck 0W26X
Nerve
Cranial 002EX
Peripheral 012YX
Omentum 0D2UX
Ovary 0U23X
Pancreas 0F2GX
Parathyroid Gland 0G2RX
Pelvic Cavity 0W2JX
Penis 0V2SX
Pericardial Cavity 0W2DX
Perineum
Female 0W2NX
Male 0W2MX
Peritoneal Cavity 0W2GX
Peritoneum 0D2WX
Pineal Body 0G21X
Pleura 0B2QX
Pleural Cavity
Left 0W2BX
Right 0W29X
Products of Conception 10207
Prostate and Seminal Vesicles 0V24X
Retroperitoneum 0W2HX
Scrotum and Tunica Vaginalis 0V28X
Sinus 092YX
Skin 0H2PX
Skull 0N20X
Spinal Canal 002UX
Spleen 072PX
Change device in *(continued)*
Subcutaneous Tissue and Fascia
Head and Neck 0J2SX
Lower Extremity 0J2WX
Trunk 0J2TX
Upper Extremity 0J2VX
Tendon
Lower 0L2YX
Upper 0L2XX
Testis 0V2DX
Thymus 072MX
Thyroid Gland 0G2KX
Trachea 0B21
Tracheobronchial Tree 0B20X
Ureter 0T29X
Urethra 0T2DX
Uterus and Cervix 0U2DXHZ
Vagina and Cul-de-sac 0U2HXGZ
Vas Deferens 0V2RX
Vulva 0U2MX
Change device in or on
Abdominal Wall 2W03X
Anorectal 2Y03X5Z
Arm
Lower
Left 2W0DX
Right 2W0CX
Upper
Left 2W0BX
Right 2W0AX
Back 2W05X
Chest Wall 2W04X
Ear 2Y02X5Z
Extremity
Lower
Left 2W0MX
Right 2W0LX
Upper
Left 2W09X
Right 2W08X
Face 2W01X
Finger
Left 2W0KX
Right 2W0JX
Foot
Left 2W0TX
Right 2W0SX
Genital Tract, Female 2Y04X5Z
Hand
Left 2W0FX
Right 2W0EX
Head 2W00X
Inguinal Region
Left 2W07X
Right 2W06X
Leg
Lower
Left 2W0RX
Right 2W0QX
Upper
Left 2W0PX
Right 2W0NX
Mouth and Pharynx 2Y00X5Z
Nasal 2Y01X5Z
Neck 2W02X
Thumb
Left 2W0HX
Right 2W0GX
Toe
Left 2W0VX
Right 2W0UX
Urethra 2Y05X5Z
Chemoembolization
see Introduction of substance in or on
Chemosurgery, Skin 3E00XTZ
Chemothalamectomy
see Destruction, Thalamus 0059
Chemotherapy, Infusion for cancer
see Introduction of substance in or on

Chest compression (CPR), external
Manual 5A12012
Mechanical 5A1221J
Chest x-ray
see Plain Radiography, Chest BW03
Chiropractic Manipulation
Abdomen 9WB9X
Cervical 9WB1X
Extremities
Lower 9WB6X
Upper 9WB7X
Head 9WB0X
Lumbar 9WB3X
Pelvis 9WB5X
Rib Cage 9WB8X
Sacrum 9WB4X
Thoracic 9WB2X
Choana
use Nasopharynx
Cholangiogram
see Plain Radiography, Hepatobiliary System and Pancreas BF0
see Fluoroscopy, Hepatobiliary System and Pancreas BF1
Cholecystectomy
see Excision, Gallbladder 0FB4
see Resection, Gallbladder 0FT4
Cholecystojejunostomy
see Bypass, Hepatobiliary System and Pancreas 0F1
see Drainage, Hepatobiliary System and Pancreas 0F9
Cholecystopexy
see Repair, Gallbladder 0FQ4
see Reposition, Gallbladder 0FS4
Cholecystoscopy 0FJ44ZZ
Cholecystostomy
see Drainage, Gallbladder 0F94
see Bypass, Gallbladder 0F14
Cholecystotomy
see Drainage, Gallbladder 0F94
Choledochectomy
see Excision, Hepatobiliary System and Pancreas 0FB
see Resection, Hepatobiliary System and Pancreas 0FT
Choledocholithotomy
see Extirpation, Duct, Common Bile 0FC9
Choledochoplasty
see Repair, Hepatobiliary System and Pancreas 0FQ
see Replacement, Hepatobiliary System and Pancreas 0FR
see Supplement, Hepatobiliary System and Pancreas 0FU
Choledochoscopy 0FJB8ZZ
Choledochotomy
see Drainage, Hepatobiliary System and Pancreas 0F9
Cholelithotomy
see Extirpation, Hepatobiliary System and Pancreas 0FC
Chondrectomy
see Excision, Lower Joints 0SB
see Excision, Upper Joints 0RB
Knee
see Excision, Lower Joints 0SB
Semilunar cartilage
see Excision, Lower Joints 0SB
Chondroglossus muscle
use Muscle, Tongue, Palate, Pharynx
Chorda tympani
use Nerve, Facial
Chordotomy
see Division, Central Nervous System and Cranial Nerves 008
Choroid plexus
use Cerebral Ventricle
Choroidectomy
see Excision, Eye 08B
see Resection, Eye 08T
Ciliary body
use Eye, Left
use Eye, Right
Ciliary ganglion
use Nerve, Head and Neck Sympathetic
cilta-cel *use* Ciltacabtagene Autoleucel
Ciltacabtagene Autoleucel XW0
Circle of Willis
use Artery, Intracranial
Circumcision 0VTTXZZ
Circumflex iliac artery
use Artery, Femoral, Left
use Artery, Femoral, Right
CivaSheet®
use Radioactive Element
CivaSheet® Brachytherapy
see Brachytherapy with qualifier Unidirectional Source
see Insertion with device Radioactive Element
Clamp and rod internal fixation system (CRIF)
use Internal Fixation Device in Lower Bones
use Internal Fixation Device in Upper Bones
Clamping
see Occlusion
Claustrum
use Basal Ganglia
Claviculectomy
see Excision, Upper Bones 0PB
see Resection, Upper Bones 0PT
Claviculotomy
see Division, Upper Bones 0P8
see Drainage, Upper Bones 0P9
Clipping, aneurysm
see Occlusion using Extraluminal Device
see Restriction using Extraluminal Device
Clitorectomy, clitoridectomy
see Excision, Clitoris 0UBJ
see Resection, Clitoris 0UTJ
Clolar
use Clofarabine
Closure
see Occlusion
see Repair
Clysis
see Introduction of substance in or on
Coagulation
see Destruction
Coagulation Factor Xa, Inactivated XW0
Coagulation Factor Xa, (Recombinant) Inactivated
use Coagulation Factor Xa, Inactivated
COALESCE® radiolucent interbody fusion device
use Interbody Fusion Device, Radiolucent Porous in New Technology
CoAxia NeuroFlo catheter
use Intraluminal Device
Cobalt/chromium head and polyethylene socket
use Synthetic Substitute, Metal on Polyethylene in 0SR
Cobalt/chromium head and socket
use Synthetic Substitute, Metal in 0SR
Coccygeal body
use Coccygeal Glomus
Coccygeus muscle
use Muscle, Trunk, Left
use Muscle, Trunk, Right
Cochlea
use Ear, Inner, Left
use Ear, Inner, Right
Cochlear implant (CI), multiple channel (electrode)
use Hearing Device, Multiple Channel Cochlear Prosthesis in 09H
Cochlear implant (CI), single channel (electrode)
use Hearing Device, Single Channel Cochlear Prosthesis in 09H
Cochlear Implant Treatment F0BZ0
Cochlear nerve
use Nerve, Acoustic
COGNIS® CRT-D
use Cardiac Resynchronization Defibrillator Pulse Generator in 0JH
COHERE® radiolucent interbody fusion device
use Interbody Fusion Device, Radiolucent Porous in New Technology
Colectomy
see Excision, Gastrointestinal System 0DB
see Resection, Gastrointestinal System 0DT
Collapse
see Occlusion
Collection from
Breast, Breast Milk 8E0HX62
Indwelling Device
Circulatory System
Blood 8C02X6K
Other Fluid 8C02X6L
Nervous System
Cerebrospinal Fluid 8C01X6J
Other Fluid 8C01X6L
Integumentary System, Breast Milk 8E0HX62
Reproductive System, Male, Sperm 8E0VX63
Colocentesis
see Drainage, Gastrointestinal System 0D9
Colofixation
see Repair, Gastrointestinal System 0DQ
see Reposition, Gastrointestinal System 0DS
Cololysis
see Release, Gastrointestinal System 0DN
Colonic Z-Stent®
use Intraluminal Device
Colonoscopy 0DJD8ZZ
Colopexy
see Repair, Gastrointestinal System 0DQ
see Reposition, Gastrointestinal System 0DS
Coloplication
see Restriction, Gastrointestinal System 0DV
Coloproctectomy
see Excision, Gastrointestinal System 0DB
see Resection, Gastrointestinal System 0DT
Coloproctostomy
see Bypass, Gastrointestinal System 0D1
see Drainage, Gastrointestinal System 0D9
Colopuncture
see Drainage, Gastrointestinal System 0D9
Colorrhaphy
see Repair, Gastrointestinal System 0DQ
Colostomy
see Bypass, Gastrointestinal System 0D1
see Drainage, Gastrointestinal System 0D9
Colpectomy
see Excision, Vagina 0UBG
see Resection, Vagina 0UTG
Colpocentesis
see Drainage, Vagina 0U9G
Colpopexy
see Repair, Vagina 0UQG
see Reposition, Vagina 0USG
Colpoplasty
see Repair, Vagina 0UQG
see Supplement, Vagina 0UUG
Colporrhaphy
see Repair, Vagina 0UQG
Colposcopy 0UJH8ZZ
Columella
use Nasal Mucosa and Soft Tissue
Common digital vein
use Vein, Foot, Left
use Vein, Foot, Right
Common facial vein
use Vein, Face, Left
use Vein, Face, Right
Common fibular nerve
use Nerve, Peroneal
Common hepatic artery
use Artery, Hepatic
Common iliac (subaortic) lymph node
use Lymphatic, Pelvis
Common interosseous artery
use Artery, Ulnar, Left
use Artery, Ulnar, Right
Common peroneal nerve
use Nerve, Peroneal
Complete (SE) stent
use Intraluminal Device
Compression
see Restriction
Abdominal Wall 2W13X
Arm
Lower
Left 2W1DX
Right 2W1CX
Upper
Left 2W1BX
Right 2W1AX
Back 2W15X
Chest Wall 2W14X
Extremity
Lower
Left 2W1MX
Right 2W1LX
Upper
Left 2W19X
Right 2W18X
Face 2W11X
Finger
Left 2W1KX
Right 2W1JX
Foot
Left 2W1TX
Right 2W1SX
Hand
Left 2W1FX
Right 2W1EX
Head 2W10X
Inguinal Region
Left 2W17X
Right 2W16X

Compression *(continued)*
- Leg
  - Lower
    - Left 2W1RX
    - Right 2W1QX
  - Upper
    - Left 2W1PX
    - Right 2W1NX
- Neck 2W12X
- Thumb
  - Left 2W1HX
  - Right 2W1GX
- Toe
  - Left 2W1VX
  - Right 2W1UX

Computer-aided Assessment, Intracranial Vascular Activity XXE0X07

Computer-aided Guidance, Transthoracic Echocardiography X2JAX47

Computer-aided Mechanical Aspiration X2C

Computer-aided Triage and Notification, Pulmonary Artery Flow XXE3X27

Computer-assisted Intermittent Aspiration
- *see* New Technology, Cardiovascular System X2C

Computer Assisted Procedure
- Extremity
  - Lower
    - No Qualifier 8E0YXBZ
    - With Computerized Tomography 8E0YXBG
    - With Fluoroscopy 8E0YXBF
    - With Magnetic Resonance Imaging 8E0YXBH
  - Upper
    - No Qualifier 8E0XXBZ
    - With Computerized Tomography 8E0XXBG
    - With Fluoroscopy 8E0XXBF
    - With Magnetic Resonance Imaging 8E0XXBH
- Head and Neck Region
  - No Qualifier 8E09XBZ
  - With Computerized Tomography 8E09XBG
  - With Fluoroscopy 8E09XBF
  - With Magnetic Resonance Imaging 8E09XBH
- Trunk Region
  - No Qualifier 8E0WXBZ
  - With Computerized Tomography 8E0WXBG
  - With Fluoroscopy 8E0WXBF
  - With Magnetic Resonance Imaging 8E0WXBH

Computerized Tomography (CT Scan)
- Abdomen BW20
  - Chest and Pelvis BW25
- Abdomen and Chest BW24
- Abdomen and Pelvis BW21
- Airway, Trachea BB2F
- Ankle
  - Left BQ2H
  - Right BQ2G
- Aorta
  - Abdominal B420
    - Intravascular Optical Coherence B420Z2Z
  - Thoracic B320
    - Intravascular Optical Coherence B320Z2Z
- Arm
  - Left BP2F
  - Right BP2E

Computerized Tomography (CT Scan) *(continued)*
- Artery
  - Celiac B421
    - Intravascular Optical Coherence B421Z2Z
  - Common Carotid
    - Bilateral B325
    - Intravascular Optical Coherence B325Z2Z
  - Coronary
    - Bypass Graft
      - Multiple B223
      - Intravascular Optical Coherence B223Z2Z
    - Multiple B221
      - Intravascular Optical Coherence B221Z2Z
  - Internal Carotid
    - Bilateral B328
    - Intravascular Optical Coherence B328Z2Z
  - Intracranial B32R
    - Intravascular Optical Coherence B32RZ2Z
  - Lower Extremity
    - Bilateral B42H
      - Intravascular Optical Coherence B42HZ2Z
    - Left B42G
      - Intravascular Optical Coherence B42GZ2Z
    - Right B42F
      - Intravascular Optical Coherence B42FZ2Z
  - Pelvic B42C
    - Intravascular Optical Coherence B42CZ2Z
  - Pulmonary
    - Left B32T
      - Intravascular Optical Coherence B32TZ2Z
    - Right B32S
      - Intravascular Optical Coherence B32SZ2Z
  - Renal
    - Bilateral B428
      - Intravascular Optical Coherence B428Z2Z
    - Transplant B42M
      - Intravascular Optical Coherence B42MZ2Z
  - Superior Mesenteric B424
    - Intravascular Optical Coherence B424Z2Z
  - Vertebral
    - Bilateral B32G
    - Intravascular Optical Coherence B32GZ2Z
- Bladder BT20
- Bone
  - Facial BN25
  - Temporal BN2F
- Brain B020
- Calcaneus
  - Left BQ2K
  - Right BQ2J
- Cerebral Ventricle B028
- Chest, Abdomen and Pelvis BW25
- Chest and Abdomen BW24
- Cisterna B027
- Clavicle
  - Left BP25
  - Right BP24
- Coccyx BR2F
- Colon BD24
- Ear B920
- Elbow
  - Left BP2H
  - Right BP2G

Computerized Tomography (CT Scan) *(continued)*
- Extremity
  - Lower
    - Left BQ2S
    - Right BQ2R
  - Upper
    - Bilateral BP2V
    - Left BP2U
    - Right BP2T
- Eye
  - Bilateral B827
  - Left B826
  - Right B825
- Femur
  - Left BQ24
  - Right BQ23
- Fibula
  - Left BQ2C
  - Right BQ2B
- Finger
  - Left BP2S
  - Right BP2R
- Foot
  - Left BQ2M
  - Right BQ2L
- Forearm
  - Left BP2K
  - Right BP2J
- Gland
  - Adrenal, Bilateral BG22
  - Parathyroid BG23
  - Parotid, Bilateral B926
  - Salivary, Bilateral B92D
  - Submandibular, Bilateral B929
  - Thyroid BG24
- Hand
  - Left BP2P
  - Right BP2N
- Hands and Wrists, Bilateral BP2Q
- Head BW28
- Head and Neck BW29
- Heart
  - Intravascular Optical Coherence B226Z2Z
  - Right and Left B226
- Hepatobiliary System, All BF2C
- Hip
  - Left BQ21
  - Right BQ20
- Humerus
  - Left BP2B
  - Right BP2A
- Intracranial Sinus B522
  - Intravascular Optical Coherence B522Z2Z
- Joint
  - Acromioclavicular, Bilateral BP23
  - Finger
    - Left BP2DZZZ
    - Right BP2CZZZ
  - Foot
    - Left BQ2Y
    - Right BQ2X
  - Hand
    - Left BP2DZZZ
    - Right BP2CZZZ
  - Sacroiliac BR2D
  - Sternoclavicular
    - Bilateral BP22
    - Left BP21
    - Right BP20
  - Temporomandibular, Bilateral BN29
  - Toe
    - Left BQ2Y
    - Right BQ2X
- Kidney
  - Bilateral BT23
  - Left BT22

Computerized Tomography (CT Scan) *(continued)*
- Kidney *(continued)*
  - Right BT21
  - Transplant BT29
- Knee
  - Left BQ28
  - Right BQ27
- Larynx B92J
- Leg
  - Left BQ2F
  - Right BQ2D
- Liver BF25
- Liver and Spleen BF26
- Lung, Bilateral BB24
- Mandible BN26
- Nasopharynx B92F
- Neck BW2F
- Neck and Head BW29
- Orbit, Bilateral BN23
- Oropharynx B92F
- Pancreas BF27
- Patella
  - Left BQ2W
  - Right BQ2V
- Pelvic Region BW2G
- Pelvis BR2C
  - Chest and Abdomen BW25
- Pelvis and Abdomen BW21
- Pituitary Gland B029
- Prostate BV23
- Ribs
  - Left BP2Y
  - Right BP2X
- Sacrum BR2F
- Scapula
  - Left BP27
  - Right BP26
- Sella Turcica B029
- Shoulder
  - Left BP29
  - Right BP28
- Sinus
  - Intracranial B522
    - Intravascular Optical Coherence B522Z2Z
  - Paranasal B922
- Skull BN20
- Spinal Cord B02B
- Spine
  - Cervical BR20
  - Lumbar BR29
  - Thoracic BR27
- Spleen and Liver BF26
- Thorax BP2W
- Tibia
  - Left BQ2C
  - Right BQ2B
- Toe
  - Left BQ2Q
  - Right BQ2P
- Trachea BB2F
- Tracheobronchial Tree
  - Bilateral BB29
  - Left BB28
  - Right BB27
- Vein
  - Pelvic (Iliac)
    - Left B52G
      - Intravascular Optical Coherence B52GZ2Z
    - Right B52F
      - Intravascular Optical Coherence B52FZ2Z
  - Pelvic (Iliac) Bilateral B52H
    - Intravascular Optical Coherence B52HZ2Z
  - Portal B52T
    - Intravascular Optical Coherence B52TZ2Z

Control bleeding in *(continued)*
Pericardial Cavity 0W3D
Perineum
Female 0W3N
Male 0W3M
Peritoneal Cavity 0W3G
Pleural Cavity
Left 0W3B
Right 0W39
Respiratory Tract 0W3Q
Retroperitoneum 0W3H
Shoulder Region
Left 0X33
Right 0X32
Wrist Region
Left 0X3H
Right 0X3G
Control bleeding using Tourniquet, External *see* Compression, Anatomical Regions 2W1
Conus arteriosus
use Ventricle, Right
Conus medullaris
use Spinal Cord, Lumbar
Convalescent Plasma (Nonautologous) *see* New Technology, Anatomical Regions XW1
Conversion
Cardiac rhythm 5A2204Z
Gastrostomy to jejunostomy feeding device
see Insertion of device in, Jejunum 0DHA
Cook Biodesign® Fistula Plug(s)
use Nonautologous Tissue Substitute
Cook Biodesign® Hernia Graft(s)
use Nonautologous Tissue Substitute
Cook Biodesign® Layered Graft(s)
use Nonautologous Tissue Substitute
Cook Zenapro™ Layered Graft(s)
use Nonautologous Tissue Substitute
Cook Zenith AAA Endovascular Graft
use Intraluminal Device
Cook Zenith® Fenestrated AAA Endovascular Graft
use Intraluminal Device, Branched or Fenestrated, One or Two Arteries in 04V
use Intraluminal Device, Branched or Fenestrated, Three or More Arteries in 04V
Coracoacromial ligament
use Bursa and Ligament, Shoulder, Left
use Bursa and Ligament, Shoulder, Right
Coracobrachialis muscle
use Muscle, Upper Arm, Left
use Muscle, Upper Arm, Right
Coracoclavicular ligament
use Bursa and Ligament, Shoulder, Left
use Bursa and Ligament, Shoulder, Right
Coracohumeral ligament
use Bursa and Ligament, Shoulder, Left
use Bursa and Ligament, Shoulder, Right
Coracoid process
use Scapula, Left
use Scapula, Right
Cordotomy
see Division, Central Nervous System and Cranial Nerves 008
Core needle biopsy
see Excision with qualifier Diagnostic
CoreValve transcatheter aortic valve
use Zooplastic Tissue in Heart and Great Vessels
Cormet Hip Resurfacing System
use Resurfacing Device in Lower Joints
Corniculate cartilage
use Larynx
CoRoent® XL
use Interbody Fusion Device in Lower Joints
Coronary arteriography
see Fluoroscopy, Heart B21
see Plain Radiography, Heart B20
Corox (OTW) Bipolar Lead
use Cardiac Lead, Defibrillator in 02H
use Cardiac Lead, Pacemaker in 02H
Corpus callosum
use Brain
Corpus cavernosum
use Penis
Corpus spongiosum
use Penis
Corpus striatum
use Basal Ganglia
Corrugator supercilii muscle
use Muscle, Facial
Cortical strip neurostimulator lead
use Neurostimulator Lead in Central Nervous System and Cranial Nerves
Corvia IASD®
use Synthetic Substitute
COSELA™ *use* Trilaciclib
Costatectomy
see Excision, Upper Bones 0PB
see Resection, Upper Bones 0PT
Costectomy
see Excision, Upper Bones 0PB
see Resection, Upper Bones 0PT
Costocervical trunk
use Artery, Subclavian, Left
use Artery, Subclavian, Right
Costochondrectomy
see Excision, Upper Bones 0PB
see Resection, Upper Bones 0PT
Costoclavicular ligament
use Bursa and Ligament, Shoulder, Left
use Bursa and Ligament, Shoulder, Right
Costosternoplasty
see Repair, Upper Bones 0PQ
see Replacement, Upper Bones 0PR
see Supplement, Upper Bones 0PU
Costotomy
see Division, Upper Bones 0P8
see Drainage, Upper Bones 0P9
Costotransverse joint
use Joint, Thoracic Vertebral
Costotransverse ligament
use Rib(s) Bursa and Ligament
Costovertebral joint
use Joint, Thoracic Vertebral
Costoxiphoid ligament
use Sternum Bursa and Ligament
Counseling
Family, for substance abuse, Other Family Counseling HZ63ZZZ
Group
12-Step HZ43ZZZ
Behavioral HZ41ZZZ
Cognitive HZ40ZZZ
Cognitive-Behavioral HZ42ZZZ
Confrontational HZ48ZZZ
Continuing Care HZ49ZZZ
Infectious Disease
Counseling *(continued)*
Group *(continued)*
Post-Test HZ4CZZZ
Pre-Test HZ4CZZZ
Interpersonal HZ44ZZZ
Motivational Enhancement HZ47ZZZ
Psychoeducation HZ46ZZZ
Spiritual HZ4BZZZ
Vocational HZ45ZZZ
Individual
12-Step HZ33ZZZ
Behavioral HZ31ZZZ
Cognitive HZ30ZZZ
Cognitive-Behavioral HZ32ZZZ
Confrontational HZ38ZZZ
Continuing Care HZ39ZZZ
Infectious Disease
Post-Test HZ3CZZZ
Pre-Test HZ3CZZZ
Interpersonal HZ34ZZZ
Motivational Enhancement HZ37ZZZ
Psychoeducation HZ36ZZZ
Spiritual HZ3BZZZ
Vocational HZ35ZZZ
Mental Health Services
Educational GZ60ZZZ
Other Counseling GZ63ZZZ
Vocational GZ61ZZZ
Countershock, cardiac 5A2204Z
Cowper's (bulbourethral) gland
use Urethra
CPAP (continuous positive airway pressure)
see Assistance, Respiratory 5A09
Craniectomy
see Excision, Head and Facial Bones 0NB
see Resection, Head and Facial Bones 0NT
Cranioplasty
see Repair, Head and Facial Bones 0NQ
see Replacement, Head and Facial Bones 0NR
see Supplement, Head and Facial Bones 0NU
Craniotomy
see Drainage, Central Nervous System and Cranial Nerves 009
see Division, Head and Facial Bones 0N8
see Drainage, Head and Facial Bones 0N9
Creation
Perineum
Female 0W4N0
Male 0W4M0
Valve
Aortic 024F0
Mitral 024G0
Tricuspid 024J0
Cremaster muscle
use Muscle, Perineum
CRESEMBA® (isavuconazonium sulfate)
use Other Anti-infective
Cribriform plate
use Bone, Ethmoid, Left
use Bone, Ethmoid, Right
Cricoid cartilage
use Trachea
Cricoidectomy
see Excision, Larynx 0CBS
Cricothyroid artery
use Artery, Thyroid, Left
use Artery, Thyroid, Right
Cricothyroid muscle
use Muscle, Neck, Left
use Muscle, Neck, Right
Crisis Intervention GZ2ZZZZ
CRRT (Continuous renal replacement therapy) 5A1D90Z
Crural fascia
use Subcutaneous Tissue and Fascia, Upper Leg, Left
use Subcutaneous Tissue and Fascia, Upper Leg, Right
Crushing, nerve
Cranial
see Destruction, Central Nervous System and Cranial Nerves 005
Peripheral
see Destruction, Peripheral Nervous System 015
Cryoablation
see Destruction
Cryotherapy
see Destruction
Cryptorchidectomy
see Excision, Male Reproductive System 0VB
see Resection, Male Reproductive System 0VT
Cryptorchiectomy
see Excision, Male Reproductive System 0VB
see Resection, Male Reproductive System 0VT
Cryptotomy
see Division, Gastrointestinal System 0D8
see Drainage, Gastrointestinal System 0D9
CT scan
see Computerized Tomography (CT Scan)
CT sialogram
see Computerized Tomography (CT Scan), Ear, Nose, Mouth and Throat B92
Cubital lymph node
use Lymphatic, Upper Extremity, Left
use Lymphatic, Upper Extremity, Right
Cubital nerve
use Nerve, Ulnar
Cuboid bone
use Tarsal, Left
use Tarsal, Right
Cuboidconavicular joint
use Joint, Tarsal, Left
use Joint, Tarsal, Right
Culdocentesis
see Drainage, Cul-de-sac 0U9F
Culdoplasty
see Repair, Cul-de-sac 0UQF
see Supplement, Cul-de-sac 0UUF
Culdoscopy 0UJH8ZZ
Culdotomy
see Drainage, Cul-de-sac 0U9F
Culmen
use Cerebellum
Cultured epidermal cell autograft
use Autologous Tissue Substitute
Cuneiform cartilage
use Larynx
Cuneonavicular joint
use Joint, Tarsal, Left
use Joint, Tarsal, Right
Cuneonavicular ligament
use Bursa and Ligament, Foot, Left
use Bursa and Ligament, Foot, Right
Curettage
see Excision
see Extraction
Cutaneous (transverse) cervical nerve
use Nerve, Cervical Plexus

CVP (central venous pressure)
see Measurement, Venous 4A04
Cyclodiathermy
see Destruction, Eye 085
Cyclophotocoagulation
see Destruction, Eye 085
CYPHER® Stent
use Intraluminal Device, Drug-eluting in Heart and Great Vessels
Cystectomy
see Excision, Bladder 0TBB
see Resection, Bladder 0TTB
Cystocele repair
see Repair, Subcutaneous Tissue and Fascia, Pelvic Region 0JQC
Cystography
see Fluoroscopy, Urinary System BT1
see Plain Radiography, Urinary System BT0
Cystolithotomy
see Extirpation, Bladder 0TCB
Cystopexy
see Repair, Bladder 0TQB
see Reposition, Bladder 0TSB
Cystoplasty
see Repair, Bladder 0TQB
see Replacement, Bladder 0TRB
see Supplement, Bladder 0TUB
Cystorrhaphy
see Repair, Bladder 0TQB
Cystoscopy 0TJB8ZZ
Cystostomy
see Bypass, Bladder 0T1B
Cystostomy tube
use Drainage Device
Cystotomy
see Drainage, Bladder 0T9B
Cystourethrography
see Fluoroscopy, Urinary System BT1
see Plain Radiography, Urinary System BT0
Cystourethroplasty
see Repair, Urinary System 0TQ
see Replacement, Urinary System 0TR
see Supplement, Urinary System 0TU
Cytarabine and Daunorubicin Liposome Antineoplastic XW0

D

DBS lead
use Neurostimulator Lead in Central Nervous System and Cranial Nerves
DeBakey Left Ventricular Assist Device
use Implantable Heart Assist System in Heart and Great Vessels
Debridement
Excisional
see Excision
Non-excisional
see Extraction
Decompression, Circulatory 6A15
Decortication, lung
see Extirpation, Respiratory System 0BC
see Release, Respiratory System 0BN
Deep brain neurostimulator lead
use Neurostimulator Lead in Central Nervous System and Cranial Nerves
Deep cervical fascia
use Subcutaneous Tissue and Fascia, Neck, Left
use Subcutaneous Tissue and Fascia, Neck, Right
Deep cervical vein
use Vein, Vertebral, Left
use Vein, Vertebral, Right
Deep circumflex iliac artery
use Artery, External Iliac, Left
use Artery, External Iliac, Right
Deep facial vein
use Vein, Face, Left
use Vein, Face, Right
Deep femoral (profunda femoris) vein
use Vein, Femoral, Left
use Vein, Femoral, Right
Deep femoral artery
use Artery, Femoral, Left
use Artery, Femoral, Right
Deep Inferior Epigastric Artery Perforator Flap
Replacement
Bilateral 0HRV077
Left 0HRU077
Right 0HRT077
Transfer
Left 0KXG
Right 0KXF
Deep palmar arch
use Artery, Hand, Left
use Artery, Hand, Right
Deep transverse perineal muscle
use Muscle, Perineum
Deferential artery
use Artery, Internal Iliac, Left
use Artery, Internal Iliac, Right
Defibrillator Generator
Abdomen 0JH8
Chest 0JH6
Defibrotide Sodium Anticoagulant XW0
Defibtech Automated Chest Compression (ACC) device 5A1221J
Defitelio
use Defibrotide Sodium Anticoagulant
Delivery
Cesarean
see Extraction, Products of Conception 10D0
Forceps
see Extraction, Products of Conception 10D0
Manually assisted 10E0XZZ
Products of Conception 10E0XZZ
Vacuum assisted
see Extraction, Products of Conception 10D0
Delta frame external fixator
use External Fixation Device, Hybrid in 0PH
use External Fixation Device, Hybrid in 0PS
use External Fixation Device, Hybrid in 0QH
use External Fixation Device, Hybrid in 0QS
Delta III Reverse shoulder prosthesis
use Synthetic Substitute, Reverse Ball and Socket in 0RR
Deltoid fascia
use Subcutaneous Tissue and Fascia, Upper Arm, Left
use Subcutaneous Tissue and Fascia, Upper Arm, Right
Deltoid ligament
use Bursa and Ligament, Ankle, Left
use Bursa and Ligament, Ankle, Right
Deltoid muscle
use Muscle, Shoulder, Left
use Muscle, Shoulder, Right
Deltopectoral (infraclavicular) lymph node
use Lymphatic, Upper Extremity, Left
use Lymphatic, Upper Extremity, Right
Denervation
Cranial nerve
see Destruction, Central Nervous System and Cranial Nerves 005
Peripheral nerve
see Destruction, Peripheral Nervous System 015
Dens
use Cervical Vertebra
Densitometry
Plain Radiography
Femur
Left BQ04ZZ1
Right BQ03ZZ1
Hip
Left BQ01ZZ1
Right BQ00ZZ1
Spine
Cervical BR00ZZ1
Lumbar BR09ZZ1
Thoracic BR07ZZ1
Whole BR0GZZ1
Ultrasonography
Elbow
Left BP4HZZ1
Right BP4GZZ1
Hand
Left BP4PZZ1
Right BP4NZZ1
Shoulder
Left BP49ZZ1
Right BP48ZZ1
Wrist
Left BP4MZZ1
Right BP4LZZ1
Denticulate (dentate) ligament
use Spinal Meninges
Depressor anguli oris muscle
use Muscle, Facial
Depressor labii inferioris muscle
use Muscle, Facial
Depressor septi nasi muscle
use Muscle, Facial
Depressor supercilii muscle
use Muscle, Facial
Dermabrasion
see Extraction, Skin and Breast 0HD
Dermis
use Skin
Descending genicular artery
use Artery, Femoral, Left
use Artery, Femoral, Right
Destruction
Acetabulum
Left 0Q55
Right 0Q54
Adenoids 0C5Q
Ampulla of Vater 0F5C
Anal Sphincter 0D5R
Anterior Chamber
Left 08533ZZ
Right 08523ZZ
Anus 0D5Q
Aorta
Abdominal 0450
Thoracic
Ascending/Arch 025X
Descending 025W
Aortic Body 0G5D
Appendix 0D5J
Destruction *(continued)*
Artery
Anterior Tibial
Left 045Q
Right 045P
Axillary
Left 0356
Right 0355
Brachial
Left 0358
Right 0357
Celiac 0451
Colic
Left 0457
Middle 0458
Right 0456
Common Carotid
Left 035J
Right 035H
Common Iliac
Left 045D
Right 045C
External Carotid
Left 035N
Right 035M
External Iliac
Left 045J
Right 045H
Face 035R
Femoral
Left 045L
Right 045K
Foot
Left 045W
Right 045V
Gastric 0452
Hand
Left 035F
Right 035D
Hepatic 0453
Inferior Mesenteric 045B
Innominate 0352
Internal Carotid
Left 035L
Right 035K
Internal Iliac
Left 045F
Right 045E
Internal Mammary
Left 0351
Right 0350
Intracranial 035G
Lower 045Y
Peroneal
Left 045U
Right 045T
Popliteal
Left 045N
Right 045M
Posterior Tibial
Left 045S
Right 045R
Pulmonary
Left 025R
Right 025Q
Pulmonary Trunk 025P
Radial
Left 035C
Right 035B
Renal
Left 045A
Right 0459
Splenic 0454
Subclavian
Left 0354
Right 0353
Superior Mesenteric 0455
Temporal
Left 035T
Right 035S

Destruction *(continued)*
- Artery *(continued)*
  - Thyroid
    - Left 035V
    - Right 035U
  - Ulnar
    - Left 035A
    - Right 0359
  - Upper 035Y
  - Vertebral
    - Left 035Q
    - Right 035P
- Atrium
  - Left 0257
  - Right 0256
- Auditory Ossicle
  - Left 095A
  - Right 0959
- Basal Ganglia 0058
- Bladder 0T5B
- Bladder Neck 0T5C
- Bone
  - Ethmoid
    - Left 0N5G
    - Right 0N5F
  - Frontal 0N51
  - Hyoid 0N5X
  - Lacrimal
    - Left 0N5J
    - Right 0N5H
  - Nasal 0N5B
  - Occipital 0N57
  - Palatine
    - Left 0N5L
    - Right 0N5K
  - Parietal
    - Left 0N54
    - Right 0N53
  - Pelvic
    - Left 0Q53
    - Right 0Q52
  - Sphenoid 0N5C
  - Temporal
    - Left 0N56
    - Right 0N55
  - Zygomatic
    - Left 0N5N
    - Right 0N5M
- Brain 0050
- Breast
  - Bilateral 0H5V
  - Left 0H5U
  - Right 0H5T
- Bronchus
  - Lingula 0B59
  - Lower Lobe
    - Left 0B5B
    - Right 0B56
  - Main
    - Left 0B57
    - Right 0B53
  - Middle Lobe, Right 0B55
  - Upper Lobe
    - Left 0B58
    - Right 0B54
- Buccal Mucosa 0C54
- Bursa and Ligament
  - Abdomen
    - Left 0M5J
    - Right 0M5H
  - Ankle
    - Left 0M5R
    - Right 0M5Q
  - Elbow
    - Left 0M54
    - Right 0M53
  - Foot
    - Left 0M5T
    - Right 0M5S
  - Hand
    - Left 0M58

Destruction *(continued)*
- Bursa and Ligament *(continued)*
  - Hand *(continued)*
    - Right 0M57
  - Head and Neck 0M50
  - Hip
    - Left 0M5M
    - Right 0M5L
  - Knee
    - Left 0M5P
    - Right 0M5N
  - Lower Extremity
    - Left 0M5W
    - Right 0M5V
  - Rib(s) 0M5G
  - Shoulder
    - Left 0M52
    - Right 0M51
  - Spine
    - Lower 0M5D
    - Upper 0M5C
  - Sternum 0M5F
  - Upper Extremity
    - Left 0M5B
    - Right 0M59
  - Wrist
    - Left 0M56
    - Right 0M55
- Carina 0B52
- Carotid Bodies, Bilateral 0G58
- Carotid Body
  - Left 0G56
  - Right 0G57
- Carpal
  - Left 0P5N
  - Right 0P5M
- Cecum 0D5H
- Cerebellum 005C
- Cerebral Hemisphere 0057
- Cerebral Meninges 0051
- Cerebral Ventricle 0056
- Cervix 0U5C
- Chordae Tendineae 0259
- Choroid
  - Left 085B
  - Right 085A
- Cisterna Chyli 075L
- Clavicle
  - Left 0P5B
  - Right 0P59
- Clitoris 0U5J
- Coccygeal Glomus 0G5B
- Coccyx 0Q5S
- Colon
  - Ascending 0D5K
  - Descending 0D5M
  - Sigmoid 0D5N
  - Transverse 0D5L
- Conduction Mechanism 0258
- Conjunctiva
  - Left 085TXZZ
  - Right 085SXZZ
- Cord
  - Bilateral 0V5H
  - Left 0V5G
  - Right 0V5F
- Cornea
  - Left 0859XZZ
  - Right 0858XZZ
- Cul-de-sac 0U5F
- Diaphragm 0B5T
- Disc
  - Cervical Vertebral 0R53
  - Cervicothoracic Vertebral 0R55
  - Lumbar Vertebral 0S52
  - Lumbosacral 0S54
  - Thoracic Vertebral 0R59
  - Thoracolumbar Vertebral 0R5B
- Duct
  - Common Bile 0F59

Destruction *(continued)*
- Duct *(continued)*
  - Cystic 0F58
  - Hepatic
    - Common 0F57
    - Left 0F56
    - Right 0F55
  - Lacrimal
    - Left 085Y
    - Right 085X
  - Pancreatic 0F5D
    - Accessory 0F5F
  - Parotid
    - Left 0C5C
    - Right 0C5B
- Duodenum 0D59
- Dura Mater 0052
- Ear
  - External
    - Left 0951
    - Right 0950
  - External Auditory Canal
    - Left 0954
    - Right 0953
  - Inner
    - Left 095E
    - Right 095D
  - Middle
    - Left 0956
    - Right 0955
- Endometrium 0U5B
- Epididymis
  - Bilateral 0V5L
  - Left 0V5K
  - Right 0V5J
- Epiglottis 0C5R
- Esophagogastric Junction 0D54
- Esophagus 0D55
  - Lower 0D53
  - Middle 0D52
  - Upper 0D51
- Eustachian Tube
  - Left 095G
  - Right 095F
- Eye
  - Left 0851XZZ
  - Right 0850XZZ
- Eyelid
  - Lower
    - Left 085R
    - Right 085Q
  - Upper
    - Left 085P
    - Right 085N
- Fallopian Tube
  - Left 0U56
  - Right 0U55
- Fallopian Tubes, Bilateral 0U57
- Femoral Shaft
  - Left 0Q59
  - Right 0Q58
- Femur
  - Lower
    - Left 0Q5C
    - Right 0Q5B
  - Upper
    - Left 0Q57
    - Right 0Q56
- Fibula
  - Left 0Q5K
  - Right 0Q5J
- Finger Nail 0H5QXZZ
- Gallbladder 0F54
- Gingiva
  - Lower 0C56
  - Upper 0C55
- Gland
  - Adrenal
    - Bilateral 0G54
    - Left 0G52
    - Right 0G53

Destruction *(continued)*
- Gland *(continued)*
  - Lacrimal
    - Left 085W
    - Right 085V
  - Minor Salivary 0C5J
  - Parotid
    - Left 0C59
    - Right 0C58
  - Pituitary 0G50
  - Sublingual
    - Left 0C5F
    - Right 0C5D
  - Submaxillary
    - Left 0C5H
    - Right 0C5G
  - Vestibular 0U5L
- Glenoid Cavity
  - Left 0P58
  - Right 0P57
- Glomus Jugulare 0G5C
- Humeral Head
  - Left 0P5D
  - Right 0P5C
- Humeral Shaft
  - Left 0P5G
  - Right 0P5F
- Hymen 0U5K
- Hypothalamus 005A
- Ileocecal Valve 0D5C
- Ileum 0D5B
- Intestine
  - Large 0D5E
    - Left 0D5G
    - Right 0D5F
  - Small 0D58
- Iris
  - Left 085D3ZZ
  - Right 085C3ZZ
- Jejunum 0D5A
- Joint
  - Acromioclavicular
    - Left 0R5H
    - Right 0R5G
  - Ankle
    - Left 0S5G
    - Right 0S5F
  - Carpal
    - Left 0R5R
    - Right 0R5Q
  - Carpometacarpal
    - Left 0R5T
    - Right 0R5S
  - Cervical Vertebral 0R51
  - Cervicothoracic Vertebral 0R54
  - Coccygeal 0S56
  - Elbow
    - Left 0R5M
    - Right 0R5L
  - Finger Phalangeal
    - Left 0R5X
    - Right 0R5W
  - Hip
    - Left 0S5B
    - Right 0S59
  - Knee
    - Left 0S5D
    - Right 0S5C
  - Lumbar Vertebral 0S50
  - Lumbosacral 0S53
  - Metacarpophalangeal
    - Left 0R5V
    - Right 0R5U
  - Metatarsal-Phalangeal
    - Left 0S5N
    - Right 0S5M
  - Occipital-cervical 0R50
  - Sacrococcygeal 0S55
  - Sacroiliac
    - Left 0S58
    - Right 0S57

Destruction *(continued)*
- Joint *(continued)*
  - Shoulder
    - Left 0R5K
    - Right 0R5J
  - Sternoclavicular
    - Left 0R5F
    - Right 0R5E
  - Tarsal
    - Left 0S5J
    - Right 0S5H
  - Tarsometatarsal
    - Left 0S5L
    - Right 0S5K
  - Temporomandibular
    - Left 0R5D
    - Right 0R5C
  - Thoracic Vertebral 0R56
  - Thoracolumbar Vertebral 0R5A
  - Toe Phalangeal
    - Left 0S5Q
    - Right 0S5P
  - Wrist
    - Left 0R5P
    - Right 0R5N
- Kidney
  - Left 0T51
  - Right 0T50
- Kidney Pelvis
  - Left 0T54
  - Right 0T53
- Larynx 0C5S
- Lens
  - Left 085K3ZZ
  - Right 085J3ZZ
- Lip
  - Lower 0C51
  - Upper 0C50
- Liver 0F50
  - Left Lobe 0F52
  - Right Lobe 0F51
- Lung
  - Bilateral 0B5M
  - Left 0B5L
  - Lower Lobe
    - Left 0B5J
    - Right 0B5F
  - Middle Lobe, Right 0B5D
  - Right 0B5K
  - Upper Lobe
    - Left 0B5G
    - Right 0B5C
- Lung Lingula 0B5H
- Lymphatic
  - Aortic 075D
  - Axillary
    - Left 0756
    - Right 0755
  - Head 0750
  - Inguinal
    - Left 075J
    - Right 075H
  - Internal Mammary
    - Left 0759
    - Right 0758
  - Lower Extremity
    - Left 075G
    - Right 075F
  - Mesenteric 075B
  - Neck
    - Left 0752
    - Right 0751
  - Pelvis 075C
  - Thoracic Duct 075K
  - Thorax 0757
  - Upper Extremity
    - Left 0754
    - Right 0753
- Mandible
  - Left 0N5V
  - Right 0N5T

Destruction *(continued)*
- Maxilla 0N5R
- Medulla Oblongata 005D
- Mesentery 0D5V
- Metacarpal
  - Left 0P5Q
  - Right 0P5P
- Metatarsal
  - Left 0Q5P
  - Right 0Q5N
- Muscle
  - Abdomen
    - Left 0K5L
    - Right 0K5K
  - Extraocular
    - Left 085M
    - Right 085L
  - Facial 0K51
  - Foot
    - Left 0K5W
    - Right 0K5V
  - Hand
    - Left 0K5D
    - Right 0K5C
  - Head 0K50
  - Hip
    - Left 0K5P
    - Right 0K5N
  - Lower Arm and Wrist
    - Left 0K5B
    - Right 0K59
  - Lower Leg
    - Left 0K5T
    - Right 0K5S
  - Neck
    - Left 0K53
    - Right 0K52
  - Papillary 025D
  - Perineum 0K5M
  - Shoulder
    - Left 0K56
    - Right 0K55
  - Thorax
    - Left 0K5J
    - Right 0K5H
  - Nasal Mucosa and Soft Tissue 095K
  - Tongue, Palate, Pharynx 0K54
  - Trunk
    - Left 0K5G
    - Right 0K5F
  - Upper Arm
    - Left 0K58
    - Right 0K57
  - Upper Leg
    - Left 0K5R
    - Right 0K5Q
- Nasal Mucosa and Soft Tissue 095K
- Nasopharynx 095N
- Nerve
  - Abdominal Sympathetic 015M
  - Abducens 005L
  - Accessory 005R
  - Acoustic 005N
  - Brachial Plexus 0153
  - Cervical 0151
  - Cervical Plexus 0150
  - Facial 005M
  - Femoral 015D
  - Glossopharyngeal 005P
  - Head and Neck Sympathetic 015K
  - Hypoglossal 005S
  - Lumbar 015B
  - Lumbar Plexus 0159
  - Lumbar Sympathetic 015N
  - Lumbosacral Plexus 015A
  - Median 0155
  - Oculomotor 005H
  - Olfactory 005F
  - Optic 005G

Destruction *(continued)*
- Nerve *(continued)*
  - Peroneal 015H
  - Phrenic 0152
  - Pudendal 015C
  - Radial 0156
  - Sacral 015R
  - Sacral Plexus 015Q
  - Sacral Sympathetic 015P
  - Sciatic 015F
  - Thoracic 0158
  - Thoracic Sympathetic 015L
  - Tibial 015G
  - Trigeminal 005K
  - Trochlear 005J
  - Ulnar 0154
  - Vagus 005Q
- Nipple
  - Left 0H5X
  - Right 0H5W
- Omentum 0D5U
- Orbit
  - Left 0N5Q
  - Right 0N5P
- Ovary
  - Bilateral 0U52
  - Left 0U51
  - Right 0U50
- Palate
  - Hard 0C52
  - Soft 0C53
- Pancreas 0F5G
- Para-aortic Body 0G59
- Paraganglion Extremity 0G5F
- Parathyroid Gland 0G5R
  - Inferior
    - Left 0G5P
    - Right 0G5N
  - Multiple 0G5Q
  - Superior
    - Left 0G5M
    - Right 0G5L
- Patella
  - Left 0Q5F
  - Right 0Q5D
- Penis 0V5S
- Pericardium 025N
- Peritoneum 0D5W
- Phalanx
  - Finger
    - Left 0P5V
    - Right 0P5T
  - Thumb
    - Left 0P5S
    - Right 0P5R
  - Toe
    - Left 0Q5R
    - Right 0Q5Q
- Pharynx 0C5M
- Pineal Body 0G51
- Pleura
  - Left 0B5P
  - Right 0B5N
- Pons 005B
- Prepuce 0V5T
- Prostate 0V50
  - Robotic Waterjet Ablation XV508A4
- Radius
  - Left 0P5J
  - Right 0P5H
- Rectum 0D5P
- Retina
  - Left 085F3ZZ
  - Right 085E3ZZ
- Retinal Vessel
  - Left 085H3ZZ
  - Right 085G3ZZ
- Rib (s)
  - 1 to 2 0P51
  - 3 or More 0P52

Destruction *(continued)*
- Sacrum 0Q51
- Scapula
  - Left 0P56
  - Right 0P55
- Sclera
  - Left 0857XZZ
  - Right 0856XZZ
- Scrotum 0V55
- Septum
  - Atrial 0255
  - Nasal 095M
  - Ventricular 025M
- Sinus
  - Accessory 095P
  - Ethmoid
    - Left 095V
    - Right 095U
  - Frontal
    - Left 095T
    - Right 095S
  - Mastoid
    - Left 095C
    - Right 095B
  - Maxillary
    - Left 095R
    - Right 095Q
  - Sphenoid
    - Left 095X
    - Right 095W
- Skin
  - Abdomen 0H57XZ
  - Back 0H56XZ
  - Buttock 0H58XZ
  - Chest 0H55XZ
  - Ear
    - Left 0H53XZ
    - Right 0H52XZ
  - Face 0H51XZ
  - Foot
    - Left 0H5NXZ
    - Right 0H5MXZ
  - Hand
    - Left 0H5GXZ
    - Right 0H5FXZ
  - Inguinal 0H5AXZ
  - Lower Arm
    - Left 0H5EXZ
    - Right 0H5DXZ
  - Lower Leg
    - Left 0H5LXZ
    - Right 0H5KXZ
  - Neck 0H54XZ
  - Perineum 0H59XZ
  - Scalp 0H50XZ
  - Upper Arm
    - Left 0H5CXZ
    - Right 0H5BXZ
  - Upper Leg
    - Left 0H5JXZ
    - Right 0H5HXZ
- Skull 0N50
- Spinal Cord
  - Cervical 005W
  - Lumbar 005Y
  - Thoracic 005X
- Spinal Meninges 005T
- Spleen 075P
- Sternum 0P50
- Stomach 0D56
  - Pylorus 0D57
- Subcutaneous Tissue and Fascia
  - Abdomen 0J58
  - Back 0J57
  - Buttock 0J59
  - Chest 0J56
  - Face 0J51
  - Foot
    - Left 0J5R
    - Right 0J5Q

Dilation *(continued)*
- Aorta
  - Abdominal 0470
  - Thoracic
    - Ascending/Arch 027X
    - Descending 027W
- Artery
  - Anterior Tibial
    - Left 047Q
      - Sustained Release Drug-eluting Intraluminal Device X27Q385
        - Four or More X27Q3C5
        - Three X27Q3B5
        - Two X27Q395
    - Right 047P
      - Sustained Release Drug-eluting Intraluminal Device X27P385
        - Four or More X27P3C5
        - Three X27P3B5
        - Two X27P395
  - Axillary
    - Left 0376
    - Right 0375
  - Brachial
    - Left 0378
    - Right 0377
  - Celiac 0471
  - Colic
    - Left 0477
    - Middle 0478
    - Right 0476
  - Common Carotid
    - Left 037J
    - Right 037H
  - Common Iliac
    - Left 047D
    - Right 047C
  - Coronary
    - Four or More Arteries 0273
    - One Artery 0270
    - Three Arteries 0272
    - Two Arteries 0271
  - External Carotid
    - Left 037N
    - Right 037M
  - External Iliac
    - Left 047J
    - Right 047H
  - Face 037R
  - Femoral
    - Left 047L
      - Sustained Release Drug-eluting Intraluminal Device X27J385
        - Four or More X27J3C5
        - Three X27J3B5
        - Two X27J395
    - Right 047K
      - Sustained Release Drug-eluting Intraluminal Device X27H385
        - Four or More X27H3C5
        - Three X27H3B5
        - Two X27H395
  - Foot
    - Left 047W
    - Right 047V
  - Gastric 0472
  - Hand
    - Left 037F
    - Right 037D
  - Hepatic 0473
  - Inferior Mesenteric 047B
  - Innominate 0372
  - Internal Carotid
    - Left 037L
    - Right 037K
  - Internal Iliac
    - Left 047F

Dilation *(continued)*
- Artery *(continued)*
  - Internal Iliac *(continued)*
    - Right 047E
  - Internal Mammary
    - Left 0371
    - Right 0370
  - Intracranial 037G
  - Lower 047Y
  - Peroneal
    - Left 047U
      - Sustained Release Drug-eluting Intraluminal Device X27U385
        - Four or More X27U3C5
        - Three X27U3B5
        - Two X27U395
    - Right 047T
      - Sustained Release Drug-eluting Intraluminal Device X27T385
        - Four or More X27T3C5
        - Three X27T3B5
        - Two X27T395
  - Popliteal
    - Left 047N
    - Left Distal
      - Sustained Release Drug-eluting Intraluminal Device X27N385
        - Four or More X27N3C5
        - Three X27N3B5
        - Two X27N395
    - Left Proximal
      - Sustained Release Drug-eluting Intraluminal Device X27L385
        - Four or More X27L3C5
        - Three X27L3B5
        - Two X27L395
    - Right 047M
    - Right Distal
      - Sustained Release Drug-eluting Intraluminal Device X27M385
        - Four or More X27M3C5
        - Three X27M3B5
        - Two X27M395
    - Right Proximal
      - Sustained Release Drug-eluting Intraluminal Device X27K385
        - Four or More X27K3C5
        - Three X27K3B5
        - Two X27K395
  - Posterior Tibial
    - Left 047S
      - Sustained Release Drug-eluting Intraluminal Device X27S385
        - Four or More X27S3C5
        - Three X27S3B5
        - Two X27S395
    - Right 047R
      - Sustained Release Drug-eluting Intraluminal Device X27R385
        - Four or More X27R3C5
        - Three X27R3B5
        - Two X27R395
  - Pulmonary
    - Left 027R
    - Right 027Q
  - Pulmonary Trunk 027P
  - Radial
    - Left 037C
    - Right 037B
  - Renal
    - Left 047A
    - Right 0479
  - Splenic 0474

Dilation *(continued)*
- Artery *(continued)*
  - Subclavian
    - Left 0374
    - Right 0373
  - Superior Mesenteric 0475
  - Temporal
    - Left 037T
    - Right 037S
  - Thyroid
    - Left 037V
    - Right 037U
  - Ulnar
    - Left 037A
    - Right 0379
  - Upper 037Y
  - Vertebral
    - Left 037Q
    - Right 037P
- Bladder 0T7B
- Bladder Neck 0T7C
- Bronchus
  - Lingula 0B79
  - Lower Lobe
    - Left 0B7B
    - Right 0B76
  - Main
    - Left 0B77
    - Right 0B73
  - Middle Lobe, Right 0B75
  - Upper Lobe
    - Left 0B78
    - Right 0B74
- Carina 0B72
- Cerebral Ventricle 0076
- Cecum 0D7H
- Cervix 0U7C
- Colon
  - Ascending 0D7K
  - Descending 0D7M
  - Sigmoid 0D7N
  - Transverse 0D7L
- Duct
  - Common Bile 0F79
  - Cystic 0F78
  - Hepatic
    - Common 0F77
    - Left 0F76
    - Right 0F75
  - Lacrimal
    - Left 087Y
    - Right 087X
  - Pancreatic 0F7D
    - Accessory 0F7F
  - Parotid
    - Left 0C7C
    - Right 0C7B
- Duodenum 0D79
- Esophagogastric Junction 0D74
- Esophagus 0D75
  - Lower 0D73
  - Middle 0D72
  - Upper 0D71
- Eustachian Tube
  - Left 097G
  - Right 097F
- Fallopian Tube
  - Left 0U76
  - Right 0U75
- Fallopian Tubes, Bilateral 0U77
- Hymen 0U7K
- Ileocecal Valve 0D7C
- Ileum 0D7B
- Intestine
  - Large 0D7E
    - Left 0D7G
    - Right 0D7F
  - Small 0D78
- Jejunum 0D7A
- Kidney Pelvis
  - Left 0T74

Dilation *(continued)*
- Kidney Pelvis *(continued)*
  - Right 0T73
- Larynx 0C7S
- Pharynx 0C7M
- Rectum 0D7P
- Stomach 0D76
  - Pylorus 0D77
- Trachea 0B71
- Ureter
  - Left 0T77
  - Right 0T76
- Ureters, Bilateral 0T78
- Urethra 0T7D
- Uterus 0U79
- Vagina 0U7G
- Valve
  - Aortic 027F
  - Mitral 027G
  - Pulmonary 027H
  - Tricuspid 027J
- Vas Deferens
  - Bilateral 0V7Q
  - Left 0V7P
  - Right 0V7N
- Vein
  - Axillary
    - Left 0578
    - Right 0577
  - Azygos 0570
  - Basilic
    - Left 057C
    - Right 057B
  - Brachial
    - Left 057A
    - Right 0579
  - Cephalic
    - Left 057F
    - Right 057D
  - Colic 0677
  - Common Iliac
    - Left 067D
    - Right 067C
  - Esophageal 0673
  - External Iliac
    - Left 067G
    - Right 067F
  - External Jugular
    - Left 057Q
    - Right 057P
  - Face
    - Left 057V
    - Right 057T
  - Femoral
    - Left 067N
    - Right 067M
  - Foot
    - Left 067V
    - Right 067T
  - Gastric 0672
  - Hand
    - Left 057H
    - Right 057G
  - Hemiazygos 0571
  - Hepatic 0674
  - Hypogastric
    - Left 067J
    - Right 067H
  - Inferior Mesenteric 0676
  - Innominate
    - Left 0574
    - Right 0573
  - Internal Jugular
    - Left 057N
    - Right 057M
  - Intracranial 057L
  - Lower 067Y
  - Portal 0678
  - Pulmonary
    - Left 027T
    - Right 027S

Dilation *(continued)*
- Vein *(continued)*
  - Renal
    - Left 067B
    - Right 0679
  - Saphenous
    - Left 067Q
    - Right 067P
  - Splenic 0671
  - Subclavian
    - Left 0576
    - Right 0575
  - Superior Mesenteric 0675
  - Upper 057Y
  - Vertebral
    - Left 057S
    - Right 057R
- Vena Cava
  - Inferior 0670
  - Superior 027V
- Ventricle
  - Left 027L
  - Right 027K

Direct Lateral Interbody Fusion (DLIF) device
- *use* Interbody Fusion Device in Lower Joints

Disarticulation
- *see* Detachment

Discectomy, diskectomy
- *see* Excision, Lower Joints 0SB
- *see* Excision, Upper Joints 0RB
- *see* Resection, Lower Joints 0ST
- *see* Resection, Upper Joints 0RT

Discography
- *see* Fluoroscopy, Axial Skeleton, Except Skull and Facial Bones BR1
- *see* Plain Radiography, Axial Skeleton, Except Skull and Facial Bones BR0

Dismembered pyeloplasty
- *see* Repair, Kidney Pelvis

Distal humerus
- *use* Humeral Shaft, Left
- *use* Humeral Shaft, Right

Distal humerus, involving joint
- *use* Joint, Elbow, Left
- *use* Joint, Elbow, Right

Distal radioulnar joint
- *use* Joint, Wrist, Left
- *use* Joint, Wrist, Right

Diversion
- *see* Bypass

Diverticulectomy
- *see* Excision, Gastrointestinal System 0DB

Division
- Acetabulum
  - Left 0Q85
  - Right 0Q84
- Anal Sphincter 0D8R
- Basal Ganglia 0088
- Bladder Neck 0T8C
- Bone
  - Ethmoid
    - Left 0N8G
    - Right 0N8F
  - Frontal 0N81
  - Hyoid 0N8X
  - Lacrimal
    - Left 0N8J
    - Right 0N8H
  - Nasal 0N8B
  - Occipital 0N87
  - Palatine
    - Left 0N8L
    - Right 0N8K
  - Parietal
    - Left 0N84
    - Right 0N83

Division *(continued)*
- Bone *(continued)*
  - Pelvic
    - Left 0Q83
    - Right 0Q82
  - Sphenoid 0N8C
  - Temporal
    - Left 0N86
    - Right 0N85
  - Zygomatic
    - Left 0N8N
    - Right 0N8M
- Brain 0080
- Bursa and Ligament
  - Abdomen
    - Left 0M8J
    - Right 0M8H
  - Ankle
    - Left 0M8R
    - Right 0M8Q
  - Elbow
    - Left 0M84
    - Right 0M83
  - Foot
    - Left 0M8T
    - Right 0M8S
  - Hand
    - Left 0M88
    - Right 0M87
  - Head and Neck 0M80
  - Hip
    - Left 0M8M
    - Right 0M8L
  - Knee
    - Left 0M8P
    - Right 0M8N
  - Lower Extremity
    - Left 0M8W
    - Right 0M8V
  - Perineum 0M8K
  - Rib(s) 0M8G
  - Shoulder
    - Left 0M82
    - Right 0M81
  - Spine
    - Lower 0M8D
    - Upper 0M8C
  - Sternum 0M8F
  - Upper Extremity
    - Left 0M8B
    - Right 0M89
  - Wrist
    - Left 0M86
    - Right 0M85
- Carpal
  - Left 0P8N
  - Right 0P8M
- Cerebral Hemisphere 0087
- Chordae Tendineae 0289
- Clavicle
  - Left 0P8B
  - Right 0P89
- Coccyx 0Q8S
- Conduction Mechanism 0288
- Esophagogastric Junction 0D84
- Femoral Shaft
  - Left 0Q89
  - Right 0Q88
- Femur
  - Lower
    - Left 0Q8C
    - Right 0Q8B
  - Upper
    - Left 0Q87
    - Right 0Q86
- Fibula
  - Left 0Q8K
  - Right 0Q8J
- Gland, Pituitary 0G80
- Glenoid Cavity
  - Left 0P88

Division *(continued)*
- Glenoid Cavity *(continued)*
  - Right 0P87
- Humeral Head
  - Left 0P8D
  - Right 0P8C
- Humeral Shaft
  - Left 0P8G
  - Right 0P8F
- Hymen 0U8K
- Kidneys, Bilateral 0T82
- Liver 0F80
  - Left Lobe 0F82
  - Right Lobe 0F81
- Mandible
  - Left 0N8V
  - Right 0N8T
- Maxilla 0N8R
- Metacarpal
  - Left 0P8Q
  - Right 0P8P
- Metatarsal
  - Left 0Q8P
  - Right 0Q8N
- Muscle
  - Abdomen
    - Left 0K8L
    - Right 0K8K
  - Facial 0K81
  - Foot
    - Left 0K8W
    - Right 0K8V
  - Hand
    - Left 0K8D
    - Right 0K8C
  - Head 0K80
  - Hip
    - Left 0K8P
    - Right 0K8N
  - Lower Arm and Wrist
    - Left 0K8B
    - Right 0K89
  - Lower Leg
    - Left 0K8T
    - Right 0K8S
  - Neck
    - Left 0K83
    - Right 0K82
  - Papillary 028D
  - Perineum 0K8M
  - Shoulder
    - Left 0K86
    - Right 0K85
  - Thorax
    - Left 0K8J
    - Right 0K8H
  - Tongue, Palate, Pharynx 0K84
  - Trunk
    - Left 0K8G
    - Right 0K8F
  - Upper Arm
    - Left 0K88
    - Right 0K87
  - Upper Leg
    - Left 0K8R
    - Right 0K8Q
- Nerve
  - Abdominal Sympathetic 018M
  - Abducens 008L
  - Accessory 008R
  - Acoustic 008N
  - Brachial Plexus 0183
  - Cervical 0181
  - Cervical Plexus 0180
  - Facial 008M
  - Femoral 018D
  - Glossopharyngeal 008P
  - Head and Neck Sympathetic 018K
  - Hypoglossal 008S
  - Lumbar 018B
  - Lumbar Plexus 0189

Division *(continued)*
- Nerve *(continued)*
  - Lumbar Sympathetic 018N
  - Lumbosacral Plexus 018A
  - Median 0185
  - Oculomotor 008H
  - Olfactory 008F
  - Optic 008G
  - Peroneal 018H
  - Phrenic 0182
  - Pudendal 018C
  - Radial 0186
  - Sacral 018R
  - Sacral Plexus 018Q
  - Sacral Sympathetic 018P
  - Sciatic 018F
  - Thoracic 0188
  - Thoracic Sympathetic 018L
  - Tibial 018G
  - Trigeminal 008K
  - Trochlear 008J
  - Ulnar 0184
  - Vagus 008Q
- Orbit
  - Left 0N8Q
  - Right 0N8P
- Ovary
  - Bilateral 0U82
  - Left 0U81
  - Right 0U80
- Pancreas 0F8G
- Patella
  - Left 0Q8F
  - Right 0Q8D
- Perineum, Female 0W8NXZZ
- Phalanx
  - Finger
    - Left 0P8V
    - Right 0P8T
  - Thumb
    - Left 0P8S
    - Right 0P8R
  - Toe
    - Left 0Q8R
    - Right 0Q8Q
- Radius
  - Left 0P8J
  - Right 0P8H
- Ribs
  - 1 to 2 0P81
  - 3 or More 0P82
- Sacrum 0Q81
- Scapula
  - Left 0P86
  - Right 0P85
- Skin
  - Abdomen 0H87XZZ
  - Back 0H86XZZ
  - Buttock 0H88XZZ
  - Chest 0H85XZZ
  - Ear
    - Left 0H83XZZ
    - Right 0H82XZZ
  - Face 0H81XZZ
  - Foot
    - Left 0H8NXZZ
    - Right 0H8MXZZ
  - Hand
    - Left 0H8GXZZ
    - Right 0H8FXZZ
  - Inguinal 0H8AXZZ
  - Lower Arm
    - Left 0H8EXZZ
    - Right 0H8DXZZ
  - Lower Leg
    - Left 0H8LXZZ
    - Right 0H8KXZZ
  - Neck 0H84XZZ
  - Perineum 0H89XZZ
  - Scalp 0H80XZZ

- **Division** *(continued)*
  - Skin *(continued)*
    - Upper Arm
      - Left 0H8CXZZ
      - Right 0H8BXZZ
    - Upper Leg
      - Left 0H8JXZZ
      - Right 0H8HXZZ
  - Skull 0N80
  - Spinal Cord
    - Cervical 008W
    - Lumbar 008Y
    - Thoracic 008X
  - Sternum 0P80
  - Stomach, Pylorus 0D87
  - Subcutaneous Tissue and Fascia
    - Abdomen 0J88
    - Back 0J87
    - Buttock 0J89
    - Chest 0J86
    - Face 0J81
    - Foot
      - Left 0J8R
      - Right 0J8Q
    - Hand
      - Left 0J8K
      - Right 0J8J
    - Head and Neck 0J8S
    - Lower Arm
      - Left 0J8H
      - Right 0J8G
    - Lower Extremity 0J8W
    - Lower Leg
      - Left 0J8P
      - Right 0J8N
    - Neck
      - Left 0J85
      - Right 0J84
    - Pelvic Region 0J8C
    - Perineum 0J8B
    - Scalp 0J80
    - Trunk 0J8T
    - Upper Arm
      - Left 0J8F
      - Right 0J8D
    - Upper Extremity 0J8V
    - Upper Leg
      - Left 0J8M
      - Right 0J8L
  - Tarsal
    - Left 0Q8M
    - Right 0Q8L
  - Tendon
    - Abdomen
      - Left 0L8G
      - Right 0L8F
    - Ankle
      - Left 0L8T
      - Right 0L8S
    - Foot
      - Left 0L8W
      - Right 0L8V
    - Hand
      - Left 0L88
      - Right 0L87
    - Head and Neck 0L80
    - Hip
      - Left 0L8K
      - Right 0L8J
    - Knee
      - Left 0L8R
      - Right 0L8Q
    - Lower Arm and Wrist
      - Left 0L86
      - Right 0L85
    - Lower Leg
      - Left 0L8P
      - Right 0L8N
    - Perineum 0L8H
    - Shoulder
      - Left 0L82

- **Division** *(continued)*
  - Tendon *(continued)*
    - Shoulder *(continued)*
      - Right 0L81
    - Thorax
      - Left 0L8D
      - Right 0L8C
    - Trunk
      - Left 0L8B
      - Right 0L89
    - Upper Arm
      - Left 0L84
      - Right 0L83
    - Upper Leg
      - Left 0L8M
      - Right 0L8L
  - Thyroid Gland Isthmus 0G8J
  - Tibia
    - Left 0Q8H
    - Right 0Q8G
  - Turbinate, Nasal 098L
  - Ulna
    - Left 0P8L
    - Right 0P8K
  - Uterine Supporting Structure 0U84
  - Vertebra
    - Cervical 0P83
    - Lumbar 0Q80
    - Thoracic 0P84
- **Doppler study**
  - *see* Ultrasonography
- **Dorsal digital nerve**
  - *use* Nerve, Radial
- **Dorsal metacarpal vein**
  - *use* Vein, Hand, Left
  - *use* Vein, Hand, Right
- **Dorsal metatarsal artery**
  - *use* Artery, Foot, Left
  - *use* Artery, Foot, Right
- **Dorsal metatarsal vein**
  - *use* Vein, Foot, Left
  - *use* Vein, Foot, Right
- **Dorsal root ganglion**
  - *use* Cervical Spinal Cord
  - *use* Lumbar Spinal Cord
  - *use* Spinal Cord
  - *use* Thoracic Spinal Cord
- **Dorsal scapular artery**
  - *use* Artery, Subclavian, Left
  - *use* Artery, Subclavian, Right
- **Dorsal scapular nerve**
  - *use* Nerve, Brachial Plexus
- **Dorsal venous arch**
  - *use* Vein, Foot, Left
  - *use* Vein, Foot, Right
- **Dorsalis pedis artery**
  - *use* Artery, Anterior Tibial, Left
  - *use* Artery, Anterior Tibial, Right
- **DownStream® System**
  - 5A0512C
  - 5A0522C
- **Drainage**
  - Abdominal Wall 0W9F
  - Acetabulum
    - Left 0Q95
    - Right 0Q94
  - Adenoids 0C9Q
  - Ampulla of Vater 0F9C
  - Anal Sphincter 0D9R
  - Ankle Region
    - Left 0Y9L
    - Right 0Y9K
  - Anterior Chamber
    - Left 0893
    - Right 0892
  - Anus 0D9Q
  - Aorta, Abdominal 0490
  - Aortic Body 0G9D
  - Appendix 0D9J

- **Drainage** *(continued)*
  - Arm
    - Lower
      - Left 0X9F
      - Right 0X9D
    - Upper
      - Left 0X99
      - Right 0X98
  - Artery
    - Anterior Tibial
      - Left 049Q
      - Right 049P
    - Axillary
      - Left 0396
      - Right 0395
    - Brachial
      - Left 0398
      - Right 0397
    - Celiac 0491
    - Colic
      - Left 0497
      - Middle 0498
      - Right 0496
    - Common Carotid
      - Left 039J
      - Right 039H
    - Common Iliac
      - Left 049D
      - Right 049C
    - External Carotid
      - Left 039N
      - Right 039M
    - External Iliac
      - Left 049J
      - Right 049H
    - Face 039R
    - Femoral
      - Left 049L
      - Right 049K
    - Foot
      - Left 049W
      - Right 049V
    - Gastric 0492
    - Hand
      - Left 039F
      - Right 039D
    - Hepatic 0493
    - Inferior Mesenteric 049B
    - Innominate 0392
    - Internal Carotid
      - Left 039L
      - Right 039K
    - Internal Iliac
      - Left 049F
      - Right 049E
    - Internal Mammary
      - Left 0391
      - Right 0390
    - Intracranial 039G
    - Lower 049Y
    - Peroneal
      - Left 049U
      - Right 049T
    - Popliteal
      - Left 049N
      - Right 049M
    - Posterior Tibial
      - Left 049S
      - Right 049R
    - Radial
      - Left 039C
      - Right 039B
    - Renal
      - Left 049A
      - Right 0499
    - Splenic 0494
    - Subclavian
      - Left 0394
      - Right 0393
    - Superior Mesenteric 0495

- **Drainage** *(continued)*
  - Artery *(continued)*
    - Temporal
      - Left 039T
      - Right 039S
    - Thyroid
      - Left 039V
      - Right 039U
    - Ulnar
      - Left 039A
      - Right 0399
    - Upper 039Y
    - Vertebral
      - Left 039Q
      - Right 039P
  - Auditory Ossicle
    - Left 099A
    - Right 0999
  - Axilla
    - Left 0X95
    - Right 0X94
  - Back
    - Lower 0W9L
    - Upper 0W9K
  - Basal Ganglia 0098
  - Bladder 0T9B
  - Bladder Neck 0T9C
  - Bone
    - Ethmoid
      - Left 0N9G
      - Right 0N9F
    - Frontal 0N91
    - Hyoid 0N9X
    - Lacrimal
      - Left 0N9J
      - Right 0N9H
    - Nasal 0N9B
    - Occipital 0N97
    - Palatine
      - Left 0N9L
      - Right 0N9K
    - Parietal
      - Left 0N94
      - Right 0N93
    - Pelvic
      - Left 0Q93
      - Right 0Q92
    - Sphenoid 0N9C
    - Temporal
      - Left 0N96
      - Right 0N95
    - Zygomatic
      - Left 0N9N
      - Right 0N9M
  - Bone Marrow 079T
  - Brain 0090
  - Breast
    - Bilateral 0H9V
    - Left 0H9U
    - Right 0H9T
  - Bronchus
    - Lingula 0B99
    - Lower Lobe
      - Left 0B9B
      - Right 0B96
    - Main
      - Left 0B97
      - Right 0B93
    - Middle Lobe, Right 0B95
    - Upper Lobe
      - Left 0B98
      - Right 0B94
  - Buccal Mucosa 0C94
  - Bursa and Ligament
    - Abdomen
      - Left 0M9J
      - Right 0M9H
    - Ankle
      - Left 0M9R
      - Right 0M9Q

Drainage *(continued)*
- Bursa and Ligament *(continued)*
  - Elbow
    - Left 0M94
    - Right 0M93
  - Foot
    - Left 0M9T
    - Right 0M9S
  - Hand
    - Left 0M98
    - Right 0M97
  - Head and Neck 200M90
  - Hip
    - Left 0M9M
    - Right 0M9L
  - Knee
    - Left 0M9P
    - Right 0M9N
  - Lower Extremity
    - Left 0M9W
    - Right 0M9V
  - Perineum 0M9K
  - Rib(s) 0M9G
  - Shoulder
    - Left 0M92
    - Right 0M91
  - Spine
    - Lower 0M9D
    - Upper 0M9C
  - Sternum 0M9F
  - Upper Extremity
    - Left 0M9B
    - Right 0M99
  - Wrist
    - Left 0M96
    - Right 0M95
- Buttock
  - Left 0Y91
  - Right 0Y90
- Carina 0B92
- Carotid Bodies, Bilateral 0G98
- Carotid Body
  - Left 0G96
  - Right 0G97
- Carpal
  - Left 0P9N
  - Right 0P9M
- Cavity, Cranial 0W91
- Cecum 0D9H
- Cerebellum 009C
- Cerebral Hemisphere 0097
- Cerebral Meninges 0091
- Cerebral Ventricle 0096
- Cervix 0U9C
- Chest Wall 0W98
- Choroid
  - Left 089B
  - Right 089A
- Cisterna Chyli 079L
- Clavicle
  - Left 0P9B
  - Right 0P99
- Clitoris 0U9J
- Coccygeal Glomus 0G9B
- Coccyx 0Q9S
- Colon
  - Ascending 0D9K
  - Descending 0D9M
  - Sigmoid 0D9N
  - Transverse 0D9L
- Conjunctiva
  - Left 089T
  - Right 089S
- Cord
  - Bilateral 0V9H
  - Left 0V9G
  - Right 0V9F
- Cornea
  - Left 0899
  - Right 0898
- Cul-de-sac 0U9F

Drainage *(continued)*
- Diaphragm 0B9T
- Disc
  - Cervical Vertebral 0R93
  - Cervicothoracic Vertebral 0R95
  - Lumbar Vertebral 0S92
  - Lumbosacral 0S94
  - Thoracic Vertebral 0R99
  - Thoracolumbar Vertebral 0R9B
- Duct
  - Common Bile 0F99
  - Cystic 0F98
  - Hepatic
    - Common 0F97
    - Left 0F96
    - Right 0F95
  - Lacrimal
    - Left 089Y
    - Right 089X
  - Pancreatic 0F9D
    - Accessory 0F9F
  - Parotid
    - Left 0C9C
    - Right 0C9B
- Duodenum 0D99
- Dura Mater 0092
- Ear
  - External
    - Left 0991
    - Right 0990
  - External Auditory Canal
    - Left 0994
    - Right 0993
  - Inner
    - Left 099E
    - Right 099D
  - Middle
    - Left 0996
    - Right 0995
- Elbow Region
  - Left 0X9C
  - Right 0X9B
- Epididymis
  - Bilateral 0V9L
  - Left 0V9K
  - Right 0V9J
- Epidural Space, Intracranial 0093
- Epiglottis 0C9R
- Esophagogastric Junction 0D94
- Esophagus 0D95
  - Lower 0D93
  - Middle 0D92
  - Upper 0D91
- Eustachian Tube
  - Left 099G
  - Right 099F
- Extremity
  - Lower
    - Left 0Y9B
    - Right 0Y99
  - Upper
    - Left 0X97
    - Right 0X96
- Eye
  - Left 0891
  - Right 0890
- Eyelid
  - Lower
    - Left 089R
    - Right 089Q
  - Upper
    - Left 089P
    - Right 089N
- Face 0W92
- Fallopian Tube
  - Left 0U96
  - Right 0U95
- Fallopian Tubes, Bilateral 0U97
- Femoral Region
  - Left 0Y98
  - Right 0Y97

Drainage *(continued)*
- Femoral Shaft
  - Left 0Q99
  - Right 0Q98
- Femur
  - Lower
    - Left 0Q9C
    - Right 0Q9B
  - Upper
    - Left 0Q97
    - Right 0Q96
- Fibula
  - Left 0Q9K
  - Right 0Q9J
- Finger Nail 0H9Q
- Foot
  - Left 0Y9N
  - Right 0Y9M
- Gallbladder 0F94
- Gingiva
  - Lower 0C96
  - Upper 0C95
- Gland
  - Adrenal
    - Bilateral 0G94
    - Left 0G92
    - Right 0G93
  - Lacrimal
    - Left 089W
    - Right 089V
  - Minor Salivary 0C9J
  - Parotid
    - Left 0C99
    - Right 0C98
  - Pituitary 0G90
  - Sublingual
    - Left 0C9F
    - Right 0C9D
  - Submaxillary
    - Left 0C9H
    - Right 0C9G
  - Vestibular 0U9L
- Glenoid Cavity
  - Left 0P98
  - Right 0P97
- Glomus Jugulare 0G9C
- Hand
  - Left 0X9K
  - Right 0X9J
- Head 0W90
- Humeral Head
  - Left 0P9D
  - Right 0P9C
- Humeral Shaft
  - Left 0P9G
  - Right 0P9F
- Hymen 0U9K
- Hypothalamus 009A
- Ileocecal Valve 0D9C
- Ileum 0D9B
- Inguinal Region
  - Left 0Y96
  - Right 0Y95
- Intestine
  - Large 0D9E
    - Left 0D9G
    - Right 0D9F
  - Small 0D98
- Iris
  - Left 089D
  - Right 089C
- Jaw
  - Lower 0W95
  - Upper 0W94
- Jejunum 0D9A
- Joint
  - Acromioclavicular
    - Left 0R9H
    - Right 0R9G

Drainage *(continued)*
- Joint *(continued)*
  - Ankle
    - Left 0S9G
    - Right 0S9F
  - Carpal
    - Left 0R9R
    - Right 0R9Q
  - Carpometacarpal
    - Left 0R9T
    - Right 0R9S
  - Cervical Vertebral 0R91
  - Cervicothoracic Vertebral 0R94
  - Coccygeal 0S96
  - Elbow
    - Left 0R9M
    - Right 0R9L
  - Finger Phalangeal
    - Left 0R9X
    - Right 0R9W
  - Hip
    - Left 0S9B
    - Right 0S99
  - Knee
    - Left 0S9D
    - Right 0S9C
  - Lumbar Vertebral 0S90
  - Lumbosacral 0S93
  - Metacarpophalangeal
    - Left 0R9V
    - Right 0R9U
  - Metatarsal-Phalangeal
    - Left 0S9N
    - Right 0S9M
  - Occipital-cervical 0R90
  - Sacrococcygeal 0S95
  - Sacroiliac
    - Left 0S98
    - Right 0S97
  - Shoulder
    - Left 0R9K
    - Right 0R9J
  - Sternoclavicular
    - Left 0R9F
    - Right 0R9E
  - Tarsal
    - Left 0S9J
    - Right 0S9H
  - Tarsometatarsal
    - Left 0S9L
    - Right 0S9K
  - Temporomandibular
    - Left 0R9D
    - Right 0R9C
  - Thoracic Vertebral 0R96
  - Thoracolumbar Vertebral 0R9A
  - Toe Phalangeal
    - Left 0S9Q
    - Right 0S9P
  - Wrist
    - Left 0R9P
    - Right 0R9N
- Kidney
  - Left 0T91
  - Right 0T90
- Kidney Pelvis
  - Left 0T94
  - Right 0T93
- Knee Region
  - Left 0Y9G
  - Right 0Y9F
- Larynx 0C9S
- Leg
  - Lower
    - Left 0Y9J
    - Right 0Y9H
  - Upper
    - Left 0Y9D
    - Right 0Y9C

Drainage *(continued)*
Subcutaneous Tissue and
Fascia *(continued)*
Neck *(continued)*
Right 0J94
Pelvic Region 0J9C
Perineum 0J9B
Scalp 0J90
Upper Arm
Left 0J9F
Right 0J9D
Upper Leg
Left 0J9M
Right 0J9L
Subdural Space, Intracranial 0094
Tarsal
Left 0Q9M
Right 0Q9L
Tendon
Abdomen
Left 0L9G
Right 0L9F
Ankle
Left 0L9T
Right 0L9S
Foot
Left 0L9W
Right 0L9V
Hand
Left 0L98
Right 0L97
Head and Neck 0L90
Hip
Left 0L9K
Right 0L9J
Knee
Left 0L9R
Right 0L9Q
Lower Arm and Wrist
Left 0L96
Right 0L95
Lower Leg
Left 0L9P
Right 0L9N
Perineum 0L9H
Shoulder
Left 0L92
Right 0L91
Thorax
Left 0L9D
Right 0L9C
Electrocautery
Right 0L99
Upper Arm
Left 0L94
Right 0L93
Upper Leg
Left 0L9M
Right 0L9L
Testis
Bilateral 0V9C
Left 0V9B
Right 0V99
Thalamus 0099
Thymus 079M
Thyroid Gland 0G9K
Left Lobe 0G9G
Right Lobe 0G9H
Tibia
Left 0Q9H
Right 0Q9G
Toe Nail 0H9R
Tongue 0C97
Tonsils 0C9P
Tooth
Lower 0C9X
Upper 0C9W
Trachea 0B91
Tunica Vaginalis
Left 0V97
Right 0V96

Drainage *(continued)*
Turbinate, Nasal 099L
Tympanic Membrane
Left 0998
Right 0997
Ulna
Left 0P9L
Right 0P9K
Ureter
Left 0T97
Right 0T96
Ureters, Bilateral 0T98
Urethra 0T9D
Uterine Supporting Structure 0U94
Uterus 0U99
Uvula 0C9N
Vagina 0U9G
Vas Deferens
Bilateral 0V9Q
Left 0V9P
Right 0V9N
Vein
Axillary
Left 0598
Right 0597
Azygos 0590
Basilic
Left 059C
Right 059B
Brachial
Left 059A
Right 0599
Cephalic
Left 059F
Right 059D
Colic 0697
Common Iliac
Left 069D
Right 069C
Esophageal 0693
External Iliac
Left 069G
Right 069F
External Jugular
Left 059Q
Right 059P
Face
Left 059V
Right 059T
Femoral
Left 069N
Right 069M
Foot
Left 069V
Right 069T
Gastric 0692
Hand
Left 059H
Right 059G
Hemiazygos 0591
Hepatic 0694
Hypogastric
Left 069J
Right 069H
Inferior Mesenteric 0696
Innominate
Left 0594
Right 0593
Internal Jugular
Left 059N
Right 059M
Intracranial 059L
Lower 069Y
Portal 0698
Renal
Left 069B
Right 0699
Saphenous
Left 069Q
Right 069P
Splenic 0691

Drainage *(continued)*
Vein *(continued)*
Subclavian
Left 0596
Right 0595
Superior Mesenteric 0695
Upper 059Y
Vertebral
Left 059S
Right 059R
Vena Cava, Inferior 0690
Vertebra
Cervical 0P93
Lumbar 0Q90
Thoracic 0P94
Vesicle
Bilateral 0V93
Left 0V92
Right 0V91
Vitreous
Left 0895
Right 0894
Vocal Cord
Left 0C9V
Right 0C9T
Vulva 0U9M
Wrist Region
Left 0X9H
Right 0X9G

Dressing
Abdominal Wall 2W23X4Z
Arm
Lower
Left 2W2DX4Z
Right 2W2CX4Z
Upper
Left 2W2BX4Z
Right 2W2AX4Z
Back 2W25X4Z
Chest Wall 2W24X4Z
Extremity
Lower
Left 2W2MX4Z
Right 2W2LX4Z
Upper
Left 2W29X4Z
Right 2W28X4Z
Face 2W21X4Z
Finger
Left 2W2KX4Z
Right 2W2JX4Z
Foot
Left 2W2TX4Z
Right 2W2SX4Z
Hand
Left 2W2FX4Z
Right 2W2EX4Z
Head 2W20X4Z
Inguinal Region
Left 2W27X4Z
Right 2W26X4Z
Leg
Lower
Left 2W2RX4Z
Right 2W2QX4Z
Upper
Left 2W2PX4Z
Right 2W2NX4Z
Neck 2W22X4Z
Thumb
Left 2W2HX4Z
Right 2W2GX4Z
Toe
Left 2W2VX4Z
Right 2W2UX4Z

Driver stent (RX) (OTW)
use Intraluminal Device

Drotrecogin alfa, infusion
see Introduction of Recombinant Human-activated Protein C

Duct of Santorini
use Duct, Pancreatic, Accessory

Duct of Wirsung
use Duct, Pancreatic

Ductogram, mammary
see Plain Radiography, Skin, Subcutaneous Tissue and Breast BH0

Ductography, mammary
see Plain Radiography, Skin, Subcutaneous Tissue and Breast BH0

Ductus deferens
use Vas Deferens
use Vas Deferens, Bilateral
use Vas Deferens, Left
use Vas Deferens, Right

Duodenal ampulla
use Ampulla of Vater

Duodenectomy
see Excision, Duodenum 0DB9
see Resection, Duodenum 0DT9

Duodenocholedochotomy
see Drainage, Gallbladder 0F94

Duodenocystostomy
see Bypass, Gallbladder 0F14
see Drainage, Gallbladder 0F94

Duodenoenterostomy
see Bypass, Gastrointestinal System 0D1
see Drainage, Gastrointestinal System 0D9

Duodenojejunal flexure
use Jejunum

Duodenolysis
see Release, Duodenum 0DN9

Duodenorrhaphy
see Repair, Duodenum 0DQ9

Duodenoscopy, single-use (aScope™ Duodeno) (EXALT™ Model D) *see* New Technology, Hepatobiliary System and Pancreas XFJ

Duodenostomy
see Bypass, Duodenum 0D19
see Drainage, Duodenum 0D99

Duodenotomy
see Drainage, Duodenum 0D99

DuraGraft® Endothelial Damage Inhibitor
use Endothelial Damage Inhibitor

DuraHeart Left Ventricular Assist System
use Implantable Heart Assist System in Heart and Great Vessels

Dural venous sinus
use Vein, Intracranial

Dura mater, intracranial
use Dura Mater

Dura mater, spinal
use Spinal Meninges

Durata® Defibrillation Lead
use Cardiac Lead, Defibrillator in 02H

Durvalumab Antineoplastic XW0

DynaNail®
use Internal Fixation Device, Sustained Compression in 0RG
use Internal Fixation Device, Sustained Compression in 0SG

DynaNail Mini®
use Internal Fixation Device, Sustained Compression in 0RG
use Internal Fixation Device, Sustained Compression in 0SG

Dynesys® Dynamic Stabilization System
use Spinal Stabilization Device, Pedicle-Based in 0RH
use Spinal Stabilization Device, Pedicle-Based in 0SH

E

E-Luminexx™ (Biliary)(Vascular) Stent
use Intraluminal Device
Earlobe
use Ear, External, Bilateral
use Ear, External, Left
use Ear, External, Right
ECCO2R (Extracorporeal Carbon Dioxide Removal) 5A0920Z
Echocardiogram
see Ultrasonography, Heart B24
Echography
see Ultrasonography
EchoTip® Insight™ Portosystemic Pressure Gradient Measurement System 4A044B2
ECMO
see Performance, Circulatory 5A15
ECMO, intraoperative
see Performance, Circulatory 5A15A
Eculizumab XW0
EDWARDS INTUITY Elite valve system
use Zooplastic Tissue, Rapid Deployment in New Technology
EEG (electroencephalogram)
see Measurement, Central Nervous 4A00
EGD (esophagogastroduodenoscopy) 0DJ08ZZ
Eighth cranial nerve
use Nerve, Acoustic
Ejaculatory duct
use Vas Deferens
use Vas Deferens, Bilateral
use Vas Deferens, Left
use Vas Deferens, Right
EKG (electrocardiogram)
see Measurement, Cardiac 4A02
EKOS™ EkoSonic® Endovascular System
see Fragmentation, Artery
Eladocagene exuparvovec XW0Q316
Electrical bone growth stimulator (EBGS)
use Bone Growth Stimulator in Head and Facial Bones
use Bone Growth Stimulator in Lower Bones
use Bone Growth Stimulator in Upper Bones
Electrical muscle stimulation (EMS) lead
use Stimulator Lead in Muscles
Electrocautery
Destruction
see Destruction
Repair
see Repair
Electroconvulsive Therapy
Bilateral-Multiple Seizure GZB3ZZZ
Bilateral-Single Seizure GZB2ZZZ
Electroconvulsive Therapy, Other GZB4ZZZ
Unilateral-Multiple Seizure GZB1ZZZ
Unilateral-Single Seizure GZB0ZZZ
Electroencephalogram (EEG)
see Measurement, Central Nervous 4A00
Electromagnetic Therapy
Central Nervous 6A22
Urinary 6A21
Electronic muscle stimulator lead
use Stimulator Lead in Muscles
Electrophysiologic stimulation (EPS)
see Measurement, Cardiac 4A02
Electroshock therapy
see Electroconvulsive Therapy
Elevation, bone fragments, skull
see Reposition, Head and Facial Bones 0NS
Eleventh cranial nerve
use Nerve, Accessory
Ellipsys® vascular access system
see New Technology, Cardiovascular System X2K
Eluvia™ Drug-Eluting Vascular Stent System
use Intraluminal Device, Sustained Release Drug-eluting in New Technology
use Intraluminal Device, Sustained Release Drug-eluting, Two in New Technology
use Intraluminal Device, Sustained Release Drug-eluting, Three in New Technology
use Intraluminal Device, Sustained Release Drug-eluting, Four or More in New Technology
ELZONRIS™
use Tagraxofusp-erzs Antineoplastic
Embolectomy
see Extirpation
Embolization
see Occlusion
see Restriction
Embolization coil(s)
use Intraluminal Device
EMG (electromyogram)
see Measurement, Musculoskeletal 4A0F
Encephalon
use Brain
Endarterectomy
see Extirpation, Lower Arteries 04C
see Extirpation, Upper Arteries 03C
Endeavor® (III)(IV) (Sprint) Zotarolimus-eluting Coronary Stent System
use Intraluminal Device, Drug-eluting in Heart and Great Vessels
EndoAVF procedure, using magnetic-guided radiofrequency
see Bypass, Upper Arteries 031
EndoAVF procedure, using thermal resistance energy
see New Technology, Cardiovascular System X2K
Endologix AFX® Endovascular AAA System
use Intraluminal Device
EndoSure® sensor
use Monitoring Device, Pressure Sensor in 02H
ENDOTAK RELIANCE® (G) Defibrillation Lead
use Cardiac Lead, Defibrillator in 02H
Endothelial damage inhibitor, applied to vein graft XY0VX83
Endotracheal tube (cuffed)(double-lumen)
use Intraluminal Device, Endotracheal Airway in Respiratory System
Endovascular fistula creation, using magnetic-guided radiofrequency
see Bypass, Upper Arteries 031
Endovascular fistula creation, using thermal resistance energy
see New Technology, Cardiovascular System X2K
Endurant® II AAA stent graft system
use Intraluminal Device
Endurant® Endovascular Stent Graft
use Intraluminal Device
Engineered Chimeric Antigen Receptor T-cell Immunotherapy
Allogeneic XW0
Autologous XW0
Enlargement
see Dilation
see Repair
EnRhythm
use Pacemaker, Dual Chamber in 0JH
ENROUTE® Transcarotid Neuroprotection System
see New Technology, Cardiovascular System X2A
ENSPRYNG™
use Satralizumab-mwge
Enterorrhaphy
see Repair, Gastrointestinal System 0DQ
Enterra gastric neurostimulator
use Stimulator Generator, Multiple Array in 0JH
Enucleation
Eyeball
see Resection, Eye 08T
Eyeball with prosthetic implant
see Replacement, Eye 08R
Ependyma
use Cerebral Ventricle
Epicel® cultured epidermal autograft
use Autologous Tissue Substitute
Epic™ Stented Tissue Valve (aortic)
use Zooplastic Tissue in Heart and Great Vessels
Epidermis
use Skin
Epididymectomy
see Excision, Male Reproductive System 0VB
see Resection, Male Reproductive System 0VT
Epididymoplasty
see Repair, Male Reproductive System 0VQ
see Supplement, Male Reproductive System 0VU
Epididymorrhaphy
see Repair, Male Reproductive System 0VQ
Epididymotomy
see Drainage, Male Reproductive System 0V9
Epidural space, spinal
use Spinal Canal
Epiphysiodesis
see Insertion of device in Lower Bones 0QH
see Insertion of device in Upper Bones 0PH
see Repair, Lower Bones 0QQ
see Repair, Upper Bones 0PQ
Epiploic foramen
use Peritoneum
Epiretinal Visual Prosthesis
Left 08H105Z
Right 08H005Z
Episiorrhaphy
see Repair, Perineum, Female 0WQN
Episiotomy
see Division, Perineum, Female 0W8N
Epithalamus
use Thalamus
Epitrochlear lymph node
use Lymphatic, Upper Extremity, Left
use Lymphatic, Upper Extremity, Right
EPS (electrophysiologic stimulation)
see Measurement, Cardiac 4A02
Eptifibatide, infusion
see Introduction of Platelet Inhibitor
ERCP (endoscopic retrograde cholangiopancreatography)
see Fluoroscopy, Hepatobiliary System and Pancreas BF1
Erdafitinib Antineoplastic XW0DXL5
Erector spinae muscle
use Muscle, Trunk, Left
use Muscle, Trunk, Right
ERLEADA™
use Apalutamide Antineoplastic
Esketamine Hydrochloride XW097M5
Esophageal artery
use Upper Artery
Esophageal obturator airway (EOA)
use Intraluminal Device, Airway in Gastrointestinal System
Esophageal plexus
use Nerve, Thoracic Sympathetic
Esophagectomy
see Excision, Gastrointestinal System 0DB
see Resection, Gastrointestinal System 0DT
Esophagocoloplasty
see Repair, Gastrointestinal System 0DQ
see Supplement, Gastrointestinal System 0DU
Esophagoenterostomy
see Bypass, Gastrointestinal System 0D1
see Drainage, Gastrointestinal System 0D9
Esophagoesophagostomy
see Bypass, Gastrointestinal System 0D1
see Drainage, Gastrointestinal System 0D9
Esophagogastrectomy
see Excision, Gastrointestinal System 0DB
see Resection, Gastrointestinal System 0DT
Esophagogastroduodenoscopy (EGD) 0DJ08ZZ
Esophagogastroplasty
see Repair, Gastrointestinal System 0DQ
see Supplement, Gastrointestinal System 0DU
Esophagogastroscopy 0DJ68ZZ
Esophagogastrostomy
see Bypass, Gastrointestinal System 0D1
see Drainage, Gastrointestinal System 0D9
Esophagojejunoplasty
see Supplement, Gastrointestinal System 0DU
Esophagojejunostomy
see Bypass, Gastrointestinal System 0D1
see Drainage, Gastrointestinal System 0D9
Esophagomyotomy
see Division, Esophagogastric Junction 0D84

Esophagoplasty
see Repair, Gastrointestinal System 0DQ
see Replacement, Esophagus 0DR5
see Supplement, Gastrointestinal System 0DU
Esophagoplication
see Restriction, Gastrointestinal System 0DV
Esophagorrhaphy
see Repair, Gastrointestinal System 0DQ
Esophagoscopy 0DJ08ZZ
Esophagotomy
see Drainage, Gastrointestinal System 0D9
Esteem® implantable hearing system
use Hearing Device in Ear, Nose, Sinus
ESWL (extracorporeal shock wave lithotripsy)
see Fragmentation
Ethmoidal air cell
use Sinus, Ethmoid, Left
use Sinus, Ethmoid, Right
Ethmoidectomy
see Excision, Ear, Nose, Sinus 09B
see Excision, Head and Facial Bones 0NB
see Resection, Ear, Nose, Sinus 09T
see Resection, Head and Facial Bones 0NT
Ethmoidotomy
see Drainage, Ear, Nose, Sinus 099
Evacuation
Hematoma
see Extirpation
Other Fluid
see Drainage
Evera (XT)(S)(DR/VR)
use Defibrillator Generator in 0JH
Everolimus-eluting coronary stent
use Intraluminal Device, Drug-eluting in Heart and Great Vessels
Evisceration
Eyeball
see Resection, Eye 08T
Eyeball with prosthetic implant
see Replacement, Eye 08R
Ex-PRESS™ mini glaucoma shunt
use Synthetic Substitute
EXALT™ Model D Single-Use Duodenoscope
see New Technology, Hepatobiliary System and Pancreas XFJ
Examination
see Inspection
Exchange
see Change device in
Excision
Abdominal Wall 0WBF
Acetabulum
Left 0QB5
Right 0QB4
Adenoids 0CBQ
Ampulla of Vater 0FBC
Anal Sphincter 0DBR
Ankle Region
Left 0YBL
Right 0YBK
Anus 0DBQ
Aorta
Abdominal 04B0
Thoracic
Ascending/Arch 02BX
Descending 02BW
Aortic Body 0GBD
Appendix 0DBJ

Excision *(continued)*
Arm
Lower
Left 0XBF
Right 0XBD
Upper
Left 0XB9
Right 0XB8
Artery
Anterior Tibial
Left 04BQ
Right 04BP
Axillary
Left 03B6
Right 03B5
Brachial
Left 03B8
Right 03B7
Celiac 04B1
Colic
Left 04B7
Middle 04B8
Right 04B6
Common Carotid
Left 03BJ
Right 03BH
Common Iliac
Left 04BD
Right 04BC
External Carotid
Left 03BN
Right 03BM
External Iliac
Left 04BJ
Right 04BH
Face 03BR
Femoral
Left 04BL
Right 04BK
Foot
Left 04BW
Right 04BV
Gastric 04B2
Hand
Left 03BF
Right 03BD
Hepatic 04B3
Inferior Mesenteric 04BB
Innominate 03B2
Internal Carotid
Left 03BL
Right 03BK
Internal Iliac
Left 04BF
Right 04BE
Internal Mammary
Left 03B1
Right 03B0
Intracranial 03BG
Lower 04BY
Peroneal
Left 04BU
Right 04BT
Popliteal
Left 04BN
Right 04BM
Posterior Tibial
Left 04BS
Right 04BR
Pulmonary
Left 02BR
Right 02BQ
Pulmonary Trunk 02BP
Radial
Left 03BC
Right 03BB
Renal
Left 04BA
Right 04B9
Splenic 04B4

Excision *(continued)*
Artery *(continued)*
Subclavian
Left 03B4
Right 03B3
Superior Mesenteric 04B5
Temporal
Left 03BT
Right 03BS
Thyroid
Left 03BV
Right 03BU
Ulnar
Left 03BA
Right 03B9
Upper 03BY
Vertebral
Left 03BQ
Right 03BP
Atrium
Left 02B7
Right 02B6
Auditory Ossicle
Left 09BA
Right 09B9
Axilla
Left 0XB5
Right 0XB4
Back
Lower 0WBL
Upper 0WBK
Basal Ganglia 00B8
Bladder 0TBB
Bladder Neck 0TBC
Bone
Ethmoid
Left 0NBG
Right 0NBF
Frontal 0NB1
Hyoid 0NBX
Lacrimal
Left 0NBJ
Right 0NBH
Nasal 0NBB
Occipital 0NB7
Palatine
Left 0NBL
Right 0NBK
Parietal
Left 0NB4
Right 0NB3
Pelvic
Left 0QB3
Right 0QB2
Sphenoid 0NBC
Temporal
Left 0NB6
Right 0NB5
Zygomatic
Left 0NBN
Right 0NBM
Brain 00B0
Breast
Bilateral 0HBV
Left 0HBU
Right 0HBT
Supernumerary 0HBY
Bronchus
Lingula 0BB9
Lower Lobe
Left 0BBB
Right 0BB6
Main
Left 0BB7
Right 0BB3
Middle Lobe, Right 0BB5
Upper Lobe
Left 0BB8
Right 0BB4
Buccal Mucosa 0CB4

Excision *(continued)*
Bursa and Ligament
Abdomen
Left 0MBJ
Right 0MBH
Ankle
Left 0MBR
Right 0MBQ
Elbow
Left 0MB4
Right 0MB3
Foot
Left 0MBT
Right 0MBS
Hand
Left 0MB8
Right 0MB7
Head and Neck 0MB0
Hip
Left 0MBM
Right 0MBL
Knee
Left 0MBP
Right 0MBN
Lower Extremity
Left 0MBW
Right 0MBV
Rib(s) 0MBG
Perineum 0MBK
Shoulder
Left 0MB2
Right 0MB1
Spine
Lower 0MBD
Upper 0MBC
Sternum 0MBF
Upper Extremity
Left 0MBB
Right 0MB9
Wrist
Left 0MB6
Right 0MB5
Buttock
Left 0YB1
Right 0YB0
Carina 0BB2
Carotid Bodies, Bilateral 0GB8
Carotid Body
Left 0GB6
Right 0GB7
Carpal
Left 0PBN
Right 0PBM
Cecum 0DBH
Cerebellum 00BC
Cerebral Hemisphere 00B7
Cerebral Meninges 00B1
Cerebral Ventricle 00B6
Cervix 0UBC
Chest Wall 0WB8
Chordae Tendineae 02B9
Choroid
Left 08BB
Right 08BA
Cisterna Chyli 07BL
Clavicle
Left 0PBB
Right 0PB9
Clitoris 0UBJ
Coccygeal Glomus 0GBB
Coccyx 0QBS
Colon
Ascending 0DBK
Descending 0DBM
Sigmoid 0DBN
Transverse 0DBL
Conduction Mechanism 02B8
Conjunctiva
Left 08BTXZ
Right 08BSXZ

Excision *(continued)*
- Cord
  - Bilateral 0VBH
  - Left 0VBG
  - Right 0VBF
- Cornea
  - Left 08B9XZ
  - Right 08B8XZ
- Cul-de-sac 0UBF
- Diaphragm 0BBT
- Disc
  - Cervical Vertebral 0RB3
  - Cervicothoracic Vertebral 0RB5
  - Lumbar Vertebral 0SB2
  - Lumbosacral 0SB4
  - Thoracic Vertebral 0RB9
  - Thoracolumbar Vertebral 0RBB
- Duct
  - Common Bile 0FB9
  - Cystic 0FB8
  - Hepatic
    - Common 0FB7
    - Left 0FB6
    - Right 0FB5
  - Lacrimal
    - Left 08BY
    - Right 08BX
  - Pancreatic 0FBD
    - Accessory 0FBF
  - Parotid
    - Left 0CBC
    - Right 0CBB
- Duodenum 0DB9
- Dura Mater 00B2
- Ear
  - External
    - Left 09B1
    - Right 09B0
  - External Auditory Canal
    - Left 09B4
    - Right 09B3
  - Inner
    - Left 09BE
    - Right 09BD
  - Middle
    - Left 09B6
    - Right 09B5
- Elbow Region
  - Left 0XBC
  - Right 0XBB
- Epididymis
  - Bilateral 0VBL
  - Left 0VBK
  - Right 0VBJ
- Epiglottis 0CBR
- Esophagogastric Junction 0DB4
- Esophagus 0DB5
  - Lower 0DB3
  - Middle 0DB2
  - Upper 0DB1
- Eustachian Tube
  - Left 09BG
  - Right 09BF
- Extremity
  - Lower
    - Left 0YBB
    - Right 0YB9
  - Upper
    - Left 0XB7
    - Right 0XB6
- Eye
  - Left 08B1
  - Right 08B0
- Eyelid
  - Lower
    - Left 08BR
    - Right 08BQ
  - Upper
    - Left 08BP
    - Right 08BN
- Face 0WB2

Excision *(continued)*
- Fallopian Tube
  - Left 0UB6
  - Right 0UB5
- Fallopian Tubes, Bilateral 0UB7
- Femoral Region
  - Left 0YB8
  - Right 0YB7
- Femoral Shaft
  - Left 0QB9
  - Right 0QB8
- Femur
  - Lower
    - Left 0QBC
    - Right 0QBB
  - Upper
    - Left 0QB7
    - Right 0QB6
- Fibula
  - Left 0QBK
  - Right 0QBJ
- Finger Nail 0HBQXZ
- Floor of mouth
  - *see* Excision, Oral Cavity and Throat 0WB3
- Foot
  - Left 0YBN
  - Right 0YBM
- Gallbladder 0FB4
- Gingiva
  - Lower 0CB6
  - Upper 0CB5
- Gland
  - Adrenal
    - Bilateral 0GB4
    - Left 0GB2
    - Right 0GB3
  - Lacrimal
    - Left 08BW
    - Right 08BV
  - Minor Salivary 0CBJ
  - Parotid
    - Left 0CB9
    - Right 0CB8
  - Pituitary 0GB0
  - Sublingual
    - Left 0CBF
    - Right 0CBD
  - Submaxillary
    - Left 0CBH
    - Right 0CBG
  - Vestibular 0UBL
- Glenoid Cavity
  - Left 0PB8
  - Right 0PB7
- Glomus Jugulare 0GBC
- Hand
  - Left 0XBK
  - Right 0XBJ
- Head 0WB0
- Humeral Head
  - Left 0PBD
  - Right 0PBC
- Humeral Shaft
  - Left 0PBG
  - Right 0PBF
- Hymen 0UBK
- Hypothalamus 00BA
- Ileocecal Valve 0DBC
- Ileum 0DBB
- Inguinal Region
  - Left 0YB6
  - Right 0YB5
- Intestine
  - Large 0DBE
    - Left 0DBG
    - Right 0DBF
  - Small 0DB8
- Iris
  - Left 08BD3Z
  - Right 08BC3Z

Excision *(continued)*
- Jaw
  - Lower 0WB5
  - Upper 0WB4
- Jejunum 0DBA
- Joint
  - Acromioclavicular
    - Left 0RBH
    - Right 0RBG
  - Ankle
    - Left 0SBG
    - Right 0SBF
  - Carpal
    - Left 0RBR
    - Right 0RBQ
  - Carpometacarpal
    - Left 0RBT
    - Right 0RBS
  - Cervical Vertebral 0RB1
  - Cervicothoracic Vertebral 0RB4
  - Coccygeal 0SB6
  - Elbow
    - Left 0RBM
    - Right 0RBL
  - Finger Phalangeal
    - Left 0RBX
    - Right 0RBW
  - Hip
    - Left 0SBB
    - Right 0SB9
  - Knee
    - Left 0SBD
    - Right 0SBC
  - Lumbar Vertebral 0SB0
  - Lumbosacral 0SB3
  - Metacarpophalangeal
    - Left 0RBV
    - Right 0RBU
  - Metatarsal-Phalangeal
    - Left 0SBN
    - Right 0SBM
  - Occipital-cervical 0RB0
  - Sacrococcygeal 0SB5
  - Sacroiliac
    - Left 0SB8
    - Right 0SB7
  - Shoulder
    - Left 0RBK
    - Right 0RBJ
  - Sternoclavicular
    - Left 0RBF
    - Right 0RBE
  - Tarsal
    - Left 0SBJ
    - Right 0SBH
  - Tarsometatarsal
    - Left 0SBL
    - Right 0SBK
  - Temporomandibular
    - Left 0RBD
    - Right 0RBC
  - Thoracic Vertebral 0RB6
  - Thoracolumbar Vertebral 0RBA
  - Toe Phalangeal
    - Left 0SBQ
    - Right 0SBP
  - Wrist
    - Left 0RBP
    - Right 0RBN
- Kidney
  - Left 0TB1
  - Right 0TB0
- Kidney Pelvis
  - Left 0TB4
  - Right 0TB3
- Knee Region
  - Left 0YBG
  - Right 0YBF
- Larynx 0CBS

Excision *(continued)*
- Leg
  - Lower
    - Left 0YBJ
    - Right 0YBH
  - Upper
    - Left 0YBD
    - Right 0YBC
- Lens
  - Left 08BK3Z
  - Right 08BJ3Z
- Lip
  - Lower 0CB1
  - Upper 0CB0
- Liver 0FB0
  - Left Lobe 0FB2
  - Right Lobe 0FB1
- Lung
  - Bilateral 0BBM
  - Left 0BBL
  - Lower Lobe
    - Left 0BBJ
    - Right 0BBF
  - Middle Lobe, Right 0BBD
  - Right 0BBK
  - Upper Lobe
    - Left 0BBG
    - Right 0BBC
- Lung Lingula 0BBH
- Lymphatic
  - Aortic 07BD
  - Axillary
    - Left 07B6
    - Right 07B5
  - Head 07B0
  - Inguinal
    - Left 07BJ
    - Right 07BH
  - Internal Mammary
    - Left 07B9
    - Right 07B8
  - Lower Extremity
    - Left 07BG
    - Right 07BF
  - Mesenteric 07BB
  - Neck
    - Left 07B2
    - Right 07B1
  - Pelvis 07BC
  - Thoracic Duct 07BK
  - Thorax 07B7
  - Upper Extremity
    - Left 07B4
    - Right 07B3
- Mandible
  - Left 0NBV
  - Right 0NBT
- Maxilla 0NBR
- Mediastinum 0WBC
- Medulla Oblongata 00BD
- Mesentery 0DBV
- Metacarpal
  - Left 0PBQ
  - Right 0PBP
- Metatarsal
  - Left 0QBP
  - Right 0QBN
- Muscle
  - Abdomen
    - Left 0KBL
    - Right 0KBK
  - Extraocular
    - Left 08BM
    - Right 08BL
  - Facial 0KB1
  - Foot
    - Left 0KBW
    - Right 0KBV
  - Hand
    - Left 0KBD
    - Right 0KBC

Excision *(continued)*
Head 0KB0
Hip
Left 0KBP
Right 0KBN
Lower Arm and Wrist
Left 0KBB
Right 0KB9
Lower Leg
Left 0KBT
Right 0KBS
Neck
Left 0KB3
Right 0KB2
Papillary 02BD
Perineum 0KBM
Shoulder
Left 0KB6
Right 0KB5
Thorax
Left 0KBJ
Right 0KBH
Tongue, Palate, Pharynx 0KB4
Trunk
Left 0KBG
Right 0KBF
Upper Arm
Left 0KB8
Right 0KB7
Upper Leg
Left 0KBR
Right 0KBQ
Nasal Mucosa and Soft Tissue 09BK
Nasopharynx 09BN
Neck 0WB6
Nerve
Abdominal Sympathetic 01BM
Abducens 00BL
Accessory 00BR
Acoustic 00BN
Brachial Plexus 01B3
Cervical 01B1
Cervical Plexus 01B0
Facial 00BM
Femoral 01BD
Glossopharyngeal 00BP
Head and Neck Sympathetic 01BK
Hypoglossal 00BS
Lumbar 01BB
Lumbar Plexus 01B9
Lumbar Sympathetic 01BN
Lumbosacral Plexus 01BA
Median 01B5
Oculomotor 00BH
Olfactory 00BF
Optic 00BG
Peroneal 01BH
Phrenic 01B2
Pudendal 01BC
Radial 01B6
Sacral 01BR
Sacral Plexus 01BQ
Sacral Sympathetic 01BP
Sciatic 01BF
Thoracic 01B8
Thoracic Sympathetic 01BL
Tibial 01BG
Trigeminal 00BK
Trochlear 00BJ
Ulnar 01B4
Vagus 00BQ
Nipple
Left 0HBX
Right 0HBW
Omentum 0DBU
Oral Cavity and Throat 0WB3
Orbit
Left 0NBQ
Right 0NBP

Excision *(continued)*
Ovary
Bilateral 0UB2
Left 0UB1
Right 0UB0
Palate
Hard 0CB2
Soft 0CB3
Pancreas 0FBG
Para-aortic Body 0GB9
Paraganglion Extremity 0GBF
Parathyroid Gland 0GBR
Inferior
Left 0GBP
Right 0GBN
Multiple 0GBQ
Superior
Left 0GBM
Right 0GBL
Patella
Left 0QBF
Right 0QBD
Penis 0VBS
Pericardium 02BN
Perineum
Female 0WBN
Male 0WBM
Peritoneum 0DBW
Phalanx
Finger
Left 0PBV
Right 0PBT
Thumb
Left 0PBS
Right 0PBR
Toe
Left 0QBR
Right 0QBQ
Pharynx 0CBM
Pineal Body 0GB1
Pleura
Left 0BBP
Right 0BBN
Pons 00BB
Prepuce 0VBT
Prostate 0VB0
Radius
Left 0PBJ
Right 0PBH
Rectum 0DBP
Retina
Left 08BF3Z
Right 08BE3Z
Retroperitoneum 0WBH
Ribs
1 to 2 0PB1
3 or More 0PB2
Sacrum 0QB1
Scapula
Left 0PB6
Right 0PB5
Sclera
Left 08B7XZ
Right 08B6XZ
Scrotum 0VB5
Septum
Atrial 02B5
Nasal 09BM
Ventricular 02BM
Shoulder Region
Left 0XB3
Right 0XB2
Sinus
Accessory 09BP
Ethmoid
Left 09BV
Right 09BU
Frontal
Left 09BT
Right 09BS

Excision *(continued)*
Sinus *(continued)*
Mastoid
Left 09BC
Right 09BB
Maxillary
Left 09BR
Right 09BQ
Sphenoid
Left 09BX
Right 09BW
Skin
Abdomen 0HB7XZ
Back 0HB6XZ
Buttock 0HB8XZ
Chest 0HB5XZ
Ear
Left 0HB3XZ
Right 0HB2XZ
Face 0HB1XZ
Foot
Left 0HBNXZ
Right 0HBMXZ
Hand
Left 0HBGXZ
Right 0HBFXZ
Inguinal 0HBAXZ
Lower Arm
Left 0HBEXZ
Right 0HBDXZ
Lower Leg
Left 0HBLXZ
Right 0HBKXZ
Neck 0HB4XZ
Perineum 0HB9XZ
Scalp 0HB0XZ
Upper Arm
Left 0HBCXZ
Right 0HBBXZ
Upper Leg
Left 0HBJXZ
Right 0HBHXZ
Skull 0NB0
Spinal Cord
Cervical 00BW
Lumbar 00BY
Thoracic 00BX
Spinal Meninges 00BT
Spleen 07BP
Sternum 0PB0
Stomach 0DB6
Pylorus 0DB7
Subcutaneous Tissue and Fascia
Abdomen 0JB8
Back 0JB7
Buttock 0JB9
Chest 0JB6
Face 0JB1
Foot
Left 0JBR
Right 0JBQ
Hand
Left 0JBK
Right 0JBJ
Lower Arm
Left 0JBH
Right 0JBG
Lower Leg
Left 0JBP
Right 0JBN
Neck
Left 0JB5
Right 0JB4
Pelvic Region 0JBC
Perineum 0JBB
Scalp 0JB0
Upper Arm
Left 0JBF
Right 0JBD
Upper Leg
Left 0JBM

Excision *(continued)*
Subcutaneous Tissue and Fascia *(continued)*
Upper Leg *(continued)*
Right 0JBL
Tarsal
Left 0QBM
Right 0QBL
Tendon
Abdomen
Left 0LBG
Right 0LBF
Ankle
Left 0LBT
Right 0LBS
Foot
Left 0LBW
Right 0LBV
Hand
Left 0LB8
Right 0LB7
Head and Neck 0LB0
Hip
Left 0LBK
Right 0LBJ
Knee
Left 0LBR
Right 0LBQ
Lower Arm and Wrist
Left 0LB6
Right 0LB5
Lower Leg
Left 0LBP
Right 0LBN
Perineum 0LBH
Shoulder
Left 0LB2
Right 0LB1
Thorax
Left 0LBD
Right 0LBC
Trunk
Left 0LBB
Right 0LB9
Upper Arm
Left 0LB4
Right 0LB3
Upper Leg
Left 0LBM
Right 0LBL
Testis
Bilateral 0VBC
Left 0VBB
Right 0VB9
Thalamus 00B9
Thymus 07BM
Thyroid Gland
Left Lobe 0GBG
Right Lobe 0GBH
Thyroid Gland Isthmus 0GBJ
Tibia
Left 0QBH
Right 0QBG
Toe Nail 0HBRXZ
Tongue 0CB7
Tonsils 0CBP
Tooth
Lower 0CBX
Upper 0CBW
Trachea 0BB1
Tunica Vaginalis
Left 0VB7
Right 0VB6
Turbinate, Nasal 09BL
Tympanic Membrane
Left 09B8
Right 09B7
Ulna
Left 0PBL
Right 0PBK

Excision *(continued)*
- Ureter
  - Left 0TB7
  - Right 0TB6
- Urethra 0TBD
- Uterine Supporting Structure 0UB4
- Uterus 0UB9
- Uvula 0CBN
- Vagina 0UBG
- Valve
  - Aortic 02BF
  - Mitral 02BG
  - Pulmonary 02BH
  - Tricuspid 02BJ
- Vas Deferens
  - Bilateral 0VBQ
  - Left 0VBP
  - Right 0VBN
- Vein
  - Axillary
    - Left 05B8
    - Right 05B7
  - Azygos 05B0
  - Basilic
    - Left 05BC
    - Right 05BB
  - Brachial
    - Left 05BA
    - Right 05B9
  - Cephalic
    - Left 05BF
    - Right 05BD
  - Colic 06B7
  - Common Iliac
    - Left 06BD
    - Right 06BC
  - Coronary 02B4
  - Esophageal 06B3
  - External Iliac
    - Left 06BG
    - Right 06BF
  - External Jugular
    - Left 05BQ
    - Right 05BP
  - Face
    - Left 05BV
    - Right 05BT
  - Femoral
    - Left 06BN
    - Right 06BM
  - Foot
    - Left 06BV
    - Right 06BT
  - Gastric 06B2
  - Hand
    - Left 05BH
    - Right 05BG
  - Hemiazygos 05B1
  - Hepatic 06B4
  - Hypogastric
    - Left 06BJ
    - Right 06BH
  - Inferior Mesenteric 06B6
  - Innominate
    - Left 05B4
    - Right 05B3
  - Internal Jugular
    - Left 05BN
    - Right 05BM
  - Intracranial 05BL
  - Lower 06BY
  - Portal 06B8
  - Pulmonary
    - Left 02BT
    - Right 02BS
  - Renal
    - Left 06BB
    - Right 06B9

Excision *(continued)*
- Vein *(continued)*
  - Saphenous
    - Left 06BQ
    - Right 06BP
  - Splenic 06B1
  - Subclavian
    - Left 05B6
    - Right 05B5
  - Superior Mesenteric 06B5
  - Upper 05BY
  - Vertebral
    - Left 05BS
    - Right 05BR
- Vena Cava
  - Inferior 06B0
  - Superior 02BV
- Ventricle
  - Left 02BL
  - Right 02BK
- Vertebra
  - Cervical 0PB3
  - Lumbar 0QB0
  - Thoracic 0PB4
- Vesicle
  - Bilateral 0VB3
  - Left 0VB2
  - Right 0VB1
- Vitreous
  - Left 08B53Z
  - Right 08B43Z
- Vocal Cord
  - Left 0CBV
  - Right 0CBT
- Vulva 0UBM
- Wrist Region
  - Left 0XBH
  - Right 0XBG

EXCLUDER® AAA Endoprosthesis
- *use* Intraluminal Device
- *use* Intraluminal Device, Branched or Fenestrated, One or Two Arteries in 04V
- *use* Intraluminal Device, Branched or Fenestrated, Three or More Arteries in 04V

EXCLUDER® IBE Endoprosthesis
- *use* Intraluminal Device, Branched or Fenestrated, One or Two Arteries in 04V

Exclusion, Left atrial appendage (LAA)
- *see* Occlusion, Atrium, Left 02L7

Exercise, rehabilitation
- *see* Motor Treatment, Rehabilitation F07

Exploration
- *see* Inspection

Express® (LD) Premounted Stent System
- *use* Intraluminal Device

Express® Biliary SD Monorail® Premounted Stent System
- *use* Intraluminal Device

Express® SD Renal Monorail® Premounted Stent System
- *use* Intraluminal Device

Extensor carpi radialis muscle
- *use* Muscle, Lower Arm and Wrist, Left

Extensor carpi radialis muscle
- *use* Muscle, Lower Arm and Wrist, Right

Extensor carpi ulnaris muscle
- *use* Muscle, Lower Arm and Wrist, Left
- *use* Muscle, Lower Arm and Wrist, Right

Extensor digitorum brevis muscle
- *use* Muscle, Foot, Left
- *use* Muscle, Foot, Right

Extensor digitorum longus muscle
- *use* Muscle, Lower Leg, Left
- *use* Muscle, Lower Leg, Right

Extensor hallucis brevis muscle
- *use* Muscle, Foot, Left
- *use* Muscle, Foot, Right

Extensor hallucis longus muscle
- *use* Muscle, Lower Leg, Left
- *use* Muscle, Lower Leg, Right

External anal sphincter
- *use* Anal Sphincter

External auditory meatus
- *use* Ear, External Auditory Canal, Left
- *use* Ear, External Auditory Canal, Right

External fixator
- *use* External Fixation Device in Head and Facial Bones
- *use* External Fixation Device in Lower Bones
- *use* External Fixation Device in Lower Joints
- *use* External Fixation Device in Upper Bones
- *use* External Fixation Device in Upper Joints

External maxillary artery
- *use* Artery, Face

External naris
- *use* Nasal Mucosa and Soft Tissue

External oblique aponeurosis
- *use* Subcutaneous Tissue and Fascia, Trunk

External oblique muscle
- *use* Muscle, Abdomen, Left
- *use* Muscle, Abdomen, Right

External popliteal nerve
- *use* Nerve, Peroneal

External pudendal artery
- *use* Artery, Femoral, Left
- *use* Artery, Femoral, Right

External pudendal vein
- *use* Vein, Saphenous, Left
- *use* Vein, Saphenous, Right

External urethral sphincter
- *use* Urethra

Extirpation
- Acetabulum
  - Left 0QC5
  - Right 0QC4
- Adenoids 0CCQ
- Ampulla of Vater 0FCC
- Anal Sphincter 0DCR
- Anterior Chamber
  - Left 08C3
  - Right 08C2
- Anus 0DCQ
- Aorta
  - Abdominal 04C0
  - Thoracic
    - Ascending/Arch 02CX
    - Descending 02CW
- Aortic Body 0GCD
- Appendix 0DCJ
- Artery
  - Anterior Tibial
    - Left 04CQ
    - Right 04CP
  - Axillary
    - Left 03C6
    - Right 03C5
  - Brachial
    - Left 03C8
    - Right 03C7
  - Celiac 04C1
  - Colic
    - Left 04C7
    - Middle 04C8
    - Right 04C6

Extirpation *(continued)*
- Artery *(continued)*
  - Common Carotid
    - Left 03CJ
    - Right 03CH
  - Common Iliac
    - Left 04CD
    - Right 04CC
  - Coronary
    - Four or More Arteries 02C3
    - One Artery 02C0
    - Three Arteries 02C2
    - Two Arteries 02C1
  - External Carotid
    - Left 03CN
    - Right 03CM
  - External Iliac
    - Left 04CJ
    - Right 04CH
  - Face 03CR
  - Femoral
    - Left 04CL
    - Right 04CK
  - Foot
    - Left 04CW
    - Right 04CV
  - Gastric 04C2
  - Hand
    - Left 03CF
    - Right 03CD
  - Hepatic 04C3
  - Inferior Mesenteric 04CB
  - Innominate 03C2
  - Internal Carotid
    - Left 03CL
    - Right 03CK
  - Internal Iliac
    - Left 04CF
    - Right 04CE
  - Internal Mammary
    - Left 03C1
    - Right 03C0
  - Intracranial 03CG
  - Lower 04CY
  - Peroneal
    - Left 04CU
    - Right 04CT
  - Popliteal
    - Left 04CN
    - Right 04CM
  - Posterior Tibial
    - Left 04CS
    - Right 04CR
  - Pulmonary
    - Left 02CR
    - Right 02CQ
  - Pulmonary Trunk 02CP
  - Radial
    - Left 03CC
    - Right 03CB
  - Renal
    - Left 04CA
    - Right 04C9
  - Splenic 04C4
  - Subclavian
    - Left 03C4
    - Right 03C3
  - Superior Mesenteric 04C5
  - Temporal
    - Left 03CT
    - Right 03CS
  - Thyroid
    - Left 03CV
    - Right 03CU
  - Ulnar
    - Left 03CA
    - Right 03C9
  - Upper 03CY
  - Vertebral
    - Left 03CQ
    - Right 03CP

Extirpation *(continued)*
- Atrium
  - Left 02C7
  - Right 02C6
- Auditory Ossicle
  - Left 09CA
  - Right 09C9
- Basal Ganglia 00C8
- Bladder 0TCB
- Bladder Neck 0TCC
- Bone
  - Ethmoid
    - Left 0NCG
    - Right 0NCF
  - Frontal 0NC1
  - Hyoid 0NCX
  - Lacrimal
    - Left 0NCJ
    - Right 0NCH
  - Nasal 0NCB
  - Occipital 0NC7
  - Palatine
    - Left 0NCL
    - Right 0NCK
  - Parietal
    - Left 0NC4
    - Right 0NC3
  - Pelvic
    - Left 0QC3
    - Right 0QC2
  - Sphenoid 0NCC
  - Temporal
    - Left 0NC6
    - Right 0NC5
  - Zygomatic
    - Left 0NCN
    - Right 0NCM
- Brain 00C0
- Breast
  - Bilateral 0HCV
  - Left 0HCU
  - Right 0HCT
- Bronchus
  - Lingula 0BC9
  - Lower Lobe
    - Left 0BCB
    - Right 0BC6
  - Main
    - Left 0BC7
    - Right 0BC3
  - Middle Lobe, Right 0BC5
  - Upper Lobe
    - Left 0BC8
    - Right 0BC4
- Buccal Mucosa 0CC4
- Bursa and Ligament
  - Abdomen
    - Left 0MCJ
    - Right 0MCH
  - Ankle
    - Left 0MCR
    - Right 0MCQ
  - Elbow
    - Left 0MC4
    - Right 0MC3
  - Foot
    - Left 0MCT
    - Right 0MCS
  - Hand
    - Left 0MC8
    - Right 0MC7
  - Head and Neck 0MC0
  - Hip
    - Left 0MCM
    - Right 0MCL
  - Knee
    - Left 0MCP
    - Right 0MCN

Extirpation *(continued)*
- Bursa and Ligament *(continued)*
  - Lower Extremity
    - Left 0MCW
    - Right 0MCV
  - Perineum 0MCK
  - Rib(s) 0MCG
  - Shoulder
    - Left 0MC2
    - Right 0MC1
  - Spine
    - Lower 0MCD
    - Upper 0MCC
  - Sternum 0MCF
  - Upper Extremity
    - Left 0MCB
    - Right 0MC9
  - Wrist
    - Left 0MC6
    - Right 0MC5
- Carina 0BC2
- Carotid Bodies, Bilateral 0GC8
- Carotid Body
  - Left 0GC6
  - Right 0GC7
- Carpal
  - Left 0PCN
  - Right 0PCM
- Cavity, Cranial 0WC1
- Cecum 0DCH
- Cerebellum 00CC
- Cerebral Hemisphere 00C7
- Cerebral Meninges 00C1
- Cerebral Ventricle 00C6
- Cervix 0UCC
- Chordae Tendineae 02C9
- Choroid
  - Left 08CB
  - Right 08CA
- Cisterna Chyli 07CL
- Clavicle
  - Left 0PCB
  - Right 0PC9
- Clitoris 0UCJ
- Coccygeal Glomus 0GCB
- Coccyx 0QCS
- Colon
  - Ascending 0DCK
  - Descending 0DCM
  - Sigmoid 0DCN
  - Transverse 0DCL
- Computer-aided Mechanical Aspiration X2C
- Conduction Mechanism 02C8
- Conjunctiva
  - Left 08CTXZZ
  - Right 08CSXZZ
- Cord
  - Bilateral 0VCH
  - Left 0VCG
  - Right 0VCF
- Cornea
  - Left 08C9XZZ
  - Right 08C8XZZ
- Cul-de-sac 0UCF
- Diaphragm 0BCT
- Disc
  - Cervical Vertebral 0RC3
  - Cervicothoracic Vertebral 0RC5
  - Lumbar Vertebral 0SC2
  - Lumbosacral 0SC4
  - Thoracic Vertebral 0RC9
  - Thoracolumbar Vertebral 0RCB
- Duct
  - Common Bile 0FC9
  - Cystic 0FC8
  - Hepatic
    - Common 0FC7
    - Left 0FC6
    - Right 0FC5

Extirpation *(continued)*
- Duct *(continued)*
  - Lacrimal
    - Left 08CY
    - Right 08CX
  - Pancreatic 0FCD
    - Accessory 0FCF
  - Parotid
    - Left 0CCC
    - Right 0CCB
- Duodenum 0DC9
- Dura Mater 00C2
- Ear
  - External
    - Left 09C1
    - Right 09C0
  - External Auditory Canal
    - Left 09C4
    - Right 09C3
  - Inner
    - Left 09CE
    - Right 09CD
  - Middle
    - Left 09C6
    - Right 09C5
- Endometrium 0UCB
- Epididymis
  - Bilateral 0VCL
  - Left 0VCK
  - Right 0VCJ
- Epidural Space, Intracranial 00C3
- Epiglottis 0CCR
- Esophagogastric Junction 0DC4
- Esophagus 0DC5
  - Lower 0DC3
  - Middle 0DC2
  - Upper 0DC1
- Eustachian Tube
  - Left 09CG
  - Right 09CF
- Eye
  - Left 08C1XZZ
  - Right 08C0XZZ
- Eyelid
  - Lower
    - Left 08CR
    - Right 08CQ
  - Upper
    - Left 08CP
    - Right 08CN
- Fallopian Tube
  - Left 0UC6
  - Right 0UC5
- Fallopian Tubes, Bilateral 0UC7
- Femoral Shaft
  - Left 0QC9
  - Right 0QC8
- Femur
  - Lower
    - Left 0QCC
    - Right 0QCB
  - Upper
    - Left 0QC7
    - Right 0QC6
- Fibula
  - Left 0QCK
  - Right 0QCJ
- Finger Nail 0HCQXZZ
- Gallbladder 0FC4
- Gastrointestinal Tract 0WCP
- Genitourinary Tract 0WCR
- Gingiva
  - Lower 0CC6
  - Upper 0CC5
- Gland
  - Adrenal
    - Bilateral 0GC4
    - Left 0GC2
    - Right 0GC3

Extirpation *(continued)*
- Gland *(continued)*
  - Lacrimal
    - Left 08CW
    - Right 08CV
  - Minor Salivary 0CCJ
  - Parotid
    - Left 0CC9
    - Right 0CC8
  - Pituitary 0GC0
  - Sublingual
    - Left 0CCF
    - Right 0CCD
  - Submaxillary
    - Left 0CCH
    - Right 0CCG
  - Vestibular 0UCL
- Glenoid Cavity
  - Left 0PC8
  - Right 0PC7
- Glomus Jugulare 0GCC
- Humeral Head
  - Left 0PCD
  - Right 0PCC
- Humeral Shaft
  - Left 0PCG
  - Right 0PCF
- Hymen 0UCK
- Hypothalamus 00CA
- Ileocecal Valve 0DCC
- Ileum 0DCB
- Intestine
  - Large 0DCE
    - Left 0DCG
    - Right 0DCF
  - Small 0DC8
- Iris
  - Left 08CD
  - Right 08CC
- Jaw
  - Lower 0WC5
  - Upper 0WC4
- Jejunum 0DCA
- Joint
  - Acromioclavicular
    - Left 0RCH
    - Right 0RCG
  - Ankle
    - Left 0SCG
    - Right 0SCF
  - Carpal
    - Left 0RCR
    - Right 0RCQ
  - Carpometacarpal
    - Left 0RCT
    - Right 0RCS
  - Cervical Vertebral 0RC1
  - Cervicothoracic Vertebral 0RC4
  - Coccygeal 0SC6
  - Elbow
    - Left 0RCM
    - Right 0RCL
  - Finger Phalangeal
    - Left 0RCX
    - Right 0RCW
  - Hip
    - Left 0SCB
    - Right 0SC9
  - Knee
    - Left 0SCD
    - Right 0SCC
  - Lumbar Vertebral 0SC0
  - Lumbosacral 0SC3
  - Metacarpophalangeal
    - Left 0RCV
    - Right 0RCU
  - Metatarsal-Phalangeal
    - Left 0SCN
    - Right 0SCM
  - Occipital-cervical 0RC0
  - Sacrococcygeal 0SC5

Extirpation *(continued)*
- Joint *(continued)*
  - Sacroiliac
    - Left 0SC8
    - Right 0SC7
  - Shoulder
    - Left 0RCK
    - Right 0RCJ
  - Sternoclavicular
    - Left 0RCF
    - Right 0RCE
  - Tarsal
    - Left 0SCJ
    - Right 0SCH
  - Tarsometatarsal
    - Left 0SCL
    - Right 0SCK
  - Temporomandibular
    - Left 0RCD
    - Right 0RCC
  - Thoracic Vertebral 0RC6
  - Thoracolumbar Vertebral 0RCA
  - Toe Phalangeal
    - Left 0SCQ
    - Right 0SCP
  - Wrist
    - Left 0RCP
    - Right 0RCN
- Kidney
  - Left 0TC1
  - Right 0TC0
- Kidney Pelvis
  - Left 0TC4
  - Right 0TC3
- Larynx 0CCS
- Lens
  - Left 08CK
  - Right 08CJ
- Lip
  - Lower 0CC1
  - Upper 0CC0
- Liver 0FC0
  - Left Lobe 0FC2
  - Right Lobe 0FC1
- Lung
  - Bilateral 0BCM
  - Left 0BCL
  - Lower Lobe
    - Left 0BCJ
    - Right 0BCF
  - Middle Lobe, Right 0BCD
  - Right 0BCK
  - Upper Lobe
    - Left 0BCG
    - Right 0BCC
- Lung Lingula 0BCH
- Lymphatic
  - Aortic 07CD
  - Axillary
    - Left 07C6
    - Right 07C5
  - Head 07C0
  - Inguinal
    - Left 07CJ
    - Right 07CH
  - Internal Mammary
    - Left 07C9
    - Right 07C8
  - Lower Extremity
    - Left 07CG
    - Right 07CF
  - Mesenteric 07CB
  - Neck
    - Left 07C2
    - Right 07C1
  - Pelvis 07CC
  - Thoracic Duct 07CK
  - Thorax 07C7
  - Upper Extremity
    - Left 07C4
    - Right 07C3

Extirpation *(continued)*
- Mandible
  - Left 0NCV
  - Right 0NCT
- Maxilla 0NCR
- Mediastinum 0WCC
- Medulla Oblongata 00CD
- Mesentery 0DCV
- Metacarpal
  - Left 0PCQ
  - Right 0PCP
- Metatarsal
  - Left 0QCP
  - Right 0QCN
- Muscle
  - Abdomen
    - Left 0KCL
    - Right 0KCK
  - Extraocular
    - Left 08CM
    - Right 08CL
  - Facial 0KC1
  - Foot
    - Left 0KCW
    - Right 0KCV
  - Hand
    - Left 0KCD
    - Right 0KCC
  - Head 0KC0
  - Hip
    - Left 0KCP
    - Right 0KCN
  - Lower Arm and Wrist
    - Left 0KCB
    - Right 0KC9
  - Lower Leg
    - Left 0KCT
    - Right 0KCS
  - Neck
    - Left 0KC3
    - Right 0KC2
  - Papillary 02CD
  - Perineum 0KCM
  - Shoulder
    - Left 0KC6
    - Right 0KC5
  - Thorax
    - Left 0KCJ
    - Right 0KCH
  - Tongue, Palate, Pharynx 0KC4
  - Trunk
    - Left 0KCG
    - Right 0KCF
  - Upper Arm
    - Left 0KC8
    - Right 0KC7
  - Upper Leg
    - Left 0KCR
    - Right 0KCQ
- Nasal Mucosa and Soft Tissue 09CK
- Nasopharynx 09CN
- Nerve
  - Abdominal Sympathetic 01CM
  - Abducens 00CL
  - Accessory 00CR
  - Acoustic 00CN
  - Brachial Plexus 01C3
  - Cervical 01C1
  - Cervical Plexus 01C0
  - Facial 00CM
  - Femoral 01CD
  - Glossopharyngeal 00CP
  - Head and Neck Sympathetic 01CK
  - Hypoglossal 00CS
  - Lumbar 01CB
  - Lumbar Plexus 01C9
  - Lumbar Sympathetic 01CN
  - Lumbosacral Plexus 01CA

Extirpation *(continued)*
- Nerve *(continued)*
  - Median 01C5
  - Oculomotor 00CH
  - Olfactory 00CF
  - Optic 00CG
  - Peroneal 01CH
  - Phrenic 01C2
  - Pudendal 01CC
  - Radial 01C6
  - Sacral 01CR
  - Sacral Plexus 01CQ
  - Sacral Sympathetic 01CP
  - Sciatic 01CF
  - Thoracic 01C8
  - Thoracic Sympathetic 01CL
  - Tibial 01CG
  - Trigeminal 00CK
  - Trochlear 00CJ
  - Ulnar 01C4
  - Vagus 00CQ
- Nipple
  - Left 0HCX
  - Right 0HCW
- Omentum 0DCU
- Oral Cavity and Throat 0WC3
- Orbit
  - Left 0NCQ
  - Right 0NCP
- Orbital Atherectomy *see* Extirpation, Heart and Great Vessels 02C
- Ovary
  - Bilateral 0UC2
  - Left 0UC1
  - Right 0UC0
- Palate
  - Hard 0CC2
  - Soft 0CC3
- Pancreas 0FCG
- Para-aortic Body 0GC9
- Paraganglion Extremity 0GCF
- Parathyroid Gland 0GCR
  - Inferior
    - Left 0GCP
    - Right 0GCN
  - Multiple 0GCQ
  - Superior
    - Left 0GCM
    - Right 0GCL
- Patella
  - Left 0QCF
  - Right 0QCD
- Pelvic Cavity 0WCJ
- Penis 0VCS
- Pericardial Cavity 0WCD
- Pericardium 02CN
- Peritoneal Cavity 0WCG
- Peritoneum 0DCW
- Phalanx
  - Finger
    - Left 0PCV
    - Right 0PCT
  - Thumb
    - Left 0PCS
    - Right 0PCR
  - Toe
    - Left 0QCR
    - Right 0QCQ
- Pharynx 0CCM
- Pineal Body 0GC1
- Pleura
  - Left 0BCP
  - Right 0BCN
- Pleural Cavity
  - Left 0WCB
  - Right 0WC9
- Pons 00CB
- Prepuce 0VCT
- Prostate 0VC0

Extirpation *(continued)*
- Radius
  - Left 0PCJ
  - Right 0PCH
- Rectum 0DCP
- Respiratory Tract 0WCQ
- Retina
  - Left 08CF
  - Right 08CE
- Retinal Vessel
  - Left 08CH
  - Right 08CG
- Retroperitoneum 0WCH
- Ribs
  - 1 to 2 0PC1
  - 3 or More 0PC2
- Sacrum 0QC1
- Scapula
  - Left 0PC6
  - Right 0PC5
- Sclera
  - Left 08C7XZZ
  - Right 08C6XZZ
- Scrotum 0VC5
- Septum
  - Atrial 02C5
  - Nasal 09CM
  - Ventricular 02CM
- Sinus
  - Accessory 09CP
  - Ethmoid
    - Left 09CV
    - Right 09CU
  - Frontal
    - Left 09CT
    - Right 09CS
  - Mastoid
    - Left 09CC
    - Right 09CB
  - Maxillary
    - Left 09CR
    - Right 09CQ
  - Sphenoid
    - Left 09CX
    - Right 09CW
- Skin
  - Abdomen 0HC7XZZ
  - Back 0HC6XZZ
  - Buttock 0HC8XZZ
  - Chest 0HC5XZZ
  - Ear
    - Left 0HC3XZZ
    - Right 0HC2XZZ
  - Face 0HC1XZZ
  - Foot
    - Left 0HCNXZZ
    - Right 0HCMXZZ
  - Hand
    - Left 0HCGXZZ
    - Right 0HCFXZZ
  - Inguinal 0HCAXZZ
  - Lower Arm
    - Left 0HCEXZZ
    - Right 0HCDXZZ
  - Lower Leg
    - Left 0HCLXZZ
    - Right 0HCKXZZ
  - Neck 0HC4XZZ
  - Perineum 0HC9XZZ
  - Scalp 0HC0XZZ
  - Upper Arm
    - Left 0HCCXZZ
    - Right 0HCBXZZ
  - Upper Leg
    - Left 0HCJXZZ
    - Right 0HCHXZZ
- Spinal Canal 00CU
- Spinal Cord
  - Cervical 00CW
  - Lumbar 00CY
  - Thoracic 00CX

Extirpation *(continued)*
- Spinal Meninges 00CT
- Spleen 07CP
- Sternum 0PC0
- Stomach 0DC6
  - Pylorus 0DC7
- Subarachnoid Space, Intracranial 00C5
- Subcutaneous Tissue and Fascia
  - Abdomen 0JC8
  - Back 0JC7
  - Buttock 0JC9
  - Chest 0JC6
  - Face 0JC1
  - Foot
    - Left 0JCR
    - Right 0JCQ
  - Hand
    - Left 0JCK
    - Right 0JCJ
  - Lower Arm
    - Left 0JCH
    - Right 0JCG
  - Lower Leg
    - Left 0JCP
    - Right 0JCN
  - Neck
    - Left 0JC5
    - Right 0JC4
  - Pelvic Region 0JCC
  - Perineum 0JCB
  - Scalp 0JC0
  - Upper Arm
    - Left 0JCF
    - Right 0JCD
  - Upper Leg
    - Left 0JCM
    - Right 0JCL
- Subdural Space, Intracranial 00C4
- Tarsal
  - Left 0QCM
  - Right 0QCL
- Tendon
  - Abdomen
    - Left 0LCG
    - Right 0LCF
  - Ankle
    - Left 0LCT
    - Right 0LCS
  - Foot
    - Left 0LCW
    - Right 0LCV
  - Hand
    - Left 0LC8
    - Right 0LC7
  - Head and Neck 0LC0
  - Hip
    - Left 0LCK
    - Right 0LCJ
  - Knee
    - Left 0LCR
    - Right 0LCQ
  - Lower Arm and Wrist
    - Left 0LC6
    - Right 0LC5
  - Lower Leg
    - Left 0LCP
    - Right 0LCN
  - Perineum 0LCH
  - Shoulder
    - Left 0LC2
    - Right 0LC1
  - Thorax
    - Left 0LCD
    - Right 0LCC
  - Trunk
    - Left 0LCB
    - Right 0LC9
  - Upper Arm
    - Left 0LC4
    - Right 0LC3

Extirpation *(continued)*
- Tendon *(continued)*
  - Upper Leg
    - Left 0LCM
    - Right 0LCL
- Testis
  - Bilateral 0VCC
  - Left 0VCB
  - Right 0VC9
- Thalamus 00C9
- Thymus 07CM
- Thyroid Gland 0GCK
  - Left Lobe 0GCG
  - Right Lobe 0GCH
- Tibia
  - Left 0QCH
  - Right 0QCG
- Toe Nail 0HCRXZZ
- Tongue 0CC7
- Tonsils 0CCP
- Tooth
  - Lower 0CCX
  - Upper 0CCW
- Trachea 0BC1
- Tunica Vaginalis
  - Left 0VC7
  - Right 0VC6
- Turbinate, Nasal 09CL
- Tympanic Membrane
  - Left 09C8
  - Right 09C7
- Ulna
  - Left 0PCL
  - Right 0PCK
- Ureter
  - Left 0TC7
  - Right 0TC6
- Urethra 0TCD
- Uterine Supporting Structure 0UC4
- Uterus 0UC9
- Uvula 0CCN
- Vagina 0UCG
- Valve
  - Aortic 02CF
  - Mitral 02CG
  - Pulmonary 02CH
  - Tricuspid 02CJ
- Vas Deferens
  - Bilateral 0VCQ
  - Left 0VCP
  - Right 0VCN
- Vein
  - Axillary
    - Left 05C8
    - Right 05C7
  - Azygos 05C0
  - Basilic
    - Left 05CC
    - Right 05CB
  - Brachial
    - Left 05CA
    - Right 05C9
  - Cephalic
    - Left 05CF
    - Right 05CD
  - Colic 06C7
  - Common Iliac
    - Left 06CD
    - Right 06CC
  - Coronary 02C4
  - Esophageal 06C3
  - External Iliac
    - Left 06CG
    - Right 06CF
  - External Jugular
    - Left 05CQ
    - Right 05CP
  - Face
    - Left 05CV
    - Right 05CT

Extirpation *(continued)*
- Vein *(continued)*
  - Femoral
    - Left 06CN
    - Right 06CM
  - Foot
    - Left 06CV
    - Right 06CT
  - Gastric 06C2
  - Hand
    - Left 05CH
    - Right 05CG
  - Hemiazygos 05C1
  - Hepatic 06C4
  - Hypogastric
    - Left 06CJ
    - Right 06CH
  - Inferior Mesenteric 06C6
  - Innominate
    - Left 05C4
    - Right 05C3
  - Internal Jugular
    - Left 05CN
    - Right 05CM
  - Intracranial 05CL
  - Lower 06CY
  - Portal 06C8
  - Pulmonary
    - Left 02CT
    - Right 02CS
  - Renal
    - Left 06CB
    - Right 06C9
  - Saphenous
    - Left 06CQ
    - Right 06CP
  - Splenic 06C1
  - Subclavian
    - Left 05C6
    - Right 05C5
  - Superior Mesenteric 06C5
  - Upper 05CY
  - Vertebral
    - Left 05CS
    - Right 05CR
- Vena Cava
  - Inferior 06C0
  - Superior 02CV
- Ventricle
  - Left 02CL
  - Right 02CK
- Vertebra
  - Cervical 0PC3
  - Lumbar 0QC0
  - Thoracic 0PC4
- Vesicle
  - Bilateral 0VC3
  - Left 0VC2
  - Right 0VC1
- Vitreous
  - Left 08C5
  - Right 08C4
- Vocal Cord
  - Left 0CCV
  - Right 0CCT
- Vulva 0UCM

Extracorporeal shock wave lithotripsy
- *see* Fragmentation

Extracranial-intracranial bypass (EC-IC)
- *see* Bypass, Upper Arteries 031

Extracorporeal Carbon Dioxide Removal (ECC02R) 5A0920Z

Extraction
- Acetabulum
  - Left 0QD50ZZ
  - Right 0QD40ZZ
- Ampulla of Vater 0FDC

Extraction *(continued)*
- Anus 0DDQ
- Appendix 0DDJ
- Auditory Ossicle
  - Left 09DA0ZZ
  - Right 09D90ZZ
- Bone
  - Ethmoid
    - Left 0NDG0ZZ
    - Right 0NDF0ZZ
  - Frontal 0ND10ZZ
  - Hyoid 0NDX0ZZ
  - Lacrimal
    - Left 0NDJ0ZZ
    - Right 0NDH0ZZ
  - Nasal 0NDB0ZZ
  - Occipital 0ND70ZZ
  - Palatine
    - Left 0NDL0ZZ
    - Right 0NDK0ZZ
  - Parietal
    - Left 0ND40ZZ
    - Right 0ND30ZZ
  - Pelvic
    - Left 0QD30ZZ
    - Right 0QD20ZZ
  - Sphenoid 0NDC0ZZ
  - Temporal
    - Left 0ND60ZZ
    - Right 0ND50ZZ
  - Zygomatic
    - Left 0NDN0ZZ
    - Right 0NDM0ZZ
- Bone Marrow 07DT
  - Iliac 07DR
  - Sternum 07DQ
  - Vertebral 07DS
- Brain 00D0
- Breast
  - Bilateral 0HDV
  - Left 0HDU
  - Right 0HDT
  - Supernumerary 0HDY
- Bronchus
  - Lingula 0BD9
  - Lower Lobe
    - Left 0BDB
    - Right 0BD6
  - Main
    - Left 0BD7
    - Right 0BD3
  - Middle Lobe, Right 0BD5
  - Upper Lobe
    - Left 0BD8
    - Right 0BD4
- Bursa and Ligament
  - Abdomen
    - Left 0MDJ
    - Right 0MDH
  - Ankle
    - Left 0MDR
    - Right 0MDQ
  - Elbow
    - Left 0MD4
    - Right 0MD3
  - Foot
    - Left 0MDT
    - Right 0MDS
  - Hand
    - Left 0MD8
    - Right 0MD7
  - Head and Neck 0MD0
  - Hip
    - Left 0MDM
    - Right 0MDL
  - Knee
    - Left 0MDP
    - Right 0MDN
  - Lower Extremity
    - Left 0MDW
    - Right 0MDV

Extraction *(continued)*
Stomach 0DD6
Pylorus 0DD7
Subcutaneous Tissue and Fascia
Abdomen 0JD8
Back 0JD7
Buttock 0JD9
Chest 0JD6
Face 0JD1
Foot
Left 0JDR
Right 0JDQ
Hand
Left 0JDK
Right 0JDJ
Lower Arm
Left 0JDH
Right 0JDG
Lower Leg
Left 0JDP
Right 0JDN
Neck
Left 0JD5
Right 0JD4
Pelvic Region 0JDC
Perineum 0JDB
Scalp 0JD0
Upper Arm
Left 0JDF
Right 0JDD
Upper Leg
Left 0JDM
Right 0JDL
Tarsal
Left 0QDM0ZZ
Right 0QDL0ZZ
Tendon
Abdomen
Left 0LDG0ZZ
Right 0LDF0ZZ
Ankle
Left 0LDT0ZZ
Right 0LDS0ZZ
Foot
Left 0LDW0ZZ
Right 0LDV0ZZ
Hand
Left 0LD80ZZ
Right 0LD70ZZ
Head and Neck
0LD00ZZ
Hip
Left 0LDK0ZZ
Right 0LDJ0ZZ
Knee
Left 0LDR0ZZ
Right 0LDQ0ZZ
Lower Arm and
Wrist
Left 0LD60ZZ
Right 0LD50ZZ
Lower Leg
Left 0LDP0ZZ
Right 0LDN0ZZ
Perineum 0LDH0ZZ
Shoulder
Left 0LD20ZZ
Right 0LD10ZZ
Thorax
Left 0LDD0ZZ
Right 0LDC0ZZ
Trunk
Left 0LDB0ZZ
Right 0LD90ZZ
Upper Arm
Left 0LD40ZZ
Right 0LD30ZZ
Upper Leg
Left 0LDM0ZZ
Right 0LDL0ZZ
Thymus 07DM

Extraction *(continued)*
Tibia
Left 0QDH0ZZ
Right 0QDG0ZZ
Toe Nail 0HDRXZZ
Tooth
Lower 0CDXXZ
Upper 0CDWXZ
Trachea 0BD1
Turbinate, Nasal 09DL
Tympanic Membrane
Left 09D8
Right 09D7
Ulna
Left 0PDL0ZZ
Right 0PDK0ZZ
Vein
Basilic
Left 05DC
Right 05DB
Brachial
Left 05DA
Right 05D9
Cephalic
Left 05DF
Right 05DD
Femoral
Left 06DN
Right 06DM
Foot
Left 06DV
Right 06DT
Hand
Left 05DH
Right 05DG
Lower 06DY
Saphenous
Left 06DQ
Right 06DP
Upper 05DY
Vertebra
Cervical 0PD30ZZ
Lumbar 0QD00ZZ
Thoracic 0PD40ZZ
Vocal Cord
Left 0CDV
Right 0CDT
Extradural space, intracranial
use Epidural Space, Intracranial
Extradural space, spinal
use Spinal Canal
EXtreme Lateral Interbody Fusion (XLIF) device
use Interbody Fusion Device in Lower Joints

F

Face lift
see Alteration, Face 0W02
Facet replacement spinal stabilization device
use Spinal Stabilization Device, Facet Replacement in 0RH
use Spinal Stabilization Device, Facet Replacement in 0SH
Facial artery
use Artery, Face
Factor Xa Inhibitor Reversal Agent, Andexanet Alfa
use Coagulation Factor Xa, Inactivated
False vocal cord
use Larynx
Falx cerebri
use Dura Mater
Fascia lata
use Subcutaneous Tissue and Fascia, Upper Leg, Left

Fascia lata *(continued)*
use Subcutaneous Tissue and Fascia, Upper Leg, Right
Fasciaplasty, fascioplasty
see Repair, Subcutaneous Tissue and Fascia 0JQ
see Replacement, Subcutaneous Tissue and Fascia 0JR
Fasciectomy
see Excision, Subcutaneous Tissue and Fascia 0JB
see Release
Fasciorrhaphy
see Repair, Subcutaneous Tissue and Fascia 0JQ
Fasciotomy
see Division, Subcutaneous Tissue and Fascia 0J8
see Drainage, Subcutaneous Tissue and Fascia 0J9
see Release
Feeding Device
Change device in
Lower 0D2DXUZ
Upper 0D20XUZ
Insertion of device in
Duodenum 0DH9
Esophagus 0DH5
Ileum 0DHB
Intestine, Small 0DH8
Jejunum 0DHA
Stomach 0DH6
Removal of device from
Esophagus 0DP5
Intestinal Tract
Lower 0DPD
Upper 0DP0
Stomach 0DP6
Revision of device in
Intestinal Tract
Lower 0DWD
Upper 0DW0
Stomach 0DW6
Femoral head
use Femur, Upper, Left
use Femur, Upper, Right
Femoral lymph node
use Lymphatic, Lower Extremity, Left
use Lymphatic, Lower Extremity, Right
Femoropatellar joint
use Joint, Knee, Left
use Joint, Knee, Left, Femoral Surface
use Joint, Knee, Right
use Joint, Knee, Right, Femoral Surface
Femorotibial joint
use Joint, Knee, Left
use Joint, Knee, Left, Tibial Surface
use Joint, Knee, Right
use Joint, Knee, Right, Tibial Surface
FETROJA®
use Cefiderocol Anti-infective
FGS (fluorescence-guided surgery)
see Fluorescence Guided Procedure
Fibular artery
use Artery, Peroneal, Left
use Artery, Peroneal, Right
Fibular sesamoid
use Metatarsal, Left
use Metatarsal, Right
Fibularis brevis muscle
use Muscle, Lower Leg, Left
use Muscle, Lower Leg, Right
Fibularis longus muscle
use Muscle, Lower Leg, Left
use Muscle, Lower Leg, Right

Fifth cranial nerve
use Nerve, Trigeminal
Filum terminale
use Spinal Meninges
Fimbriectomy
see Excision, Female Reproductive System 0UB
see Resection, Female Reproductive System 0UT
Fine needle aspiration
Fluid or gas
see Drainage
Tissue biopsy
see Excision
see Extraction
First cranial nerve
use Nerve, Olfactory
First intercostal nerve
use Nerve, Brachial Plexus
Fistulization
see Bypass
see Drainage
see Repair
Fitting
Arch bars, for fracture reduction
see Reposition, Mouth and Throat 0CS
Arch bars, for immobilization
see Immobilization, Face 2W31
Artificial limb
see Device Fitting, Rehabilitation F0D
Hearing aid
see Device Fitting, Rehabilitation F0D
Ocular prosthesis F0DZ8UZ
Prosthesis, limb
see Device Fitting, Rehabilitation F0D
Prosthesis, ocular F0DZ8UZ
Fixation, bone
External, with fracture reduction
see Reposition
External, without fracture reduction
see Insertion
Internal, with fracture reduction
see Reposition
Internal, without fracture reduction
see Insertion
FLAIR® Endovascular Stent Graft
use Intraluminal Device
Flexible Composite Mesh
use Synthetic Substitute
Flexor carpi radialis muscle
use Muscle, Lower Arm and Wrist, Left
use Muscle, Lower Arm and Wrist, Right
Flexor carpi ulnaris muscle
use Muscle, Lower Arm and Wrist, Left
use Muscle, Lower Arm and Wrist, Right
Flexor digitorum brevis muscle
use Muscle, Foot, Left
use Muscle, Foot, Right
Flexor digitorum longus muscle
use Muscle, Lower Leg, Left
use Muscle, Lower Leg, Right
Flexor hallucis brevis muscle
use Muscle, Foot, Left
use Muscle, Foot, Right
Flexor hallucis longus muscle
use Muscle, Lower Leg, Left
use Muscle, Lower Leg, Right
Flexor pollicis longus muscle
use Muscle, Lower Arm and Wrist, Left
use Muscle, Lower Arm and Wrist, Right

- **Flow Diverter embolization device**
  - *use* Intraluminal Device, Flow Diverter in 03V
- **FlowSense Noninvasive Thermal Sensor**
  - *see* Measurement, Central Nervous Cerebrospinal Fluid Shunt
- **Fluorescence Guided Procedure**
  - Extremity
    - Lower 8E0Y
    - Upper 8E0X
  - Head and Neck Region 8E09
    - Aminolevulinic Acid 8E09
    - No Qualifier 8E09
  - Trunk Region 8E0W
- **Fluorescent Pyrazine, Kidney**
  - XT25XE5
- **Fluoroscopy**
  - Abdomen and Pelvis BW11
  - Airway, Upper BB1DZZZ
  - Ankle
    - Left BQ1
    - Right BQ1G
  - Aorta
    - Abdominal B410
      - Laser, Intraoperative B410
    - Thoracic B310
      - Laser, Intraoperative B310
    - Thoraco-Abdominal B31P
      - Laser, Intraoperative B31P
  - Aorta and Bilateral Lower Extremity Arteries B41D
    - Laser, Intraoperative B41D
  - Arm
    - Left BP1FZZZ
    - Right BP1EZZZ
  - Artery
    - Brachiocephalic-Subclavian
      - Right B311
      - Laser, Intraoperative B311
    - Bronchial B31L
      - Laser, Intraoperative B31L
    - Bypass Graft, Other B21F
    - Cervico-Cerebral Arch B31Q
      - Laser, Intraoperative B31Q
    - Common Carotid
      - Bilateral B315
        - Laser, Intraoperative B315
      - Left B314
        - Laser, Intraoperative B314
      - Right B313
        - Laser, Intraoperative B313
    - Coronary
      - Bypass Graft
        - Multiple B213
          - Laser, Intraoperative B213
        - Single B212
          - Laser, Intraoperative B212
      - Multiple B211
        - Laser, Intraoperative B211
      - Single B210
        - Laser, Intraoperative B210
    - External Carotid
      - Bilateral B31C
        - Laser, Intraoperative B31C
      - Left B31B
        - Laser, Intraoperative B31B
      - Right B319
        - Laser, Intraoperative B319
    - Hepatic B412
      - Laser, Intraoperative B412
    - Inferior Mesenteric B415
      - Laser, Intraoperative B415
    - Intercostal B31L
      - Laser, Intraoperative B31L
    - Internal Carotid
      - Bilateral B318
        - Laser, Intraoperative B318
      - Left B317
        - Laser, Intraoperative B317

Fluoroscopy *(continued)*
  - Artery *(continued)*
    - Internal Carotid *(continued)*
      - Right B316
        - Laser, Intraoperative B316
    - Internal Mammary Bypass Graft
      - Left B218
      - Right B217
    - Intra-Abdominal
      - Laser, Intraoperative B41B
      - Other B41B
    - Intracranial B31R
      - Laser, Intraoperative B31R
    - Lower
      - Laser, Intraoperative B41J
      - Other B41J
    - Lower Extremity
      - Bilateral and Aorta B41D
        - Laser, Intraoperative B41D
      - Left B41G
        - Laser, Intraoperative B41G
      - Right B41F
        - Laser, Intraoperative B41F
    - Lumbar B419
      - Laser, Intraoperative B419
    - Pelvic B41C
      - Laser, Intraoperative B41C
    - Pulmonary
      - Left B31T
        - Laser, Intraoperative B31T
      - Right B31S
        - Laser, Intraoperative B31S
    - Pulmonary Trunk B31U
      - Laser, Intraoperative B31U
    - Renal
      - Bilateral B418
        - Laser, Intraoperative B418
      - Left B417
        - Laser, Intraoperative B417
      - Right B416
        - Laser, Intraoperative B416
    - Spinal B31M
      - Laser, Intraoperative B31M
    - Splenic B413
      - Laser, Intraoperative B413
    - Subclavian
      - Laser, Intraoperative B312
      - Left B312
    - Superior Mesenteric B414
      - Laser, Intraoperative B414
    - Upper
      - Laser, Intraoperative B31N
      - Other B31N
    - Upper Extremity
      - Bilateral B31K
        - Laser, Intraoperative B31K
      - Left B31J
        - Laser, Intraoperative B31J
      - Right B31H
        - Laser, Intraoperative B31H
    - Vertebral
      - Bilateral B31G
        - Laser, Intraoperative B31G
      - Left B31F
        - Laser, Intraoperative B31F
      - Right B31D
        - Laser, Intraoperative B31D
  - Bile Duct BF10
    - Pancreatic Duct and Gallbladder BF14
  - Bile Duct and Gallbladder BF13
  - Biliary Duct BF11
  - Bladder BT10
    - Kidney and Ureter BT14
      - Left BT1F
      - Right BT1D
  - Bladder and Urethra BT1B
  - Bowel, Small BD1

Fluoroscopy *(continued)*
  - Calcaneus
    - Left BQ1KZZZ
    - Right BQ1JZZZ
  - Clavicle
    - Left BP15ZZZ
    - Right BP14ZZZ
  - Coccyx BR1F
  - Colon BD14
  - Corpora Cavernosa BV10
  - Dialysis Fistula B51W
  - Dialysis Shunt B51W
  - Diaphragm BB16ZZZ
  - Disc
    - Cervical BR11
    - Lumbar BR13
    - Thoracic BR12
  - Duodenum BD19
  - Elbow
    - Left BP1H
    - Right BP1G
  - Epiglottis B91G
  - Esophagus BD11
  - Extremity
    - Lower BW1C
    - Upper BW1J
  - Facet Joint
    - Cervical BR14
    - Lumbar BR16
    - Thoracic BR15
  - Fallopian Tube
    - Bilateral BU12
    - Left BU11
    - Right BU10
  - Fallopian Tube and Uterus BU18
  - Femur
    - Left BQ14ZZZ
    - Right BQ13ZZZ
  - Finger
    - Left BP1SZZZ
    - Right BP1RZZZ
  - Foot
    - Left BQ1MZZZ
    - Right BQ1LZZZ
  - Forearm
    - Left BP1KZZZ
    - Right BP1JZZZ
  - Gallbladder BF12
    - Bile Duct and Pancreatic Duct BF14
  - Gallbladder and Bile Duct BF13
  - Gastrointestinal, Upper BD1
  - Hand
    - Left BP1PZZZ
    - Right BP1NZZZ
  - Head and Neck BW19
  - Heart
    - Left B215
    - Right B214
    - Right and Left B216
  - Hip
    - Left BQ11
    - Right BQ10
  - Humerus
    - Left BP1BZZZ
    - Right BP1AZZZ
  - Ileal Diversion Loop BT1C
  - Ileal Loop, Ureters and Kidney BT1G
  - Intracranial Sinus B512
  - Joint
    - Acromioclavicular, Bilateral BP13ZZZ
    - Finger
      - Left BP1D
      - Right BP1C
    - Foot
      - Left BQ1Y
      - Right BQ1X

Fluoroscopy *(continued)*
  - Joint *(continued)*
    - Hand
      - Left BP1D
      - Right BP1C
    - Lumbosacral BR1B
    - Sacroiliac BR1D
    - Sternoclavicular
      - Bilateral BP12ZZZ
      - Left BP11ZZZ
      - Right BP10ZZZ
    - Temporomandibular
      - Bilateral BN19
      - Left BN18
      - Right BN17
    - Thoracolumbar BR18
    - Toe
      - Left BQ1Y
      - Right BQ1X
  - Kidney
    - Bilateral BT13
    - Ileal Loop and Ureter BT1G
    - Left BT12
    - Right BT11
    - Ureter and Bladder BT14
      - Left BT1F
      - Right BT1D
  - Knee
    - Left BQ18
    - Right BQ17
  - Larynx B91J
  - Leg
    - Left BQ1FZZZ
    - Right BQ1DZZZ
  - Liver BF15
  - Lung
    - Bilateral BB14ZZZ
    - Left BB13ZZZ
    - Right BB12ZZZ
  - Mediastinum BB1CZZZ
  - Mouth BD1B
  - Neck and Head BW19
  - Oropharynx BD1B
  - Pancreatic Duct BF1
    - Gallbladder and Bile Buct BF14
  - Patella
    - Left BQ1WZZZ
    - Right BQ1VZZZ
  - Pelvis BR1C
  - Pelvis and Abdomen BW11
  - Pharynx B91G
  - Ribs
    - Left BP1YZZZ
    - Right BP1XZZZ
  - Sacrum BR1F
  - Scapula
    - Left BP17ZZZ
    - Right BP16ZZZ
  - Shoulder
    - Left BP19
    - Right BP18
  - Sinus, Intracranial B512
  - Spinal Cord B01B
  - Spine
    - Cervical BR10
    - Lumbar BR19
    - Thoracic BR17
    - Whole BR1G
  - Sternum BR1H
  - Stomach BD12
  - Toe
    - Left BQ1QZZZ
    - Right BQ1PZZZ
  - Tracheobronchial Tree
    - Bilateral BB19YZZ
    - Left BB18YZZ
    - Right BB17YZZ
  - Ureter
    - Ileal Loop and Kidney BT1G

Fluoroscopy *(continued)*
Ureter *(continued)*
Kidney and Bladder BT14
Left BT1F
Right BT1D
Left BT17
Right BT16
Urethra BT15
Urethra and Bladder BT1B
Uterus BU16
Uterus and Fallopian Tube BU18
Vagina BU19
Vasa Vasorum BV18
Vein
Cerebellar B511
Cerebral B511
Epidural B510
Jugular
Bilateral B515
Left B514
Right B513
Lower Extremity
Bilateral B51D
Left B51C
Right B51B
Other B51V
Pelvic (Iliac)
Left B51G
Right B51F
Pelvic (Iliac) Bilateral B51H
Portal B51T
Pulmonary
Bilateral B51S
Left B51R
Right B51Q
Renal
Bilateral B51L
Left B51K
Right B51J
Spanchnic B51T
Subclavian
Left B517
Right B516
Upper Extremity
Bilateral B51P
Left B51N
Right B51M
Vena Cava
Inferior B519
Superior B518
Wrist
Left BP1M
Right BP1L
Fluoroscopy, laser intraoperative
Fluoroscopy, Heart B21
Fluoroscopy, Lower Arteries B41
Fluoroscopy, Upper Arteries B31
Flushing
see Irrigation
Foley catheter
use Drainage Device
Fontan completion procedure Stage II
see Bypass, Vena Cava, Inferior 0610
Foramen magnum
use Occipital Bone
Foramen of Monro (intraventricular)
use Cerebral Ventricle
Foreskin
use Prepuce
Formula™ Balloon-Expandable Renal Stent System
use Intraluminal Device
Fosfomycin Anti-infective
XW0
Fosfomycin injection
use Fosfomycin Anti-infective
Fossa of Rosenmuller
use Nasopharynx
Fourth cranial nerve
use Nerve, Trochlear
Fourth ventricle
use Cerebral Ventricle
Fovea
use Retina, Left
use Retina, Right
Fragmentation
Ampulla of Vater 0FFC
Anus 0DFQ
Appendix 0DFJ
Artery
Anterior Tibial
Left 04FQ3Z
Right 04FP3Z
Axillary
Left 03F63Z
Right 03F53Z
Brachial
Left 03F83Z
Right 03F73Z
Common Illiac
Left 04FD3Z
Right 04FC3Z
Coronary
Four or More Arteries 02F33ZZ
One Artery 02F03ZZ
Three Arteries 02F23ZZ
Two Arteries 02F13ZZ
External Illiac
Left 04FJ3Z
Right 04FH3Z
Femoral
Left 04FL3Z
Right 04FK3Z
Innominate 03F23Z
Internal Illiac
Left 04FF3Z
Right 04FE3Z
Intracranial 03FG3Z
Lower 04FY3Z
Peroneal
Left 04FU3Z
Right 04FT3Z
Popliteal
Left 04FN3Z
Right 04FM3Z
Posterior Tibial
Left 04FS3Z
Right 04FR3Z
Pulmonary
Left 02FR3Z
Right 02FQ3Z
Pulmonary Trunk 02FP3Z
Radial
Left 03FC3Z
Right 03FB3Z
Subclavian
Left 03F43Z
Right 03F33Z
Ulnar
Left 03FA3Z
Right 03F93Z
Upper 03FY3Z
Bladder 0TFB
Bladder Neck 0TFC
Bronchus
Lingula 0BF9
Lower Lobe
Left 0BFB
Right 0BF6
Main
Left 0BF7
Right 0BF3
Middle Lobe, Right 0BF5
Upper Lobe
Left 0BF8
Right 0BF4
Carina 0BF2
Cavity, Cranial 0WF1
Fragmentation *(continued)*
Cecum 0DFH
Cerebral Ventricle 00F6
Colon
Ascending 0DFK
Descending 0DFM
Sigmoid 0DFN
Transverse 0DFL
Duct
Common Bile 0FF9
Cystic 0FF8
Hepatic
Common 0FF7
Left 0FF6
Right 0FF5
Pancreatic 0FFD
Accessory 0FFF
Parotid
Left 0CFC
Right 0CFB
Duodenum 0DF9
Epidural Space, Intracranial 00F3
Esophagus 0DF5
Fallopian Tube
Left 0UF6
Right 0UF5
Fallopian Tubes, Bilateral 0UF7
Gallbladder 0FF4
Gastrointestinal Tract 0WFP
Genitourinary Tract 0WFR
Ileum 0DFB
Intestine
Large 0DFE
Left 0DFG
Right 0DFF
Small 0DF8
Jejunum 0DFA
Kidney Pelvis
Left 0TF4
Right 0TF3
Mediastinum 0WFC
Oral Cavity and Throat 0WF3
Pelvic Cavity 0WFJ
Pericardial Cavity 0WFD
Pericardium 02FN
Peritoneal Cavity 0WFG
Pleural Cavity
Left 0WFB
Right 0WF9
Rectum 0DFP
Respiratory Tract 0WFQ
Spinal Canal 00FU
Stomach 0DF6
Subarachnoid Space, Intracranial 00F5
Subdural Space, Intracranial 00F4
Trachea 0BF1
Ureter
Left 0TF7
Right 0TF6
Urethra 0TFD
Uterus 0UF9
Vein
Axillary
Left 05F83Z
Right 05F73Z
Basilic
Left 05FC3Z
Right 05FB3Z
Brachial
Left 05FA3Z
Right 05F93Z
Cephalic
Left 05FF3Z
Right 05FD3Z
Common Iliac
Left 06FD3Z
Right 06FC3Z
External Iliac
Left 06FG3Z
Right 06FF3Z
Fragmentation *(continued)*
Vein *(continued)*
Femoral
Left 06FN3Z
Right 06FM3Z
Hypogastric
Left 06FJ3Z
Right 06FH3Z
Innominate
Left 05F43Z
Right 05F33Z
Lower 06FY3Z
Pulmonary
Left 02FT3Z
Right 02FS3Z
Saphenous
Left 06FQ3Z
Right 06FP3Z
Subclavian
Left 05F63Z
Right 05F53Z
Upper 05FY3Z
Vitreous
Left 08F5
Right 08F4
Fragmentation, Ultrasonic
see Fragmentation, Artery
Freestyle (Stentless) Aortic Root Bioprosthesis
use Zooplastic Tissue in Heart and Great Vessels
Frenectomy
see Excision, Mouth and Throat 0CB
see Resection, Mouth and Throat 0CT
Frenoplasty, frenuloplasty
see Repair, Mouth and Throat 0CQ
see Replacement, Mouth and Throat 0CR
see Supplement, Mouth and Throat 0CU
Frenotomy
see Drainage, Mouth and Throat 0C9
see Release, Mouth and Throat 0CN
Frenulotomy
see Drainage, Mouth and Throat 0C9
see Release, Mouth and Throat 0CN
Frenulum labii inferioris
use Lip, Lower
Frenulum labii superioris
use Lip, Upper
Frenulum linguae
use Tongue
Frenulumectomy
see Excision, Mouth and Throat 0CB
see Resection, Mouth and Throat 0CT
Frontal lobe
use Cerebral Hemisphere
Frontal vein
use Vein, Face, Left
use Vein, Face, Right
Frozen elephant trunk (FET) technique, aortic arch replacement
see New Technology, Cardiovascular System X2R
see Replacement, Heart and Great Vessels 02R
Frozen elephant trunk (FET) technique, thoracic aorta restriction
see New Technology, Cardiovascular System X2V
see Restriction, Heart and Great Vessels 02V

FUJIFILM EP-7000X System for Oxygen Saturation Endoscopic Imaging (OXEI)
see New Technology, Gastrointestinal System XD2
Fulguration
see Destruction
Fundoplication, gastroesophageal
see Restriction, Esophagogastric Junction 0DV4
Fundus uteri
use Uterus
Fusion
Acromioclavicular
Left 0RGH
Right 0RGG
Ankle
Left 0SGG
Right 0SGF
Carpal
Left 0RGR
Right 0RGQ
Carpometacarpal
Left 0RGT
Right 0RGS
Cervical Vertebral 0RG1
2 or more 0RG2
Interbody Fusion Device
Nanotextured Surface XRG2092
Radiolucent Porous XRG20F3
Interbody Fusion Device, Nanotextured Surface XRG1092
Radiolucent Porous XRG10F3
Cervicothoracic Vertebral 0RG4
Interbody Fusion Device
Nanotextured Surface XRG4092
Radiolucent Porous XRG40F3
Coccygeal 0SG6
Elbow
Left 0RGM
Right 0RGL
Finger Phalangeal
Left 0RGX
Right 0RGW
Hip
Left 0SGB
Right 0SG9
Knee
Left 0SGD
Right 0SGC
Lumbar Vertebral 0SG0
2 or more 0SG1
Interbody Fusion Device
Customizable XRGC
Nanotextured Surface XRGC092
Radiolucent Porous XRGC0F3
Interbody Fusion Device
Customizable XRGB
Nanotextured Surface XRGB092
Radiolucent Porous XRGB0F3
Lumbosacral 0SG3
Interbody Fusion Device
Customizable XRGD
Nanotextured Surface XRGD092
Radiolucent Porous XRGD0F3
Metacarpophalangeal
Left 0RGV
Right 0RGU
Metatarsal-Phalangeal
Left 0SGN
Right 0SGM

Fusion *(continued)*
Occipital-cervical 0RG0
Interbody Fusion Device
Nanotextured Surface XRG0092
Radiolucent Porous XRG00F3
Sacrococcygeal 0SG5
Sacroiliac
Left 0SG8
Right 0SG7
Shoulder
Left 0RGK
Right 0RGJ
Sternoclavicular
Left 0RGF
Right 0RGE
Tarsal
Left 0SGJ
Right 0SGH
Tarsometatarsal
Left 0SGL
Right 0SGK
Temporomandibular
Left 0RGD
Right 0RGC
Thoracic Vertebral 0RG6
2 to 7 0RG7
Interbody Fusion Device Nanotextured Surface XRG7092
Radiolucent Porous XRG70F3
8 or more 0RG8
Interbody Fusion Device
Nanotextured Surface XRG8092
Radiolucent Porous XRG80F3
Interbody Fusion Device
Nanotextured Surface XRG6092
Radiolucent Porous XRG60F3
Thoracolumbar Vertebral 0RGA
Interbody Fusion Device
Customizable XRGA
Nanotextured Surface XRGA092
Radiolucent Porous XRGA0F3
Toe Phalangeal
Left 0SGQ
Right 0SGP
Wrist
Left 0RGP
Right 0RGN
Fusion screw (compression)(lag)(locking)
use Internal Fixation Device in Lower Joints
use Internal Fixation Device in Upper Joints

G

Gait training
see Motor Treatment, Rehabilitation F07
Galea aponeurotica
use Subcutaneous Tissue and Fascia, Scalp
Gammaglobulin
use Globulin
GammaTile™
use Radioactive Element, Cesium-131 Collagen Implant in 00H
GAMUNEX-C, for COVID-19 treatment
use High-Dose Intravenous Immune Globulin
Ganglion impar (ganglion of Walther)
use Nerve, Sacral Sympathetic
Ganglionectomy
Destruction of lesion
see Destruction
Excision of lesion
see Excision
Gasserian ganglion
use Nerve, Trigeminal
Gastrectomy
Partial
see Excision, Stomach 0DB6
Total
see Resection, Stomach 0DT6
Vertical (sleeve)
see Excision, Stomach 0DB6
Gastric electrical stimulation (GES) lead
use Stimulator Lead in Gastrointestinal System
Gastric lymph node
use Lymphatic, Aortic
Gastric pacemaker lead
use Stimulator Lead in Gastrointestinal System
Gastric plexus
use Nerve, Abdominal Sympathetic
Gastrocnemius muscle
use Muscle, Lower Leg, Left
use Muscle, Lower Leg, Right
Gastrocolic ligament
use Omentum
Gastrocolic omentum
use Omentum
Gastrocolostomy
see Bypass, Gastrointestinal System 0D1
see Drainage, Gastrointestinal System 0D9
Gastroduodenal artery
use Artery, Hepatic
Gastroduodenectomy
see Excision, Gastrointestinal System 0DB
see Resection, Gastrointestinal System 0DT
Gastroduodenoscopy 0DJ08ZZ
Gastroenteroplasty
see Repair, Gastrointestinal System 0DQ
see Supplement, Gastrointestinal System 0DU
Gastroenterostomy
see Bypass, Gastrointestinal System 0D1
see Drainage, Gastrointestinal System 0D9
Gastroesophageal (GE) junction
use Esophagogastric Junction
Gastrogastrostomy
see Bypass, Stomach 0D16
see Drainage, Stomach 0D96
Gastrohepatic omentum
use Omentum
Gastrojejunostomy
see Bypass, Stomach 0D16
see Drainage, Stomach 0D96
Gastrolysis
see Release, Stomach 0DN6
Gastropexy
see Repair, Stomach 0DQ6
see Reposition, Stomach 0DS6
Gastrophrenic ligament
use Omentum
Gastroplasty
see Repair, Stomach 0DQ6
see Supplement, Stomach 0DU6
Gastroplication
see Restriction, Stomach 0DV6
Gastropylorectomy
see Excision, Gastrointestinal System 0DB
Gastrorrhaphy
see Repair, Stomach 0DQ6
Gastroscopy 0DJ68ZZ
Gastrosplenic ligament
use Omentum
Gastrostomy
see Bypass, Stomach 0D16
see Drainage, Stomach 0D96
Gastrotomy
see Drainage, Stomach 0D96
Gemellus muscle
use Muscle, Hip, Left
use Muscle, Hip, Right
Geniculate ganglion
use Nerve, Facial
Geniculate nucleus
use Thalamus
Genioglossus muscle
use Muscle, Tongue, Palate, Pharynx
Genioplasty
see Alteration, Jaw, Lower 0W05
Genitofemoral nerve
use Nerve, Lumbar Plexus
GIAPREZA™
use Synthetic Human Angiotensin II
Gilteritinib Antineoplastic XW0DXV5
Gingivectomy
see Excision, Mouth and Throat 0CB
Gingivoplasty
see Repair, Mouth and Throat 0CQ
see Replacement, Mouth and Throat 0CR
see Supplement, Mouth and Throat 0CU
Glans penis
use Prepuce
Glenohumeral joint
use Joint, Shoulder, Left
use Joint, Shoulder, Right
Glenohumeral ligament
use Bursa and Ligament, Shoulder, Left
use Bursa and Ligament, Shoulder, Right
Glenoid fossa (of scapula)
use Glenoid Cavity, Left
use Glenoid Cavity, Right
Glenoid ligament (labrum)
use Shoulder Joint, Left
use Shoulder Joint, Right
Globus pallidus
use Basal Ganglia
Glomectomy
see Excision, Endocrine System 0GB
see Resection, Endocrine System 0GT
Glossectomy
see Excision, Tongue 0CB7
see Resection, Tongue 0CT7
Glossoepiglottic fold
use Epiglottis
Glossopexy
see Repair, Tongue 0CQ7
see Reposition, Tongue 0CS7
Glossoplasty
see Repair, Tongue 0CQ7
see Replacement, Tongue 0CR7
see Supplement, Tongue 0CU7
Glossorrhaphy
see Repair, Tongue 0CQ7
Glossotomy
see Drainage, Tongue 0C97
Glottis
use Larynx

Gluteal Artery Perforator Flap
Replacement
Bilateral 0HRV079
Left 0HRU079
Right 0HRT079
Transfer
Left 0KXG
Right 0KXF
Gluteal lymph node
use Lymphatic, Pelvis
Gluteal vein
use Vein, Hypogastric, Left
use Vein, Hypogastric, Right
Gluteus maximus muscle
use Muscle, Hip, Left
use Muscle, Hip, Right
Gluteus medius muscle
use Muscle, Hip, Left
use Muscle, Hip, Right
Gluteus minimus muscle
use Muscle, Hip, Left
use Muscle, Hip, Right
GORE® DUALMESH®
use Synthetic Substitute
GORE EXCLUDER® AAA Endoprosthesis
use Intraluminal Device
use Intraluminal Device, Branched or Fenestrated, One or Two Arteries in 04V
use Intraluminal Device, Branched or Fenestrated, Three or More Arteries in 04V
GORE EXCLUDER® IBE Endoprosthesis
use Intraluminal Device, Branched or Fenestrated, One or Two Arteries in 04V
GORE TAG® Thoracic Endoprosthesis
use Intraluminal Device
Gracilis muscle
use Muscle, Upper Leg, Left
use Muscle, Upper Leg, Right
Graft
see Replacement
see Supplement
Great auricular nerve
use Nerve, Cervical Plexus
Great cerebral vein
use Vein, Intracranial
Great(er) saphenous vein
use Vein, Saphenous, Left
use Vein, Saphenous, Right
Greater alar cartilage
use Nasal Mucosa and Soft Tissue
Greater occipital nerve
use Nerve, Cervical
Greater Omentum
use Omentum
Greater splanchnic nerve
use Nerve, Thoracic Sympathetic
Greater superficial petrosal nerve
use Nerve, Facial
Greater trochanter
use Femur, Upper, Left
use Femur, Upper, Right
Greater tuberosity
use Humeral Head, Left
use Humeral Head, Right
Greater vestibular (Bartholin's) gland
use Gland, Vestibular
Greater wing
use Bone, Sphenoid
GS-5734 *use* Remdesivir Anti-infective
Guedel airway
use Intraluminal Device, Airway in Mouth and Throat
Guidance, catheter placement
EKG
see Measurement, Physiological Systems 4A0
Fluoroscopy
see Fluoroscopy, Veins B51
Ultrasound
see Ultrasonography, Veins B54

H

Hallux
use Toe, 1st, Left
use Toe, 1st, Right
Hamate bone
use Carpal, Left
use Carpal, Right
Hancock Bioprosthesis (aortic) (mitral) valve
use Zooplastic Tissue in Heart and Great Vessels
Hancock Bioprosthetic Valved Conduit
use Zooplastic Tissue in Heart and Great Vessels
Harmony™ transcatheter pulmonary valve (TPV) placement 02RH38M
Harvesting, stem cells
see Pheresis, Circulatory 6A55
hdIVIG (high-dose intravenous immunoglobin), for COVID-19 treatment
use High-Dose Intravenous Immune Globulin
Head of fibula
use Fibula, Left
use Fibula, Right
Hearing Aid Assessment F14Z
Hearing Assessment F13Z
Hearing Device
Bone Conduction
Left 09HE
Right 09HD
Insertion of device in
Left 0NH6
Right 0NH5
Multiple Channel Cochlear Prosthesis
Left 09HE
Right 09HD
Removal of device from, Skull 0NP0
Revision of device in, Skull 0NW0
Single Channel Cochlear Prosthesis
Left 09HE
Right 09HD
Hearing Treatment F09Z
Heart Assist System
Implantable
Insertion of device in, Heart 02HA
Removal of device from, Heart 02PA
Revision of device in, Heart 02WA
Short-term External
Insertion of device in, Heart 02HA
Removal of device from, Heart 02PA
Revision of device in, Heart 02WA
HeartMate II® Left Ventricular Assist Device (LVAD)
use Implantable Heart Assist System in Heart and Great Vessels
HeartMate 3™ LVAS
use Implantable Heart Assist System in Heart and Great Vessels
HeartMate XVE® Left Ventricular Assist Device (LVAD)
use Implantable Heart Assist System in Heart and Great Vessels
HeartMate® implantable heart assist system
see Insertion of device in, Heart 02HA
Helix
use Ear, External, Bilateral
use Ear, External, Left
use Ear, External, Right
Hematopoietic cell transplant (HCT)
see Transfusion, Circulatory 302
Hemicolectomy
see Resection, Gastrointestinal System 0DT
Hemicystectomy
see Excision, Urinary System 0TB
Hemigastrectomy
see Excision, Gastrointestinal System 0DB
Hemiglossectomy
see Excision, Mouth and Throat 0CB
Hemilaminectomy
see Excision, Lower Bones 0QB
see Excision, Upper Bones 0PB
Hemilaminotomy
see Drainage, Lower Bones 0Q9
see Drainage, Upper Bones 0P9
see Excision, Lower Bones 0QB
see Excision, Upper Bones 0PB
see Release, Central Nervous System and Cranial Nerves 00N
see Release, Lower Bones 0QN
see Release, Peripheral Nervous System 01N
see Release, Upper Bones 0PN
Hemilaryngectomy
see Excision, Larynx 0CBS
Hemimandibulectomy
see Excision, Head and Facial Bones 0NB
Hemimaxillectomy
see Excision, Head and Facial Bones 0NB
Hemipylorectomy
see Excision, Gastrointestinal System 0DB
Hemispherectomy
see Excision, Central Nervous System and Cranial Nerves 00B
see Resection, Central Nervous System and Cranial Nerves 00T
Hemithyroidectomy
see Resection, Endocrine System 0GT
see Excision, Endocrine System 0GB
Hemodialysis
see Performance, Urinary 5A1D
Hemolung® Respiratory Assist System (RAS) 5A0920Z
Hemospray® Endoscopic Hemostat
use Mineral-based Topical Hemostatic Agent
Hepatectomy
see Excision, Hepatobiliary System and Pancreas 0FB
see Resection, Hepatobiliary System and Pancreas 0FT
Hepatic artery proper
use Artery, Hepatic
Hepatic flexure
use Colon, Transverse
Hepatic lymph node
use Lymphatic, Aortic
Hepatic plexus
use Nerve, Abdominal Sympathetic
Hepatic portal vein
use Vein, Portal
Hepaticoduodenostomy
see Bypass, Hepatobiliary System and Pancreas 0F1
see Drainage, Hepatobiliary System and Pancreas 0F9
Hepaticotomy
see Drainage, Hepatobiliary System and Pancreas 0F9
Hepatocholedochostomy
see Drainage, Duct, Common Bile 0F99
Hepatogastric ligament
use Omentum
Hepatopancreatic ampulla
use Ampulla of Vater
Hepatopexy
see Repair, Hepatobiliary System and Pancreas 0FQ
see Reposition, Hepatobiliary System and Pancreas 0FS
Hepatorrhaphy
see Repair, Hepatobiliary System and Pancreas 0FQ
Hepatotomy
see Drainage, Hepatobiliary System and Pancreas 0F9
Herculink (RX) Elite Renal Stent System
use Intraluminal Device
Herniorrhaphy
see Repair, Anatomical Regions, General 0WQ
see Repair, Anatomical Regions, Lower Extremities 0YQ
With synthetic substitute
see Supplement, Anatomical Regions, General 0WU
see Supplement, Anatomical Regions, Lower Extremities 0YU
HIG (hyperimmune globulin), for COVID-19 treatment
use Hyperimmune Globulin
High-Dose intravenous Immune Globulin, for COVID-19 treatment XW1
High-dose intravenous immunoglobulin (hdIVIG), for COVID-19 treatment
use High-Dose Intravenous Immune Globulin
Hip (joint) liner
use Liner in Lower Joints
HIPEC (hyperthermic intraperitoneal chemotherapy) 3E0M30Y
hIVIG (hyperimmune intravenous immunoglobulin), for COVID-19 treatment,
use Hyperimmune Globulin
Holter monitoring 4A12X45
Holter valve ventricular shunt
use Synthetic Substitute
Human angiotensin II, synthetic
use Synthetic Human Angiotensin II
Humeroradial joint
use Joint, Elbow, Left
use Joint, Elbow, Right
Humeroulnar joint
use Joint, Elbow, Left
use Joint, Elbow, Right
Humerus, distal
use Humeral Shaft, Left
use Humeral Shaft, Right
Hydrocelectomy
see Excision, Male Reproductive System 0VB
Hydrotherapy
Assisted exercise in pool
see Motor Treatment, Rehabilitation F07
Whirlpool
see Activities of Daily Living Treatment, Rehabilitation F08
Hymenectomy
see Excision, Hymen 0UBK
see Resection, Hymen 0UTK

Hymenoplasty
see Repair, Hymen 0UQK
see Supplement, Hymen 0UUK
Hymenorrhaphy
see Repair, Hymen 0UQK
Hymenotomy
see Division, Hymen 0U8K
see Drainage, Hymen 0U9K
Hyoglossus muscle
use Muscle, Tongue, Palate, Pharynx
Hyoid artery
use Artery, Thyroid, Left
use Artery, Thyroid, Right
Hyperalimentation
see Introduction of substance in or on
Hyperbaric oxygenation
Decompression sickness treatment
see Decompression, Circulatory 6A15
Wound treatment
see Assistance, Circulatory 5A05
Hyperimmune globulin
use Globulin
Hyperimmune globulin, for COVID-19 treatment XW1
Hyperimmune intravenous immunoglobulin (hIVIG), for COVID-19 treatment
use Hyperimmune Globulin
Hyperthermia
Radiation Therapy
Abdomen DWY38ZZ
Adrenal Gland DGY28ZZ
Bile Ducts DFY28ZZ
Bladder DTY28ZZ
Bone, Other DPYC8ZZ
Bone Marrow D7Y08ZZ
Brain D0Y08ZZ
Brain Stem D0Y18ZZ
Breast
Left DMY08ZZ
Right DMY18ZZ
Bronchus DBY18ZZ
Cervix DUY18ZZ
Chest DWY28ZZ
Chest Wall DBY78ZZ
Colon DDY58ZZ
Diaphragm DBY88ZZ
Duodenum DDY28ZZ
Ear D9Y08ZZ
Esophagus DDY08ZZ
Eye D8Y08ZZ
Femur DPY98ZZ
Fibula DPYB8ZZ
Gallbladder DFY18ZZ
Gland
Adrenal DGY28ZZ
Parathyroid DGY48ZZ
Pituitary DGY08ZZ
Thyroid DGY58ZZ
Glands, Salivary D9Y68ZZ
Head and Neck DWY18ZZ
Hemibody DWY48ZZ
Humerus DPY68ZZ
Hypopharynx D9Y38ZZ
Ileum DDY48ZZ
Jejunum DDY38ZZ
Kidney DTY08ZZ
Larynx D9YB8ZZ
Liver DFY08ZZ
Lung DBY28ZZ
Lymphatics
Abdomen D7Y68ZZ
Axillary D7Y48ZZ
Inguinal D7Y88ZZ
Neck D7Y38ZZ
Pelvis D7Y78ZZ
Thorax D7Y58ZZ
Mandible DPY38ZZ

Hyperthermia *(continued)*
Radiation Therapy *(continued)*
Maxilla DPY28ZZ
Mediastinum DBY68ZZ
Mouth D9Y48ZZ
Nasopharynx D9YD8ZZ
Neck and Head DWY18ZZ
Nerve, Peripheral D0Y78ZZ
Nose D9Y18ZZ
Oropharynx D9YF8ZZ
Ovary DUY08ZZ
Palate
Hard D9Y88ZZ
Soft D9Y98ZZ
Pancreas DFY38ZZ
Parathyroid Gland DGY48ZZ
Pelvic Bones DPY88ZZ
Pelvic Region DWY68ZZ
Pineal Body DGY18ZZ
Pituitary Gland DGY08ZZ
Pleura DBY58ZZ
Prostate DVY08ZZ
Radius DPY78ZZ
Rectum DDY78ZZ
Rib DPY58ZZ
Sinuses D9Y78ZZ
Skin
Abdomen DHY88ZZ
Arm DHY48ZZ
Back DHY78ZZ
Buttock DHY98ZZ
Chest DHY68ZZ
Face DHY28ZZ
Leg DHYB8ZZ
Neck DHY38ZZ
Skull DPY08ZZ
Spinal Cord D0Y68ZZ
Spleen D7Y28ZZ
Sternum DPY48ZZ
Stomach DDY18ZZ
Testis DVY18ZZ
Thymus D7Y18ZZ
Thyroid Gland DGY58ZZ
Tibia DPYB8ZZ
Tongue D9Y58ZZ
Trachea DBY08ZZ
Ulna DPY78ZZ
Ureter DTY18ZZ
Urethra DTY38ZZ
Uterus DUY28ZZ
Whole Body DWY58ZZ
Whole Body 6A3Z
Hyperthermic intraperitoneal chemotherapy (HIPEC) 3E0M30Y
Hypnosis GZFZZZZ
Hypogastric artery
use Artery, Internal Iliac, Left
use Artery, Internal Iliac, Right
Hypopharynx
use Pharynx
Hypophysectomy
see Excision, Gland, Pituitary 0GB0
see Resection, Gland, Pituitary 0GT0
Hypophysis
use Gland, Pituitary
Hypothalamotomy
see Destruction, Thalamus 0059
Hypothenar muscle
use Muscle, Hand, Left
use Muscle, Hand, Right
Hypothermia, Whole Body 6A4Z
Hysterectomy
Supracervical
see Resection, Uterus 0UT9
Total
see Resection, Uterus 0UT9
Hysterolysis
see Release, Uterus 0UN9

Hysteropexy
see Repair, Uterus 0UQ9
see Reposition, Uterus 0US9
Hysteroplasty
see Repair, Uterus 0UQ9
Hysterorrhaphy
see Repair, Uterus 0UQ9
Hysteroscopy 0UJD8ZZ
Hysterotomy
see Drainage, Uterus 0U99
Hysterotrachelectomy
see Resection, Cervix 0UTC
see Resection, Uterus 0UT9
Hysterotracheloplasty
see Repair, Uterus 0UQ9
Hysterotrachelorrhaphy
see Repair, Uterus 0UQ9

I

IABP (Intra-aortic balloon pump)
see Assistance, Cardiac 5A02
IAEMT (Intraoperative anesthetic effect monitoring and titration)
see Monitoring, Central Nervous 4A10
IASD® (InterAtrial Shunt Device), Corvia
use Synthetic Substitute
Idarucizumab, Pradaxa® (dabigatran) reversal agent
use Other Therapeutic Substance
Ide-cel
use Idecabtagene Vicleucel Immunotherapy
Idecabtagene Vicleucel
use Idecabtagene Vicleucel Immunotherapy
Idecabtagene Vicleucel Immunotherapy XW0
IGIV-C, for COVID-19 treatment
use Hyperimmune Globulin
IHD (Intermittent hemodialysis) 5A1D70Z
Ileal artery
use Artery, Superior Mesenteric
Ileectomy
see Excision, Ileum 0DBB
see Resection, Ileum 0DTB
Ileocolic artery
use Artery, Superior Mesenteric
Ileocolic vein
use Vein, Colic
Ileopexy
see Repair, Ileum 0DQB
see Reposition, Ileum 0DSB
Ileorrhaphy
see Repair, Ileum 0DQB
Ileoscopy 0DJD8ZZ
Ileostomy
see Bypass, Ileum 0D1B
see Drainage, Ileum 0D9B
Ileotomy
see Drainage, Ileum 0D9B
Ileoureterostomy
see Bypass, Urinary System 0T1
Iliac crest
use Bone, Pelvic, Left
use Bone, Pelvic, Right
Iliac fascia
use Subcutaneous Tissue and Fascia, Upper Leg, Left
use Subcutaneous Tissue and Fascia, Upper Leg, Right
Iliac lymph node
use Lymphatic, Pelvis
Iliacus muscle
use Muscle, Hip, Left
use Muscle, Hip, Right
Iliofemoral ligament
use Bursa and Ligament, Hip, Left
use Bursa and Ligament, Hip, Right

Iliohypogastric nerve
use Nerve, Lumbar Plexus
Ilioinguinal nerve
use Nerve, Lumbar Plexus
Iliolumbar artery
use Artery, Internal Iliac, Left
use Artery, Internal Iliac, Right
Iliolumbar ligament
use Bursa and Ligament, Lower Spine
Iliotibial tract (band)
use Subcutaneous Tissue and Fascia, Upper Leg, Left
use Subcutaneous Tissue and Fascia, Upper Leg, Right
Ilium
use Bone, Pelvic, Left
use Bone, Pelvic, Right
Ilizarov external fixator
use External Fixation Device, Ring in 0PH
use External Fixation Device, Ring in 0PS
use External Fixation Device, Ring in 0QH
use External Fixation Device, Ring in 0QS
Ilizarov-Vecklich device
use External Fixation Device, Limb Lengthening in 0QH
use External Fixation Device, Limb Lengthening in 0PH
Imaging, diagnostic
see Computerized Tomography (CT Scan)
see Fluoroscopy
see Magnetic Resonance Imaging (MRI)
see Plain Radiography
see Ultrasonography
Imdevimab (REGN10987) and Casirivimab (REGN10933)
use REGN-COV2 Monoclonal Antibody
IMFINZI®
use Durvalumab Antineoplastic
IMI/REL
use Imipenem-cilastatin-relebactam Anti-infective
Imipenem-cilastatin-relebactam Anti-infective XW0
Immobilization
Abdominal Wall 2W33X
Arm
Lower
Left 2W3DX
Right 2W3CX
Upper
Left 2W3BX
Right 2W3AX
Back 2W35X
Chest Wall 2W34X
Extremity
Lower
Left 2W3MX
Right 2W3LX
Upper
Left 2W39X
Right 2W38X
Face 2W31X
Finger
Left 2W3KX
Right 2W3JX
Foot
Left 2W3TX
Right 2W3SX
Hand
Left 2W3FX
Right 2W3EX
Head 2W30X

Immobilization *(continued)*
Inguinal Region
Left 2W37X
Right 2W36X
Leg
Lower
Left 2W3RX
Right 2W3QX
Upper
Left 2W3PX
Right 2W3NX
Neck 2W32X
Thumb
Left 2W3H
Right 2W3GX
Toe
Left 2W3VX
Right 2W3UX
Immunization
see Introduction of Serum, Toxoid, and Vaccine
Immunoglobulin
use Globulin
Immunotherapy
see Introduction of Immunotherapeutic Substance
Immunotherapy, antineoplastic
Interferon
see Introduction of Low-dose Interleukin-2
Interleukin-2, high-dose
see Introduction of High-dose Interleukin-2
Interleukin-2, low-dose
see Introduction of Low-dose Interleukin-2
Monoclonal antibody
see Introduction of Monoclonal Antibody
Proleukin, high-dose
see Introduction of High-dose Interleukin-2
Proleukin, low-dose
see Introduction of Low-dose Interleukin-2
Impella® heart pump
use Short-term External Heart Assist System in Heart and Great Vessels
Impeller Pump
Continuous, Output 5A0221D
Intermittent, Output 5A0211D
Implantable cardioverter-defibrillator (ICD)
use Defibrillator Generator in 0JH
Implantable drug infusion pump (anti-spasmodic)(chemotherapy)(pain)
use Infusion Device, Pump in Subcutaneous Tissue and Fascia
Implantable glucose monitoring device
use Monitoring Device
Implantable hemodynamic monitor (IHM)
use Monitoring Device, Hemodynamic in 0JH
Implantable hemodynamic monitoring system (IHMS)
use Monitoring Device, Hemodynamic in 0JH
Implantable Miniature Telescope™ (IMT)
use Synthetic Substitute, Intraocular Telescope in 08R
Implantation
see Insertion
see Replacement
Implanted (venous)(access) port
use Vascular Access Device, Totally Implantable in Subcutaneous Tissue and Fascia
IMV (intermittent mandatory ventilation)
see Assistance, Respiratory 5A09
In Vitro Fertilization 8E0ZXY1
Incision, abscess
see Drainage
Incudectomy
see Excision, Ear, Nose, Sinus 09B
see Resection, Ear, Nose, Sinus 09T
Incudopexy
see Reposition, Ear, Nose, Sinus 09S
see Repair, Ear, Nose, Sinus 09Q
Incus
use Auditory Ossicle, Left
use Auditory Ossicle, Right
Induction of labor
Artificial rupture of membranes
see Drainage, Pregnancy 109
Oxytocin
see Introduction of Hormone
InDura, intrathecal catheter (1P) (spinal)
use Infusion Device
Inferior cardiac nerve
use Nerve, Thoracic Sympathetic
Inferior cerebellar vein
use Vein, Intracranial
Inferior cerebral vein
use Vein, Intracranial
Inferior epigastric artery
use Artery, External Iliac, Left
use Artery, External Iliac, Right
Inferior epigastric lymph node
use Lymphatic, Pelvis
Inferior genicular artery
use Artery, Popliteal, Left
use Artery, Popliteal, Right
Inferior gluteal artery
use Artery, Internal Iliac, Left
use Artery, Internal Iliac, Right
Inferior gluteal nerve
use Nerve, Sacral Plexus
Inferior hypogastric plexus
use Nerve, Abdominal Sympathetic
Inferior labial artery
use Artery, Face
Inferior longitudinal muscle
use Muscle, Tongue, Palate, Pharynx
Inferior mesenteric ganglion
use Nerve, Abdominal Sympathetic
Inferior mesenteric lymph node
use Lymphatic, Mesenteric
Inferior mesenteric plexus
use Nerve, Abdominal Sympathetic
Inferior oblique muscle
use Muscle, Extraocular, Left
use Muscle, Extraocular, Right
Inferior pancreaticoduodenal artery
use Artery, Superior Mesenteric
Inferior phrenic artery
use Aorta, Abdominal
Inferior rectus muscle
use Muscle, Extraocular, Left
use Muscle, Extraocular, Right
Inferior suprarenal artery
use Artery, Renal, Left
use Artery, Renal, Right
Inferior tarsal plate
use Eyelid, Lower, Left
use Eyelid, Lower, Right
Inferior thyroid vein
use Vein, Innominate, Left
use Vein, Innominate, Right
Inferior tibiofibular joint
use Joint, Ankle, Left
use Joint, Ankle, Right
Inferior turbinate
use Turbinate, Nasal
Inferior ulnar collateral artery
use Artery, Brachial, Left
use Artery, Brachial, Right
Inferior vesical artery
use Artery, Internal Iliac, Left
use Artery, Internal Iliac, Right
Infraauricular lymph node
use Lymphatic, Head
Infraclavicular (deltopectoral) lymph node
use Lymphatic, Upper Extremity, Left
use Lymphatic, Upper Extremity, Right
Infrahyoid muscle
use Muscle, Neck, Left
use Muscle, Neck, Right
Infraparotid lymph node
use Lymphatic, Head
Infraspinatus fascia
use Subcutaneous Tissue and Fascia, Upper Arm, Left
use Subcutaneous Tissue and Fascia, Upper Arm, Right
Infraspinatus muscle
use Muscle, Shoulder, Left
use Muscle, Shoulder, Right
Infundibulopelvic ligament
use Uterine Supporting Structure
Infusion
see Introduction of substance in or on
Infusion Device, Pump
Insertion of device in
Abdomen 0JH8
Back 0JH7
Chest 0JH6
Lower Arm
Left 0JHH
Right 0JHG
Lower Leg
Left 0JHP
Right 0JHN
Trunk 0JHT
Upper Arm
Left 0JHF
Right 0JHD
Upper Leg
Left 0JHM
Right 0JHL
Removal of device from
Lower Extremity 0JPW
Trunk 0JPT
Upper Extremity 0JPV
Revision of device in
Lower Extremity 0JWW
Trunk 0JWT
Upper Extremity 0JWV
Infusion, glucarpidase
Central vein 3E043GQ
Peripheral vein 3E033GQ
Inguinal canal
use Inguinal Region, Bilateral
use Inguinal Region, Left
use Inguinal Region, Right
Inguinal triangle
use Inguinal Region, Bilateral
use Inguinal Region, Left
use Inguinal Region, Right
Injection
see Introduction of substance in or on
Injection, Concentrated Bone Marrow Aspirate (CBMA), intramuscular XK02303
Injection reservoir, port
use Vascular Access Device, Totally Implantable in Subcutaneous Tissue and Fascia
Injection reservoir, pump
use Infusion Device, Pump in Subcutaneous Tissue and Fascia
Insemination, artificial 3E0P7LZ
Insertion
Antimicrobial envelope
see Introduction of Anti-infective
Aqueous drainage shunt
see Bypass, Eye 081
see Drainage, Eye 089
Products of Conception 10H0
Spinal Stabilization Device
see Insertion of device in, Upper Joints 0RH
see Insertion of device in, Lower Joints 0SH
Insertion of device in
Abdominal Wall 0WHF
Acetabulum
Left 0QH5
Right 0QH4
Anal Sphincter 0DHR
Ankle Region
Left 0YHL
Right 0YHK
Anus 0DHQ
Aorta
Abdominal 04H0
Thoracic
Ascending/Arch 02HX
Descending 02HW
Arm
Lower
Left 0XHF
Right 0XHD
Upper
Left 0XH9
Right 0XH8
Artery
Anterior Tibial
Left 04HQ
Right 04HP
Axillary
Left 03H6
Right 03H5
Brachial
Left 03H8
Right 03H7
Celiac 04H1
Colic
Left 04H7
Middle 04H8
Right 04H6
Common Carotid
Left 03HJ
Right 03HH
Common Iliac
Left 04HD
Right 04HC
Coronary
Four or More Arteries 02H3
One Artery 02H0
Three Arteries 02H2
Two Arteries 02H1
External Carotid
Left 03HN
Right 03HM
External Iliac
Left 04HJ
Right 04HH
Face 03HR
Femoral
Left 04HL
Right 04HK
Foot
Left 04HW
Right 04HV
Gastric 04H2
Hand
Left 03HF
Right 03HD
Hepatic 04H3

Insertion of device in *(continued)*

- Artery *(continued)*
  - Inferior Mesenteric 04HB
  - Innominate 03H2
  - Internal Carotid
    - Left 03HL
    - Right 03HK
  - Internal Iliac
    - Left 04HF
    - Right 04HE
  - Internal Mammary
    - Left 03H1
    - Right 03H0
  - Intracranial 03HG
  - Lower 04HY
  - Peroneal
    - Left 04HU
    - Right 04HT
  - Popliteal
    - Left 04HN
    - Right 04HM
  - Posterior Tibial
    - Left 04HS
    - Right 04HR
  - Pulmonary
    - Left 02HR
    - Right 02HQ
  - Pulmonary Trunk 02HP
  - Radial
    - Left 03HC
    - Right 03HB
  - Renal
    - Left 04HA
    - Right 04H9
  - Splenic 04H4
  - Subclavian
    - Left 03H4
    - Right 03H3
  - Superior Mesenteric 04H5
  - Temporal
    - Left 03HT
    - Right 03HS
  - Thyroid
    - Left 03HV
    - Right 03HU
  - Ulnar
    - Left 03HA
    - Right 03H9
  - Upper 03HY
  - Vertebral
    - Left 03HQ
    - Right 03HP
- Atrium
  - Left 02H7
  - Right 02H6
- Axilla
  - Left 0XH5
  - Right 0XH4
- Back
  - Lower 0WHL
  - Upper 0WHK
- Bladder 0THB
- Bladder Neck 0THC
- Bone
  - Ethmoid
    - Left 0NHG
    - Right 0NHF
  - Facial 0NHW
  - Frontal 0NH1
  - Hyoid 0NHX
  - Lacrimal
    - Left 0NHJ
    - Right 0NHH
  - Lower 0QHY
  - Nasal 0NHB
  - Occipital 0NH7
  - Palatine
    - Left 0NHL
    - Right 0NHK
  - Parietal
    - Left 0NH4

Insertion of device in *(continued)*

- Bone *(continued)*
  - Parietal *(continued)*
    - Right 0NH3
  - Pelvic
    - Left 0QH3
    - Right 0QH2
  - Sphenoid 0NHC
  - Temporal
    - Left 0NH6
    - Right 0NH5
  - Upper 0PHY
  - Zygomatic
    - Left 0NHN
    - Right 0NHM
- Bone Marrow 07HT
- Brain 00H0
- Breast
  - Bilateral 0HHV
  - Left 0HHU
  - Right 0HHT
- Bronchus
  - Lingula 0BH9
  - Lower Lobe
    - Left 0BHB
    - Right 0BH6
  - Main
    - Left 0BH7
    - Right 0BH3
  - Middle Lobe, Right 0BH5
  - Upper Lobe
    - Left 0BH8
    - Right 0BH4
- Bursa and Ligament
  - Lower 0MHY
  - Upper 0MHX
- Buttock
  - Left 0YH1
  - Right 0YH0
- Carpal
  - Left 0PHN
  - Right 0PHM
- Cavity, Cranial 0WH1
- Cerebral Ventricle 00H6
- Cervix 0UHC
- Chest Wall 0WH8
- Cisterna Chyli 07HL
- Clavicle
  - Left 0PHB
  - Right 0PH9
- Coccyx 0QHS
- Cul-de-sac 0UHF
- Diaphragm 0BHT
- Disc
  - Cervical Vertebral 0RH3
  - Cervicothoracic Vertebral 0RH5
  - Lumbar Vertebral 0SH2
  - Lumbosacral 0SH4
  - Thoracic Vertebral 0RH9
  - Thoracolumbar Vertebral 0RHB
- Duct
  - Hepatobiliary 0FHB
  - Pancreatic 0FHD
- Duodenum 0DH9
- Ear
  - Inner
    - Left 09HE
    - Right 09HD
  - Left 09HJ
  - Right 09HH
- Elbow Region
  - Left 0XHC
  - Right 0XHB
- Epididymis and Spermatic Cord 0VHM
- Esophagus 0DH5
- Extremity
  - Lower
    - Left 0YHB
    - Right 0YH9

Insertion of device in *(continued)*

- Extremity *(continued)*
  - Upper
    - Left 0XH7
    - Right 0XH6
- Eye
  - Left 08H1
  - Right 08H0
- Face 0WH2
- Fallopian Tube 0UH8
- Femoral Region
  - Left 0YH8
  - Right 0YH7
- Femoral Shaft
  - Left 0QH9
  - Right 0QH8
- Femur
  - Lower
    - Left 0QHC
    - Right 0QHB
  - Upper
    - Left 0QH7
    - Right 0QH6
- Fibula
  - Left 0QHK
  - Right 0QHJ
- Foot
  - Left 0YHN
  - Right 0YHM
- Gallbladder 0FH4
- Gastrointestinal Tract 0WHP
- Genitourinary Tract 0WHR
- Gland
  - Endocrine 0GHS
  - Salivary 0CHA
- Glenoid Cavity
  - Left 0PH8
  - Right 0PH7
- Hand
  - Left 0XHK
  - Right 0XHJ
- Head 0WH0
- Heart 02HA
- Humeral Head
  - Left 0PHD
  - Right 0PHC
- Humeral Shaft
  - Left 0PHG
  - Right 0PHF
- Ileum 0DHB
- Inguinal Region
  - Left 0YH6
  - Right 0YH5
- Intestinal Tract
  - Lower 0DHD
  - Upper 0DH0
- Intestine
  - Large 0DHE
  - Small 0DH8
- Jaw
  - Lower 0WH5
  - Upper 0WH4
- Jejunum 0DHA
- Joint
  - Acromioclavicular
    - Left 0RHH
    - Right 0RHG
  - Ankle
    - Left 0SHG
    - Right 0SHF
  - Carpal
    - Left 0RHR
    - Right 0RHQ
  - Carpometacarpal
    - Left 0RHT
    - Right 0RHS
  - Cervical Vertebral 0RH1
  - Cervicothoracic Vertebral 0RH4
  - Coccygeal 0SH6

Insertion of device in *(continued)*

- Joint *(continued)*
  - Elbow
    - Left 0RHM
    - Right 0RHL
  - Finger Phalangeal
    - Left 0RHX
    - Right 0RHW
  - Hip
    - Left 0SHB
    - Right 0SH9
  - Knee
    - Left 0SHD
    - Right 0SHC
  - Lumbar Vertebral 0SH0
  - Lumbosacral 0SH3
  - Metacarpophalangeal
    - Left 0RHV
    - Right 0RHU
  - Metatarsal-Phalangeal
    - Left 0SHN
    - Right 0SHM
  - Occipital-cervical 0RH0
  - Sacrococcygeal 0SH5
  - Sacroiliac
    - Left 0SH8
    - Right 0SH7
  - Shoulder
    - Left 0RHK
    - Right 0RHJ
  - Sternoclavicular
    - Left 0RHF
    - Right 0RHE
  - Tarsal
    - Left 0SHJ
    - Right 0SHH
  - Tarsometatarsal
    - Left 0SHL
    - Right 0SHK
  - Temporomandibular
    - Left 0RHD
    - Right 0RHC
  - Thoracic Vertebral 0RH6
  - Thoracolumbar Vertebral
  - Toe Phalangeal
    - Left 0SHQ
    - Right 0SHP
  - Wrist
    - Left 0RHP
    - Right 0RHN
- Kidney 0TH5
- Knee Region
  - Left 0YHG
  - Right 0YHF
- Larynx 0CHS
- Leg
  - Lower
    - Left 0YHJ
    - Right 0YHH
  - Upper
    - Left 0YHD
    - Right 0YHC
- Liver 0FH0
  - Left Lobe 0FH2
  - Right Lobe 0FH1
- Lung
  - Left 0BHL
  - Right 0BHK
- Lymphatic 07HN3
  - Thoracic Duct 07HK
- Mandible
  - Left 0NHV
  - Right 0NHT
- Maxilla 0NHR
- Mediastinum 0WHC
- Metacarpal
  - Left 0PHQ
  - Right 0PHP
- Metatarsal
  - Left 0QHP
  - Right 0QHN

Insertion of device in *(continued)*
- Mouth and Throat 0CHY
- Muscle
  - Lower 0KHY
  - Upper 0KHX
- Nasal Mucosa and Soft Tissue 09HK
- Nasopharynx 09HN
- Neck 0WH6
- Nerve
  - Cranial 00HE
  - Peripheral 01HY
- Nipple
  - Left 0HHX
  - Right 0HHW
- Oral Cavity and Throat 0WH3
- Orbit
  - Left 0NHQ
  - Right 0NHP
- Ovary 0UH3
- Pancreas 0FHG
- Patella
  - Left 0QHF
  - Right 0QHD
- Pelvic Cavity 0WHJ
- Penis 0VHS
- Pericardial Cavity 0WHD
- Pericardium 02HN
- Perineum
  - Female 0WHN
  - Male 0WHM
- Peritoneal Cavity 0WHG
- Phalanx
  - Finger
    - Left 0PHV
    - Right 0PHT
  - Thumb
    - Left 0PHS
    - Right 0PHR
  - Toe
    - Left 0QHR
    - Right 0QHQ
- Pleura 0BHQ
- Pleural Cavity
  - Left 0WHB
  - Right 0WH9
- Prostate 0VH0
- Prostate and Seminal Vesicles 0VH4
- Radius
  - Left 0PHJ
  - Right 0PHH
- Rectum 0DHP
- Respiratory Tract 0WHQ
- Retroperitoneum 0WHH
- Ribs
  - 1 to 2 0PH1
  - 3 or More 0PH2
- Sacrum 0QH1
- Scapula
  - Left 0PH6
  - Right 0PH5
- Scrotum and Tunica Vaginalis 0VH8
- Shoulder Region
  - Left 0XH3
  - Right 0XH2
- Sinus 09HY
- Skin 0HHPXYZ
- Skull 0NH0
- Spinal Canal 00HU
- Spinal Cord 00HV
- Spleen 07HP
- Sternum 0PH0
- Stomach 0DH6
- Subcutaneous Tissue and Fascia
  - Abdomen 0JH8
  - Back 0JH7
  - Buttock 0JH9
  - Chest 0JH6

Insertion of device in *(continued)*
- Subcutaneous Tissue and Fascia *(continued)*
  - Face 0JH1
  - Foot
    - Left 0JHR
    - Right 0JHQ
  - Hand
    - Left 0JHK
    - Right 0JHJ
  - Head and Neck 0JHS
  - Lower Arm
    - Left 0JHH
    - Right 0JHG
  - Lower Extremity 0JHW
  - Lower Leg
    - Left 0JHP
    - Right 0JHN
  - Neck
    - Left 0JH5
    - Right 0JH4
  - Pelvic Region 0JHC
  - Perineum 0JHB
  - Scalp 0JH0
  - Trunk 0JHT
  - Upper Arm
    - Left 0JHF
    - Right 0JHD
  - Upper Extremity 0JHV
  - Upper Leg
    - Left 0JHM
    - Right 0JHL
- Tarsal
  - Left 0QHM
  - Right 0QHL
- Tendon
  - Lower 0LHY
  - Upper 0LHX
- Testis 0VHD
- Thymus 07HM
- Tibia
  - Left 0QHH
  - Right 0QHG
- Tongue 0CH7
- Trachea 0BH1
- Tracheobronchial Tree 0BH0
- Ulna
  - Left 0PHL
  - Right 0PHK
- Ureter 0TH9
- Urethra 0THD
- Uterus 0UH9
- Uterus and Cervix 0UHD
- Vagina 0UHG
- Vagina and Cul-de-sac 0UHH
- Vas Deferens 0VHR
- Vein
  - Axillary
    - Left 05H8
    - Right 05H7
  - Azygos 05H0
  - Basilic
    - Left 05HC
    - Right 05HB
  - Brachial
    - Left 05HA
    - Right 05H9
  - Cephalic
    - Left 05HF
    - Right 05HD
  - Colic 06H7
  - Common Iliac
    - Left 06HD
    - Right 06HC
  - Coronary 02H4
  - Esophageal 06H3
  - External Iliac
    - Left 06HG
    - Right 06HF
  - External Jugular
    - Left 05HQ

Insertion of device in *(continued)*
- Vein *(continued)*
  - External Jugular *(continued)*
    - Right 05HP
  - Face
    - Left 05HV
    - Right 05HT
  - Femoral
    - Left 06HN
    - Right 06HM
  - Foot
    - Left 06HV
    - Right 06HT
  - Gastric 06H2
  - Hand
    - Left 05HH
    - Right 05HG
  - Hemiazygos 05H1
  - Hepatic 06H4
  - Hypogastric
    - Left 06HJ
    - Right 06HH
  - Inferior Mesenteric 06H6
  - Innominate
    - Left 05H4
    - Right 05H3
  - Internal Jugular
    - Left 05HN
    - Right 05HM
  - Intracranial 05HL
  - Lower 06HY
  - Portal 06H8
  - Pulmonary
    - Left 02HT
    - Right 02HS
  - Renal
    - Left 06HB
    - Right 06H9
  - Saphenous
    - Left 06HQ
    - Right 06HP
  - Splenic 06H1
  - Subclavian
    - Left 05H6
    - Right 05H5
  - Superior Mesenteric 06H5
  - Upper 05HY
  - Vertebral
    - Left 05HS
    - Right 05HR
- Vena Cava
  - Inferior 06H0
  - Superior 02HV
- Ventricle
  - Left 02HL
  - Right 02HK
- Vertebra
  - Cervical 0PH3
  - Lumbar 0QH0
  - Thoracic 0PH4
- Wrist Region
  - Left 0XHH
  - Right 0XHG

Inspection
- Abdominal Wall 0WJF
- Ankle Region
  - Left 0YJL
  - Right 0YJK
- Arm
  - Lower
    - Left 0XJF
    - Right 0XJD
  - Upper
    - Left 0XJ9
    - Right 0XJ8
- Artery
  - Lower 04JY
  - Upper 03JY
- Axilla
  - Left 0XJ5
  - Right 0XJ4

Inspection *(continued)*
- Back
  - Lower 0WJL
  - Upper 0WJK
- Bladder 0TJB
- Bone
  - Facial 0NJW
  - Lower 0QJY
  - Nasal 0NJB
  - Upper 0PJY
- Bone Marrow 07JT
- Brain 00J0
- Breast
  - Left 0HJU
  - Right 0HJT
- Bursa and Ligament
  - Lower 0MJY
  - Upper 0MJX
- Buttock
  - Left 0YJ1
  - Right 0YJ0
- Cavity, Cranial 0WJ1
- Chest Wall 0WJ8
- Cisterna Chyli 07JL
- Diaphragm 0BJT
- Disc
  - Cervical Vertebral 0RJ3
  - Cervicothoracic Vertebral 0RJ5
  - Lumbar Vertebral 0SJ2
  - Lumbosacral 0SJ4
  - Thoracic Vertebral 0RJ9
  - Thoracolumbar Vertebral 0RJB
- Duct
  - Hepatobiliary 0FJB
  - Pancreatic 0FJD
- Ear
  - Inner
    - Left 09JE
    - Right 09JD
  - Left 09JJ
  - Right 09JH
- Elbow Region
  - Left 0XJC
  - Right 0XJB
- Epididymis and Spermatic Cord 0VJM
- Extremity
  - Lower
    - Left 0YJB
    - Right 0YJ9
  - Upper
    - Left 0XJ7
    - Right 0XJ6
- Eye
  - Left 08J1XZZ
  - Right 08J0XZZ
- Face 0WJ2
- Fallopian Tube 0UJ8
- Femoral Region
  - Bilateral 0YJE
  - Left 0YJ8
  - Right 0YJ7
- Finger Nail 0HJQXZZ
- Foot
  - Left 0YJN
  - Right 0YJM
- Gallbladder 0FJ4
- Gastrointestinal Tract 0WJP
- Genitourinary Tract 0WJR
- Gland
  - Adrenal 0GJ5
  - Endocrine 0GJS
  - Pituitary 0GJ0
  - Salivary 0CJA
- Great Vessel 02JY
- Hand
  - Left 0XJK
  - Right 0XJJ
- Head 0WJ0
- Heart 02JA

Inspection *(continued)*
Inguinal Region
Bilateral 0YJA
Left 0YJ6
Right 0YJ5
Intestinal Tract
Lower 0DJD
Upper 0DJ0
Jaw
Lower 0WJ5
Upper 0WJ4
Joint
Acromioclavicular
Left 0RJH
Right 0RJG
Ankle
Left 0SJG
Right 0SJF
Carpal
Left 0RJR
Right 0RJQ
Carpometacarpal
Left 0RJT
Right 0RJS
Cervical Vertebral 0RJ1
Cervicothoracic Vertebral 0RJ4
Coccygeal 0SJ6
Elbow
Left 0RJM
Right 0RJL
Finger Phalangeal
Left 0RJX
Right 0RJW
Hip
Left 0SJB
Right 0SJ9
Knee
Left 0SJD
Right 0SJC
Lumbar Vertebral 0SJ0
Lumbosacral 0SJ3
Metacarpophalangeal
Left 0RJV
Right 0RJU
Metatarsal-Phalangeal
Left 0SJN
Right 0SJM
Occipital-cervical 0RJ0
Sacrococcygeal 0SJ5
Sacroiliac
Left 0SJ8
Right 0SJ7
Shoulder
Left 0RJK
Right 0RJJ
Sternoclavicular
Left 0RJF
Right 0RJE
Tarsal
Left 0SJJ
Right 0SJH
Tarsometatarsal
Left 0SJL
Right 0SJK
Temporomandibular
Left 0RJD
Right 0RJC
Thoracic Vertebral 0RJ6
Thoracolumbar Vertebral 0RJA
Toe Phalangeal
Left 0SJQ
Right 0SJP
Wrist
Left 0RJP
Right 0RJN
Kidney 0TJ5
Knee Region
Left 0YJG
Right 0YJF
Larynx 0CJS

Inspection *(continued)*
Leg
Lower
Left 0YJJ
Right 0YJH
Upper
Left 0YJD
Right 0YJC
Lens
Left 08JKXZZ
Right 08JJXZZ
Liver 0FJ0
Lung
Left 0BJL
Right 0BJK
Lymphatic 07JN
Thoracic Duct 07JK
Mediastinum 0WJC
Mesentery 0DJV
Mouth and Throat 0CJY
Muscle
Extraocular
Left 08JM
Right 08JL
Lower 0KJY
Upper 0KJX
Nasal Mucosa and Soft Tissue 09JK
Neck 0WJ6
Nerve
Cranial 00JE
Peripheral 01JY
Omentum 0DJU
Oral Cavity and Throat 0WJ3
Ovary 0UJ3
Pancreas 0FJG
Parathyroid Gland 0GJR
Pelvic Cavity 0WJJ
Penis 0VJS
Pericardial Cavity 0WJD
Perineum
Female 0WJN
Male 0WJM
Peritoneal Cavity 0WJG
Peritoneum 0DJW
Pineal Body 0GJ1
Pleura 0BJQ
Pleural Cavity
Left 0WJB
Right 0WJ9
Products of Conception 10J0
Ectopic 10J2
Retained 10J1
Prostate and Seminal Vesicles 0VJ4
Respiratory Tract 0WJQ
Retroperitoneum 0WJH
Scrotum and Tunica Vaginalis 0VJ8
Shoulder Region
Left 0XJ3
Right 0XJ2
Sinus 09JY
Skin 0HJPXZZ
Skull 0NJ0
Spinal Canal 00JU
Spinal Cord 00JV
Spleen 07JP
Stomach 0DJ6
Subcutaneous Tissue and Fascia
Head and Neck 0JJS
Lower Extremity 0JJW
Trunk 0JJT
Upper Extremity 0JJV
Tendon
Lower 0LJY
Upper 0LJX
Testis 0VJD
Thymus 07JM
Thyroid Gland 0GJK
Toe Nail 0HJRX
Trachea 0BJ1

Inspection *(continued)*
Tracheobronchial Tree 0BJ0
Tympanic Membrane
Left 09J8
Right 09J7
Ureter 0TJ9
Urethra 0TJD
Uterus and Cervix 0UJD
Vagina and Cul-de-sac 0UJH
Vas Deferens 0VJR
Vein
Lower 06JY
Upper 05JY
Vulva 0UJM
Wrist Region
Left 0XJH
Right 0XJG
Instillation
see Introduction of substance in or on
Insufflation
see Introduction of substance in or on
Interatrial septum
use Septum, Atrial
InterAtrial Shunt Device IASD®, Corvia
use Synthetic Substitute
Interbody fusion (spine) cage
use Interbody Fusion Device in Lower Joints
use Interbody Fusion Device in Upper Joints
Interbody Fusion Device
Customizable
Lumbar Vertebral XRGB
2 or more XRGC
Lumbosacral XRGD
Thoracolumbar Vertebral XRGA
Nanotextured Surface
Cervical Vertebral XRG1092
2 or more XRG2092
Cervicothoracic Vertebral XRG4092
Lumbar Vertebral XRGB092
2 or more XRGC092
Lumbosacral XRGD092
Occipital-cervical XRG0092
Thoracic Vertebral XRG6092
2 to 7 XRG7092
8 or more XRG8092
Thoracolumbar Vertebral XRGA092
Radiolucent Porous
Cervical Vertebral XRG10F3
2 or more XRG20F3
Cervicothoracic Vertebral XRG40F3
Lumbar Vertebral XRGB0F3
2 or more XRGC0F3
Lumbosacral XRGD0F3
Occipital-cervical XRG00F3
Thoracic Vertebral XRG60F3
2 to 7 XRG70F3
8 or more XRG80F3
Thoracolumbar Vertebral XRGA0F3
Intercarpal joint
use Joint, Carpal, Left
use Joint, Carpal, Right
Intercarpal ligament
use Bursa and Ligament, Hand, Left
use Bursa and Ligament, Hand, Right
INTERCEPT Blood System for Plasma Pathogen Reduced Cryoprecipitated Fibrinogen Complex
use Pathogen Reduced Cryoprecipitated Fibrinogen Complex

INTERCEPT Fibrinogen Complex
use Pathogen Reduced Cryoprecipitated Fibrinogen Complex
Interclavicular ligament
use Bursa and Ligament, Shoulder, Left
use Bursa and Ligament, Shoulder, Right
Intercostal lymph node
use Lymphatic, Thorax
Intercostal muscle
use Muscle, Thorax, Left
use Muscle, Thorax, Right
Intercostal nerve
use Nerve, Thoracic
Intercostobrachial nerve
use Nerve, Thoracic
Intercuneiform joint
use Joint, Tarsal, Left
use Joint, Tarsal, Right
Intercuneiform ligament
use Bursa and Ligament, Foot, Left
use Bursa and Ligament, Foot, Right
Intermediate bronchus
use Main Bronchus, Right
Intermediate cuneiform bone
use Tarsal, Left
use Tarsal, Right
Intermittent hemodialysis (IHD) 5A1D70Z
Intermittent mandatory ventilation
see Assistance, Respiratory 5A09
Intermittent Negative Airway Pressure
24-96 Consecutive Hours, Ventilation 5A0945B
Greater than 96 Consecutive Hours, Ventilation 5A0955B
Less than 24 Consecutive Hours, Ventilation 5A0935B
Intermittent Positive Airway Pressure
24-96 Consecutive Hours, Ventilation 5A09458
Greater than 96 Consecutive Hours, Ventilation 5A09558
Less than 24 Consecutive Hours, Ventilation 5A09358
Intermittent positive pressure breathing
see Assistance, Respiratory 5A09
Internal anal sphincter
use Anal Sphincter
Internal (basal) cerebral vein
use Vein, Intracranial
Internal carotid artery, intracranial portion
use Intracranial Artery
Internal carotid plexus
use Nerve, Head and Neck Sympathetic
Internal iliac vein
use Vein, Hypogastric, Left
use Vein, Hypogastric, Right
Internal maxillary artery
use Artery, External Carotid, Left
use Artery, External Carotid, Right
Internal naris
use Nasal Mucosa and Soft Tissue
Internal oblique muscle
use Muscle, Abdomen, Left
use Muscle, Abdomen, Right
Internal pudendal artery
use Artery, Internal Iliac, Left
use Artery, Internal Iliac, Right
Internal pudendal vein
use Vein, Hypogastric, Left
use Vein, Hypogastric, Right

Internal thoracic artery
use Artery, Internal Mammary, Left
use Artery, Internal Mammary, Right
use Artery, Subclavian, Left
use Artery, Subclavian, Right
Internal urethral sphincter
use Urethra
Interphalangeal (IP) joint
use Joint, Finger Phalangeal, Left
use Joint, Finger Phalangeal, Right
use Joint, Toe Phalangeal, Left
use Joint, Toe Phalangeal, Right
Interphalangeal ligament
use Bursa and Ligament, Foot, Left
use Bursa and Ligament, Foot, Right
use Bursa and Ligament, Hand, Left
use Bursa and Ligament, Hand, Right
Interrogation, cardiac rhythm related device
Interrogation only
see Measurement, Cardiac 4B02
With cardiac function testing
see Measurement, Cardiac 4A02
Interruption
see Occlusion
Interspinalis muscle
use Muscle, Trunk, Left
use Muscle, Trunk, Right
Interspinous ligament, cervical
use Head and Neck Bursa and Ligament
Interspinous ligament, lumbar
use Lower Spine Bursa and Ligament
Interspinous ligament, thoracic
use Upper Spine Bursa and Ligament
Interspinous process spinal stabilization device
use Spinal Stabilization Device, Interspinous Process in 0RH
use Spinal Stabilization Device, Interspinous Process in 0SH
InterStim® Therapy lead
use Neurostimulator Lead in Peripheral Nervous System
InterStim® II Therapy neurostimulator
use Stimulator Generator, Single Array in 0JH
InterStim™ Micro Therapy neurostimulator
use Stimulator Generator, Single Array Rechargeable in 0JH
Intertransversarius muscle
use Muscle, Trunk, Left
use Muscle, Trunk, Right
Intertransverse ligament, cervical
use Head and Neck Bursa and Ligament
Intertransverse ligament, lumbar
use Lower Spine Bursa and Ligament
Intertransverse ligament, thoracic
use Upper Spine Bursa and Ligament
Interventricular foramen (Monro)
use Cerebral Ventricle
Interventricular septum
use Septum, Ventricular
Intestinal lymphatic trunk
use Cisterna Chyli
Intracranial Arterial Flow, Whole Blood mRNA XXE5XT7
Intraluminal Device
Airway
Esophagus 0DH5
Mouth and Throat 0CHY
Intraluminal Device *(continued)*
Airway *(continued)*
Nasopharynx 09HN
Bioactive
Occlusion
Common Carotid
Left 03LJ
Right 03LH
External Carotid
Left 03LN
Right 03LM
Internal Carotid
Left 03LL
Right 03LK
Intracranial 03LG
Vertebral
Left 03LQ
Right 03LP
Restriction
Common Carotid
Left 03VJ
Right 03VH
External Carotid
Left 03VN
Right 03VM
Internal Carotid
Left 03VL
Right 03VK
Intracranial 03VG
Vertebral
Left 03VQ
Right 03VP
Endobronchial Valve
Lingula 0BH9
Lower Lobe
Left 0BHB
Right 0BH6
Main
Left 0BH7
Right 0BH3
Middle Lobe, Right 0BH5
Upper Lobe
Left 0BH8
Right 0BH4
Endotracheal Airway
Change device in, Trachea 0B21XEZ
Insertion of device in, Trachea 0BH1
Pessary
Change device in, Vagina and Cul-de-sac 0U2HXGZ
Insertion of device in
Cul-de-sac 0UHF
Vagina 0UHG
Intramedullary (IM) rod (nail)
use Internal Fixation Device, Intramedullary in Lower Bones
use Internal Fixation Device, Intramedullary in Upper Bones
Intramedullary skeletal kinetic distractor (ISKD)
use Internal Fixation Device, Intramedullary in Lower Bones
use Internal Fixation Device, Intramedullary in Upper Bones
Intraocular Telescope
Left 08RK30Z
Right 08RJ30Z
Intra.OX 8E02XDZ
Intraoperative Radiation Therapy (IORT)
Anus DDY8CZZ
Bile Ducts DFY2CZZ
Bladder DTY2CZZ
Brain D0Y0CZZ
Brain Stem D0Y1CZZ
Cervix DUY1CZZ
Colon DDY5CZZ
Duodenum DDY2CZZ
Intraoperative Radiation Therapy (IORT) *(continued)*
Gallbladder DFY1CZZ
Ileum DDY4CZZ
Jejunum DDY3CZZ
Kidney DTY0CZZ
Larynx D9YBCZZ
Liver DFY0CZZ
Mouth D9Y4CZZ
Nasopharynx D9YDCZZ
Nerve, Peripheral D0Y7CZZ
Ovary DUY0CZZ
Pancreas DFY3CZZ
Pharynx D9YCCZZ
Prostate DVY0CZZ
Rectum DDY7CZZ
Spinal Cord D0Y6CZZ
Stomach DDY1CZZ
Ureter DTY1CZZ
Urethra DTY3CZZ
Uterus DUY2CZZ
Intrauterine device (IUD)
use Contraceptive Device in Female Reproductive System
Intravascular fluorescence angiography (IFA)
see Monitoring, Physiological Systems 4A1
Intravascular Lithotripsy (IVL)
see Fragmentation
Intravascular ultrasound assisted thrombolysis
see Fragmentation, Artery
Introduction of substance in or on
Artery
Central 3E06
Analgesics 3E06
Anesthetic, Intracirculatory 3E06
Anti-infective 3E06
Anti-inflammatory 3E06
Antiarrhythmic 3E06
Antineoplastic 3E06
Destructive Agent 3E06
Diagnostic Substance, Other 3E06
Electrolytic Substance 3E06
Hormone 3E06
Hypnotics 3E06
Immunotherapeutic 3E06
Nutritional Substance 3E06
Platelet Inhibitor 3E06
Radioactive Substance 3E06
Sedatives 3E06
Serum 3E06
Thrombolytic 3E06
Toxoid 3E06
Vaccine 3E06
Vasopressor 3E06
Water Balance Substance 3E06
Coronary 3E07
Diagnostic Substance, Other 3E07
Platelet Inhibitor 3E07
Thrombolytic 3E07
Peripheral 3E05
Analgesics 3E05
Anesthetic, Intracirculatory 3E05
Anti-infective 3E052
Anti-inflammatory 3E05
Antiarrhythmic 3E05
Antineoplastic 3E05
Destructive Agent 3E05
Diagnostic Substance, Other 3E05
Introduction of substance in or on *(continued)*
Artery *(continued)*
Peripheral 3E05 *(continued)*
Electrolytic Substance 3E05
Hormone 3E05
Hypnotics 3E05
Immunotherapeutic 3E05
Nutritional Substance 3E05
Platelet Inhibitor 3E05
Radioactive Substance 3E05
Sedatives 3E05
Serum 3E05
Thrombolytic 3E05
Toxoid 3E05
Vaccine 3E05
Vasopressor 3E05
Water Balance Substance 3E05
Biliary Tract 3E0J
Analgesics 3E0J
Anesthetic, Agent 3E0J
Anti-infective 3E0J
Anti-inflammatory 3E0J
Antineoplastic 3E0J
Destructive Agent 3E0J
Diagnostic Substance, Other 3E0J
Electrolytic Substance 3E0J
Gas 3E0J
Hypnotics 3E0J
Islet Cells, Pancreatic 3E0J
Nutritional Substance 3E0J
Radioactive Substance 3E0J
Sedatives 3E0J
Water Balance Substance 3E0J
Bone 3E0V
Analgesics 3E0V3NZ
Anesthetic, Agent 3E0V3BZ
Anti-infective 3E0V32
Anti-inflammatory 3E0V33Z
Antineoplastic 3E0V30
Destructive Agent 3E0V3TZ
Diagnostic Substance, Other 3E0V3KZ
Electrolytic Substance 3E0V37Z
Hypnotics 3E0V3NZ
Nutritional Substance 3E0V36Z
Radioactive Substance 3E0V3HZ
Sedatives 3E0V3NZ
Water Balance Substance 3E0V37Z
Bone Marrow 3E0A3GC
Antineoplastic 3E0A30
Brain 3E0Q
Analgesics 3E0Q
Anesthetic, Agent 3E0Q
Anti-infective 3E0Q
Anti-inflammatory 3E0Q
Antineoplastic 3E0Q
Destructive Agent 3E0Q
Diagnostic Substance, Other 3E0Q
Electrolytic Substance 3E0Q
Gas 3E0Q
Hypnotics 3E0Q
Nutritional Substance 3E0Q
Radioactive Substance 3E0Q
Sedatives 3E0Q
Stem Cells
Embryonic 3E0Q
Somatic 3E0Q
Water Balance Substance 3E0Q
Cranial Cavity 3E0Q
Analgesics 3E0Q
Anesthetic Agent 3E0Q
Anti-infective 3E0Q

Introduction of substance in or on *(continued)*
- Cranial Cavity 3E0Q *(continued)*
  - Anti-inflammatory 3E0Q
  - Antineoplastic 3E0Q
  - Destructive Agent 3E0Q
  - Diagnostic Substance, Other 3E0Q
  - Electrolytic Substance 3E0Q
  - Gas 3E0Q
  - Hypnotics 3E0Q
  - Nutritional Substance 3E0Q
  - Radioactive Substance 3E0Q
  - Sedatives 3E0Q
  - Stem Cells
    - Embryonic 3E0Q
    - Somatic 3E0Q
  - Water Balance Substance 3E0Q
- Ear 3E0B
  - Analgesics 3E0B
  - Anesthetic Agentl 3E0B
  - Anti-infective 3E0B
  - Anti-inflammatory 3E0B
  - Antineoplastic 3E0B
  - Destructive Agent 3E0B
  - Diagnostic Substance, Other 3E0B
  - Hypnotics 3E0B
  - Radioactive Substance 3E0B
  - Sedatives 3E0B
- Epidural Space 3E0S3GC
  - Analgesics 3E0S3NZ
  - Anesthetic Agent 3E0S3BZ
  - Anti-infective 3E0S32
  - Anti-inflammatory 3E0S33Z
  - Antineoplastic 3E0S30
  - Destructive Agent 3E0S3TZ
  - Diagnostic Substance, Other 3E0S3KZ
  - Electrolytic Substance 3E0S37Z
  - Gas 3E0S
  - Hypnotics 3E0S3NZ
  - Nutritional Substance 3E0S36Z
  - Radioactive Substance 3E0S3HZ
  - Sedatives 3E0S3NZ
  - Water Balance Substance 3E0S37Z
- Eye 3E0C
  - Analgesics 3E0C
  - Anesthetic Agent 3E0C
  - Anti-infective 3E0C
  - Anti-inflammatory 3E0C
  - Antineoplastic 3E0C
  - Destructive Agent 3E0C
  - Diagnostic Substance, Other 3E0C
  - Gas 3E0C
  - Hypnotics 3E0C
  - Pigment 3E0C
  - Radioactive Substance 3E0C
  - Sedatives 3E0C
- Gastrointestinal Tract
  - Lower 3E0H
    - Analgesics 3E0H
    - Anesthetic Agent 3E0H
    - Anti-infective 3E0H
    - Anti-inflammatory 3E0H
    - Antineoplastic 3E0H
    - Destructive Agent 3E0H
    - Diagnostic Substance, Other 3E0H
    - Electrolytic Substance 3E0H
    - Gas 3E0H
    - Hypnotics 3E0H
    - Nutritional Substance 3E0H
    - Radioactive Substance 3E0H
    - Sedatives 3E0H
    - Water Balance Substance 3E0H

Introduction of substance in or on *(continued)*
- Gastrointestinal Tract *(continued)*
  - Upper 3E0G
    - Analgesics 3E0G
    - Anesthetic Agent 3E0G
    - Anti-infective 3E0G
    - Anti-inflammatory 3E0G
    - Antineoplastic 3E0G
    - Destructive Agent 3E0G
    - Diagnostic Substance, Other 3E0G
    - Electrolytic Substance 3E0G
    - Gas 3E0G
    - Hypnotics 3E0G
    - Nutritional Substance 3E0G
    - Radioactive Substance 3E0G
    - Sedatives 3E0G
    - Water Balance Substance 3E0G
- Genitourinary Tract 3E0K
  - Analgesics 3E0K
  - Anesthetic Agent 3E0K
  - Anti-infective 3E0K
  - Anti-inflammatory 3E0K
  - Antineoplastic 3E0K
  - Destructive Agent 3E0K
  - Diagnostic Substance, Other 3E0K
  - Electrolytic Substance 3E0K
  - Gas 3E0K
  - Hypnotics 3E0K
  - Nutritional Substance 3E0K
  - Radioactive Substance 3E0K
  - Sedatives 3E0K
  - Water Balance Substance 3E0K
- Heart 3E08
  - Diagnostic Substance, Other 3E08
  - Platelet Inhibitor 3E08
  - Thrombolytic 3E08
- Joint 3E0U
  - Analgesics 3E0U3NZ
  - Anesthetic Agent 3E0U3BZ
  - Anti-infective 3E0U
  - Anti-inflammatory 3E0U33Z
  - Antineoplastic 3E0U30
  - Destructive Agent 3E0U3TZ
  - Diagnostic Substance, Other 3E0U3KZ
  - Electrolytic Substance 3E0U37Z
  - Gas 3E0U3SF
  - Hypnotics 3E0U3NZ
  - Nutritional Substance 3E0U36Z
  - Radioactive Substance 3E0U3HZ
  - Sedatives 3E0U3NZ
  - Water Balance Substance 3E0U37Z
- Lymphatic 3E0W3GC
  - Analgesics 3E0W3NZ
  - Anesthetic Agent 3E0W3BZ
  - Anti-infective 3E0W32
  - Anti-inflammatory 3E0W33Z
  - Antineoplastic 3E0W30
  - Destructive Agent 3E0W3TZ
  - Diagnostic Substance, Other 3E0W3KZ
  - Electrolytic Substance 3E0W37Z
  - Hypnotics 3E0W3NZ
  - Nutritional Substance 3E0W36Z
  - Radioactive Substance 3E0W3HZ
  - Sedatives 3E0W3NZ
  - Water Balance Substance 3E0W37Z
- Mouth 3E0D
  - Analgesics 3E0D
  - Anesthetic Agent 3E0D
  - Anti-infective 3E0D
  - Anti-inflammatory 3E0D
  - Antiarrhythmic 3E0D

Introduction of substance in or on *(continued)*
- Mouth 3E0D *(continued)*
  - Antineoplastic 3E0D
  - Destructive Agent 3E0D
  - Diagnostic Substance, Other 3E0D
  - Electrolytic Substance 3E0D
  - Hypnotics 3E0D
  - Nutritional Substance 3E0D
  - Radioactive Substance 3E0D
  - Sedatives 3E0D
  - Serum 3E0D
  - Toxoid 3E0D
  - Vaccine 3E0D
  - Water Balance Substance 3E0D
- Mucous Membrane 3E00XGC
  - Analgesics 3E00XNZ
  - Anesthetic Agent 3E00XBZ
  - Anti-infective 3E00X2
  - Anti-inflammatory 3E00X3Z
  - Antineoplastic 3E00X0
  - Destructive Agent 3E00XTZ
  - Diagnostic Substance, Other 3E00XKZ
  - Hypnotics 3E00XNZ
  - Pigment 3E00XMZ
  - Sedatives 3E00XNZ
  - Serum 3E00X4Z
  - Toxoid 3E00X4Z
  - Vaccine 3E00X4Z
- Muscle 3E023GC
  - Analgesics 3E023NZ
  - Anesthetic Agent 3E023BZ
  - Anti-infective 3E0232
  - Anti-inflammatory 3E0233Z
  - Antineoplastic 3E0230
  - Destructive Agent 3E023TZ
  - Diagnostic Substance, Other 3E023KZ
  - Electrolytic Substance 3E0237Z
  - Hypnotics 3E023NZ
  - Nutritional Substance 3E0236Z
  - Radioactive Substance 3E023HZ
  - Sedatives 3E023NZ
  - Serum 3E0234Z
  - Toxoid 3E0234Z
  - Vaccine 3E0234Z
  - Water Balance Substance 3E0237Z
- Nerve
  - Cranial 3E0X3GC
    - Anesthetic Agent 3E0X3BZ
    - Anti-inflammatory 3E0X33Z
    - Destructive Agent 3E0X3TZ
  - Peripheral 3E0T3GC
    - Anesthetic Agent 3E0T3BZ
    - Anti-inflammatory 3E0T33Z
    - Destructive Agent 3E0T3TZ
  - Plexus 3E0T3GC Agent 3E0T3BZ
    - Anti-inflammatory 3E0T33Z
    - Destructive Agent 3E0T3TZ
- Nose 3E09
  - Analgesics 3E09
  - Anesthetic Agent 3E09
  - Anti-infective 3E09
  - Anti-inflammatory 3E09
  - Antineoplastic 3E09
  - Destructive Agent 3E09
  - Diagnostic Substance, Other 3E09
  - Hypnotics 3E09
  - Radioactive Substance 3E09
  - Sedatives 3E09
  - Serum 3E09
  - Toxoid 3E09
  - Vaccine 3E09
- Pancreatic Tract 3E0J
  - Analgesics 3E0J
  - Anesthetic Agent 3E0J

Introduction of substance in or on *(continued)*
- Pancreatic Tract 3E0J *(continued)*
  - Anti-infective 3E0J
  - Anti-inflammatory 3E0J
  - Antineoplastic 3E0J0
  - Destructive Agent 3E0J
  - Diagnostic Substance, Other 3E0J
  - Electrolytic Substance 3E0J
  - Gas 3E0J
  - Hypnotics 3E0J
  - Islet Cells, Pancreatic 3E0JU
  - Nutritional Substance 3E0J
  - Radioactive Substance 3E0J
  - Sedatives 3E0J
  - Water Balance Substance 3E0J
- Pericardial Cavity 3E0Y
  - Analgesics 3E0Y3NZ
  - Anesthetic Agent 3E0Y3BZ
  - Anti-infective 3E0Y32
  - Anti-inflammatory 3E0Y33Z
  - Antineoplastic 3E0Y
  - Destructive Agent 3E0Y3TZ
  - Diagnostic Substance, Other 3E0Y3KZ
  - Electrolytic Substance 3E0Y37Z
  - Gas 3E0Y
  - Hypnotics 3E0Y3NZ
  - Nutritional Substance 3E0Y36Z
  - Radioactive Substance 3E0Y3HZ
  - Sedatives 3E0Y3NZ
  - Water Balance Substance 3E0Y37Z
- Peritoneal Cavity 3E0M
  - Adhesion Barrier 3E0M
  - Analgesics 3E0M3NZ
  - Anesthetic Agent 3E0M3BZ
  - Anti-infective 3E0M32
  - Anti-inflammatory 3E0M33Z
  - Antineoplastic 3E0M
  - Destructive Agent 3E0M3TZ
  - Diagnostic Substance, Other 3E0M3KZ
  - Electrolytic Substance 3E0M37Z
  - Gas 3E0M
  - Hypnotics 3E0M3NZ
  - Nutritional Substance 3E0M36Z
  - Radioactive Substance 3E0M3HZ
  - Sedatives 3E0M3NZ
  - Water Balance Substance 3E0M37Z
- Pharynx 3E0D
  - Analgesics 3E0D
  - Anesthetic Agent 3E0D
  - Anti-infective 3E0D
  - Anti-inflammatory 3E0D
  - Antiarrhythmic 3E0D
  - Antineoplastic 3E0D
  - Destructive Agent 3E0D
  - Diagnostic Substance, Other 3E0D
  - Electrolytic Substance 3E0D
  - Hypnotics 3E0D
  - Nutritional Substance 3E0D
  - Radioactive Substance 3E0D
  - Sedatives 3E0D
  - Serum 3E0D
  - Toxoid 3E0D
  - Vaccine 3E0D
  - Water Balance Substance 3E0D
- Pleural Cavity 3E0L
  - Adhesion Barrier 3E0L
  - Analgesics 3E0L3NZ
  - Anesthetic Agent 3E0L3BZ
  - Anti-infective 3E0L32
  - Anti-inflammatory 3E0L33Z
  - Antineoplastic 3E0L
  - Destructive Agent 3E0L3TZ
  - Diagnostic Substance, Other 3E0L3KZ

Introduction of substance in or on *(continued)*
Pleural Cavity 3E0L *(continued)*
Electrolytic Substance 3E0L37Z
Gas 3E0L
Hypnotics 3E0L3NZ
Nutritional Substance 3E0L36Z
Radioactive Substance 3E0L3HZ
Sedatives 3E0L3NZ
Water Balance Substance 3E0L37Z
Products of Conception 3E0E
Analgesics 3E0E
Anesthetic Agent 3E0E
Anti-infective 3E0E2
Anti-inflammatory 3E0E
Antineoplastic 3E0E0
Destructive Agent 3E0E
Diagnostic Substance, Other 3E0E
Electrolytic Substance 3E0E
Gas 3E0E
Hypnotics 3E0E
Nutritional Substance 3E0E
Radioactive Substance 3E0E
Sedatives 3E0E
Water Balance Substance 3E0E
Reproductive
Female 3E0P
Adhesion Barrier 3E0P0
Analgesics 3E0P
Anesthetic Agent 3E0P
Anti-infective 3E0P
Anti-inflammatory 3E0P
Antineoplastic 3E0P
Destructive Agent 3E0P
Diagnostic Substance, Other 3E0P
Electrolytic Substance 3E0P
Gas 3E0P
Hormone 3E0P
Hypnotics 3E0P
Nutritional Substance 3E0P
Ovum, Fertilized 3E0P
Radioactive Substance 3E0P
Sedatives 3E0P
Sperm 3E0P
Water Balance Substance 3E0P
Male 3E0N
Analgesics 3E0N
Anesthetic Agent 3E0N
Anti-infective 3E0N
Anti-inflammatory 3E0N
Antineoplastic 3E0N0
Destructive Agent 3E0N
Diagnostic Substance, Other 3E0N
Electrolytic Substance 3E0N
Gas 3E0N
Hypnotics 3E0N
Nutritional Substance 3E0N
Radioactive Substance 3E0N
Sedatives 3E0N
Water Balance Substance 3E0N
Respiratory Tract 3E0F
Analgesics 3E0F
Anesthetic Agent 3E0F
Anti-infective 3E0F
Anti-inflammatory 3E0F
Antineoplastic 3E0F
Destructive Agent 3E0F
Diagnostic Substance, Other 3E0F
Electrolytic Substance 3E0F
Gas 3E0F
Hypnotics 3E0F
Nutritional Substance 3E0F
Radioactive Substance 3E0F
Sedatives 3E0F
Water Balance Substance 3E0F

Introduction of substance in or on *(continued)*
Skin 3E00XGC
Analgesics 3E00XNZ
Anesthetic Agent 3E00XBZ
Anti-infective 3E00X2
Anti-inflammatory 3E00X3Z
Antineoplastic 3E00X0
Destructive Agent 3E00XTZ
Diagnostic Substance, Other 3E00XKZ
Hypnotics 3E00XNZ
Pigment 3E00XMZ
Sedatives 3E00XNZ
Serum 3E00X4Z
Toxoid 3E00X4Z
Vaccine 3E00X4Z
Spinal Canal 3E0R3GC
Analgesics 3E0R3NZ
Anesthetic Agent 3E0R3BZ
Anti-infective 3E0R32
Anti-inflammatory 3E0R33Z
Antineoplastic 3E0R30
Destructive Agent 3E0R3TZ
Diagnostic Substance, Other 3E0R3KZ
Electrolytic Substance 3E0R37Z
Gas 3E0R
Hypnotics 3E0R3NZ
Nutritional Substance 3E0R36Z
Radioactive Substance 3E0R3HZ
Sedatives 3E0R3NZ
Stem Cells
Embryonic 3E0R
Somatic 3E0R
Water Balance Substance 3E0R37Z
Subcutaneous Tissue 3E013GC
Analgesics 3E013NZ
Anesthetic Agent 3E013BZ
Anti-infective 3E01
Anti-inflammatory 3E0133Z
Antineoplastic 3E0130
Destructive Agent 3E013TZ
Diagnostic Substance, Other 3E013KZ
Electrolytic Substance 3E0137Z
Hormone 3E013V
Hypnotics 3E013NZ
Nutritional Substance 3E0136Z
Radioactive Substance 3E013HZ
Sedatives 3E013NZ
Serum 3E0134Z
Toxoid 3E0134Z
Vaccine 3E0134Z
Water Balance Substance 3E0137Z
Vein
Central 3E04
Analgesics 3E04
Anesthetic, Intracirculatory 3E04
Anti-infective 3E04
Anti-inflammatory 3E04
Antiarrhythmic 3E04
Antineoplastic 3E04
Destructive Agent 3E04
Diagnostic Substance, Other 3E04
Electrolytic Substance 3E04
Hormone 3E04
Hypnotics 3E04
Immunotherapeutic 3E04
Nutritional Substance 3E04
Platelet Inhibitor 3E04
Radioactive Substance 3E04
Sedatives 3E04
Serum 3E04
Thrombolytic 3E04
Toxoid 3E04
Vaccine 3E04

Introduction of substance in or on *(continued)*
Vein *(continued)*
Central 3E04 *(continued)*
Vasopressor 3E04
Water Balance Substance 3E04
Peripheral 3E03
Analgesics 3E03
Anesthetic, Intracirculatory 3E03
Anti-infective 3E03
Anti-inflammatory 3E03
Antiarrhythmic 3E03
Antineoplastic 3E03
Destructive Agent 3E03
Diagnostic Substance, Other 3E03
Electrolytic Substance 3E03
Hormone 3E03
Hypnotics 3E03
Immunotherapeutic 3E03
Islet Cells, Pancreatic 3E03
Nutritional Substance 3E03
Platelet Inhibitor 3E03
Radioactive Substance 3E03
Sedatives 3E03
Serum 3E03
Thrombolytic 3E03
Toxoid 3E03
Vaccine 3E03
Vasopressor 3E03
Water Balance Substance 3E03
Intubation
Airway
see Insertion of device in, Esophagus 0DH5
see Insertion of device in, Mouth and Throat 0CHY
see Insertion of device in, Trachea 0BH1
Drainage device
see Drainage
Feeding Device
see Insertion of device in, Gastrointestinal System 0DH
INTUITY Elite valve system, EDWARDS
use Zooplastic Tissue, Rapid Deployment Technique in New Technology
Iobenguane I-131 Antineoplastic XW0
Iobenguane I-131, High Specific Activity (HSA)
use Iobenguane I-131 Antineoplastic
IPPB (intermittent positive pressure breathing)
see Assistance, Respiratory 5A09
IRE (Irreversible Electroporation)
see Destruction, Hepatobiliary System and Pancreas 0F5
Iridectomy
see Excision, Eye 08B
see Resection, Eye 08T
Iridoplasty
see Repair, Eye 08Q
see Replacement, Eye 08R
see Supplement, Eye 08U
Iridotomy
see Drainage, Eye 089
Irreversible Electroporation (IRE)
see Destruction, Hepatobiliary System and Pancreas 0F5
Irrigation
Biliary Tract, Irrigating Substance 3E1J
Brain, Irrigating Substance 3E1Q38Z

Irrigation *(continued)*
Cranial Cavity, Irrigating Substance 3E1Q38Z
Ear, Irrigating Substance 3E1B
Epidural Space, Irrigating Substance 3E1S38Z
Eye, Irrigating Substance 3E1C
Gastrointestinal Tract
Lower, Irrigating Substance 3E1H
Upper, Irrigating Substance 3E1G
Genitourinary Tract, Irrigating Substance 3E1K
Irrigating Substance 3C1ZX8Z
Joint, Irrigating Substance 3E1U
Mucous Membrane, Irrigating Substance 3E10
Nose, Irrigating Substance 3E19
Pancreatic Tract, Irrigating Substance 3E1J
Pericardial Cavity, Irrigating Substance 3E1Y38Z
Peritoneal Cavity
Dialysate 3E1M39Z
Irrigating Substance 3E1M
Pleural Cavity, Irrigating Substance 3E1L38Z
Reproductive
Female, Irrigating Substance 3E1P
Male, Irrigating Substance 3E1N
Respiratory Tract, Irrigating Substance 3E1F
Skin, Irrigating Substance 3E10
Spinal Canal, Irrigating Substance 3E1R38Z
Isavuconazole (isavuconazonium sulfate)
use Other Anti-Infective
ISC-REST kit
ISCDx XXE5XT7
QIAGEN Access Anti-SARS-CoV-2 Total Test XXE5XV7
QIAstat-Dx Respiratory SARS-CoV-2 Panel XXE97U7
Ischiatic nerve
use Nerve, Sciatic
Ischiocavernosus muscle
use Muscle, Perineum
Ischiofemoral ligament
use Bursa and Ligament, Hip, Left
use Bursa and Ligament, Hip, Right
Ischium
use Bone, Pelvic, Left
use Bone, Pelvic, Right
Isolation 8E0ZXY6
Isotope Administration, Other Radiation, Whole Body DWY5G
Itrel (3)(4) neurostimulator
use Stimulator Generator, Single Array in 0JH

J

Jakafi®
use Ruxolitinib
Jejunal artery
use Artery, Superior Mesenteric
Jejunectomy
see Excision, Jejunum 0DBA
see Resection, Jejunum 0DTA
Jejunocolostomy
see Bypass, Gastrointestinal System 0D1
see Drainage, Gastrointestinal System 0D9
Jejunopexy
see Repair, Jejunum 0DQA
see Reposition, Jejunum 0DSA

Jejunostomy
see Bypass, Jejunum 0D1A
see Drainage, Jejunum 0D9A
Jejunotomy
see Drainage, Jejunum 0D9A
Joint fixation plate
use Internal Fixation Device in Lower Joints
use Internal Fixation Device in Upper Joints
Joint liner (insert)
use Liner in Lower Joints
Joint spacer (antibiotic)
use Spacer in Lower Joints
use Spacer in Upper Joints
Jugular body
use Glomus Jugulare
Jugular lymph node
use Lymphatic, Neck, Left
use Lymphatic, Neck, Right

K

Kappa
use Pacemaker, Dual Chamber in 0JH
Kcentra
use 4-Factor Prothrombin Complex Concentrate
Keratectomy, kerectomy
see Excision, Eye 08B
see Resection, Eye 08T
Keratocentesis
see Drainage, Eye 089
Keratoplasty
see Repair, Eye 08Q
see Replacement, Eye 08R
see Supplement, Eye 08U
Keratotomy
see Drainage, Eye 089
see Repair, Eye 08Q
KEVZARA® *use* Sarilumab
Keystone Heart TriGuard 3™ CEPD (cerebral embolic protection device) X2A6325
Kirschner wire (K-wire)
use Internal Fixation Device in Head and Facial Bones
use Internal Fixation Device in Lower Bones
use Internal Fixation Device in Lower Joints
use Internal Fixation Device in Upper Bones
use Internal Fixation Device in Upper Joints
Knee (implant) insert
use Liner in Lower Joints
KUB x-ray
see Plain Radiography, Kidney, Ureter and Bladder BT04
Kuntscher nail
use Internal Fixation Device, Intramedullary in Lower Bones
use Internal Fixation Device, Intramedullary in Upper Bones
KYMRIAH®
use Tisagenlecleucel Immunotherapy

L

Labia majora
use Vulva
Labia minora
use Vulva
Labial gland
use Lip, Lower
use Lip, Upper
Labiectomy
see Excision, Female Reproductive System 0UB
see Resection, Female Reproductive System 0UT
see Release, Central Nervous System 00N
see Release, Peripheral Nervous System 01N
Lacrimal canaliculus
use Duct, Lacrimal, Left
use Duct, Lacrimal, Right
Lacrimal punctum
use Duct, Lacrimal, Left
use Duct, Lacrimal, Right
Lacrimal sac
use Duct, Lacrimal, Left
use Duct, Lacrimal, Right
LAGB (laparoscopic adjustable gastric banding)
Initial procedure 0DV64CZ
Surgical correction
see Revision of device in, Stomach 0DW6
Laminectomy
see Excision, Lower Bones 0QB
see Excision, Upper Bones 0PB
see Release, Central Nervous System and Cranial Nerves 00N
see Release, Peripheral Nervous System 01N
Laminotomy
see Drainage, Lower Bones 0Q9
see Drainage, Upper Bones 0P9
see Excision, Lower Bones 0QB
see Excision, Upper Bones 0PB
see Release, Central Nervous System and Cranial Nerves 00N
see Release, Lower Bones 0QN
see Release, Peripheral Nervous System 01N
see Release, Upper Bones 0PN
LAP-BAND® adjustable gastric banding system
use Extraluminal Device
Laparoscopic-assisted transanal pull-through
see Excision, Gastrointestinal System 0DB
see Resection, Gastrointestinal System 0DT
Laparoscopy
see Inspection
Laparotomy
Drainage
see Drainage, Peritoneal Cavity 0W9G
Exploratory
see Inspection, Peritoneal Cavity 0WJG
Laryngectomy
see Excision, Larynx 0CBS
see Resection, Larynx 0CTS
Laryngocentesis
see Drainage, Larynx 0C9S
Laryngogram
see Fluoroscopy, Larynx B91J
Laryngopexy
see Repair, Larynx 0CQS
Laryngopharynx
use Pharynx
Laryngoplasty
see Repair, Larynx 0CQS
see Replacement, Larynx 0CRS
see Supplement, Larynx 0CUS
Laryngorrhaphy
see Repair, Larynx 0CQS
Laryngoscopy 0CJS8ZZ
Laryngotomy
see Drainage, Larynx 0C9S
Laser Interstitial Thermal Therapy
Adrenal Gland DGY2KZZ
Anus DDY8KZZ
Bile Ducts DFY2KZZ
Brain D0Y0KZZ
Brain Stem D0Y1KZZ
Breast
Left DMY0KZZ
Right DMY1KZZ
Bronchus DBY1KZZ
Chest Wall DBY7KZZ
Colon DDY5KZZ
Diaphragm DBY8KZZ
Duodenum DDY2KZZ
Esophagus DDY0KZZ
Gallbladder DFY1KZZ
Gland
Adrenal DGY2KZZ
Parathyroid DGY4KZZ
Pituitary DGY0KZZ
Thyroid DGY5KZZ
Ileum DDY4KZZ
Jejunum DDY3KZZ
Liver DFY0KZZ
Lung DBY2KZZ
Mediastinum DBY6KZZ
Nerve, Peripheral D0Y7KZZ
Pancreas DFY3KZZ
Parathyroid Gland DGY4KZZ
Pineal Body DGY1KZZ
Pituitary Gland DGY0KZZ
Pleura DBY5KZZ
Prostate DVY0KZZ
Rectum DDY7KZZ
Spinal Cord D0Y6KZZ
Stomach DDY1KZZ
Thyroid Gland DGY5KZZ
Trachea DBY0KZZ
Lateral (brachial) lymph node
use Lymphatic, Axillary, Left
use Lymphatic, Axillary, Right
Lateral canthus
use Eyelid, Upper, Left
use Eyelid, Upper, Right
Lateral collateral ligament (LCL)
use Bursa and Ligament, Knee, Left
use Bursa and Ligament, Knee, Right
Lateral condyle of femur
use Femur, Lower, Left
use Femur, Lower, Right
Lateral condyle of tibia
use Tibia, Left
use Tibia, Right
Lateral cuneiform bone
use Tarsal, Left
use Tarsal, Right
Lateral epicondyle of femur
use Femur, Lower, Left
use Femur, Lower, Right
Lateral epicondyle of humerus
use Humeral Shaft, Left
use Humeral Shaft, Right
Lateral femoral cutaneous nerve
use Nerve, Lumbar Plexus
Lateral malleolus
use Fibula, Left
use Fibula, Right
Lateral meniscus
use Joint, Knee, Left
use Joint, Knee, Right
Lateral nasal cartilage
use Nasal Mucosa and Soft Tissue
Lateral plantar artery
use Artery, Foot, Left
use Artery, Foot, Right
Lateral plantar nerve
use Nerve, Tibial
Lateral rectus muscle
use Muscle, Extraocular, Left
use Muscle, Extraocular, Right
Lateral sacral artery
use Artery, Internal Iliac, Left
use Artery, Internal Iliac, Right
Lateral sacral vein
use Vein, Hypogastric, Left
use Vein, Hypogastric, Right
Lateral sural cutaneous nerve
use Nerve, Peroneal
Lateral tarsal artery
use Artery, Foot, Left
use Artery, Foot, Right
Lateral temporomandibular ligament
use Bursa and Ligament, Head and Neck
Lateral thoracic artery
use Artery, Axillary, Left
use Artery, Axillary, Right
Latissimus dorsi muscle
use Muscle, Trunk, Left
use Muscle, Trunk, Right
Latissimus Dorsi Myocutaneous Flap
Replacement
Bilateral 0HRV075
Left 0HRU075
Right 0HRT075
Transfer
Left 0KXG
Right 0KXF
Lavage
see Irrigation
Bronchial alveolar, diagnostic
see Drainage, Respiratory System 0B9
Least splanchnic nerve
use Nerve, Thoracic Sympathetic
Lefamulin Anti-infective XW0
Left ascending lumbar vein
use Vein, Hemiazygos
Left atrioventricular valve
use Valve, Mitral
Left auricular appendix
use Atrium, Left
Left colic vein
use Vein, Colic
Left coronary sulcus
use Heart, Left
Left gastric artery
use Artery, Gastric
Left gastroepiploic artery
use Artery, Splenic
Left gastroepiploic vein
use Vein, Splenic
Left inferior phrenic vein
use Vein, Renal, Left
Left inferior pulmonary vein
use Vein, Pulmonary, Left
Left jugular trunk
use Lymphatic, Thoracic Duct
Left lateral ventricle
use Cerebral Ventricle
Left ovarian vein
use Vein, Renal, Left
Left second lumbar vein
use Vein, Renal, Left
Left subclavian trunk
use Lymphatic, Thoracic Duct
Left subcostal vein
use Vein, Hemiazygos
Left superior pulmonary vein
use Vein, Pulmonary, Left
Left suprarenal vein
use Vein, Renal, Left
Left testicular vein
use Vein, Renal, Left
Lengthening
Bone, with device
see Insertion of Limb Lengthening Device
Muscle, by incision
see Division, Muscles 0K8

Lengthening *(continued)*
Tendon, by incision
see Division, Tendons 0L8
Leptomeninges, intracranial
use Cerebral Meninges
Leptomeninges, spinal
use Spinal Meninges
Lesser alar cartilage
use Nasal Mucosa and Soft Tissue
Lesser occipital nerve
use Nerve, Cervical Plexus
Lesser Omentum
use Omentum
Lesser saphenous vein
use Saphenous Vein, Left
use Saphenous Vein, Right
Lesser splanchnic nerve
use Nerve, Thoracic Sympathetic
Lesser trochanter
use Femur, Upper, Left
use Femur, Upper, Right
Lesser tuberosity
use Humeral Head, Left
use Humeral Head, Right
Lesser wing
use Bone, Sphenoid
Leukopheresis, therapeutic
see Pheresis, Circulatory 6A55
Levator anguli oris muscle
use Muscle, Facial
Levator ani muscle
use Perineum Muscle
Levator labii superioris alaeque nasi muscle
use Muscle, Facial
Levator labii superioris muscle
use Muscle, Facial
Levator palpebrae superioris muscle
use Eyelid, Upper, Left
use Eyelid, Upper, Right
Levator scapulae muscle
use Muscle, Neck, Left
use Muscle, Neck, Right
Levator veli palatini muscle
use Muscle, Tongue, Palate, Pharynx
Levatores costarum muscle
use Muscle, Thorax, Left
use Muscle, Thorax, Right
Lifeline ARM Automated Chest Compression (ACC) device 5A1221J
LifeStent® (Flexstar)(XL) Vascular Stent System
use Intraluminal Device
Lifileucel *use* Lifileucel Immunotherapy
Lifileucel Immunotherapy XW0
Ligament of head of fibula
use Bursa and Ligament, Knee, Left
use Bursa and Ligament, Knee, Right
Ligament of the lateral malleolus
use Bursa and Ligament, Ankle, Left
use Bursa and Ligament, Ankle, Right
Ligamentum flavum, cervical
use Head and Neck Bursa and Ligament
Ligamentum flavum, lumbar
use Lower Spine Bursa and Ligament
Ligamentum flavum, thoracic
use Upper Spine Bursa and Ligament
Ligation
see Occlusion
Ligation, hemorrhoid
see Occlusion, Lower Veins, Hemorrhoidal Plexus
Light Therapy GZJZZZZ
Liner
Removal of device from
Hip
Left 0SPB09Z
Right 0SP909Z
Knee
Left 0SPD09Z
Right 0SPC09Z
Revision of device in
Hip
Left 0SWB09Z
Right 0SW909Z
Knee
Left 0SWD09Z
Right 0SWC09Z
Supplement
Hip
Left 0SUB09Z
Acetabular Surface 0SUE09Z
Femoral Surface 0SUS09Z
Right 0SU909Z
Acetabular Surface 0SUA09Z
Femoral Surface 0SUR09Z
Knee
Left 0SUD09
Femoral Surface 0SUU09Z
Tibial Surface 0SUW09Z
Right 0SUC09
Femoral Surface 0SUT09Z
Tibial Surface 0SUV09Z
Lingual artery
use Artery, External Carotid, Left
use Artery, External Carotid, Right
Lingual tonsil
use Pharynx
Lingulectomy, lung
see Excision, Lung Lingula 0BBH
see Resection, Lung Lingula 0BTH
Lisocabtagene Maraleucel
use Lisacabtagene Maraleucel Immunotherapy
Lisocabtagene Maraleucel Immunotherapy XW0
Lithoplasty
see Fragmentation
Lithotripsy
see Fragmentation
With removal of fragments
see Extirpation
LITT (laser interstitial thermal therapy)
see Laser Interstitial Thermal Therapy
LIVIAN™ CRT-D
use Cardiac Resynchronization Defibrillator Pulse Generator in 0JH
Lobectomy
see Excision, Central Nervous System and Cranial Nerves 00B
see Excision, Endocrine System 0GB
see Excision, Hepatobiliary System and Pancreas 0FB
see Excision, Respiratory System 0BB
see Resection, Endocrine System 0GT
see Resection, Hepatobiliary System and Pancreas 0FT
see Resection, Respiratory System 0BT
Lobotomy
see Division, Brain 0080
Localization
see Map
see Imaging
Locus ceruleus
use Pons
Long thoracic nerve
use Nerve, Brachial Plexus
Loop ileostomy
see Bypass, Ileum 0D1B
Loop recorder, implantable
use Monitoring Device
Lower GI series
see Fluoroscopy, Colon BD14
Lower Respiratory Fluid Nucleic Acid-base Microbial Detection XXEBXQ6
LTX Regional Anticoagulant
use Nafamostat Anticoagulant
LUCAS® Chest Compression System 5A1221J
Lumbar artery
use Aorta, Abdominal
Lumbar facet joint
use Joint, Lumbar Vertebral
Lumbar ganglion
use Nerve, Lumbar Sympathetic
Lumbar lymph node
use Lymphatic, Aortic
Lumbar lymphatic trunk
use Cisterna Chyli
Lumbar splanchnic nerve
use Nerve, Lumbar Sympathetic
Lumbosacral facet joint
use Joint, Lumbosacral
Lumbosacral trunk
use Nerve, Lumbar
Lumpectomy
see Excision
Lunate bone
use Carpal, Left
use Carpal, Right
Lunotriquetral ligament
use Bursa and Ligament, Hand, Left
use Bursa and Ligament, Hand, Right
Lurbinectedin XW0
Lymphadenectomy
see Excision, Lymphatic and Hemic Systems 07B
see Resection, Lymphatic and Hemic Systems 07T
Lymphadenotomy
see Drainage, Lymphatic and Hemic Systems 079
Lymphangiectomy
see Excision, Lymphatic and Hemic Systems 07B
see Resection, Lymphatic and Hemic Systems 07T
Lymphangiogram
see Plain Radiography, Lymphatic System B70
Lymphangioplasty
see Repair, Lymphatic and Hemic Systems 07Q
see Supplement, Lymphatic and Hemic Systems 07U
Lymphangiorrhaphy
see Repair, Lymphatic and Hemic Systems 07Q
Lymphangiotomy
see Drainage, Lymphatic and Hemic Systems 079
Lysis
see Release

M

Macula
use Retina, Left
use Retina, Right
MAGEC® Spinal Bracing and Distraction System
use Magnetically Controlled Growth Rod(s) in New Technology
Magnet extraction, ocular foreign body
see Extirpation, Eye 08C
Magnetic-guided radiofrequency endovascular fistula
Radial Artery, Left 031C
Radial Artery, Right 031B
Ulnar Artery, Left 031A
Ulnar Artery, Right 0319
Magnetic Resonance Imaging (MRI)
Abdomen BW30
Ankle
Left BQ3H
Right BQ3G
Aorta
Abdominal B430
Thoracic B330
Arm
Left BP3F
Right BP3E
Artery
Celiac B431
Cervico-Cerebral Arch B33Q
Common Carotid, Bilateral B335
Coronary
Bypass Graft, Multiple B233
Multiple B231
Internal Carotid, Bilateral B338
Intracranial B33R
Lower Extremity
Bilateral B43H
Left B43G
Right B43F
Pelvic B43C
Renal, Bilateral B438
Spinal B33M
Superior Mesenteric B434
Upper Extremity
Bilateral B33K
Left B33J
Right B33H
Vertebral, Bilateral B33G
Bladder BT30
Brachial Plexus BW3P
Brain B030
Breast
Bilateral BH32
Left BH31
Right BH30
Calcaneus
Left BQ3K
Right BQ3J
Chest BW33Y
Coccyx BR3F
Connective Tissue
Lower Extremity BL31
Upper Extremity BL30
Corpora Cavernosa BV30
Disc
Cervical BR31
Lumbar BR33
Thoracic BR32
Ear B930
Elbow
Left BP3H
Right BP3G
Eye
Bilateral B837
Left B836
Right B835
Femur
Left BQ34
Right BQ33
Fetal Abdomen BY33
Fetal Extremity BY35
Fetal Head BY30
Fetal Heart BY31
Fetal Spine BY34
Fetal Thorax BY32
Fetus, Whole BY36

Magnetic Resonance Imaging (MRI) *(continued)*
- Foot
  - Left BQ3M
  - Right BQ3L
- Forearm
  - Left BP3K
  - Right BP3J
- Gland
  - Adrenal, Bilateral BG32
  - Parathyroid BG33
  - Parotid, Bilateral B936
  - Salivary, Bilateral B93D
  - Submandibular, Bilateral B939
  - Thyroid BG34
- Head BW38
- Heart, Right and Left B236
- Hip
  - Left BQ31
  - Right BQ30
- Intracranial Sinus B532
- Joint
  - Finger
    - Left BP3D
    - Right BP3C
  - Hand
    - Left BP3D
    - Right BP3C
  - Temporomandibular, Bilateral BN39
- Kidney
  - Bilateral BT33
  - Left BT32
  - Right BT31
  - Transplant BT39
- Knee
  - Left BQ38
  - Right BQ37
- Larynx B93J
- Leg
  - Left BQ3F
  - Right BQ3D
- Liver BF35
- Liver and Spleen BF36
- Lung Apices BB3G
- Nasopharynx B93F
- Neck BW3F
- Nerve
  - Acoustic B03C
  - Brachial Plexus BW3P
- Oropharynx B93F
- Ovary
  - Bilateral BU35
  - Left BU34
  - Right BU33
- Ovary and Uterus BU3C
- Pancreas BF37
- Patella
  - Left BQ3W
  - Right BQ3V
- Pelvic Region BW3G
- Pelvis BR3C
- Pituitary Gland B039
- Plexus, Brachial BW3P
- Prostate BV33
- Retroperitoneum BW3H
- Sacrum BR3F
- Scrotum BV34
- Sella Turcica B039
- Shoulder
  - Left BP39
  - Right BP38
- Sinus
  - Intracranial B532
  - Paranasal B932
- Spinal Cord B03B
- Spine
  - Cervical BR30
  - Lumbar BR39
  - Thoracic BR37
- Spleen and Liver BF36

Magnetic Resonance Imaging (MRI) *(continued)*
- Subcutaneous Tissue
  - Abdomen BH3H
  - Extremity
    - Lower BH3J
    - Upper BH3F
  - Head BH3D
  - Neck BH3D
  - Pelvis BH3H
  - Thorax BH3G
- Tendon
  - Lower Extremity BL33
  - Upper Extremity BL32
- Testicle
  - Bilateral BV37
  - Left BV36
  - Right BV35
- Toe
  - Left BQ3Q
  - Right BQ3P
- Uterus BU36
  - Pregnant BU3B
- Uterus and Ovary BU3C
- Vagina BU39
- Vein
  - Cerebellar B531
  - Cerebral B531
  - Jugular, Bilateral B535
  - Lower Extremity
    - Bilateral B53D
    - Left B53C
    - Right B53B
  - Other B53V
  - Pelvic (Iliac) Bilateral B53H
  - Portal B53T
  - Pulmonary, Bilateral B53S
  - Renal, Bilateral B53L
  - Spanchnic B53T
  - Upper Extremity
    - Bilateral B53P
    - Left B53N
    - Right B53M
- Vena Cava
  - Inferior B539
  - Superior B538
- Wrist
  - Left BP3M
  - Right BP3L

Magnetically Controlled Growth Rod(s)
- Cervical XNS3
- Lumbar XNS0
- Thoracic XNS4

Malleotomy
- *see* Drainage, Ear, Nose, Sinus 099

Malleus
- *use* Auditory Ossicle, Left
- *use* Auditory Ossicle, Right

Mammaplasty, mammoplasty
- *see* Alteration, Skin and Breast 0H0
- *see* Repair, Skin and Breast 0HQ
- *see* Replacement, Skin and Breast 0HR
- *see* Supplement, Skin and Breast 0HU

Mammary duct
- *use* Breast, Bilateral
- *use* Breast, Left
- *use* Breast, Right

Mammary gland
- *use* Breast, Bilateral
- *use* Breast, Left
- *use* Breast, Right

Mammectomy
- *see* Excision, Skin and Breast 0HB
- *see* Resection, Skin and Breast 0HT

Mammillary body
- *use* Hypothalamus

Mammography
- *see* Plain Radiography, Skin, Subcutaneous Tissue and Breast BH0

Mammotomy
- *see* Drainage, Skin and Breast 0H9

Mandibular nerve
- *use* Nerve, Trigeminal

Mandibular notch
- *use* Mandible, Left
- *use* Mandible, Right

Mandibulectomy
- *see* Excision, Head and Facial Bones 0NB
- *see* Resection, Head and Facial Bones 0NT

Manipulation
- Adhesions
  - *see* Release
- Chiropractic
  - *see* Chiropractic Manipulation

Manual removal, retained placenta
- *see* Extraction, Products of Conception, Retained 10D1

Manubrium
- *use* Sternum

Map
- Basal Ganglia 00K8
- Brain 00K0
- Cerebellum 00KC
- Cerebral Hemisphere 00K7
- Conduction Mechanism 02K8
- Hypothalamus 00KA
- Medulla Oblongata 00KD
- Pons 00KB
- Thalamus 00K9

Mapping
- Doppler ultrasound
  - *see* Ultrasonography
- Electrocardiogram only
  - *see* Measurement, Cardiac 4A02

Mark IV Breathing Pacemaker System
- *use* Stimulator Generator in Subcutaneous Tissue and Fascia

Marsupialization
- *see* Drainage
- *see* Excision

Massage, cardiac
- External 5A12012
- Open 02QA0ZZ

Masseter muscle
- *use* Muscle, Head

Masseteric fascia
- *use* Subcutaneous Tissue and Fascia, Face

Mastectomy
- *see* Excision, Skin and Breast 0HB
- *see* Resection, Skin and Breast 0HT

Mastoid (postauricular) lymph node
- *use* Lymphatic, Neck, Left
- *use* Lymphatic, Neck, Right

Mastoid air cells
- *use* Sinus, Mastoid, Left
- *use* Sinus, Mastoid, Right

Mastoid process
- *use* Bone, Temporal, Left
- *use* Bone, Temporal, Right

Mastoidectomy
- *see* Excision, Ear, Nose, Sinus 09B
- *see* Resection, Ear, Nose, Sinus 09T

Mastoidotomy
- *see* Drainage, Ear, Nose, Sinus 099

Mastopexy
- *see* Repair, Skin and Breast 0HQ
- *see* Reposition, Skin and Breast 0HS

Mastorrhaphy
- *see* Repair, Skin and Breast 0HQ

Mastotomy
- *see* Drainage, Skin and Breast 0H9

Maxillary artery
- *use* Artery, External Carotid, Left
- *use* Artery, External Carotid, Right

Maxillary nerve
- *use* Nerve, Trigeminal

Maximo II DR (VR)
- *use* Defibrillator Generator in 0JH

Maximo II DR CRT-D
- *use* Cardiac Resynchronization Defibrillator Pulse Generator in 0JH

Measurement
- Arterial
  - Flow
    - Coronary 4A03
    - Intracranial 4A03X5D
    - Peripheral 4A03
    - Pulmonary 4A03
  - Pressure
    - Coronary 4A03
    - Peripheral 4A03
    - Pulmonary 4A03
    - Thoracic, Other 4A03
  - Pulse
    - Coronary 4A03
    - Peripheral 4A03
    - Pulmonary 4A03
  - Saturation, Peripheral 4A03
  - Sound, Peripheral 4A03
- Biliary
  - Flow 4A0C
  - Pressure 4A0C
- Cardiac
  - Action Currents 4A02
  - Defibrillator 4B02XTZ
  - Electrical Activity 4A02
    - Guidance 4A02X4A
    - No Qualifier 4A02X4Z
  - Output 4A02
  - Pacemaker 4B02XSZ
  - Rate 4A02
  - Rhythm 4A02
  - Sampling and Pressure
    - Bilateral 4A02
    - Left Heart 4A02
    - Right Heart 4A02
  - Sound 4A02
  - Total Activity, Stress 4A02XM4
- Central Nervous
  - Cerebrospinal Fluid Shunt, Wireless Sensor 4B00XW0
  - Conductivity 4A00
  - Electrical Activity 4A00
  - Pressure 4A000BZ
    - Intracranial 4A00
  - Saturation, Intracranial 4A00
  - Stimulator 4B00XVZ
  - Temperature, Intracranial 4A00
- Circulatory, Volume 4A05XLZ
- Gastrointestinal
  - Motility 4A0B
  - Pressure 4A0B
  - Secretion 4A0B
- Lower Respiratory Fluid Nucleic Acid-base Microbial Detection XXEBXQ6
- Lymphatic
  - Flow 4A06
  - Pressure 4A06
- Metabolism 4A0Z
- Musculoskeletal
  - Contractility 4A0F
  - Pressure 4A0F3BE
  - Stimulator 4B0FXVZ
- Olfactory, Acuity 4A08X0Z
- Peripheral Nervous
  - Conductivity
    - Motor 4A01
    - Sensory 4A01

Measurement *(continued)*
Peripheral Nervous *(continued)*
Electrical Activity 4A01
Stimulator 4B01XVZ
Positive Blood Culture Fluorescence Hybridization for Organism Identification, Concentration and Susceptibility XXE5XN6
Products of Conception
Cardiac
Electrical Activity 4A0H
Rate 4A0H
Rhythm 4A0H
Sound 4A0HH
Nervous
Conductivity 4A0J
Electrical Activity 4A0J
Pressure 4A0J
Respiratory
Capacity 4A09
Flow 4A09
Pacemaker 4B09X
Rate 4A09
Resistance 4A09
Total Activity 4A09
Volume 4A09
Sleep 4A0ZXQZ
Temperature 4A0Z
Urinary
Contractility 4A0D
Flow 4A0D
Pressure 4A0D
Resistance 4A0D
Volume 4A0D
Venous
Flow
Central 4A04
Peripheral 4A04
Portal 4A04
Pulmonary 4A04
Pressure
Central 4A04
Peripheral 4A04
Portal 4A04
Pulmonary 4A04
Pulse
Central 4A04
Peripheral 4A04
Portal 4A04
Pulmonary 4A04
Saturation, Peripheral 4A04
Visual
Acuity 4A07X0Z
Mobility 4A07X7Z
Pressure 4A07XBZ
Whole Blood Nucleic Acid-base Microbial Detection XXE5XM5
Meatoplasty, urethra
see Repair, Urethra 0TQD
Meatotomy
see Drainage, Urinary System 0T9
Mechanical chest compression (mCPR) 5A1221J
Mechanical Initial Specimen Diversion Technique Using Active Negative Pressure (blood collection) XXE5XR7
Mechanical ventilation
see Performance, Respiratory 5A19
Medial canthus
use Eyelid, Lower, Left
use Eyelid, Lower, Right
Medial collateral ligament (MCL)
use Bursa and Ligament, Knee, Left
use Bursa and Ligament, Knee, Right
Medial condyle of femur
use Femur, Lower, Left
use Femur, Lower, Right
Medial condyle of tibia
use Tibia, Left
use Tibia, Right
Medial cuneiform bone
use Tarsal, Left
use Tarsal, Right
Medial epicondyle of femur
use Femur, Lower, Left
use Femur, Lower, Right
Medial epicondyle of humerus
use Humeral Shaft, Left
use Humeral Shaft, Right
Medial malleolus
use Tibia, Left
use Tibia, Right
Medial meniscus
use Joint, Knee, Left
use Joint, Knee, Right
Medial plantar artery
use Artery, Foot, Left
use Artery, Foot, Right
Medial plantar nerve
use Nerve, Tibial
Medial popliteal nerve
use Nerve, Tibial
Medial rectus muscle
use Muscle, Extraocular, Left
use Muscle, Extraocular, Right
Medial sural cutaneous nerve
use Nerve, Tibial
Median antebrachial vein
use Vein, Basilic, Left
use Vein, Basilic, Right
Median cubital vein
use Vein, Basilic, Left
use Vein, Basilic, Right
Median sacral artery
use Aorta, Abdominal
Mediastinal cavity
use Mediastinum
Mediastinal lymph node
use Lymphatic, Thorax
Mediastinal space
use Mediastinum
Mediastinoscopy 0WJC4ZZ
Medication Management GZ3ZZZZ
for substance abuse
Antabuse HZ83ZZZ
Bupropion HZ87ZZZ
Clonidine HZ86ZZZ
Levo-alpha-acetyl-methadol (LAAM) HZ82ZZZ
Methadone Maintenance HZ81ZZZ
Naloxone HZ85ZZZ
Naltrexone HZ84ZZZ
Nicotine Replacement HZ80ZZZ
Other Replacement Medication HZ89ZZZ
Psychiatric Medication HZ88ZZZ
Meditation 8E0ZXY5
Medtronic Endurant® II AAA stent graft system
use Intraluminal Device
Meissner's (submucous) plexus
use Nerve, Abdominal Sympathetic
Melody® transcatheter pulmonary valve
use Zooplastic Tissue in Heart and Great Vessels
Membranous urethra
use Urethra
Meningeorrhaphy
see Repair, Cerebral Meninges 00Q1
see Repair, Spinal Meninges 00QT
Meniscectomy, knee
see Excision, Joint, Knee, Left 0SBD
see Excision, Joint, Knee, Right 0SBC
Mental foramen
use Mandible, Left
use Mandible, Right
Mentalis muscle
use Muscle, Facial
Mentoplasty
see Alteration, Jaw, Lower 0W05
Meropenem-vaborbactam Anti-infective XW0
Mesenterectomy
see Excision, Mesentery 0DBV
Mesenteriorrhaphy, mesenterorrhaphy
see Repair, Mesentery 0DQV
Mesenteriplication
see Repair, Mesentery 0DQV
Mesoappendix
use Mesentery
Mesocolon
use Mesentery
Metacarpal ligament
use Bursa and Ligament, Hand, Left
use Bursa and Ligament, Hand, Right
Metacarpophalangeal ligament
use Bursa and Ligament, Hand, Left
use Bursa and Ligament, Hand, Right
Metal on metal bearing surface
use Synthetic Substitute, Metal in 0SR
Metatarsal ligament
use Bursa and Ligament, Foot, Left
use Bursa and Ligament, Foot, Right
Metatarsectomy
see Excision, Lower Bones 0QB
see Resection, Lower Bones 0QT
Metatarsophalangeal (MTP) joint
use Joint, Metatarsal-Phalangeal, Left
use Joint, Metatarsal-Phalangeal, Right
Metatarsophalangeal ligament
use Bursa and Ligament, Foot, Left
use Bursa and Ligament, Foot, Right
Metathalamus
use Thalamus
Micro-Driver stent (RX) (OTW)
use Intraluminal Device
MicroMed HeartAssist
use Implantable Heart Assist System in Heart and Great Vessels
Micrus CERECYTE microcoil
use Intraluminal Device, Bioactive in Upper Arteries
Midcarpal joint
use Joint, Carpal, Left
use Joint, Carpal, Right
Middle cardiac nerve
use Nerve, Thoracic Sympathetic
Middle cerebral artery
use Artery, Intracranial
Middle cerebral vein
use Vein, Intracranial
Middle colic vein
use Vein, Colic
Middle genicular artery
use Artery, Popliteal, Left
use Artery, Popliteal, Right
Middle hemorrhoidal vein
use Vein, Hypogastric, Left
use Vein, Hypogastric, Right
Middle rectal artery
use Artery, Internal Iliac, Left
use Artery, Internal Iliac, Right
Middle suprarenal artery
use Aorta, Abdominal
Middle temporal artery
use Artery, Temporal, Left
use Artery, Temporal, Right
Middle turbinate
use Turbinate, Nasal
Mineral-based Topical Hemostatic Agent XW0
MIRODERM™ Biologic Wound Matrix
use Skin Substitute, Porcine Liver Derived in New Technology
MitraClip valve repair system
use Synthetic Substitute
Mitral annulus
use Valve, Mitral
Mitroflow® Aortic Pericardial Heart Valve
use Zooplastic Tissue in Heart and Great Vessels
Mobilization, adhesions
see Release
Molar gland
use Buccal Mucosa
MolecuLight i:X® wound imaging
see Other Imaging, Anatomical Regions BW5
Monitoring
Arterial
Flow
Coronary 4A13
Peripheral 4A13
Pulmonary 4A13
Pressure
Coronary 4A13
Peripheral 4A13
Pulmonary 4A13
Pulse
Coronary 4A13
Peripheral 4A13
Pulmonary 4A13
Saturation, Peripheral 4A13
Sound, Peripheral 4A13
Cardiac
Electrical Activity 4A12
Ambulatory 4A12X45
No Qualifier 4A12X4Z
Output 4A12
Rate 4A12
Rhythm 4A12
Sound 4A12
Total Activity, Stress 4A12XM4
Vascular Perfusion, Indocyanine Green Dye 4A12XSH
Central Nervous
Conductivity 4A10
Electrical Activity
Intraoperative 4A10
No Qualifier 4A10
Pressure 4A100BZ
Intracranial 4A10
Saturation, Intracranial 4A10
Temperature, Intracranial 4A10
Gastrointestinal
Motility 4A1B
Pressure 4A1B
Secretion 4A1B
Vascular Perfusion, Indocyanine Green Dye 4A1BXSH
Kidney, Fluorescent Pyrazine XT25XE5
Lymphatic
Flow
Indocyanine Green Dye 4A16
No Qualifier A416
Pressure 4A16
Oxygen Saturation Endoscopic Imaging (OXEI) XD2

Monitoring *(continued)*
Peripheral Nervous
Conductivity
Motor 4A11
Sensory 4A11
Electrical Activity
Intraoperative 4A11
No Qualifier 4A11
Products of Conception
Cardiac
Electrical Activity 4A1H
Rate 4A1H
Rhythm 4A1H
Sound 4A1H
Nervous
Conductivity 4A1J
Electrical Activity 4A1J
Pressure 4A1J
Respiratory
Capacity 4A19
Flow 4A19
Rate 4A19
Resistance 4A19
Volume 4A19
Skin and Breast
Vascular Perfusion, Indocyanine Green Dye 4A1GXSH
Sleep 4A1ZXQZ
Temperature 4A1Z
Urinary
Contractility 4A1D
Flow 4A1D
Pressure 4A1D
Resistance 4A1D
Volume 4A1D
Venous
Flow
Central 4A14
Peripheral 4A14
Portal 4A14
Pulmonary 4A14
Pressure
Central 4A14
Peripheral 4A14
Portal 4A14
Pulmonary 4A14
Pulse
Central 4A14
Peripheral 4A14
Portal 4A14
Pulmonary 4A14
Saturation
Central 4A14
Portal 4A14
Pulmonary 4A14
Monitoring Device, Hemodynamic
Abdomen 0JH8
Chest 0JH6
Mosaic Bioprosthesis (aortic) (mitral) valve
use Zooplastic Tissue in Heart and Great Vessels
Motor Function Assessment F01
Motor Treatment F07
MR Angiography
see Magnetic Resonance Imaging (MRI), Heart B23
see Magnetic Resonance Imaging (MRI), Lower Arteries B43
see Magnetic Resonance Imaging (MRI), Upper Arteries B33
MULTI-LINK (VISION)(MINI-VISION)(ULTRA) Coronary Stent System
use Intraluminal Device
Multiple sleep latency test 4A0ZXQZ
Musculocutaneous nerve
use Nerve, Brachial Plexus
Musculopexy
see Repair, Muscles 0KQ
see Reposition, Muscles 0KS
Musculophrenic artery
use Artery, Internal Mammary, Left
use Artery, Internal Mammary, Right
Musculoplasty
see Repair, Muscles 0KQ
see Supplement, Muscles 0KU
Musculorrhaphy
see Repair, Muscles 0KQ
Musculospiral nerve
use Nerve, Radial
Myectomy
see Excision, Muscles 0KB
see Resection, Muscles 0KT
Myelencephalon
use Medulla Oblongata
Myelogram
CT
see Computerized Tomography (CT Scan), Central Nervous System B02
MRI
see Magnetic Resonance Imaging (MRI), Central Nervous System B03
Myenteric (Auerbach's) plexus
use Nerve, Abdominal Sympathetic
Myocardial Bridge Release
see Release, Artery, Coronary
Myomectomy
see Excision, Female Reproductive System 0UB
Myometrium
use Uterus
Myopexy
see Repair, Muscles 0KQ
see Reposition, Muscles 0KS
Myoplasty
see Repair, Muscles 0KQ
see Supplement, Muscles 0KU
Myorrhaphy
see Repair, Muscles 0KQ
Myoscopy
see Inspection, Muscles 0KJ
Myotomy
see Division, Muscles 0K8
see Drainage, Muscles 0K9
Myringectomy
see Excision, Ear, Nose, Sinus 09B
see Resection, Ear, Nose, Sinus 09T
Myringoplasty
see Repair, Ear, Nose, Sinus 09Q
see Replacement, Ear, Nose, Sinus 09R
see Supplement, Ear, Nose, Sinus 09U
Myringostomy
see Drainage, Ear, Nose, Sinus 099
Myringotomy
see Drainage, Ear, Nose, Sinus 099

N

NA-1 (Nerinitide)
use Nerinitide
Nafamostat Anticoagulant XY0YX37
Nail bed
use Finger Nail
use Toe Nail
Nail plate
use Finger Nail
use Toe Nail
nanoLOCK™ interbody fusion device
use Interbody Fusion Device, Nanotextured Surface in New Technology
Narcosynthesis GZGZZZZ
Narsoplimab Monoclonal Antibody XW0
Nasal cavity
use Nasal Mucosa and Soft Tissue
Nasal concha
use Turbinate, Nasal
Nasalis muscle
use Muscle, Facial
Nasolacrimal duct
use Duct, Lacrimal, Left
use Duct, Lacrimal, Right
Nasopharyngeal airway (NPA)
use Intraluminal Device, Airway in Ear, Nose, Sinus
Navicular bone
use Tarsal, Left
use Tarsal, Right
Near Infrared Spectroscopy, Circulatory System 8E02
Neck of femur
use Femur, Upper, Left
use Femur, Upper, Right
Neck of humerus (anatomical) (surgical)
use Humeral Head, Left
use Humeral Head, Right
Neovasc Reducer™
use Reduction Device in New Technology
Nephrectomy
see Excision, Urinary System 0TB
see Resection, Urinary System 0TT
Nephrolithotomy
see Extirpation, Urinary System 0TC
Nephrolysis
see Release, Urinary System 0TN
Nephropexy
see Repair, Urinary System 0TQ
see Reposition, Urinary System 0TS
Nephroplasty
see Repair, Urinary System 0TQ
see Supplement, Urinary System 0TU
Nephropyeloureterostomy
see Bypass, Urinary System 0T1
see Drainage, Urinary System 0T9
Nephrorrhaphy
see Repair, Urinary System 0TQ
Nephroscopy, transurethral 0TJ58ZZ
Nephrostomy
see Bypass, Urinary System 0T1
see Drainage, Urinary System 0T9
Nephrotomography
see Fluoroscopy, Urinary System BT1
see Plain Radiography, Urinary System BT0
Nephrotomy
see Division, Urinary System 0T8
see Drainage, Urinary System 0T9
Nerinitide XW0
Nerve conduction study
see Measurement, Central Nervous 4A00
see Measurement, Peripheral Nervous 4A01
Nerve Function Assessment F01
Nerve to the stapedius
use Nerve, Facial
Nesiritide
use Human B-type Natriuretic Peptide
Neurectomy
see Excision, Central Nervous System and Cranial Nerves 00B
see Excision, Peripheral Nervous System 01B
Neurexeresis
see Extraction, Central Nervous System and Cranial Nerves 00D
see Extraction, Peripheral Nervous System 01D
Neurohypophysis
use Gland, Pituitary
Neurolysis
see Release, Central Nervous System and Cranial Nerves 00N
see Release, Peripheral Nervous System 01N
Neuromuscular electrical stimulation (NEMS) lead
use Stimulator Lead in Muscles
Neurophysiologic monitoring
see Monitoring, Central Nervous 4A10
Neuroplasty
see Repair, Central Nervous System and Cranial Nerves 00Q
see Repair, Peripheral Nervous System 01Q
see Supplement, Central Nervous System and Cranial Nerves 00U
see Supplement, Peripheral Nervous System 01U
Neurorrhaphy
see Repair, Central Nervous System and Cranial Nerves 00Q
see Repair, Peripheral Nervous System 01Q
Neurostimulator Generator
Insertion of device in, Skull 0NH00NZ
Removal of device from, Skull 0NP00NZ
Revision of device in, Skull 0NW00NZ
Neurostimulator generator, multiple channel
use Stimulator Generator, Multiple Array in 0JH
Neurostimulator generator, multiple channel rechargeable
use Stimulator Generator, Multiple Array Rechargeable in 0JH
Neurostimulator generator, single channel
use Stimulator Generator, Single Array in 0JH
Neurostimulator generator, single channel rechargeable
use Stimulator Generator, Single Array Rechargeable in 0JH
Neurostimulator Lead
Insertion of device in
Brain 00H0
Cerebral Ventricle 00H6
Nerve
Cranial 00HE
Peripheral 01HY
Spinal Canal 00HU
Spinal Cord 00HV
Vein
Azygos 05H0
Innominate
Left 05H4
Right 05H3
Removal of device from
Brain 00P0
Cerebral Ventricle 00P6

Neurostimulator Lead *(continued)*
Removal of device from *(continued)*
Nerve
Cranial 00PE
Peripheral 01PY
Spinal Canal 00PU
Spinal Cord 00PV
Vein
Azygos 05P0
Innominate
Left 05P4
Right 05HP3
Revision of device in
Brain 00W0
Cerebral Ventricle 00W6
Nerve
Cranial 00WE
Peripheral 01WY
Spinal Canal 00WU
Spinal Cord 00WV
Vein
Azygos 05W0
Innominate
Left 05W4
Right 05HW3
Neurostimulator Lead in Oropharynx XWHD7Q7
Neurotomy
see Division, Central Nervous System and Cranial Nerves 008
see Division, Peripheral Nervous System and Cranial Nerves 018
Neurotripsy
see Destruction, Central Nervous System and Cranial Nerves 005
see Destruction, Peripheral Nervous System 015
Neutralization plate
use Internal Fixation Device in Head and Facial Bones
use Internal Fixation Device in Lower Bones
use Internal Fixation Device in Upper Bones
New Technology
Amivantamab Monoclonal Antibody XW0
Antibiotic-eluting Bone Void Filler XW0V0P7
Aorta
Thoracic Arch using Branched Synthetic Substitute with Intraluminal Device X2RX0N7
Thoracic Descending using Branched Synthetic Substitute with Intraluminal Device X2VW0N7
Apalutamide Antineoplstic XW0DJX5
Atezolizumab Antineoplastic XW0
Axicabtagene Ciloleucel Immunotherapy XW0
Bezlotoxumab Monoclonal Antibody XW0
Bioengineered Allogeneic Construct, Skin XHRPXF7
Brexanolone XW0
Brexucabtagene Autoleucel Immunotherapy XW0
Bromelain-enriched Proteolytic Enzyme XW0
Caplacizumab XW0
Cefiderocol Anti-infective XW0
Ceftolozane/Tazobactam Anti-infective XW0
Cerebral Embolic Filtration
Dual Filter X2A5312
Extracorporeal Flow Reversal Circuit X2A
Single Deflection Filter X2A6325

New Technology *(continued)*
Ciltacabtagene Autoleucel XW0
Coagulation Factor Xa, Inactivated XW0
Computer-aided Assessment, Intracranial Vascular Activity XXE0X07
Computer-aided Guidance, Transthoracic Echocardiography X2JAX47
Computer-aided Mechanical Aspiration X2C
Computer-aided Triage and Notification, Pulmonary Artery Flow XXE3X27
Concentrated Bone Marrow Aspirate XK02303
Coronary Sinus, Reduction Device X2V73Q7
Cytarabine and Daunorubicin Liposome Antineoplastic XW0
Defibrotide Sodium Anticoagulant XW0
Destruction, Prostate, Robotic Waterjet Ablation XV508A4
Dilation
Anterior Tibial
Left
Sustained Release Drug-eluting Intraluminal Device X27Q385
Four or More X27Q3C5
Three X27Q3B5
Two X27Q395
Right
Sustained Release Drug-eluting Intraluminal Device X27P385
Four or More X27P3C5
Three X27P3B5
Two X27P395
Femoral
Left
Sustained Release Drug-eluting Intraluminal Device X27J385
Four or More X27J3C5
Three X27J3B5
Two X27J395
Right
Sustained Release Drug-eluting Intraluminal Device X27H385
Four or More X27H3C5
Three X27H3B5
Two X27H395
Peroneal
Left
Sustained Release Drug-eluting Intraluminal Device X27U385
Four or More X27U3C5
Three X27U3B5
Two X27U395
Right
Sustained Release Drug-eluting Intraluminal Device X27T385
Four or More X27T3C5
Three X27T3B5
Two X27T395
Popliteal
Left Distal
Sustained Release Drug-eluting Intraluminal Device X27N385
Four or More X27N3C5
Three X27N3B5
Two X27N395

New Technology *(continued)*
Dilation *(continued)*
Popliteal *(continued)*
Left Proximal
Sustained Release Drug-eluting Intraluminal Device X27L385
Four or More X27L3C5
Three X27L3B5
Two X27L395
Right Distal
Sustained Release Drug-eluting Intraluminal Device X27M385
Four or More X27M3C5
Three X27M3B5
Two X27M395
Right Proximal
Sustained Release Drug-eluting Intraluminal Device X27K385
Four or More X27K3C5
Three X27QK3B5
Two X27K395
Posterior Tibial
Left
Sustained Release Drug-eluting Intraluminal Device X27S385
Four or More X27S3C5
Three X27S3B5
Two X27S395
Right
Sustained Release Drug-eluting Intraluminal Device X27R385
Four or More X27R3C5
Three X27R3B5
Two X27R395
Durvalumab Antineoplastic XW0
Eculizumab XW0
Eladocagene exuparvovec XW0Q316
Endothelial Damage Inhibitor XY0VX83
Engineered Chimeric Antigen Receptor T-cell Immunotherapy
Allogeneic XW0
Autologous XW0
Erdafitinib Antineoplastic XW0DXL5
Esketamine Hydrochloride XW097M5
Fosfomycin Anti-infective XW0
Fusion
Cervical Vertebral
2 or more
Nanotextured Surface XRG2092
Radiolucent Porous XRG20F3
Interbody Fusion Device
Nanotextured Surface XRG1092
Radiolucent Porous XRG10F3
Cervicothoracic Vertebral
Nanotextured Surface XRG4092
Radiolucent Porous XRG40F3
Lumbar Vertebral
2 or more
Customizable XRGC
Nanotextured Surface XRGC092
Radiolucent Porous XRGC0F3
Interbody Fusion Device
Customizable XRGB
Nanotextured Surface XRGB092
Radiolucent Porous XRGB0F3

New Technology *(continued)*
Fusion *(continued)*
Lumbosacral
Customizable XRGD
Nanotextured Surface XRGD092
Radiolucent Porous XRGD0F3
Occipital-cervical
Nanotextured Surface XRG0092
Radiolucent Porous XRG00F3
Thoracic Vertebral
2 to 7
Nanotextured Surface XRG7092
Radiolucent Porous XRG70F3
8 or more
Nanotextured Surface XRG8092
Radiolucent Porous XRG80F3
Interbody Fusion Device
Nanotextured Surface XRG6092
Radiolucent Porous XRG60F3
Thoracolumbar Vertebral
Customizable XRGA
Nanotextured Surface XRGA092
Radiolucent Porous XRGA0F3
Gilteritinib Antineoplastic XW0DXV5
High-Dose Intravenous Immune Globulin, for COVID-19 treatment XW1
Hyperimmune Globulin, for COVID-19 treatment XW1
Idecabtagene Vicleucel Immunotherapy XW0
Imipenem-cilastatin-relebactam Anti-infective XW0
Intracranial Arterial Flow, Whole Blood mRNA XXE5XT7
Iobenguane I-131 Antineoplastic XW0
Kidney, Fluorescent Pyrazine XT25XE5
Lefamulin Anti-infective XW0
Lifileucel Immunotherapy XW0
Lisocabtagene Maraleucel Immunotherapy XW0
Lower Respiratory Fluid Nucleic Acid-base Microbial Detection XXEBXQ6
Lurbinectedin XW0
Mechanical Initial Specimen Diversion Technique Using Active Negative Pressure (blood collection) XXE5XR7
Meropenem-vaborbactam Anti-infective XW0
Mineral-based Topical Hemostatic Agent XW0
Nafamostat Anticoagulant XY0YX37
Narsoplimab Monoclonal Antibody XW0
Nerinitide XW0
Neurostimulator Lead in Oropharynx XWHD7Q7
Omadacycline Anti-infective XW0
Other New Technology Therapeutic Substance XW0
Oxygen Saturation Endoscopic Imaging (OXEI) XD2
Plasma, Convalescent (Nonautologous) XW1
Plazomicin Anti-infective XW0

New Technology *(continued)*
- Positive Blood Culture Fluorescence Hybridization for Organism Identification, Concentration and Susceptibility XXE5XN6
- Radial artery aeriovenous fistula, using Thermal Resistance Energy X2K
- Remdesivir Anti-infective XW0
- Replacement
  - Skin Substitute, Porcine Liver Derived XHRPXL2
  - Zooplastic Tissue, Rapid Deployment Technique X2RF
- Reposition
  - Cervical, Magnetically Controlled Growth Rod(s) XNS3
  - Lumbar
    - Magnetically Controlled Growth Rod(s) XNS0
    - Posterior (Dynamic) Distraction Device XNS0
  - Thoracic
    - Magnetically Controlled Growth Rod(s) XNS4
    - Posterior (Dynamic) Distraction Device XNS4
- Ruxolitinib XW0DXT5
- Sarilumab XW0
- SARS-CoV-2 Antibody Detection, Serum/Plasma Nanoparticle Fluorescence XXE5XV7
- SARS-CoV-2 Polymerase Chain Reaction, Nasopharyngeal Fluid XXE97U7
- Satralizumab-mwge XW01397
- Single-use Duodenoscope XFJ
- Single-use Oversleeve with Intraoperative Colonic Irrigation XDPH8K7
- Supplement
  - Lumbar, Mechanically Expandable (Paired) Synthetic Substitute XNU0356
  - Thoracic, Mechanically Expandable (Paired) Synthetic Substitute XNU4356
- Synthetic Human Angiotensin II XW0
- Tagraxofusp-erzs Antineoplastic XW0
- Terlipressin XW0
- Tisagenlecleucel Immunotherapy XW0
- Tocilizumab XW0
- Trilaciclib XW0
- Uridine Triacetate XW0DX82
- Venetoclax Antineoplastic XW0DXR5
- Whole Blood Nucleic Acid-base Microbial Detection XXE5XM5

NexoBrid™
- *use* Bromelain-enriched Proteolytic Enzyme

Ninth cranial nerve
- *use* Nerve, Glossopharyngeal

NIRS (Near Infrared Spectroscopy)
- *see* Physiological Systems and Anatomical Regions 8E0

Nitinol framed polymer mesh
- *use* Synthetic Substitute

Niyad™
- *use* Nafamostat Anticoagulant

Non-tunneled central venous catheter
- *use* Infusion Device

Nonimaging Nuclear Medicine Assay
- Bladder, Kidneys and Ureters CT63
- Blood C763
- Kidneys, Ureters and Bladder CT63
- Lymphatics and Hematologic System C76YYZZ
- Ureters, Kidneys and Bladder CT63
- Urinary System CT6YYZZ

Nonimaging Nuclear Medicine Probe
- Abdomen CW50
- Abdomen and Chest CW54
- Abdomen and Pelvis CW51
- Brain C050
- Central Nervous System C05YYZZ
- Chest CW53ZZ
- Chest and Abdomen CW54
- Chest and Neck CW56
- Extremity
  - Lower CP5PZZZ
  - Upper CP5NZZZ
- Head and Neck CW5B
- Heart C25YYZZ
  - Right and Left C256
- Lymphatics
  - Head C75J
  - Head and Neck C755
  - Lower Extremity C75P
  - Neck C75K
  - Pelvic C75D
  - Trunk C75M
  - Upper Chest C75L
  - Upper Extremity C75N
- Lymphatics and Hematologic System C75YYZZ
- Musculoskeletal System, Other CP5YYZZ
- Neck and Chest CW56
- Neck and Head CW5B
- Pelvic Region CW5J
- Pelvis and Abdomen CW51
- Spine CP55ZZZ

Nonimaging Nuclear Medicine Uptake
- Endocrine System CG4YYZZ
- Gland, Thyroid CG42

Nostril
- *use* Nasal Mucosa and Soft Tissue

Novacor Left Ventricular Assist Device
- *use* Implantable Heart Assist System in Heart and Great Vessels

Novation® Ceramic AHS® (Articulation Hip System)
- *use* Synthetic Substitute, Ceramic in 0SR

Nuclear medicine
- *see* Nonimaging Nuclear Medicine Assay
- *see* Nonimaging Nuclear Medicine Probe
- *see* Nonimaging Nuclear Medicine Uptake
- *see* Planar Nuclear Medicine Imaging
- *see* Positron Emission Tomographic (PET) Imaging
- *see* Systemic Nuclear Medicine Therapy
- *see* Tomographic (Tomo) Nuclear Medicine Imaging

Nuclear scintigraphy
- *see* Nuclear Medicine

Nutrition, concentrated substances
- Enteral infusion 3E0G36Z
- Parenteral (peripheral) infusion
  - *see* Introduction of Nutritional Substance

NUZYRA™
- *use* Omadacycline Anti-infective

O

Obliteration
- *see* Destruction

Obturator artery
- *use* Artery, Internal Iliac, Left
- *use* Artery, Internal Iliac, Right

Obturator lymph node
- *use* Lymphatic, Pelvis

Obturator muscle
- *use* Muscle, Hip, Left
- *use* Muscle, Hip, Right

Obturator nerve
- *use* Nerve, Lumbar Plexus

Obturator vein
- *use* Vein, Hypogastric, Left
- *use* Vein, Hypogastric, Right

Obtuse margin
- *use* Heart, Left

Occipital artery
- *use* Artery, External Carotid, Left
- *use* Artery, External Carotid, Right

Occipital lobe
- *use* Cerebral Hemisphere

Occipital lymph node
- *use* Lymphatic, Neck, Left
- *use* Lymphatic, Neck, Right

Occipitofrontalis muscle
- *use* Muscle, Facial

Occlusion
- Ampulla of Vater 0FLC
- Anus 0DLQ
- Aorta
  - Abdominal 04L0
  - Thoracic, Descending 02LW3DJ
- Artery
  - Anterior Tibial
    - Left 04LQ
    - Right 04LP
  - Axillary
    - Left 03L6
    - Right 03L5
  - Brachial
    - Left 03L8
    - Right 03L7
  - Celiac 04L1
  - Colic
    - Left 04L7
    - Middle 04L8
    - Right 04L6
  - Common Carotid
    - Left 03LJ
    - Right 03LH
  - Common Iliac
    - Left 04LD
    - Right 04LC
  - External Carotid
    - Left 03LN
    - Right 03LM
  - External Iliac
    - Left 04LJ
    - Right 04LH
  - Face 03LR
  - Femoral
    - Left 04LL
    - Right 04LK
  - Foot
    - Left 04LW
    - Right 04LV
  - Gastric 04L2
  - Hand
    - Left 03LF
    - Right 03LD
  - Hepatic 04L3
  - Inferior Mesenteric 04LB
  - Innominate 03L2

Occlusion *(continued)*
- Artery *(continued)*
  - Internal Carotid
    - Left 03LL
    - Right 03LK
  - Internal Iliac
    - Left 04LF
    - Right 04LE
  - Internal Mammary
    - Left 03L1
    - Right 03L0
  - Intracranial 03LG
  - Lower 04LY
  - Peroneal
    - Left 04LU
    - Right 04LT
  - Popliteal
    - Left 04LN
    - Right 04LM
  - Posterior Tibial
    - Left 04LS
    - Right 04LR
  - Pulmonary
    - Left 02LR
    - Right 02LQ
  - Pulmonary Trunk 02LP
  - Radial
    - Left 03LC
    - Right 03LB
  - Renal
    - Left 04LA
    - Right 04L9
  - Splenic 04L4
  - Subclavian
    - Left 03L4
    - Right 03L3
  - Superior Mesenteric 04L5
  - Temporal
    - Left 03LT
    - Right 03LS
  - Thyroid
    - Left 03LV
    - Right 03LU
  - Ulnar
    - Left 03LA
    - Right 03L9
  - Upper 03LY
  - Vertebral
    - Left 03LQ
    - Right 03LP
- Atrium, Left 02L7
- Bladder 0TLB
- Bladder Neck 0TLC
- Bronchus
  - Lingula 0BL9
  - Lower Lobe
    - Left 0BLB
    - Right 0BL6
  - Main
    - Left 0BL7
    - Right 0BL3
  - Middle Lobe, Right 0BL5
  - Upper Lobe
    - Left 0BL8
    - Right 0BL4
- Carina 0BL2
- Cecum 0DLH
- Cisterna Chyli 07LL
- Colon
  - Ascending 0DLK
  - Descending 0DLM
  - Sigmoid 0DLN
  - Transverse 0DLL
- Cord
  - Bilateral 0VLH
  - Left 0VLG
  - Right 0VLF
- Cul-de-sac 0ULF
- Duct
  - Common Bile 0FL9
  - Cystic 0FL8

Occlusion *(continued)*
Duct *(continued)*
  Hepatic
    Common 0FL7
    Left 0FL6
    Right 0FL5
  Lacrimal
    Left 08LY
    Right 08LX
  Pancreatic 0FLD
    Accessory 0FLF
  Parotid
    Left 0CLC
    Right 0CLB
Duodenum 0DL9
Esophagogastric Junction 0DL4
Esophagus 0DL5
  Lower 0DL3
  Middle 0DL2
  Upper 0DL1
Fallopian Tube
  Left 0UL6
  Right 0UL5
Fallopian Tubes, Bilateral 0UL7
Ileocecal Valve 0DLC
Ileum 0DLB
Intestine
  Large 0DLE
    Left 0DLG
    Right 0DLF
  Small 0DL8
Jejunum 0DLA
Kidney Pelvis
  Left 0TL4
  Right 0TL3
Left atrial appendage (LAA)
  see Occlusion, Atrium, Left 02L7
Lymphatic
  Aortic 07LD
  Axillary
    Left 07L6
    Right 07L5
  Head 07L0
  Inguinal
    Left 07LJ
    Right 07LH
  Internal Mammary
    Left 07L9
    Right 07L8
  Lower Extremity
    Left 07LG
    Right 07LF
  Mesenteric 07LB
  Neck
    Left 07L2
    Right 07L1
  Pelvis 07LC
  Thoracic Duct 07LK
  Thorax 07L7
  Upper Extremity
    Left 07L4
    Right 07L3
Rectum 0DLP
Stomach 0DL6
  Pylorus 0DL7
Trachea 0BL1
Ureter
  Left 0TL7
  Right 0TL6
Urethra 0TLD
Vagina 0ULG
Valve, Pulmonary 02LH
Vas Deferens
  Bilateral 0VLQ
  Left 0VLP
  Right 0VLN
Vein
  Axillary
    Left 05L8
    Right 05L7

Occlusion *(continued)*
Vein *(continued)*
  Azygos 05L0
  Basilic
    Left 05LC
    Right 05LB
  Brachial
    Left 05LA
    Right 05L9
  Cephalic
    Left 05LF
    Right 05LD
  Colic 06L7
  Common Iliac
    Left 06LD
    Right 06LC
  Esophageal 06L3
  External Iliac
    Left 06LG
    Right 06LF
  External Jugular
    Left 05LQ
    Right 05LP
  Face
    Left 05LV
    Right 05LT
  Femoral
    Left 06LN
    Right 06LM
  Foot
    Left 06LV
    Right 06LT
  Gastric 06L2
  Hand
    Left 05LH
    Right 05LG
  Hemiazygos 05L1
  Hepatic 06L4
  Hypogastric
    Left 06LJ
    Right 06LH
  Inferior Mesenteric 06L6
  Innominate
    Left 05L4
    Right 05L3
  Internal Jugular
    Left 05LN
    Right 05LM
  Intracranial 05LL
  Lower 06LY
  Portal 06L8
  Pulmonary
    Left 02LT
    Right 02LS
  Renal
    Left 06LB
    Right 06L9
  Saphenous
    Left 06LQ
    Right 06LP
  Splenic 06L1
  Subclavian
    Left 05L6
    Right 05L5
  Superior Mesenteric 06L5
  Upper 05LY
  Vertebral
    Left 05LS
    Right 05LR
Vena Cava
  Inferior 06L0
  Superior 02LV
Occlusion, REBOA (resuscitative endovascular balloon occlusion of the aorta)
02LW3DJ
04L03DJ
Occupational therapy
  see Activities of Daily Living Treatment, Rehabilitation F08
Octagam 10%, for COVID-19 treatment
  use High-Dose Intravenous Immune Globulin
Odentectomy
  see Excision, Mouth and Throat 0CB
  see Resection, Mouth and Throat 0CT
Odontoid process
  use Cervical Vertebra
Olecranon bursa
  use Bursa and Ligament, Elbow, Left
  use Bursa and Ligament, Elbow, Right
Olecranon process
  use Ulna, Left
  use Ulna, Right
Olfactory bulb
  use Nerve, Olfactory
Omadacycline Anti-infective XW0
Omentectomy, omentumectomy
  see Excision, Gastrointestinal System 0DB
  see Resection, Gastrointestinal System 0DT
Omentofixation
  see Repair, Gastrointestinal System 0DQ
Omentoplasty
  see Repair, Gastrointestinal System 0DQ
  see Replacement, Gastrointestinal System 0DR
  see Supplement, Gastrointestinal System 0DU
Omentorrhaphy
  see Repair, Gastrointestinal System 0DQ
Omentotomy
  see Drainage, Gastrointestinal System 0D9
Omnilink Elite Vascular Balloon Expandable Stent System
  use Intraluminal Device
Onychectomy
  see Excision, Skin and Breast 0HB
  see Resection, Skin and Breast 0HT
Onychoplasty
  see Repair, Skin and Breast 0HQ
  see Replacement, Skin and Breast 0HR
Onychotomy
  see Drainage, Skin and Breast 0H9
Oophorectomy
  see Excision, Female Reproductive System 0UB
  see Resection, Female Reproductive System 0UT
Oophoropexy
  see Repair, Female Reproductive System 0UQ
  see Reposition, Female Reproductive System 0US
Oophoroplasty
  see Repair, Female Reproductive System 0UQ
  see Supplement, Female Reproductive System 0UU
Oophororrhaphy
  see Repair, Female Reproductive System 0UQ
Oophorostomy
  see Drainage, Female Reproductive System 0U9
Oophorotomy
  see Drainage, Female Reproductive System 0U9
  see Division, Female Reproductive System 0U8
Oophorrhaphy
  see Repair, Female Reproductive System 0UQ
Open Pivot (mechanical) valve
  use Synthetic Substitute
Open Pivot Aortic Valve Graft (AVG)
  use Synthetic Substitute
Ophthalmic artery
  use Intracranial Artery
Ophthalmic nerve
  use Nerve, Trigeminal
Ophthalmic vein
  use Vein, Intracranial
Opponensplasty
  Tendon replacement
    see Replacement, Tendons 0LR
  Tendon transfer
    see Transfer, Tendons 0LX
Optic chiasma
  use Nerve, Optic
Optic disc
  use Retina, Left
  use Retina, Right
Optic foramen
  use Bone, Sphenoid
Optical coherence tomography, intravascular
  see Computerized Tomography (CT Scan)
Optimizer™ III implantable pulse generator
  use Contractility Modulation Device in 0JH
Orbicularis oculi muscle
  use Eyelid, Upper, Left
  use Eyelid, Upper, Right
Orbicularis oris muscle
  use Muscle, Facial
Orbital Atherectomy
  see Extirpation, Heart and Great Vessels 02C
Orbital fascia
  use Subcutaneous Tissue and Fascia, Face
Orbital portion of ethmoid bone
  use Orbit, Left
  use Orbit, Right
Orbital portion of frontal bone
  use Orbit, Left
  use Orbit, Right
Orbital portion of lacrimal bone
  use Orbit, Left
  use Orbit, Right
Orbital portion of maxilla
  use Orbit, Left
  use Orbit, Right
Orbital portion of palatine bone
  use Orbit, Left
  use Orbit, Right
Orbital portion of sphenoid bone
  use Orbit, Left
  use Orbit, Right
Orbital portion of zygomatic bone
  use Orbit, Left
  use Orbit, Right
Orchectomy, orchidectomy, orchiectomy
  see Excision, Male Reproductive System 0VB
  see Resection, Male Reproductive System 0VT
Orchidoplasty, orchioplasty
  see Repair, Male Reproductive System 0VQ
  see Replacement, Male Reproductive System 0VR
  see Supplement, Male Reproductive System 0VU
Orchidorrhaphy, orchiorrhaphy
  see Repair, Male Reproductive System 0VQ

Orchidotomy, orchiotomy, orchotomy
see Drainage, Male Reproductive System 0V9
Orchiopexy
see Repair, Male Reproductive System 0VQ
see Reposition, Male Reproductive System 0VS
Oropharyngeal airway (OPA)
use Intraluminal Device, Airway in Mouth and Throat
Oropharynx
use Pharynx
Ossiculectomy
see Excision, Ear, Nose, Sinus 09B
see Resection, Ear, Nose, Sinus 09T
Ossiculotomy
see Drainage, Ear, Nose, Sinus 099
Ostectomy
see Excision, Head and Facial Bones 0NB
see Excision, Lower Bones 0QB
see Excision, Upper Bones 0PB
see Resection, Head and Facial Bones 0NT
see Resection, Lower Bones 0QT
see Resection, Upper Bones 0PT
Osteoclasis
see Division, Head and Facial Bones 0N8
see Division, Lower Bones 0Q8
see Division, Upper Bones 0P8
Osteolysis
see Release, Head and Facial Bones 0NN
see Release, Lower Bones 0QN
see Release, Upper Bones 0PN
Osteopathic Treatment
Abdomen 7W09X
Cervical 7W01X
Extremity
Lower 7W06X
Upper 7W07X
Head 7W00X
Lumbar 7W03X
Pelvis 7W05X
Rib Cage 7W08X
Sacrum 7W04X
Thoracic 7W02X
Osteopexy
see Repair, Head and Facial Bones 0NQ
see Repair, Lower Bones 0QQ
see Repair, Upper Bones 0PQ
see Reposition, Head and Facial Bones 0NS
see Reposition, Lower Bones 0QS
see Reposition, Upper Bones 0PS
Osteoplasty
see Repair, Head and Facial Bones 0NQ
see Repair, Lower Bones 0QQ
see Repair, Upper Bones 0PQ
see Replacement, Head and Facial Bones 0NR
see Replacement, Lower Bones 0QR
see Replacement, Upper Bones 0PR
see Supplement, Head and Facial Bones 0NU
see Supplement, Lower Bones 0QU
see Supplement, Upper Bones 0PU
Osteorrhaphy
see Repair, Head and Facial Bones 0NQ
see Repair, Lower Bones 0QQ
see Repair, Upper Bones 0PQ
Osteotomy, ostotomy
see Division, Head and Facial Bones 0N8
see Division, Lower Bones 0Q8
see Division, Upper Bones 0P8
see Drainage, Head and Facial Bones 0N9
see Drainage, Lower Bones 0Q9
see Drainage, Upper Bones 0P9
Other Imaging
Bile Duct, Indocyanine Green Dye, Intraoperative BF50200
Bile Duct and Gallbladder, Indocyanine Green Dye, Intraoperative BF53200
Extremity
Lower BW5CZ1Z
Upper BW5JZ1Z
Gallbladder, Indocyanine Green Dye, Intraoperative BF52200
Gallbladder and Bile Duct, Indocyanine Green Dye, Intraoperative BF53200
Head and Neck BW59Z1Z
Hepatobiliary System, All, Indocyanine Green Dye, Intraoperative BF5C200
Liver, Indocyanine Green Dye, Intraoperative BF55200
Liver and Spleen, Indocyanine Green Dye, Intraoperative BF56200
Neck and Head BW59Z1Z
Pancreas, Indocyanine Green Dye, Intraoperative BF57200
Spleen and Liver, Indocyanine Green Dye, Intraoperative BF56200
Trunk BW52Z1Z
Other New Technology Therapeutic Substance XW0
Otic ganglion
use Nerve, Head and Neck Sympathetic
OTL-101
use Hematopoietic Stem/Progenitor Cells, Genetically Modified
OTL-103
use Hematopoietic Stem/Progenitor Cells, Genetically Modified
OTL-200
use Hematopoietic Stem/Progenitor Cells, Genetically Modified
Otoplasty
see Repair, Ear, Nose, Sinus 09Q
see Replacement, Ear, Nose, Sinus 09R
see Supplement, Ear, Nose, Sinus 09U
Otoscopy
see Inspection, Ear, Nose, Sinus 09J
Oval window
use Ear, Middle, Left
use Ear, Middle, Right
Ovarian artery
use Aorta, Abdominal
Ovarian ligament
use Uterine Supporting Structure
Ovariectomy
see Excision, Female Reproductive System 0UB
see Resection, Female Reproductive System 0UT
Ovariocentesis
see Drainage, Female Reproductive System 0U9
Ovariopexy
see Repair, Female Reproductive System 0UQ
see Reposition, Female Reproductive System 0US
Ovariotomy
see Division, Female Reproductive System 0U8
see Drainage, Female Reproductive System 0U9
Ovatio™ CRT-D
use Cardiac Resynchronization Defibrillator Pulse Generator in 0JH
Oversewing
Gastrointestinal ulcer
see Repair, Gastrointestinal System 0DQ
Pleural bleb
see Repair, Respiratory System 0BQ
Oviduct
use Fallopian Tube, Left
use Fallopian Tube, Right
Oximetry, Fetal pulse 10H073Z
OXINIUM
use Synthetic Substitute, Oxidized Zirconium on Polyethylene in 0SR
Oxygen Saturation Endoscopic Imaging (OXEI) XD2
Oxygenation
Extracorporeal membrane (ECMO)
see Performance, Circulatory 5A15
Hyperbaric
see Assistance, Circulatory 5A05
Supersaturated
see Assistance, Circulatory 5A05

P

Pacemaker
Dual Chamber
Abdomen 0JH8
Chest 0JH6
Intracardiac
Insertion of device in
Atrium
Left 02H7
Right 02H6
Vein, Coronary 02H4
Ventricle
Left 02HL
Right 02HK
Removal of device from
Heart 02PA
Revision of device in
Heart 02WA
Single Chamber
Abdomen 0JH8
Chest 0JH6
Single Chamber Rate Responsive
Abdomen 0JH8
Chest 0JH6
Packing
Abdominal Wall 2W43X5Z
Anorectal 2Y43X5Z
Arm
Lower
Left 2W4DX5Z
Right 2W4CX5Z
Upper
Left 2W4BX5Z
Right 2W4AX5Z
Back 2W45X5Z
Chest Wall 2W44X5Z
Ear 2Y42X5Z
Extremity
Lower
Left 2W4MX5Z
Right 2W4LX5Z
Upper
Left 2W49X5Z
Right 2W48X5Z
Face 2W41X5Z
Packing *(continued)*
Finger
Left 2W4KX5Z
Right 2W4JX5Z
Foot
Left 2W4TX5Z
Right 2W4SX5Z
Genital Tract, Female 2Y44X5Z
Hand
Left 2W4FX5Z
Right 2W4EX5Z
Head 2W40X5Z
Inguinal Region
Left 2W47X5Z
Right 2W46X5Z
Leg
Lower
Left 2W4RX5Z
Right 2W4QX5Z
Upper
Left 2W4PX5Z
Right 2W4NX5Z
Mouth and Pharynx 2Y40X5Z
Nasal 2Y41X5Z
Neck 2W42X5Z
Thumb
Left 2W4HX5Z
Right 2W4GX5Z
Toe
Left 2W4VX5Z
Right 2W4UX5Z
Urethra 2Y45X5Z
Paclitaxel-eluting coronary stent
use Intraluminal Device, Drug-eluting in Heart and Great Vessels
Paclitaxel-eluting peripheral stent
use Intraluminal Device, Drug-eluting in Lower Arteries
use Intraluminal Device, Drug-eluting in Upper Arteries
Palatine gland
use Buccal Mucosa
Palatine tonsil
use Tonsils
Palatine uvula
use Uvula
Palatoglossal muscle
use Muscle, Tongue, Palate, Pharynx
Palatopharyngeal muscle
use Muscle, Tongue, Palate, Pharynx
Palatoplasty
see Repair, Mouth and Throat 0CQ
see Replacement, Mouth and Throat 0CR
see Supplement, Mouth and Throat 0CU
Palatorrhaphy
see Repair, Mouth and Throat 0CQ
Palmar (volar) digital vein
use Vein, Hand, Left
use Vein, Hand, Right
Palmar (volar) metacarpal vein
use Vein, Hand, Left
use Vein, Hand, Right
Palmar cutaneous nerve
use Nerve, Median
use Nerve, Radial
Palmar fascia (aponeurosis)
use Subcutaneous Tissue and Fascia, Hand, Left
use Subcutaneous Tissue and Fascia, Hand, Right
Palmar interosseous muscle
use Muscle, Hand, Left
use Muscle, Hand, Right

Palmar ulnocarpal ligament
use Bursa and Ligament, Wrist, Left
use Bursa and Ligament, Wrist, Right
Palmaris longus muscle
use Muscle, Lower Arm and Wrist, Left
use Muscle, Lower Arm and Wrist, Right
Pancreatectomy
see Excision, Pancreas 0FBG
see Resection, Pancreas 0FTG
Pancreatic artery
use Artery, Splenic
Pancreatic plexus
use Nerve, Abdominal Sympathetic
Pancreatic vein
use Vein, Splenic
Pancreaticoduodenostomy
see Bypass, Hepatobiliary System and Pancreas 0F1
Pancreaticosplenic lymph node
use Lymphatic, Aortic
Pancreatogram, endoscopic retrograde
see Fluoroscopy, Pancreatic Duct BF18
Pancreatolithotomy
see Extirpation, Pancreas 0FCG
Pancreatotomy
see Division, Pancreas 0F8G
see Drainage, Pancreas 0F9G
Panniculectomy
see Excision, Skin, Abdomen 0HB7
see Excision, Subcutaneous Tissue and Fascia, Abdomen 0JB8
Paraaortic lymph node
use Lymphatic, Aortic
Paracentesis
Eye
see Drainage, Eye 089
Peritoneal Cavity
see Drainage, Peritoneal Cavity 0W9G
Tympanum
see Drainage, Ear, Nose, Sinus 099
Parapharyngeal space
use Neck
Pararectal lymph node
use Lymphatic, Mesenteric
Parasternal lymph node
use Lymphatic, Thorax
Parathyroidectomy
see Excision, Endocrine System 0GB
see Resection, Endocrine System 0GT
Paratracheal lymph node
use Lymphatic, Thorax
Paraurethral (Skene's) gland
use Gland, Vestibular
Parenteral nutrition, total
see Introduction of Nutritional Substance
Parietal lobe
use Cerebral Hemisphere
Parotid lymph node
use Lymphatic, Head
Parotid plexus
use Nerve, Facial
Parotidectomy
see Excision, Mouth and Throat 0CB
see Resection, Mouth and Throat 0CT
Pars flaccida
use Tympanic Membrane, Left
use Tympanic Membrane, Right
Partial joint replacement
Hip
see Replacement, Lower Joints 0SR
Knee
see Replacement, Lower Joints 0SR
Shoulder
see Replacement, Upper Joints 0RR
Partially absorbable mesh
use Synthetic Substitute
Patch, blood, spinal 3E0R3GC
Patellapexy
see Repair, Lower Bones 0QQ
see Reposition, Lower Bones 0QS
Patellaplasty
see Repair, Lower Bones 0QQ
see Replacement, Lower Bones 0QR
see Supplement, Lower Bones 0QU
Patellar ligament
use Bursa and Ligament, Knee, Left
use Bursa and Ligament, Knee, Right
Patellar tendon
use Tendon, Knee, Left
use Tendon, Knee, Right
Patellectomy
see Excision, Lower Bones 0QB
see Resection, Lower Bones 0QT
Patellofemoral joint
use Joint, Knee, Left
use Joint, Knee, Left, Femoral Surface
use Joint, Knee, Right
use Joint, Knee, Right, Femoral Surface
pAVF (percutaneous arteriovenous fistula), using magnetic-guided radiofrequency
see Bypass, Upper Arteries 031
pAVF (percutaneous arteriovenous fistula), using thermal resistance energy
see New Technology, Cardiovascular System X2K
Pectineus muscle
use Muscle, Upper Leg, Left
use Muscle, Upper Leg, Right
Pectoral (anterior) lymph node
use Lymphatic, Axillary, Left
use Lymphatic, Axillary, Right
Pectoral fascia
use Subcutaneous Tissue and Fascia, Chest
Pectoralis major muscle
use Muscle, Thorax, Left
use Muscle, Thorax, Right
Pectoralis minor muscle
use Muscle, Thorax, Left
use Muscle, Thorax, Right
Pedicle-based dynamic stabilization device
use Spinal Stabilization Device, Pedicle-Based in 0RH
use Spinal Stabilization Device, Pedicle-Based in 0SH
PEEP (positive end expiratory pressure)
see Assistance, Respiratory 5A09
PEG (percutaneous endoscopic gastrostomy) 0DH63UZ
PEJ (percutaneous endoscopic jejunostomy) 0DHA3UZ
Pelvic splanchnic nerve
use Nerve, Abdominal Sympathetic
use Nerve, Sacral Sympathetic
Penectomy
see Excision, Male Reproductive System 0VB
see Resection, Male Reproductive System 0VT
Penile urethra
use Urethra
Penumbra Indigo® Aspiration System
see New Technology, Cardiovascular System X2C
PERCEPT™ neurostimulator
use Stimulator Generator, Multiple Array in 0JH
Perceval sutureless valve
use Zooplastic Tissue, Rapid Deployment Technique in New Technology
Percutaneous endoscopic gastrojejunostomy (PEG/J) tube
use Feeding Device in Gastrointestinal System
Percutaneous endoscopic gastrostomy (PEG) tube
use Feeding Device in Gastrointestinal System
Percutaneous nephrostomy catheter
use Drainage Device
Percutaneous transluminal coronary angioplasty (PTCA)
see Dilation, Heart and Great Vessels 027
Performance
Biliary
Multiple, Filtration 5A1C60Z
Single, Filtration 5A1C00Z
Cardiac
Continuous
Output 5A1221Z
Pacing 5A1223Z
Intermittent, Pacing 5A1213Z
Single, Output, Manual 5A12012
Circulatory
Continuous
Central Membrane 5A1522F
Peripheral Veno-arterial Membrane 5A1522G
Peripheral Veno-venous Membrane 5A1522H
Intraoperative
Central Membrane 5A15A2F
Peripheral Veno-arterial Membrane 5A15A2G
Peripheral Veno-venous Membrane 5A15A2H
Respiratory
24-96 Consecutive Hours, Ventilation 5A1945Z
Greater than 96 Consecutive Hours, Ventilation 5A1955Z
Less than 24 Consecutive Hours, Ventilation 5A1935Z
Single, Ventilation, Nonmechanical5A19054
Urinary
Continuous, Greater than 18 hours per day, Filtration 5A1D90Z
Intermittent, Less than 6 hours per day, Filtration 5A1D70Z
Prolonged Intermittent, 6-18 hours per day, Filtration 5A1D80Z
Perfusion
see Introduction of substance in or on
Perfusion, donor organ
Heart 6AB50BZ
Kidney(s) 6ABT0BZ
Liver 6ABF0BZ
Lung(s) 6ABB0BZ
Pericardiectomy
see Excision, Pericardium 02BN
see Resection, Pericardium 02TN
Pericardiocentesis
see Drainage, Pericardial Cavity 0W9D
Pericardiolysis
see Release, Pericardium 02NN
Pericardiophrenic artery
use Artery, Internal Mammary, Left
use Artery, Internal Mammary, Right
Pericardioplasty
see Repair, Pericardium 02QN
see Replacement, Pericardium 02RN
see Supplement, Pericardium 02UN
Pericardiorrhaphy
see Repair, Pericardium 02QN
Pericardiostomy
see Drainage, Pericardial Cavity 0W9D
Pericardiotomy
see Drainage, Pericardial Cavity 0W9D
Perimetrium
use Uterus
Peripheral Intravascular Lithotripsy (Peripheral IVL)
see Fragmentation
Peripheral parenteral nutrition
see Introduction of Nutritional Substance
Peripherally inserted central catheter (PICC)
use Infusion Device
Peritoneal dialysis 3E1M39Z
Peritoneocentesis
see Drainage, Peritoneal Cavity 0W9G
see Drainage, Peritoneum 0D9W
Peritoneoplasty
see Repair, Peritoneum 0DQW
see Replacement, Peritoneum 0DRW
see Supplement, Peritoneum 0DUW
Peritoneoscopy 0DJW4ZZ
Peritoneotomy
see Drainage, Peritoneum 0D9W
Peritoneumectomy
see Excision, Peritoneum 0DBW
Peroneus brevis muscle
use Muscle, Lower Leg, Left
use Muscle, Lower Leg, Right
Peroneus longus muscle
use Muscle, Lower Leg, Left
use Muscle, Lower Leg, Right
Pessary ring
use Intraluminal Device, Pessary in Female Reproductive System
PET scan
see Positron Emission Tomographic (PET) Imaging
Petrous part of temoporal bone
use Bone, Temporal, Left
use Bone, Temporal, Right
Phacoemulsification, lens
With IOL implant
see Replacement, Eye 08R
Without IOL implant
see Extraction, Eye 08D
Phagenyx® System XWHD7Q7
Phalangectomy
see Excision, Lower Bones 0QB
see Excision, Upper Bones 0PB
see Resection, Lower Bones 0QT
see Resection, Upper Bones 0PT

Phallectomy
see Excision, Penis 0VBS
see Resection, Penis 0VTS
Phalloplasty
see Repair, Penis 0VQS
see Supplement, Penis 0VUS
Phallotomy
see Drainage, Penis 0V9S
Pharmacotherapy, for substance abuse
Antabuse HZ93ZZZ
Bupropion HZ97ZZZ
Clonidine HZ96ZZZ
Levo-alpha-acetyl-methadol (LAAM) HZ92ZZZ
Methadone Maintenance HZ91ZZZ
Naloxone HZ95ZZZ
Naltrexone HZ94ZZZ
Nicotine Replacement HZ90ZZZ
Psychiatric Medication HZ98ZZZ
Replacement Medication, Other HZ99ZZZ
Pharyngeal constrictor muscle
use Muscle, Tongue, Palate, Pharynx
Pharyngeal plexus
use Nerve, Vagus
Pharyngeal recess
use Nasopharynx
Pharyngeal tonsil
use Adenoids
Pharyngogram
see Fluoroscopy, Pharynix B91G
Pharyngoplasty
see Repair, Mouth and Throat 0CQ
see Replacement, Mouth and Throat 0CR
see Supplement, Mouth and Throat 0CU
Pharyngorrhaphy
see Repair, Mouth and Throat 0CQ
Pharyngotomy
see Drainage, Mouth and Throat 0C9
Pharyngotympanic tube
use Eustachian Tube, Left
use Eustachian Tube, Right
Pheresis
Erythrocytes 6A55
Leukocytes 6A55
Plasma 6A55
Platelets 6A55
Stem Cells
Cord Blood 6A55
Hematopoietic 6A55
Phlebectomy
see Excision, Lower Veins 06B
see Excision, Upper Veins 05B
see Extraction, Lower Veins 06D
see Extraction, Upper Veins 05D
Phlebography
see Plain Radiography, Veins B50
Impedance 4A04X51
Phleborrhaphy
see Repair, Lower Veins 06Q
see Repair, Upper Veins 05Q
Phlebotomy
see Drainage, Lower Veins 069
see Drainage, Upper Veins 059
Photocoagulation
For Destruction
see Destruction
For Repair
see Repair
Photopheresis, therapeutic
see Phototherapy, Circulatory 6A65
Phototherapy
Circulatory 6A65
Skin 6A60

Phototherapy *(continued)*
Ultraviolet light
see Ultraviolet Light Therapy, Physiological Systems 6A8
Phrenectomy, phrenoneurectomy
see Excision, Nerve, Phrenic 01B2
Phrenemphraxis
see Destruction, Nerve, Phrenic 0152
Phrenic nerve stimulator generator
use Stimulator Generator in Subcutaneous Tissue and Fascia
Phrenic nerve stimulator lead
use Diaphragmatic Pacemaker Lead in Respiratory System
Phreniclasis
see Destruction, Nerve, Phrenic 0152
Phrenicoexeresis
see Extraction, Nerve, Phrenic 01D2
Phrenicotomy
see Division, Nerve, Phrenic 0182
Phrenicotripsy
see Destruction, Nerve, Phrenic 0152
Phrenoplasty
see Repair, Respiratory System 0BQ
see Supplement, Respiratory System 0BU
Phrenotomy
see Drainage, Respiratory System 0B9
Physiatry
see Motor Treatment, Rehabilitation F07
Physical medicine
see Motor Treatment, Rehabilitation F07
Physical therapy
see Motor Treatment, Rehabilitation F07
PHYSIOMESH™ Flexible Composite Mesh
use Synthetic Substitute
Pia mater, intracranial
use Cerebral Meninges
Pia mater, spinal
use Spinal Meninges
Pinealectomy
see Excision, Pineal Body 0GB1
see Resection, Pineal Body 0GT1
Pinealoscopy 0GJ14ZZ
Pinealotomy
see Drainage, Pineal Body 0G91
Pinna
use Ear, External, Bilateral
use Ear, External, Left
use Ear, External, Right
Pipeline™ (Flex) embolization device
use Intraluminal Device, Flow Diverter in 03V
Piriform recess (sinus)
use Pharynx
Piriformis muscle
use Muscle, Hip, Right
use Muscle, Hip, Left
PIRRT (Prolonged intermittent renal replacement therapy) 5A1D80Z
Pisiform bone
use Carpal, Left
use Carpal, Right
Pisohamate ligament
use Bursa and Ligament, Hand, Left
use Bursa and Ligament, Hand, Right

Pisometacarpal ligament
use Bursa and Ligament, Hand, Left
use Bursa and Ligament, Hand, Right
Pituitectomy
see Excision, Gland, Pituitary 0GB0
see Resection, Gland, Pituitary 0GT0
Plain film radiology
see Plain Radiography
Plain Radiography
Abdomen BW00ZZZ
Abdomen and Pelvis BW01ZZZ
Abdominal Lymphatic
Bilateral B701
Unilateral B700
Airway, Upper BB0DZZZ
Ankle
Left BQ0H
Right BQ0G
Aorta
Abdominal B400
Thoracic B300
Thoraco-Abdominal B30P
Aorta and Bilateral Lower Extremity Arteries B40D
Arch
Bilateral BN0DZZZ
Left BN0CZZZ
Right BN0BZZZ
Arm
Left BP0FZZZ
Right BP0EZZZ
Artery
Brachiocephalic-Subclavian, Right B301
Bronchial B30L
Bypass Graft, Other B20F
Cervico-Cerebral Arch B30Q
Common Carotid
Bilateral B305
Left B304
Right B303
Coronary
Bypass Graft
Multiple B203
Single B202
Multiple B201
Single B200
External Carotid
Bilateral B30C
Left B30B
Right B309
Hepatic B402
Inferior Mesenteric B405
Intercostal B30L
Internal Carotid
Bilateral B308
Left B307
Right B306
Internal Mammary Bypass Graft
Left B208
Right B207
Intra-Abdominal, Other B40B
Intracranial B30R
Lower, Other B40J
Lower Extremity
Bilateral and Aorta B40D
Left B40G
Right B40F
Lumbar B409
Pelvic B40C
Pulmonary
Left B30T
Right B30S
Renal
Bilateral B408
Left B407
Right B406
Transplant B40M

Plain Radiography *(continued)*
Artery *(continued)*
Spinal B30M
Splenic B403
Subclavian, Left B302
Superior Mesenteric B404
Upper, Other B30N
Upper Extremity
Bilateral B30K
Left B30J
Right B30H
Vertebral
Bilateral B30G
Left B30F
Right B30D
Bile Duct BF00
Bile Duct and Gallbladder BF03
Bladder BT00
Kidney and Ureter BT04
Bladder and Urethra BT0B
Bone
Facial BN05ZZZ
Nasal BN04ZZZ
Bones, Long, All BW0BZZZ
Breast
Bilateral BH02ZZZ
Left BH01ZZZ
Right BH00ZZZ
Calcaneus
Left BQ0KZZZ
Right BQ0JZZZ
Chest BW03ZZZ
Clavicle
Left BP05ZZZ
Right BP04ZZZ
Coccyx BR0FZZZ
Corpora Cavernosa BV00
Dialysis Fistula B50W
Dialysis Shunt B50W
Disc
Cervical BR01
Lumbar BR03
Thoracic BR02
Duct
Lacrimal
Bilateral B802
Left B801
Right B800
Mammary
Multiple
Left BH06
Right BH05
Single
Left BH04
Right BH03
Elbow
Left BP0H
Right BP0G
Epididymis
Left BV02
Right BV01
Extremity
Lower BW0CZZZ
Upper BW0JZZZ
Eye
Bilateral B807ZZZ
Left B806ZZZ
Right B805ZZZ
Facet Joint
Cervical BR04
Lumbar BR06
Thoracic BR05
Fallopian Tube
Bilateral BU02
Left BU01
Right BU00
Fallopian Tube and Uterus BU08
Femur
Left, Densitometry BQ04ZZ1
Right, Densitometry BQ03ZZ1

Plain Radiography *(continued)*
- Finger
  - Left BP0SZZZ
  - Right BP0RZZZ
- Foot
  - Left BQ0MZZZ
  - Right BQ0LZZZ
- Forearm
  - Left BP0KZZZ
  - Right BP0JZZZ
- Gallbladder and Bile Duct BF03
- Gland
  - Parotid
    - Bilateral B906
    - Left B905
    - Right B904
  - Salivary
    - Bilateral B90D
    - Left B90C
    - Right B90B
  - Submandibular
    - Bilateral B909
    - Left B908
    - Right B907
- Hand
  - Left BP0PZZZ
  - Right BP0NZZZ
- Heart
  - Left B205
  - Right B204
  - Right and Left B206
- Hepatobiliary System, All BF0C
- Hip
  - Left BQ01
    - Densitometry BQ01ZZ1
  - Right BQ00
    - Densitometry BQ00ZZ1
- Humerus
  - Left BP0BZZZ
  - Right BP0AZZZ
- Ileal Diversion Loop BT0C
- Intracranial Sinus B502
- Joint
  - Acromioclavicular, Bilateral BP03ZZZ
  - Finger
    - Left BP0D
    - Right BP0C
  - Foot
    - Left BQ0Y
    - Right BQ0X
  - Hand
    - Left BP0D
    - Right BP0C
  - Lumbosacral BR0BZZZ
  - Sacroiliac BR0D
  - Sternoclavicular
    - Bilateral BP02ZZZ
    - Left BP01ZZZ
    - Right BP00ZZZ
  - Temporomandibular
    - Bilateral BN09
    - Left BN08
    - Right BN07
  - Thoracolumbar BR08ZZZ
  - Toe
    - Left BQ0Y
    - Right BQ0X
- Kidney
  - Bilateral BT03
  - Left BT02
  - Right BT01
  - Ureter and Bladder BT04
- Knee
  - Left BQ08
  - Right BQ07
- Leg
  - Left BQ0FZZZ
  - Right BQ0DZZZ

Plain Radiography *(continued)*
- Lymphatic
  - Head B704
  - Lower Extremity
    - Bilateral B70B
    - Left B709
    - Right B708
  - Neck B704
  - Pelvic B70C
  - Upper Extremity
    - Bilateral B707
    - Left B706
    - Right B705
- Mandible BN06ZZZ
- Mastoid B90HZZZ
- Nasopharynx B90FZZZ
- Optic Foramina
  - Left B804ZZZ
  - Right B803ZZZ
- Orbit
  - Bilateral BN03ZZZ
  - Left BN02ZZZ
  - Right BN01ZZZ
- Oropharynx B90FZZZ
- Patella
  - Left BQ0WZZZ
  - Right BQ0VZZZ
- Pelvis BR0CZZZ
- Pelvis and Abdomen BW01ZZZ
- Prostate BV03
- Retroperitoneal Lymphatic
  - Bilateral B701
  - Unilateral B700
- Ribs
  - Left BP0YZZZ
  - Right BP0XZZZ
- Sacrum BR0FZZZ
- Scapula
  - Left BP07ZZZ
  - Right BP06ZZZ
- Shoulder
  - Left BP09
  - Right BP08
- Sinus
  - Intracranial B502
  - Paranasal B902ZZZ
- Skull BN00ZZZ
- Spinal Cord B00B
- Spine
  - Cervical, Densitometry BR00ZZ1
  - Lumbar, Densitometry BR09ZZ1
  - Thoracic, Densitometry BR07ZZ1
  - Whole, Densitometry BR0GZZ1
- Sternum BR0HZZZ
- Teeth
  - All BN0JZZZ
  - Multiple BN0HZZZ
- Testicle
  - Left BV06
  - Right BV05
- Toe
  - Left BQ0QZZZ
  - Right BQ0PZZZ
- Tooth, Single BN0GZZZ
- Tracheobronchial Tree
  - Bilateral BB09YZZ
  - Left BB08Y
  - Right BB07Y
- Ureter
  - Bilateral BT08
  - Kidney and Bladder BT04
  - Left BT07
  - Right BT06
- Urethra BT05
- Urethra and Bladder BT0B
- Uterus BU06
- Uterus and Fallopian Tube BU08
- Vagina BU09
- Vasa Vasorum BV08

Plain Radiography *(continued)*
- Vein
  - Cerebellar B501
  - Cerebral B501
  - Epidural B500
  - Jugular
    - Bilateral B505
    - Left B504
    - Right B503
  - Lower Extremity
    - Bilateral B50D
    - Left B50C
    - Right B50B
  - Other B50V
  - Pelvic (Iliac)
    - Left B50G
    - Right B50F
  - Pelvic (Iliac) Bilateral B50H
  - Portal B50T
  - Pulmonary
    - Bilateral B50S
    - Left B50R
    - Right B50Q
  - Renal
    - Bilateral B50L
    - Left B50K
    - Right B50J
  - Spanchnic B50T
  - Subclavian
    - Left B507
    - Right B506
  - Upper Extremity
    - Bilateral B50P
    - Left B50N
    - Right B50M
- Vena Cava
  - Inferior B509
  - Superior B508
- Whole Body BW0KZZZ
  - Infant BW0MZZZ
- Whole Skeleton BW0LZZZ
- Wrist
  - Left BP0M
  - Right BP0L

Planar Nuclear Medicine Imaging
- Abdomen CW10
- Abdomen and Chest CW14
- Abdomen and Pelvis CW11
- Anatomical Regions, Multiple CW1YYZZ
- Anatomical Region, Other CW1ZZZZ
- Bladder, Kidneys and Ureters CT13
- Bladder and Ureters CT1H
- Blood C713
- Bone Marrow C710
- Brain C010
- Breast CH1YYZZ
  - Bilateral CH12
  - Left CH11
  - Right CH10
- Bronchi and Lungs CB12
- Central Nervous System C01YYZZ
- Cerebrospinal Fluid C015
- Chest CW13
- Chest and Abdomen CW14
- Chest and Neck CW16
- Digestive System CD1YYZZ
- Ducts, Lacrimal, Bilateral C819
- Ear, Nose, Mouth and Throat C91YYZZ
- Endocrine System CG1YYZZ
- Extremity
  - Lower CW1D
    - Bilateral CP1F
    - Left CP1D
    - Right CP1C
  - Upper CW1M
    - Bilateral CP1B
    - Left CP19
    - Right CP18

Planar Nuclear Medicine Imaging *(continued)*
- Eye C81YYZZ
- Gallbladder CF14
- Gastrointestinal Tract CD17
  - Upper CD15
- Gland
  - Adrenal, Bilateral CG14
  - Parathyroid CG11
  - Thyroid CG12
- Glands, Salivary, Bilateral C91B
- Head and Neck CW1B
- Heart C21YYZZ
  - Right and Left C216
- Hepatobiliary System, All CF1C
- Hepatobiliary System and Pancreas CF1YYZZ
- Kidneys, Ureters and Bladder CT13
- Liver CF15
- Liver and Spleen CF16
- Lungs and Bronchi CB12
- Lymphatics
  - Head C71J
  - Head and Neck C715
  - Lower Extremity C71P
  - Neck C71K
  - Pelvic C71D
  - Trunk C71M
  - Upper Chest C71L
  - Upper Extremity C71N
- Lymphatics and Hematologic System C71YYZZ
- Musculoskeletal System
  - All CP1Z
  - Other CP1YYZZ
- Myocardium C21G
- Neck and Chest CW16
- Neck and Head CW1B
- Pancreas and Hepatobiliary System CF1YYZZ
- Pelvic Region CW1J
- Pelvis CP16
- Pelvis and Abdomen CW11
- Pelvis and Spine CP17
- Reproductive System, Male CV1YYZZ
- Respiratory System CB1YYZZ
- Skin CH1YYZZ
- Skull CP11
- Spine CP15
- Spine and Pelvis CP17
- Spleen C712
- Spleen and Liver CF16
- Subcutaneous Tissue CH1YYZZ
- Testicles, Bilateral CV19
- Thorax CP14
- Ureters, Kidneys and Bladder CT13
- Ureters and Bladder CT1H
- Urinary System CT1YYZZ
- Veins C51YYZZ
  - Central C51R
  - Lower Extremity
    - Bilateral C51D
    - Left C51C
    - Right C51B
  - Upper Extremity
    - Bilateral C51Q
    - Left C51P
    - Right C51N
- Whole Body CW1N

Plantar digital vein
- *use* Vein, Foot, Left
- *use* Vein, Foot, Right

Plantar fascia (aponeurosis)
- *use* Subcutaneous Tissue and Fascia, Foot, Left
- *use* Subcutaneous Tissue and Fascia, Foot, Right

Plantar metatarsal vein
use Vein, Foot, Left
use Vein, Foot, Right
Plantar venous arch
use Vein, Foot, Left
use Vein, Foot, Right
Plaque Radiation
Abdomen DWY3FZZ
Adrenal Gland DGY2FZZ
Anus DDY8FZZ
Bile Ducts DFY2FZZ
Bladder DTY2FZZ
Bone, Other DPYCFZZ
Bone Marrow D7Y0FZZ
Brain D0Y0FZZ
Brain Stem D0Y1FZZ
Breast
Left DMY0FZZ
Right DMY1FZZ
Bronchus DBY1FZZ
Cervix DUY1FZZ
Chest DWY2FZZ
Chest Wall DBY7FZZ
Colon DDY5FZZ
Diaphragm DBY8FZZ
Duodenum DDY2FZZ
Ear D9Y0FZZ
Esophagus DDY0FZZ
Eye D8Y0FZZ
Femur DPY9FZZ
Fibula DPYBFZZ
Gallbladder DFY1FZZ
Gland
Adrenal DGY2FZZ
Parathyroid DGY4FZZ
Pituitary DGY0FZZ
Thyroid DGY5FZZ
Glands, Salivary D9Y6FZZ
Head and Neck DWY1FZZ
Hemibody DWY4FZZ
Humerus DPY6FZZ
Ileum DDY4FZZ
Jejunum DDY3FZZ
Kidney DTY0FZZ
Larynx D9YBFZZ
Liver DFY0FZZ
Lung DBY2FZZ
Lymphatics
Abdomen D7Y6FZZ
Axillary D7Y4FZZ
Inguinal D7Y8FZZ
Neck D7Y3FZZ
Pelvis D7Y7FZZ
Thorax D7Y5FZZ
Mandible DPY3FZZ
Maxilla DPY2FZZ
Mediastinum DBY6FZZ
Mouth D9Y4FZZ
Nasopharynx D9YDFZZ
Neck and Head DWY1FZZ
Nerve, Peripheral D0Y7FZZ
Nose D9Y1FZZ
Ovary DUY0FZZ
Palate
Hard D9Y8FZZ
Soft D9Y9FZZ
Pancreas DFY3FZZ
Parathyroid Gland DGY4FZZ
Pelvic Bones DPY8FZZ
Pelvic Region DWY6FZZ
Pharynx D9YCFZZ
Pineal Body DGY1FZZ
Pituitary Gland DGY0FZZ
Pleura DBY5FZZ
Prostate DVY0FZZ
Radius DPY7FZZ
Rectum DDY7FZZ
Rib DPY5FZZ
Sinuses D9Y7FZZ
Skin
Abdomen DHY8FZZ
Plaque Radiation *(continued)*
Skin *(continued)*
Arm DHY4FZZ
Back DHY7FZZ
Buttock DHY9FZZ
Chest DHY6FZZ
Face DHY2FZZ
Foot DHYCFZZ
Hand DHY5FZZ
Leg DHYBFZZ
Neck DHY3FZZ
Skull DPY0FZZ
Spinal Cord D0Y6FZZ
Spleen D7Y2FZZ
Sternum DPY4FZZ
Stomach DDY1FZZ
Testis DVY1FZZ
Thymus D7Y1FZZ
Thyroid Gland DGY5FZZ
Tibia DPYBFZZ
Tongue D9Y5FZZ
Trachea DBY0FZZ
Ulna DPY7FZZ
Ureter DTY1FZZ
Urethra DTY3FZZ
Uterus DUY2FZZ
Whole Body DWY5FZZ
Plasma, Convalescent (Nonautologous) XW1
Plasmapheresis, therapeutic
see Pheresis, Physiological Systems 6A5
Plateletpheresis, therapeutic
see Pheresis, Physiological Systems 6A5
Platysma muscle
use Muscle, Neck, Left
use Muscle, Neck, Right
Plazomicin Anti-infective XW0
Pleurectomy
see Excision, Respiratory System 0BB
see Resection, Respiratory System 0BT
Pleurocentesis
see Drainage, Anatomical Regions, General 0W9
Pleurodesis, pleurosclerosis
Chemical injection
see Introduction of substance in or on, Pleural Cavity 3E0L
Surgical
see Destruction, Respiratory System 0B5
Pleurolysis
see Release, Respiratory System 0BN
Pleuroscopy 0BJQ4ZZ
Pleurotomy
see Drainage, Respiratory System 0B9
Plica semilunaris
use Conjunctiva, Left
use Conjunctiva, Right
Plication
see Restriction
Pneumectomy
see Excision, Respiratory System 0BB
see Resection, Respiratory System 0BT
Pneumocentesis
see Drainage, Respiratory System 0B9
Pneumogastric nerve
use Nerve, Vagus
Pneumolysis
see Release, Respiratory System 0BN
Pneumonectomy
see Resection, Respiratory System 0BT
Pneumonolysis
see Release, Respiratory System 0BN
Pneumonopexy
see Repair, Respiratory System 0BQ
see Reposition, Respiratory System 0BS
Pneumonorrhaphy
see Repair, Respiratory System 0BQ
Pneumonotomy
see Drainage, Respiratory System 0B9
Pneumotaxic center
use Pons
Pneumotomy
see Drainage, Respiratory System 0B9
Pollicization
see Transfer, Anatomical Regions, Upper Extremities 0XX
Polyclonal hyperimmune globulin
use Globulin
Polyethylene socket
use Synthetic Substitute, Polyethylene in 0SR
Polymethylmethacrylate (PMMA)
use Synthetic Substitute
Polypectomy, gastrointestinal
see Excision, Gastrointestinal System 0DB
Polypropylene mesh
use Synthetic Substitute
Polysomnogram 4A1ZXQZ
Pontine tegmentum
use Pons
Popliteal ligament
use Bursa and Ligament, Knee, Left
use Bursa and Ligament, Knee, Right
Popliteal lymph node
use Lymphatic, Lower Extremity, Left
use Lymphatic, Lower Extremity, Right
Popliteal vein
use Vein, Femoral, Left
use Vein, Femoral, Right
Popliteus muscle
use Muscle, Lower Leg, Left
use Muscle, Lower Leg, Right
Porcine (bioprosthetic) valve
use Zooplastic Tissue in Heart and Great Vessels
Positive Blood Culture Fluorescence Hybridization for Organism Identification, Concentration and Susceptibility XXE5XN6
Positive end expiratory pressure
see Performance, Respiratory 5A19
Positron Emission Tomographic (PET) Imaging
Brain C030
Bronchi and Lungs CB32
Central Nervous System C03YYZZ
Heart C23YYZZ
Lungs and Bronchi CB32
Myocardium C23G
Respiratory System CB3YYZZ
Whole Body CW3NYZZ
Positron emission tomography
see Positron Emission Tomographic (PET) Imaging
Postauricular (mastoid) lymph node
use Lymphatic, Neck, Left
use Lymphatic, Neck, Right
Postcava
use Vena Cava, Inferior
Posterior (subscapular) lymph node
use Lymphatic, Axillary, Left
use Lymphatic, Axillary, Right
Posterior auricular artery
use Artery, External Carotid, Left
use Artery, External Carotid, Right
Posterior auricular nerve
use Nerve, Facial
Posterior auricular vein
use Vein, External Jugular, Left
use Vein, External Jugular, Right
Posterior cerebral artery
use Artery, Intracranial
Posterior chamber
use Eye, Left
use Eye, Right
Posterior circumflex humeral artery
use Artery, Axillary, Left
use Artery, Axillary, Right
Posterior communicating artery
use Artery, Intracranial
Posterior cruciate ligament (PCL)
use Bursa and Ligament, Knee, Left
use Bursa and Ligament, Knee, Right
Posterior (Dynamic) Distraction Device
Lumbar XNS0
Thoracic XNS4
Posterior facial (retromandibular) vein
use Vein, Face, Left
use Vein, Face, Right
Posterior femoral cutaneous nerve
use Nerve, Sacral Plexus
Posterior inferior cerebellar artery (PICA)
use Artery, Intracranial
Posterior interosseous nerve
use Nerve, Radial
Posterior labial nerve
use Nerve, Pudendal
Posterior scrotal nerve
use Nerve, Pudendal
Posterior spinal artery
use Artery, Vertebral, Left
use Artery, Vertebral, Right
Posterior tibial recurrent artery
use Artery, Anterior Tibial, Left
use Artery, Anterior Tibial, Right
Posterior ulnar recurrent artery
use Artery, Ulnar, Left
use Artery, Ulnar, Right
Posterior vagal trunk
use Nerve, Vagus
PPN (peripheral parenteral nutrition)
see Introduction of Nutritional Substance
Praxbind® (idarucizumab), Pradaxa® (dabigatran) reversal agent
use Other Therapeutic Substance
Preauricular lymph node
use Lymphatic, Head
Precava
use Vena Cava, Superior
PRECICE intramedullary limb lengthening system
use Internal Fixation Device, Intramedullary Limb Lengthening in 0PH
use Internal Fixation Device, Intramedullary Limb Lengthening in 0QH
Prepatellar bursa
use Bursa and Ligament, Knee, Left
use Bursa and Ligament, Knee, Right

Preputiotomy
see Drainage, Male Reproductive System 0V9
Pressure support ventilation
see Performance, Respiratory 5A19
PRESTIGE® Cervical Disc
use Synthetic Substitute
Pretracheal fascia
use Subcutaneous Tissue and Fascia, Neck, Left
use Subcutaneous Tissue and Fascia, Neck, Right
Prevertebral fascia
use Subcutaneous Tissue and Fascia, Neck, Left
use Subcutaneous Tissue and Fascia, Neck, Right
PrimeAdvanced neurostimulator (SureScan)(MRI Safe)
use Stimulator Generator, Multiple Array in 0JH
Princeps pollicis artery
use Artery, Hand, Left
use Artery, Hand, Right
Probing, duct
Diagnostic
see Inspection
Dilation
see Dilation
PROCEED™ Ventral Patch
use Synthetic Substitute
Procerus muscle
use Muscle, Facial
Proctectomy
see Excision, Rectum 0DBP
see Resection, Rectum 0DTP
Proctoclysis
see Introduction of substance in or on, Gastrointestinal Tract, Lower 3E0H
Proctocolectomy
see Excision, Gastrointestinal System 0DB
see Resection, Gastrointestinal System 0DT
Proctocolpoplasty
see Repair, Gastrointestinal System 0DQ
see Supplement, Gastrointestinal System 0DU
Proctoperineoplasty
see Repair, Gastrointestinal System 0DQ
see Supplement, Gastrointestinal System 0DU
Proctoperineorrhaphy
see Repair, Gastrointestinal System 0DQ
Proctopexy
see Repair, Rectum 0DQP
see Reposition, Rectum 0DSP
Proctoplasty
see Repair, Rectum 0DQP
see Supplement, Rectum 0DUP
Proctorrhaphy
see Repair, Rectum 0DQP
Proctoscopy 0DJD8ZZ
Proctosigmoidectomy
see Excision, Gastrointestinal System 0DB
see Resection, Gastrointestinal System 0DT
Proctosigmoidoscopy 0DJD8ZZ
Proctostomy
see Drainage, Rectum 0D9P
Proctotomy
see Drainage, Rectum 0D9P
Prodisc-C
use Synthetic Substitute
Prodisc-L
use Synthetic Substitute
Production, atrial septal defect
see Excision, Septum, Atrial 02B5
Profunda brachii
use Artery, Brachial, Left
use Artery, Brachial, Right
Profunda femoris (deep femoral) vein
use Vein, Femoral, Left
use Vein, Femoral, Right
PROLENE Polypropylene Hernia System (PHS)
use Synthetic Substitute
Prolonged intermittent renal replacement therapy (PIRRT) 5A1D80Z
Pronator quadratus muscle
use Muscle, Lower Arm and Wrist, Left
use Muscle, Lower Arm and Wrist, Right
Pronator teres muscle
use Muscle, Lower Arm and Wrist, Left
use Muscle, Lower Arm and Wrist, Right
Prostatectomy
see Excision, Prostate 0VB0
see Resection, Prostate 0VT0
Prostatic urethra
use Urethra
Prostatomy, prostatotomy
see Drainage, Prostate 0V90
Protecta XT CRT-D
use Cardiac Resynchronization Defibrillator Pulse Generator in 0JH
Protecta XT DR (XT VR)
use Defibrillator Generator in 0JH
Protégé® RX Carotid Stent System
use Intraluminal Device
Proximal radioulnar joint
use Joint, Elbow, Left
use Joint, Elbow, Right
Psoas muscle
use Muscle, Hip, Left
use Muscle, Hip, Right
PSV (pressure support ventilation)
see Performance, Respiratory 5A19
Psychoanalysis GZ54ZZZ
Psychological Tests
Cognitive Status GZ14ZZZ
Developmental GZ10ZZZ
Intellectual and Psychoeducational GZ12ZZZ
Neurobehavioral Status GZ14ZZZ
Neuropsychological GZ13ZZZ
Personality and Behavioral GZ11ZZZ
Psychotherapy
Family, Mental Health Services GZ72ZZZ
Group GZHZZZZ
Mental Health Services GZHZZZZ
Individual
see Psychotherapy, Individual, Mental Health Services for substance abuse
12-Step HZ53ZZZ
Behavioral HZ51ZZZ
Cognitive HZ50ZZZ
Cognitive-Behavioral HZ52ZZZ
Confrontational HZ58ZZZ
Interactive HZ55ZZZ
Psychotherapy *(continued)*
Individual *(continued)*
see Psychotherapy, Individual, Mental Health Services *(continued)*
Interpersonal HZ54ZZZ
Motivational Enhancement HZ57ZZZ
Psychoanalysis HZ5BZZZ
Psychodynamic HZ5CZZZ
Psychoeducation HZ56ZZZ
Psychophysiological HZ5DZZZ
Supportive HZ59ZZZ
Mental Health Services
Behavioral GZ51ZZZ
Cognitive GZ52ZZZ
Cognitive-Behavioral GZ58ZZZ
Interactive GZ50ZZZ
Interpersonal GZ53ZZZ
Psychoanalysis GZ54ZZZ
Psychodynamic GZ55ZZZ
Psychophysiological GZ59ZZZ
Supportive GZ56ZZZ
PTCA (percutaneous transluminal coronary angioplasty)
see Dilation, Heart and Great Vessels 027
Pterygoid muscle
use Muscle, Head
Pterygoid process
use Bone, Sphenoid
Pterygopalatine (sphenopalatine) ganglion
use Nerve, Head and Neck Sympathetic
Pubis
use Bone, Pelvic, Left
use Bone, Pelvic, Right
Pubofemoral ligament
use Bursa and Ligament, Hip, Left
use Bursa and Ligament, Hip, Right
Pudendal nerve
use Nerve, Sacral Plexus
Pull-through, laparoscopic-assisted transanal
see Excision, Gastrointestinal System 0DB
see Resection, Gastrointestinal System 0DT
Pull-through, rectal
see Resection, Rectum 0DTP
Pulmoaortic canal
use Artery, Pulmonary, Left
Pulmonary annulus
use Valve, Pulmonary
Pulmonary artery wedge monitoring
see Monitoring, Arterial 4A13
Pulmonary plexus
use Nerve, Thoracic Sympathetic
use Nerve, Vagus
Pulmonic valve
use Valve, Pulmonary
Pulpectomy
see Excision, Mouth and Throat 0CB
Pulverization
see Fragmentation
Pulvinar
use Thalamus
Pump reservoir
use Infusion Device, Pump in Subcutaneous Tissue and Fascia
Punch biopsy
see Excision with qualifier Diagnostic
Puncture
see Drainage
Puncture, lumbar
see Drainage, Spinal Canal 009U
Pure-Vu® System XDPH8K7
Pyelography
see Fluoroscopy, Urinary System BT1
see Plain Radiography, Urinary System BT0
Pyeloileostomy, urinary diversion
see Bypass, Urinary System 0T1
Pyeloplasty
see Repair, Urinary System 0TQ
see Replacement, Urinary System 0TR
see Supplement, Urinary System 0TU
Pyeloplasty, dismembered
see Repair, Kidney Pelvis
Pyelorrhaphy
see Repair, Urinary System 0TQ
Pyeloscopy 0TJ58ZZ
Pyelostomy
see Drainage, Urinary System 0T9
see Bypass, Urinary System 0T1
Pyelotomy
see Drainage, Urinary System 0T9
Pylorectomy
see Excision, Stomach, Pylorus 0DB7
see Resection, Stomach, Pylorus 0DT7
Pyloric antrum
use Stomach, Pylorus
Pyloric canal
use Stomach, Pylorus
Pyloric sphincter
use Stomach, Pylorus
Pylorodiosis
see Dilation, Stomach, Pylorus 0D77
Pylorogastrectomy
see Excision, Gastrointestinal System 0DB
see Resection, Gastrointestinal System 0DT
Pyloroplasty
see Repair, Stomach, Pylorus 0DQ7
see Supplement, Stomach, Pylorus 0DU7
Pyloroscopy 0DJ68ZZ
Pylorotomy
see Drainage, Stomach, Pylorus 0D97
Pyramidalis muscle
use Muscle, Abdomen, Left
use Muscle, Abdomen, Right

Q

Quadrangular cartilage
use Septum, Nasal
Quadrant resection of breast
see Excision, Skin and Breast 0HB
Quadrate lobe
use Liver
Quadratus femoris muscle
use Muscle, Hip, Left
use Muscle, Hip, Right
Quadratus lumborum muscle
use Muscle, Trunk, Left
use Muscle, Trunk, Right
Quadratus plantae muscle
use Muscle, Foot, Left
use Muscle, Foot, Right

Quadriceps (femoris)
use Muscle, Upper Leg, Left
use Muscle, Upper Leg, Right
Quarantine 8E0ZXY6

R

Radial artery arteriovenous fistula, using Thermal Resistance Energy X2K
Radial collateral carpal ligament
use Bursa and Ligament, Wrist, Left
use Bursa and Ligament, Wrist, Right
Radial collateral ligament
use Bursa and Ligament, Elbow, Left
use Bursa and Ligament, Elbow, Right
Radial notch
use Ulna, Left
use Ulna, Right
Radial recurrent artery
use Artery, Radial, Left
use Artery, Radial, Right
Radial vein
use Vein, Brachial, Left
use Vein, Brachial, Right
Radialis indicis
use Artery, Hand, Left
use Artery, Hand, Right
Radiation Therapy
see Beam Radiation
see Brachytherapy
see Other Radiation
see Stereotactic Radiosurgery
Radiation treatment
see Radiation Therapy
Radiocarpal joint
use Joint, Wrist, Left
use Joint, Wrist, Right
Radiocarpal ligament
use Bursa and Ligament, Wrist, Left
use Bursa and Ligament, Wrist, Right
Radiography
see Plain Radiography
Radiology, analog
see Plain Radiography
Radiology, diagnostic
see Imaging, Diagnostic
Radioulnar ligament
use Bursa and Ligament, Wrist, Left
use Bursa and Ligament, Wrist, Right
Range of motion testing
see Motor Function Assessment, Rehabilitation F01
Rapid ASPECTS XXE0X07
REALIZE® Adjustable Gastric Band
use Extraluminal Device
Reattachment
Abdominal Wall 0WMF0ZZ
Ampulla of Vater 0FMC
Ankle Region
Left 0YML0ZZ
Right 0YMK0ZZ
Arm
Lower
Left 0XMF0ZZ
Right 0XMD0ZZ
Upper
Left 0XM90ZZ
Right 0XM80ZZ
Axilla
Left 0XM50ZZ
Right 0XM40ZZ
Back
Lower 0WML0ZZ
Upper 0WMK0ZZ

Reattachment *(continued)*
Bladder 0TMB
Bladder Neck 0TMC
Breast
Bilateral 0HMVXZZ
Left 0HMUXZZ
Right 0HMTXZZ
Bronchus
Lingula 0BM90ZZ
Lower Lobe
Left 0BMB0ZZ
Right 0BM60ZZ
Main
Left 0BM70ZZ
Right 0BM30ZZ
Middle Lobe, Right 0BM50ZZ
Upper Lobe
Left 0BM80ZZ
Right 0BM40ZZ
Bursa and Ligament
Abdomen
Left 0MMJ
Right 0MMH
Ankle
Left 0MMR
Right 0MMQ
Elbow
Left 0MM4
Right 0MM3
Foot
Left 0MMT
Right 0MMS
Hand
Left 0MM8
Right 0MM7
Head and Neck 0MM0
Hip
Left 0MMM
Right 0MML
Knee
Left 0MMP
Right 0MMN
Lower Extremity
Left 0MMW
Right 0MMV
Perineum 0MMK
Rib(s) 0MMG
Shoulder
Left 0MM2
Right 0MM1
Spine
Lower 0MMD
Upper 0MMC
Sternum 0MMF
Upper Extremity
Left 0MMB
Right 0MM9
Wrist
Left 0MM6
Right 0MM5
Buttock
Left 0YM10ZZ
Right 0YM00ZZ
Carina 0BM20ZZ
Cecum 0DMH
Cervix 0UMC
Chest Wall 0WM80ZZ
Clitoris 0UMJXZZ
Colon
Ascending 0DMK
Descending 0DMM
Sigmoid 0DMN
Transverse 0DML
Cord
Bilateral 0VMH
Left 0VMG
Right 0VMF
Cul-de-sac 0UMF
Diaphragm 0BMT0ZZ

Reattachment *(continued)*
Duct
Common Bile 0FM9
Cystic 0FM8
Hepatic
Common 0FM7
Left 0FM6
Right 0FM5
Pancreatic 0FMD
Accessory 0FMF
Duodenum 0DM9
Ear
Left 09M1XZZ
Right 09M0XZZ
Elbow Region
Left 0XMC0ZZ
Right 0XMB0ZZ
Esophagus 0DM5
Extremity
Lower
Left 0YMB0ZZ
Right 0YM90ZZ
Upper
Left 0XM70ZZ
Right 0XM60ZZ
Eyelid
Lower
Left 08MRXZZ
Right 08MQXZZ
Upper
Left 08MPXZZ
Right 08MNXZZ
Face 0WM20ZZ
Fallopian Tube
Left 0UM6
Right 0UM5
Fallopian Tubes, Bilateral 0UM7
Femoral Region
Left 0YM80ZZ
Right 0YM70ZZ
Finger
Index
Left 0XMP0ZZ
Right 0XMN0ZZ
Little
Left 0XMW0ZZ
Right 0XMV0ZZ
Middle
Left 0XMR0ZZ
Right 0XMQ0ZZ
Ring
Left 0XMT0ZZ
Right 0XMS0ZZ
Foot
Left 0YMN0ZZ
Right 0YMM0ZZ
Forequarter
Left 0XM10ZZ
Right 0XM00ZZ
Gallbladder 0FM4
Gland
Left 0GM2
Right 0GM3
Hand
Left 0XMK0ZZ
Right 0XMJ0ZZ
Hindquarter
Bilateral 0YM40ZZ
Left 0YM30ZZ
Right 0YM20ZZ
Hymen 0UMK
Ileum 0DMB
Inguinal Region
Left 0YM60ZZ
Right 0YM50ZZ
Intestine
Large 0DME
Left 0DMG
Right 0DMF
Small 0DM8

Reattachment *(continued)*
Jaw
Lower 0WM50ZZ
Upper 0WM40ZZ
Jejunum 0DMA
Kidney
Left 0TM1
Right 0TM0
Kidney Pelvis
Left 0TM4
Right 0TM3
Kidneys, Bilateral 0TM2
Knee Region
Left 0YMG0ZZ
Right 0YMF0ZZ
Leg
Lower
Left 0YMJ0ZZ
Right 0YMH0ZZ
Upper
Left 0YMD0ZZ
Right 0YMC0ZZ
Lip
Lower 0CM10ZZ
Upper 0CM00ZZ
Liver 0FM0
Left Lobe 0FM2
Right Lobe 0FM1
Lung
Left 0BML0ZZ
Lower Lobe
Left 0BMJ0ZZ
Right 0BMF0ZZ
Middle Lobe, Right 0BMD0ZZ
Right 0BMK0ZZ
Upper Lobe
Left 0BMG0ZZ
Right 0BMC0ZZ
Lung Lingula 0BMH0ZZ
Muscle
Abdomen
Left 0KML
Right 0KMK
Facial 0KM1
Foot
Left 0KMW
Right 0KMV
Hand
Left 0KMD
Right 0KMC
Head 0KM0
Hip
Left 0KMP
Right 0KMN
Lower Arm and Wrist
Left 0KMB
Right 0KM9
Lower Leg
Left 0KMT
Right 0KMS
Neck
Left 0KM3
Right 0KM2
Perineum 0KMM
Shoulder
Left 0KM6
Right 0KM5
Thorax
Left 0KMJ
Right 0KMH
Tongue, Palate, Pharynx 0KM4
Trunk
Left 0KMG
Right 0KMF
Upper Arm
Left 0KM8
Right 0KM7
Upper Leg
Left 0KMR
Right 0KMQ

Reattachment *(continued)*
Nasal Mucosa and Soft Tissue 09MKXZZ
Neck 0WM60ZZ
Nipple
Left 0HMXXZZ
Right 0HMWXZZ
Ovary
Bilateral 0UM2
Left 0UM1
Right 0UM0
Palate, Soft 0CM30ZZ
Pancreas 0FMG
Parathyroid Gland 0GMR
Inferior
Left 0GMP
Right 0GMN
Multiple 0GMQ
Superior
Left 0GMM
Right 0GML
Penis 0VMSXZZ
Perineum
Female 0WMN0ZZ
Male 0WMM0ZZ
Rectum 0DMP
Scrotum 0VM5XZZ
Shoulder Region
Left 0XM30ZZ
Right 0XM20ZZ
Skin
Abdomen 0HM7XZZ
Back 0HM6XZZ
Buttock 0HM8XZZ
Chest 0HM5XZZ
Ear
Left 0HM3XZZ
Right 0HM2XZZ
Face 0HM1XZZ
Foot
Left 0HMNXZZ
Right 0HMMXZZ
Hand
Left 0HMGXZZ
Right 0HMFXZZ
Inguinal 0HMAXZZ
Lower Arm
Left 0HMEXZZ
Right 0HMDXZZ
Lower Leg
Left 0HMLXZZ
Right 0HMKXZZ
Neck 0HM4XZZ
Perineum 0HM9XZZ
Scalp 0HM0XZZ
Upper Arm
Left 0HMCXZZ
Right 0HMBXZZ
Upper Leg
Left 0HMJXZZ
Right 0HMHXZZ
Stomach 0DM6
Tendon
Abdomen
Left 0LMG
Right 0LMF
Ankle
Left 0LMT
Right 0LMS
Foot
Left 0LMW
Right 0LMV
Hand
Left 0LM8
Right 0LM7
Head and Neck 0LM0
Hip
Left 0LMK
Right 0LMJ

Reattachment *(continued)*
Tendon *(continued)*
Knee
Left 0LMR
Right 0LMQ
Lower Arm and Wrist
Left 0LM6
Right 0LM5
Lower Leg
Left 0LMP
Right 0LMN
Perineum 0LMH
Shoulder
Left 0LM2
Right 0LM1
Thorax
Left 0LMD
Right 0LMC
Trunk
Left 0LMB
Right 0LM9
Upper Arm
Left 0LM4
Right 0LM3
Upper Leg
Left 0LMM
Right 0LML
Testis
Bilateral 0VMC
Left 0VMB
Right 0VM9
Thumb
Left 0XMM0ZZ
Right 0XML0ZZ
Thyroid Gland
Left Lobe 0GMG
Right Lobe 0GMH
Toe
1st
Left 0YMQ0ZZ
Right 0YMP0ZZ
2nd
Left 0YMS0ZZ
Right 0YMR0ZZ
3rd
Left 0YMU0ZZ
Right 0YMT0ZZ
4th
Left 0YMW0ZZ
Right 0YMV0ZZ
5th
Left 0YMY0ZZ
Right 0YMX0ZZ
Tongue 0CM70ZZ
Tooth
Lower 0CMX
Upper 0CMW
Trachea 0BM10ZZ
Tunica Vaginalis
Left 0VM7
Right 0VM6
Ureter
Left 0TM7
Right 0TM6
Ureters, Bilateral 0TM8
Urethra 0TMD
Uterine Supporting Structure 0UM4
Uterus 0UM9
Uvula 0CMN0ZZ
Vagina 0UMG
Vulva 0UMMXZZ
Wrist Region
Left 0XMH0ZZ
Right 0XMG0ZZ
REBOA (resuscitative endovascular balloon occlusion of the aorta)
02LW3DJ
04L03DJ

Rebound HRD® (Hernia Repair Device)
use Synthetic Substitute
RECELL® cell suspension autograft
see Replacement, Skin and Breast 0HR
Recession
see Repair
see Reposition
Reclosure, disrupted abdominal wall
0WQFXZZ
Reconstruction
see Repair
see Replacement
see Supplement
Rectectomy
see Excision, Rectum 0DBP
see Resection, Rectum 0DTP
Rectocele repair
see Repair, Subcutaneous Tissue and Fascia, Pelvic Region 0JQC
Rectopexy
see Repair, Gastrointestinal System 0DQ
see Reposition, Gastrointestinal System 0DS
Rectoplasty
see Repair, Gastrointestinal System 0DQ
see Supplement, Gastrointestinal System 0DU
Rectorrhaphy
see Repair, Gastrointestinal System 0DQ
Rectoscopy 0DJD8ZZ
Rectosigmoid junction
use Colon, Sigmoid
Rectosigmoidectomy
see Excision, Gastrointestinal System 0DB
see Resection, Gastrointestinal System 0DT
Rectostomy
see Drainage, Rectum 0D9P
Rectotomy
see Drainage, Rectum 0D9P
Rectus abdominis muscle
use Muscle, Abdomen, Left
use Muscle, Abdomen, Right
Rectus femoris muscle
use Muscle, Upper Leg, Left
use Muscle, Upper Leg, Right
Recurrent laryngeal nerve
use Nerve, Vagus
Reducer® System
use Reduction Device in New Technology
Reduction
Dislocation
see Reposition
Fracture
see Reposition
Intussusception, intestinal
see Reposition, Gastrointestinal System 0DS
Mammoplasty
see Excision, Skin and Breast 0HB
Prolapse
see Reposition
Torsion
see Reposition
Volvulus, gastrointestinal
see Reposition, Gastrointestinal System 0DS
Reduction Device, Coronary Sinus
X2V73Q7
Refusion
see Fusion

Rehabilitation
see Activities of Daily Living Assessment, Rehabilitation F02
see Activities of Daily Living Treatment, Rehabilitation F08
see Caregiver Training, Rehabilitation F0F
see Cochlear Implant Treatment, Rehabilitation F0B
see Device Fitting, Rehabilitation F0D
see Hearing Treatment, Rehabilitation F09
see Motor Function Assessment, Rehabilitation F01
see Motor Treatment, Rehabilitation F07
see Speech Assessment, Rehabilitation F00
see Speech Treatment, Rehabilitation F06
see Vestibular Treatment, Rehabilitation F0C
Reimplantation
see Reattachment
see Reposition
see Transfer
Reinforcement
see Repair
see Supplement
Relaxation, scar tissue
see Release
Release
Acetabulum
Left 0QN5
Right 0QN4
Adenoids 0CNQ
Ampulla of Vater 0FNC
Anal Sphincter 0DNR
Anterior Chamber
Left 08N33ZZ
Right 08N23ZZ
Anus 0DNQ
Aorta
Abdominal 04N0
Thoracic
Ascending/Arch 02NX
Descending 02NW
Aortic Body 0GND
Appendix 0DNJ
Artery
Anterior Tibial
Left 04NQ
Right 04NP
Axillary
Left 03N6
Right 03N5
Brachial
Left 03N8
Right 03N7
Celiac 04N1
Colic
Left 04N7
Middle 04N8
Right 04N6
Common Carotid
Left 03NJ
Right 03NH
Common Iliac
Left 04ND
Right 04NC
Coronary
Four or More Arteries 02N3
One Artery 02N0
Three Arteries 02N2
Two Arteries 02N1
External Carotid
Left 03NN
Right 03NM

Release *(continued)*
Artery *(continued)*
External Iliac
Left 04NJ
Right 04NH
Face 03NR
Femoral
Left 04NL
Right 04NK
Foot
Left 04NW
Right 04NV
Gastric 04N2
Hand
Left 03NF
Right 03ND
Hepatic 04N3
Inferior Mesenteric
04NB
Innominate 03N2
Internal Carotid
Left 03NL
Right 03NK
Internal Iliac
Left 04NF
Right 04NE
Internal Mammary
Left 03N1
Right 03N0
Intracranial 03NG
Lower 04NY
Peroneal
Left 04NU
Right 04NT
Popliteal
Left 04NN
Right 04NM
Posterior Tibial
Left 04NS
Right 04NR
Pulmonary
Left 02NR
Right 02NQ
Pulmonary Trunk
02NP
Radial
Left 03NC
Right 03NB
Renal
Left 04NA
Right 04N9
Splenic 04N4
Subclavian
Left 03N4
Right 03N3
Superior Mesenteric 04N5
Temporal
Left 03NT
Right 03NS
Thyroid
Left 03NV
Right 03NU
Ulnar
Left 03NA
Right 03N9
Upper 03NY
Vertebral
Left 03NQ
Right 03NP
Atrium
Left 02N7
Right 02N6
Auditory Ossicle
Left 09NA
Right 09N9
Basal Ganglia 00N8
Bladder 0TNB
Bladder Neck 0TNC
Bone
Ethmoid
Left 0NNG

Release *(continued)*
Bone *(continued)*
Ethmoid *(continued)*
Right 0NNF
Frontal 0NN1
Hyoid 0NNX
Lacrimal
Left 0NNJ
Right 0NNH
Nasal 0NNB
Occipital 0NN7
Palatine
Left 0NNL
Right 0NNK
Parietal
Left 0NN4
Right 0NN3
Pelvic
Left 0QN3
Right 0QN2
Sphenoid 0NNC
Temporal
Left 0NN6
Right 0NN5
Zygomatic
Left 0NNN
Right 0NNM
Brain 00N0
Breast
Bilateral 0HNV
Left 0HNU
Right 0HNT
Bronchus
Lingula 0BN9
Lower Lobe
Left 0BNB
Right 0BN6
Main
Left 0BN7
Right 0BN3
Middle Lobe, Right
0BN5
Upper Lobe
Left 0BN8
Right 0BN4
Buccal Mucosa 0CN4
Bursa and Ligament
Abdomen
Left 0MNJ
Right 0MNH
Ankle
Left 0MNR
Right 0MNQ
Elbow
Left 0MN4
Right 0MN3
Foot
Left 0MNT
Right 0MNS
Hand
Left 0MN8
Right 0MN7
Head and Neck 0MN0
Hip
Left 0MNM
Right 0MNL
Knee
Left 0MNP
Right 0MNN
Lower Extremity
Left 0MNW
Right 0MNV
Perineum 0MNK
Rib(s) 0MNG
Shoulder
Left 0MN2
Right 0MN1
Spine
Lower 0MND
Upper 0MNC
Sternum 0MNF

Release *(continued)*
Bursa and Ligament *(continued)*
Upper Extremity
Left 0MNB
Right 0MN9
Wrist
Left 0MN6
Right 0MN5
Carina 0BN2
Carotid Bodies, Bilateral 0GN8
Carotid Body
Left 0GN6
Right 0GN7
Carpal
Left 0PNN
Right 0PNM
Cecum 0DNH
Cerebellum 00NC
Cerebral Hemisphere 00N7
Cerebral Meninges 00N1
Cerebral Ventricle 00N6
Cervix 0UNC
Chordae Tendineae 02N9
Choroid
Left 08NB
Right 08NA
Cisterna Chyli 07NL
Clavicle
Left 0PNB
Right 0PN9
Clitoris 0UNJ
Coccygeal Glomus 0GNB
Coccyx 0QNS
Colon
Ascending 0DNK
Descending 0DNM
Sigmoid 0DNN
Transverse 0DNL
Conduction Mechanism 02N8
Conjunctiva
Left 08NTXZZ
Right 08NSXZZ
Cord
Bilateral 0VNH
Left 0VNG
Right 0VNF
Cornea
Left 08N9XZZ
Right 08N8XZZ
Cul-de-sac 0UNF
Diaphragm 0BNT
Disc
Cervical Vertebral 0RN3
Cervicothoracic Vertebral
0RN5
Lumbar Vertebral 0SN2
Lumbosacral 0SN4
Thoracic Vertebral 0RN9
Thoracolumbar Vertebral
0RNB
Duct
Common Bile 0FN9
Cystic 0FN8
Hepatic
Common 0FN7
Left 0FN6
Right 0FN5
Lacrimal
Left 08NY
Right 08NX
Pancreatic 0FND
Accessory 0FNF
Parotid
Left 0CNC
Right 0CNB
Duodenum 0DN9
Dura Mater 00N2
Ear
External
Left 09N1
Right 09N0

Release *(continued)*
Ear *(continued)*
External Auditory Canal
Left 09N4
Right 09N3
Inner
Left 09NE
Right 09ND
Middle
Left 09N6
Right 09N5
Epididymis
Bilateral 0VNL
Left 0VNK
Right 0VNJ
Epiglottis 0CNR
Esophagogastric Junction
0DN4
Esophagus 0DN5
Lower 0DN3
Middle 0DN2
Upper 0DN1
Eustachian Tube
Left 09NG
Right 09NF
Eye
Left 08N1XZZ
Right 08N0XZZ
Eyelid
Lower
Left 08NR
Right 08NQ
Upper
Left 08NP
Right 08NN
Fallopian Tube
Left 0UN6
Right 0UN5
Fallopian Tubes, Bilateral
0UN7
Femoral Shaft
Left 0QN9
Right 0QN8
Femur
Lower
Left 0QNC
Right 0QNB
Upper
Left 0QN7
Right 0QN6
Fibula
Left 0QNK
Right 0QNJ
Finger Nail 0HNQXZZ
Gallbladder 0FN4
Gingiva
Lower 0CN6
Upper 0CN5
Gland
Adrenal
Bilateral 0GN4
Left 0GN2
Right 0GN3
Lacrimal
Left 08NW
Right 08NV
Minor Salivary 0CNJ
Parotid
Left 0CN9
Right 0CN8
Pituitary 0GN0
Sublingual
Left 0CNF
Right 0CND
Submaxillary
Left 0CNH
Right 0CNG
Vestibular 0UNL
Glenoid Cavity
Left 0PN8
Right 0PN7

Release *(continued)*
- Glomus Jugulare 0GNC
- Humeral Head
  - Left 0PND
  - Right 0PNC
- Humeral Shaft
  - Left 0PNG
  - Right 0PNF
- Hymen 0UNK
- Hypothalamus 00NA
- Ileocecal Valve 0DNC
- Ileum 0DNB
- Intestine
  - Large 0DNE
    - Left 0DNG
    - Right 0DNF
  - Small 0DN8
- Iris
  - Left 08ND3
  - Right 08NC3
- Jejunum 0DNA
- Joint
  - Acromioclavicular
    - Left 0RNH
    - Right 0RNG
  - Ankle
    - Left 0SNG
    - Right 0SNF
  - Carpal
    - Left 0RNR
    - Right 0RNQ
  - Carpometacarpal
    - Left 0RNT
    - Right 0RNS
  - Cervical Vertebral 0RN1
  - Cervicothoracic Vertebral 0RN4
  - Coccygeal 0SN6
  - Elbow
    - Left 0RNM
    - Right 0RNL
  - Finger Phalangeal
    - Left 0RNX
    - Right 0RNW
  - Hip
    - Left 0SNB
    - Right 0SN9
  - Knee
    - Left 0SND
    - Right 0SNC
  - Lumbar Vertebral 0SN0
  - Lumbosacral 0SN3
  - Metacarpophalangeal
    - Left 0RNV
    - Right 0RNU
  - Metatarsal-Phalangeal
    - Left 0SNN
    - Right 0SNM
  - Occipital-cervical 0RN0
  - Sacrococcygeal 0SN5
  - Sacroiliac
    - Left 0SN8
    - Right 0SN7
  - Shoulder
    - Left 0RNK
    - Right 0RNJ
  - Sternoclavicular
    - Left 0RNF
    - Right 0RNE
  - Tarsal
    - Left 0SNJ
    - Right 0SNH
  - Tarsometatarsal
    - Left 0SNL
    - Right 0SNK
  - Temporomandibular
    - Left 0RND
    - Right 0RNC
  - Thoracic Vertebral 0RN6

Release *(continued)*
- Joint *(continued)*
  - Thoracolumbar Vertebral 0RNA
  - Toe Phalangeal
    - Left 0SNQ
    - Right 0SNP
  - Wrist
    - Left 0RNP
    - Right 0RNN
- Kidney
  - Left 0TN1
  - Right 0TN0
- Kidney Pelvis
  - Left 0TN4
  - Right 0TN3
- Larynx 0CNS
- Lens
  - Left 08NK3ZZ
  - Right 08NJ3ZZ
- Lip
  - Lower 0CN1
  - Upper 0CN0
- Liver 0FN0
  - Left Lobe 0FN2
  - Right Lobe 0FN1
- Lung
  - Bilateral 0BNM
  - Left 0BNL
  - Lower Lobe
    - Left 0BNJ
    - Right 0BNF
  - Middle Lobe, Right 0BND
  - Right 0BNK
  - Upper Lobe
    - Left 0BNG
    - Right 0BNC
- Lung Lingula 0BNH
- Lymphatic
  - Aortic 07ND
  - Axillary
    - Left 07N6
    - Right 07N5
  - Head 07N0
  - Inguinal
    - Left 07NJ
    - Right 07NH
  - Internal Mammary
    - Left 07N9
    - Right 07N8
  - Lower Extremity
    - Left 07NG
    - Right 07NF
  - Mesenteric 07NB
  - Neck
    - Left 07N2
    - Right 07N1
  - Pelvis 07NC
  - Thoracic Duct 07NK
  - Thorax 07N7
  - Upper Extremity
    - Left 07N4
    - Right 07N3
- Mandible
  - Left 0NNV
  - Right 0NNT
- Maxilla 0NNR
- Medulla Oblongata 00ND
- Mesentery 0DNV
- Metacarpal
  - Left 0PNQ
  - Right 0PNP
- Metatarsal
  - Left 0QNP
  - Right 0QNN
- Muscle
  - Abdomen
    - Left 0KNL
    - Right 0KNK

Release *(continued)*
- Muscle *(continued)*
  - Extraocular
    - Left 08NM
    - Right 08NL
  - Facial 0KN1
  - Foot
    - Left 0KNW
    - Right 0KNV
  - Hand
    - Left 0KND
    - Right 0KNC
  - Head 0KN0
  - Hip
    - Left 0KNP
    - Right 0KNN
  - Lower Arm and Wrist
    - Left 0KNB
    - Right 0KN9
  - Lower Leg
    - Left 0KNT
    - Right 0KNS
  - Neck
    - Left 0KN3
    - Right 0KN2
  - Papillary 02ND
  - Perineum 0KNM
  - Shoulder
    - Left 0KN6
    - Right 0KN5
  - Thorax
    - Left 0KNJ
    - Right 0KNH
  - Tongue, Palate, Pharynx 0KN4
  - Trunk
    - Left 0KNG
    - Right 0KNF
  - Upper Arm
    - Left 0KN8
    - Right 0KN7
  - Upper Leg
    - Left 0KNR
    - Right 0KNQ
- Myocardial Bridge
  - *see* Release, Artery, Coronary
- Nasal Mucosa and Soft Tissue 09NK
- Nasopharynx 09NN
- Nerve
  - Abdominal Sympathetic 01NM
  - Abducens 00NL
  - Accessory 00NR
  - Acoustic 00NN
  - Brachial Plexus 01N3
  - Cervical 01N1
  - Cervical Plexus 01N0
  - Facial 00NM
  - Femoral 01ND
  - Glossopharyngeal 00NP
  - Head and Neck Sympathetic 01NK
  - Hypoglossal 00NS
  - Lumbar 01NB
  - Lumbar Plexus 01N9
  - Lumbar Sympathetic 01NN
  - Lumbosacral Plexus 01NA
  - Median 01N5
  - Oculomotor 00NH
  - Olfactory 00NF
  - Optic 00NG
  - Peroneal 01NH
  - Phrenic 01N2
  - Pudendal 01NC
  - Radial 01N6
  - Sacral 01NR
  - Sacral Plexus 01NQ
  - Sacral Sympathetic 01NP
  - Sciatic 01NF
  - Thoracic 01N8

Release *(continued)*
- Nerve *(continued)*
  - Thoracic Sympathetic 01NL
  - Tibial 01NG
  - Trigeminal 00NK
  - Trochlear 00NJ
  - Ulnar 01N4
  - Vagus 00NQ
- Nipple
  - Left 0HNX
  - Right 0HNW
- Nose 09NKZZ
- Omentum 0DNU
- Orbit
  - Left 0NNQ
  - Right 0NNP
- Ovary
  - Bilateral 0UN2
  - Left 0UN1
  - Right 0UN0
- Palate
  - Hard 0CN2
  - Soft 0CN3
- Pancreas 0FNG
- Para-aortic Body 0GN9
- Paraganglion Extremity 0GNF
- Parathyroid Gland 0GNR
  - Inferior
    - Left 0GNP
    - Right 0GNN
  - Multiple 0GNQ
  - Superior
    - Left 0GNM
    - Right 0GNL
- Patella
  - Left 0QNF
  - Right 0QND
- Penis 0VNSZZ
- Pericardium 02NN
- Peritoneum 0DNW
- Phalanx
  - Finger
    - Left 0PNV
    - Right 0PNT
  - Thumb
    - Left 0PNS
    - Right 0PNR
  - Toe
    - Left 0QNR
    - Right 0QNQ
- Pharynx 0CNM
- Pineal Body 0GN1
- Pleura
  - Left 0BNP
  - Right 0BNN
- Pons 00NB
- Prepuce 0VNT
- Prostate 0VN0
- Radius
  - Left 0PNJ
  - Right 0PNH
- Rectum 0DNP
- Retina
  - Left 08NF3ZZ
  - Right 08NE3ZZ
- Retinal Vessel
  - Left 08NH3ZZ
  - Right 08NG3ZZ
- Ribs
  - 1 to 2 0PN1
  - 3 or More 0PN2
- Sacrum 0QN1
- Scapula
  - Left 0PN6
  - Right 0PN5
- Sclera
  - Left 08N7XZZ
  - Right 08N6XZZ
- Scrotum 0VN5

Removal *(continued)*
- Inguinal Region *(continued)*
  - Right 2W56X
- Leg
  - Lower
    - Left 2W5RX
    - Right 2W5QX
  - Upper
    - Left 2W5PX
    - Right 2W5NX
- Mouth and Pharynx 2Y50X5Z
- Nasal 2Y51X5Z
- Neck 2W52X
- Thumb
  - Left 2W5HX
  - Right 2W5GX
- Toe
  - Left 2W5VX
  - Right 2W5UX
- Urethra 2Y55X5Z

Removal of device from
- Abdominal Wall 0WPF
- Acetabulum
  - Left 0QP5
  - Right 0QP4
- Anal Sphincter 0DPR
- Anus 0DPQ
- Artery
  - Lower 04PY
  - Upper 03PY
- Back
  - Lower 0WPL
  - Upper 0WPK
- Bladder 0TPB
- Bone
  - Facial 0NPW
  - Lower 0QPY
  - Nasal 0NPB
  - Pelvic
    - Left 0QP3
    - Right 0QP2
  - Upper 0PPY
- Bone Marrow 07PT
- Brain 00P0
- Breast
  - Left 0HPU
  - Right 0HPT
- Bursa and Ligament
  - Lower 0MPY
  - Upper 0MPX
- Carpal
  - Left 0PPN
  - Right 0PPM
- Cavity, Cranial 0WP1
- Cerebral Ventricle 00P6
- Chest Wall 0WP8
- Cisterna Chyli 07PL
- Clavicle
  - Left 0PPB
  - Right 0PP9
- Coccyx 0QPS
- Diaphragm 0BPT
- Disc
  - Cervical Vertebral 0RP3
  - Cervicothoracic Vertebral 0RP5
  - Lumbar Vertebral 0SP2
  - Lumbosacral 0SP4
  - Thoracic Vertebral 0RP9
  - Thoracolumbar Vertebral 0RPB
- Duct
  - Hepatobiliary 0FPB
  - Pancreatic 0FPD
- Ear
  - Inner
    - Left 09PE
    - Right 09PD
  - Left 09PJ
  - Right 09PH
- Epididymis and Spermatic Cord 0VPM

Removal of device from *(continued)*
- Esophagus 0DP5
- Extremity
  - Lower
    - Left 0YPB
    - Right 0YP9
  - Upper
    - Left 0XP7
    - Right 0XP6
- Eye
  - Left 08P1
  - Right 08P0
- Face 0WP2
- Fallopian Tube 0UP8
- Femoral Shaft
  - Left 0QP9
  - Right 0QP8
- Femur
  - Lower
    - Left 0QPC
    - Right 0QPB
  - Upper
    - Left 0QP7
    - Right 0QP6
- Fibula
  - Left 0QPK
  - Right 0QPJ
- Finger Nail 0HPQX
- Gallbladder 0FP4
- Gastrointestinal Tract 0WPP
- Genitourinary Tract 0WPR
- Gland
  - Adrenal 0GP5
  - Endocrine 0GPS
  - Pituitary 0GP0
  - Salivary 0CPA
- Glenoid Cavity
  - Left 0PP8
  - Right 0PP7
- Great Vessel 02PY
- Hair 0HPSX
- Head 0WP0
- Heart 02PA
- Humeral Head
  - Left 0PPD
  - Right 0PPC
- Humeral Shaft
  - Left 0PPG
  - Right 0PPF
- Intestinal Tract
  - Lower 0DPD
  - Upper 0DP0
- Jaw
  - Lower 0WP5
  - Upper 0WP4
- Joint
  - Acromioclavicular
    - Left 0RPH
    - Right 0RPG
  - Ankle
    - Left 0SPG
    - Right 0SPF
  - Carpal
    - Left 0RPR
    - Right 0RPQ
  - Carpometacarpal
    - Left 0RPT
    - Right 0RPS
  - Cervical Vertebral 0RP1
  - Cervicothoracic Vertebral 0RP4
  - Coccygeal 0SP6
  - Elbow
    - Left 0RPM
    - Right 0RPL
  - Finger Phalangeal
    - Left 0RPX
    - Right 0RPW
  - Hip
    - Left 0SPB
      - Acetabular Surface 0SPE
      - Femoral Surface 0SPS

Removal of device from *(continued)*
- Joint *(continued)*
  - Hip *(continued)*
    - Right 0SP9
      - Acetabular Surface 0SPA
      - Femoral Surface 0SPR
  - Knee
    - Left 0SPD
      - Femoral Surface 0SPU
      - Tibial Surface 0SPW
    - Right 0SPC
      - Femoral Surface 0SPT
      - Tibial Surface 0SPV
  - Lumbar Vertebral 0SP0
  - Lumbosacral 0SP3
  - Metacarpophalangeal
    - Left 0RPV
    - Right 0RPU
  - Metatarsal-Phalangeal
    - Left 0SPN
    - Right 0SPM
  - Occipital-cervical 0RP0
  - Sacrococcygeal 0SP5
  - Sacroiliac
    - Left 0SP8
    - Right 0SP7
  - Shoulder
    - Left 0RPK
    - Right 0RPJ
  - Sternoclavicular
    - Left 0RPF
    - Right 0RPE
  - Tarsal
    - Left 0SPJ
    - Right 0SPH
  - Tarsometatarsal
    - Left 0SPL
    - Right 0SPK
  - Temporomandibular
    - Left 0RPD
    - Right 0RPC
  - Thoracic Vertebral 0RP6
  - Thoracolumbar Vertebral 0RPA
  - Toe Phalangeal
    - Left 0SPQ
    - Right 0SPP
  - Wrist
    - Left 0RPP
    - Right 0RPN
- Kidney 0TP5
- Larynx 0CPS
- Lens
  - Left 08PK3
  - Right 08PJ3
- Liver 0FP0
- Lung
  - Left 0BPL
  - Right 0BPK
- Lymphatic 07PN
  - Thoracic Duct 07PK
- Mediastinum 0WPC
- Mesentery 0DPV
- Metacarpal
  - Left 0PPQ
  - Right 0PPP
- Metatarsal
  - Left 0QPP
  - Right 0QPN
- Mouth and Throat 0CPY
- Muscle
  - Extraocular
    - Left 08PM
    - Right 08PL
  - Lower 0KPY
  - Upper 0KPX
- Nasal Mucosa and Soft Tissue 09PK
- Neck 0WP6
- Nerve
  - Cranial 00PE
  - Peripheral 01PY

Removal of device from *(continued)*
- Omentum 0DPU
- Ovary 0UP3
- Pancreas 0FPGZ
- Parathyroid Gland 0GPR0
- Patella
  - Left 0QPF
  - Right 0QPD
- Pelvic Cavity 0WPJ
- Penis 0VPS
- Pericardial Cavity 0WPD
- Perineum
  - Female 0WPN
  - Male 0WPM
- Peritoneal Cavity 0WPG
- Peritoneum 0DPW
- Phalanx
  - Finger
    - Left 0PPV
    - Right 0PPT
  - Thumb
    - Left 0PPS
    - Right 0PPR
  - Toe
    - Left 0QPR
    - Right 0QPQ
- Pineal Body 0GP10
- Pleura 0BPQ
- Pleural Cavity
  - Left 0WPB
  - Right 0WP9
- Products of Conception 10P0
- Prostate and Seminal Vesicles 0VP4
- Radius
  - Left 0PPJ
  - Right 0PPH
- Rectum 0DPP1
- Respiratory Tract 0WPQZ
- Retroperitoneum 0WPH
- Ribs
  - 1 to 2 0PP1
  - 3 or More 0PP2
- Sacrum 0QP1
- Scapula
  - Left 0PP6
  - Right 0PP5
- Scrotum and Tunica Vaginalis 0VP8
- Sinus 09PY0
- Skin 0HPPX
- Skull 0NP0
- Spinal Canal 00PU
- Spinal Cord 00PV
- Spleen 07PP
- Sternum 0PP0
- Stomach 0DP6
- Subcutaneous Tissue and Fascia
  - Head and Neck 0JPS
  - Lower Extremity 0JPW
  - Trunk 0JPT
  - Upper Extremity 0JPV
- Tarsal
  - Left 0QPM
  - Right 0QPL
- Tendon
  - Lower 0LPY
  - Upper 0LPX
- Testis 0VPD
- Thymus 07PM
- Thyroid Gland 0GPK0
- Tibia
  - Left 0QPH
  - Right 0QPG
- Toe Nail 0HPRXZ
- Trachea 0BP1
- Tracheobronchial Tree 0BP0
- Tympanic Membrane
  - Left 09P80
  - Right 09P70

Removal of device from *(continued)*
- Ulna
  - Left 0PPL
  - Right 0PPK
- Ureter 0TP9
- Urethra 0TPD
- Uterus and Cervix 0UPD
- Vagina and Cul-de-sac 0UPH
- Vas Deferens 0VPR
- Vein
  - Azygos 05P0
  - Innominate
    - Left 05P4
    - Right 05P3
  - Lower 06PY
  - Upper 05PY
- Vertebra
  - Cervical 0PP3
  - Lumbar 0QP0
  - Thoracic 0PP4
- Vulva 0UPM

Renal calyx
- *use* Kidney
- *use* Kidneys, Bilateral
- *use* Kidney, Left
- *use* Kidney, Right

Renal capsule
- *use* Kidney
- *use* Kidneys, Bilateral
- *use* Kidney, Left
- *use* Kidney, Right

Renal cortex
- *use* Kidney
- *use* Kidneys, Bilateral
- *use* Kidney, Left
- *use* Kidney, Right

Renal dialysis
- *see* Performance, Urinary 5A1D

Renal nerve
- *use* Abdominal Sympathetic Nerve

Renal plexus
- *use* Nerve, Abdominal Sympathetic

Renal segment
- *use* Kidney
- *use* Kidneys, Bilateral
- *use* Kidney, Left
- *use* Kidney, Right

Renal segmental artery
- *use* Artery, Renal, Left
- *use* Artery, Renal, Right

Reopening, operative site
- Control of bleeding
  - *see* Control bleeding in
- Inspection only
  - *see* Inspection

Repair
- Abdominal Wall 0WQF
- Acetabulum
  - Left 0QQ5
  - Right 0QQ4
- Adenoids 0CQQ
- Ampulla of Vater 0FQC
- Anal Sphincter 0DQR
- Ankle Region
  - Left 0YQL
  - Right 0YQK
- Anterior Chamber
  - Left 08Q33
  - Right 08Q23
- Anus 0DQQ
- Aorta
  - Abdominal 04Q0
  - Thoracic
    - Ascending/Arch 02QX
    - Descending 02QW
- Aortic Body 0GQD
- Appendix 0DQJ

Repair *(continued)*
- Arm
  - Lower
    - Left 0XQF
    - Right 0XQD
  - Upper
    - Left 0XQ9
    - Right 0XQ8
- Artery
  - Anterior Tibial
    - Left 04QQ
    - Right 04QP
  - Axillary
    - Left 03Q6
    - Right 03Q5
  - Brachial
    - Left 03Q8
    - Right 03Q7
  - Celiac 04Q1
  - Colic
    - Left 04Q7
    - Middle 04Q8
    - Right 04Q6
  - Common Carotid
    - Left 03QJ
    - Right 03QH
  - Common Iliac
    - Left 04QD
    - Right 04QC
  - Coronary
    - Four or More Arteries 02Q3
    - One Artery 02Q0
    - Three Arteries 02Q2
    - Two Arteries 02Q1
  - External Carotid
    - Left 03QN
    - Right 03QM
  - External Iliac
    - Left 04QJ
    - Right 04QH
  - Face 03QR
  - Femoral
    - Left 04QL
    - Right 04QK
  - Foot
    - Left 04QW
    - Right 04QV
  - Gastric 04Q2
  - Hand
    - Left 03QF
    - Right 03QD
  - Hepatic 04Q3
  - Inferior Mesenteric 04QB
  - Innominate 03Q2
  - Internal Carotid
    - Left 03QL
    - Right 03QK
  - Internal Iliac
    - Left 04QF
    - Right 04QE
  - Internal Mammary
    - Left 03Q1
    - Right 03Q0
  - Intracranial 03QG
  - Lower 04QY
  - Peroneal
    - Left 04QU
    - Right 04QT
  - Popliteal
    - Left 04QN
    - Right 04QM
  - Posterior Tibial
    - Left 04QS
    - Right 04QR
  - Pulmonary
    - Left 02QR
    - Right 02QQ
  - Pulmonary Trunk 02QP

Repair *(continued)*
- Artery *(continued)*
  - Radial
    - Left 03QC
    - Right 03QB
  - Renal
    - Left 04QA
    - Right 04Q9
  - Splenic 04Q4
  - Subclavian
    - Left 03Q4
    - Right 03Q3
  - Superior Mesenteric 04Q5
  - Temporal
    - Left 03QT
    - Right 03QS
  - Thyroid
    - Left 03QV
    - Right 03QU
  - Ulnar
    - Left 03QA
    - Right 03Q9
  - Upper 03QY
  - Vertebral
    - Left 03QQ
    - Right 03QP
- Atrium
  - Left 02Q7
  - Right 02Q6
- Auditory Ossicle
  - Left 09QA
  - Right 09Q9
- Axilla
  - Left 0XQ5
  - Right 0XQ4
- Back
  - Lower 0WQL
  - Upper 0WQK
- Basal Ganglia 00Q8
- Bladder 0TQB
- Bladder Neck 0TQC
- Bone
  - Ethmoid
    - Left 0NQG
    - Right 0NQF
  - Frontal 0NQ1
  - Hyoid 0NQX
  - Lacrimal
    - Left 0NQJ
    - Right 0NQH
  - Nasal 0NQB
  - Occipital 0NQ7
  - Palatine
    - Left 0NQL
    - Right 0NQK
  - Parietal
    - Left 0NQ4
    - Right 0NQ3
  - Pelvic
    - Left 0QQ3
    - Right 0QQ2
  - Sphenoid 0NQC
  - Temporal
    - Left 0NQ6
    - Right 0NQ
  - Zygomatic
    - Left 0NQN
    - Right 0NQM
- Brain 00Q0
- Breast
  - Bilateral 0HQV
  - Left 0HQU
  - Right 0HQT
  - Supernumerary 0HQY
- Bronchus
  - Lingula 0BQ9
  - Lower Lobe
    - Left 0BQB

Repair *(continued)*
- Bronchus *(continued)*
  - Lower Lobe *(continued)*
    - Right 0BQ6
  - Main
    - Left 0BQ7
    - Right 0BQ3
  - Middle Lobe, Right 0BQ5
  - Upper Lobe
    - Left 0BQ8
    - Right 0BQ4
- Buccal Mucosa 0CQ4
- Bursa and Ligament
  - Abdomen
    - Left 0MQJ
    - Right 0MQH
  - Ankle
    - Left 0MQR
    - Right 0MQQ
  - Elbow
    - Left 0MQ4
    - Right 0MQ3
  - Foot
    - Left 0MQT
    - Right 0MQS
  - Hand
    - Left 0MQ8
    - Right 0MQ7
  - Head and Neck 0MQ0
  - Hip
    - Left 0MQM
    - Right 0MQL
  - Knee
    - Left 0MQP
    - Right 0MQN
  - Lower Extremity
    - Left 0MQW
    - Right 0MQV
  - Perineum 0MQK
  - Rib(s) 0MQG
  - Shoulder
    - Left 0MQ2
    - Right 0MQ1
  - Spine
    - Lower 0MQD
    - Upper 0MQC
  - Sternum 0MQF
  - Upper Extremity
    - Left 0MQB
    - Right 0MQ9
  - Wrist
    - Left 0MQ6
    - Right 0MQ5
- Buttock
  - Left 0YQ1
  - Right 0YQ0
- Carina 0BQ2
- Carotid Bodies, Bilateral 0GQ8
- Carotid Body
  - Left 0GQ6
  - Right 0GQ7
- Carpal
  - Left 0PQN
  - Right 0PQM
- Cecum 0DQH
- Cerebellum 00QC
- Cerebral Hemisphere 00Q7
- Cerebral Meninges 00Q1
- Cerebral Ventricle 00Q6
- Cervix 0UQC
- Chest Wall 0WQ8
- Chordae Tendineae 02Q9
- Choroid
  - Left 08QB
  - Right 08QA
- Cisterna Chyli 07QL
- Clavicle
  - Left 0PQB
  - Right 0PQ9

Repair *(continued)*
- Clitoris 0UQJ
- Coccygeal Glomus 0GQB
- Coccyx 0QQS
- Colon
  - Ascending 0DQK
  - Descending 0DQM
  - Sigmoid 0DQN
  - Transverse 0DQL
- Conduction Mechanism 02Q8
- Conjunctiva
  - Left 08QTXZZ
  - Right 08QSXZZ
- Cord
  - Bilateral 0VQH
  - Left 0VQG
  - Right 0VQF
- Cornea
  - Left 08Q9XZZ
  - Right 08Q8XZZ
- Cul-de-sac 0UQF
- Diaphragm 0BQT
- Disc
  - Cervical Vertebral 0RQ3
  - Cervicothoracic Vertebral 0RQ5
  - Lumbar Vertebral 0SQ2
  - Lumbosacral 0SQ4
  - Thoracic Vertebral 0RQ9
  - Thoracolumbar Vertebral 0RQB
- Duct
  - Common Bile 0FQ9
  - Cystic 0FQ8
  - Hepatic
    - Common 0FQ7
    - Left 0FQ6
    - Right 0FQ5
  - Lacrimal
    - Left 08QY
    - Right 08QX
  - Pancreatic 0FQD
    - Accessory 0FQF
  - Parotid
    - Left 0CQC
    - Right 0CQB
- Duodenum 0DQ9
- Dura Mater 00Q2
- Ear
  - External
    - Bilateral 09Q2
    - Left 09Q1
    - Right 09Q0
  - External Auditory Canal
    - Left 09Q4
    - Right 09Q3
  - Inner
    - Left 09QE
    - Right 09QD
  - Middle
    - Left 09Q6
    - Right 09Q5
- Elbow Region
  - Left 0XQC
  - Right 0XQB
- Epididymis
  - Bilateral 0VQL
  - Left 0VQK
  - Right 0VQJ
- Epiglottis 0CQR
- Esophagogastric Junction 0DQ4
- Esophagus 0DQ5
  - Lower 0DQ3
  - Middle 0DQ2
  - Upper 0DQ1

Repair *(continued)*
- Eustachian Tube
  - Left 09QG
  - Right 09QF
- Extremity
  - Lower
    - Left 0YQB
    - Right 0YQ9
  - Upper
    - Left 0XQ7
    - Right 0XQ6
- Eye
  - Left 08Q1XZZ
  - Right 08Q0XZZ
- Eyelid
  - Lower
    - Left 08QR
    - Right 08QQ
  - Upper
    - Left 08QP
    - Right 08QN
- Face 0WQ2
- Fallopian Tube
  - Left 0UQ6
  - Right 0UQ5
- Fallopian Tubes, Bilateral 0UQ7
- Femoral Region
  - Bilateral 0YQE
  - Left 0YQ8
  - Right 0YQ7
- Femoral Shaft
  - Left 0QQ9
  - Right 0QQ8
- Femur
  - Lower
    - Left 0QQC
    - Right 0QQB
  - Upper
    - Left 0QQ7
    - Right 0QQ6
- Fibula
  - Left 0QQK
  - Right 0QQJ
- Finger
  - Index
    - Left 0XQP
    - Right 0XQN
  - Little
    - Left 0XQW
    - Right 0XQV
  - Middle
    - Left 0XQR
    - Right 0XQQ
  - Ring
    - Left 0XQT
    - Right 0XQS
- Finger Nail 0HQQXZZ
- Floor of mouth
  - *see* Repair, Oral Cavity and Throat 0WQ3
- Foot
  - Left 0YQN
  - Right 0YQM
- Gallbladder 0FQ4
- Gingiva
  - Lower 0CQ6
  - Upper 0CQ5
- Gland
  - Adrenal
    - Bilateral 0GQ4
    - Left 0GQ2
    - Right 0GQ3
  - Lacrimal
    - Left 08QW
    - Right 08QV
  - Minor Salivary 0CQJ
  - Parotid
    - Left 0CQ9
    - Right 0CQ8
  - Pituitary 0GQ0

Repair *(continued)*
- Gland *(continued)*
  - Sublingual
    - Left 0CQF
    - Right 0CQD
  - Submaxillary
    - Left 0CQH
    - Right 0CQG
  - Vestibular 0UQL
- Glenoid Cavity
  - Left 0PQ8
  - Right 0PQ7
- Glomus Jugulare 0GQC
- Hand
  - Left 0XQK
  - Right 0XQJ
- Head 0WQ0
- Heart 02QA
  - Left 02QC
  - Right 02QB
- Humeral Head
  - Left 0PQD
  - Right 0PQC
- Humeral Shaft
  - Left 0PQG
  - Right 0PQF
- Hymen 0UQK
- Hypothalamus 00QA
- Ileocecal Valve 0DQC
- Ileum 0DQB
- Inguinal Region
  - Bilateral 0YQA
  - Left 0YQ6
  - Right 0YQ5
- Intestine
  - Large 0DQE
    - Left 0DQG
    - Right 0DQF
  - Small 0DQ8
- Iris
  - Left 08QD3ZZ
  - Right 08QC3ZZ
- Jaw
  - Lower 0WQ5
  - Upper 0WQ4
- Jejunum 0DQA
- Joint
  - Acromioclavicular
    - Left 0RQH
    - Right 0RQG
  - Ankle
    - Left 0SQG
    - Right 0SQF
  - Carpal
    - Left 0RQR
    - Right 0RQQ
  - Carpometacarpal
    - Left 0RQT
    - Right 0RQS
  - Cervical Vertebral 0RQ1
  - Cervicothoracic Vertebral 0RQ4
  - Coccygeal 0SQ6
  - Elbow
    - Left 0RQM
    - Right 0RQL
  - Finger Phalangeal
    - Left 0RQX
    - Right 0RQW
  - Hip
    - Left 0SQB
    - Right 0SQ9
  - Knee
    - Left 0SQD
    - Right 0SQC
  - Lumbar Vertebral 0SQ0
  - Lumbosacral 0SQ3
  - Metacarpophalangeal
    - Left 0RQV
    - Right 0RQU

Repair *(continued)*
- Joint *(continued)*
  - Metatarsal-Phalangeal
    - Left 0SQN
    - Right 0SQM
  - Occipital-cervical 0RQ0
  - Sacrococcygeal 0SQ5
  - Sacroiliac
    - Left 0SQ8
    - Right 0SQ7
  - Shoulder
    - Left 0RQK
    - Right 0RQJ
  - Sternoclavicular
    - Left 0RQF
    - Right 0RQE
  - Tarsal
    - Left 0SQJ
    - Right 0SQH
  - Tarsometatarsal
    - Left 0SQL
    - Right 0SQK
  - Temporomandibular
    - Left 0RQD
    - Right 0RQC
  - Thoracic Vertebral 0RQ6
  - Thoracolumbar Vertebral 0RQA
  - Toe Phalangeal
    - Left 0SQQ
    - Right 0SQP
  - Wrist
    - Left 0RQP
    - Right 0RQN
- Kidney
  - Left 0TQ1
  - Right 0TQ0
- Kidney Pelvis
  - Left 0TQ4
  - Right 0TQ3
- Knee Region
  - Left 0YQG
  - Right 0YQF
- Larynx 0CQS
- Leg
  - Lower
    - Left 0YQJ
    - Right 0YQH
  - Upper
    - Left 0YQD
    - Right 0YQC
- Lens
  - Left 08QK3ZZ
  - Right 08QJ3ZZ
- Lip
  - Lower 0CQ1
  - Upper 0CQ0
- Liver 0FQ0
  - Left Lobe 0FQ2
  - Right Lobe 0FQ1
- Lung
  - Bilateral 0BQM
  - Left 0BQL
  - Lower Lobe
    - Left 0BQJ
    - Right 0BQF
  - Middle Lobe, Right 0BQD
  - Right 0BQK
  - Upper Lobe
    - Left 0BQG
    - Right 0BQC
- Lung Lingula 0BQH
- Lymphatic
  - Aortic 07QD
  - Axillary
    - Left 07Q6
    - Right 07Q5
  - Head 07Q0
  - Inguinal
    - Left 07QJ
    - Right 07QH

Repair *(continued)*
Tendon *(continued)*
Lower Arm and Wrist
Left 0LQ6
Right 0LQ5
Lower Leg
Left 0LQP
Right 0LQN
Perineum 0LQH
Shoulder
Left 0LQ2
Right 0LQ1
Thorax
Left 0LQD
Right 0LQC
Trunk
Left 0LQB
Right 0LQ9
Upper Arm
Left 0LQ4
Right 0LQ3
Upper Leg
Left 0LQM
Right 0LQL
Testis
Bilateral 0VQC
Left 0VQB
Right 0VQ9
Thalamus 00Q9
Thumb
Left 0XQM
Right 0XQL
Thymus 07QM
Thyroid Gland 0GQK
Left Lobe 0GQG
Right Lobe 0GQH
Thyroid Gland Isthmus 0GQJ
Tibia
Left 0QQH
Right 0QQG
Toe
1st
Left 0YQQ
Right 0YQP
2nd
Left 0YQS
Right 0YQR
3rd
Left 0YQU
Right 0YQT
4th
Left 0YQW
Right 0YQV
5th
Left 0YQY
Right 0YQX
Toe Nail 0HQRXZZ
Tongue 0CQ7
Tonsils 0CQP
Tooth
Lower 0CQX
Upper 0CQW
Trachea 0BQ1
Tunica Vaginalis
Left 0VQ7
Right 0VQ6
Turbinate, Nasal 09QL
Tympanic Membrane
Left 09Q8
Right 09Q7
Ulna
Left 0PQL
Right 0PQK
Ureter
Left 0TQ7
Right 0TQ6
Urethra 0TQD
Uterine Supporting Structure 0UQ4

Repair *(continued)*
Uterus 0UQ9
Uvula 0CQN
Vagina 0UQG
Valve
Aortic 02QF
Mitral 02QG
Pulmonary 02QH
Tricuspid 02QJ
Vas Deferens
Bilateral 0VQQ
Left 0VQP
Right 0VQN
Vein
Axillary
Left 05Q8
Right 05Q7
Azygos 05Q0
Basilic
Left 05QC
Right 05QB
Brachial
Left 05QA
Right 05Q9
Cephalic
Left 05QF
Right 05QD
Colic 06Q7
Common Iliac
Left 06QD
Right 06QC
Coronary 02Q4
Esophageal 06Q3
External Iliac
Left 06QG
Right 06QF
External Jugular
Left 05QQ
Right 05QP
Face
Left 05QV
Right 05QT
Femoral
Left 06QN
Right 06QM
Foot
Left 06QV
Right 06QT
Gastric 06Q2
Hand
Left 05QH
Right 05QG
Hemiazygos 05Q1
Hepatic 06Q4
Hypogastric
Left 06QJ
Right 06QH
Inferior Mesenteric 06Q6
Innominate
Left 05Q4
Right 05Q3
Internal Jugular
Left 05QN
Right 05QM
Intracranial 05QL
Lower 06QY
Portal 06Q8
Pulmonary
Left 02QT
Right 02QS
Renal
Left 06QB
Right 06Q9
Saphenous
Left 06QQ
Right 06QP
Splenic 06Q1
Subclavian
Left 05Q6
Right 05Q5

Repair *(continued)*
Vein *(continued)*
Superior Mesenteric 06Q5
Upper 05QY
Vertebral
Left 05QS
Right 05QR
Vena Cava
Inferior 06Q0
Superior 02QV
Ventricle
Left 02QL
Right 02QK
Vertebra
Cervical 0PQ3
Lumbar 0QQ0
Thoracic 0PQ4
Vesicle
Bilateral 0VQ3
Left 0VQ2
Right 0VQ1
Vitreous
Left 08Q53ZZ
Right 08Q43ZZ
Vocal Cord
Left 0CQV
Right 0CQT
Vulva 0UQM
Wrist Region
Left 0XQH
Right 0XQG
Repair, obstetric laceration, periurethral 0UQMXZZ
Replacement
Acetabulum
Left 0QR5
Right 0QR4
Ampulla of Vater 0FRC
Anal Sphincter 0DRR
Aorta
Abdominal 04R0
Thoracic
Ascending/Arch 02RX
Descending 02RW
Artery
Anterior Tibial
Left 04RQ
Right 04RP
Axillary
Left 03R6
Right 03R5
Brachial
Left 03R8
Right 03R7
Celiac 04R1
Colic
Left 04R7
Middle 04R8
Right 04R6
Common Carotid
Left 03RJ
Right 03RH
Common Iliac
Left 04RD
Right 04RC
External Carotid
Left 03RN
Right 03RM
External Iliac
Left 04RJ
Right 04RH
Face 03RR
Femoral
Left 04RL
Right 04RK
Foot
Left 04RW
Right 04RV
Gastric 04R2

Replacement *(continued)*
Artery *(continued)*
Hand
Left 03RF
Right 03RD
Hepatic 04R3
Inferior Mesenteric 04R B
Innominate 03R2
Internal Carotid
Left 03RL
Right 03RK
Internal Iliac
Left 04RF
Right 04RE
Internal Mammary
Left 03R1
Right 03R0
Intracranial 03RG
Lower 04RY
Peroneal
Left 04RU
Right 04RT
Popliteal
Left 04RN
Right 04RM
Posterior Tibial
Left 04RS
Right 04RR
Pulmonary
Left 02RR
Right 02RQ
Pulmonary Trunk 02RP
Radial
Left 03RC
Right 03RB
Renal
Left 04RA
Right 04R9
Splenic 04R4
Subclavian
Left 03R4
Right 03R3
Superior Mesenteric 04R5
Temporal
Left 03RT
Right 03RS
Thyroid
Left 03RV
Right 03RU
Ulnar
Left 03RA
Right 03R9
Upper 03RY
Vertebral
Left 03RQ
Right 03RP
Atrium
Left 02R
Right 02R6
Auditory Ossicle
Left 09RA0
Right 09R90
Bladder 0TRB
Bladder Neck 0TRC
Bone
Ethmoid
Left 0NRG
Right 0NRF
Frontal 0NR1
Hyoid 0NRX
Lacrimal
Left 0NRJ
Right 0NRH
Nasal 0NRB
Occipital 0NR7
Palatine
Left 0NRL
Right 0NRK

Replacement *(continued)*
- Bone *(continued)*
  - Parietal
    - Left 0NR4
    - Right 0NR3
  - Pelvic
    - Left 0QR3
    - Right 0QR2
  - Sphenoid 0NRC
  - Temporal
    - Left 0NR6
    - Right 0NR5
  - Zygomatic
    - Left 0NRN
    - Right 0NRM
- Breast
  - Bilateral 0HRV
  - Left 0HRU
  - Right 0HRT
- Bronchus
  - Lingula 0BR9
  - Lower Lobe
    - Left 0BRB
    - Right 0BR6
  - Main
    - Left 0BR7
    - Right 0BR3
  - Middle Lobe, Right 0BR5
  - Upper Lobe
    - Left 0BR8
    - Right 0BR4
- Buccal Mucosa 0CR4
- Bursa and Ligament
  - Abdomen
    - Left 0MRJ
    - Right 0MRH
  - Ankle
    - Left 0MRR
    - Right 0MRQ
  - Elbow
    - Left 0MR4
    - Right 0MR3
  - Foot
    - Left 0MRT
    - Right 0MRS
  - Hand
    - Left 0MR8
    - Right 0MR7
  - Head and Neck 0MR0
  - Hip
    - Left 0MRM
    - Right 0MRL
  - Knee
    - Left 0MRP
    - Right 0MRN
  - Lower Extremity
    - Left 0MRW
    - Right 0MRV
  - Perineum 0MRK
  - Rib(s) 0MRG
  - Shoulder
    - Left 0MR2
    - Right 0MR1
  - Spine
    - Lower 0MRD
    - Upper 0MRC
  - Sternum 0MRF
  - Upper Extremity
    - Left 0MRB
    - Right 0MR9
  - Wrist
    - Left 0MR6
    - Right 0MR5
- Carina 0BR2
- Carpal
  - Left 0PRN
  - Right 0PRM
- Cerebral Meninges 00R1
- Cerebral Ventricle 00R6

Replacement *(continued)*
- Chordae Tendineae 02R9
- Choroid
  - Left 08RB
  - Right 08RA
- Clavicle
  - Left 0PRB
  - Right 0PR9
- Coccyx 0QRS
- Conjunctiva
  - Left 08RTX
  - Right 08RSX
- Cornea
  - Left 08R9
  - Right 08R8
- Diaphragm 0BRT
- Disc
  - Cervical Vertebral 0RR30
  - Cervicothoracic Vertebral 0RR50
  - Lumbar Vertebral 0SR20
  - Lumbosacral 0SR40
  - Thoracic Vertebral 0RR90
  - Thoracolumbar Vertebral 0RRB0
- Duct
  - Common Bile 0FR9
  - Cystic 0FR8
  - Hepatic
    - Common 0FR7
    - Left 0FR6
    - Right 0FR5
  - Lacrimal
    - Left 08RY
    - Right 08RX
  - Pancreatic 0FRD
    - Accessory 0FRF
  - Parotid
    - Left 0CRC
    - Right 0CRB
- Dura Mater 00R2
- Ear
  - External
    - Bilateral 09R2
    - Left 09R1
    - Right 09R0
  - Inner
    - Left 09RE0
    - Right 09RD0
  - Middle
    - Left 09R60
    - Right 09R50
- Epiglottis 0CRR
- Esophagus 0DR5
- Eye
  - Left 08R1
  - Right 08R0
- Eyelid
  - Lower
    - Left 08RR
    - Right 08RQ
  - Upper
    - Left 08RP
    - Right 08RN
- Femoral Shaft
  - Left 0QR9
  - Right 0QR8
- Femur
  - Lower
    - Left 0QRC
    - Right 0QRB
  - Upper
    - Left 0QR7
    - Right 0QR6
- Fibula
  - Left 0QRK
  - Right 0QRJ
- Finger Nail 0HRQX
- Gingiva
  - Lower 0CR6
  - Upper 0CR5

Replacement *(continued)*
- Glenoid Cavity
  - Left 0PR8
  - Right 0PR7
- Hair 0HRSX
- Heart 02RA0
- Humeral Head
  - Left 0PRD
  - Right 0PRC
- Humeral Shaft
  - Left 0PRG
  - Right 0PRF
- Iris
  - Left 08RD3
  - Right 08RC3
- Joint
  - Acromioclavicular
    - Left 0RRH0
    - Right 0RRG0
  - Ankle
    - Left 0SRG
    - Right 0SRF
  - Carpal
    - Left 0RRR0
    - Right 0RRQ0
  - Carpometacarpal
    - Left 0RRT0
    - Right 0RRS0
  - Cervical Vertebral 0RR10
  - Cervicothoracic Vertebral 0RR40
  - Coccygeal 0SR60
  - Elbow
    - Left 0RRM0
    - Right 0RRL0
  - Finger Phalangeal
    - Left 0RRX0
    - Right 0RRW0
  - Hip
    - Left 0SRB
      - Acetabular Surface 0SRE
      - Femoral Surface 0SRS
    - Right 0SR9
      - Acetabular Surface 0SRA
      - Femoral Surface 0SRR
  - Knee
    - Left 0SRD
      - Femoral Surface 0SRU
      - Tibial Surface 0SRW
    - Right 0SRC
      - Femoral Surface 0SRT
      - Tibial Surface 0SRV
  - Lumbar Vertebral 0SR00
  - Lumbosacral 0SR30
  - Metacarpophalangeal
    - Left 0RRV0
    - Right 0RRU0
  - Metatarsal-Phalangeal
    - Left 0SRN0
    - Right 0SRM0
  - Occipital-cervical 0RR00
  - Sacrococcygeal 0SR50
  - Sacroiliac
    - Left 0SR80
    - Right 0SR70
  - Shoulder
    - Left 0RRK
    - Right 0RRJ
  - Sternoclavicular
    - Left 0RRF0
    - Right 0RRE0
  - Tarsal
    - Left 0SRJ0
    - Right 0SRH0
  - Tarsometatarsal
    - Left 0SRL0
    - Right 0SRK0
  - Temporomandibular
    - Left 0RRD0
    - Right 0RRC0

Replacement *(continued)*
- Joint *(continued)*
  - Thoracic Vertebral 0RR60
  - Thoracolumbar Vertebral 0RRA0
  - Toe Phalangeal
    - Left 0SRQ0
    - Right 0SRP0
  - Wrist
    - Left 0RRP0
    - Right 0RRN0
- Kidney Pelvis
  - Left 0TR4
  - Right 0TR3
- Larynx 0CRS
- Lens
  - Left 08RK30Z
  - Right 08RJ30Z
- Lip
  - Lower 0CR1
  - Upper 0CR0
- Mandible
  - Left 0NRV
  - Right 0NRT
- Maxilla 0NRR
- Mesentery 0DRV
- Metacarpal
  - Left 0PRQ
  - Right 0PRP
- Metatarsal
  - Left 0QRP
  - Right 0QR
- Muscle
  - Abdomen
    - Left 0KRL
    - Right 0KRK
  - Facial 0KR1
  - Foot
    - Left 0KRW
    - Right 0KRV
  - Hand
    - Left 0KRD
    - Right 0KRC
  - Head 0KR0
  - Hip
    - Left 0KRP
    - Right 0KRN
  - Lower Arm and Wrist
    - Left 0KRB
    - Right 0KR9
  - Lower Leg
    - Left 0KRT
    - Right 0KRS
  - Neck
    - Left 0KR3
    - Right 0KR2
  - Papillary 02RD
  - Perineum 0KRM
  - Shoulder
    - Left 0KR6
    - Right 0KR5
  - Thorax
    - Left 0KRJ
    - Right 0KRH
  - Tongue, Palate, Pharynx 0KR4
  - Trunk
    - Left 0KRG
    - Right 0KRF
  - Upper Arm
    - Left 0KR8
    - Right 0KR7
  - Upper Leg
    - Left 0KRR
    - Right 0KRQ
- Nasal Mucosa and Soft Tissue 09RK
- Nasopharynx 09RN
- Nerve
  - Abducens 00RL

Reposition *(continued)*
- Joint *(continued)*
  - Finger Phalangeal
    - Left 0RSX
    - Right 0RSW
  - Hip
    - Left 0SSB
    - Right 0SS9
  - Knee
    - Left 0SSD
    - Right 0SSC
  - Lumbar Vertebral 0SS0
  - Lumbosacral 0SS3
  - Metacarpophalangeal
    - Left 0RSV
    - Right 0RSU
  - Metatarsal-Phalangeal
    - Left 0SSN
    - Right 0SSM
  - Occipital-cervical 0RS0
  - Sacrococcygeal 0SS5
  - Sacroiliac
    - Left 0SS8
    - Right 0SS7
  - Shoulder
    - Left 0RSK
    - Right 0RSJ
  - Sternoclavicular
    - Left 0RSF
    - Right 0RSE
  - Tarsal
    - Left 0SSJ
    - Right 0SSH
  - Tarsometatarsal
    - Left 0SSL
    - Right 0SSK
  - Temporomandibular
    - Left 0RSD
    - Right 0RSC
  - Thoracic Vertebral 0RS6
  - Thoracolumbar Vertebral 0RSA
  - Toe Phalangeal
    - Left 0SSQ
    - Right 0SSP
  - Wrist
    - Left 0RSP
    - Right 0RSN
- Kidney
  - Left 0TS1
  - Right 0TS0
- Kidney Pelvis
  - Left 0TS4
  - Right 0TS3
- Kidneys, Bilateral 0TS2
- Lens
  - Left 08SK3ZZ
  - Right 08SJ3ZZ
- Lip
  - Lower 0CS1
  - Upper 0CS0
- Liver 0FS0
- Lung
  - Left 0BSL0ZZ
  - Lower Lobe
    - Left 0BSJ0ZZ
    - Right 0BSF0ZZ
  - Middle Lobe, Right 0BSD0ZZ
  - Right 0BSK0ZZ
  - Upper Lobe
    - Left 0BSG0ZZ
    - Right 0BSC0ZZ
- Lung Lingula 0BSH0ZZ
- Mandible
  - Left 0NSV
  - Right 0NST
- Maxilla 0NSR
- Metacarpal
  - Left 0PSQ
  - Right 0PSP
- Metatarsal
  - Left 0QSP

Reposition *(continued)*
- Metatarsal *(continued)*
  - Right 0QSN
- Muscle
  - Abdomen
    - Left 0KSL
    - Right 0KSK
  - Extraocular
    - Left 08SM
    - Right 08SL
  - Facial 0KS1
  - Foot
    - Left 0KSW
    - Right 0KSV
  - Hand
    - Left 0KSD
    - Right 0KSC
  - Head 0KS0
  - Hip
    - Left 0KSP
    - Right 0KSN
  - Lower Arm and Wrist
    - Left 0KSB
    - Right 0KS9
  - Lower Leg
    - Left 0KST
    - Right 0KSS
  - Neck
    - Left 0KS3
    - Right 0KS2
  - Perineum 0KSM
  - Shoulder
    - Left 0KS6
    - Right 0KS5
  - Thorax
    - Left 0KSJ
    - Right 0KSH
  - Tongue, Palate, Pharynx 0KS4
  - Trunk
    - Left 0KSG
    - Right 0KSF
  - Upper Arm
    - Left 0KS8
    - Right 0KS7
  - Upper Leg
    - Left 0KSR
    - Right 0KSQ
- Nasal Mucosa and Soft Tissue 09SK
- Nerve
  - Abducens 00SL
  - Accessory 00SR
  - Acoustic 00SN
  - Brachial Plexus 01S3
  - Cervical 01S1
  - Cervical Plexus 01S0
  - Facial 00SM
  - Femoral 01SD
  - Glossopharyngeal 00SP
  - Hypoglossal 00SS
  - Lumbar 01SB
  - Lumbar Plexus 01S9
  - Lumbosacral Plexus 01SA
  - Median 01S5
  - Oculomotor 00SH
  - Olfactory 00SF
  - Optic 00SG
  - Peroneal 01SH
  - Phrenic 01S2
  - Pudendal 01SC
  - Radial 01S6
  - Sacral 01SR
  - Sacral Plexus 01SQ
  - Sciatic 01SF
  - Thoracic 01S8
  - Tibial 01SG
  - Trigeminal 00SK
  - Trochlear 00SJ
  - Ulnar 01S4
  - Vagus 00SQ
- Nipple
  - Left 0HSXXZZ

Reposition *(continued)*
- Nipple *(continued)*
  - Right 0HSWXZZ
- Orbit
  - Left 0NSQ
  - Right 0NSP
- Ovary
  - Bilateral 0US2
  - Left 0US1
  - Right 0US0
- Palate
  - Hard 0CS2
  - Soft 0CS3
- Pancreas 0FSG
- Parathyroid Gland 0GSR
  - Inferior
    - Left 0GSP
    - Right 0GSN
  - Multiple 0GSQ
  - Superior
    - Left 0GSM
    - Right 0GSL
- Patella
  - Left 0QSF
  - Right 0QSD
- Phalanx
  - Finger
    - Left 0PSV
    - Right 0PST
  - Thumb
    - Left 0PSS
    - Right 0PSR
  - Toe
    - Left 0QSR
    - Right 0QSQ
- Products of Conception 10S0
  - Ectopic 10S2
- Radius
  - Left 0PSJ
  - Right 0PSH
- Rectum 0DSP
- Retinal Vessel
  - Left 08SH3ZZ
  - Right 08SG3ZZ
- Ribs
  - 1 to 2 0PS1
  - 3 or More 0PS2
- Sacrum 0QS1
- Scapula
  - Left 0PS6
  - Right 0PS5
- Septum, Nasal 09SM
- Sesamoid Bone(s) 1st Toe
  - *see* Reposition, Metatarsal, Right 0QSN
  - *see* Reposition, Metatarsal, Left 0QSP
- Skull 0NS0
- Spinal Cord
  - Cervical 00SW
  - Lumbar 00SY
  - Thoracic 00SX
- Spleen 07SP0ZZ
- Sternum 0PS0
- Stomach 0DS6
- Tarsal
  - Left 0QSM
  - Right 0QSL
- Tendon
  - Abdomen
    - Left 0LSG
    - Right 0LSF
  - Ankle
    - Left 0LST
    - Right 0LSS
  - Foot
    - Left 0LSW
    - Right 0LSV
  - Hand
    - Left 0LS8
    - Right 0LS7

Reposition *(continued)*
- Tendon *(continued)*
  - Head and Neck 0LS0
  - Hip
    - Left 0LSK
    - Right 0LSJ
  - Knee
    - Left 0LSR
    - Right 0LSQ
  - Lower Arm and Wrist
    - Left 0LS6
    - Right 0LS5
  - Lower Leg
    - Left 0LSP
    - Right 0LSN
  - Perineum 0LSH
  - Shoulder
    - Left 0LS2
    - Right 0LS1
  - Thorax
    - Left 0LSD
    - Right 0LSC
  - Trunk
    - Left 0LSB
    - Right 0LS9
  - Upper Arm
    - Left 0LS4
    - Right 0LS3
  - Upper Leg
    - Left 0LSM
    - Right 0LSL
- Testis
  - Bilateral 0VSC
  - Left 0VSB
  - Right 0VS9
- Thymus 07SM0ZZ
- Thyroid Gland
  - Left Lobe 0GSG
  - Right Lobe 0GSH
- Tibia
  - Left 0QSH
  - Right 0QSG
- Tongue 0CS7
- Tooth
  - Lower 0CSX
  - Upper 0CSW
- Trachea 0BS10ZZ
- Turbinate, Nasal 09SL
- Tympanic Membrane
  - Left 09S8
  - Right 09S7
- Ulna
  - Left 0PSL
  - Right 0PSK
- Ureter
  - Left 0TS7
  - Right 0TS6
- Ureters, Bilateral 0TS8
- Urethra 0TSD
- Uterine Supporting Structure 0US4
- Uterus 0US9
- Uvula 0CSN
- Vagina 0USG
- Vein
  - Axillary
    - Left 05S8
    - Right 05S7
  - Azygos 05S0
  - Basilic
    - Left 05SC
    - Right 05SB
  - Brachial
    - Left 05SA
    - Right 05S9
  - Cephalic
    - Left 05SF
    - Right 05SD

Reposition *(continued)*
- Vein *(continued)*
  - Colic 06S7
  - Common Iliac
    - Left 06SD
    - Right 06SC
  - Esophageal 06S3
  - External Iliac
    - Left 06SG
    - Right 06SF
  - External Jugular
    - Left 05SQ
    - Right 05SP
  - Face
    - Left 05SV
    - Right 05ST
  - Femoral
    - Left 06SN
    - Right 06SM
  - Foot
    - Left 06SV
    - Right 06ST
  - Gastric 06S2
  - Hand
    - Left 05SH
    - Right 05SG
  - Hemiazygos 05S1
  - Hepatic 06S4
  - Hypogastric
    - Left 06SJ
    - Right 06SH
  - Inferior Mesenteric 06S6
  - Innominate
    - Left 05S4
    - Right 05S3
  - Internal Jugular
    - Left 05SN
    - Right 05SM
  - Intracranial 05SL
  - Lower 06SY
  - Portal 06S8
  - Pulmonary
    - Left 02ST0ZZ
    - Right 02SS0ZZ
  - Renal
    - Left 06SB
    - Right 06S9
  - Saphenous
    - Left 06SQ
    - Right 06SP
  - Splenic 06S1
  - Subclavian
    - Left 05S6
    - Right 05S5
  - Superior Mesenteric 06S5
  - Upper 05SY
  - Vertebral
    - Left 05SS
    - Right 05SR
- Vena Cava
  - Inferior 06S0
  - Superior 02SV0ZZ
- Vertebra
  - Cervical 0PS3
    - Magnetically Controlled Growth Rod(s) XNS3
  - Lumbar 0QS0
    - Magnetically Controlled Growth Rod(s) XNS0
    - Posterior (Dynamic) Distraction Device XNS0
  - Thoracic 0PS4
    - Magnetically Controlled Growth Rod(s) XNS4
    - Posterior (Dynamic) Distraction Device XNS4
- Vocal Cord
  - Left 0CSV
  - Right 0CST

Resection
- Acetabulum
  - Left 0QT50ZZ
  - Right 0QT40ZZ
- Adenoids 0CTQ
- Ampulla of Vater 0FTC
- Anal Sphincter 0DTR
- Anus 0DTQ
- Aortic Body 0GTD
- Appendix 0DTJ
- Auditory Ossicle
  - Left 09TA
  - Right 09T9
- Bladder 0TTB
- Bladder Neck 0TTC
- Bone
  - Ethmoid
    - Left 0NTG0ZZ
    - Right 0NTF0ZZ
  - Frontal 0NT10ZZ
  - Hyoid 0NTX0ZZ
  - Lacrimal
    - Left 0NTJ0ZZ
    - Right 0NTH0ZZ
  - Nasal 0NTB0ZZ
  - Occipital 0NT70ZZ
  - Palatine
    - Left 0NTL0ZZ
    - Right 0NTK0ZZ
  - Parietal
    - Left 0NT40ZZ
    - Right 0NT30ZZ
  - Pelvic
    - Left 0QT30ZZ
    - Right 0QT20ZZ
  - Sphenoid 0NTC0ZZ
  - Temporal
    - Left 0NT60ZZ
    - Right 0NT50ZZ
  - Zygomatic
    - Left 0NTN0ZZ
    - Right 0NTM0ZZ
- Breast
  - Bilateral 0HTV0ZZ
  - Left 0HTU0ZZ
  - Right 0HTT0ZZ
  - Supernumerary 0HTY0ZZ
- Bronchus
  - Lingula 0BT9
  - Lower Lobe
    - Left 0BTB
    - Right 0BT6
  - Main
    - Left 0BT7
    - Right 0BT3
  - Middle Lobe, Right 0BT5
  - Upper Lobe
    - Left 0BT8
    - Right 0BT4
- Bursa and Ligament
  - Abdomen
    - Left 0MTJ
    - Right 0MTH
  - Ankle
    - Left 0MTR
    - Right 0MTQ
  - Elbow
    - Left 0MT4
    - Right 0MT3
  - Foot
    - Left 0MTT
    - Right 0MTS
  - Hand
    - Left 0MT8
    - Right 0MT7
  - Head and Neck 0MT0
  - Hip
    - Left 0MTM
    - Right 0MTL

Resection *(continued)*
- Bursa and Ligament *(continued)*
  - Knee
    - Left 0MTP
    - Right 0MTN
  - Lower Extremity
    - Left 0MTW
    - Right 0MTV
  - Perineum 0MTK
  - Rib(s) 0MTG
  - Shoulder
    - Left 0MT2
    - Right 0MT1
  - Spine
    - Lower 0MTD
    - Upper 0MTC
  - Sternum 0MTF
  - Upper Extremity
    - Left 0MTB
    - Right 0MT9
  - Wrist
    - Left 0MT6
    - Right 0MT5
- Carina 0BT2
- Carotid Bodies, Bilateral 0GT8
- Carotid Body
  - Left 0GT6
  - Right 0GT7
- Carpal
  - Left 0PTN0ZZ
  - Right 0PTM0ZZ
- Cecum 0DTH
- Cerebral Hemisphere 00T7
- Cervix 0UTC
- Chordae Tendineae 02T9
- Cisterna Chyli 07TL
- Clavicle
  - Left 0PTB0ZZ
  - Right 0PT90ZZ
- Clitoris 0UTJ
- Coccygeal Glomus 0GTB
- Coccyx 0QTS0ZZ
- Colon
  - Ascending 0DTK
  - Descending 0DTM
  - Sigmoid 0DTN
  - Transverse 0DTL
- Conduction Mechanism 02T8
- Cord
  - Bilateral 0VTH
  - Left 0VTG
  - Right 0VTF
- Cornea
  - Left 08T9XZZ
  - Right 08T8XZZ
- Cul-de-sac 0UTF
- Diaphragm 0BTT
- Disc
  - Cervical Vertebral 0RT30ZZ
  - Cervicothoracic Vertebral 0RT50ZZ
  - Lumbar Vertebral 0ST20ZZ
  - Lumbosacral 0ST40ZZ
  - Thoracic Vertebral 0RT90ZZ
  - Thoracolumbar Vertebral 0RTB0ZZ
- Duct
  - Common Bile 0FT9
  - Cystic 0FT8
  - Hepatic
    - Common 0FT7
    - Left 0FT6
    - Right 0FT5
  - Lacrimal
    - Left 08TY
    - Right 08TX
  - Pancreatic 0FTD
    - Accessory 0FTF
  - Parotid
    - Left 0CTC0ZZ
    - Right 0CTB0ZZ

Resection *(continued)*
- Duodenum 0DT9
- Ear
  - External
    - Left 09T1
    - Right 09T0
  - Inner
    - Left 09TE
    - Right 09TD
  - Middle
    - Left 09T6
    - Right 09T5
- Epididymis
  - Bilateral 0VTL
  - Left 0VTK
  - Right 0VTJ
- Epiglottis 0CTR
- Esophagogastric Junction 0DT4
- Esophagus 0DT5
  - Lower 0DT3
  - Middle 0DT2
  - Upper 0DT1
- Eustachian Tube
  - Left 09TG
  - Right 09TF
- Eye
  - Left 08T1XZZ
  - Right 08T0XZZ
- Eyelid
  - Lower
    - Left 08TR
    - Right 08TQ
  - Upper
    - Left 08TP
    - Right 08TN
- Fallopian Tube
  - Left 0UT6
  - Right 0UT5
- Fallopian Tubes, Bilateral 0UT7
- Femoral Shaft
  - Left 0QT90ZZ
  - Right 0QT80ZZ
- Femur
  - Lower
    - Left 0QTC0ZZ
    - Right 0QTB0ZZ
  - Upper
    - Left 0QT70ZZ
    - Right 0QT60ZZ
- Fibula
  - Left 0QTK0ZZ
  - Right 0QTJ0ZZ
- Finger Nail 0HTQXZZ
- Gallbladder 0FT4
- Gland
  - Adrenal
    - Bilateral 0GT4
    - Left 0GT2
    - Right 0GT3
  - Lacrimal
    - Left 08TW
    - Right 08TV
  - Minor Salivary 0CTJ0ZZ
  - Parotid
    - Left 0CT90ZZ
    - Right 0CT80ZZ
  - Pituitary 0GT0
  - Sublingual
    - Left 0CTF0ZZ
    - Right 0CTD0ZZ
  - Submaxillary
    - Left 0CTH0ZZ
    - Right 0CTG0ZZ
  - Vestibular 0UTL
- Glenoid Cavity
  - Left 0PT80ZZ
  - Right 0PT70ZZ
- Glomus Jugulare 0GTC
- Humeral Head
  - Left 0PTD0ZZ
  - Right 0PTC0ZZ

Resection *(continued)*
- Humeral Shaft
  - Left 0PTG0ZZ
  - Right 0PTF0ZZ
- Hymen 0UTK
- Ileocecal Valve 0DTC
- Ileum 0DTB
- Intestine
  - Large 0DTE
    - Left 0DTG
    - Right 0DTF
  - Small 0DT8
- Iris
  - Left 08TD3ZZ
  - Right 08TC3ZZ
- Jejunum 0DTA
- Joint
  - Acromioclavicular
    - Left 0RTH0ZZ
    - Right 0RTG0ZZ
  - Ankle
    - Left 0STG0ZZ
    - Right 0STF0ZZ
  - Carpal
    - Left 0RTR0ZZ
    - Right 0RTQ0ZZ
  - Carpometacarpal
    - Left 0RTT0ZZ
    - Right 0RTS0ZZ
  - Cervicothoracic Vertebral 0RT40ZZ
  - Coccygeal 0ST60ZZ
  - Elbow
    - Left 0RTM0ZZ
    - Right 0RTL0ZZ
  - Finger Phalangeal
    - Left 0RTX0ZZ
    - Right 0RTW0ZZ
  - Hip
    - Left 0STB0ZZ
    - Right 0ST90ZZ
  - Knee
    - Left 0STD0ZZ
    - Right 0STC0ZZ
  - Metacarpophalangeal
    - Left 0RTV0ZZ
    - Right 0RTU0ZZ
  - Metatarsal-Phalangeal
    - Left 0STN0ZZ
    - Right 0STM0ZZ
  - Sacrococcygeal 0ST50ZZ
  - Sacroiliac
    - Left 0ST80ZZ
    - Right 0ST70ZZ
  - Shoulder
    - Left 0RTK0ZZ
    - Right 0RTJ0ZZ
  - Sternoclavicular
    - Left 0RTF0ZZ
    - Right 0RTE0ZZ
  - Tarsal
    - Left 0STJ0ZZ
    - Right 0STH0ZZ
  - Tarsometatarsal
    - Left 0STL0ZZ
    - Right 0STK0ZZ
  - Temporomandibular
    - Left 0RTD0ZZ
    - Right 0RTC0ZZ
  - Toe Phalangeal
    - Left 0STQ0ZZ
    - Right 0STP0ZZ
  - Wrist
    - Left 0RTP0ZZ
    - Right 0RTN0ZZ
- Kidney
  - Left 0TT1
  - Right 0TT0

Resection *(continued)*
- Kidney Pelvis
  - Left 0TT4
  - Right 0TT3
- Kidneys, Bilateral 0TT2
- Larynx 0CTS
- Lens
  - Left 08TK3ZZ
  - Right 08TJ3ZZ
- Lip
  - Lower 0CT1
  - Upper 0CT0
- Liver 0FT0
  - Left Lobe 0FT2
  - Right Lobe 0FT1
- Lung
  - Bilateral 0BTM
  - Left 0BTL
  - Lower Lobe
    - Left 0BTJ
    - Right 0BTF
  - Middle Lobe, Right 0BTD
  - Right 0BTK
  - Upper Lobe
    - Left 0BTG
    - Right 0BTC
- Lung Lingula 0BTH
- Lymphatic
  - Aortic 07TD
  - Axillary
    - Left 07T6
    - Right 07T5
  - Head 07T0
  - Inguinal
    - Left 07TJ
    - Right 07TH
  - Internal Mammary
    - Left 07T9
    - Right 07T8
  - Lower Extremity
    - Left 07TG
    - Right 07TF
  - Mesenteric 07TB
  - Neck
    - Left 07T2
    - Right 07T1
  - Pelvis 07TC
  - Thoracic Duct 07TK
  - Thorax 07T7
  - Upper Extremity
    - Left 07T4
    - Right 07T3
- Mandible
  - Left 0NTV0ZZ
  - Right 0NTT0ZZ
- Maxilla 0NTR0ZZ
- Metacarpal
  - Left 0PTQ0ZZ
  - Right 0PTP0ZZ
- Metatarsal
  - Left 0QTP0ZZ
  - Right 0QTN0ZZ
- Muscle
  - Abdomen
    - Left 0KTL
    - Right 0KTK
  - Extraocular
    - Left 08TM
    - Right 08TL
  - Facial 0KT1
  - Foot
    - Left 0KTW
    - Right 0KTV
  - Hand
    - Left 0KTD
    - Right 0KTC
  - Head 0KT0
  - Hip
    - Left 0KTP
    - Right 0KTN

Resection *(continued)*
- Muscle *(continued)*
  - Lower Arm and Wrist
    - Left 0KTB
    - Right 0KT9
  - Lower Leg
    - Left 0KTT
    - Right 0KTS
  - Neck
    - Left 0KT3
    - Right 0KT2
  - Papillary 02TD
  - Perineum 0KTM
  - Shoulder
    - Left 0KT6
    - Right 0KT5
  - Thorax
    - Left 0KTJ
    - Right 0KTH
  - Tongue, Palate, Pharynx 0KT4
  - Trunk
    - Left 0KTG
    - Right 0KTF
  - Upper Arm
    - Left 0KT8
    - Right 0KT7
  - Upper Leg
    - Left 0KTR
    - Right 0KTQ
- Nasal Mucosa and Soft Tissue 09TK
- Nasopharynx 09TN
- Nipple
  - Left 0HTXXZZ
  - Right 0HTWXZZ
- Omentum 0DTU
- Orbit
  - Left 0NTQ0ZZ
  - Right 0NTP0ZZ
- Ovary
  - Bilateral 0UT2
  - Left 0UT1
  - Right 0UT0
- Palate
  - Hard 0CT2
  - Soft 0CT3
- Pancreas 0FTG
- Para-aortic Body 0GT9
- Paraganglion Extremity 0GTF
- Parathyroid Gland 0GTR
  - Inferior
    - Left 0GTP
    - Right 0GTN
  - Multiple 0GTQ
  - Superior
    - Left 0GTM
    - Right 0GTL
- Patella
  - Left 0QTF0ZZ
  - Right 0QTD0ZZ
- Penis 0VTS
- Pericardium 02TN
- Phalanx
  - Finger
    - Left 0PTV0ZZ
    - Right 0PTT0ZZ
  - Thumb
    - Left 0PTS0ZZ
    - Right 0PTR0ZZ
  - Toe
    - Left 0QTR0ZZ
    - Right 0QTQ0ZZ
- Pharynx 0CTM
- Pineal Body 0GT1
- Prepuce 0VTT
- Products of Conception, Ectopic 10T2
- Prostate 0VT0
- Radius
  - Left 0PTJ0ZZ
  - Right 0PTH0ZZ

Resection *(continued)*
- Rectum 0DTP
- Ribs
  - 1 to 2 0PT10ZZ
  - 3 or More 0PT20ZZ
- Scapula
  - Left 0PT60ZZ
  - Right 0PT50ZZ
- Scrotum 0VT5
- Septum
  - Atrial 02T5
  - Nasal 09TM
  - Ventricular 02TM
- Sinus
  - Accessory 09TP
  - Ethmoid
    - Left 09TV
    - Right 09TU
  - Frontal
    - Left 09TT
    - Right 09TS
  - Mastoid
    - Left 09TC
    - Right 09TB
  - Maxillary
    - Left 09TR
    - Right 09TQ
  - Sphenoid
    - Left 09TX
    - Right 09TW
- Spleen 07TP
- Sternum 0PT00ZZ
- Stomach 0DT6
  - Pylorus 0DT7
- Tarsal
  - Left 0QTM0ZZ
  - Right 0QTL0ZZ
- Tendon
  - Abdomen
    - Left 0LTG
    - Right 0LTF
  - Ankle
    - Left 0LTT
    - Right 0LTS
  - Foot
    - Left 0LTW
    - Right 0LTV
  - Hand
    - Left 0LT8
    - Right 0LT7
  - Head and Neck 0LT0
  - Hip
    - Left 0LTK
    - Right 0LTJ
  - Knee
    - Left 0LTR
    - Right 0LTQ
  - Lower Arm and Wrist
    - Left 0LT6
    - Right 0LT5
  - Lower Leg
    - Left 0LTP
    - Right 0LTN
  - Perineum 0LTH
  - Shoulder
    - Left 0LT2
    - Right 0LT1
  - Thorax
    - Left 0LTD
    - Right 0LTC
  - Trunk
    - Left 0LTB
    - Right 0LT9
  - Upper Arm
    - Left 0LT4
    - Right 0LT3
  - Upper Leg
    - Left 0LTM
    - Right 0LTL

Resection *(continued)*
Testis
Bilateral 0VTC
Left 0VTB
Right 0VT9
Thymus 07TM
Thyroid Gland 0GTK
Left Lobe 0GTG
Right Lobe 0GTH
Thyroid Gland Isthmus 0GTJ
Tibia
Left 0QTH0ZZ
Right 0QTG0ZZ
Toe Nail 0HTRXZZ
Tongue 0CT7
Tonsils 0CTP
Tooth
Lower 0CTX0Z
Upper 0CTW0Z
Trachea 0BT1
Tunica Vaginalis
Left 0VT7
Right 0VT6
Turbinate, Nasal 09TL
Tympanic Membrane
Left 09T8
Right 09T7
Ulna
Left 0PTL0ZZ
Right 0PTK0ZZ
Ureter
Left 0TT7
Right 0TT6
Urethra 0TTD
Uterine Supporting Structure 0UT4
Uterus 0UT9
Uvula 0CTN
Vagina 0UTG
Valve, Pulmonary 02TH
Vas Deferens
Bilateral 0VTQ
Left 0VTP
Right 0VTN
Vesicle
Bilateral 0VT3
Left 0VT2
Right 0VT1
Vitreous
Left 08T53ZZ
Right 08T43ZZ
Vocal Cord
Left 0CTV
Right 0CTT
Vulva 0UTM
Resection, Left ventricular outflow tract obstruction (LVOT)
see Dilation, Ventricle, Left 027L
Resection, Subaortic membrane (Left ventricular outflow tract obstruction)
see Dilation, Ventricle, Left 027L
Restoration, Cardiac, Single, Rhythm 5A2204Z
RestoreAdvanced neurostimulator (SureScan)(MRI Safe)
use Stimulator Generator, Multiple Array Rechargeable in 0JH
RestoreSensor neurostimulator (SureScan)(MRI Safe)
use Stimulator Generator, Multiple Array Rechargeable in 0JH
RestoreUltra neurostimulator (SureScan)(MRI Safe)
use Stimulator Generator, Multiple Array Rechargeable in 0JH
Restriction
Ampulla of Vater 0FVC
Anus 0DVQ

Restriction *(continued)*
Aorta
Abdominal 04V0
Intraluminal Device, Branched or Fenestrated 04V0
Thoracic
Ascending/Arch, Intraluminal Device, Branched or Fenestrated 02VX
Descending, Intraluminal Device, Branched or Fenestrated 02VW
Artery
Anterior Tibial
Left 04VQ
Right 04VP
Axillary
Left 03V6
Right 03V5
Brachial
Left 03V8
Right 03V7
Celiac 04V1
Colic
Left 04V7
Middle 04V8
Right 04V6
Common Carotid
Left 03VJ
Right 03VH
Common Iliac
Left 04VD
Right 04VC
External Carotid
Left 03VN
Right 03VM
External Iliac
Left 04VJ
Right, 04VHZ
Face 03VR
Femoral
Left 04VL
Right 04VK
Foot
Left 04VW
Right 04VV
Gastric 04V2
Hand
Left 03VF
Right 03VD
Hepatic 04V3
Inferior Mesenteric 04VB
Innominate 03V2
Internal Carotid
Left 03VL
Right 03VK
Internal Iliac
Left 04VF
Right 04VE
Internal Mammary
Left 03V1
Right 03V0
Intracranial 03VG
Lower 04VY
Peroneal
Left 04VU
Right 04VT
Popliteal
Left 04VN
Right 04VM
Posterior Tibial
Left 04VS
Right 04VR
Pulmonary
Left 02VR
Right 02VQ
Pulmonary Trunk 02VP
Radial
Left 03VC
Right 03VB

Restriction *(continued)*
Artery *(continued)*
Renal
Left 04VA
Right 04V9
Splenic 04V4
Subclavian
Left 03V4
Right 03V3
Superior Mesenteric 04V5
Temporal
Left 03VT
Right 03VS
Thyroid
Left 03VV
Right 03VU
Ulnar
Left 03VA
Right 03V9
Upper 03VY
Vertebral
Left 03VQ
Right 03VP
Bladder 0TVB
Bladder Neck 0TVC
Bronchus
Lingula 0BV9
Lower Lobe
Left 0BVB
Right 0BV6
Main
Left 0BV7
Right 0BV3
Middle Lobe, Right 0BV5
Upper Lobe
Left 0BV8
Right 0BV4
Carina 0BV2
Cecum 0DVH
Cervix 0UVC
Cisterna Chyli 07VL
Colon
Ascending 0DVK
Descending 0DVM
Sigmoid 0DVN
Transverse 0DVL
Duct
Common Bile 0FV9
Cystic 0FV8
Hepatic
Common 0FV7
Left 0FV6
Right 0FV5
Lacrimal
Left 08VY
Right 08VX
Pancreatic 0FVD
Accessory 0FVF
Parotid
Left 0CVC
Right 0CVB
Duodenum 0DV9
Esophagogastric Junction 0DV4
Esophagus 0DV5
Lower 0DV3
Middle 0DV2
Upper 0DV1
Heart 02VA
Ileocecal Valve 0DVC
Ileum 0DVB
Intestine
Large 0DVE
Left 0DVG
Right 0DVF
Small 0DV8
Jejunum 0DVA
Kidney Pelvis
Left 0TV4

Restriction *(continued)*
Kidney Pelvis *(continued)*
Right 0TV3
Lymphatic
Aortic 07VD
Axillary
Left 07V6
Right 07V5
Head 07V0
Inguinal
Left 07VJ
Right 07VH
Internal Mammary
Left 07V9
Right 07V8
Lower Extremity
Left 07VG
Right 07VF
Mesenteric 07VB
Neck
Left 07V2
Right 07V1
Pelvis 07VC
Thoracic Duct 07VK
Thorax 07V7
Upper Extremity
Left 07V4
Right 07V3
Rectum 0DVP
Stomach 0DV6
Pylorus 0DV7
Trachea 0BV1
Ureter
Left 0TV7
Right 0TV6
Urethra 0TVD
Valve, Mitral 02VG
Vein
Axillary
Left 05V8
Right 05V7
Azygos 05V0
Basilic
Left 05VC
Right 05VB
Brachial
Left 05VA
Right 05V9
Cephalic
Left 05VF
Right 05VD
Colic 06V7Z
Common Iliac
Left 06VD
Right 06VC
Esophageal 06V3
External Iliac
Left 06VG
Right 06VF
External Jugular
Left 05VQ
Right 05VP
Face
Left 05VV
Right 05VT
Femoral
Left 06VN
Right 06VM
Foot
Left 06VV
Right 06VT
Gastric 06V2
Hand
Left 05VH
Right 05VG
Hemiazygos 05V1
Hepatic 06V4
Hypogastric
Left 06VJ
Right 06VH

Revision of device in *(continued)*
Lung
Left 0BWL
Right 0BWK
Lymphatic 07WN
Thoracic Duct 07WK
Mediastinum 0WWC
Mesentery 0DWV
Metacarpal
Left 0PWQ
Right 0PWP
Metatarsal
Left 0QWP
Right 0QWN
Mouth and Throat 0CWY
Muscle
Extraocular
Left 08WM
Right 08WL
Lower 0KWY
Upper 0KWX
Nasal Mucosa and Soft Tissue 09WK
Neck 0WW6
Nerve
Cranial 00WE
Peripheral 01WY
Omentum 0DWU
Ovary 0UW3
Pancreas 0FWG
Parathyroid Gland 0GWR
Patella
Left 0QWF
Right 0QWD
Pelvic Cavity 0WWJ
Penis 0VWS
Pericardial Cavity 0WWD
Perineum
Female 0WWN
Male 0WWM
Peritoneal Cavity 0WWG
Peritoneum 0DWW
Phalanx
Finger
Left 0PWV
Right 0PWT
Thumb
Left 0PWS
Right 0PWR
Toe
Left 0QWR
Right 0QWQ
Pineal Body 0GW10
Pleura 0BWQ
Pleural Cavity
Left 0WWB
Right 0WW9
Prostate and Seminal Vesicles 0VW4
Radius
Left 0PWJ
Right 0PWH
Respiratory Tract 0WWQ
Retroperitoneum 0WWH
Ribs
1 to 2 0PW1
3 or More 0PW2
Sacrum 0QW1
Scapula
Left 0PW6
Right 0PW5
Scrotum and Tunica Vaginalis 0VW8
Septum
Atrial 02W5
Ventricular 02WM
Sinus 09WY0
Skin 0HWPX
Skull 0NW0
Spinal Canal 00WU
Spinal Cord 00WV

Revision of device in *(continued)*
Spleen 07WP
Sternum 0PW0
Stomach 0DW6
Subcutaneous Tissue and Fascia
Head and Neck 0JWS
Lower Extremity 0JWW
Trunk 0JWT
Upper Extremity 0JWV
Tarsal
Left 0QWM
Right 0QWL
Tendon
Lower 0LWY
Upper 0LWX
Testis 0VWD
Thymus 07WM
Thyroid Gland 0GWK0
Tibia
Left 0QWH
Right 0QWG
Toe Nail 0HWRX
Trachea 0BW1F
Tracheobronchial Tree 0BW0
Tympanic Membrane
Left 09W8
Right 09W7
Ulna
Left 0PWL
Right 0PWK
Ureter 0TW9M
Urethra 0TWD
Uterus and Cervix 0UWD
Vagina and Cul-de-sac 0UWH
Valve
Aortic 02WF
Mitral 02WG
Pulmonary 02WH
Tricuspid 02WJ
Vas Deferens 0VWR
Vein
Azygos 05W0
Innominate
Left 05W4
Right 05W3
Lower 06WY
Upper 05WY
Vertebra
Cervical 0PW3
Lumbar 0QW0
Thoracic 0PW4
Vulva 0UWM

Revo MRI™ SureScan® pacemaker
use Pacemaker, Dual Chamber in 0JH
rhBMP-2
use Recombinant Bone Morphogenetic Protein
Rheos® System device
use Stimulator Generator in Subcutaneous Tissue and Fascia
Rheos® System lead
use Stimulator Lead in Upper Arteries
Rhinopharynx
use Nasopharynx
Rhinoplasty
see Alteration, Nasal Mucosa and Soft Tissue 090K
see Repair, Nasal Mucosa and Soft Tissue 09QK
see Replacement, Nasal Mucosa and Soft Tissue 09RK
see Supplement, Nasal Mucosa and Soft Tissue 09UK
Rhinorrhaphy
see Repair, Nasal Mucosa and Soft Tissue 09QK
Rhinoscopy 09JKXZZ
Rhizotomy
see Division, Central Nervous System and Cranial Nerves 008
see Division, Peripheral Nervous System 018
Rhomboid major muscle
use Muscle, Trunk, Left
use Muscle, Trunk, Right
Rhomboid minor muscle
use Muscle, Trunk, Left
use Muscle, Trunk, Right
Rhythm electrocardiogram
see Measurement, Cardiac 4A02
Rhytidectomy
see Alteration, Face 0W02
Right ascending lumbar vein
use Vein, Azygos
Right atrioventricular valve
use Valve, Tricuspid
Right auricular appendix
use Atrium, Right
Right colic vein
use Vein, Colic
Right coronary sulcus
use Heart, Right
Right gastric artery
use Artery, Gastric
Right gastroepiploic vein
use Vein, Superior Mesenteric
Right inferior phrenic vein
use Vena Cava, Inferior
Right inferior pulmonary vein
use Vein, Pulmonary, Right
Right jugular trunk
use Lymphatic, Neck, Right
Right lateral ventricle
use Cerebral Ventricle
Right lymphatic duct
use Lymphatic, Neck, Right
Right ovarian vein
use Vena Cava, Inferior
Right second lumbar vein
use Vena Cava, Inferior
Right subclavian trunk
use Lymphatic, Neck, Right
Right subcostal vein
use Vein, Azygos
Right superior pulmonary vein
use Vein, Pulmonary, Right
Right suprarenal vein
use Vena Cava, Inferior
Right testicular vein
use Vena Cava, Inferior
Rima glottidis
use Larynx
Risorius muscle
use Muscle, Facial
RNS System lead
use Neurostimulator Lead in Central Nervous System and Cranial Nerves
RNS system neurostimulator generator
use Neurostimulator Generator in Head and Facial Bones
Robotic Assisted Procedure
Extremity
Lower 8E0Y
Upper 8E0X
Head and Neck Region 8E09
Trunk Region 8E0W
Robotic Waterjet Ablation, Destruction, Prostate XV508A4
Rotation of fetal head
Forceps 10S07ZZ
Manual 10S0XZZ
Round ligament of uterus
use Uterine Supporting Structure
Round window
use Ear, Inner, Left
use Ear, Inner, Right
Roux-en-Y operation
see Bypass, Gastrointestinal System 0D1
see Bypass, Hepatobiliary System and Pancreas 0F1
Rupture
Adhesions
see Release
Fluid collection
see Drainage
Ruxolitinib XW0DXT5

S

S-ICD™ lead
use SubutaneousDifibrillator Lead in Subcutaneous Tissue and Fascia
Sacral ganglion
use Nerve, Sacral Sympathetic
Sacral lymph node
use Lymphatic, Pelvis
Sacral nerve modulation (SNM) lead
use Stimulator Lead in Urinary System
Sacral neuromodulation lead
use Stimulator Lead in Urinary System
Sacral splanchnic nerve
use Nerve, Sacral Sympathetic
Sacrectomy
see Excision, Lower Bones 0QB
Sacrococcygeal ligament
use Bursa and Ligament, Lower Spine
Sacrococcygeal symphysis
use Joint, Sacrococcygeal
Sacroiliac ligament
use Bursa and Ligament, Lower Spine
Sacrospinous ligament
use Bursa and Ligament, Lower Spine
Sacrotuberous ligament
use Bursa and Ligament, Lower Spine
Salpingectomy
see Excision, Female Reproductive System 0UB
see Resection, Female Reproductive System 0UT
Salpingolysis
see Release, Female Reproductive System 0UN
Salpingopexy
see Repair, Female Reproductive System 0UQ
see Reposition, Female Reproductive System 0US
Salpingopharyngeus muscle
use Muscle, Tongue, Palate, Pharynx
Salpingoplasty
see Repair, Female Reproductive System 0UQ
see Supplement, Female Reproductive System 0UU
Salpingorrhaphy
see Repair, Female Reproductive System 0UQ
Salpingoscopy 0UJ88ZZ
Salpingostomy
see Drainage, Female Reproductive System 0U9

Salpingotomy
see Drainage, Female Reproductive System 0U9
Salpinx
use Fallopian Tube, Left
use Fallopian Tube, Right
Saphenous nerve
use Nerve, Femoral
SAPIEN transcatheter aortic valve
use Zooplastic Tissue in Heart and Great Vessels
Sarilumab XW0
SARS-CoV-2 Antibody Detection, Serum/Plasma Nanoparticle Fluorescence XXE5XV7
SARS-CoV-2 Polymerase Chain Reaction, Nasopharyngeal Fluid XXE97U7
Sartorius muscle
use Muscle, Upper Leg, Left
use Muscle, Upper Leg, Right
Satralizumab-mwge XW01397
SAVAL below-the-knee (BTK) drug-eluting stent system
use Intraluminal Device, Sustained Release Drug-eluting in New Technology
use Intraluminal Device, Sustained Release Drug-eluting, Four or More in New Technology
use Intraluminal Device, Sustained Release Drug-eluting, Three in New Technology
use Intraluminal Device, Sustained Release Drug-eluting, Two in New Technology
Scalene muscle
use Muscle, Neck, Left
use Muscle, Neck, Right
Scan
Computerized Tomography (CT)
see Computerized Tomography (CT Scan)
Radioisotope
see Planar Nuclear Medicine Imaging
Scaphoid bone
use Carpal, Left
use Carpal, Right
Scapholunate ligament
use Bursa and Ligament, Wrist, Left
use Bursa and Ligament, Wrist, Right
Scaphotrapezium ligament
use Bursa and Ligament, Hand, Left
use Bursa and Ligament, Hand, Right
Scapulectomy
see Excision, Upper Bones 0PB
see Resection, Upper Bones 0PT
Scapulopexy
see Repair, Upper Bones 0PQ
see Reposition, Upper Bones 0PS
Scarpa's (vestibular) ganglion
use Nerve, Acoustic
Sclerectomy
see Excision, Eye 08B
Sclerotherapy, mechanical
see Destruction
Sclerotherapy, via injection of sclerosing agent
see Introduction, Destructive Agent
Sclerotomy
see Drainage, Eye 089
Scrotectomy
see Excision, Male Reproductive System 0VB
see Resection, Male Reproductive System 0VT
Scrotoplasty
see Repair, Male Reproductive System 0VQ
see Supplement, Male Reproductive System 0VU
Scrotorrhaphy
see Repair, Male Reproductive System 0VQ
Scrototomy
see Drainage, Male Reproductive System 0V9
Sebaceous gland
use Skin
Second cranial nerve
use Nerve, Optic
Section, cesarean
see Extraction, Pregnancy 10D
Secura (DR) (VR)
use Defibrillator Generator in 0JH
Sella Turcica
use Bone, Sphenoid
Semicircular canal
use Ear, Inner, Left
use Ear, Inner, Right
Semimembranosus muscle
use Muscle, Upper Leg, Left
use Muscle, Upper Leg, Right
Semitendinosus muscle
use Muscle, Upper Leg, Left
use Muscle, Upper Leg, Right
Sentinel™ Cerebral Protection System (CPS) X2A5312
Seprafilm
use Adhesion Barrier
Septal cartilage
use Septum, Nasal
Septectomy
see Excision, Ear, Nose, Sinus 09B
see Excision, Heart and Great Vessels 02B
see Resection, Ear, Nose, Sinus 09T
see Resection, Heart and Great Vessels 02T
Septoplasty
see Repair, Ear, Nose, Sinus 09Q
see Repair, Heart and Great Vessels 02Q
see Replacement, Ear, Nose, Sinus 09R
see Replacement, Heart and Great Vessels 02R
see Reposition, Ear, Nose, Sinus 09S
see Supplement, Ear, Nose, Sinus 09U
see Supplement, Heart and Great Vessels 02U
Septostomy, balloon atrial 02163Z7
Septotomy
see Drainage, Ear, Nose, Sinus 099
Sequestrectomy, bone
see Extirpation
Serratus anterior muscle
use Muscle, Thorax, Left
use Muscle, Thorax, Right
Serratus posterior muscle
use Muscle, Trunk, Left
use Muscle, Trunk, Right
Seventh cranial nerve
use Nerve, Facial
Sheffield hybrid external fixator
use External Fixation Device, Hybrid in 0PH
use External Fixation Device, Hybrid in 0PS
use External Fixation Device, Hybrid in 0QH
use External Fixation Device, Hybrid in 0QS
Sheffield ring external fixator
use External Fixation Device, Ring in 0PH
use External Fixation Device, Ring in 0PS
use External Fixation Device, Ring in 0QH
use External Fixation Device, Ring in 0QS
Shirodkar cervical cerclage 0UVC7ZZ
Shockwave Intravascular Lithotripsy (Shockwave IVL)
see Fragmentation
Shock Wave Therapy, Musculoskeletal 6A93
Short gastric artery
use Artery, Splenic
Shortening
see Excision
see Repair
see Reposition
Shunt creation
see Bypass
Sialoadenectomy
Complete
see Resection, Mouth and Throat 0CT
Partial
see Excision, Mouth and Throat 0CB
Sialodochoplasty
see Repair, Mouth and Throat 0CQ
see Replacement, Mouth and Throat 0CR
see Supplement, Mouth and Throat 0CU
Sialoectomy
see Excision, Mouth and Throat 0CB
see Resection, Mouth and Throat 0CT
Sialography
see Plain Radiography, Ear, Nose, Mouth and Throat B90
Sialolithotomy
see Extirpation, Mouth and Throat 0CC
Sigmoid artery
use Artery, Inferior Mesenteric
Sigmoid flexure
use Colon, Sigmoid
Sigmoid vein
use Vein, Inferior Mesenteric
Sigmoidectomy
see Excision, Gastrointestinal System 0DB
see Resection, Gastrointestinal System 0DT
Sigmoidorrhaphy
see Repair, Gastrointestinal System 0DQ
Sigmoidoscopy 0DJD8ZZ
Sigmoidotomy
see Drainage, Gastrointestinal System 0D9
Single lead pacemaker (atrium) (ventricle)
use Pacemaker, Single Chamber in 0JH
Single lead rate responsive pacemaker (atrium)(ventricle)
use Pacemaker, Single Chamber Rate Responsive in 0JH
Single-use Duodenoscope XFJ
Single-use Oversleeve with Intraoperative Colonic Irrigation XDPH8K7
Sinoatrial node
use Conduction Mechanism
Sinogram
Abdominal Wall
see Fluoroscopy, Abdomen and Pelvis BW11
Chest Wall
see Plain Radiography, Chest BW03
Retroperitoneum
see Fluoroscopy, Abdomen and Pelvis BW11
Sinusectomy
see Excision, Ear, Nose, Sinus 09B
see Resection, Ear, Nose, Sinus 09T
Sinusoscopy 09JY4ZZ
Sinusotomy
see Drainage, Ear, Nose, Sinus 099
Sinus venosus
use Atrium, Right
Sirolimus-eluting coronary stent
use Intraluminal Device, Drug-eluting in Heart and Great Vessels
Sixth cranial nerve
use Nerve, Abducens
Size reduction, breast
see Excision, Skin and Breast 0HB
SJM Biocor® Stented Valve System
use Zooplastic Tissue in Heart and Great Vessels
Skene's (paraurethral) gland
use Gland, Vestibular
Skin Substitute, Porcine Liver Derived, Replacement XHRPXL2
Sling
Fascial, orbicularis muscle (mouth)
see Supplement, Muscle, Facial 0KU1
Levator muscle, for urethral suspension
see Reposition, Bladder Neck 0TSC
Pubococcygeal, for urethral suspension
see Reposition, Bladder Neck 0TSC
Rectum
see Reposition, Rectum 0DSP
Small bowel series
see Fluoroscopy, Bowel, Small BD13
Small saphenous vein
use Vein, Saphenous, Left
use Vein, Saphenous, Right
Snapshot_NIR 8E02XDZ
Snaring, polyp, colon
see Excision, Gastrointestinal System 0DB
Solar (celiac) plexus
use Nerve, Abdominal Sympathetic
Soleus muscle
use Muscle, Lower Leg, Left
use Muscle, Lower Leg, Right
Soliris®
see Eculizumab
Spacer
Insertion of device in
Disc
Lumbar Vertebral 0SH2
Lumbosacral 0SH4
Joint
Acromioclavicular
Left 0RHH
Right 0RHG
Ankle
Left 0SHG
Right 0SHF

Spacer *(continued)*
Insertion of device in *(continued)*
Joint*(continued)*
Carpal
Left 0RHR
Right 0RHQ
Carpometacarpal
Left 0RHT
Right 0RHS
Cervical Vertebral 0RH1
Cervicothoracic Vertebral 0RH4
Coccygeal 0SH6
Elbow
Left 0RHM
Right 0RHL
Finger Phalangeal
Left 0RHX
Right 0RHW
Hip
Left 0SHB
Right 0SH9
Knee
Left 0SHD
Right 0SHC
Lumbar Vertebral 0SH0
Lumbosacral 0SH3
Metacarpophalangeal
Left 0RHV
Right 0RHU
Metatarsal-Phalangeal
Left 0SHN
Right 0SHM
Occipital-cervical 0RH0
Sacrococcygeal 0SH5
Sacroiliac
Left 0SH8
Right 0SH7
Shoulder
Left 0RHK
Right 0RHJ
Sternoclavicular
Left 0RHF
Right 0RHE
Tarsal
Left 0SHJ
Right 0SHH
Tarsometatarsal
Left 0SHL
Right 0SHK
Temporomandibular
Left 0RHD
Right 0RHC
Thoracic Vertebral 0RH6
Thoracolumbar Vertebral 0RHA
Toe Phalangeal
Left 0SHQ
Right 0SHP
Wrist
Left 0RHP
Right 0RHN
Removal of device from
Acromioclavicular
Left 0RPH
Right 0RPG
Ankle
Left 0SPG
Right 0SPF
Carpal
Left 0RPR
Right 0RPQ
Carpometacarpal
Left 0RPT
Right 0RPS
Cervical Vertebral 0RP1
Cervicothoracic Vertebral 0RP4
Coccygeal 0SP6
Elbow
Left 0RPM

Spacer *(continued)*
Removal of device from *(continued)*
Elbow *(continued)*
Right 0RPL
Finger Phalangeal
Left 0RPX
Right 0RPW
Hip
Left 0SPB
Right 0SP9
Knee
Left 0SPD
Right 0SPC
Lumbar Vertebral 0SP0
Lumbosacral 0SP3
Metacarpophalangeal
Left 0RPV
Right 0RPU
Metatarsal-Phalangeal
Left 0SPN
Right 0SPM
Occipital-cervical 0RP0
Sacrococcygeal 0SP5
Sacroiliac
Left 0SP8
Right 0SP7
Shoulder
Left 0RPK
Right 0RPJ
Sternoclavicular
Left 0RPF
Right 0RPE
Tarsal
Left 0SPJ
Right 0SPH
Tarsometatarsal
Left 0SPL
Right 0SPK
Temporomandibular
Left 0RPD
Right 0RPC
Thoracic Vertebral 0RP6
Thoracolumbar Vertebral 0RPA
Toe Phalangeal
Left 0SPQ
Right 0SPP
Wrist
Left 0RPP
Right 0RPN
Revision of device in
Acromioclavicular
Left 0RWH
Right 0RWG
Ankle
Left 0SWG
Right 0SWF
Carpal
Left 0RWR
Right 0RWQ
Carpometacarpal
Left 0RWT
Right 0RWS
Cervical Vertebral 0RW1
Cervicothoracic Vertebral 0RW4
Coccygeal 0SW6
Elbow
Left 0RWM
Right 0RWL
Finger Phalangeal
Left 0RWX
Right 0RWW
Hip
Left 0SWB
Right 0SW9
Knee
Left 0SWD
Right 0SWC
Lumbar Vertebral 0SW0
Lumbosacral 0SW3

Spacer *(continued)*
Revision of device in *(continued)*
Metacarpophalangeal
Left 0RWV
Right 0RWU
Metatarsal-Phalangeal
Left 0SWN
Right 0SWM
Occipital-cervical 0RW0
Sacrococcygeal 0SW5
Sacroiliac
Left 0SW8
Right 0SW7
Shoulder
Left 0RWK
Right 0RWJ
Sternoclavicular
Left 0RWF
Right 0RWE
Tarsal
Left 0SWJ
Right 0SWH
Tarsometatarsal
Left 0SWL
Right 0SWK
Temporomandibular
Left 0RWD
Right 0RWC
Thoracic Vertebral 0RW6
Thoracolumbar Vertebral 0RWA
Toe Phalangeal
Left 0SWQ
Right 0SWP
Wrist
Left 0RWP
Right 0RWN

Spacer, Articulating (Antibiotic)
use Articulating Spacer in Lower Joints

Spacer, Static (Antibiotic)
use Spacer in Lower Joints

Spectroscopy
Intravascular Near Infrared 8E023DZ
Near Infrared
see Physiological Systems and Anatomical Regions 8E0

Speech Assessment F00

Speech therapy
see Speech Treatment, Rehabilitation F06

Speech Treatment F06

Sphenoidectomy
see Excision, Ear, Nose, Sinus 09B
see Excision, Head and Facial Bones 0NB
see Resection, Ear, Nose, Sinus 09T
see Resection, Head and Facial Bones 0NT

Sphenoidotomy
see Drainage, Ear, Nose, Sinus 099

Sphenomandibular ligament
use Bursa and Ligament, Head and Neck

Sphenopalatine (pterygopalatine) ganglion
use Nerve, Head and Neck Sympathetic

Sphincterorrhaphy, anal
see Repair, Anal Sphincter 0DQR

Sphincterotomy, anal
see Division, Anal Sphincter 0D8R
see Drainage, Anal Sphincter 0D9R

Spinal cord neurostimulator lead
use Neurostimulator Lead in Central Nervous System and Cranial Nerves

Spinal growth rod(s), magnetically controlled
use Magnetically Controlled Growth Rod(s) in New Technology

Spinal nerve, cervical
use Nerve, Cervical

Spinal nerve, lumbar
use Nerve, Lumbar

Spinal nerve, sacral
use Nerve, Sacral

Spinal nerve, thoracic
use Nerve, Thoracic

Spinal Stabilization Device
Facet Replacement
Cervical Vertebral 0RH1
Cervicothoracic Vertebral 0RH4
Lumbar Vertebral 0SH0
Lumbosacral 0SH3
Occipital-cervical 0RH0
Thoracic Vertebral 0RH6
Thoracolumbar Vertebral 0RHA
Interspinous Process
Cervical Vertebral 0RH1
Cervicothoracic Vertebral 0RH4
Lumbar Vertebral 0SH0
Lumbosacral 0SH3
Occipital-cervical 0RH0
Thoracic Vertebral 0RH6
Thoracolumbar Vertebral 0RHA
Pedicle-Based
Cervical Vertebral 0RH1
Cervicothoracic Vertebral 0RH4
Lumbar Vertebral 0SH0
Lumbosacral 0SH3
Occipital-cervical 0RH0
Thoracic Vertebral 0RH6
Thoracolumbar Vertebral 0RHA

SpineJack® system
use Synthetic Substitute, Mechanically Expandable (Paired) in New Technology

Spinous process
use Vertebra, Cervical
use Vertebra, Lumbar
use Vertebra, Thoracic

Spiral ganglion
use Nerve, Acoustic

Spiration IBV™ Valve System
use Intraluminal Device, Endobronchial Valve in Respiratory System

Splenectomy
see Excision, Lymphatic and Hemic Systems 07B
see Resection, Lymphatic and Hemic Systems 07T

Splenic flexure
use Colon, Transverse

Splenic plexus
use Nerve, Abdominal Sympathetic

Splenius capitis muscle
use Muscle, Head

Splenius cervicis muscle
use Muscle, Neck, Left
use Muscle, Neck, Right

Splenolysis
see Release, Lymphatic and Hemic Systems 07N

Splenopexy
see Repair, Lymphatic and Hemic Systems 07Q
see Reposition, Lymphatic and Hemic Systems 07S

Splenoplasty
see Repair, Lymphatic and Hemic Systems 07Q

Splenorrhaphy
see Repair, Lymphatic and Hemic Systems 07Q

Splenotomy
see Drainage, Lymphatic and Hemic Systems 079

Splinting, musculoskeletal
see Immobilization, Anatomical Regions 2W3
SPRAVATO™
use Esketamine Hydrochloride
SPY system intravascular fluorescence angiography
see Monitoring, Physiological Systems 4A1
SPY PINPOINT fluorescence imaging system
see Monitoring, Physiological Systems 4A1
see Other Imaging, Hepatobiliary System and Pancreas BF5
SPY system intraoperative fluorescence cholangiography
see Other Imaging, Hepatobiliary System and Pancreas BF5
Staged hepatectomy
see Division, Hepatobiliary System and Pancreas 0F8
see Resection, Hepatobiliary System and Pancreas 0FT
Stapedectomy
see Excision, Ear, Nose, Sinus 09B
see Resection, Ear, Nose, Sinus 09T
Stapediolysis
see Release, Ear, Nose, Sinus 09N
Stapedioplasty
see Repair, Ear, Nose, Sinus 09Q
see Replacement, Ear, Nose, Sinus 09R
see Supplement, Ear, Nose, Sinus 09U
Stapedotomy
see Drainage, Ear, Nose, Sinus 099
Stapes
use Auditory Ossicle, Left
use Auditory Ossicle, Right
Static Spacer (Antibiotic)
use Spacer in Lower Joints
STELARA®
use Other New Technology Therapeutic Substance
Stellate ganglion
use Nerve, Head and Neck Sympathetic
Stem cell transplant
see Transfusion, Circulatory 302
Stensen's duct
use Duct, Parotid, Left
use Duct, Parotid, Right
Stent retriever thrombectomy
see Extirpation, Upper Arteries 03C
Stent, intraluminal (cardiovascular)(gastrointestinal)(hepatobiliary)(urinary)
use Intraluminal Device
Stented tissue valve
use Zooplastic Tissue in Heart and Great Vessels
Stereotactic Radiosurgery
Abdomen DW23
Adrenal Gland DG22
Bile Ducts DF22
Bladder DT22
Bone Marrow D720
Brain D020
Brain Stem D021
Breast
Left DM20
Right DM21
Bronchus DB21
Cervix DU21
Chest DW22
Chest Wall DB27
Colon DD25
Diaphragm DB28
Duodenum DD22
Ear D920
Esophagus DD20

Stereotactic Radiosurgery *(continued)*
Eye D820
Gallbladder DF21
Gamma Beam
Abdomen DW23JZZ
Adrenal Gland DG22JZZ
Bile Ducts DF22JZZ
Bladder DT22JZZ
Bone Marrow D720JZZ
Brain D020JZZ
Brain Stem D021JZZ
Breast
Left DM20JZZ
Right DM21JZZ
Bronchus DB21JZZ
Cervix DU21JZZ
Chest DW22JZZ
Chest Wall DB27JZZ
Colon DD25JZZ
Diaphragm DB28JZZ
Duodenum DD22JZZ
Ear D920JZZ
Esophagus DD20JZZ
Eye D820JZZ
Gallbladder DF21JZZ
Gland
Adrenal DG22JZZ
Parathyroid DG24JZZ
Pituitary DG20JZZ
Thyroid DG25JZZ
Glands, Salivary D926JZZ
Head and Neck DW21JZZ
Ileum DD24JZZ
Jejunum DD23JZZ
Kidney DT20JZZ
Larynx D92BJZZ
Liver DF20JZZ
Lung DB22JZZ
Lymphatics
Abdomen D726JZZ
Axillary D724JZZ
Inguinal D728JZZ
Neck D723JZZ
Pelvis D727JZZ
Thorax D725JZZ
Mediastinum DB26JZZ
Mouth D924JZZ
Nasopharynx D92DJZZ
Neck and Head DW21JZZ
Nerve, Peripheral D027JZZ
Nose D921JZZ
Ovary DU20JZZ
Palate
Hard D928JZZ
Soft D929JZZ
Pancreas DF23JZZ
Parathyroid Gland DG24JZZ
Pelvic Region DW26JZZ
Pharynx D92CJZZ
Pineal Body DG21JZZ
Pituitary Gland DG20JZZ
Pleura DB25JZZ
Prostate DV20JZZ
Rectum DD27JZZ
Sinuses D927JZZ
Spinal Cord D026JZZ
Spleen D722JZZ
Stomach DD21JZZ
Testis DV21JZZ
Thymus D721JZZ
Thyroid Gland DG25JZZ
Tongue D925JZZ
Trachea DB20JZZ
Ureter DT21JZZ
Urethra DT23JZZ
Uterus DU22JZZ
Gland
Adrenal DG22
Parathyroid DG24
Pituitary DG20

Stereotactic Radiosurgery *(continued)*
Gland *(continued)*
Thyroid DG25
Glands, Salivary D926
Head and Neck DW21
Ileum DD24
Jejunum DD23
Kidney DT20
Larynx D92B
Liver DF20
Lung DB22
Lymphatics
Abdomen D726
Axillary D724
Inguinal D728
Neck D723
Pelvis D727
Thorax D725
Mediastinum DB26
Mouth D924
Nasopharynx D92D
Neck and Head DW21
Nerve, Peripheral D027
Nose D921
Other Photon
Abdomen DW23DZZ
Adrenal Gland DG22DZZ
Bile Ducts DF22DZZ
Bladder DT22DZZ
Bone Marrow D720DZZ
Brain D020DZZ
Brain Stem D021DZZ
Breast
Left DM20DZZ
Right DM21DZZ
Bronchus DB21DZZ
Cervix DU21DZZ
Chest DW22DZZ
Chest Wall DB27DZZ
Colon DD25DZZ
Diaphragm DB28DZZ
Duodenum DD22DZZ
Ear D920DZZ
Esophagus DD20DZZ
Eye D820DZZ
Gallbladder DF21DZZ
Gland
Adrenal DG22DZZ
Parathyroid DG24DZZ
Pituitary DG20DZZ
Thyroid DG25DZZ
Glands, Salivary D926DZZ
Head and Neck DW21DZZ
Ileum DD24DZZ
Jejunum DD23DZZ
Kidney DT20DZZ
Larynx D92BDZZ
Liver DF20DZZ
Lung DB22DZZ
Lymphatics
Abdomen D726DZZ
Axillary D724DZZ
Inguinal D728DZZ
Neck D723DZZ
Pelvis D727DZZ
Thorax D725DZZ
Mediastinum DB26DZZ
Mouth D924DZZ
Nasopharynx D92DDZZ
Neck and Head DW21DZZ
Nerve, Peripheral D027DZZ
Nose D921DZZ
Ovary DU20DZZ
Palate
Hard D928DZZ
Soft D929DZZ
Pancreas DF23DZZ
Parathyroid Gland DG24DZZ
Pelvic Region DW26DZZ
Pharynx D92CDZZ

Stereotactic Radiosurgery *(continued)*
Other Photon *(continued)*
Pineal Body DG21DZZ
Pituitary Gland DG20DZZ
Pleura DB25DZZ
Prostate DV20DZZ
Rectum DD27DZZ
Sinuses D927DZZ
Spinal Cord D026DZZ
Spleen D722DZZ
Stomach DD21DZZ
Testis DV21DZZ
Thymus D721DZZ
Thyroid Gland DG25DZZ
Tongue D925DZZ
Trachea DB20DZZ
Ureter DT21DZZ
Urethra DT23DZZ
Uterus DU22DZZ
Ovary DU20
Palate
Hard D928
Soft D929
Pancreas DF23
Parathyroid Gland DG24
Particulate
Abdomen DW23HZZ
Adrenal Gland DG22HZZ
Bile Ducts DF22HZZ
Bladder DT22HZZ
Bone Marrow D720HZZ
Brain D020HZZ
Brain Stem D021HZZ
Breast
Left DM20HZZ
Right DM21HZZ
Bronchus DB21HZZ
Cervix DU21HZZ
Chest DW22HZZ
Chest Wall DB27HZZ
Colon DD25HZZ
Diaphragm DB28HZZ
Duodenum DD22HZZ
Ear D920HZZ
Esophagus DD20HZZ
Eye D820HZZ
Gallbladder DF21HZZ
Gland
Adrenal DG22HZZ
Parathyroid DG24HZZ
Pituitary DG20HZZ
Thyroid DG25HZZ
Glands, Salivary D926HZZ
Head and Neck DW21HZZ
Ileum DD24HZZ
Jejunum DD23HZZ
Kidney DT20HZZ
Larynx D92BHZZ
Liver DF20HZZ
Lung DB22HZZ
Lymphatics
Abdomen D726HZZ
Axillary D724HZZ
Inguinal D728HZZ
Neck D723HZZ
Pelvis D727HZZ
Thorax D725HZZ
Mediastinum DB26HZZ
Mouth D924HZZ
Nasopharynx D92DHZZ
Neck and Head DW21HZZ
Nerve, Peripheral D027HZZ
Nose D921HZZ
Ovary DU20HZZ
Palate
Hard D928HZZ
Soft D929HZZ
Pancreas DF23HZZ
Parathyroid Gland DG24HZZ
Pelvic Region DW26HZZ

Stereotactic Radiosurgery *(continued)*
Particulate *(continued)*
Pharynx D92CHZZ
Pineal Body DG21HZZ
Pituitary Gland DG20HZZ
Pleura DB25HZZ
Prostate DV20HZZ
Rectum DD27HZZ
Sinuses D927HZZ
Spinal Cord D026HZZ
Spleen D722HZZ
Stomach DD21HZZ
Testis DV21HZZ
Thymus D721HZZ
Thyroid Gland DG25HZZ
Tongue D925HZZ
Trachea DB20HZZ
Ureter DT21HZZ
Urethra DT23HZZ
Uterus DU22HZZ
Pelvic Region DW26
Pharynx D92C
Pineal Body DG21
Pituitary Gland DG20
Pleura DB25
Prostate DV20
Rectum DD27
Sinuses D927
Spinal Cord D026
Spleen D722
Stomach DD21
Testis DV21
Thymus D721
Thyroid Gland DG25
Tongue D925
Trachea SB20
Ureter DT21
Urethra DT23
Uterus DU22
Steripath® Micro™ Blood Collection System XXE5XR7
Sternoclavicular ligament
use Bursa and Ligament, Shoulder, Left
use Bursa and Ligament, Shoulder, Right
Sternocleidomastoid artery
use Artery, Thyroid, Left
use Artery, Thyroid, Right
Sternocleidomastoid muscle
use Muscle, Neck, Left
use Muscle, Neck, Right
Sternocostal ligament
use Sternum Bursa and Ligament
Sternotomy
see Division, Sternum 0P80
see Drainage, Sternum 0P90
Stimulation, cardiac
Cardioversion 5A2204Z
Electrophysiologic testing
see Measurement, Cardiac 4A02
Stimulator Generator
Insertion of device in
Abdomen 0JH8
Back 0JH7
Chest 0JH6
Multiple Array
Abdomen 0JH8
Back 0JH7
Chest 0JH6
Multiple Array Rechargeable
Abdomen 0JH8
Back 0JH7
Chest 0JH6
Removal of device from, Subcutaneous Tissue and Fascia, Trunk 0JPT
Revision of device in, Subcutaneous Tissue and Fascia, Trunk 0JWT
Stimulator Generator *(continued)*
Single Array
Abdomen 0JH8
Back 0JH7
Chest 0JH6
Single Array Rechargeable
Abdomen 0JH8
Back 0JH7
Chest 0JH6
Stimulator Lead
Insertion of device in
Anal Sphincter 0DHR
Artery
Left 03HL
Right 03HK
Bladder 0THB
Muscle
Lower 0KHY
Upper 0KHX
Stomach 0DH6
Ureter 0TH9
Removal of device from
Anal Sphincter 0DPR
Artery, Upper 03PY
Bladder 0TPB
Muscle
Lower 0KPY
Upper 0KPX
Stomach 0DP6
Ureter 0TP9
Revision of device in
Anal Sphincter 0DWR
Artery, Upper 03WY
Bladder 0TWB
Muscle
Lower 0KWY
Upper 0KWX
Stomach 0DW6
Ureter 0TW9
Stoma
Excision
Abdominal Wall 0WBFXZ2
Neck 0WB6XZ2
Repair
Abdominal Wall 0WQFXZ2
Neck 0WQ6XZ2
Stomatoplasty
see Repair, Mouth and Throat 0CQ
see Replacement, Mouth and Throat 0CR
see Supplement, Mouth and Throat 0CU
Stomatorrhaphy
see Repair, Mouth and Throat 0CQ
StrataGraft®
use Bioengineered Allogeneic Construct
Stratos LV
use Cardiac Resynchronization Pacemaker Pulse Generator in 0JH
Stress test
4A02XM4
4A12XM4
Stripping
see Extraction
Study
Electrophysiologic stimulation, cardiac
see Measurement, Cardiac 4A02
Ocular motility 4A07X7Z
Pulmonary airway flow measurement
see Measurement, Respiratory 4A09
Visual acuity 4A07X0Z
Styloglossus muscle
use Muscle, Tongue, Palate, Pharynx
Stylomandibular ligament
use Bursa and Ligament, Head and Neck
Stylopharyngeus muscle
use Muscle, Tongue, Palate, Pharynx
Subacromial bursa
use Bursa and Ligament, Shoulder, Left
use Bursa and Ligament, Shoulder, Right
Subaortic (common iliac) lymph node
use Lymphatic, Pelvis
Subarachnoid space, spinal
use Spinal Canal
Subclavicular (apical) lymph node
use Lymphatic, Axillary, Left
use Lymphatic, Axillary, Right
Subclavius muscle
use Muscle, Thorax, Left
use Muscle, Thorax, Right
Subclavius nerve
use Nerve, Brachial Plexus
Subcostal artery
use Upper Artery
Subcostal muscle
use Muscle, Thorax, Left
use Muscle, Thorax, Right
Subcostal nerve
use Nerve, Thoracic
Subcutaneous injection reservoir, port
use Vascular Access Device, Totally Implantable in Subcutaneous Tissue and Fascia
Subcutaneous Defibrillator Lead
Insertion of device in, Subcutaneous Tissue and Fascia, Chest 0JH6
Removal of device from, Subcutaneous Tissue and Fascia, Trunk 0JPT
Revision of device in, Subcutaneous Tissue and Fascia, Trunk 0JWT
Subcutaneous injection reservoir, pump
use Infusion Device, Pump in Subcutaneous Tissue and Fascia
Subdermal progesterone implant
use Contraceptive Device in Subcutaneous Tissue and Fascia
Subdural space, spinal
use Spinal Canal
Submandibular ganglion
use Nerve, Facial
use Nerve, Head and Neck Sympathetic
Submandibular gland
use Gland, Submaxillary, Left
use Gland, Submaxillary, Right
Submandibular lymph node
use Lymphatic, Head
Submandibular space
use Subcutaneous Tissue and Fascia, Face
Submaxillary ganglion
use Nerve, Head and Neck Sympathetic
Submaxillary lymph node
use Lymphatic, Head
Submental artery
use Artery, Face
Submental lymph node
use Lymphatic, Head
Submucous (Meissner's) plexus
use Nerve, Abdominal Sympathetic
Suboccipital nerve
use Nerve, Cervical
Suboccipital venous plexus
use Vein, Vertebral, Left
use Vein, Vertebral, Right
Subparotid lymph node
use Lymphatic, Head
Subscapular (posterior) lymph node
use Lymphatic, Axillary, Left
use Lymphatic, Axillary, Right
Subscapular aponeurosis
use Subcutaneous Tissue and Fascia, Upper Arm, Left
use Subcutaneous Tissue and Fascia, Upper Arm, Right
Subscapular artery
use Artery, Axillary, Left
use Artery, Axillary, Right
Subscapularis muscle
use Muscle, Shoulder, Left
use Muscle, Shoulder, Right
Substance Abuse Treatment
Counseling
Family, for substance abuse, Other Family Counseling HZ63ZZZ
Group
12-Step HZ43ZZZ
Behavioral HZ41ZZZ
Cognitive HZ40ZZZ
Cognitive-Behavioral HZ42ZZZ
Confrontational HZ48ZZZ
Continuing Care HZ49ZZZ
Infectious Disease
Post-Test HZ4CZZZ
Pre-Test HZ4CZZZ
Interpersonal HZ44ZZZ
Motivational Enhancement HZ47ZZZ
Psychoeducation HZ46ZZZ
Spiritual HZ4BZZZ
Vocational HZ45ZZZ
Individual
12-Step HZ33ZZZ
Behavioral HZ31ZZZ
Cognitive HZ30ZZZ
Cognitive-Behavioral HZ32ZZZ
Confrontational HZ38ZZZ
Continuing Care HZ39ZZZ
Infectious Disease
Post-Test HZ3CZZZ
Pre-Test HZ3CZZZ
Interpersonal HZ34ZZZ
Motivational Enhancement HZ37ZZZ
Psychoeducation HZ36ZZZ
Spiritual HZ3BZZZ
Vocational HZ35ZZZ
Detoxification Services, for substance abuse HZ2ZZZZ
Medication Management
Antabuse HZ83ZZZ
Bupropion HZ87ZZZ
Clonidine HZ86ZZZ
Levo-alpha-acetyl-methadol (LAAM) HZ82ZZZ
Methadone Maintenance HZ81ZZZ
Naloxone HZ85ZZZ
Naltrexone HZ84ZZZ
Nicotine Replacement HZ80ZZZ
Other Replacement Medication HZ89ZZZ
Psychiatric Medication HZ88ZZZ
Pharmacotherapy
Antabuse HZ93ZZZ
Bupropion HZ97ZZZ
Clonidine HZ96ZZZ
Levo-alpha-acetyl-methadol (LAAM) HZ92ZZZ
Methadone Maintenance HZ91ZZZ
Naloxone HZ95ZZZ
Naltrexone HZ94ZZZ
Nicotine Replacement HZ90ZZZ

Substance Abuse Treatment *(continued)*
Pharmacotherapy *(continued)*
Psychiatric Medication HZ98ZZZ
Replacement Medication, Other HZ99ZZZ
Psychotherapy
12-Step HZ53ZZZ
Behavioral HZ51ZZZ
Cognitive HZ50ZZZ
Cognitive-Behavioral HZ52ZZZ
Confrontational HZ58ZZZ
Interactive HZ55ZZZ
Interpersonal HZ54ZZZ
Motivational Enhancement HZ57ZZZ
Psychoanalysis HZ5BZZZ
Psychodynamic HZ5CZZZ
Psychoeducation HZ56ZZZ
Psychophysiological HZ5DZZZ
Supportive HZ59ZZZ
Substantia nigra
use Basal Ganglia
Subtalar (talocalcaneal) joint
use Joint, Tarsal, Left
use Joint, Tarsal, Right
Subtalar ligament
use Bursa and Ligament, Foot, Left
use Bursa and Ligament, Foot, Right
Subthalamic nucleus
use Basal Ganglia
Suction curettage (D&C), nonobstetric
see Extraction, Endometrium 0UDB
Suction curettage, obstetric post-delivery
see Extraction, Products of Conception, Retained 10D1
Superficial circumflex iliac vein
use Vein, Saphenous, Left
use Vein, Saphenous, Right
Superficial epigastric artery
use Artery, Femoral, Left
use Artery, Femoral, Right
Superficial epigastric vein
use Vein, Saphenous, Left
use Vein, Saphenous, Right
Superficial Inferior Epigastric Artery Flap
Replacement
Bilateral 0HRV078
Left 0HRU078
Right 0HRT078
Transfer
Left 0KXG
Right 0KXF
Superficial palmar arch
use Artery, Hand, Left
use Artery, Hand, Right
Superficial palmar venous arch
use Vein, Hand, Left
use Vein, Hand, Right
Superficial temporal artery
use Artery, Temporal, Left
use Artery, Temporal, Right
Superficial transverse perineal muscle
use Muscle, Perineum
Superior cardiac nerve
use Nerve, Thoracic Sympathetic
Superior cerebellar vein
use Vein, Intracranial
Superior cerebral vein
use Vein, Intracranial
Superior clunic (cluneal) nerve
use Nerve, Lumbar
Superior epigastric artery
use Artery, Internal Mammary, Left
use Artery, Internal Mammary, Right
Superior genicular artery
use Artery, Popliteal, Left
use Artery, Popliteal, Right
Superior gluteal artery
use Artery, Internal Iliac, Left
use Artery, Internal Iliac, Right
Superior gluteal nerve
use Nerve, Lumbar Plexus
Superior hypogastric plexus
use Nerve, Abdominal Sympathetic
Superior labial artery
use Artery, Face
Superior laryngeal artery
use Artery, Thyroid, Left
use Artery, Thyroid, Right
Superior laryngeal nerve
use Nerve, Vagus
Superior longitudinal muscle
use Muscle, Tongue, Palate, Pharynx
Superior mesenteric ganglion
use Nerve, Abdominal Sympathetic
Superior mesenteric lymph node
use Lymphatic, Mesenteric
Superior mesenteric plexus
use Nerve, Abdominal Sympathetic
Superior oblique muscle
use Muscle, Extraocular, Left
use Muscle, Extraocular, Right
Superior olivary nucleus
use Pons
Superior rectal artery
use Artery, Inferior Mesenteric
Superior rectal vein
use Vein, Inferior Mesenteric
Superior rectus muscle
use Muscle, Extraocular, Left
use Muscle, Extraocular, Right
Superior tarsal plate
use Eyelid, Upper, Left
use Eyelid, Upper, Right
Superior thoracic artery
use Artery, Axillary, Left
use Artery, Axillary, Right
Superior thyroid artery
use External Carotid Artery, Left
use External Carotid Artery, Right
use Thyroid, Left
use Thyroid, Right
Superior turbinate
use Turbinate, Nasal
Superior ulnar collateral artery
use Artery, Brachial, Left
use Artery, Brachial, Right
Supersaturated Oxygen therapy
5A0512C
5A0522C
Supplement
Abdominal Wall 0WUF
Acetabulum
Left 0QU5
Right 0QU4
Ampulla of Vater 0FUC
Anal Sphincter 0DUR
Ankle Region
Left 0YUL
Right 0YUK
Anus 0DUQ
Aorta
Abdominal 04U0
Thoracic
Ascending/Arch 02UX
Descending 02UW
Arm
Lower
Left 0XUF
Right 0XUD
Upper
Left 0XU9
Right 0XU8
Supplement *(continued)*
Artery
Anterior Tibial
Left 04UQ
Right 04UP
Axillary
Left 03U6
Right 03U5
Brachial
Left 03U8
Right 03U7
Celiac 04U1
Colic
Left 04U7
Middle 04U8
Right 04U6
Common Carotid
Left 03UJ
Right 03UH
Common Iliac
Left 04UD
Right 04UC
Coronary
Four or More Arteries 02U3
One Artery 02U0
Three Arteries 02U2
Two Arteries 02U1
External Carotid
Left 03UN
Right 03UM
External Iliac
Left 04UJ
Right 04UH
Face 03UR
Femoral
Left 04UL
Right 04UK
Foot
Left 04UW
Right 04UV
Gastric 04U2
Hand
Left 03UF
Right 03UD
Hepatic 04U3
Inferior Mesenteric 04UB
Innominate 03U2
Internal Carotid
Left 03UL
Right 03UK
Internal Iliac
Left 04UF
Right 04UE
Internal Mammary
Left 03U1
Right 03U0
Intracranial 03UG
Lower 04UY
Peroneal
Left 04UU
Right 04UT
Popliteal
Left 04UN
Right 04UM
Posterior Tibial
Left 04US
Right 04UR
Pulmonary
Left 02UR
Right 02UQ
Pulmonary Trunk 02UP
Radial
Left 03UC
Right 03UB
Renal
Left 04UA
Right 04U9
Splenic 04U4
Subclavian
Left 03U4
Right 03U3
Supplement *(continued)*
Artery *(continued)*
Superior Mesenteric 04U5
Temporal
Left 03UT
Right 03US
Thyroid
Left 03UV
Right 03UU
Ulnar
Left 03UA
Right 03U9
Upper 03UY
Vertebral
Left 03UQ
Right 03UP
Atrium
Left 02U7
Right 02U6
Auditory Ossicle
Left 09UA
Right 09U9
Axilla
Left 0XU5
Right 0XU4
Back
Lower 0WUL
Upper 0WUK
Bladder 0TUB
Bladder Neck 0TUC
Bone
Ethmoid
Left 0NUG
Right 0NUF
Frontal 0NU1
Hyoid 0NUX
Lacrimal
Left 0NUJ
Right 0NUH
Nasal 0NUB
Occipital 0NU7
Palatine
Left 0NUL
Right 0NUK
Parietal
Left 0NU4
Right 0NU3
Pelvic
Left 0QU3
Right 0QU2
Sphenoid 0NUC
Temporal
Left 0NU6
Right 0NU5
Zygomatic
Left 0NUN
Right 0NUM
Breast
Bilateral 0HUV
Left 0HUU
Right 0HUT
Bronchus
Lingula 0BU9
Lower Lobe
Left 0BUB
Right 0BU6
Main
Left 0BU7
Right 0BU3
Middle Lobe, Right 0BU5
Upper Lobe
Left 0BU8
Right 0BU4
Buccal Mucosa 0CU4
Bursa and Ligament
Abdomen
Left 0MUJ
Right 0MUH

Supplement *(continued)*
- Bursa and Ligament *(continued)*
  - Ankle
    - Left 0MUR
    - Right 0MUQ
  - Elbow
    - Left 0MU4
    - Right 0MU3
  - Foot
    - Left 0MUT
    - Right 0MUS
  - Hand
    - Left 0MU8
    - Right 0MU7
  - Head and Neck 0MU0
  - Hip
    - Left 0MUM
    - Right 0MUL
  - Knee
    - Left 0MUP
    - Right 0MUN
  - Lower Extremity
    - Left 0MUW
    - Right 0MUV
  - Perineum 0MUK
  - Rib(s) 0MUC
  - Shoulder
    - Left 0MU2
    - Right 0MU1
  - Spine
    - Lower 0MUD
    - Upper 0MUC
  - Sternum 0MUF
  - Upper Extremity
    - Left 0MUB
    - Right 0MU9
  - Wrist
    - Left 0MU6
    - Right 0MU5
- Buttock
  - Left 0YU1
  - Right 0YU0
- Carina 0BU2
- Carpal
  - Left 0PUN
  - Right 0PUM
- Cecum 0DUH
- Cerebral Meninges 00U1
- Cerebral Ventricle 00U6
- Chest Wall 0WU8
- Chordae Tendineae 02U9
- Cisterna Chyli 07UL
- Clavicle
  - Left 0PUB
  - Right 0PU9
- Clitoris 0UUJ
- Coccyx 0QUS
- Colon
  - Ascending 0DUK
  - Descending 0DUM
  - Sigmoid 0DUN
  - Transverse 0DUL
- Cord
  - Bilateral 0VUH
  - Left 0VUG
  - Right 0VUF
- Cornea
  - Left 08U9
  - Right 08U8
- Cul-de-sac 0UUF
- Diaphragm 0BUT
- Disc
  - Cervical Vertebral 0RU3
  - Cervicothoracic Vertebral 0RU5
  - Lumbar Vertebral 0SU2
  - Lumbosacral 0SU4
  - Thoracic Vertebral 0RU9
  - Thoracolumbar Vertebral 0RUB

Supplement *(continued)*
- Duct
  - Common Bile 0FU9
  - Cystic 0FU8
  - Hepatic
    - Common 0FU7
    - Left 0FU6
    - Right 0FU5
  - Lacrimal
    - Left 08UY
    - Right 08UX
  - Pancreatic 0FUD
    - Accessory 0FUF
- Duodenum 0DU9
- Dura Mater 00U2
- Ear
  - External
    - Bilateral 09U2
    - Left 09U1
    - Right 09U0
  - Inner
    - Left 09UE
    - Right 09UD
  - Middle
    - Left 09U6
    - Right 09U5
- Elbow Region
  - Left 0XUC
  - Right 0XUB
- Epididymis
  - Bilateral 0VUL
  - Left 0VUK
  - Right 0VUJ
- Epiglottis 0CUR
- Esophagogastric Junction 0DU4
- Esophagus 0DU5
  - Lower 0DU3
  - Middle 0DU2
  - Upper 0DU1
- Extremity
  - Lower
    - Left 0YUB
    - Right 0YU9
  - Upper
    - Left 0XU7
    - Right 0XU6
- Eye
  - Left 08U1
  - Right 08U0
- Eyelid
  - Lower
    - Left 08UR
    - Right 08UQ
  - Upper
    - Left 08UP
    - Right 08UN
- Face 0WU2
- Fallopian Tube
  - Left 0UU6
  - Right 0UU5
- Fallopian Tubes, Bilateral 0UU7
- Femoral Region
  - Bilateral 0YUE
  - Left 0YU8
  - Right 0YU7
- Femoral Shaft
  - Left 0QU9
  - Right 0QU8
- Femur
  - Lower
    - Left 0QUC
    - Right 0QUB
  - Upper
    - Left 0QU7
    - Right 0QU6
- Fibula
  - Left 0QUK
  - Right 0QUJ

Supplement *(continued)*
- Finger
  - Index
    - Left 0XUP
    - Right 0XUN
  - Little
    - Left 0XUW
    - Right 0XUV
  - Middle
    - Left 0XUR
    - Right 0XUQ
  - Ring
    - Left 0XUT
    - Right 0XUS
- Foot
  - Left 0YUN
  - Right 0YUM
- Gingiva
  - Lower 0CU6
  - Upper 0CU5
- Glenoid Cavity
  - Left 0PU8
  - Right 0PU7
- Hand
  - Left 0XUK
  - Right 0XUJ
- Head 0WU0
- Heart 02UA
- Humeral Head
  - Left 0PUD
  - Right 0PUC
- Humeral Shaft
  - Left 0PUG
  - Right 0PUF
- Hymen 0UUK
- Ileocecal Valve 0DUC
- Ileum 0DUB
- Inguinal Region
  - Bilateral 0YUA
  - Left 0YU6
  - Right 0YU5
- Intestine
  - Large 0DUE
    - Left 0DUG
    - Right 0DUF
  - Small 0DU8
- Iris
  - Left 08UD
  - Right 08UC
- Jaw
  - Lower 0WU5
  - Upper 0WU4
- Jejunum 0DUA
- Joint
  - Acromioclavicular
    - Left 0RUH
    - Right 0RUG
  - Ankle
    - Left 0SUG
    - Right 0SUF
  - Carpal
    - Left 0RUR
    - Right 0RUQ
  - Carpometacarpal
    - Left 0RUT
    - Right 0RUS
  - Cervical Vertebral 0RU1
  - Cervicothoracic Vertebral 0RU4
  - Coccygeal 0SU6
  - Elbow
    - Left 0RUM
    - Right 0RUL
  - Finger Phalangeal
    - Left 0RUX
    - Right 0RUW
  - Hip
    - Left 0SUB
      - Acetabular Surface 0SUE
      - Femoral Surface 0SUS

Supplement *(continued)*
- Joint *(continued)*
  - Hip *(continued)*
    - Right 0SU9
      - Acetabular Surface 0SUA
      - Femoral Surface 0SUR
  - Knee
    - Left 0SUD
      - Femoral Surface 0SUU09Z
      - Tibial Surface 0SUW09Z
    - Right 0SUC
      - Femoral Surface 0SUT09Z
      - Tibial Surface 0SUV09Z
  - Lumbar Vertebral 0SU0
  - Lumbosacral 0SU3
  - Metacarpophalangeal
    - Left 0RUV
    - Right 0RUU
  - Metatarsal-Phalangeal
    - Left 0SUN
    - Right 0SUM
  - Occipital-cervical 0RU0
  - Sacrococcygeal 0SU5
  - Sacroiliac
    - Left 0SU8
    - Right 0SU7
  - Shoulder
    - Left 0RUK
    - Right 0RUJ
  - Sternoclavicular
    - Left 0RUF
    - Right 0RUE
  - Tarsal
    - Left 0SUJ
    - Right 0SUH
  - Tarsometatarsal
    - Left 0SUL
    - Right 0SUK
  - Temporomandibular
    - Left 0RUD
    - Right 0RUC
  - Thoracic Vertebral 0RU6
  - Thoracolumbar Vertebral 0RUA
  - Toe Phalangeal
    - Left 0SUQ
    - Right 0SUP
  - Wrist
    - Left 0RUP
    - Right 0RUN
- Kidney Pelvis
  - Left 0TU4
  - Right 0TU3
- Knee Region
  - Left 0YUG
  - Right 0YUF
- Larynx 0CUS
- Leg
  - Lower
    - Left 0YUJ
    - Right 0YUH
  - Upper
    - Left 0YUD
    - Right 0YUC
- Lip
  - Lower 0CU1
  - Upper 0CU0
- Lymphatic
  - Aortic 07UD
  - Axillary
    - Left 07U6
    - Right 07U5
  - Head 07U0
  - Inguinal
    - Left 07UJ
    - Right 07UH
  - Internal Mammary
    - Left 07U9
    - Right 07U8

Supplement *(continued)*
- Vein *(continued)*
  - Basilic
    - Left 05UC
    - Right 05UB
  - Brachial
    - Left 05UA
    - Right 05U9
  - Cephalic
    - Left 05UF
    - Right 05UD
  - Colic 06U7
  - Common Iliac
    - Left 06UD
    - Right 06UC
  - Esophageal 06U3
  - External Iliac
    - Left 06UG
    - Right 06UF
  - External Jugular
    - Left 05UQ
    - Right 05UP
  - Face
    - Left 05UV
    - Right 05UT
  - Femoral
    - Left 06UN
    - Right 06UM
  - Foot
    - Left 06UV
    - Right 06UT
  - Gastric 06U2
  - Hand
    - Left 05UH
    - Right 05UG
  - Hemiazygos 05U1
  - Hepatic 06U4
  - Hypogastric
    - Left 06UJ
    - Right 06UH
  - Inferior Mesenteric 06U6
  - Innominate
    - Left 05U4
    - Right 05U3
  - Internal Jugular
    - Left 05UN
    - Right 05UM
  - Intracranial 05UL
  - Lower 06UY
  - Portal 06U8
  - Pulmonary
    - Left 02UT
    - Right 02US
  - Renal
    - Left 06UB
    - Right 06U9
  - Saphenous
    - Left 06UQ
    - Right 06UP
  - Splenic 06U1
  - Subclavian
    - Left 05U6
    - Right 05U5
  - Superior Mesenteric 06U5
  - Upper 05UY
  - Vertebral
    - Left 05US
    - Right 05UR
- Vena Cava
  - Inferior 06U0
  - Superior 02UV
- Ventricle
  - Left 02UL
  - Right 02UK
- Vertebra
  - Cervical 0PU3
  - Lumbar 0QU0
    - Mechanically Expandable (Paired) Synthetic Substitute XNU0356

Supplement *(continued)*
- Vertebra *(continued)*
  - Thoracic 0PU4
    - Mechanically Expandable (Paired) Synthetic Substitute XNU4356
- Vesicle
  - Bilateral 0VU3
  - Left 0VU2
  - Right 0VU1
- Vocal Cord
  - Left 0CUV
  - Right 0CUT
- Vulva 0UUM
- Wrist Region
  - Left 0XUH
  - Right 0XUG

Supraclavicular (Virchow's) lymph node
- *use* Lymphatic, Neck, Left
- *use* Lymphatic, Neck, Right

Supraclavicular nerve
- *use* Nerve, Cervical Plexus

Suprahyoid lymph node
- *use* Lymphatic, Head

Suprahyoid muscle
- *use* Muscle, Neck, Left
- *use* Muscle, Neck, Right

Suprainguinal lymph node
- *use* Lymphatic, Pelvis

Supraorbital vein
- *use* Vein, Face, Left
- *use* Vein, Face, Right

Suprarenal gland
- *use* Gland, Adrenal
- *use* Gland, Adrenal, Bilateral
- *use* Gland, Adrenal, Left
- *use* Gland, Adrenal, Right

Suprarenal plexus
- *use* Nerve, Abdominal Sympathetic

Suprascapular nerve
- *use* Nerve, Brachial Plexus

Supraspinatus fascia
- *use* Subcutaneous Tissue and Fascia, Upper Arm, Left
- *use* Subcutaneous Tissue and Fascia, Upper Arm, Right

Supraspinatus muscle
- *use* Muscle, Shoulder, Left
- *use* Muscle, Shoulder, Right

Supraspinous ligament
- *use* Bursa and Ligament, Lower Spine
- *use* Bursa and Ligament, Upper Spine

Suprasternal notch
- *use* Sternum

Supratrochlear lymph node
- *use* Lymphatic, Upper Extremity, Left
- *use* Lymphatic, Upper Extremity, Right

Sural artery
- *use* Artery, Popliteal, Left
- *use* Artery, Popliteal, Right

Surpass Streamline™ Flow Diverter
- *use* Intraluminal Device, Flow Diverter in 03V

Suspension
- Bladder Neck
  - *see* Reposition, Bladder Neck 0TSC
- Kidney
  - *see* Reposition, Urinary System 0TS
- Urethra
  - *see* Reposition, Urinary System 0TS
- Urethrovesical
  - *see* Reposition, Bladder Neck 0TSC
- Uterus
  - *see* Reposition, Uterus 0US9

Suspension *(continued)*
- Uterus *(continued)*
  - Vagina
  - *see* Reposition, Vagina 0USG

Sustained Release Drug-eluting Intraluminal Device
- Dilation
  - Anterior Tibial
    - Left X27Q385
    - Right X27P385
  - Femoral
    - Left X27J385
    - Right X27H385
  - Peroneal
    - Left X27U385
    - Right X27T385
  - Popliteal
    - Left Distal X27N385
    - Left Proximal X27L385
    - Right Distal X27M385
    - Right Proximal X27K385
  - Posterior Tibial
    - Left X27S385
    - Right X27R385
- Four or More
  - Anterior Tibial
    - Left X27Q3C5
    - Right X27P3C5
  - Femoral
    - Left X27J3C5
    - Right X27H3C5
  - Peroneal
    - Left X27U3C5
    - Right X27T3C5
  - Popliteal
    - Left Distal X27N3C5
    - Left Proximal X27L3C5
    - Right Distal X27M3C5
    - Right Proximal X27K3C5
  - Posterior Tibial
    - Left X27S3C5
    - Right X27R3C5
- Three
  - Anterior Tibial
    - Left X27Q3B5
    - Right X27P3B5
  - Femoral
    - Left X27J3B5
    - Right X27H3B5
  - Peroneal
    - Left X27U3B5
    - Right X27T3B5
  - Popliteal
    - Left Distal X27N3B5
    - Left Proximal X27L3B5
    - Right Distal X27M3B5
    - Right Proximal X27K3B5
  - Posterior Tibial
    - Left X27S3B5
    - Right X27R3B5
- Two
  - Anterior Tibial
    - Left X27Q395
    - Right X27P395
  - Femoral
    - Left X27J395
    - Right X27H395
  - Peroneal
    - Left X27U395
    - Right X27T395
  - Popliteal
    - Left Distal X27N395
    - Left Proximal X27L395
    - Right Distal X27M395
    - Right Proximal X27K395
  - Posterior Tibial
    - Left X27S395
    - Right X27R395

Suture
- Laceration repair
  - *see* Repair

Suture *(continued)*
- Ligation
  - *see* Occlusion

Suture Removal
- Extremity
  - Lower 8E0YXY8
  - Upper 8E0XXY8
- Head and Neck Region 8E09XY8
- Trunk Region 8E0WXY8

Sutureless valve, Perceval
- *use* Zooplastic Tissue, Rapid Deployment Technique in New Technology

Sweat gland
- *use* Skin

Sympathectomy
- *see* Excision, Peripheral Nervous System 01B

SynCardia Total Artificial Heart
- *use* Synthetic Substitute

SynCardia (temporary) total artificial heart (TAH) *use* Synthetic Substitute, Pneumatic in 02R

Synchra CRT-P
- *use* Cardiac Resynchronization Pacemaker Pulse Generator in 0JH

SynchroMed pump
- *use* Infusion Device, Pump in Subcutaneous Tissue and Fascia

Synechiotomy, iris
- *see* Release, Eye 08N

Synovectomy
- Lower joint
  - *see* Excision, Lower Joints 0SB
- Upper joint
  - *see* Excision, Upper Joints 0RB

Systemic Nuclear Medicine Therapy
- Abdomen CW70
- Anatomical Regions, Multiple CW7YYZZ
- Chest CW73
- Thyroid CW7G
- Whole Body CW7N

Synthetic Human Angiotensin II XW0

T

Tagraxofusp-erzs Antineoplastic XW0

Takedown
- Arteriovenous shunt
  - *see* Removal of device from, Upper Arteries 03P
- Arteriovenous shunt, with creation of new shunt
  - *see* Bypass, Upper Arteries 031
- Stoma
  - *see* Excision
  - *see* Reposition

Talent® Converter
- *use* Intraluminal Device

Talent® Occluder
- *use* Intraluminal Device

Talent® Stent Graft (abdominal) (thoracic)
- *use* Intraluminal Device

Talocalcaneal (subtalar) joint
- *use* Joint, Tarsal, Left
- *use* Joint, Tarsal, Right

Talocalcaneal ligament
- *use* Bursa and Ligament, Foot, Left
- *use* Bursa and Ligament, Foot, Right

Talocalcaneonavicular joint
- *use* Joint, Tarsal, Left
- *use* Joint, Tarsal, Right

Talocalcaneonavicular ligament
- *use* Bursa and Ligament, Foot, Left

Talocalcaneonavicular ligament *(continued)*
use Bursa and Ligament, Foot, Right
Talocrural joint
use Joint, Ankle, Left
use Joint, Ankle, Right
Talofibular ligament
use Bursa and Ligament, Ankle, Left
use Bursa and Ligament, Ankle, Right
Talus bone
use Tarsal, Left
use Tarsal, Right
TandemHeart® System
use Short-term External Heart Assist System in Heart and Great Vessels
Tarsectomy
see Excision, Lower Bones 0QB
see Resection, Lower Bones 0QT
Tarsometatarsal ligament
use Bursa and Ligament, Foot, Left
use Bursa and Ligament, Foot, Right
Tarsorrhaphy
see Repair, Eye 08Q
Tattooing
Cornea 3E0CXMZ
Skin
see Introduction of substance in or on, Skin 3E00
TAXUS® Liberté® Paclitaxel-eluting Coronary Stent System
use Intraluminal Device, Drug-eluting in Heart and Great Vessels
TBNA (transbronchial needle aspiration)
Fluid or gas
see Drainage, Respiratory System 0B9
Tissue biopsy
see Extraction, Respiratory System 0BD
Tecartus™
use Brexucabtagene Autoleucel Immunotherapy
TECENTRIQ®
use Atezolizumab Antineoplastic
Telemetry 4A12X4Z
Ambulatory 4A12X45
Temperature gradient study 4A0ZXKZ
Temporal lobe
use Cerebral Hemisphere
Temporalis muscle
use Muscle, Head
Temporoparietalis muscle
use Muscle, Head
Tendolysis
see Release, Tendons 0LN
Tendonectomy
see Excision, Tendons 0LB
see Resection, Tendons 0LT
Tendonoplasty, tenoplasty
see Repair, Tendons 0LQ
see Replacement, Tendons 0LR
see Supplement, Tendons 0LU
Tendorrhaphy
see Repair, Tendons 0LQ
Tendototomy
see Division, Tendons 0L8
see Drainage, Tendons 0L9
Tenectomy, tenonectomy
see Excision, Tendons 0LB
see Resection, Tendons 0LT
Tenolysis
see Release, Tendons 0LN
Tenontorrhaphy
see Repair, Tendons 0LQ
Tenontotomy
see Division, Tendons 0L8
see Drainage, Tendons 0L9
Tenorrhaphy
see Repair, Tendons 0LQ
Tenosynovectomy
see Excision, Tendons 0LB
see Resection, Tendons 0LT
Tenotomy
see Division, Tendons 0L8
see Drainage, Tendons 0L9
Tensor fasciae latae muscle
use Muscle, Hip, Left
use Muscle, Hip, Right
Tensor veli palatini muscle
use Muscle, Tongue, Palate, Pharynx
Tenth cranial nerve
use Nerve, Vagus
Tentorium cerebelli
use Dura Mater
Teres major muscle
use Muscle, Shoulder, Left
use Muscle, Shoulder, Right
Teres minor muscle
use Muscle, Shoulder, Left
use Muscle, Shoulder, Right
Terlipressin XW0
TERLIVAZ®
use Terlipressin
Termination of pregnancy
Aspiration curettage 10A07ZZ
Dilation and curettage 10A07ZZ
Hysterotomy 10A00ZZ
Intra-amniotic injection 10A03ZZ
Laminaria 10A07ZW
Vacuum 10A07Z6
Testectomy
see Excision, Male Reproductive System 0VB
see Resection, Male Reproductive System 0VT
Testicular artery
use Aorta, Abdominal
Testing
Glaucoma 4A07XBZ
Hearing
see Hearing Assessment, Diagnostic Audiology F13
Mental health
see Psychological Tests
Muscle function, electromyography (EMG)
see Measurement, Musculoskeletal 4A0F
Muscle function, manual
see Motor Function Assessment, Rehabilitation F01
Neurophysiologic monitoring, intra-operative
see Monitoring, Physiological Systems 4A1
Range of motion
see Motor Function Assessment, Rehabilitation F01
Vestibular function
see Vestibular Assessment, Diagnostic Audiology F15
Thalamectomy
see Excision, Thalamus 00B9
Thalamotomy
see Drainage, Thalamus 0099
Thenar muscle
use Muscle, Hand, Left
use Muscle, Hand, Right
Therapeutic Massage
Musculoskeletal System 8E0KX1Z
Reproductive System
Prostate 8E0VX1C
Rectum 8E0VX1D
Therapeutic occlusion coil(s)
use Intraluminal Device
Thermography 4A0ZXKZ
Thermotherapy, prostate
see Destruction, Prostate 0V50
Third cranial nerve
use Nerve, Oculomotor
Third occipital nerve
use Nerve, Cervical
Third ventricle
use Cerebral Ventricle
Thoracectomy
see Excision, Anatomical Regions, General 0WB
Thoracentesis
see Drainage, Anatomical Regions, General 0W9
Thoracic aortic plexus
use Nerve, Thoracic Sympathetic
Thoracic esophagus
use Esophagus, Middle
Thoracic facet joint
use Joint, Thoracic Vertebral
Thoracic ganglion
use Nerve, Thoracic Sympathetic
Thoracoacromial artery
use Artery, Axillary, Left
use Artery, Axillary, Right
Thoracocentesis
see Drainage, Anatomical Regions, General 0W9
Thoracolumbar facet joint
use Joint, Thoracolumbar Vertebral
Thoracoplasty
see Repair, Anatomical Regions, General 0WQ
see Supplement, Anatomical Regions, General 0WU
Thoracostomy tube
use Drainage Device
Thoracostomy, for lung collapse
see Drainage, Respiratory System 0B9
Thoracotomy
see Drainage, Anatomical Regions, General 0W9
Thoraflex™ Hybrid device *use* Branched Synthetic Substitute with Intraluminal Device in New Technology
Thoratec IVAD (Implantable Ventricular Assist Device)
use Implantable Heart Assist System in Heart and Great Vessels
Thoratec Paracorporeal Ventricular Assist Device
use Short-term External Heart Assist System in Heart and Great Vessels
Thrombectomy
see Extirpation
Thrombolysis, Ultrasound assisted
see Fragmentation, Artery
Thymectomy
see Excision, Lymphatic and Hemic Systems 07B
see Resection, Lymphatic and Hemic Systems 07T
Thymopexy
see Repair, Lymphatic and Hemic Systems 07Q
see Reposition, Lymphatic and Hemic Systems 07S
Thymus gland
use Thymus
Thyroarytenoid muscle
use Muscle, Neck, Left
use Muscle, Neck, Right
Thyrocervical trunk
use Artery, Thyroid, Left
use Artery, Thyroid, Right
Thyroid cartilage
use Larynx
Thyroidectomy
see Excision, Endocrine System 0GB
see Resection, Endocrine System 0GT
Thyroidorrhaphy
see Repair, Endocrine System 0GQ
Thyroidoscopy 0GJK4ZZ
Thyroidotomy
see Drainage, Endocrine System 0G9
Tibial insert
use Liner in Lower Joints
Tibial sesamoid
use Metatarsal, Left
use Metatarsal, Right
Tibialis anterior muscle
use Muscle, Lower Leg, Left
use Muscle, Lower Leg, Right
Tibialis posterior muscle
use Muscle, Lower Leg, Left
use Muscle, Lower Leg, Right
Tibiofemoral joint
use Joint, Knee, Left
use Joint, Knee, Left, Tibial Surface
use Joint, Knee, Right
use Joint, Knee, Right, Tibial Surface
Tibioperoneal trunk
use Popliteal Artery, Left
use Popliteal Artery, Right
Tisagenlecleucel
use Tisagenlecleucel Immunotherapy
Tisagenlecleucel Immunotherapy XW0
Tissue bank graft
use Nonautologous Tissue Substitute
Tissue Expander
Insertion of device in
Breast
Bilateral 0HHV
Left 0HHU
Right 0HHT
Nipple
Left 0HHX
Right 0HHW
Subcutaneous Tissue and Fascia
Abdomen 0JH8
Back 0JH7
Buttock 0JH9
Chest 0JH6
Face 0JH1
Foot
Left 0JHR
Right 0JHQ
Hand
Left 0JHK
Right 0JHJ
Lower Arm
Left 0JHH
Right 0JHG
Lower Leg
Left 0JHP
Right 0JHN
Neck
Left 0JH5
Right 0JH4
Pelvic Region 0JHC
Perineum 0JHB
Scalp 0JH0
Upper Arm
Left 0JHF
Right 0JHD
Upper Leg
Left 0JHM
Right 0JHL

Tissue Expander *(continued)*
Removal of device from
Breast
Left 0HPU
Right 0HPT
Subcutaneous Tissue and Fascia
Head and Neck 0JPS
Lower Extremity 0JPW
Trunk 0JPT
Upper Extremity 0JPV
Revision of device in
Breast
Left 0HWU
Right 0HWT
Subcutaneous Tissue and Fascia
Head and Neck 0JWS
Lower Extremity 0JWW
Trunk 0JWT
Upper Extremity 0JWV
Tissue expander (inflatable) (injectable)
use Tissue Expander in Skin and Breast
use Tissue Expander in Subcutaneous Tissue and Fascia
Tissue Plasminogen Activator (tPA) (r-tPA)
use Thrombolytic Other
Titanium Sternal Fixation System (TSFS)
use Internal Fixation Device, Rigid Plate in 0PS
use Internal Fixation Device, Rigid Plate in 0PH
Tocilizumab XW0
Tomographic (Tomo) Nuclear Medicine Imaging
Abdomen CW20
Abdomen and Chest CW24
Abdomen and Pelvis CW21
Anatomical Regions, Multiple CW2YYZZ
Bladder, Kidneys and Ureters CT23
Brain C020
Breast CH2YYZZ
Bilateral CH22
Left CH21
Right CH20
Bronchi and Lungs CB22
Central Nervous System C02YYZZ
Cerebrospinal Fluid C025
Chest CW23
Chest and Abdomen CW24
Chest and Neck CW26
Digestive System CD2YYZZ
Endocrine System CG2YYZZ
Extremity
Lower CW2D
Bilateral CP2F
Left CP2D
Right CP2C
Upper CW2M
Bilateral CP2B
Left CP29
Right CP28
Gallbladder CF24
Gastrointestinal Tract CD27
Gland, Parathyroid CG21
Head and Neck CW2B
Heart C22YYZZ
Right and Left C226
Hepatobiliary System and Pancreas CF2YYZZ
Kidneys, Ureters and Bladder CT23
Liver CF25
Liver and Spleen CF26
Lungs and Bronchi CB22
Lymphatics and Hematologic System C72YYZZ
Musculoskeletal System, Other CP2YYZZ
Tomographic (Tomo) Nuclear Medicine Imaging *(continued)*
Myocardium C22G
Neck and Chest CW26
Neck and Head CW2B
Pancreas and Hepatobiliary System CF2YYZZ
Pelvic Region CW2J
Pelvis CP26
Pelvis and Abdomen CW21
Pelvis and Spine CP27
Respiratory System CB2YYZZ
Skin CH2YYZZ
Skull CP21
Skull and Cervical Spine CP23
Spine
Cervical CP22
Cervical and Skull CP23
Lumbar CP2H
Thoracic CP2G
Thoracolumbar CP2J
Spine and Pelvis CP27
Spleen C722
Spleen and Liver CF26
Subcutaneous Tissue CH2YYZZ
Thorax CP24
Ureters, Kidneys and Bladder CT23
Urinary System CT2YYZZ
Tomography, computerized
see Computerized Tomography (CT Scan)
Tongue, base of
use Pharynx
Tonometry 4A07XBZ
Tonsillectomy
see Excision, Mouth and Throat 0CB
see Resection, Mouth and Throat 0CT
Tonsillotomy
see Drainage, Mouth and Throat 0C9
Total Anomalous Pulmonary Venous Return (TAPVR) repair
see Bypass, Atrium, Left 0217
see Bypass, Vena Cava, Superior 021V
Total artificial (replacement) heart
use Synthetic Substitute
Total parenteral nutrition (TPN)
see Introduction of Nutritional Substance
Tourniquet, External
see Compression, Anatomical Regions 2W1
Trachectomy
see Excision, Trachea 0BB1
see Resection, Trachea 0BT1
Trachelectomy
see Excision, Cervix 0UBC
see Resection, Cervix 0UTC
Trachelopexy
see Repair, Cervix 0UQC
see Reposition, Cervix 0USC
Tracheloplasty
see Repair, Cervix 0UQC
Trachelorrhaphy
see Repair, Cervix 0UQC
Trachelotomy
see Drainage, Cervix 0U9C
Tracheobronchial lymph node
use Lymphatic, Thorax
Tracheoesophageal fistulization 0B110D6
Tracheolysis
see Release, Respiratory System 0BN
Tracheoplasty
see Repair, Respiratory System 0BQ
see Supplement, Respiratory System 0BU
Tracheorrhaphy
see Repair, Respiratory System 0BQ
Tracheoscopy 0BJ18ZZ
Tracheostomy
see Bypass, Respiratory System 0B1
Tracheostomy Device
Bypass, Trachea 0B11
Change device in, Trachea 0B21XFZ
Removal of device from, Trachea 0BP1
Revision of device in, Trachea 0BW1
Tracheostomy tube
use Tracheostomy Device in Respiratory System
Tracheotomy
see Drainage, Respiratory System 0B9
Traction
Abdominal Wall 2W63X
Arm
Lower
Left 2W6DX
Right 2W6CX
Upper
Left 2W6BX
Right 2W6AX
Back 2W65X
Chest Wall 2W64X
Extremity
Lower
Left 2W6MX
Right 2W6LX
Upper
Left 2W69X
Right 2W68X
Face 2W61X
Finger
Left 2W6KX
Right 2W6JX
Foot
Left 2W6TX
Right 2W6SX
Hand
Left 2W6FXZ
Right 2W6EXZ
Head 2W60X
Inguinal Region
Left 2W67X
Right 2W66X
Leg
Lower
Left 2W6RX
Right 2W6QX
Upper
Left 2W6PX
Right 2W6NX
Neck 2W62X
Thumb
Left 2W6HX
Right 2W6GX
Toe
Left 2W6VX
Right 2W6UX
Tractotomy
see Division, Central Nervous System and Cranial Nerves 008
Tragus
use Ear, External, Bilateral
use Ear, External, Left
use Ear, External, Right
Training, caregiver
see Caregiver Training
TRAM (transverse rectus abdominis myocutaneous) flap reconstruction
Free
see Replacement, Skin and Breast 0HR
Pedicled
see Transfer, Muscles 0KX
Transcatheter Pulmonary Valve (TPV) placement
In conduit 02RH38L
Native site 02RH38M
Transdermal Glomerular Filtration Rate (GFR) Measurement System XT25XE5
Transection
see Division
Transfer
Buccal Mucosa 0CX4
Bursa and Ligament
Abdomen
Left 0MXJ
Right 0MXH
Ankle
Left 0MXR
Right 0MXQ
Elbow
Left 0MX4
Right 0MX3
Foot
Left 0MXT
Right 0MXS
Hand
Left 0MX8
Right 0MX7
Head and Neck 0MX0
Hip
Left 0MXM
Right 0MXL
Knee
Left 0MXP
Right 0MXN
Lower Extremity
Left 0MXW
Right 0MXV
Perineum 0MXK
Rib(s) 0MXG
Shoulder
Left 0MX2
Right 0MX1
Spine
Lower 0MXD
Upper 0MXC
Sternum 0MXF
Upper Extremity
Left 0MXB
Right 0MX9
Wrist
Left 0MX6
Right 0MX5
Finger
Left 0XXP0ZM
Right 0XXN0ZL
Gingiva
Lower 0CX6
Upper 0CX5
Immunotherapy
see New Technology, Anatomical Regions XW2
Intestine
Large 0DXE
Small 0DX8
Lip
Lower 0CX1
Upper 0CX0
Muscle
Abdomen
Left 0KXL
Right 0KXK
Extraocular
Left 08XM
Right 08XL
Facial 0KX1
Foot
Left 0KXW
Right 0KXV
Hand
Left 0KXD

- **Transfer** *(continued)*
  - Muscle *(continued)*
    - Hand *(continued)*
      - Right 0KXC
    - Head 0KX0
    - Hip
      - Left 0KXP
      - Right 0KXN
    - Lower Arm and Wrist
      - Left 0KXB
      - Right 0KX9
    - Lower Leg
      - Left 0KXT
      - Right 0KXS
    - Neck
      - Left 0KX3
      - Right 0KX2
    - Perineum 0KXM
    - Shoulder
      - Left 0KX6
      - Right 0KX5
    - Thorax
      - Left 0KXJ
      - Right 0KXH
    - Tongue, Palate, Pharynx 0KX4
    - Trunk
      - Left 0KXG
      - Right 0KXF
    - Upper Arm
      - Left 0KX8
      - Right 0KX7
    - Upper Leg
      - Left 0KXR
      - Right 0KXQ
  - Nerve
    - Abducens 00XL
    - Accessory 00XR
    - Acoustic 00XN
    - Cervical 01X1
    - Facial 00XM
    - Femoral 01XD
    - Glossopharyngeal 00XP
    - Hypoglossal 00XS
    - Lumbar 01XB
    - Median 01X5
    - Oculomotor 00XH
    - Olfactory 00XF
    - Optic 00XG
    - Peroneal 01XH
    - Phrenic 01X2
    - Pudendal 01XC
    - Radial 01X6
    - Sciatic 01XF
    - Thoracic 01X8
    - Tibial 01XG
    - Trigeminal 00XK
    - Trochlear 00XJ
    - Ulnar 01X4
    - Vagus 00XQ
  - Palate, Soft 0CX3
  - Prepuce 0VXT
  - Skin
    - Abdomen 0HX7XZZ
    - Back 0HX6XZZ
    - Buttock 0HX8XZZ
    - Chest 0HX5XZZ
    - Ear
      - Left 0HX3XZZ
      - Right 0HX2XZZ
    - Face 0HX1XZZ
    - Foot
      - Left 0HXNXZZ
      - Right 0HXMXZZ
    - Hand
      - Left 0HXGXZZ
      - Right 0HXFXZZ
    - Inguinal 0HXAXZZ
    - Lower Arm
      - Left 0HXEXZZ
      - Right 0HXDXZZ
- **Transfer** *(continued)*
  - Skin *(continued)*
    - Lower Leg
      - Left 0HXLXZZ
      - Right 0HXKXZZ
    - Neck 0HX4XZZ
    - Perineum 0HX9XZZ
    - Scalp 0HX0XZZ
    - Upper Arm
      - Left 0HXCXZZ
      - Right 0HXBXZZ
    - Upper Leg
      - Left 0HXJXZZ
      - Right 0HXHXZZ
  - Stomach 0DX6
  - Subcutaneous Tissue and Fascia
    - Abdomen 0JX8
    - Back 0JX7
    - Buttock 0JX9
    - Chest 0JX6
    - Face 0JX1
    - Foot
      - Left 0JXR
      - Right 0JXQ
    - Hand
      - Left 0JXK
      - Right 0JXJ
    - Lower Arm
      - Left 0JXH
      - Right 0JXG
    - Lower Leg
      - Left 0JXP
      - Right 0JXN
    - Neck
      - Left 0JX5
      - Right 0JX4
    - Pelvic Region 0JXC
    - Perineum 0JXB
    - Scalp 0JX0
    - Upper Arm
      - Left 0JXF
      - Right 0JXD
    - Upper Leg
      - Left 0JXM
      - Right 0JXL
  - Tendon
    - Abdomen
      - Left 0LXG
      - Right 0LXF
    - Ankle
      - Left 0LXT
      - Right 0LXS
    - Foot
      - Left 0LXW
      - Right 0LXV
    - Hand
      - Left 0LX8
      - Right 0LX7
    - Head and Neck 0LX0
    - Hip
      - Left 0LXK
      - Right 0LXJ
    - Knee
      - Left 0LXR
      - Right 0LXQ
    - Lower Arm and Wrist
      - Left 0LX6
      - Right 0LX5
    - Lower Leg
      - Left 0LXP
      - Right 0LXN
    - Perineum 0LXH
    - Shoulder
      - Left 0LX2
      - Right 0LX1
    - Thorax
      - Left 0LXD
      - Right 0LXC
    - Trunk
      - Left 0LXB
      - Right 0LX9
- **Transfer** *(continued)*
  - Tendon *(continued)*
    - Upper Arm
      - Left 0LX4
      - Right 0LX3
    - Upper Leg
      - Left 0LXM
      - Right 0LXL
  - Tongue 0CX7
- **Transfusion**
  - Immunotherapy *see* New Technology, Anatomical Regions XW2
  - Products of Conception
    - Antihemophilic Factors 3027
    - Blood
      - Platelets 3027
      - Red Cells 3027
        - Frozen 3027
      - White Cells 3027
      - Whole 3027
    - Factor IX 3027
    - Fibrinogen 3027
    - Globulin 3027
    - Plasma
      - Fresh 3027
      - Frozen 3027
    - Plasma Cryoprecipitate 3027
    - Serum Albumin 3027
  - Vein
    - 4-Factor Prothrombin Complex Concentrate 30283B1
    - Central
      - Antihemophilic Factors 30243V
      - Blood
        - Platelets 30243R
        - Red Cells 30243N
          - Frozen 30243P
        - White Cells 30243Q
        - Whole 30243H
      - Bone Marrow 30243G
      - Factor IX 30243W
      - Fibrinogen 30243T
      - Globulin 30243S
      - Hematopoietic Stem/Progenitor Cells (HSPC), Genetically Modified 30243C0
      - Pathogen Reduced Cryoprecipitated Fibrinogen Complex 30243D1
      - Plasma
        - Fresh 30243L
        - Frozen 30243K
      - Plasma Cryoprecipitate 30243M
      - Serum Albumin 30243J
      - Stem Cells
        - Cord Blood 30243X
        - Embryonic 30243AZ
        - Hematopoietic 30243Y
        - T-cell Depleted Hematopoietic 30243U
    - Peripheral
      - Antihemophilic Factors 30233V
      - Blood
        - Platelets 30233R
        - Red Cells 30233N
          - Frozen 30233P
        - White Cells 30233Q
        - Whole 30233H
      - Bone Marrow 30233G
      - Factor IX 30233W
      - Fibrinogen 30233T
      - Globulin 30233S
- **Transfusion** *(continued)*
  - Vein *(continued)*
    - Peripheral *(continued)*
      - Hematopoietic Stem/Progenitor Cells (HSPC), Genetically Modified 30233C0
      - Pathogen Reduced Cryoprecipitated Fibrinogen Complex 30233D1
      - Plasma
        - Fresh 30233L
        - Frozen 30233K
      - Plasma Cryoprecipitate 30233M
      - Serum Albumin 30233J
      - Stem Cells
        - Cord Blood 30233X
        - Embryonic 30233AZ
        - Hematopoietic 30233Y
        - T-cell Depleted Hematopoietic 30233U
- **Transplant**
  - *see* Transplantation
- **Transplantation**
  - Bone marrow
    - *see* Transfusion, Circulatory 302
  - Esophagus 0DY50Z
  - Face 0WY20Z
  - Hand
    - Left 0XYK0Z
    - Right 0XYJ0Z
  - Heart 02YA0Z
  - Hematopoietic cell
    - *see* Transfusion, Circulatory 302
  - Intestine
    - Large 0DYE0Z
    - Small 0DY80Z
  - Kidney
    - Left 0TY10Z
    - Right 0TY00Z
  - Liver 0FY00Z
  - Lung
    - Bilateral 0BYM0Z
    - Left 0BYL0Z
    - Lower Lobe
      - Left 0BYJ0Z
      - Right 0BYF0Z
    - Middle Lobe, Right 0BYD0Z
    - Right 0BYK0Z
    - Upper Lobe
      - Left 0BYG0Z
      - Right 0BYC0Z
  - Lung Lingula 0BYH0Z
  - Ovary
    - Left 0UY10Z
    - Right 0UY00Z
  - Pancreas 0FYG0Z
  - Penis 0VYS0Z
  - Products of Conception 10Y0
  - Scrotum 0VY50Z
  - Spleen 07YP0Z
  - Stem cell
    - *see* Transfusion, Circulatory 302
  - Stomach 0DY60Z
  - Thymus 07YM0Z
  - Uterus 0UY90Z
- **Transposition**
  - *see* Bypass
  - *see* Reposition
  - *see* Transfer
- **Transversalis fascia**
  - *use* Subcutaneous Tissue and Fascia, Trunk
- **Transverse acetabular ligament**
  - *use* Bursa and Ligament, Hip, Left
  - *use* Bursa and Ligament, Hip, Right
- **Transverse (cutaneous) cervical nerve**
  - *use* Nerve, Cervical Plexus

Transverse facial artery
use Artery, Temporal, Left
use Artery, Temporal, Right
Transverse foramen
use Cervical Vertebra
Transverse humeral ligament
use Bursa and Ligament, Shoulder, Left
use Bursa and Ligament, Shoulder, Right
Transverse ligament of atlas
use Bursa and Ligament, Head and Neck
Transverse process
use Cervical Vertebra
use Thoracic Vertebra
use Lumbar Vertebra
Transverse Rectus Abdominis Myocutaneous Flap
Replacement
Bilateral 0HRV076
Left 0HRU076
Right 0HRT076
Transfer
Left 0KXL
Right 0KXK
Transverse scapular ligament
use Bursa and Ligament, Shoulder, Left
use Bursa and Ligament, Shoulder, Right
Transverse thoracis muscle
use Muscle, Thorax, Left
use Muscle, Thorax, Right
Transversospinalis muscle
use Muscle, Trunk, Left
use Muscle, Trunk, Right
Transversus abdominis muscle
use Muscle, Abdomen, Left
use Muscle, Abdomen, Right
Trapezium bone
use Carpal, Left
use Carpal, Right
Trapezius muscle
use Muscle, Trunk, Left
use Muscle, Trunk, Right
Trapezoid bone
use Carpal, Left
use Carpal, Right
Triceps brachii muscle
use Muscle, Upper Arm, Left
use Muscle, Upper Arm, Right
Tricuspid annulus
use Valve, Tricuspid
Trifacial nerve
use Nerve, Trigeminal
Trifecta™ Valve (aortic)
use Zooplastic Tissue in Heart and Great Vessels
Trigone of bladder
use Bladder
TriGuard 3™ CEPD (cerebral embolic protection device)
X2A6325
Trilaciclib XW0
Trimming, excisional
see Excision
Triquetral bone
use Carpal, Left
use Carpal, Right
Trochanteric bursa
use Bursa and Ligament, Hip, Left
use Bursa and Ligament, Hip, Right
TUMT (Transurethral microwave thermotherapy of prostate)
0V507ZZ
TUNA (transurethral needle ablation of prostate)
0V507ZZ
Tunneled central venous catheter
use Vascular Access Device Tunneled in Subcutaneous Tissue and Fascia
Tunneled spinal (intrathecal) catheter
use Infusion Device
Turbinectomy
see Excision, Ear, Nose, Sinus 09B
see Resection, Ear, Nose, Sinus 09T
Turbinoplasty
see Repair, Ear, Nose, Sinus 09Q
see Replacement, Ear, Nose, Sinus 09R
see Supplement, Ear, Nose, Sinus 09U
Turbinotomy
see Division, Ear, Nose, Sinus 098
see Drainage, Ear, Nose, Sinus 099
TURP (transurethral resection of prostate)
see Excision, Prostate 0VB0
see Resection, Prostate 0VT0
Twelfth cranial nerve
use Nerve, Hypoglossal
Two lead pacemaker
use Pacemaker, Dual Chamber in 0JH
Tympanic cavity
use Ear, Middle, Left
use Ear, Middle, Right
Tympanic nerve
use Nerve, Glossopharyngeal
Tympanic part of temoporal bone
use Bone, Temporal, Left
use Bone, Temporal, Right
Tympanogram
see Hearing Assessment, Diagnostic Audiology F13
Tympanoplasty
see Repair, Ear, Nose, Sinus 09Q
see Replacement, Ear, Nose, Sinus 09R
see Supplement, Ear, Nose, Sinus 09U
Tympanosympathectomy
see Excision, Nerve, Head and Neck Sympathetic 01BK
Tympanotomy
see Drainage, Ear, Nose, Sinus 099
TYRX Antibacterial Envelope
use Anti-infective Envelope

U

Ulnar collateral carpal ligament
use Bursa and Ligament, Wrist, Left
use Bursa and Ligament, Wrist, Right
Ulnar collateral ligament
use Bursa and Ligament, Elbow, Left
use Bursa and Ligament, Elbow, Right
Ulnar notch
use Radius, Left
use Radius, Right
Ulnar vein
use Vein, Brachial, Left
use Vein, Brachial, Right
Ultrafiltration
Hemodialysis
see Performance, Urinary 5A1D
Therapeutic plasmapheresis
see Pheresis, Circulatory 6A55
Ultraflex™ Precision Colonic Stent System
use Intraluminal Device
ULTRAPRO Hernia System (UHS)
use Synthetic Substitute
ULTRAPRO Partially Absorbable Lightweight Mesh
use Synthetic Substitute
ULTRAPRO Plug
use Synthetic Substitute
Ultrasonic osteogenic stimulator
use Bone Growth Stimulator in Head and Facial Bones
use Bone Growth Stimulator in Lower Bones
use Bone Growth Stimulator in Upper Bones
Ultrasonography
Abdomen BW40ZZZ
Abdomen and Pelvis BW41ZZZ
Abdominal Wall BH49ZZZ
Aorta
Abdominal, Intravascular B440ZZ3
Thoracic, Intravascular B340ZZ3
Appendix BD48ZZZ
Artery
Brachiocephalic-Subclavian, Right, Intravascular B341ZZ3
Celiac and Mesenteric, Intravascular B44KZZ3
Common Carotid
Bilateral, Intravascular B345ZZ3
Left, Intravascular B344ZZ3
Right, Intravascular B343ZZ3
Coronary
Multiple B241YZZ
Intravascular B241ZZ3
Transesophageal B241ZZ4
Single B240YZZ
Intravascular B240ZZ3
Transesophageal B240ZZ4
Femoral, Intravascular B44LZZ3
Inferior Mesenteric, Intravascular B445ZZ3
Internal Carotid
Bilateral, Intravascular B348ZZ3
Left, Intravascular B347ZZ3
Right, Intravascular B346ZZ3
Intra-Abdominal, Other, Intravascular B44BZZ3
Intracranial, Intravascular B34RZZ3
Lower Extremity
Bilateral, Intravascular B44HZZ3
Left, Intravascular B44GZZ3
Right, Intravascular B44FZZ3
Mesenteric and Celiac, Intravascular B44KZZ3
Ophthalmic, Intravascular B34VZZ3
Penile, Intravascular B44NZZ3
Pulmonary
Left, Intravascular B34TZZ3
Right, Intravascular B34SZZ3
Renal
Bilateral, Intravascular B448ZZ3
Left, Intravascular B447ZZ3
Right, Intravascular B446ZZ3
Subclavian, Left, Intravascular B342ZZ3
Superior Mesenteric, Intravascular B444ZZ3
Upper Extremity
Bilateral, Intravascular B34KZZ3
Left, Intravascular B34JZZ3
Right, Intravascular B34HZZ3
Ultrasonography *(continued)*
Bile Duct BF40ZZZ
Bile Duct and Gallbladder BF43ZZZ
Bladder BT40ZZZ
and Kidney BT4JZZZ
Brain B040ZZZ
Breast
Bilateral BH42ZZZ
Left BH41ZZZ
Right BH40ZZZ
Chest Wall BH4BZZZ
Coccyx BR4FZZZ
Connective Tissue
Lower Extremity BL41ZZZ
Upper Extremity BL40ZZZ
Duodenum BD49ZZZ
Elbow
Left, Densitometry BP4HZZ1
Right, Densitometry BP4GZZ1
Esophagus BD41ZZZ
Extremity
Lower BH48ZZZ
Upper BH47ZZZ
Eye
Bilateral B847ZZZ
Left B846ZZZ
Right B845ZZZ
Fallopian Tube
Bilateral BU42
Left BU41
Right BU40
Fetal Umbilical Cord BY47ZZZ
Fetus
First Trimester, Multiple Gestation BY4BZZZ
Second Trimester, Multiple Gestation BY4DZZZ
Single
First Trimester BY49ZZZ
Second Trimester BY4CZZZ
Third Trimester BY4FZZZ
Third Trimester, Multiple Gestation BY4GZZZ
Gallbladder BF42ZZZ
Gallbladder and Bile Duct BF43ZZZ
Gastrointestinal Tract BD47ZZZ
Gland
Adrenal
Bilateral BG42ZZZ
Left BG41ZZZ
Right BG40ZZZ
Parathyroid BG43ZZZ
Thyroid BG44ZZZ
Hand
Left, Densitometry BP4PZZ1
Right, Densitometry BP4NZZ1
Head and Neck BH4CZZZ
Heart
Left B245YZZ
Intravascular B245ZZ3
Transesophageal B245ZZ4
Pediatric B24DYZZ
Intravascular B24DZZ3
Transesophageal B24DZZ4
Right B244YZZ
Intravascular B244ZZ3
Transesophageal B244ZZ4
Right and Left B246YZZ
Intravascular B246ZZ3
Transesophageal B246ZZ4
Heart with Aorta B24BYZZ
Intravascular B24BZZ3
Transesophageal B24BZZ4
Hepatobiliary System, All BF4CZZZ
Hip
Bilateral BQ42ZZZ

Ultrasonography *(continued)*
Hip *(continued)*
Left BQ41ZZZ
Right BQ40ZZZ
Kidney
and Bladder BT4JZZZ
Bilateral BT43ZZZ
Left BT42ZZZ
Right BT41ZZZ
Transplant BT49ZZZ
Knee
Bilateral BQ49ZZZ
Left BQ48ZZZ
Right BQ47ZZZ
Liver BF45ZZZ
Liver and Spleen BF46ZZZ
Mediastinum BB4CZZZ
Neck BW4FZZZ
Ovary
Bilateral BU45
Left BU44
Right BU43
Ovary and Uterus BU4C
Pancreas BF47ZZZ
Pelvic Region BW4GZZZ
Pelvis and Abdomen BW41ZZZ
Penis BV4BZZZ
Pericardium B24CYZZ
Intravascular B24CZZ3
Transesophageal B24CZZ4
Placenta BY48ZZZ
Pleura BB4BZZZ
Prostate and Seminal Vesicle BV49ZZZ
Rectum BD4CZZZ
Sacrum BR4FZZZ
Scrotum BV44ZZZ
Seminal Vesicle and Prostate BV49ZZZ
Shoulder
Left, Densitometry BP49ZZ1
Right, Densitometry BP48ZZ1
Spinal Cord B04BZZZ
Spine
Cervical BR40ZZZ
Lumbar BR49ZZZ
Thoracic BR47ZZZ
Spleen and Liver BF46ZZZ
Stomach BD42ZZZ
Tendon
Lower Extremity BL43ZZZ
Upper Extremity BL42ZZZ
Ureter
Bilateral BT48ZZZ
Left BT47ZZZ
Right BT46ZZZ
Urethra BT45ZZZ
Uterus BU46
Uterus and Ovary BU4C
Vein
Jugular
Left, Intravascular B544ZZ3
Right, Intravascular B543ZZ3
Lower Extremity
Bilateral, Intravascular B54DZZ3
Left, Intravascular B54CZZ3
Right, Intravascular B54BZZ3
Portal, Intravascular B54TZZ3
Renal
Bilateral, Intravascular B54LZZ3
Left, Intravascular B54KZZ3
Right, Intravascular B54JZZ3
Spanchnic, Intravascular B54TZZ3
Subclavian
Left, Intravascular B547ZZ3
Right, Intravascular B546ZZ3

Ultrasonography *(continued)*
Vein *(continued)*
Upper Extremity
Bilateral, Intravascular B54PZZ3
Left, Intravascular B54NZZ3
Right, Intravascular B54MZZ3
Vena Cava
Inferior, Intravascular B549ZZ3
Superior, Intravascular B548ZZ3
Wrist
Left, Densitometry BP4MZZ1
Right, Densitometry BP4LZZ1
Ultrasound bone healing system
use Bone Growth Stimulator in Head and Facial Bones
use Bone Growth Stimulator in Lower Bones
use Bone Growth Stimulator in Upper Bones
Ultrasound Therapy
Heart 6A75
No Qualifier 6A75
Vessels
Head and Neck 6A75
Other 6A75
Peripheral 6A75
Ultraviolet Light Therapy, Skin 6A80
Umbilical artery
use Artery, Internal Iliac, Left
use Artery, Internal Iliac, Right
use Artery, Lower
Uniplanar external fixator
use External Fixation Device, Monoplanar in 0PH
use External Fixation Device, Monoplanar in 0PS
use External Fixation Device, Monoplanar in 0QH
use External Fixation Device, Monoplanar in 0QS
Upper GI series
see Fluoroscopy, Gastrointestinal, Upper BD15
Ureteral orifice
use Ureter
use Ureter, Left
use Ureter, Right
use Ureters, Bilateral
Ureterectomy
see Excision, Urinary System 0TB
see Resection, Urinary System 0TT
Ureterocolostomy
see Bypass, Urinary System 0T1
Ureterocystostomy
see Bypass, Urinary System 0T1
Ureteroenterostomy
see Bypass, Urinary System 0T1
Ureteroileostomy
see Bypass, Urinary System 0T1
Ureterolithotomy
see Extirpation, Urinary System 0TC
Ureterolysis
see Release, Urinary System 0TN
Ureteroneocystostomy
see Bypass, Urinary System 0T1
see Reposition, Urinary System 0TS
Ureteropelvic junction (UPJ)
use Kidney Pelvis, Left
use Kidney Pelvis, Right
Ureteropexy
see Repair, Urinary System 0TQ
see Reposition, Urinary System 0TS

Ureteroplasty
see Repair, Urinary System 0TQ
see Replacement, Urinary System 0TR
see Supplement, Urinary System 0TU
Ureteroplication
see Restriction, Urinary System 0TV
Ureteropyelography
see Fluoroscopy, Urinary System BT1
Ureterorrhaphy
see Repair, Urinary System 0TQ
Ureteroscopy 0TJ98ZZ
Ureterostomy
see Bypass, Urinary System 0T1
see Drainage, Urinary System 0T9
Ureterotomy
see Drainage, Urinary System 0T9
Ureteroureterostomy
see Bypass, Urinary System 0T1
Ureterovesical orifice
use Ureter
use Ureters, Bilateral
use Ureter, Left
use Ureter, Right
Urethral catheterization, indwelling 0T9B70Z
Urethrectomy
see Excision, Urethra 0TBD
see Resection, Urethra 0TTD
Urethrolithotomy
see Extirpation, Urethra 0TCD
Urethrolysis
see Release, Urethra 0TND
Urethropexy
see Repair, Urethra 0TQD
see Reposition, Urethra 0TSD
Urethroplasty
see Repair, Urethra 0TQD
see Replacement, Urethra 0TRD
see Supplement, Urethra 0TUD
Urethrorrhaphy
see Repair, Urethra 0TQD
Urethroscopy 0TJD8ZZ
Urethrotomy
see Drainage, Urethra 0T9D
Uridine Triacetate XW0DX82
Urinary incontinence stimulator lead
use Stimulator Lead in Urinary System
Urography
see Fluoroscopy, Urinary System BT1
Ustekinumab
use Other New Technology Therapeutic Substance
Uterine Artery
use Artery, Internal Iliac, Left
use Artery, Internal Iliac, Right
Uterine artery embolization (UAE)
see Occlusion, Lower Arteries 04L
Uterine cornu
use Uterus
Uterine tube
use Fallopian Tube, Left
use Fallopian Tube, Right
Uterine vein
use Vein, Hypogastric, Left
use Vein, Hypogastric, Right
Uvulectomy
see Excision, Uvula 0CBN
see Resection, Uvula 0CTN
Uvulorrhaphy
see Repair, Uvula 0CQN

Uvulotomy
see Drainage, Uvula 0C9N

V

V-Wave Interatrial Shunt System
use Synthetic Substitute
Vabomere™
use Meropenem-vaboractam Anti-infective
Vaccination
see Introduction of Serum, Toxoid, and Vaccine
Vacuum extraction, obstetric 10D07Z6
Vaginal artery
use Artery, Internal Iliac, Left
use Artery, Internal Iliac, Right
Vaginal pessary
use Intraluminal Device, Pessary in Female Reproductive System
Vaginal vein
use Vein, Hypogastric, Left
use Vein, Hypogastric, Right
Vaginectomy
see Excision, Vagina 0UBG
see Resection, Vagina 0UTG
Vaginofixation
see Repair, Vagina 0UQG
see Reposition, Vagina 0USG
Vaginoplasty
see Repair, Vagina 0UQG
see Supplement, Vagina 0UUG
Vaginorrhaphy
see Repair, Vagina 0UQG
Vaginoscopy 0UJH8ZZ
Vaginotomy
see Drainage, Female Reproductive System 0U9
Vagotomy
see Division, Nerve, Vagus 008Q
Valiant Thoracic Stent Graft
use Intraluminal Device
Valvotomy, valvulotomy
see Division, Heart and Great Vessels 028
see Release, Heart and Great Vessels 02N
Valvuloplasty
see Repair, Heart and Great Vessels 02Q
see Replacement, Heart and Great Vessels 02R
see Supplement, Heart and Great Vessels 02U
Valvuloplasty, Alfieri Stitch
see Restriction, Valve, Mitral 02VG
Vascular Access Device
Totally Implantable
Insertion of device in
Abdomen 0JH8
Chest 0JH6
Lower Arm
Left 0JHH
Right 0JHG
Lower Leg
Left 0JHP
Right 0JHN
Upper Arm
Left 0JHF
Right 0JHD
Upper Leg
Left 0JHM
Right 0JHL
Removal of device from
Lower Extremity 0JPW
Trunk 0JPT
Upper Extremity 0JPV
Revision of device in

Vascular Access Device *(continued)*
Totally Implantable *(continued)*
Lower Extremity 0JWW
Trunk 0JWT
Upper Extremity 0JWV
Tunneled
Insertion of device in
Abdomen 0JH8
Chest 0JH6
Lower Arm
Left 0JHH
Right 0JHG
Lower Leg
Left 0JHP
Right 0JHN
Upper Arm
Left 0JHF
Right 0JHD
Upper Leg
Left 0JHM
Right 0JHL
Removal of device from
Lower Extremity 0JPW
Trunk 0JPT
Upper Extremity 0JPV
Revision of device in
Lower Extremity 0JWW
Trunk 0JWT
Upper Extremity 0JWV
Vasectomy
see Excision, Male Reproductive System 0VB
Vasography
see Fluoroscopy, Male Reproductive System BV1
see Plain Radiography, Male Reproductive System BV0
Vasoligation
see Occlusion, Male Reproductive System 0VL
Vasorrhaphy
see Repair, Male Reproductive System 0VQ
Vasostomy
see Bypass, Male Reproductive System 0V1
Vasotomy
Drainage
see Drainage, Male Reproductive System 0V9
see Occlusion, Male Reproductive System 0VL
With ligation
Vasovasostomy
see Repair, Male Reproductive System 0VQ
Vastus intermedius muscle
use Muscle, Upper Leg, Left
use Muscle, Upper Leg, Right
Vastus lateralis muscle
use Muscle, Upper Leg, Left
use Muscle, Upper Leg, Right
Vastus medialis muscle
use Muscle, Upper Leg, Left
use Muscle, Upper Leg, Right
VCG (vectorcardiogram)
see Measurement, Cardiac 4A02
Vectra® Vascular Access Graft
use Vascular Access Device, Tunneled in Subcutaneous Tissue and Fascia
Veklury *use* Remdesivir Anti-infective
Venclexta®
use Venetoclax Antineoplastic
Venetoclax Antineoplastic XW0DXR5
Venectomy
see Excision, Lower Veins 06B
see Excision, Upper Veins 05B
Venography
see Fluoroscopy, Veins B51
see Plain Radiography, Veins B50
Venorrhaphy
see Repair, Lower Veins 06Q
see Repair, Upper Veins 05Q
Venotripsy
see Occlusion, Lower Veins 06L
see Occlusion, Upper Veins 05L
Ventricular fold
use Larynx
Ventriculoatriostomy
see Bypass, Central Nervous System and Cranial Nerves 001
Ventriculocisternostomy
see Bypass, Central Nervous System and Cranial Nerves 001
Ventriculogram, cardiac
Combined left and right heart
see Fluoroscopy, Heart, Right and Left B216
Left ventricle
see Fluoroscopy, Heart, Left B215
Right ventricle
see Fluoroscopy, Heart, Right B214
Ventriculopuncture, through previously implanted catheter 8C01X6J
Ventriculoscopy 00J04ZZ
Ventriculostomy
External drainage
see Drainage, Cerebral Ventricle 0096
Internal shunt
see Bypass, Cerebral Ventricle 0016
Ventriculovenostomy
see Bypass, Cerebral Ventricle 0016
Ventrio™ Hernia Patch
use Synthetic Substitute
VEP (visual evoked potential) 4A07X0Z
Vermiform appendix
use Appendix
Vermilion border
use Lip, Lower
use Lip, Upper
Versa
use Pacemaker, Dual Chamber in 0JH
Version, obstetric
External 10S0XZZ
Internal 10S07ZZ
Vertebral arch
use Vertebra, Cervical
use Vertebra, Lumbar
use Vertebra, Thoracic
Vertebral body
use Cervical Vertebra
use Thoracic Vertebra
use Lumbar Vertebra
Vertebral canal
use Spinal Canal
Vertebral foramen
use Vertebra, Cervical
use Vertebra, Lumbar
use Vertebra, Thoracic
Vertebral lamina
use Vertebra, Cervical
use Vertebra, Lumbar
use Vertebra, Thoracic
Vertebral pedicle
use Vertebra, Cervical
use Vertebra, Lumbar
use Vertebra, Thoracic
Vesical vein
use Vein, Hypogastric, Left
use Vein, Hypogastric, Right
Vesicotomy
see Drainage, Urinary System 0T9
Vesiculectomy
see Excision, Male Reproductive System 0VB
see Resection, Male Reproductive System 0VT
Vesiculogram, seminal
see Plain Radiography, Male Reproductive System BV0
Vesiculotomy
see Drainage, Male Reproductive System 0V9
Vestibular (Scarpa's) ganglion
use Nerve, Acoustic
Vestibular Assessment F15Z
Vestibular nerve
use Nerve, Acoustic
Vestibular Treatment F0C
Vestibulocochlear nerve
use Nerve, Acoustic
VH-IVUS (virtual histology intravascular ultrasound)
see Ultrasonography, Heart B24
Virchow's (supraclavicular) lymph node
use Lymphatic, Neck, Left
use Lymphatic, Neck, Right
Virtuoso (II) (DR) (VR)
use Defibrillator Generator in 0JH
Vistogard®
use Uridine Triacetate
Vitrectomy
see Excision, Eye 08B
see Resection, Eye 08T
Vitreous body
use Vitreous, Left
use Vitreous, Right
Viva (XT)(S)
use Cardiac Resynchronization Defibrillator Pulse Generator in 0JH
Vocal fold
use Vocal Cord, Left
use Vocal Cord, Right
Vocational
Assessment
Retraining
see Activities of Daily Living Assessment, Rehabilitation F02
see Activities of Daily Living Treatment, Rehabilitation F08
Volar (palmar) digital vein
use Vein, Hand, Left
use Vein, Hand, Right
Volar (palmar) metacarpal vein
use Vein, Hand, Left
use Vein, Hand, Right
Vomer bone
use Septum, Nasal
Vomer of nasal septum
use Bone, Nasal
Voraxaze
Glucarpidase
Vulvectomy
see Excision, Female Reproductive System 0UB
see Resection, Female Reproductive System 0UT
VYXEOS™
use Cytarabine and Daunorubicin Liposome Antineoplastic

W

WALLSTENT® Endoprosthesis
use Intraluminal Device
Washing
see Irrigation
WavelinQ EndoAVF system
Radial Artery, Left 031C
Radial Artery, Right 031B
Ulnar Artery, Left 031A
Ulnar Artery, Right 0319
Wedge resection, pulmonary
see Excision, Respiratory System 0BB
Whole Blood Nucleic Acid-base Microbial Detection XXE5XM5
Window
see Drainage
Wiring, dental 2W31X9Z

X

X-ray
see Plain Radiography
X-STOP® Spacer
use Spinal Stabilization Device, Interspinous Process in 0RH
use Spinal Stabilization Device, Interspinous Process in 0SH
Xact Carotid Stent System
use Intraluminal Device
XENLETA™
use Lefamulin Anti-infective
Xenograft
use Zooplastic Tissue in Heart and Great Vessels
XIENCE Everolimus Eluting Coronary Stent System
use Intraluminal Device, Drug-eluting in Heart and Great Vessels
Xiphoid process
use Sternum
XLIF® System
use Interbody Fusion Device in Lower Joints
XOSPATA®
use Gilteritinib Antineoplastic

Y

Yescarta®
use Axicabtagene Ciloleucel Immunotherapy
Yoga Therapy 8E0ZXY4

Z

Z-plasty, skin for scar contracture
see Release, Skin and Breast 0HN
Zenith AAA Endovascular Graft
use Intraluminal Device
Zenith® Fenestrated AAA Endovascular Graft
use Intraluminal Device, Branched or Fenestrated, One or Two Arteries in 04V
use Intraluminal Device, Branched or Fenestrated, Three or More Arteries in 04V
Zenith Flex® AAA Endovascular Graft
use Intraluminal Device
Zenith TX2® TAA Endovascular Graft
use Intraluminal Device
Zenith® Renu™ AAA Ancillary Graft
use Intraluminal Device
ZEPZELCA™ *use* Lurbinectedin
ZERBAXA®
use Ceftolozane/Tazobactam Anti-infective

Zilver® PTX® (paclitaxel) Drug-Eluting Peripheral Stent
use Intraluminal Device, Drug-eluting in Lower Arteries
use Intraluminal Device, Drug-eluting in Upper Arteries
Zimmer® NexGen® LPS Mobile Bearing Knee
use Synthetic Substitute
Zimmer® NexGen® LPS-Flex Mobile Knee
use Synthetic Substitute
ZINPLAVA™
use Bezlotoxumab Monoclonal AntibodyZonule of Zinn
Zonule of Zinn
use Lens, Left
use Lens, Right
Zooplastic Tissue, Rapid Deployment Technique, Replacement X2RF
Zotarolimus-eluting coronary stent
use Intraluminal Device, Drug-eluting in Heart and Great Vessels
ZULRESSO™
use Brexanolone
Zygomatic process of frontal bone
use Bone, Frontal
Zygomatic process of temporal bone
use Bone, Temporal, Left
use Bone, Temporal, Right
Zygomaticus muscle
use Muscle, Facial
Zyvox
use Oxazolidinones

Medical and Surgical (001–0YW)

Within each section of ICD-10-PCS the characters have different meanings. The seven character meanings for the Medical and Surgical section are illustrated here through the procedure example of *Percutaneous needle core biopsy of the right kidney*.

Section	Body System	Root Operation	Body Part	Approach	Device	Qualifier
Med/Surg	Urinary	Excision	Kidney, Right	Percutaneous	None	Diagnostic
0	T	B	0	3	Z	X

Section (Character 1)

All Medical and Surgical procedure codes have a first character value of 0.

Body System (Character 2)

The alphanumeric character for the body system is placed in the second position. The following are the body systems applicable to the Medical and Surgical section.

Character Value	Character Value Description
0	Central Nervous System and Cranial Nerves
1	Peripheral Nervous System
2	Heart and Great Vessels
3	Upper Arteries
4	Lower Arteries
5	Upper Veins
6	Lower Veins
7	Lymphatic and Hemic Systems
8	Eye
9	Ear, Nose, Sinus
B	Respiratory System
C	Mouth and Throat
D	Gastrointestinal System
F	Hepatobiliary System and Pancreas
G	Endocrine System
H	Skin and Breast
J	Subcutaneous Tissue and Fascia
K	Muscles
L	Tendons
M	Bursae and Ligaments
N	Head and Facial Bones
P	Upper Bones
Q	Lower Bones
R	Upper Joints
S	Lower Joints
T	Urinary System
U	Female Reproductive System
V	Male Reproductive System
W	Anatomical Regions, General
X	Anatomical Regions, Upper Extremities
Y	Anatomical Regions, Lower Extremities

Root Operations (Character 3)

The alphanumeric character value for root operations is placed in the third position. Listed below are the root operations applicable to the Medical and Surgical section with their associated meaning.

Character Value	Root Operation	Root Operation Definition
0	Alteration	Modifying the anatomic structure of a body part without affecting the function of the body part
1	Bypass	Altering the route of passage of the contents of a tubular body part
2	Change	Taking out or off a device from a body part and putting back an identical or similar device in or on the same body part without cutting or puncturing the skin or a mucous membrane
3	Control	Stopping, or attempting to stop, postprocedural or other acute bleeding
4	Creation	Making a new genital structure that does not take over the function of a body part
5	Destruction	Physical eradication of all or a portion of a body part by the direct use of energy, force, or a destructive agent
6	Detachment	Cutting off all or a portion of the upper or lower extremities
7	Dilation	Expanding an orifice or the lumen of a tubular body part
8	Division	Cutting into a body part, without draining fluids and/or gases from the body part, in order to separate or transect a body part
9	Drainage	Taking or letting out fluids and/or gases from a body part
B	Excision	Cutting out or off, without replacement, a portion of a body part
C	Extirpation	Taking or cutting out solid matter from a body part
D	Extraction	Pulling or stripping out or off all or a portion of a body part by the use of force
F	Fragmentation	Breaking solid matter in a body part into pieces
G	Fusion	Joining together portions of an articular body part rendering the articular body part immobile
H	Insertion	Putting in a nonbiological appliance that monitors, assists, performs, or prevents a physiological function but does not physically take the place of a body part
J	Inspection	Visually and/or manually exploring a body part
K	Map	Locating the route of passage of electrical impulses and/or locating functional areas in a body part
L	Occlusion	Completely closing an orifice or the lumen of a tubular body part
M	Reattachment	Putting back in or on all or a portion of a separated body part to its normal location or other suitable location
N	Release	Freeing a body part from an abnormal physical constraint by cutting or by the use of force
P	Removal	Taking out or off a device from a body part
Q	Repair	Restoring, to the extent possible, a body part to its normal anatomic structure and function
R	Replacement	Putting in or on biological or synthetic material that physically takes the place and/or function of all or a portion of a body part
S	Reposition	Moving to its normal location, or other suitable location, all or a portion of a body part
T	Resection	Cutting out or off, without replacement, all of a body part
V	Restriction	Partially closing an orifice or the lumen of a tubular body part
W	Revision	Correcting, to the extent possible, a portion of a malfunctioning device or the position of a displaced device
U	Supplement	Putting in or on biological or synthetic material that physically reinforces and/or augments the function of a portion of a body part
X	Transfer	Moving, without taking out, all or a portion of a body part to another location to take over the function of all or a portion of a body part
Y	Transplantation	Putting in or on all or a portion of a living body part taken from another individual or animal to physically take the place and/or function of all or a portion of a similar body part

Body Part (Character 4)

For each body system the applicable body part character values will be available for procedure code construction. An example of a body part for this section is the Large Intestines.

Approach (Character 5)

The approach is the technique used to reach the procedure site. The following are the approach character values for the Medical and Surgical section with the associated definitions.

Character Value	Approach	Approach Definition
0	Open	Cutting through the skin or mucous membrane and any other body layers necessary to expose the site of the procedure
3	Percutaneous	Entry, by puncture or minor incision, of instrumentation through the skin or mucous membrane and any other body layers necessary to reach the site of the procedure
4	Percutaneous Endoscopic	Entry, by puncture or minor incision, of instrumentation through the skin or mucous membrane and any other body layers necessary to reach and visualize the site of the procedure
7	Via Natural or Artificial Opening	Entry of instrumentation through a natural or artificial external opening to reach the site of the procedure
8	Via Natural or Artificial Opening Endoscopic	Entry of instrumentation through a natural or artificial external opening to reach and visualize the site of the procedure
F	Via Natural or Artificial Opening Percutaneous Endoscopic	Entry of instrumentation through a natural or artificial external opening to reach and visualize the site of the procedure, and entry, by puncture or minor incision, of instrumentation through the skin or mucous membrane and any other body layers necessary to aid in the performance of the procedure
X	External	Procedures performed directly on the skin or mucous membrane and procedures performed indirectly by the application of external force through the skin or mucous membrane

Device (Character 6)

Depending on the procedure performed there may or may not be a device used. There are several types of devices included in the Medical and Surgical section that fall into one of the four following categories.

- Electronic Appliances
- Grafts and Prostheses
- Implants
- Simple or Mechanical Appliances

When a device is not utilized during the procedure, the character value of Z should be reported.

If a coder is unsure of which option to select for the device utilized during the procedure, Appendix E can be used to guide the selection. For example, if the coder is in Table 02R (replacement of heart and great vessels) the coder can locate the device categories in Appendix E (Autologous Tissue Substitute, Zooplastic Tissue, Synthetic Substitute, and Nonautologous Tissue Substitue). For each of these categories brand name devices and other devices are listed. The coder should select the category in which the device utilized during the procedure is listed.

Qualifier (Character 7)

The qualifier represents an additional attribute for the procedure when applicable. In the preceding example of *Percutaneous needle core biopsy of the right kidney*, the qualifier of X was used to report that the biopsy procedure was diagnostic in nature. If there is no qualifier for a procedure, the Z character value should be reported.

Important Definitions for the Medical and Surgical Section

Medical Surgical Root Operation	Qualifier	Definition
Detachment of Upper and Lower Extremities (0X6 and 0Y6) Arms and Legs	1 – High	Amputation at the proximal portion of the shaft of the humerus or femur
	2 – Mid	Amputation at the middle portion of the shaft of the humerus or femur
	3 – Low	Amputation at the distal portion of the shaft of the humerus or femur
Detachment of Upper and Lower Extremities (0X6 and 0Y6) Fingers, Thumbs, and Toes	0 – Complete	Amputation at the metacarpophalangeal/metatarsal-phalangeal joint
	1 – High	Amputation anywhere along the proximal phalanx
	2 – Mid	Amputation through the proximal interphalangeal joint or anywhere along the middle phalanx
	3 – Low	Amputation through the distal interphalangeal joint or anywhere along the distal phalanx
Transplantation	0 – Allogeneic	Being genetically different although belonging to or obtained from the same species*
	1 – Syngeneic	Genetically identical or closely related, so as to allow tissue transplant; immunologically compatible*
	2 – Zooplastic	Surgical transfer of tissue from an animal to a human*

*Taken from The Free Dictionary by Farlex at www.thefreedictionary.com

Official Coding Guidelines for the Medical and Surgical Section

Medical and Surgical Section Guidelines (section 0)

B2. Body System

General guidelines

B2.1a The procedure codes in Anatomical Regions, General, Anatomical Regions, Upper Extremities and Anatomical Regions, Lower Extremities can be used when the procedure is performed on an anatomical region rather than a specific body part, or on the rare occasion when no information is available to support assignment of a code to a specific body part.

Examples: Chest tube drainage of the pleural cavity is coded to the root operation Drainage found in the body system Anatomical Regions, General. Suture repair of the abdominal wall is coded to the root operation Repair in the body system Anatomical Regions, General. Amputation of the foot is coded to the root operation Detachment in the body system Anatomical Regions, Lower Extremities.

B2.1b Where the general body part values "upper" and "lower" are provided as an option in the Upper Arteries, Lower Arteries, Upper Veins, Lower Veins, Muscles and Tendons body systems, "upper" or "lower" specifies body parts located above or below the diaphragm respectively.

Example: Vein body parts above the diaphragm are found in the Upper Veins body system; vein body parts below the diaphragm are found in the Lower Veins body system.

B3. Root Operation

General guidelines

B3.1a In order to determine the appropriate root operation, the full definition of the root operation as contained in the PCS Tables must be applied.

B3.1b Components of a procedure specified in the root operation definition or explanation as integral to that root operation are not coded separately. Procedural steps necessary to reach the operative site and close the operative site, including anastomosis of a tubular body part, are also not coded separately.

Examples: Resection of a joint as part of a joint replacement procedure is included in the root operation definition of Replacement and is not coded separately. Laparotomy performed to reach the site of an open liver biopsy is not coded separately. In a resection of sigmoid colon with anastomosis of descending colon to rectum, the anastomosis is not coded separately.

Multiple procedures

B3.2 During the same operative episode, multiple procedures are coded if:

a. The same root operation is performed on different body parts as defined by distinct values of the body part character.

Examples: Diagnostic excision of liver and pancreas are coded separately. Excision of lesion in the ascending colon and excision of lesion in the transverse colon are coded separately.

b. The same root operation is repeated at different body sites that are included in the same body part value.

Examples: Excision of the sartorius muscle and excision of the gracilis muscle are both included in the upper leg muscle body part value, and multiple procedures are coded. Extraction of multiple toenails are coded separately.

c. Multiple root operations with distinct objectives are performed on the same body part.

Example: Destruction of sigmoid lesion and bypass of sigmoid colon are coded separately.

d. The intended root operation is attempted using one approach but is converted to a different approach.

Example: Laparoscopic cholecystectomy converted to an open cholecystectomy is coded as percutaneous endoscopic Inspection and open Resection.

Discontinued or incomplete procedures

B3.3 If the intended procedure is discontinued or otherwise not complete, code the procedure to the root operation performed. If a procedure is discontinued before any other root operation is performed, code the root operation Inspection of the body part or anatomical region inspected.

Example: A planned aortic valve replacement procedure is discontinued after the initial thoracotomy and before any incision is made in the heart muscle, when the patient becomes hemodynamically unstable. This procedure is coded as an open Inspection of the mediastinum.

Biopsy procedures

B3.4a Biopsy procedures are coded using the root operations Excision, Extraction, or Drainage and the qualifier Diagnostic.

Examples: Fine needle aspiration biopsy of lung is coded to the root operation Drainage with the qualifier Diagnostic. Biopsy of bone marrow is coded to the root operation Extraction with the qualifier Diagnostic. Lymph node sampling for biopsy is coded to the root operation Excision with the qualifier Diagnostic.

Biopsy followed by more definitive treatment

B3.4b If a diagnostic Excision, Extraction, or Drainage procedure (biopsy) is followed by a more definitive procedure, such as Destruction, Excision or Resection at the same procedure site, both the biopsy and the more definitive treatment are coded.

Example: Biopsy of breast followed by partial mastectomy at the same procedure site, both the biopsy and the partial mastectomy procedure are coded.

Overlapping body layers

B3.5 If root operations Excision, Extraction, Repair or Inspection are performed on overlapping layers of the musculoskeletal system, the body part specifying the deepest layer is coded.

Example: Excisional debridement that includes skin and subcutaneous tissue and muscle is coded to the muscle body part.

Bypass procedures

B3.6a Bypass procedures are coded by identifying the body part bypassed "from" and the body part bypassed "to." The fourth character body part specifies the body part bypassed from, and the qualifier specifies the body part bypassed to.

Example: Bypass from stomach to jejunum, stomach is the body part and jejunum is the qualifier.

B3.6b Coronary artery bypass procedures are coded differently than other bypass procedures as described in the previous guideline. Rather than identifying the body part bypassed from, the body part identifies the number of coronary artery sites bypassed to, and the qualifier specifies the vessel bypassed from.

Example: Aortocoronary artery bypass of the left anterior descending coronary artery and the obtuse marginal coronary artery is classified in the body part axis of classification as two coronary arteries and the qualifier specifies the aorta as the body part bypassed from.

B3.6c If multiple coronary arteries are bypassed, a separate procedure is coded for each coronary artery that uses a different device and/or qualifier.

Example: Aortocoronary artery bypass and internal mammary coronary artery bypass are coded separately.

Control vs. more definitive root operations

B3.7 The root operation Control is defined as, "Stopping, or attempting to stop, postprocedural or other acute bleeding." Control is the root operation coded when the procedure performed to achieve hemostasis, beyond what would be considered integral to a procedure, utilizes techniques (e.g. cautery, application of substances or pressure, suturing or ligation or clipping of bleeding points at the site) that are not described by a more specific root operation definition, such as Bypass, Detachment, Excision, Extraction, Reposition, Replacement, or Resection. If a more specific root operation definition applies to the procedure performed, then the more specific root operation is coded instead of Control.

Examples: Silver nitrate cautery to treat acute nasal bleeding is coded to the root operation Control. Liquid embolization of the right internal iliac artery to treat acute hematoma by stopping blood flow is coded to the root operation Occlusion. Suctioning of residual blood to achieve hemostasis during a transbronchial cryobiopsy is considered integral to the cryobiopsy procedure and is not coded separately.

Excision vs. Resection

B3.8 PCS contains specific body parts for anatomical subdivisions of a body part, such as lobes of the lungs or liver and regions of the intestine. Resection of the specific body part is coded whenever all of the body part is cut out or off, rather than coding Excision of a less specific body part.

Example: Left upper lung lobectomy is coded to Resection of Upper Lung Lobe, Left rather than Excision of Lung, Left.

Excision for graft

B3.9 If an autograft is obtained from a different procedure site in order to complete the objective of the procedure, a separate procedure is coded, except when the seventh character qualifier value in the ICD-10-PCS table fully specifies the site from which the autograft was obtained.

Examples: Coronary bypass with excision of saphenous vein graft, excision of saphenous vein is coded separately. Replacement of breast with autologous deep inferior epigastric artery perforator (DIEP) flap, excision of the DIEP flap is not coded separately. The seventh character qualifier value Deep Inferior Epigastric Artery Perforator Flap in the Replacement table fully specifies the site of the autograft harvest.

Fusion procedures of the spine

B3.10a The body part coded for a spinal vertebral joint(s) rendered immobile by a spinal fusion procedure is classified by the level of the spine (e.g. thoracic). There are distinct body part values for a single vertebral joint and for multiple vertebral joints at each spinal level.

Example: Body part values specify Lumbar Vertebral Joint, Lumbar Vertebral Joints, 2 or More and Lumbosacral Vertebral Joint.

B3.10b If multiple vertebral joints are fused, a separate procedure is coded for each vertebral joint that uses a different device and/or qualifier.

Example: Fusion of lumbar vertebral joint, posterior approach, anterior column and fusion of lumbar vertebral joint, posterior approach, posterior column are coded separately.

B3.10c Combinations of devices and materials are often used on a vertebral joint to render the joint immobile. When combinations of devices are used on the same vertebral joint, the device value coded for the procedure is as follows:

- If an interbody fusion device is used to render the joint immobile (containing bone graft or bone graft substitute), the procedure is coded with the device value Interbody Fusion Device
- If bone graft is the only device used to render the joint immobile, the procedure is coded with the device value Nonautologous Tissue Substitute or Autologous Tissue Substitute
- If a mixture of autologous and nonautologous bone graft (with or without biological or synthetic extenders or binders) is used to render the joint immobile, code the procedure with the device value Autologous Tissue Substitute

Examples: Fusion of a vertebral joint using a cage style interbody fusion device containing morsellized bone graft is coded to the device Interbody Fusion Device. Fusion of a vertebral joint using a bone dowel interbody fusion device made of cadaver bone and packed with a mixture of local morsellized bone and demineralized bone matrix is coded to the device Interbody Fusion Device. Fusion of a vertebral joint using both autologous bone graft and bone bank bone graft is coded to the device Autologous Tissue Substitute.

Inspection procedures

B3.11a Inspection of a body part(s) performed in order to achieve the objective of a procedure is not coded separately.

Example: Fiberoptic bronchoscopy performed for irrigation of bronchus, only the irrigation procedure is coded.

B3.11b If multiple tubular body parts are inspected, the most distal body part inspected is coded. If multiple non-tubular body parts in a region are inspected, the body part that specifies the entire area inspected is coded.

Examples: Cystoureteroscopy with inspection of bladder and ureters is coded to the ureter body part value. Exploratory laparotomy with general inspection of abdominal contents is coded to the peritoneal cavity body part value.

B3.11c When both an Inspection procedure and another procedure are performed on the same body part during the same episode, if the Inspection procedure is performed using a different approach than the other procedure, the Inspection procedure is coded separately.

Example: Endoscopic Inspection of the duodenum is coded separately when open Excision of the duodenum is performed during the same procedural episode.

Occlusion vs. Restriction for vessel embolization procedures

B3.12 If the objective of an embolization procedure is to completely close a vessel, the root operation Occlusion is coded. If the objective of an embolization procedure is to narrow the lumen of a vessel, the root operation Restriction is coded.

Examples: Tumor embolization is coded to the root operation Occlusion, because the objective of the procedure is to cut off the blood supply to the vessel. Embolization of a cerebral aneurysm is coded to the root operation Restriction, because the objective of the procedure is not to close off the vessel entirely, but to narrow the lumen of the vessel at the site of the aneurysm where it is abnormally wide.

Release procedures

B3.13 In the root operation Release, the body part value coded is the body part being freed and not the tissue being manipulated or cut to free the body part.

Example: Lysis of intestinal adhesions is coded to the specific intestine body part value.

Release vs. Division

B3.14 If the sole objective of the procedure is freeing a body part without cutting the body part, the root operation is Release. If the sole objective of the procedure is separating or transecting a body part, the root operation is Division.

Example: Freeing a nerve root from surrounding scar tissue to relieve pain is coded to the root operation Release. Severing a nerve root to relieve pain is coded to the root operation Division.

Reposition for fracture treatment

B3.15 Reduction of a displaced fracture is coded to the root operation Reposition and the application of a cast or splint in conjunction with the Reposition procedure is not coded separately. Treatment of a nondisplaced fracture is coded to the procedure performed.

Examples: Putting a pin in a nondisplaced fracture is coded to the root operation Insertion. Casting of a nondisplaced fracture is coded to the root operation Immobilization in the Placement section.

Transplantation vs. Administration

B3.16 Putting in a mature and functioning living body part taken from another individual or animal is coded to the root operation Transplantation. Putting in autologous or nonautologous cells is coded to the Administration section.

Example: Putting in autologous or nonautologous bone marrow, pancreatic islet cells or stem cells is coded to the Administration section.

Transfer procedures using multiple tissue layers

B3.17 The root operation Transfer contains qualifiers that can be used to specify when a transfer flap is composed of more than one tissue layer, such as a musculocutaneous flap. For procedures involving transfer of multiple tissue layers including skin, subcutaneous tissue, fascia or muscle, the procedure is coded to the body part value that describes the deepest tissue layer in the flap, and the qualifier can be used to describe the other tissue layer(s) in the transfer flap.

Example: A musculocutaneous flap transfer is coded to the appropriate body part value in the body system Muscles, and the qualifier is used to describe the additional tissue layer(s) in the transfer flap.

Excision/Resection followed by replacement

B3.18 If an Excision or Resection of a body part is followed by a Replacement procedure, code both procedures to identify each distinct objective, except when the Excision or Resection is considered integral and preparatory for the Replacement procedure.

Examples: Mastectomy followed by reconstruction, both Resection and Replacement of the breast are coded to fully capture the distinct objectives of the procedures performed. Maxillectomy with obturator reconstruction, both Excision and Replacement of the maxilla are coded to fully capture the distinct objectives of the procedures performed. Excisional debridement of tendon with skin graft, both the Excision of the tendon and the Replacement of the skin with a graft are coded to fully capture the distinct objectives of the procedures performed. Esophagectomy followed by reconstruction with colonic interposition, both the Resection and the Transfer of the large intestine to function as the esophagus are coded to fully capture the distinct objectives of the procedures performed.

Examples: Resection of a joint as part of a joint replacement procedure is considered integral and preparatory for the Replacement of the joint and the Resection is not coded separately. Resection of a valve as part of a valve replacement procedure is considered integral and preparatory for the valve Replacement and the Resection is not coded separately.

B4. Body Part

General guidelines

B4.1a If a procedure is performed on a portion of a body part that does not have a separate body part value, code the body part value corresponding to the whole body part.

Example: A procedure performed on the alveolar process of the mandible is coded to the mandible body part.

B4.1b If the prefix "peri" is combined with a body part to identify the site of the procedure, and the site of the procedure is not further specified, then the procedure is coded to the body part named. This guideline applies only when a more specific body part value is not available.

Examples: A procedure site identified as perirenal is coded to the kidney body part when the site of the procedure is not further specified. A procedure site described in the documentation as peri-urethral tissue, and the documentation also indicates that it is the vulvar tissue and not the urethral tissue that is the site of the procedure, then the procedure is coded to the vulva body part. A procedure site documented as involving the periosteum is coded to the corresponding bone body part.

B4.1c If a procedure is performed on a continuous section of a tubular body part, code the body part value corresponding to the anatomically most proximal (closest to the heart) portion of the tubular body part.

Examples: A procedure performed on a continuous section of artery from the femoral artery to the external iliac artery with the point of entry at the femoral artery is coded to the external iliac body part. A procedure performed on a continuous section of artery from the femoral artery to the external iliac artery with the point of entry at the external iliac artery is also coded to the external iliac artery body part.

Branches of body parts

B4.2 Where a specific branch of a body part does not have its own body part value in PCS, the body part is typically coded to the closest proximal branch that has a specific body part value. In the cardiovascular body systems, if a general body part is available in the correct root operation table, and coding to a proximal branch would require assigning a code in a different body system, the procedure is coded using the general body part value.

Examples: A procedure performed on the mandibular branch of the trigeminal nerve is coded to the trigeminal nerve body part value. Occlusion of the bronchial artery is coded to the body part value Upper Artery in the body system Upper Arteries, and not to the body part value Thoracic Aorta, Descending in the body system Heart and Great Vessels.

Bilateral body part values

B4.3 Bilateral body part values are available for a limited number of body parts. If the identical procedure is performed on contralateral body parts, and a bilateral body part value exists for that body part, a single procedure is coded using the bilateral body part value. If no bilateral body part value exists, each procedure is coded separately using the appropriate body part value.

Examples: The identical procedure performed on both fallopian tubes is coded once using the body part value Fallopian Tube, Bilateral. The identical procedure performed on both knee joints is coded twice using the body part values Knee Joint, Right and Knee Joint, Left.

Coronary arteries

B4.4 The coronary arteries are classified as a single body part that is further specified by number of arteries treated. One procedure code specifying multiple arteries is used when the same procedure is performed, including the same device and qualifier values.

Examples: Angioplasty of two distinct coronary arteries with placement of two stents is coded as Dilation of Coronary Artery, Two Arteries, with Two Intraluminal Devices. Angioplasty of two distinct coronary arteries, one with stent placed and one without, is coded separately as Dilation of Coronary Artery, One Artery with Intraluminal Device, and Dilation of Coronary Artery, One Artery with no device.

Tendons, ligaments, bursae and fascia near a joint

B4.5 Procedures performed on tendons, ligaments, bursae and fascia supporting a joint are coded to the body part in the respective body system that is the focus of the procedure. Procedures performed on joint structures themselves are coded to the body part in the joint body systems.

Examples: Repair of the anterior cruciate ligament of the knee is coded to the knee bursae and ligament body part in the Bursae and Ligaments body system. Knee arthroscopy with shaving of articular cartilage is coded to the knee joint body part in the Lower Joints body system.

Skin, subcutaneous tissue and fascia overlying a joint

B4.6 If a procedure is performed on the skin, subcutaneous tissue or fascia overlying a joint, the procedure is coded to the following body part:

- Shoulder is coded to Upper Arm
- Elbow is coded to Lower Arm
- Wrist is coded to Lower Arm
- Hip is coded to Upper Leg
- Knee is coded to Lower Leg
- Ankle is coded to Foot

Fingers and toes

B4.7 If a body system does not contain a separate body part value for fingers, procedures performed on the fingers are coded to the body part value for the hand. If a body system does not contain a separate body part value for toes, procedures performed on the toes are coded to the body part value for the foot.

Example: Excision of finger muscle is coded to one of the hand muscle body part values in the Muscles body system.

Upper and lower intestinal tract

B4.8 In the Gastrointestinal body system, the general body part values Upper Intestinal Tract and Lower Intestinal Tract are provided as an option for the root operations such as Change, Insertion, Inspection, Removal and Revision. Upper Intestinal Tract includes the portion of the gastrointestinal tract from the esophagus down to and including the duodenum, and Lower Intestinal Tract includes the portion of the gastrointestinal tract from the jejunum down to and including the rectum and anus.

Example: In the root operation Change table, change of a device in the jejunum is coded using the body part Lower Intestinal Tract.

B5. Approach

Open approach with percutaneous endoscopic assistance

B5.2a Procedures performed using the open approach with percutaneous endoscopic assistance are coded to the approach Open.

Example: Laparoscopic-assisted sigmoidectomy is coded to the approach Open.

Percutaneous endoscopic approach with extension of incision

B5.2b Procedures performed using the percutaneous endoscopic approach, with incision or extension of an incision to assist in the removal of all or a portion of a body part or to anastomose a tubular body part to complete the procedure, are coded to the approach value Percutaneous Endoscopic.

Examples: Laparoscopic sigmoid colectomy with extension of stapling port for removal of specimen and direct anastomosis is coded to the approach value Percutaneous Endoscopic. Laparoscopic nephrectomy with midline incision for removing the resected kidney is coded to the approach value Percutaneous Endoscopic. Robotic-assisted laparoscopic prostatectomy with extension of incision for removal of the resected prostate is coded to the approach value Percutaneous Endoscopic.

External approach

B5.3a Procedures performed within an orifice on structures that are visible without the aid of any instrumentation are coded to the approach External.

Example: Resection of tonsils is coded to the approach External.

B5.3b Procedures performed indirectly by the application of external force through the intervening body layers are coded to the approach External.

Example: Closed reduction of fracture is coded to the approach External.

Percutaneous procedure via device

B5.4 Procedures performed percutaneously via a device placed for the procedure are coded to the approach Percutaneous.

Example: Fragmentation of kidney stone performed via percutaneous nephrostomy is coded to the approach Percutaneous.

B6. Device

General guidelines

B6.1a A device is coded only if a device remains after the procedure is completed. If no device remains, the device value No Device is coded. In limited root operations, the classification provides the qualifier values Temporary and Intraoperative, for specific procedures involving clinically significant devices, where the purpose of the device is to be utilized for a brief duration during the procedure or current inpatient stay. If a device that is intended to remain after the procedure is completed requires removal before the end of the operative episode in which it was inserted (for example, the device size is inadequate or a complication occurs), both the insertion and removal of the device should be coded.

B6.1b Materials such as sutures, ligatures, radiological markers and temporary post-operative wound drains are considered integral to the performance of a procedure and are not coded as devices.

B6.1c Procedures performed on a device only and not on a body part are specified in the root operations Change, Irrigation, Removal and Revision, and are coded to the procedure performed.

Example: Irrigation of percutaneous nephrostomy tube is coded to the root operation Irrigation of indwelling device in the Administration section.

Drainage device

B6.2 A separate procedure to put in a drainage device is coded to the root operation Drainage with the device value Drainage Device.

Coding Guidelines Reference

Coding Guidelines References

The tables below link ICD-10-PCS coding guidelines to Medical and Surgical section root operations, specific body system tables, and body systems. The guidelines identified in each table are provided in order to remind users to reference the coding guidelines prior to code reporting. The tables provide coding guideline references at the body system and root operation level. It is imperative to review the ICD-10-PCS coding guidelines to ensure the procedure code being reported is accurate and complete.

Root Operation References

Root Operation	Character Value	Coding Guideline(s)
Bypass	1	B3.6a
Change	2	B6.1c
Control	3	B3.7
Division	8	B3.14
Drainage	9	B3.4a, B3.4b, B6.2

Continued →

Root Operation	Character Value	Coding Guideline(s)
Excision	B	B3.4a, B3.4b, B3.8, B3.9, B3.18
Extraction	D	B3.4a, B3.4b
Inspection	J	B3.11a, B3.11b, B3.11c
Occlusion	L	B3.12
Release	N	B3.13, B3.14
Removal	P	B6.1c
Replacement	R	B3.18
Resection	T	B3.8, B3.18
Restriction	V	B3.12
Revision	W	B6.1c
Transplantation	Y	B3.16

Table References

Table	Body System	Root Operation	Coding Guideline(s)
021	Heart and Great Vessels	Bypass	B3.6b, B3.6c, B4.4
027	Heart and Great Vessels	Dilation	B4.4
02C	Heart and Great Vessels	Extirpation	B4.4
02Q	Heart and Great Vessels	Repair	B4.4
0HB	Skin and Breast	Excision	B3.5
0HJ	Skin and Breast	Inspection	B3.5
0HQ	Skin and Breast	Repair	B3.5
0HX	Skin and Breast	Transfer	B3.17
0JB	Subcutaneous Tissue and Fascia	Excision	B3.5
0JJ	Subcutaneous Tissue and Fascia	Inspection	B3.5
0JQ	Subcutaneous Tissue and Fascia	Repair	B3.5
0JX	Subcutaneous Tissue and Fascia	Transfer	B3.17
0KB	Muscles	Excision	B3.5
0KJ	Muscles	Inspection	B3.5
0KQ	Muscles	Repair	B3.5
0KX	Muscles	Transfer	B3.17
0LB	Tendons	Excision	B3.5
0LJ	Tendons	Inspection	B3.5
0LQ	Tendons	Repair	B3.5
0MB	Bursae and Ligaments	Excision	B3.5
0MJ	Bursae and Ligaments	Inspection	B3.5
0MQ	Bursae and Ligaments	Repair	B3.5
0NB	Head and Facial Bones	Excision	B3.5
0NJ	Head and Facial Bones	Inspection	B3.5
0NQ	Head and Facial Bones	Repair	B3.5
0NS	Head and Facial Bones	Reposition	B3.15
0PB	Upper Bones	Excision	B3.5
0PJ	Upper Bones	Inspection	B3.5
0PQ	Upper Bones	Repair	B3.5
0PS	Upper Bones	Reposition	B3.15
0QB	Lower Bones	Excision	B3.5
0QJ	Lower Bones	Inspection	B3.5
0QQ	Lower Bones	Repair	B3.5
0QS	Lower Bones	Reposition	B3.15
0RB	Upper Joints	Excision	B3.5

Continued →

Table	Body System	Root Operation	Coding Guideline(s)
0RG	Upper Joints	Fusion	B3.10a, B3.10b, B3.10c
0RJ	Upper Joints	Inspection	B3.5
0RQ	Upper Joints	Repair	B3.5
0SB	Lower Joints	Excision	B3.5
0SG	Lower Joints	Fusion	B3.10a, B3.10b, B3.10c
0SJ	Lower Joints	Inspection	B3.5
0SQ	Lower Joints	Repair	B3.5
0UD	Female Reproductive System	Extraction	C2

Body System References

Body System	Character Value	Coding Guideline(s)
Gastrointestinal System	D	B4.8
Subcutaneous Tissue and Fascia	J	B4.5, B4.6
Tendons	L	B4.5
Bursae and Ligaments	M	B4.5
Upper Joints	R	B4.5
Lower Joints	S	B4.5

Medial Views of Cerebrum

Sagittal section of brain in situ

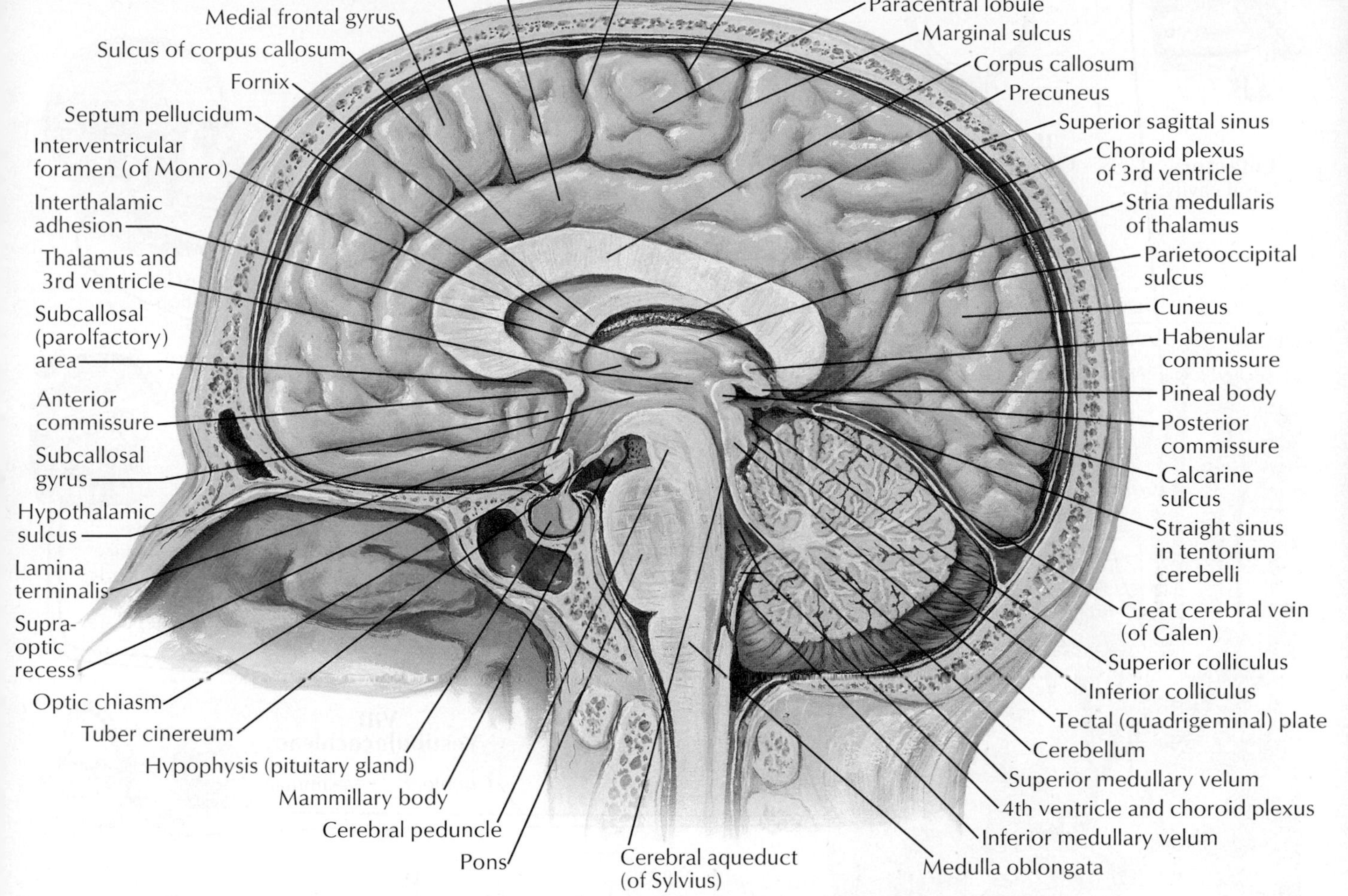
Cingulate gyrus
Cingulate sulcus
Medial frontal gyrus
Sulcus of corpus callosum
Fornix
Septum pellucidum
Interventricular foramen (of Monro)
Interthalamic adhesion
Thalamus and 3rd ventricle
Subcallosal (parolfactory) area
Anterior commissure
Subcallosal gyrus
Hypothalamic sulcus
Lamina terminalis
Supra-optic recess
Optic chiasm
Tuber cinereum
Hypophysis (pituitary gland)
Mammillary body
Cerebral peduncle
Pons
Cerebral aqueduct (of Sylvius)
Paracentral sulcus
Central sulcus (of Rolando)
Paracentral lobule
Marginal sulcus
Corpus callosum
Precuneus
Superior sagittal sinus
Choroid plexus of 3rd ventricle
Stria medullaris of thalamus
Parietooccipital sulcus
Cuneus
Habenular commissure
Pineal body
Posterior commissure
Calcarine sulcus
Straight sinus in tentorium cerebelli
Great cerebral vein (of Galen)
Superior colliculus
Inferior colliculus
Tectal (quadrigeminal) plate
Cerebellum
Superior medullary velum
4th ventricle and choroid plexus
Inferior medullary velum
Medulla oblongata

Medial surface of cerebral hemisphere: brainstem excised

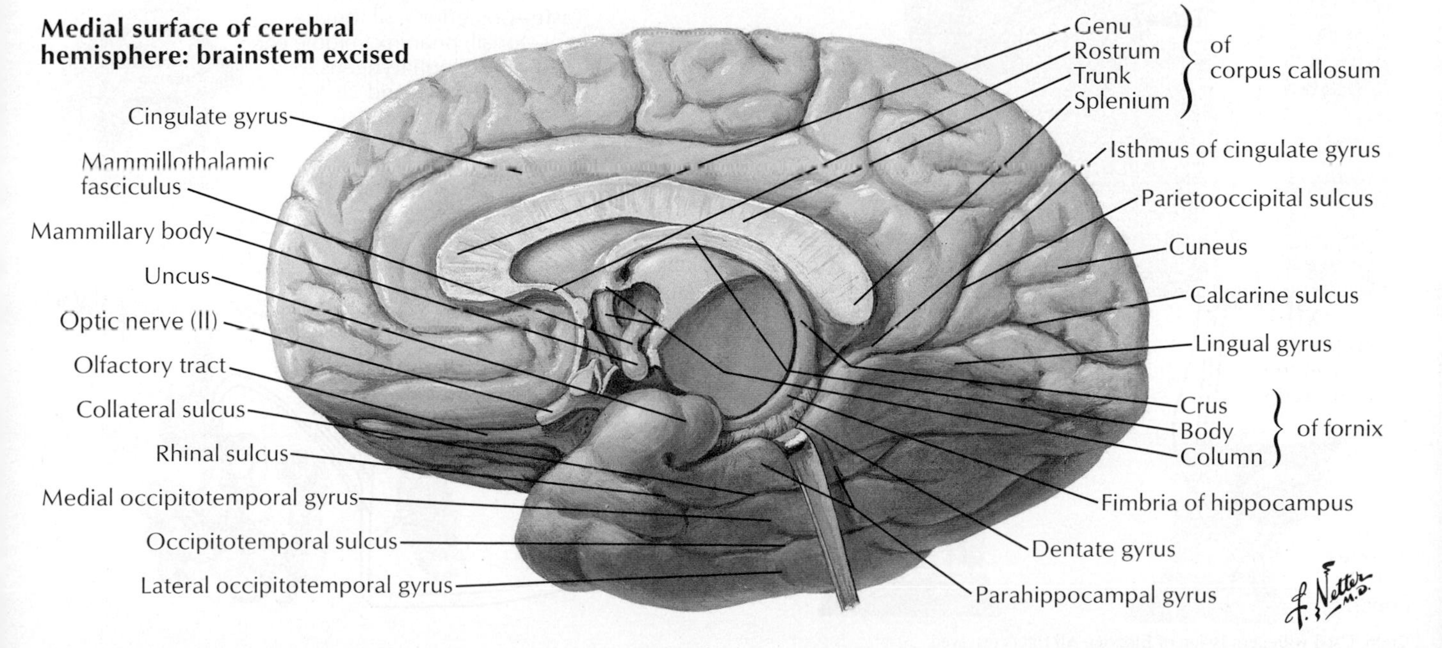
Cingulate gyrus
Mammillothalamic fasciculus
Mammillary body
Uncus
Optic nerve (II)
Olfactory tract
Collateral sulcus
Rhinal sulcus
Medial occipitotemporal gyrus
Occipitotemporal sulcus
Lateral occipitotemporal gyrus
Genu
Rostrum
Trunk
Splenium
of corpus callosum
Isthmus of cingulate gyrus
Parietooccipital sulcus
Cuneus
Calcarine sulcus
Lingual gyrus
Crus
Body
Column
of fornix
Fimbria of hippocampus
Dentate gyrus
Parahippocampal gyrus
F. Netter M.D.

Cranial Nerves: Schema

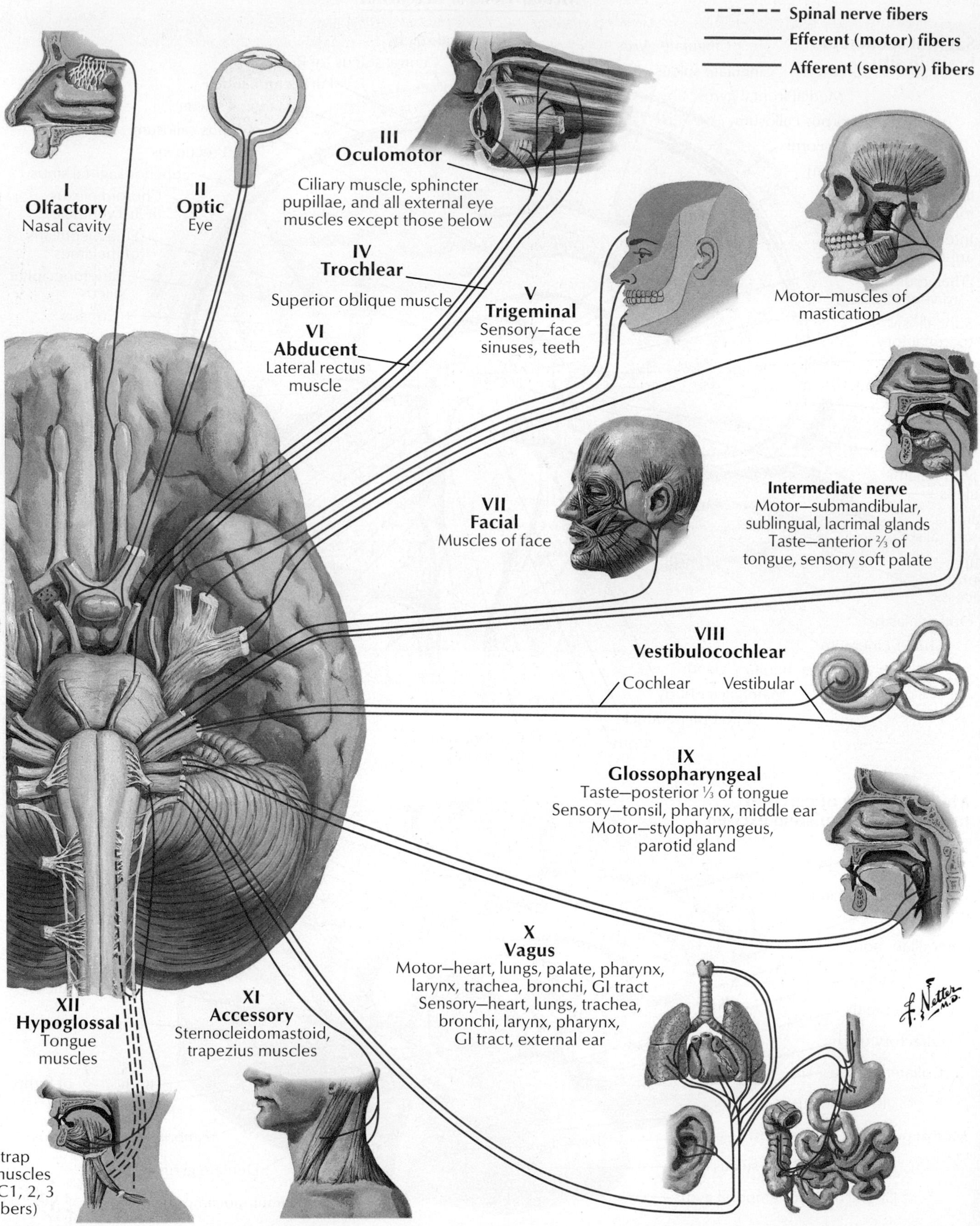

Spinal nerve fibers
Efferent (motor) fibers
Afferent (sensory) fibers
I
Olfactory
Nasal cavity
II
Optic
Eye
III
Oculomotor
Ciliary muscle, sphincter pupillae, and all external eye muscles except those below
IV
Trochlear
Superior oblique muscle
V
Trigeminal
Sensory—face sinuses, teeth
Motor—muscles of mastication
VI
Abducent
Lateral rectus muscle
VII
Facial
Muscles of face
Intermediate nerve
Motor—submandibular, sublingual, lacrimal glands
Taste—anterior ⅔ of tongue, sensory soft palate
VIII
Vestibulocochlear
Cochlear
Vestibular
IX
Glossopharyngeal
Taste—posterior ⅓ of tongue
Sensory—tonsil, pharynx, middle ear
Motor—stylopharyngeus, parotid gland
X
Vagus
Motor—heart, lungs, palate, pharynx, larynx, trachea, bronchi, GI tract
Sensory—heart, lungs, trachea, bronchi, larynx, pharynx, GI tract, external ear
XI
Accessory
Sternocleidomastoid, trapezius muscles
XII
Hypoglossal
Tongue muscles
Strap muscles (C1, 2, 3 fibers)
F. Netter M.D.

Section 0 **Medical and Surgical**
Body System 0 **Central Nervous System and Cranial Nerves**
Operation 1 **Bypass:** Altering the route of passage of the contents of a tubular body part

Body Part (4th)	Approach (5th)	Device (6th)	Qualifier (7th)
6 Cerebral Ventricle	**0** Open **3** Percutaneous **4** Percutaneous Endoscopic	**7** Autologous Tissue Substitute **J** Synthetic Substitute **K** Nonautologous Tissue Substitute	**0** Nasopharynx **1** Mastoid Sinus **2** Atrium **3** Blood Vessel **4** Pleural Cavity **5** Intestine **6** Peritoneal Cavity **7** Urinary Tract **8** Bone Marrow **A** Subgaleal Space **B** Cerebral Cisterns
6 Cerebral Ventricle	**0** Open **3** Percutaneous **4** Percutaneous Endoscopic	**Z** No Device	**B** Cerebral Cisterns
U Spinal Canal	**0** Open **3** Percutaneous **4** Percutaneous Endoscopic	**7** Autologous Tissue Substitute **J** Synthetic Substitute **K** Nonautologous Tissue Substitute	**2** Atrium **4** Pleural Cavity **6** Peritoneal Cavity **7** Urinary Tract **9** Fallopian Tube

Section 0 **Medical and Surgical**
Body System 0 **Central Nervous System and Cranial Nerves**
Operation 2 **Change:** Taking out or off a device from a body part and putting back an identical or similar device in or on the same body part without cutting or puncturing the skin or a mucous membrane

Body Part (4th)	Approach (5th)	Device (6th)	Qualifier (7th)
0 Brain **E** Cranial Nerve **U** Spinal Canal	**X** External	**0** Drainage Device **Y** Other Device	**Z** No Qualifier

Section 0 **Medical and Surgical**
Body System 0 **Central Nervous System and Cranial Nerves**
Operation 5 **Destruction:** Physical eradication of all or a portion of a body part by the direct use of energy, force, or a destructive agent

Body Part (4th)	Approach (5th)	Device (6th)	Qualifier (7th)
0 Brain **1** Cerebral Meninges **2** Dura Mater **6** Cerebral Ventricle **7** Cerebral Hemisphere **8** Basal Ganglia **9** Thalamus **A** Hypothalamus **B** Pons **C** Cerebellum **D** Medulla Oblongata **F** Olfactory Nerve **G** Optic Nerve **H** Oculomotor Nerve **J** Trochlear Nerve **K** Trigeminal Nerve **L** Abducens Nerve **M** Facial Nerve **N** Acoustic Nerve **P** Glossopharyngeal Nerve **Q** Vagus Nerve **R** Accessory Nerve **S** Hypoglossal Nerve **T** Spinal Meninges **W** Cervical Spinal Cord **X** Thoracic Spinal Cord **Y** Lumbar Spinal Cord	**0** Open **3** Percutaneous **4** Percutaneous Endoscopic	**Z** No Device	**Z** No Qualifier

Section 0 **Medical and Surgical**
Body System 0 **Central Nervous System and Cranial Nerves**
Operation 7 **Dilation:** Expanding an orifice or the lumen of a tubular body part

Body Part (4th)	Approach (5th)	Device (6th)	Qualifier (7th)
6 Cerebral Ventricle	**0** Open **3** Percutaneous **4** Percutaneous Endoscopic	**Z** No Device	**Z** No Qualifie

Section 0 **Medical and Surgical**
Body System 0 **Central Nervous System and Cranial Nerves**
Operation 8 **Division:** Cutting into a body part, without draining fluids and/or gases from the body part, in order to separate or transect a body part

Body Part (4th)	Approach (5th)	Device (6th)	Qualifier (7th)
0 Brain **7** Cerebral Hemisphere **8** Basal Ganglia **F** Olfactory Nerve **G** Optic Nerve **H** Oculomotor Nerve **J** Trochlear Nerve **K** Trigeminal Nerve **L** Abducens Nerve **M** Facial Nerve **N** Acoustic Nerve **P** Glossopharyngeal Nerve **Q** Vagus Nerve **R** Accessory Nerve **S** Hypoglossal Nerve **W** Cervical Spinal Cord **X** Thoracic Spinal Cord **Y** Lumbar Spinal Cord	**0** Open **3** Percutaneous **4** Percutaneous Endoscopic	**Z** No Device	**Z** No Qualifier

Section 0 **Medical and Surgical**
Body System 0 **Central Nervous System and Cranial Nerves**
Operation 9 **Drainage:** Taking or letting out fluids and/or gases from a body part

Body Part (4th)	Approach (5th)	Device (6th)	Qualifier (7th)
0 Brain **1** Cerebral Meninges **2** Dura Mater **3** Epidural Space, Intracranial **4** Subdural Space, Intracranial **5** Subarachnoid Space, Intracranial **6** Cerebral Ventricle **7** Cerebral Hemisphere **8** Basal Ganglia **9** Thalamus **A** Hypothalamus **B** Pons **C** Cerebellum **D** Medulla Oblongata **F** Olfactory Nerve **G** Optic Nerve **H** Oculomotor Nerve **J** Trochlear Nerve **K** Trigeminal Nerve **L** Abducens Nerve **M** Facial Nerve **N** Acoustic Nerve **P** Glossopharyngeal Nerve **Q** Vagus Nerve **R** Accessory Nerve **S** Hypoglossal Nerve **T** Spinal Meninges **U** Spinal Canal **W** Cervical Spinal Cord **X** Thoracic Spinal Cord **Y** Lumbar Spinal Cord	**0** Open **3** Percutaneous **4** Percutaneous Endoscopic	**0** Drainage Device	**Z** No Qualifier
0 Brain **1** Cerebral Meninges **2** Dura Mater **3** Epidural Space, Intracranial **4** Subdural Space, Intracranial **5** Subarachnoid Space, Intracranial **6** Cerebral Ventricle **7** Cerebral Hemisphere **8** Basal Ganglia **9** Thalamus **A** Hypothalamus **B** Pons **C** Cerebellum **D** Medulla Oblongata **F** Olfactory Nerve **G** Optic Nerve **H** Oculomotor Nerve **J** Trochlear Nerve **K** Trigeminal Nerve **L** Abducens Nerve **M** Facial Nerve **N** Acoustic Nerve **P** Glossopharyngeal Nerve **Q** Vagus Nerve **R** Accessory Nerve **S** Hypoglossal Nerve **T** Spinal Meninges **U** Spinal Canal **W** Cervical Spinal Cord **X** Thoracic Spinal Cord **Y** Lumbar Spinal Cord	**0** Open **3** Percutaneous **4** Percutaneous Endoscopic	**Z** No Device	**X** Diagnostic **Z** No Qualifier

Section 0 **Medical and Surgical**
Body System 0 **Central Nervous System and Cranial Nerves**
Operation B **Excision:** Cutting out or off, without replacement, a portion of a body part

Body Part (4th)	Approach (5th)	Device (6th)	Qualifier (7th)
0 Brain **1** Cerebral Meninges **2** Dura Mater **6** Cerebral Ventricle **7** Cerebral Hemisphere **8** Basal Ganglia **9** Thalamus **A** Hypothalamus **B** Pons **C** Cerebellum **D** Medulla Oblongata **F** Olfactory Nerve **G** Optic Nerve **H** Oculomotor Nerve **J** Trochlear Nerve **K** Trigeminal Nerve **L** Abducens Nerve **M** Facial Nerve **N** Acoustic Nerve **P** Glossopharyngeal Nerve **Q** Vagus Nerve **R** Accessory Nerve **S** Hypoglossal Nerve **T** Spinal Meninges **W** Cervical Spinal Cord **X** Thoracic Spinal Cord **Y** Lumbar Spinal Cord	**0** Open **3** Percutaneous **4** Percutaneous Endoscopic	**Z** No Device	**X** Diagnostic **Z** No Qualifier

Section	**0**	**Medical and Surgical**
Body System	**0**	**Central Nervous System and Cranial Nerves**
Operation	**C**	**Extirpation:** Taking or cutting out solid matter from a body part

Body Part (4th)	Approach (5th)	Device (6th)	Qualifier (7th)
0 Brain **1** Cerebral Meninges **2** Dura Mater **3** Epidural Space, Intracranial **4** Subdural Space, Intracranial **5** Subarachnoid Space, Intracranial **6** Cerebral Ventricle **7** Cerebral Hemisphere **8** Basal Ganglia **9** Thalamus **A** Hypothalamus **B** Pons **C** Cerebellum **D** Medulla Oblongata **F** Olfactory Nerve **G** Optic Nerve **H** Oculomotor Nerve **J** Trochlear Nerve **K** Trigeminal Nerve **L** Abducens Nerve **M** Facial Nerve **N** Acoustic Nerve **P** Glossopharyngeal Nerve **Q** Vagus Nerve **R** Accessory Nerve **S** Hypoglossal Nerve **T** Spinal Meninges **U** Spinal Canal **W** Cervical Spinal Cord **X** Thoracic Spinal Cord **Y** Lumbar Spinal Cord	**0** Open **3** Percutaneous **4** Percutaneous Endoscopic	**Z** No Device	**Z** No Qualifier

Section	**0**	**Medical and Surgical**
Body System	**0**	**Central Nervous System and Cranial Nerves**
Operation	**D**	**Extraction:** Pulling or stripping out or off all or a portion of a body part by the use of force

Body Part (4th)	Approach (5th)	Device (6th)	Qualifier (7th)
0 Brain **1** Cerebral Meninges **2** Dura Mater **7** Cerebral Hemisphere **F** Olfactory Nerve **G** Optic Nerve **H** Oculomotor Nerve **J** Trochlear Nerve **K** Trigeminal Nerve **L** Abducens Nerve **M** Facial Nerve **N** Acoustic Nerve **P** Glossopharyngeal Nerve **Q** Vagus Nerve **R** Accessory Nerve **S** Hypoglossal Nerve **T** Spinal Meninges	**0** Open **3** Percutaneous **4** Percutaneous Endoscopic	**Z** No Device	**Z** No Qualifier

Section 0 **Medical and Surgical**
Body System 0 **Central Nervous System and Cranial Nerves**
Operation F **Fragmentation:** Breaking solid matter in a body part into pieces

Body Part (4th)	Approach (5th)	Device (6th)	Qualifier (7th)
3 Epidural Space, Intracranial **4** Subdural Space, Intracranial **5** Subarachnoid Space, Intracranial **6** Cerebral Ventricle **U** Spinal Canal	**0** Open **3** Percutaneous **4** Percutaneous Endoscopic **X** External	**Z** No Device	**Z** No Qualifier

Section 0 **Medical and Surgical**
Body System 0 **Central Nervous System and Cranial Nerves**
Operation H **Insertion:** Putting in a nonbiological appliance that monitors, assists, performs, or prevents a physiological function but does not physically take the place of a body part

Body Part (4th)	Approach (5th)	Device (6th)	Qualifier (7th)
0 Brain	**0** Open	**1** Radioactive Element **2** Monitoring Device **3** Infusion Device **4** Radioactive Element, Cesium-131 Collagen Implant **M** Neurostimulator Lead **Y** Other Device	**Z** No Qualifier
0 Brain	**3** Percutaneous **4** Percutaneous Endoscopic	**1** Radioactive Element **2** Monitoring Device **3** Infusion Device **M** Neurostimulator Lead **Y** Other Device	**Z** No Qualifier
6 Cerebral Ventricle **E** Cranial Nerve **U** Spinal Canal **V** Spinal Cord	**0** Open **3** Percutaneous **4** Percutaneous Endoscopic	**1** Radioactive Element **2** Monitoring Device **3** Infusion Device **M** Neurostimulator Lead **Y** Other Device	**Z** No Qualifier

Section 0 **Medical and Surgical**
Body System 0 **Central Nervous System and Cranial Nerves**
Operation J **Inspection:** Visually and/or manually exploring a body part

Body Part (4th)	Approach (5th)	Device (6th)	Qualifier (7th)
0 Brain **E** Cranial Nerve **U** Spinal Canal **V** Spinal Cord	**0** Open **3** Percutaneous **4** Percutaneous Endoscopic	**Z** No Device	**Z** No Qualifier

Section 0 **Medical and Surgical**
Body System 0 **Central Nervous System and Cranial Nerves**
Operation K **Map:** Locating the route of passage of electrical impulses and/or locating functional areas in a body part

Body Part (4th)	Approach (5th)	Device (6th)	Qualifier (7th)
0 Brain **7** Cerebral Hemisphere **8** Basal Ganglia **9** Thalamus **A** Hypothalamus **B** Pons **C** Cerebellum **D** Medulla Oblongata	**0** Open **3** Percutaneous **4** Percutaneous Endoscopic	**Z** No Device	**Z** No Qualifier

Section 0 **Medical and Surgical**
Body System 0 **Central Nervous System and Cranial Nerves**
Operation N **Release:** Freeing a body part from an abnormal physical constraint by cutting or by the use of force

Body Part (4th)	Approach (5th)	Device (6th)	Qualifier (7th)
0 Brain **1** Cerebral Meninges **2** Dura Mater **6** Cerebral Ventricle **7** Cerebral Hemisphere **8** Basal Ganglia **9** Thalamus **A** Hypothalamus **B** Pons **C** Cerebellum **D** Medulla Oblongata **F** Olfactory Nerve **G** Optic Nerve **H** Oculomotor Nerve **J** Trochlear Nerve **K** Trigeminal Nerve **L** Abducens Nerve **M** Facial Nerve **N** Acoustic Nerve **P** Glossopharyngeal Nerve **Q** Vagus Nerve **R** Accessory Nerve **S** Hypoglossal Nerve **T** Spinal Meninges **W** Cervical Spinal Cord **X** Thoracic Spinal Cord **Y** Lumbar Spinal Cord	**0** Open **3** Percutaneous **4** Percutaneous Endoscopic	**Z** No Device	**Z** No Qualifier

Section 0 **Medical and Surgical**
Body System 0 **Central Nervous System and Cranial Nerves**
Operation P **Removal:** Taking out or off a device from a body part

Body Part (4th)	Approach (5th)	Device (6th)	Qualifier (7th)
0 Brain **V** Spinal Cord	**0** Open **3** Percutaneous **4** Percutaneous Endoscopic	**0** Drainage Device **2** Monitoring Device **3** Infusion Device **7** Autologous Tissue Substitute **J** Synthetic Substitute **K** Nonautologous Tissue Substitute **M** Neurostimulator Lead **Y** Other Device	**Z** No Qualifier
0 Brain **V** Spinal Cord	**X** External	**0** Drainage Device **2** Monitoring Device **3** Infusion Device **M** Neurostimulator Lead	**Z** No Qualifier
6 Cerebral Ventricle **U** Spinal Canal	**0** Open **3** Percutaneous **4** Percutaneous Endoscopic	**0** Drainage Device **2** Monitoring Device **3** Infusion Device **J** Synthetic Substitute **M** Neurostimulator Lead **Y** Other Device	**Z** No Qualifier
6 Cerebral Ventricle **U** Spinal Canal	**X** External	**0** Drainage Device **2** Monitoring Device **3** Infusion Device **M** Neurostimulator Lead	**Z** No Qualifier

Continued →

Section 0 **Medical and Surgical**
Body System 0 **Central Nervous System and Cranial Nerves**
Operation P **Removal:** Taking out or off a device from a body part

Body Part (4th)	Approach (5th)	Device (6th)	Qualifier (7th)
E Cranial Nerve	0 Open 3 Percutaneous 4 Percutaneous Endoscopic	0 Drainage Device 2 Monitoring Device 3 Infusion Device 7 Autologous Tissue Substitute M Neurostimulator Lead Y Other Device	Z No Qualifier
E Cranial Nerve	X External	0 Drainage Device 2 Monitoring Device 3 Infusion Device M Neurostimulator Lead	Z No Qualifier

Section 0 **Medical and Surgical**
Body System 0 **Central Nervous System and Cranial Nerves**
Operation Q **Repair:** Restoring, to the extent possible, a body part to its normal anatomic structure and function

Body Part (4th)	Approach (5th)	Device (6th)	Qualifier (7th)
0 Brain 1 Cerebral Meninges 2 Dura Mater 6 Cerebral Ventricle 7 Cerebral Hemisphere 8 Basal Ganglia 9 Thalamus A Hypothalamus B Pons C Cerebellum D Medulla Oblongata F Olfactory Nerve G Optic Nerve H Oculomotor Nerve J Trochlear Nerve K Trigeminal Nerve L Abducens Nerve M Facial Nerve N Acoustic Nerve P Glossopharyngeal Nerve Q Vagus Nerve R Accessory Nerve S Hypoglossal Nerve T Spinal Meninges W Cervical Spinal Cord X Thoracic Spinal Cord Y Lumbar Spinal Cord	0 Open 3 Percutaneous 4 Percutaneous Endoscopic	Z No Device	Z No Qualifier

Section 0 **Medical and Surgical**
Body System 0 **Central Nervous System and Cranial Nerves**
Operation R **Replacement:** Putting in or on biological or synthetic material that physically takes the place and/or function of all or a portion of a body part

Body Part (4th)	Approach (5th)	Device (6th)	Qualifier (7th)
1 Cerebral Meninges **2** Dura Mater **6** Cerebral Ventricle **F** Olfactory Nerve **G** Optic Nerve **H** Oculomotor Nerve **J** Trochlear Nerve **K** Trigeminal Nerve **L** Abducens Nerve **M** Facial Nerve **N** Acoustic Nerve **P** Glossopharyngeal Nerve **Q** Vagus Nerve **R** Accessory Nerve **S** Hypoglossal Nerve **T** Spinal Meninges	**0** Open **4** Percutaneous Endoscopic	**7** Autologous Tissue Substitute **J** Synthetic Substitute **K** Nonautologous Tissue Substitute	**Z** No Qualifier

Section 0 **Medical and Surgical**
Body System 0 **Central Nervous System and Cranial Nerves**
Operation S **Reposition:** Moving to its normal location, or other suitable location, all or a portion of a body part

Body Part (4th)	Approach (5th)	Device (6th)	Qualifier (7th)
F Olfactory Nerve **G** Optic Nerve **H** Oculomotor Nerve **J** Trochlear Nerve **K** Trigeminal Nerve **L** Abducens Nerve **M** Facial Nerve **N** Acoustic Nerve **P** Glossopharyngeal Nerve **Q** Vagus Nerve **R** Accessory Nerve **S** Hypoglossal Nerve **W** Cervical Spinal Cord **X** Thoracic Spinal Cord **Y** Lumbar Spinal Cord	**0** Open **3** Percutaneous **4** Percutaneous Endoscopic	**Z** No Device	**Z** No Qualifier

Section 0 **Medical and Surgical**
Body System 0 **Central Nervous System and Cranial Nerves**
Operation T **Resection:** Cutting out or off, without replacement, all of a body part

Body Part (4th)	Approach (5th)	Device (6th)	Qualifier (7th)
7 Cerebral Hemisphere	**0** Open **3** Percutaneous **4** Percutaneous Endoscopic	**Z** No Device	**Z** No Qualifier

Section 0 **Medical and Surgical**
Body System 0 **Central Nervous System and Cranial Nerves**
Operation U **Supplement:** Putting in or on biological or synthetic material that physically reinforces and/or augments the function of a portion of a body part

Body Part (4th)	Approach (5th)	Device (6th)	Qualifier (7th)
1 Cerebral Meninges **2** Dura Mater **6** Cerebral Ventricle **F** Olfactory Nerve **G** Optic Nerve **H** Oculomotor Nerve **J** Trochlear Nerve **K** Trigeminal Nerve **L** Abducens Nerve **M** Facial Nerve **N** Acoustic Nerve **P** Glossopharyngeal Nerve **Q** Vagus Nerve **R** Accessory Nerve **S** Hypoglossal Nerve **T** Spinal Meninges	**0** Open **3** Percutaneous **4** Percutaneous Endoscopic	**7** Autologous Tissue Substitute **J** Synthetic Substitute **K** Nonautologous Tissue Substitute	**Z** No Qualifier

Section 0 **Medical and Surgical**
Body System 0 **Central Nervous System and Cranial Nerves**
Operation W **Revision:** Correcting, to the extent possible, a portion of a malfunctioning device or the position of a displaced device

Body Part (4th)	Approach (5th)	Device (6th)	Qualifier (7th)
0 Brain **V** Spinal Cord	**0** Open **3** Percutaneous **4** Percutaneous Endoscopic	**0** Drainage Device **2** Monitoring Device **3** Infusion Device **7** Autologous Tissue Substitute **J** Synthetic Substitute **K** Nonautologous Tissue Substitute **M** Neurostimulator Lead **Y** Other Device	**Z** No Qualifier
0 Brain **V** Spinal Cord	**X** External	**0** Drainage Device **2** Monitoring Device **3** Infusion Device **7** Autologous Tissue Substitute **J** Synthetic Substitute **K** Nonautologous Tissue Substitute **M** Neurostimulator Lead	**Z** No Qualifier
6 Cerebral Ventricle **U** Spinal Canal	**0** Open **3** Percutaneous **4** Percutaneous Endoscopic	**0** Drainage Device **2** Monitoring Device **3** Infusion Device **J** Synthetic Substitute **M** Neurostimulator Lead **Y** Other Device	**Z** No Qualifier
6 Cerebral Ventricle **U** Spinal Canal	**X** External	**0** Drainage Device **2** Monitoring Device **3** Infusion Device **J** Synthetic Substitute **M** Neurostimulator Lead	**Z** No Qualifier

Continued →

Section 0 **Medical and Surgical**
Body System 0 **Central Nervous System and Cranial Nerves**
Operation W **Revision:** Correcting, to the extent possible, a portion of a malfunctioning device or the position of a displaced device

Body Part (4th)	Approach (5th)	Device (6th)	Qualifier (7th)
E Cranial Nerve	**0** Open **3** Percutaneous **4** Percutaneous Endoscopic	**0** Drainage Device **2** Monitoring Device **3** Infusion Device **7** Autologous Tissue Substitute **M** Neurostimulator Lead **Y** Other Device	**Z** No Qualifier
E Cranial Nerve	**X** External	**0** Drainage Device **2** Monitoring Device **3** Infusion Device **7** Autologous Tissue Substitute **M** Neurostimulator Lead	**Z** No Qualifier

Section 0 **Medical and Surgical**
Body System 0 **Central Nervous System and Cranial Nerves**
Operation X **Transfer:** Moving, without taking out, all or a portion of a body part to another location to take over the function of all or a portion of a body part

Body Part (4th)	Approach (5th)	Device (6th)	Qualifier (7th)
F Olfactory Nerve **G** Optic Nerve **H** Oculomotor Nerve **J** Trochlear Nerve **K** Trigeminal Nerve **L** Abducens Nerve **M** Facial Nerve **N** Acoustic Nerve **P** Glossopharyngeal Nerve **Q** Vagus Nerve **R** Accessory Nerve **S** Hypoglossal Nerve	**0** Open **4** Percutaneous Endoscopic	**Z** No Device	**F** Olfactory Nerve **G** Optic Nerve **H** Oculomotor Nerve **J** Trochlear Nerve **K** Trigeminal Nerve **L** Abducens Nerve **M** Facial Nerve **N** Acoustic Nerve **P** Glossopharyngeal Nerve **Q** Vagus Nerve **R** Accessory Nerve **S** Hypoglossal Nerve

AHA Coding Clinic

00163J6 Bypass Cerebral Ventricle to Peritoneal Cavity with Synthetic Substitute, Percutaneous Approach—AHA CC: 2Q, 2013, 36-37; 2Q, 2021, 19-20

00163JA Bypass Cerebral Ventricle to Subgaleal Space with Synthetic Substitute, Percutaneous Approach—AHA CC: 4Q, 2019, 22

001U0J2 Bypass Spinal Canal to Atrium with Synthetic Substitute, Open Approach—AHA CC: 4Q, 2018, 86

005W0ZZ Destruction of Cervical Spinal Cord, Open Approach—AHA CC: 2Q, 2021, 17-18

005X0ZZ Destruction of Thoracic Spinal Cord, Open Approach—AHA CC: 2Q, 2021, 17-18

00764AA Dilation of Cerebral Ventricle, Percutaneous Endoscopic Approach—AHA CC: 4Q, 2017, 40-41

009430Z Drainage of Intracranial Subdural Space with Drainage Device, Percutaneous Approach—AHA CC: 3Q, 2015, 11-12

009630Z Drainage of Cerebral Ventricle with Drainage Device, Percutaneous Approach—AHA CC: 3Q, 2015, 12-13

009U00Z Drainage of Spinal Canal with Drainage Device, Open Approach—AHA CC: 4Q, 2018, 85

009U3ZX Drainage of Spinal Canal, Percutaneous Approach, Diagnostic—AHA CC: 1Q, 2014, 8

009W00Z Drainage of Cervical Spinal Cord with Drainage Device, Open Approach—AHA CC: 2Q, 2015, 30

00B00ZX Excision of Brain, Open Approach, Diagnostic—AHA CC: 1Q, 2015, 12-13

00B70ZZ Excision of Cerebral Hemisphere, Open Approach—AHA CC: 4Q, 2014, 34-35; 2Q, 2016, 18

00BM0ZZ Excision of Facial Nerve, Open Approach—AHA CC: 2Q, 2016, 12-14

00BR0ZZ Excision of Accessory Nerve, Open Approach—AHA CC: 2Q, 2016, 12-14

00BS0ZZ Excision of Hypoglossal Nerve, Open Approach—AHA CC: 2Q, 2016, 12-14

00BY0ZZ Excision of Lumbar Spinal Cord, Open Approach—AHA CC: 3Q, 2014, 24

00C00ZZ Extirpation of Matter from Brain, Open Approach—AHA CC: 1Q, 2015, 12-13; 4Q, 2016, 27-28

00C04ZZ Extirpation of Matter from Brain, Percutaneous Endoscopic Approach—AHA CC: 2Q, 2019, 36-37

00C40ZZ Extirpation of Matter from Intracranial Subdural Space, Open Approach—AHA CC: 3Q, 2015, 10-11; 2Q, 2016, 29; 3Q, 2019, 4-5

00C74ZZ Extirpation of Matter from Cerebral Hemisphere, Percutaneous Endoscopic Approach—AHA CC: 3Q, 2015, 13

00CU0ZZ Extirpation of Matter from Spinal Canal, Open Approach—AHA CC: 4Q, 2017, 48

00D20ZZ Extraction of Dura Mater, Open Approach—AHA CC: 3Q, 2015, 13-14

00H633Z Insertion of Infusion Device into Cerebral Ventricle, Percutaneous Approach—AHA CC: 2Q, 2020, 15-16

00HU03Z Insertion of Infusion Device into Spinal Canal, Open Approach—AHA CC: 2Q, 2020, 16-17

00HU33Z Insertion of Infusion Device into Spinal Canal, Percutaneous Approach—AHA CC: 3Q, 2014, 19-20

00J00ZZ Inspection of Brain, Open Approach—AHA CC: 2Q, 2019, 36-37

00J04ZZ Inspection of Brain, Percutaneous Endoscopic Approach—AHA CC: 2Q, 2021, 19-20

00JU3ZZ Inspection of Spinal Canal, Percutaneous Approach—AHA CC: 1Q, 2017, 50

00N00ZZ Release Brain, Open Approach—AHA CC: 2Q, 2016, 29

00N70ZZ Release Cerebral Hemisphere, Open Approach—AHA CC: 3Q, 2018, 30

00NC0ZZ Release Cerebellum, Open Approach—AHA CC: 3Q, 2017, 10-11

00NM4ZZ Release Facial Nerve, Percutaneous Endoscopic Approach—AHA CC: 4Q, 2018, 10

00NW0ZZ Release Cervical Spinal Cord, Open Approach—AHA CC: 2Q, 2015, 20-22; 2Q, 2017, 23-24

00NW3ZZ Release Cervical Spinal Cord, Percutaneous Approach—AHA CC: 2Q, 2019, 19-20

00NY0ZZ Release Lumbar Spinal Cord, Open Approach—AHA CC: 3Q, 2014, 24; 1Q, 2019, 28-29

00PU03Z Removal of Infusion Device from Spinal Canal, Open Approach—AHA CC: 3Q, 2014, 19-20

00Q20ZZ Repair Dura Mater, Open Approach—AHA CC: 3Q, 2013, 25; 3Q, 2014, 7-8

00SM0ZZ Reposition Facial Nerve, Open Approach—AHA CC: 4Q, 2014, 35

00U20KZ Supplement Dura Mater with Nonautologous Tissue Substitute, Open Approach—AHA CC: 3Q, 2017, 10-11; 1Q, 2018, 9

00UT0KZ Supplement Spinal Meninges with Nonautologous Tissue Substitute, Open Approach—AHA CC: 3Q, 2014, 24

Peripheral Nervous System

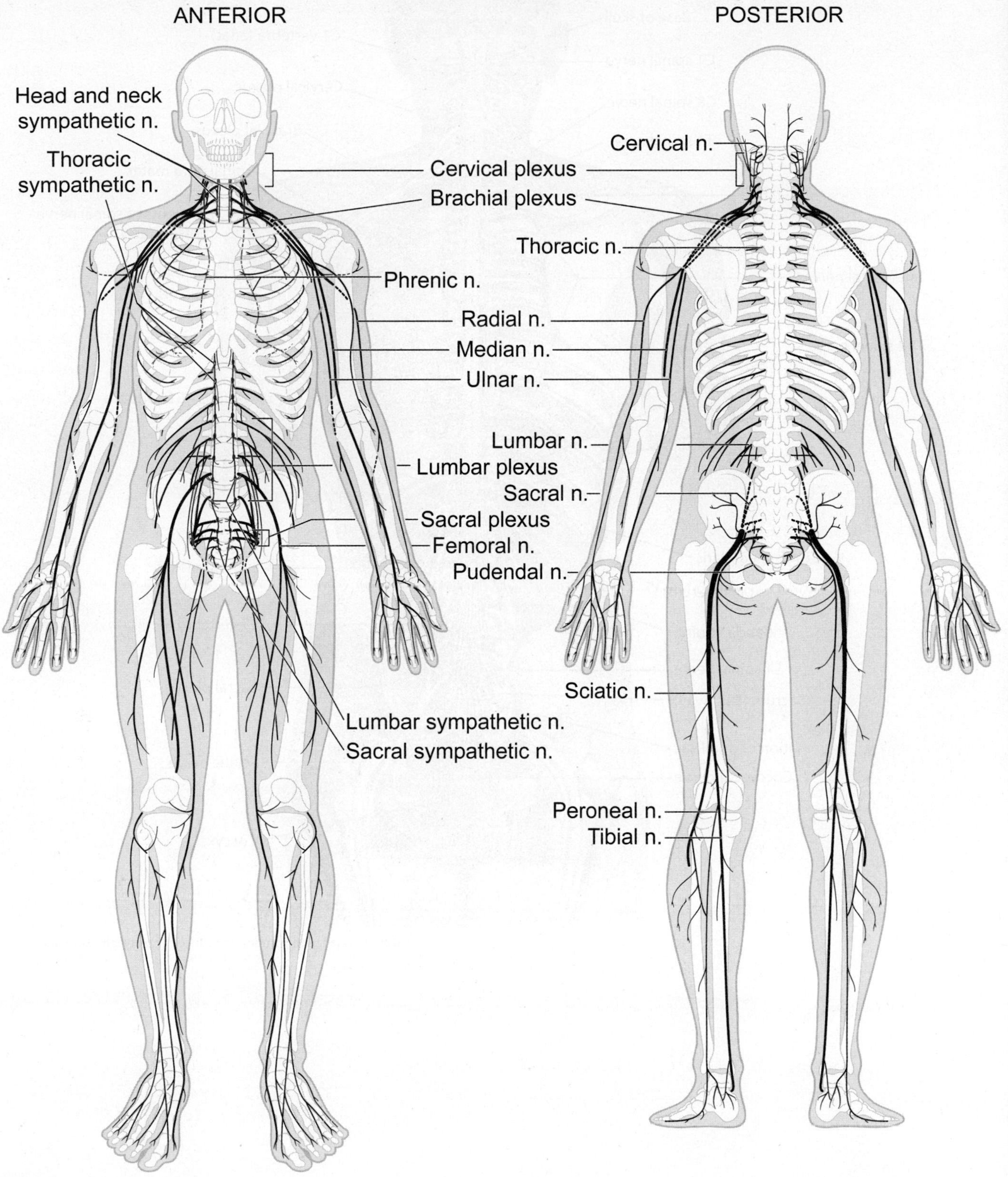
ANTERIOR
POSTERIOR
Head and neck sympathetic n.
Thoracic sympathetic n.
Cervical n.
Cervical plexus
Brachial plexus
Thoracic n.
Phrenic n.
Radial n.
Median n.
Ulnar n.
Lumbar n.
Lumbar plexus
Sacral n.
Sacral plexus
Femoral n.
Pudendal n.
Sciatic n.
Lumbar sympathetic n.
Sacral sympathetic n.
Peroneal n.
Tibial n.

Spinal Column

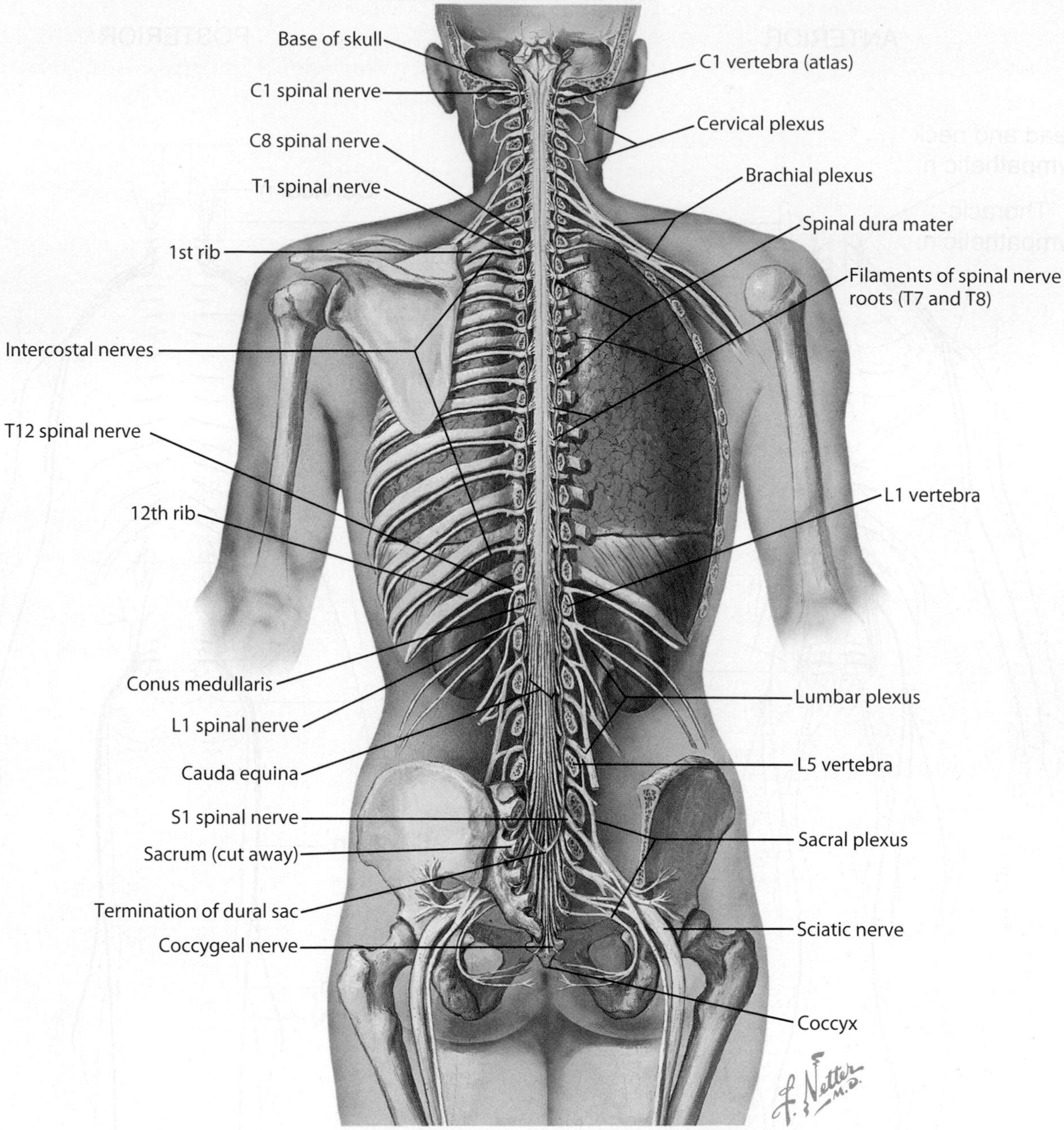

Base of skull
C1 vertebra (atlas)
C1 spinal nerve
Cervical plexus
C8 spinal nerve
Brachial plexus
T1 spinal nerve
Spinal dura mater
1st rib
Filaments of spinal nerve roots (T7 and T8)
Intercostal nerves
T12 spinal nerve
L1 vertebra
12th rib
Conus medullaris
Lumbar plexus
L1 spinal nerve
Cauda equina
L5 vertebra
S1 spinal nerve
Sacral plexus
Sacrum (cut away)
Termination of dural sac
Sciatic nerve
Coccygeal nerve
Coccyx
F. Netter M.D.

Section 0 **Medical and Surgical**
Body System 1 **Peripheral Nervous System**
Operation 2 **Change:** Taking out or off a device from a body part and putting back an identical or similar device in or on the same body part without cutting or puncturing the skin or a mucous membrane

Body Part (4th)	Approach (5th)	Device (6th)	Qualifier (7th)
Y Peripheral Nerve	**X** External	**0** Drainage Device **Y** Other Device	**Z** No Qualifier

Section 0 **Medical and Surgical**
Body System 1 **Peripheral Nervous System**
Operation 5 **Destruction:** Physical eradication of all or a portion of a body part by the direct use of energy, force, or a destructive agent

Body Part (4th)	Approach (5th)	Device (6th)	Qualifier (7th)
0 Cervical Plexus **1** Cervical Nerve **2** Phrenic Nerve **3** Brachial Plexus **4** Ulnar Nerve **5** Median Nerve **6** Radial Nerve **8** Thoracic Nerve **9** Lumbar Plexus **A** Lumbosacral Plexus **B** Lumbar Nerve **C** Pudendal Nerve **D** Femoral Nerve **F** Sciatic Nerve **G** Tibial Nerve **H** Peroneal Nerve **K** Head and Neck Sympathetic Nerve **L** Thoracic Sympathetic Nerve **M** Abdominal Sympathetic Nerve **N** Lumbar Sympathetic Nerve **P** Sacral Sympathetic Nerve **Q** Sacral Plexus **R** Sacral Nerve	**0** Open **3** Percutaneous **4** Percutaneous Endoscopic	**Z** No Device	**Z** No Qualifier

Section 0 **Medical and Surgical**
Body System 1 **Peripheral Nervous System**
Operation 8 **Division:** Cutting into a body part, without draining fluids and/or gases from the body part, in order to separate or transect a body part

Body Part (4th)	Approach (5th)	Device (6th)	Qualifier (7th)
0 Cervical Plexus **1** Cervical Nerve **2** Phrenic Nerve **3** Brachial Plexus **4** Ulnar Nerve **5** Median Nerve **6** Radial Nerve **8** Thoracic Nerve **9** Lumbar Plexus **A** Lumbosacral Plexus **B** Lumbar Nerve **C** Pudendal Nerve **D** Femoral Nerve **F** Sciatic Nerve **G** Tibial Nerve **H** Peroneal Nerve **K** Head and Neck Sympathetic Nerve **L** Thoracic Sympathetic Nerve **M** Abdominal Sympathetic Nerve **N** Lumbar Sympathetic Nerve **P** Sacral Sympathetic Nerve **Q** Sacral Plexus **R** Sacral Nerve	**0** Open **3** Percutaneous **4** Percutaneous Endoscopic	**Z** No Device	**Z** No Qualifier

Section 0 **Medical and Surgical**
Body System 1 **Peripheral Nervous System**
Operation 9 **Drainage:** Taking or letting out fluids and/or gases from a body part

Body Part (4th)	Approach (5th)	Device (6th)	Qualifier (7th)
0 Cervical Plexus **1** Cervical Nerve **2** Phrenic Nerve **3** Brachial Plexus **4** Ulnar Nerve **5** Median Nerve **6** Radial Nerve **8** Thoracic Nerve **9** Lumbar Plexus **A** Lumbosacral Plexus **B** Lumbar Nerve **C** Pudendal Nerve **D** Femoral Nerve **F** Sciatic Nerve **G** Tibial Nerve **H** Peroneal Nerve **K** Head and Neck Sympathetic Nerve **L** Thoracic Sympathetic Nerve **M** Abdominal Sympathetic Nerve **N** Lumbar Sympathetic Nerve **P** Sacral Sympathetic Nerve **Q** Sacral Plexus **R** Sacral Nerve	**0** Open **3** Percutaneous **4** Percutaneous Endoscopic	**0** Drainage Device	**Z** No Qualifier

Continued →

Section 0 **Medical and Surgical**
Body System 1 **Peripheral Nervous System**
Operation 9 **Drainage:** Taking or letting out fluids and/or gases from a body part

Body Part (4th)	Approach (5th)	Device (6th)	Qualifier (7th)
0 Cervical Plexus **1** Cervical Nerve **2** Phrenic Nerve **3** Brachial Plexus **4** Ulnar Nerve **5** Median Nerve **6** Radial Nerve **8** Thoracic Nerve **9** Lumbar Plexus **A** Lumbosacral Plexus **B** Lumbar Nerve **C** Pudendal Nerve **D** Femoral Nerve **F** Sciatic Nerve **G** Tibial Nerve **H** Peroneal Nerve **K** Head and Neck Sympathetic Nerve **L** Thoracic Sympathetic Nerve **M** Abdominal Sympathetic Nerve **N** Lumbar Sympathetic Nerve **P** Sacral Sympathetic Nerve **Q** Sacral Plexus **R** Sacral Nerve	**0** Open **3** Percutaneous **4** Percutaneous Endoscopic	**Z** No Device	**X** Diagnostic **Z** No Qualifier

Section 0 **Medical and Surgical**
Body System 1 **Peripheral Nervous System**
Operation B **Excision:** Cutting out or off, without replacement, a portion of a body part

Body Part (4th)	Approach (5th)	Device (6th)	Qualifier (7th)
0 Cervical Plexus **1** Cervical Nerve **2** Phrenic Nerve **3** Brachial Plexus **4** Ulnar Nerve **5** Median Nerve **6** Radial Nerve **8** Thoracic Nerve **9** Lumbar Plexus **A** Lumbosacral Plexus **B** Lumbar Nerve **C** Pudendal Nerve **D** Femoral Nerve **F** Sciatic Nerve **G** Tibial Nerve **H** Peroneal Nerve **K** Head and Neck Sympathetic Nerve **L** Thoracic Sympathetic Nerve **M** Abdominal Sympathetic Nerve **N** Lumbar Sympathetic Nerve **P** Sacral Sympathetic Nerve **Q** Sacral Plexus **R** Sacral Nerve	**0** Open **3** Percutaneous **4** Percutaneous Endoscopic	**Z** No Device	**X** Diagnostic **Z** No Qualifier

Section 0 **Medical and Surgical**
Body System 1 **Peripheral Nervous System**
Operation C **Extirpation:** Taking or cutting out solid matter from a body part

Body Part (4th)	Approach (5th)	Device (6th)	Qualifier (7th)
0 Cervical Plexus **1** Cervical Nerve **2** Phrenic Nerve **3** Brachial Plexus **4** Ulnar Nerve **5** Median Nerve **6** Radial Nerve **8** Thoracic Nerve **9** Lumbar Plexus **A** Lumbosacral Plexus **B** Lumbar Nerve **C** Pudendal Nerve **D** Femoral Nerve **F** Sciatic Nerve **G** Tibial Nerve **H** Peroneal Nerve **K** Head and Neck Sympathetic Nerve **L** Thoracic Sympathetic Nerve **M** Abdominal Sympathetic Nerve **N** Lumbar Sympathetic Nerve **P** Sacral Sympathetic Nerve **Q** Sacral Plexus **R** Sacral Nerve	**0** Open **3** Percutaneous **4** Percutaneous Endoscopic	**Z** No Device	**Z** No Qualifier

Section 0 **Medical and Surgical**
Body System 1 **Peripheral Nervous System**
Operation D **Extraction:** Pulling or stripping out or off all or a portion of a body part by the use of force

Body Part (4th)	Approach (5th)	Device (6th)	Qualifier (7th)
0 Cervical Plexus **1** Cervical Nerve **2** Phrenic Nerve **3** Brachial Plexus **4** Ulnar Nerve **5** Median Nerve **6** Radial Nerve **8** Thoracic Nerve **9** Lumbar Plexus **A** Lumbosacral Plexus **B** Lumbar Nerve **C** Pudendal Nerve **D** Femoral Nerve **F** Sciatic Nerve **G** Tibial Nerve **H** Peroneal Nerve **K** Head and Neck Sympathetic Nerve **L** Thoracic Sympathetic Nerve **M** Abdominal Sympathetic Nerve **N** Lumbar Sympathetic Nerve **P** Sacral Sympathetic Nerve **Q** Sacral Plexus **R** Sacral Nerve	**0** Open **3** Percutaneous **4** Percutaneous Endoscopic	**Z** No Device	**Z** No Qualifier

Section 0 **Medical and Surgical**
Body System 1 **Peripheral Nervous System**
Operation H **Insertion:** Putting in a nonbiological appliance that monitors, assists, performs, or prevents a physiological function but does not physically take the place of a body part

Body Part (4th)	Approach (5th)	Device (6th)	Qualifier (7th)
Y Peripheral Nerve	**0** Open **3** Percutaneous **4** Percutaneous Endoscopic	**1** Radioactive Element **2** Monitoring Device **M** Neurostimulator Lead **Y** Other Device	**Z** No Qualifier

Section 0 **Medical and Surgical**
Body System 1 **Peripheral Nervous System**
Operation J **Inspection:** Visually and/or manually exploring a body part

Body Part (4th)	Approach (5th)	Device (6th)	Qualifier (7th)
Y Peripheral Nerve	**0** Open **3** Percutaneous **4** Percutaneous Endoscopic	**Z** No Device	**Z** No Qualifier

Section 0 **Medical and Surgical**
Body System 1 **Peripheral Nervous System**
Operation N **Release:** Freeing a body part from an abnormal physical constraint by cutting or by the use of force

Body Part (4th)	Approach (5th)	Device (6th)	Qualifier (7th)
0 Cervical Plexus **1** Cervical Nerve **2** Phrenic Nerve **3** Brachial Plexus **4** Ulnar Nerve **5** Median Nerve **6** Radial Nerve **8** Thoracic Nerve **9** Lumbar Plexus **A** Lumbosacral Plexus **B** Lumbar Nerve **C** Pudendal Nerve **D** Femoral Nerve **F** Sciatic Nerve **G** Tibial Nerve **H** Peroneal Nerve **K** Head and Neck Sympathetic Nerve **L** Thoracic Sympathetic Nerve **M** Abdominal Sympathetic Nerve **N** Lumbar Sympathetic Nerve **P** Sacral Sympathetic Nerve **Q** Sacral Plexus **R** Sacral Nerve	**0** Open **3** Percutaneous **4** Percutaneous Endoscopic	**Z** No Device	**Z** No Qualifier

Section 0 **Medical and Surgical**
Body System 1 **Peripheral Nervous System**
Operation P **Removal:** Taking out or off a device from a body part

Body Part (4th)	Approach (5th)	Device (6th)	Qualifier (7th)
Y Peripheral Nerve	**0** Open **3** Percutaneous **4** Percutaneous Endoscopic	**0** Drainage Device **2** Monitoring Device **7** Autologous Tissue Substitute **M** Neurostimulator Lead **Y** Other Device	**Z** No Qualifier
Y Peripheral Nerve	**X** External	**0** Drainage Device **2** Monitoring Device **M** Neurostimulator Lead	**Z** No Qualifier

Section 0 **Medical and Surgical**
Body System 1 **Peripheral Nervous System**
Operation Q **Repair:** Restoring, to the extent possible, a body part to its normal anatomic structure and function

Body Part (4th)	Approach (5th)	Device (6th)	Qualifier (7th)
0 Cervical Plexus 1 Cervical Nerve 2 Phrenic Nerve 3 Brachial Plexus 4 Ulnar Nerve 5 Median Nerve 6 Radial Nerve 8 Thoracic Nerve 9 Lumbar Plexus A Lumbosacral Plexus B Lumbar Nerve C Pudendal Nerve D Femoral Nerve F Sciatic Nerve G Tibial Nerve H Peroneal Nerve K Head and Neck Sympathetic Nerve L Thoracic Sympathetic Nerve M Abdominal Sympathetic Nerve N Lumbar Sympathetic Nerve P Sacral Sympathetic Nerve Q Sacral Plexus R Sacral Nerve	0 Open 3 Percutaneous 4 Percutaneous Endoscopic	Z No Device	Z No Qualifier

Section 0 **Medical and Surgical**
Body System 1 **Peripheral Nervous System**
Operation R **Replacement:** Putting in or on biological or synthetic material that physically takes the place and/or function of all or a portion of a body part

Body Part (4th)	Approach (5th)	Device (6th)	Qualifier (7th)
1 Cervical Nerve 2 Phrenic Nerve 4 Ulnar Nerve 5 Median Nerve 6 Radial Nerve 8 Thoracic Nerve B Lumbar Nerve C Pudendal Nerve D Femoral Nerve F Sciatic Nerve G Tibial Nerve H Peroneal Nerve R Sacral Nerve	0 Open 4 Percutaneous Endoscopic	7 Autologous Tissue Substitute J Synthetic Substitute K Nonautologous Tissue Substitute	Z No Qualifier

Section 0 **Medical and Surgical**
Body System 1 **Peripheral Nervous System**
Operation S **Reposition:** Moving to its normal location, or other suitable location, all or a portion of a body part

Body Part (4th)	Approach (5th)	Device (6th)	Qualifier (7th)
0 Cervical Plexus **1** Cervical Nerve **2** Phrenic Nerve **3** Brachial Plexus **4** Ulnar Nerve **5** Median Nerve **6** Radial Nerve **8** Thoracic Nerve **9** Lumbar Plexus **A** Lumbosacral Plexus **B** Lumbar Nerve **C** Pudendal Nerve **D** Femoral Nerve **F** Sciatic Nerve **G** Tibial Nerve **H** Peroneal Nerve **Q** Sacral Plexus **R** Sacral Nerve	**0** Open **3** Percutaneous **4** Percutaneous Endoscopic	**Z** No Device	**Z** No Qualifier

Section 0 **Medical and Surgical**
Body System 1 **Peripheral Nervous System**
Operation U **Supplement:** Putting in or on biological or synthetic material that physically reinforces and/or augments the function of a portion of a body part

Body Part (4th)	Approach (5th)	Device (6th)	Qualifier (7th)
1 Cervical Nerve **2** Phrenic Nerve **4** Ulnar Nerve **5** Median Nerve **6** Radial Nerve **8** Thoracic Nerve **B** Lumbar Nerve **C** Pudendal Nerve **D** Femoral Nerve **F** Sciatic Nerve **G** Tibial Nerve **H** Peroneal Nerve **R** Sacral Nerve	**0** Open **3** Percutaneous **4** Percutaneous Endoscopic	**7** Autologous Tissue Substitute **J** Synthetic Substitute **K** Nonautologous Tissue Substitute	**Z** No Qualifier

Section 0 **Medical and Surgical**
Body System 1 **Peripheral Nervous System**
Operation W **Revision:** Correcting, to the extent possible, a portion of a malfunctioning device or the position of a displaced device

Body Part (4th)	Approach (5th)	Device (6th)	Qualifier (7th)
Y Peripheral Nerve	**0** Open **3** Percutaneous **4** Percutaneous Endoscopic	**0** Drainage Device **2** Monitoring Device **7** Autologous Tissue Substitute **M** Neurostimulator Lead **Y** Other Device	**Z** No Qualifier
Y Peripheral Nerve	**X** External	**0** Drainage Device **2** Monitoring Device **7** Autologous Tissue Substitute **M** Neurostimulator Lead	**Z** No Qualifier

Section 0 **Medical and Surgical**
Body System 1 **Peripheral Nervous System**
Operation X **Transfer:** Moving, without taking out, all or a portion of a body part to another location to take over the function of all or a portion of a body part

Body Part (4th)	Approach (5th)	Device (6th)	Qualifier (7th)
1 Cervical Nerve **2** Phrenic Nerve	**0** Open **4** Percutaneous Endoscopic	**Z** No Device	**1** Cervical Nerve **2** Phrenic Nerve
4 Ulnar Nerve **5** Median Nerve **6** Radial Nerve	**0** Open **4** Percutaneous Endoscopic	**Z** No Device	**4** Ulnar Nerve **5** Median Nerve **6** Radial Nerve
8 Thoracic Nerve	**0** Open **4** Percutaneous Endoscopic	**Z** No Device	**8** Thoracic Nerve
B Lumbar Nerve **C** Pudendal Nerve	**0** Open **4** Percutaneous Endoscopic	**Z** No Device	**B** Lumbar Nerve **C** Perineal Nerve
D Femoral Nerve **F** Sciatic Nerve **G** Tibial Nerve **H** Peroneal Nerve	**0** Open **4** Percutaneous Endoscopic	**Z** No Device	**D** Femoral Nerve **F** Sciatic Nerve **G** Tibial Nerve **H** Peroneal Nerve

AHA Coding Clinic

01BL0ZZ Excision of Thoracic Sympathetic Nerve, Open Approach—AHA CC: 2Q, 2017, 19-20
01N10ZZ Release Cervical Nerve, Open Approach—AHA CC: 2Q, 2016, 17
01N30ZZ Release Brachial Plexus, Open Approach—AHA CC: 2Q, 2016, 23
01N50ZZ Release Median Nerve, Open Approach—AHA CC: 3Q, 2014, 33-34
01NB0ZZ Release Lumbar Nerve, Open Approach—AHA CC: 2Q, 2015, 34; 2Q, 2016, 16; 2Q, 2018, 22-23; 1Q, 2019, 28-29
01NR0ZZ Release Sacral Nerve, Open Approach—AHA CC: 1Q, 2019, 28-29
01U50KZ Supplement Median Nerve with Nonautologous Tissue Substitute, Open Approach—AHA CC: 4Q, 2017, 62
01U80KZ Supplement Thoracic Nerve with Nonautologous Tissue Substitute, Open Approach—AHA CC: 3Q, 2019, 32-33

Atria, Ventricles and Interventricular Septum

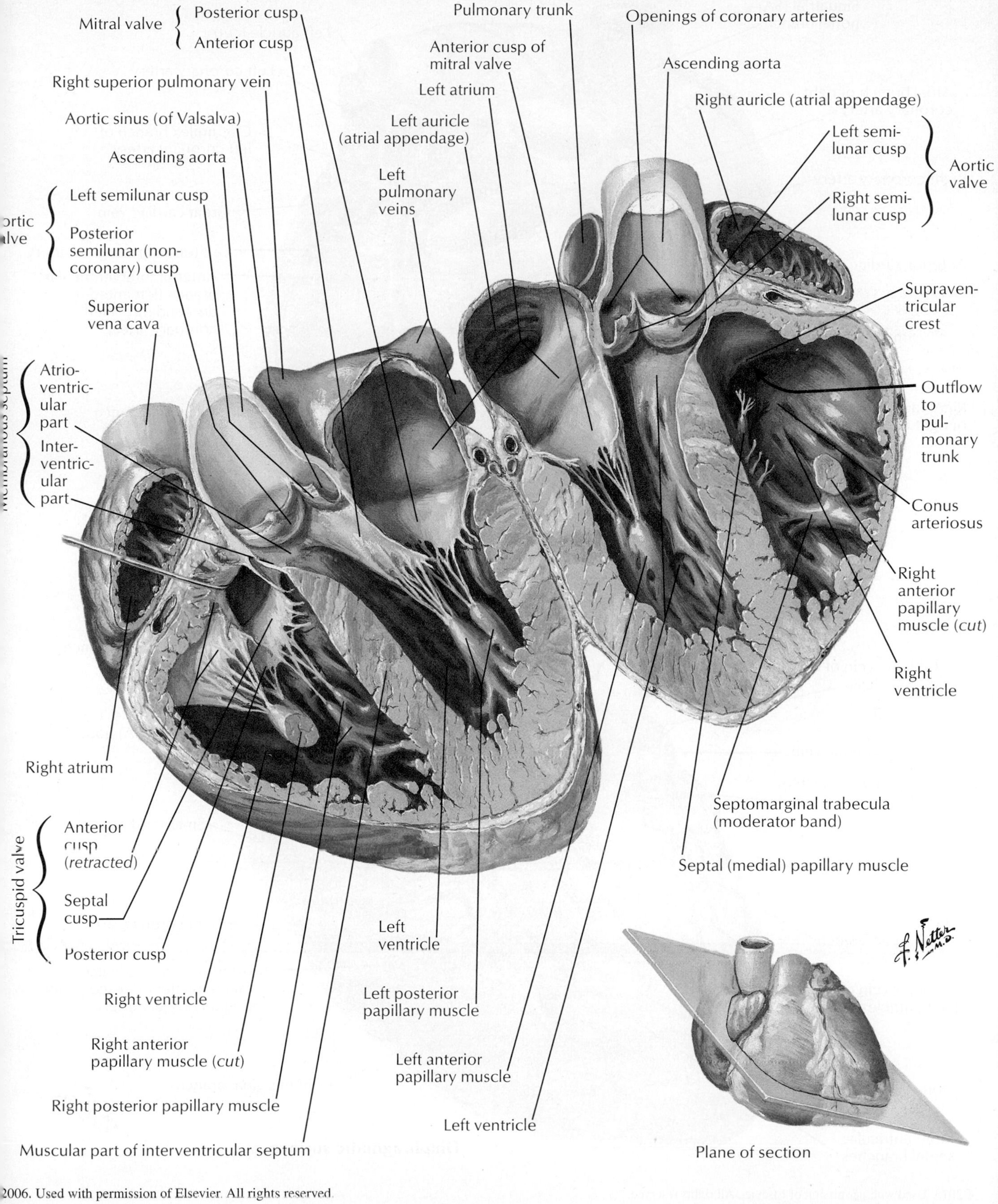
Mitral valve
Posterior cusp
Anterior cusp
Right superior pulmonary vein
Aortic sinus (of Valsalva)
Ascending aorta
Left semilunar cusp
Posterior semilunar (non-coronary) cusp
Superior vena cava
Atrio-ventric-ular part
Inter-ventric-ular part
Pulmonary trunk
Anterior cusp of mitral valve
Left atrium
Left auricle (atrial appendage)
Left pulmonary veins
Openings of coronary arteries
Ascending aorta
Right auricle (atrial appendage)
Left semi-lunar cusp
Right semi-lunar cusp
Aortic valve
Supraven-tricular crest
Outflow to pul-monary trunk
Conus arteriosus
Right anterior papillary muscle (*cut*)
Right ventricle
Septomarginal trabecula (moderator band)
Septal (medial) papillary muscle
Right atrium
Tricuspid valve
Anterior cusp (*retracted*)
Septal cusp
Posterior cusp
Right ventricle
Right anterior papillary muscle (*cut*)
Right posterior papillary muscle
Muscular part of interventricular septum
Left ventricle
Left posterior papillary muscle
Left anterior papillary muscle
Left ventricle
Plane of section

Arteries and Veins of the Heart; Arteries and Cardiac Veins

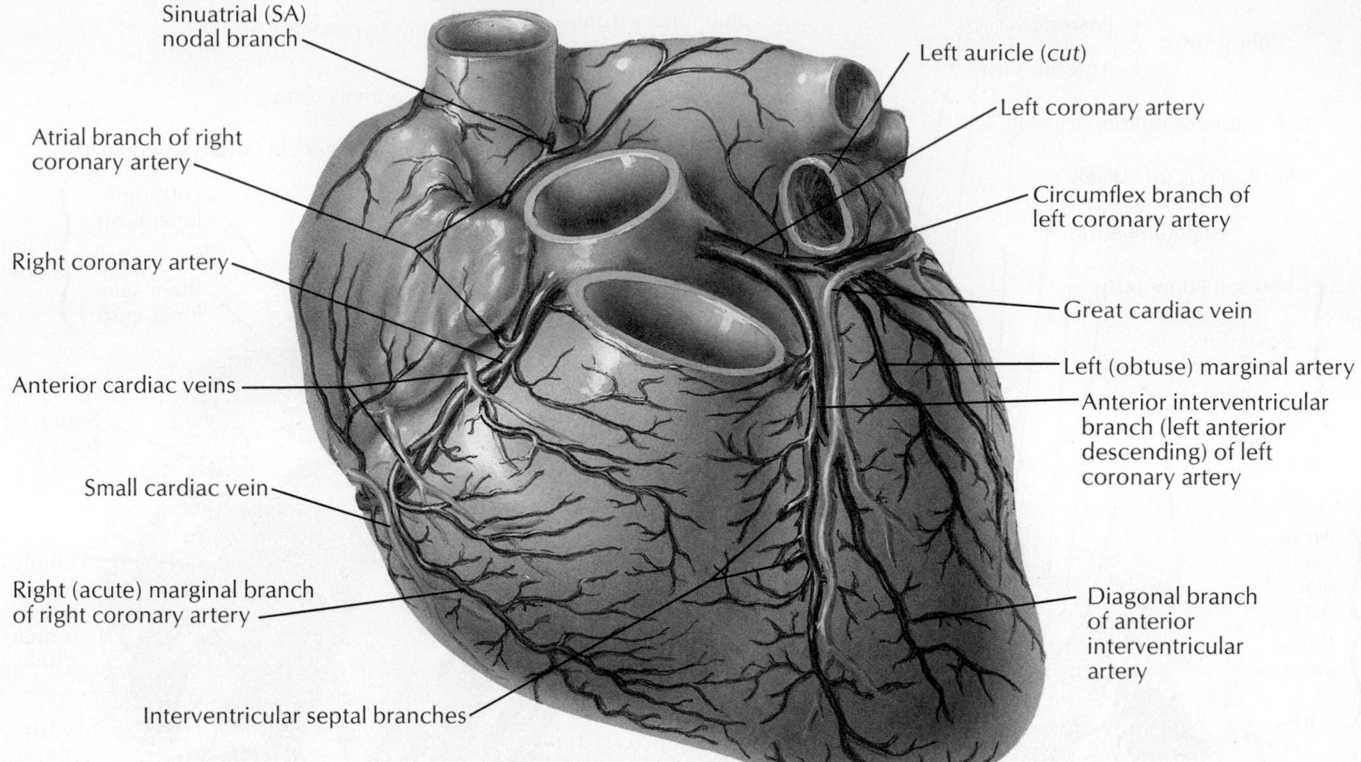
Sinuatrial (SA) nodal branch
Left auricle (cut)
Left coronary artery
Atrial branch of right coronary artery
Circumflex branch of left coronary artery
Right coronary artery
Great cardiac vein
Left (obtuse) marginal artery
Anterior cardiac veins
Anterior interventricular branch (left anterior descending) of left coronary artery
Small cardiac vein
Right (acute) marginal branch of right coronary artery
Diagonal branch of anterior interventricular artery
Interventricular septal branches

Sternocostal surface

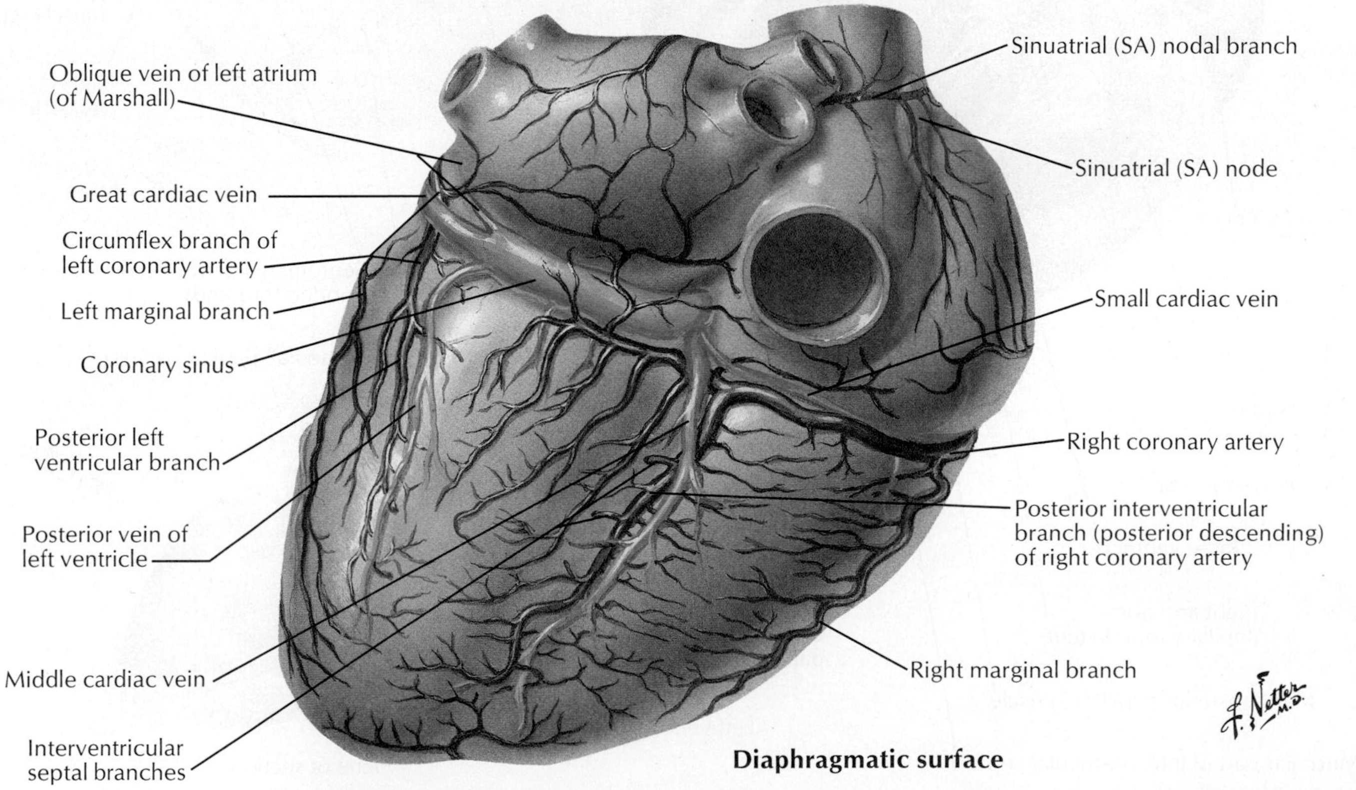
Sinuatrial (SA) nodal branch
Oblique vein of left atrium (of Marshall)
Sinuatrial (SA) node
Great cardiac vein
Circumflex branch of left coronary artery
Left marginal branch
Small cardiac vein
Coronary sinus
Posterior left ventricular branch
Right coronary artery
Posterior vein of left ventricle
Posterior interventricular branch (posterior descending) of right coronary artery
Middle cardiac vein
Right marginal branch
Interventricular septal branches
F. Netter M.D.

Diaphragmatic surface

Right Coronary Artery – Segmental Replacement

Right coronary-artery segmental replacement

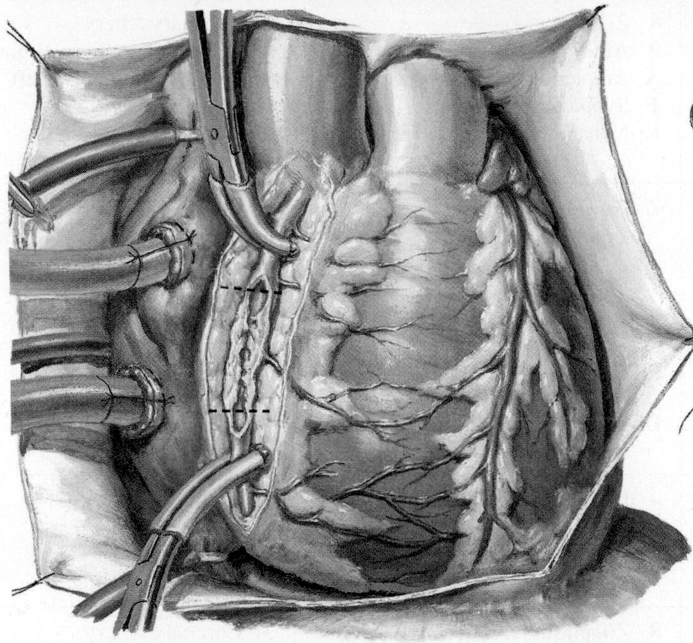

A. Diseased segment of right coronary artery widely exposed, clamped, and incised; portion between broken lines to be excised

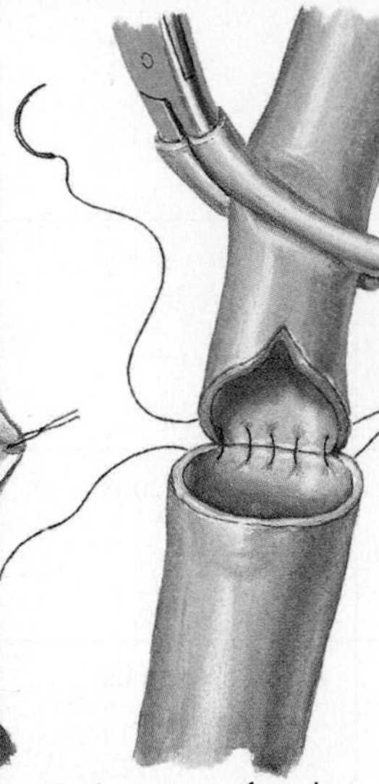

B. Segment of saphenous vein being sutured to proximal end of transected coronary artery

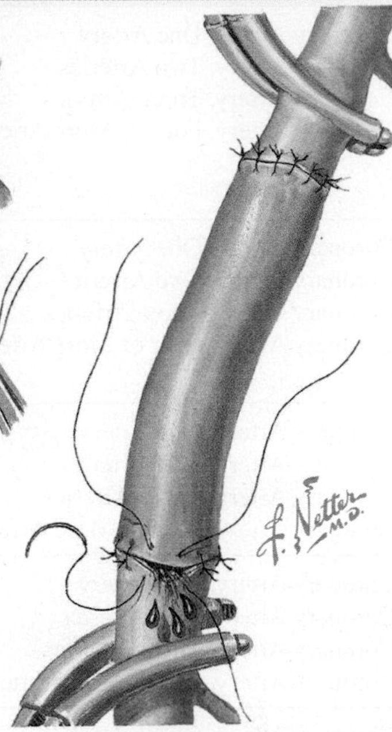

C. Lower end of saphenous graft sutured to distal portion of artery; blood and air allowed to escape by loosening distal clamp prior to final closure

Right coronary-artery bypass

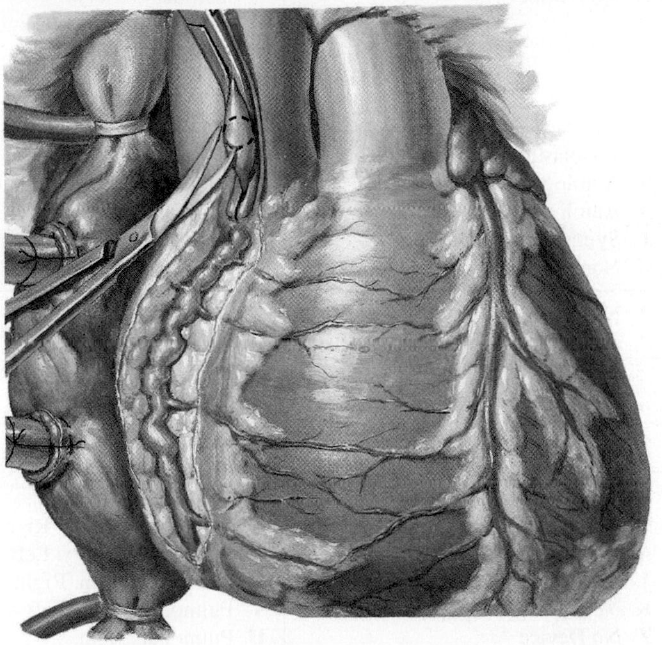

A′. Small area of aorta longitudinally isolated by clamp above right coronary orifice, and ostium created therein

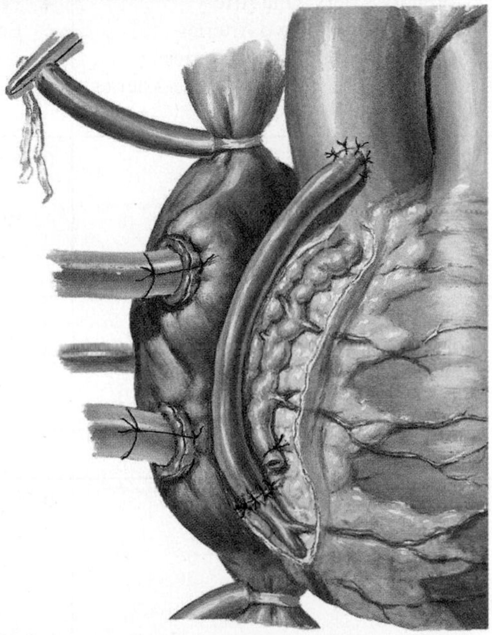

B′. Segment of saphenous vein implanted into new aortic ostium and anastomosed to end of divided right coronary artery distal to diseased area; proximal end of artery ligated

Heart and Great Vessels Tables 021–02Y

Section 0 **Medical and Surgical**
Body System 2 **Heart and Great Vessels**
Operation 1 **Bypass:** Altering the route of passage of the contents of a tubular body part

Body Part (4th)	Approach (5th)	Device (6th)	Qualifier (7th)
0 Coronary Artery, One Artery **1** Coronary Artery, Two Arteries **2** Coronary Artery, Three Arteries **3** Coronary Artery, Four or More Arteries	**0** Open	**8** Zooplastic Tissue **9** Autologous Venous Tissue **A** Autologous Arterial Tissue **J** Synthetic Substitute **K** Nonautologous Tissue Substitute	**3** Coronary Artery **8** Internal Mammary, Right **9** Internal Mammary, Left **C** Thoracic Artery **F** Abdominal Artery **W** Aorta
0 Coronary Artery, One Artery **1** Coronary Artery, Two Arteries **2** Coronary Artery, Three Arteries **3** Coronary Artery, Four or More Arteries	**0** Open	**Z** No Device	**3** Coronary Artery **8** Internal Mammary, Right **9** Internal Mammary, Left **C** Thoracic Artery **F** Abdominal Artery
0 Coronary Artery, One Artery **1** Coronary Artery, Two Arteries **2** Coronary Artery, Three Arteries **3** Coronary Artery, Four or More Arteries	**3** Percutaneous	**4** Intraluminal Device, Drug-eluting **D** Intraluminal Device	**4** Coronary Vein
0 Coronary Artery, One Artery **1** Coronary Artery, Two Arteries **2** Coronary Artery, Three Arteries **3** Coronary Artery, Four or More Arteries	**4** Percutaneous Endoscopic	**4** Intraluminal Device, Drug-eluting **D** Intraluminal Device	**4** Coronary Vein
0 Coronary Artery, One Artery **1** Coronary Artery, Two Arteries **2** Coronary Artery, Three Arteries **3** Coronary Artery, Four or More Arteries	**4** Percutaneous Endoscopic	**8** Zooplastic Tissue **9** Autologous Venous Tissue **A** Autologous Arterial Tissue **J** Synthetic Substitute **K** Nonautologous Tissue Substitute	**3** Coronary Artery **8** Internal Mammary, Right **9** Internal Mammary, Left **C** Thoracic Artery **F** Abdominal Artery **W** Aorta
0 Coronary Artery, One Artery **1** Coronary Artery, Two Arteries **2** Coronary Artery, Three Arteries **3** Coronary Artery, Four or More Arteries	**4** Percutaneous Endoscopic	**Z** No Device	**3** Coronary Artery **8** Internal Mammary, Right **9** Internal Mammary, Left **C** Thoracic Artery **F** Abdominal Artery
6 Atrium, Right	**0** Open **4** Percutaneous Endoscopic	**8** Zooplastic Tissue **9** Autologous Venous Tissue **A** Autologous Arterial Tissue **J** Synthetic Substitute **K** Nonautologous Tissue Substitute	**P** Pulmonary Trunk **Q** Pulmonary Artery, Right **R** Pulmonary Artery, Left
6 Atrium, Right	**0** Open **4** Percutaneous Endoscopic	**Z** No Device	**7** Atrium, Left **P** Pulmonary Trunk **Q** Pulmonary Artery, Right **R** Pulmonary Artery, Left
6 Atrium, Right	**3** Percutaneous	**Z** No Device	**7** Atrium, Left
7 Atrium, Left	**0** Open **4** Percutaneous Endoscopic	**8** Zooplastic Tissue **9** Autologous Venous Tissue **A** Autologous Arterial Tissue **J** Synthetic Substitute **K** Nonautologous Tissue Substitute **Z** No Device	**P** Pulmonary Trunk **Q** Pulmonary Artery, Right **R** Pulmonary Artery, Left **S** Pulmonary Vein, Right **T** Pulmonary Vein, Left **U** Pulmonary Vein, Confluence
7 Atrium	**3** Percutaneous	**J** Synthetic Substitute	**6** Atrium, Right
K Ventricle, Right **L** Ventricle, Left	**0** Open **4** Percutaneous Endoscopic	**8** Zooplastic Tissue **9** Autologous Venous Tissue **A** Autologous Arterial Tissue **J** Synthetic Substitute **K** Nonautologous Tissue Substitute	**P** Pulmonary Trunk **Q** Pulmonary Artery, Right **R** Pulmonary Artery, Left

Continued →

Section 0 **Medical and Surgical**
Body System 2 **Heart and Great Vessels**
Operation 1 **Bypass:** Altering the route of passage of the contents of a tubular body part

Body Part (4th)	Approach (5th)	Device (6th)	Qualifier (7th)
K Ventricle, Right **L** Ventricle, Left	**0** Open **4** Percutaneous Endoscopic	**Z** No Device	**5** Coronary Circulation **8** Internal Mammary, Right **9** Internal Mammary, Left **C** Thoracic Artery **F** Abdominal Artery **P** Pulmonary Trunk **Q** Pulmonary Artery, Right **R** Pulmonary Artery, Left **W** Aorta
P Pulmonary Trunk **Q** Right Pulmonary Artery **R** Left Pulmonary Artery	**0** Open **4** Percutaneous Endoscopic	**8** Zooplastic Tissue **9** Autologous Venous Tissue **A** Autologous Arterial Tissue **J** Synthetic Substitute **K** Nonautologous Tissue Substitute	**A** Innominate Artery **B** Subclavin **D** Carotid
V Superior Vena Cava	**0** Open **4** Percutaneous Endoscopic	**8** Zooplastic Tissue **9** Autologous Venous Tissue **A** Autologous Arterial Tissue **J** Synthetic Substitute **K** Nonautologous Tissue Substitute **Z** No Device	**P** Pulmonary Trunk **Q** Pulmonary Artery, Right **R** Pulmonary Artery, Left **S** Pulmonary Vein, Right **T** Pulmonary Vein, Left **U** Pulmonary Vein, Confluence
W Thoracic Aorta, Descending	**0** Open	**8** Zooplastic Tissue **9** Autologous Venous Tissue **A** Autologous Arterial Tissue **J** Synthetic Substitute **K** Nonautologous Tissue Substitute	**A** Innominate Artery **B** Subclavian **D** Carotid **F** Abdominal Artery **G** Axillary Artery **H** Brachial Artery **P** Pulmonary Trunk **Q** Pulmonary Artery, Right **R** Pulmonary Artery, Left **V** Lower Extremity Artery
W Thoracic Aorta, Descending	**0** Open	**Z** No Device	**A** Innominate Artery **B** Subclavian **D** Carotid **P** Pulmonary Trunk **Q** Pulmonary Artery, Right **R** Pulmonary Artery, Left
W Thoracic Aorta, Descending	**4** Percutaneous Endoscopic	**8** Zooplastic Tissue **9** Autologous Venous Tissue **A** Autologous Arterial Tissue **J** Synthetic Substitute **K** Nonautologous Tissue Substitute **Z** No Device	**A** Innominate Artery **B** Subclavian **D** Carotid **P** Pulmonary Trunk **Q** Pulmonary Artery, Right **R** Pulmonary Artery, Left
X Thoracic Aorta, Ascending/Arch	**0** Open **4** Percutaneous Endoscopic	**8** Zooplastic Tissue **9** Autologous Venous Tissue **A** Autologous Arterial Tissue **J** Synthetic Substitute **K** Nonautologous Tissue Substitute **Z** No Device	**A** Innominate Artery **B** Subclavian **D** Carotid **P** Pulmonary Trunk **Q** Pulmonary Artery, Right **R** Pulmonary Artery, Left

Section 0 **Medical and Surgical**
Body System 2 **Heart and Great Vessels**
Operation 4 **Creation:** Putting in or on biological or synthetic material to form a new body part that to the extent possible replicates the anatomic structure or function of an absent body part

Body Part (4th)	Approach (5th)	Device (6th)	Qualifier (7th)
F Aortic Valve	**0** Open	**7** Autologous Tissue Substitute **8** Zooplastic Tissue **J** Synthetic Substitute **K** Nonautologous Tissue Substitute	**J** Truncal Valve
G Mitral Valve **J** Tricuspid Valve	**0** Open	**7** Autologous Tissue Substitute **8** Zooplastic Tissue **J** Synthetic Substitute **K** Nonautologous Tissue Substitute	**2** Common Atrioventricular Valve

Section 0 **Medical and Surgical**
Body System 2 **Heart and Great Vessels**
Operation 5 **Destruction:** Physical eradication of all or a portion of a body part by the direct use of energy, force, or a destructive agent

Body Part (4th)	Approach (5th)	Device (6th)	Qualifier (7th)
4 Coronary Vein **5** Atrial Septum **6** Atrium, Right **8** Conduction Mechanism **9** Chordae Tendineae **D** Papillary Muscle **F** Aortic Valve **G** Mitral Valve **H** Pulmonary Valve **J** Tricuspid Valve **K** Ventricle, Right **L** Ventricle, Left **M** Ventricular Septum **N** Pericardium **P** Pulmonary Trunk **Q** Pulmonary Artery, Right **R** Pulmonary Artery, Left **S** Pulmonary Vein, Right **T** Pulmonary Vein, Left **V** Superior Vena Cava **W** Thoracic Aorta, Descending **X** Thoracic Aorta, Ascending/Arch	**0** Open **3** Percutaneous **4** Percutaneous Endoscopic	**Z** No Device	**Z** No Qualifier
7 Atrium, Left	**0** Open **3** Percutaneous **4** Percutaneous Endoscopic	**Z** No Device	**K** Left Atrial Appendage **Z** No Qualifier

Section 0 **Medical and Surgical**
Body System 2 **Heart and Great Vessels**
Operation 7 **Dilation:** Expanding an orifice or the lumen of a tubular body part

Body Part (4th)	Approach (5th)	Device (6th)	Qualifier (7th)
0 Coronary Artery, One Artery **1** Coronary Artery, Two Arteries **2** Coronary Artery, Three Arteries **3** Coronary Artery, Four or More Arteries	**0** Open **3** Percutaneous **4** Percutaneous Endoscopic	**4** Intraluminal Device, Drug-eluting **5** Intraluminal Device, Drug-eluting, Two **6** Intraluminal Device, Drug-eluting, Three **7** Intraluminal Device, Drug-eluting, Four or More **D** Intraluminal Device **E** Intraluminal Devices, Two **F** Intraluminal Devices, Three **G** Intraluminal Devices, Four or More **T** Intraluminal Device, Radioactive **Z** No Device	**6** Bifurcation **Z** No Qualifier
F Aortic Valve **G** Mitral Valve **H** Pulmonary Valve **J** Tricuspid Valve **K** Ventricle, Right **L** Ventricle, Left **P** Pulmonary Trunk **Q** Pulmonary Artery, Right **S** Pulmonary Vein, Right **T** Pulmonary Vein, Left **V** Superior Vena Cava **W** Thoracic Aorta, Descending **X** Thoracic Aorta, Ascending/Arch	**0** Open **3** Percutaneous **4** Percutaneous Endoscopic	**4** Intraluminal Device, Drug-eluting **D** Intraluminal Device **Z** No Device	**Z** No Qualifier
R Pulmonary Artery, Left	**0** Open **3** Percutaneous **4** Percutaneous Endoscopic	**4** Intraluminal Device, Drug-eluting **D** Intraluminal Device **Z** No Device	**T** Ductus Arteriosus **Z** No Qualifier

Section 0 **Medical and Surgical**
Body System 2 **Heart and Great Vessels**
Operation 8 **Division:** Cutting into a body part, without draining fluids and/or gases from the body part, in order to separate or transect a body part

Body Part (4th)	Approach (5th)	Device (6th)	Qualifier (7th)
8 Conduction Mechanism **9** Chordae Tendineae **D** Papillary Muscle	**0** Open **3** Percutaneous **4** Percutaneous Endoscopic	**Z** No Device	**Z** No Qualifier

Section 0 **Medical and Surgical**
Body System 2 **Heart and Great Vessels**
Operation B **Excision:** Cutting out or off, without replacement, a portion of a body part

Body Part (4th)	Approach (5th)	Device (6th)	Qualifier (7th)
4 Coronary Vein **5** Atrial Septum **6** Atrium, Right **8** Conduction Mechanism **9** Chordae Tendineae **D** Papillary Muscle **F** Aortic Valve **G** Mitral Valve **H** Pulmonary Valve **J** Tricuspid Valve **K** Ventricle, Right **L** Ventricle, Left **M** Ventricular Septum **N** Pericardium **P** Pulmonary Trunk **Q** Pulmonary Artery, Right **R** Pulmonary Artery, Left **S** Pulmonary Vein, Right **T** Pulmonary Vein, Left **V** Superior Vena Cava **W** Thoracic Aorta, Descending **X** Thoracic Aorta, Ascending/Arch	**0** Open **3** Percutaneous **4** Percutaneous Endoscopic	**Z** No Device	**X** Diagnostic **Z** No Qualifier
7 Atrium, Left	**0** Open **3** Percutaneous **4** Percutaneous Endoscopic	**Z** No Device	**K** Left Atrial Appendage **X** Diagnostic **Z** No Qualifier

Section 0 **Medical and Surgical**
Body System 2 **Heart and Great Vessels**
Operation C **Extirpation:** Taking or cutting out solid matter from a body part

Body Part (4th)	Approach (5th)	Device (6th)	Qualifier (7th)
0 Coronary Artery, One Artery **1** Coronary Artery, Two Arteries **2** Coronary Artery, Three Arteries **3** Coronary Artery, Four or More Arteries	**0** Open **4** Percutaneous Endoscopic	**Z** No Device	**6** Bifurcation **Z** No Qualifier
0 Coronary Artery, One Artery **1** Coronary Artery, Two Arteries **2** Coronary Artery, Three Arteries **3** Coronary Artery, Four or More Arteries	**3** Percutaneous	**Z** No Device	**6** Bifurcation **7** Orbital Atherectomy Technique **Z** No Qualifier

Continued →

Section 0 **Medical and Surgical**
Body System 2 **Heart and Great Vessels**
Operation C **Extirpation:** Taking or cutting out solid matter from a body part

Body Part (4th)	Approach (5th)	Device (6th)	Qualifier (7th)
4 Coronary Vein **5** Atrial Septum **6** Atrium, Right **7** Atrium, Left **8** Conduction Mechanism **9** Chordae Tendineae **D** Papillary Muscle **F** Aortic Valve **G** Mitral Valve **H** Pulmonary Valve **J** Tricuspid Valve **K** Ventricle, Right **L** Ventricle, Left **M** Ventricular Septum **N** Pericardium **P** Pulmonary Trunk **Q** Pulmonary Artery, Right **R** Pulmonary Artery, Left **S** Pulmonary Vein, Right **T** Pulmonary Vein, Left **V** Superior Vena Cava **W** Thoracic Aorta, Descending **X** Thoracic Aorta, Ascending/Arch	**0** Open **3** Percutaneous **4** Percutaneous Endoscopic	**Z** No Device	**Z** No Qualifier

Section 0 **Medical and Surgical**
Body System 2 **Heart and Great Vessels**
Operation F **Fragmentation:** Breaking solid matter in a body part into pieces

Body Part (4th)	Approach (5th)	Device (6th)	Qualifier (7th)
0 Coronary Artery, One Artery **1** Coronary Artery, Two Arteries **2** Coronary Artery, Three Arteries **3** Coronary Artery, Four or More Arteries	**3** Percutaneous	**Z** No Device	**Z** No Qualifier
N Pericardium	**0** Open **3** Percutaneous **4** Percutaneous Endoscopic **X** External	**Z** No Device	**Z** No Qualifier
P Pulmonary Trunk **Q** Pulmonary Artery, Right **R** Pulmonary Artery, Left **S** Pulmonary Vein, Right **T** Pulmonary Vein, Left	**3** Percutaneous	**Z** No Device	**0** Ultrasonic **Z** No Qualifier

Section 0 **Medical and Surgical**
Body System 2 **Heart and Great Vessels**
Operation H **Insertion:** Putting in a nonbiological appliance that monitors, assists, performs, or prevents a physiological function but does not physically take the place of a body part

Body Part (4th)	Approach (5th)	Device (6th)	Qualifier (7th)
0 Coronary Artery, One Artery **1** Coronary Artery, Two Arteries **2** Coronary Artery, Three Arteries **3** Coronary Artery, Four or More Arteries	**0** Open **3** Percutaneous **4** Percutaneous Endoscopic	**D** Intraluminal Device **Y** Other Device	**Z** No Qualifier

Continued →

Section 0 **Medical and Surgical**
Body System 2 **Heart and Great Vessels**
Operation H **Insertion:** Putting in a nonbiological appliance that monitors, assists, performs, or prevents a physiological function but does not physically take the place of a body part

Body Part (4th)	Approach (5th)	Device (6th)	Qualifier (7th)
4 Coronary Vein **6** Atrium, Right **7** Atrium, Left **K** Ventricle, Right **L** Ventricle, Left	**0** Open **3** Percutaneous **4** Percutaneous Endoscopic	**0** Monitoring Device, Pressure Sensor **2** Monitoring Device **3** Infusion Device **D** Intraluminal Device **J** Cardiac Lead, Pacemaker **K** Cardiac Lead, Defibrillator **M** Cardiac Lead **N** Intracardiac Pacemaker **Y** Other Device	**Z** No Qualifier
A Heart	**0** Open **3** Percutaneous **4** Percutaneous Endoscopic	**Q** Implantable Heart Assist System **Y** Other Device	**Z** No Qualifier
A Heart	**0** Open **3** Percutaneous **4** Percutaneous Endoscopic	**R** Short-term External Heart Assist System	**J** Intraoperative **S** Biventricular **Z** No Qualifier
N Pericardium	**0** Open **3** Percutaneous **4** Percutaneous Endoscopic	**0** Monitoring Device, Pressure Sensor **2** Monitoring Device **J** Cardiac Lead, Pacemaker **K** Cardiac Lead, Defibrillator **M** Cardiac Lead **Y** Other Device	**Z** No Qualifier
P Pulmonary Trunk **Q** Pulmonary Artery, Right **R** Pulmonary Artery, Left **S** Pulmonary Vein, Right **T** Pulmonary Vein, Left **V** Superior Vena Cava **W** Thoracic Aorta, Descending	**0** Open **3** Percutaneous **4** Percutaneous Endoscopic	**0** Monitoring Device, Pressure Sensor **2** Monitoring Device **3** Infusion Device **D** Intraluminal Device **Y** Other Device	**Z** No Qualifier
X Thoracic Aorta, Ascending/Arch	**0** Open **3** Percutaneous **4** Percutaneous Endoscopic	**0** Monitoring Device, Pressure Sensor **2** Monitoring Device **3** Infusion Device **D** Intraluminal Device	**Z** No Qualifier

Section 0 **Medical and Surgical**
Body System 2 **Heart and Great Vessels**
Operation J **Inspection:** Visually and/or manually exploring a body part

Body Part (4th)	Approach (5th)	Device (6th)	Qualifier (7th)
A Heart **Y** Great Vessel	**0** Open **3** Percutaneous **4** Percutaneous Endoscopic	**Z** No Device	**Z** No Qualifier

Section 0 **Medical and Surgical**
Body System 2 **Heart and Great Vessels**
Operation K **Map:** Locating the route of passage of electrical impulses and/or locating functional areas in a body part

Body Part (4th)	Approach (5th)	Device (6th)	Qualifier (7th)
8 Conduction Mechanism	**0** Open **3** Percutaneous **4** Percutaneous Endoscopic	**Z** No Device	**Z** No Qualifier

Section 0 **Medical and Surgical**
Body System 2 **Heart and Great Vessels**
Operation L **Occlusion:** Completely closing an orifice or the lumen of a tubular body part

Body Part (4th)	Approach (5th)	Device (6th)	Qualifier (7th)
7 Atrium, Left	**0** Open **3** Percutaneous **4** Percutaneous Endoscopic	**C** Extraluminal Device **D** Intraluminal Device **Z** No Device	**K** Left Atrial Appendage
H Pulmonary Valve **P** Pulmonary Trunk **Q** Pulmonary Artery, Right **S** Pulmonary Vein, Right **T** Pulmonary Vein, Left **V** Superior Vena Cava	**0** Open **3** Percutaneous **4** Percutaneous Endoscopic	**C** Extraluminal Device **D** Intraluminal Device **Z** No Device	**Z** No Qualifier
R Pulmonary Artery, Left	**0** Open **3** Percutaneous **4** Percutaneous Endoscopic	**C** Extraluminal Device **D** Intraluminal Device **Z** No Device	**T** Ductus Arteriosus **Z** No Qualifier
W Thoracic Aorta, Descending	**3** Percutaneous	**D** Intraluminal Device	**J** Temporary

Section 0 **Medical and Surgical**
Body System 2 **Heart and Great Vessels**
Operation N **Release:** Freeing a body part from an abnormal physical constraint by cutting or by the use of force

Body Part (4th)	Approach (5th)	Device (6th)	Qualifier (7th)
0 Coronary Artery, One Artery **1** Coronary Artery, Two Arteries **2** Coronary Artery, Three Arteries **3** Coronary Artery, Four or More Arteries **4** Coronary Vein **5** Atrial Septum **6** Atrium, Right **7** Atrium, Left **8** Conduction Mechanism **9** Chordae Tendineae **D** Papillary Muscle **F** Aortic Valve **G** Mitral Valve **H** Pulmonary Valve **J** Tricuspid Valve **K** Ventricle, Right **L** Ventricle, Left **M** Ventricular Septum **N** Pericardium **P** Pulmonary Trunk **Q** Pulmonary Artery, Right **R** Pulmonary Artery, Left **S** Pulmonary Vein, Right **T** Pulmonary Vein, Left **V** Superior Vena Cava **W** Thoracic Aorta, Descending **X** Thoracic Aorta, Ascending/Arch	**0** Open **3** Percutaneous **4** Percutaneous Endoscopic	**Z** No Device	**Z** No Qualifier

Section 0 **Medical and Surgical**
Body System 2 **Heart and Great Vessels**
Operation P **Removal:** Taking out or off a device from a body part

Body Part (4th)	Approach (5th)	Device (6th)	Qualifier (7th)
A Heart	**0** Open **3** Percutaneous **4** Percutaneous Endoscopic	**2** Monitoring Device **3** Infusion Device **7** Autologous Tissue Substitute **8** Zooplastic Tissue **C** Extraluminal Device **D** Intraluminal Device **J** Synthetic Substitute **K** Nonautologous Tissue Substitute **M** Cardiac Lead **N** Intracardiac Pacemaker **Q** Implantable Heart Assist System **Y** Other Device	**Z** No Qualifier
A Heart	**0** Open **3** Percutaneous **4** Percutaneous Endoscopic	**R** Short-term External Heart Assist System	**S** Biventricular **Z** No Qualifier
A Heart	**X** External	**2** Monitoring Device **3** Infusion Device **D** Intraluminal Device **M** Cardiac Lead	**Z** No Qualifier
Y Great Vessel	**0** Open **3** Percutaneous **4** Percutaneous Endoscopic	**2** Monitoring Device **3** Infusion Device **7** Autologous Tissue Substitute **8** Zooplastic Tissue **C** Extraluminal Device **D** Intraluminal Device **J** Synthetic Substitute **K** Nonautologous Tissue Substitute **Y** Other Device	**Z** No Qualifier
Y Great Vessel	**X** External	**2** Monitoring Device **3** Infusion Device **D** Intraluminal Device	**Z** No Qualifier

Section 0 **Medical and Surgical**
Body System 2 **Heart and Great Vessels**
Operation Q **Repair:** Restoring, to the extent possible, a body part to its normal anatomic structure and function

Body Part (4th)	Approach (5th)	Device (6th)	Qualifier (7th)
0 Coronary Artery, One Artery **1** Coronary Artery, Two Arteries **2** Coronary Artery, Three Arteries **3** Coronary Artery, Four or More Arteries **4** Coronary Vein **5** Atrial Septum **6** Atrium, Right **7** Atrium, Left **8** Conduction Mechanism **9** Chordae Tendineae **A** Heart **B** Heart, Right **C** Heart, Left **D** Papillary Muscle **H** Pulmonary Valve **K** Ventricle, Right **L** Ventricle, Left **M** Ventricular Septum **N** Pericardium **P** Pulmonary Trunk **Q** Pulmonary Artery, Right **R** Pulmonary Artery, Left **S** Pulmonary Vein, Right	**0** Open **3** Percutaneous **4** Percutaneous Endoscopic	**Z** No Device	**Z** No Qualifier

Continued →

Section 0 Medical and Surgical
Body System 2 Heart and Great Vessels
Operation Q **Removal:** Taking out or off a device from a body part

Body Part (4th)	Approach (5th)	Device (6th)	Qualifier (7th)
T Pulmonary Vein, Left **V** Superior Vena Cava **W** Thoracic Aorta, Descending **X** Thoracic Aorta, Ascending/Arch			
F Aortic Valve	**0** Open **3** Percutaneous **4** Percutaneous Endoscopic	**Z** No Device	**J** Truncal Valve **Z** No Qualifier
G Mitral Valve	**0** Open **3** Percutaneous **4** Percutaneous Endoscopic	**Z** No Device	**E** Atrioventricular Valve, Left **Z** No Qualifier
J Tricuspid Valve	**0** Open **3** Percutaneous **4** Percutaneous Endoscopic	**Z** No Device	**G** Atrioventricular Valve, Right **Z** No Qualifier

Section 0 Medical and Surgical
Body System 2 Heart and Great Vessels
Operation R **Replacement:** Putting in or on biological or synthetic material that physically takes the place and/or function of all or a portion of a body part

Body Part (4th)	Approach (5th)	Device (6th)	Qualifier (7th)
5 Atrial Septum **6** Atrium, Right **7** Atrium, Left **9** Chordae Tendineae **D** Papillary Muscle **K** Ventricle, Right **L** Ventricle, Left **M** Ventricular Septum **N** Pericardium **P** Pulmonary Trunk **Q** Pulmonary Artery, Right **R** Pulmonary Artery, Left **S** Pulmonary Vein, Right **T** Pulmonary Vein, Left **V** Superior Vena Cava **W** Thoracic Aorta, Descending **X** Thoracic Aorta, Ascending/Arch	**0** Open **4** Percutaneous Endoscopic	**7** Autologous Tissue Substitute **8** Zooplastic Tissue **J** Synthetic Substitute **K** Nonautologous Tissue Substitute	**Z** No Qualifier
A Heart	**0** Open	**L** Biologic with Synthetic Substitute, Autoregulated Electrohydraulic **M** Synthetic Substitute, Pneumatic	**Z** No Qualifier

Continued →

ection 0 **Medical and Surgical**
Body System 2 **Heart and Great Vessels**
Operation R **Replacement:** Putting in or on biological or synthetic material that physically takes the place and/or function of all or a portion of a body part

Body Part (4th)	Approach (5th)	Device (6th)	Qualifier (7th)
F Aortic Valve **G** Mitral Valve **J** Tricuspid Valve	**0** Open **4** Percutaneous Endoscopic	**7** Autologous Tissue Substitute **8** Zooplastic Tissue **J** Synthetic Substitute **K** Nonautologous Tissue Substitute	**Z** No Qualifier
F Aortic Valve **G** Mitral Valve **J** Tricuspid Valve	**3** Percutaneous	**7** Autologous Tissue Substitute **8** Zooplastic Tissue **J** Synthetic Substitute **K** Nonautologous Tissue Substitute	**H** Transapical **Z** No Qualifier
H Pulmonary Valve	**0** Open **4** Percutaneous Endoscopic	**7** Autologous Tissue Substitute **8** Zooplastic Tissue **J** Synthetic Substitute **K** Nonautologous Tissue Substitute	**Z** No Qualifier
H Pulmonary Valve	**3** Percutaneous	**7** Autologous Tissue Substitute **J** Synthetic Substitute **K** Nonautologous Tissue Substitute	**H** Transapical **Z** No Qualifier
H Pulmonary Valve	**3** Percutaneous	**8** Zooplastic Tissue	**H** Transapical **L** In Exisiting Conduit **M** Native Site **Z** No Qualifier

Section 0 **Medical and Surgical**
Body System 2 **Heart and Great Vessels**
Operation S **Reposition:** Moving to its normal location, or other suitable location, all or a portion of a body part

Body Part (4th)	Approach (5th)	Device (6th)	Qualifier (7th)
0 Coronary Artery, One Artery **1** Coronary Artery, Two Arteries **P** Pulmonary Trunk **Q** Pulmonary Artery, Right **R** Pulmonary Artery, Left **S** Pulmonary Vein, Right **T** Pulmonary Vein, Left **V** Superior Vena Cava **W** Thoracic Aorta, Descending **X** Thoracic Aorta, Ascending/Arch	**0** Open	**Z** No Device	**Z** No Qualifier

Section 0 **Medical and Surgical**
Body System 2 **Heart and Great Vessels**
Operation T **Resection:** Cutting out or off, without replacement, all of a body part

Body Part (4th)	Approach (5th)	Device (6th)	Qualifier (7th)
5 Atrial Septum **8** Conduction Mechanism **9** Chordae Tendineae **D** Papillary Muscle **H** Pulmonary Valve **M** Ventricular Septum **N** Pericardium	**0** Open **3** Percutaneous **4** Percutaneous Endoscopic	**Z** No Device	**Z** No Qualifier

Section 0 **Medical and Surgical**
Body System 2 **Heart and Great Vessels**
Operation U **Supplement:** Putting in or on biological or synthetic material that physically reinforces and/or augments the function of a portion of a body part

Body Part (4th)	Approach (5th)	Device (6th)	Qualifier (7th)
0 Coronary Artery, One Artery **1** Coronary Artery, Two Arteries **2** Coronary Artery, Three Arteries **3** Coronary Artery, Four or More Arteries **5** Atrial Septum **6** Atrium, Right **7** Atrium, Left **9** Chordae Tendineae **A** Heart **D** Papillary Muscle **H** Pulmonary Valve **K** Ventricle, Right **L** Ventricle, Left **M** Ventricular Septum **N** Pericardium **P** Pulmonary Trunk **Q** Pulmonary Artery, Right **R** Pulmonary Artery, Left **S** Pulmonary Vein, Right **T** Pulmonary Vein, Left **V** Superior Vena Cava **W** Thoracic Aorta, Descending **X** Thoracic Aorta, Ascending/Arch	**0** Open **3** Percutaneous **4** Percutaneous Endoscopic	**7** Autologous Tissue Substitute **8** Zooplastic Tissue **J** Synthetic Substitute **K** Nonautologous Tissue Substitute	**Z** No Qualifier
F Aortic Valve	**0** Open **3** Percutaneous **4** Percutaneous Endoscopic	**7** Autologous Tissue Substitute **8** Zooplastic Tissue **J** Synthetic Substitute **K** Nonautologous Tissue Substitute	**J** Truncal Valve **Z** No Qualifier
G Mitral Valve	**0** Open **4** Percutaneous Endoscopic	**7** Autologous Tissue Substitute **8** Zooplastic Tissue **J** Synthetic Substitute **K** Nonautologous Tissue Substitute	**E** Atrioventricular Valve, Left **Z** No Qualifier
G Mitral Valve	**3** Percutaneous	**7** Autologous Tissue Substitute **8** Zooplastic Tissue **K** Nonautologous Tissue Substitute	**E** Atrioventricular Valve, Left **Z** No Qualifier
G Mitral Valve	**3** Percutaneous	**J** Synthetic Substitute	**E** Atrioventricular Valve, Left **H** Transapical **Z** No Qualifier
J Tricuspid Valve	**0** Open **3** Percutaneous **4** Percutaneous Endoscopic	**7** Autologous Tissue Substitute **8** Zooplastic Tissue **J** Synthetic Substitute **K** Nonautologous Tissue Substitute	**G** Atrioventricular Valve, Right **Z** No Qualifier

Section 0 **Medical and Surgical**
Body System 2 **Heart and Great Vessels**
Operation V **Restriction:** Partially closing an orifice or the lumen of a tubular body part

Body Part (4th)	Approach (5th)	Device (6th)	Qualifier (7th)
A Heart	**0** Open **3** Percutaneous **4** Percutaneous Endoscopic	**C** Extraluminal Device **Z** No Device	**Z** No Qualifier
G Mitral Valve	**0** Open **3** Percutaneous **4** Percutaneous Endoscopic	**Z** No Device	**Z** No Qualifier
L Ventricle, Left **P** Pulmonary Trunk **Q** Pulmonary Artery, Right **S** Pulmonary Vein, Right **T** Pulmonary Vein, Left **V** Superior Vena Cava	**0** Open **3** Percutaneous **4** Percutaneous Endoscopic	**C** Extraluminal Device **D** Intraluminal Device **Z** No Device	**Z** No Qualifier
R Pulmonary Artery, Left	**0** Open **3** Percutaneous **4** Percutaneous Endoscopic	**C** Extraluminal Device **D** Intraluminal Device **Z** No Device	**T** Ductus Arteriosus **Z** No Qualifier
W Thoracic Aorta, Descending **X** Thoracic Aorta, Ascending/Arch	**0** Open **3** Percutaneous **4** Percutaneous Endoscopic	**C** Extraluminal Device **D** Intraluminal Device **E** Intraluminal Device, Branched or Fenestrated, One or Two Arteries **F** Intraluminal Device, Branched or Fenestrated, Three or More Arteries **Z** No Device	**Z** No Qualifier

Section 0 **Medical and Surgical**
Body System 2 **Heart and Great Vessels**
Operation W **Revision:** Correcting, to the extent possible, a portion of a malfunctioning device or the position of a displaced device

Body Part (4th)	Approach (5th)	Device (6th)	Qualifier (7th)
5 Atrial Septum **M** Ventricular Septum	**0** Open **4** Percutaneous Endoscopic	**J** Synthetic Substitute	**Z** No Qualifier
A Heart	**0** Open **3** Percutaneous **4** Percutaneous Endoscopic	**2** Monitoring Device **3** Infusion Device **7** Autologous Tissue Substitute **8** Zooplastic Tissue **C** Extraluminal Device **D** Intraluminal Device **J** Synthetic Substitute **K** Nonautologous Tissue Substitute **M** Cardiac Lead **N** Intracardiac Pacemaker **Q** Implantable Heart Assist System **Y** Other Device	**Z** No Qualifier
A Heart	**0** Open **3** Percutaneous **4** Percutaneous Endoscopic	**R** Short-term External Heart Assist System	**S** Biventricular **Z** No Qualifier

Continued →

Section 0 **Medical and Surgical**
Body System 2 **Heart and Great Vessels**
Operation W **Revision:** Correcting, to the extent possible, a portion of a malfunctioning device or the position of a displaced device

Body Part (4th)	Approach (5th)	Device (6th)	Qualifier (7th)
A Heart	**X** External	**2** Monitoring Device **3** Infusion Device **7** Autologous Tissue Substitute **8** Zooplastic Tissue **C** Extraluminal Device **D** Intraluminal Device **J** Synthetic Substitute **K** Nonautologous Tissue Substitute **M** Cardiac Lead **N** Intracardiac Pacemaker **Q** Implantable Heart Assist System	**Z** No Qualifier
A Heart	**X** External	**R** Short-term External Heart Assist System	**S** Biventricular **Z** No Qualifier
F Aortic Valve **G** Mitral Valve **H** Pulmonary Valve **J** Tricuspid Valve	**0** Open **3** Percutaneous **4** Percutaneous Endoscopic	**7** Autologous Tissue Substitute **8** Zooplastic Tissue **J** Synthetic Substitute **K** Nonautologous Tissue Substitute	**Z** No Qualifier
Y Great Vessel	**0** Open **3** Percutaneous **4** Percutaneous Endoscopic	**2** Monitoring Device **3** Infusion Device **7** Autologous Tissue Substitute **8** Zooplastic Tissue **C** Extraluminal Device **D** Intraluminal Device **J** Synthetic Substitute **K** Nonautologous Tissue Substitute **Y** Other Device	**Z** No Qualifier
Y Great Vessel	**X** External	**2** Monitoring Device **3** Infusion Device **7** Autologous Tissue Substitute **8** Zooplastic Tissue **C** Extraluminal Device **D** Intraluminal Device **J** Synthetic Substitute **K** Nonautologous Tissue Substitute	**Z** No Qualifier

Section 0 **Medical and Surgical**
Body System 2 **Heart and Great Vessels**
Operation Y **Transplantation:** Putting in or on all or a portion of a living body part taken from another individual or animal to physically take the place and/or function of all or a portion of a similar body part

Body Part (4th)	Approach (5th)	Device (6th)	Qualifier (7th)
A Heart	**0** Open	**Z** No Device	**0** Allogeneic **1** Syngeneic **2** Zooplastic

AHA Coding Clinic

0210098 Bypass Coronary Artery, One Artery from Right Internal Mammary with Autologous Venous Tissue, Open Approach—AHA CC: 3Q, 2018, 8-9

021009W Bypass Coronary Artery, One Artery from Aorta with Autologous Venous Tissue, Open Approach—AHA CC: 1Q, 2014, 10-11

02100AW Bypass Coronary Artery, One Artery from Aorta with Autologous Arterial Tissue, Open Approach—AHA CC: 4Q, 2016, 83-84

02100Z9 Bypass Coronary Artery, One Artery from Left Internal Mammary, Open Approach—AHA CC: 3Q, 2014, 8, 20-21; 1Q, 2016, 27-28; 4Q, 2016, 83-84

021109W Bypass Coronary Artery, Two Arteries from Aorta with Autologous VenousTissue, Open Approach—AHA CC: 3Q, 2014, 20-21; 4Q, 2016, 83-84

021209W Bypass Coronary Artery, Three Arteries from Aorta with Autologous Venous Tissue, Open Approach—AHA CC: 1Q, 2016, 27-28

02160JQ Bypass Right Atrium to Right Pulmonary Artery with Synthetic Substitute, Open Approach—AHA CC: 3Q, 2014, 29

02163Z7 Bypass Right Atrium to Left Atrium, Percutaneous Approach—AHA CC: 4Q, 2017, 56

02170ZU Bypass Left Atrium to Pulmonary Vein Confluence, Open Approach—AHA CC: 4Q, 2016, 108-109

02173J6 Bypass Left Atrium to Right Atrium with Synthetic Substitute, Percutaneous Approach—AHA CC: 4Q, 2020, 44-45

021K0JP Bypass Right Ventricle to Pulmonary Trunk with Synthetic Substitute, Open Approach—AHA CC: 1Q, 2017, 19-20; 1Q, 2020, 24-25

021K0JQ Bypass Right Ventricle to Right Pulmonary Artery with Synthetic Substitute, Open Approach—AHA CC: 3Q, 2014, 30

021K0KP Bypass Right Ventricle to Pulmonary Trunk with Nonautologous Tissue Substitute, Open Approach—AHA CC: 3Q, 2015, 16-17; 4Q, 2015. 22-23, 25

021V08S Bypass Superior Vena Cava to Right Pulmonary Vein with Zooplastic Tissue, Open Approach—AHA CC: 4Q, 2016, 145

021V09S Bypass Superior Vena Cava to Right Pulmonary Vein with Autologous Venous Tissue, Open Approach—AHA CC: 4Q, 2016, 144

021W0JQ Bypass Thoracic Aorta, Descending to Right Pulmonary Artery with Synthetic Substitute, Open Approach—AHA CC: 3Q, 2014, 3

021W0JV Bypass Thoracic Aorta, Descending to Lower Extremity Artery with Synthetic Substitute, Open Approach—AHA CC: 4Q, 2018, 46

021X0JA Bypass Thoracic Aorta, Ascending/Arch to Innominate Artery with Synthetic Substitute, Open Approach—AHA CC: 3Q, 2019, 30-31; 4Q, 2019, 23; 1Q, 2020, 37

021X0JD Bypass Thoracic Aorta, Ascending/Arch to Carotid with Synthetic Substitute, Open Approach—AHA CC: 3Q, 2019, 30-31

02570ZK Destruction of Left Atrial Appendage, Open Approach—AHA CC: 3Q, 2014, 20-21

02580ZZ Destruction of Conduction Mechanism, Open Approach—AHA CC: 3Q, 2016, 44

02583ZZ Destruction of Conduction Mechanism, Percutaneous Approach—AHA CC: 3Q, 2014, 19; 4Q, 2014, 47-48; 3Q, 2016, 43-44; 1Q, 2020, 32-33

02584ZZ Destruction of Conduction Mechanism, Percutaneous Endoscopic Approach—AHA CC: 1Q, 2020, 32-33

025M3ZZ Destruction of Ventricular Septum, Percutaneous Approach—AHA CC: 3Q, 2018, 27

025N0ZZ Destruction of Pericardium, Open Approach—AHA CC: 2Q, 2016, 17-18

0270346 Dilation of Coronary Artery, One Artery, Bifurcation, with Drug-eluting Intraluminal Device, Percutaneous Approach—AHA CC: 2Q, 2015, 4-5; 4Q, 2016, 88

027034Z Dilation of Coronary Artery, One Artery with Drug-eluting Intraluminal Device, Percutaneous Approach—AHA CC: 2Q, 2014, 4; 2Q, 2015, 3-4; 4Q, 2015, 13-14; 4Q, 2019, 39-40

027037Z Dilation of Coronary Artery, One Artery with Four or More Drug-eluting Intraluminal Devices, Percutaneous Approach—AHA CC: 4Q, 2016, 85-86

02703DZ Dilation of Coronary Artery, One Artery with Intraluminal Device, Percutaneous Approach—AHA CC: 2Q, 2015, 4

02703EZ Dilation of Coronary Artery, One Artery with Two Intraluminal Devices, Percutaneous Approach—AHA CC: 4Q, 2016, 84-85

02703ZZ Dilation of Coronary Artery, One Artery, Percutaneous Approach—AHA CC: 3Q, 2015, 10; 4Q, 2016, 88, 3Q, 2018, 7-8

027134Z Dilation of Coronary Artery, Two Arteries with Drug-eluting Intraluminal Device, Percutaneous Approach—AHA CC: 2Q, 2015, 5

0271356 Dilation of Coronary Artery, Two Arteries, Bifurcation, with Two Drug-eluting Intraluminal Devices, Percutaneous Approach—AHA CC: 4Q, 2016, 87

027136Z Dilation of Coronary Artery, Two Arteries with Three Drug-eluting Intraluminal Devices, Percutaneous Approach—AHA CC: 4Q, 2016, 84-85

027234Z Dilation of Coronary Artery, Three Arteries with Drug-eluting Intraluminal Device, Percutaneous Approach—AHA CC: 2Q, 2015, 3

027H0ZZ Dilation of Pulmonary Valve, Open Approach—AHA CC: 1Q, 2016, 16-17

027L0ZZ Dilation of Left Ventricle, Open Approach—AHA CC: 4Q, 2017, 33

027Q0DZ Dilation of Right Pulmonary Artery with Intraluminal Device, Open Approach—AHA CC: 3Q, 2015, 16-17

027V3ZZ Dilation of Superior Vena Cava, Percutaneous Approach—AHA CC: 3Q, 2018, 10

02BG0ZZ Excision of Mitral Valve, Open Approach—AHA CC: 2Q, 2015, 23-24

02BK3ZX Excision of Right Ventricle, Percutaneous Approach, Diagnostic—AHA CC: 3Q, 2019, 32

02BN0ZZ Excision of Pericardium, Open Approach—AHA CC: 2Q, 2019, 20-21

02CG0ZZ Extirpation of Matter from Mitral Valve, Open Approach—AHA CC: 2Q, 2016, 24-25

02H13DZ Insertion of Intraluminal Device into Coronary Artery, Two Arteries, Percutaneous Approach—AHA CC: 4Q, 2019, 24

02H633Z Insertion of Infusion Device into Right Atrium, Percutaneous Approach—AHA CC: 2Q, 2016, 15-16; 2Q, 2017, 24-26

02H63KZ Insertion of Cardiac Lead into Right Atrium, Percutaneous Approach—AHA CC: 2Q, 2018, 19

02H73DZ Insertion of Intraluminal Device into Left Atrium, Percutaneous Approach—AHA CC: 4Q, 2017, 104-105

02HA0QZ Insertion of Implantable Heart Assist System into Heart, Open Approach—AHA CC: 1Q, 2019, 24

02HA3RJ Insertion of Short-term External Heart Assist System into Heart, Intraoperative, Percutaneous Approach—AHA CC: 4Q, 2017, 43-44

02HA3RS Insertion of Biventricular Short-term External Heart Assist System into Heart, Percutaneous Approach—AHA CC: 4Q, 2016, 138-139

02HA3RZ Insertion of Short-term External Heart Assist System into Heart, Percutaneous Approach—AHA CC: 1Q, 2017, 11-12; 4Q, 2017, 44-45

02HK3DZ Insertion of Intraluminal Device into Right Ventricle, Percutaneous Approach—AHA CC: 2Q, 2015, 31-32

02HL0DZ Insertion of Intraluminal Device into Left Ventricle, Open Approach—AHA CC: 3Q, 2019, 19-20

02HL3JZ Insertion of Pacemaker Lead into Left Ventricle, Percutaneous Approach—AHA CC: 3Q, 2019, 23

02HP32Z Insertion of Monitoring Device into Pulmonary Trunk, Percutaneous Approach—AHA CC: 3Q, 2015, 35

02HV33Z Insertion of Infusion Device into Superior Vena Cava, Percutaneous Approach—AHA CC: 3Q, 2013, 18; 2Q, 2015, 33-34; 4Q, 2015, 14-15, 28-32; 4Q, 2017, 63-64

02JA3ZZ Inspection of Heart, Percutaneous Approach—AHA CC: 3Q, 2015, 9

02L70CK Occlusion of Left Atrial Appendage with Extraluminal Device, Open Approach—AHA CC: 3Q, 2014, 20-21

02L73DK Occlusion of Left Atrial Appendage with Intraluminal Device, Percutaneous Approach—AHA CC: 4Q, 2018, 94

02LQ3DZ Occlusion of Right Pulmonary Artery with Intraluminal Device, Percutaneous Approach—AHA CC: 4Q, 2017, 34

02LR0ZT Occlusion of Ductus Arteriosus, Open Approach—AHA CC: 4Q, 2015, 23-24

02LS3DZ Occlusion of Right Pulmonary Vein with Intraluminal Device, Percutaneous Approach—AHA CC: 2Q, 2016, 26; 4Q, 2017, 34

02N00ZZ Release Coronary Artery, One Artery, Open Approach—AHA CC: 2Q, 2019, 13-14

02NK0ZZ Release Right Ventricle, Open Approach—AHA CC: 3Q, 2014, 16-17

02NN0ZZ Release Pericardium, Open Approach—AHA CC: 2Q, 2019, 20-21

02PA0QZ Removal of Implantable Heart Assist System from Heart, Open Approach—AHA CC: 1Q, 2019, 24

02PA0RZ Removal of Short-term External Heart Assist System from Heart, Open Approach—AHA CC: 1Q, 2017, 13-14

02PA3DZ Removal of Intraluminal Device from Heart, Percutaneous Approach—AHA CC: 4Q, 2017, 104-105

02PA3MZ Removal of Cardiac Lead from Heart, Percutaneous Approach—AHA CC: 3Q, 2015, 33

02PA3NZ Removal of Intracardiac Pacemaker from Heart, Percutaneous Approach—AHA CC: 4Q, 2016, 96-97

02PA3RZ Removal of Short-term External Heart Assist System from Heart, Percutaneous Approach—AHA CC: 4Q, 2016, 139; 1Q, 2017, 11-12; 4Q, 2017, 44-45; 4Q, 2018, 54

02PY33Z Removal of Infusion Device from Great Vessel, Percutaneous Approach—AHA CC: 4Q, 2015, 31-32; 2Q, 2016, 15-16; 2Q, 2017, 24-26

02PY3JZ Removal of Synthetic Substitute from Great Vessel, Percutaneous Approach—AHA CC: 4Q, 2018, 85

02PYX3Z Removal of Infusion Device from Great Vessel, External Approach—AHA CC: 3Q, 2016, 19

02Q50ZZ Repair Atrial Septum, Open Approach—AHA CC: 4Q, 2015, 23-24

02QS0ZZ Repair Right Pulmonary Vein, Open Approach—AHA CC: 1Q, 2017, 18-19

02QT0ZZ Repair Left Pulmonary Vein, Open Approach—AHA CC: 1Q, 2017, 18-19

02QW0ZZ Repair Thoracic Aorta, Descending, Open Approach—AHA CC: 3Q, 2015, 16

02RF38Z Replacement of Aortic Valve with Zooplastic Tissue, Percutaneous Approach—AHA CC: 1Q, 2019, 31-32

02RF3JZ Replacement of Aortic Valve with Synthetic Substitute, Percutaneous Approach—AHA CC: 4Q, 2019, 24

02RG08Z Replacement of Mitral Valve with Zooplastic Tissue, Open Approach—AHA CC: 3Q, 2019, 23-24

02RJ3JZ Replacement of Tricuspid Valve with Synthetic Substitute, Percutaneous Approach—AHA CC: 4Q, 2017, 56

02RJ48Z Replacement of Tricuspid Valve with Zooplastic Tissue, Percutaneous Endoscopic Approach—AHA CC: 3Q, 2016, 32

02RK0JZ Replacement of Right Ventricle with Synthetic Substitute, Open Approach—AHA CC: 1Q, 2017, 13-14

02RL0JZ Replacement of Left Ventricle with Synthetic Substitute, Open Approach—AHA CC: 1Q, 2017, 13-14

02RW0KZ Replacement of Thoracic Aorta, Descending with Nonautologous Tissue Substitute, Open Approach—AHA CC: 1Q, 2014, 10-11

02RX0JZ Replacement of Thoracic Aorta, Ascending/Arch with Synthetic Substitute, Open Approach—AHA CC: 3Q, 2019, 24; 1Q, 2020, 25-26

02S10ZZ Reposition Coronary Artery, Two Arteries, Open Approach—AHA CC: 4Q, 2016, 103-104

02SP0ZZ Reposition Pulmonary Trunk, Open Approach—AHA CC: 4Q, 2015, 23-24; 4Q, 2016, 103-104

02SW0ZZ Reposition Thoracic Aorta, Descending, Open Approach—AHA CC: 4Q, 2015, 23-24

02SX0ZZ Reposition Thoracic Aorta, Ascending/Arch, Open Approach—AHA CC: 4Q, 2016, 103-104

02U03JZ Supplement Coronary Artery, One Artery with Synthetic Substitute, Percutaneous Approach—AHA CC: 4Q, 2019, 25-26

02U607Z Supplement Right Atrium with Autologous Tissue Substitute, Open Approach—AHA CC: 3Q, 2017, 7-8

02U707Z Supplement Left Atrium with Autologous Tissue Substitute, Open Approach— AHA CC: 3Q, 2017, 7-8

02UF08Z Supplement Aortic Valve with Zooplastic Tissue, Open Approach—AHA CC: 4Q, 2015, 25

02UG08Z Supplement Mitral Valve with Zooplastic Tissue, Open Approach—AHA CC: 4Q, 2017, 36

02UG0JZ Supplement Mitral Valve with Synthetic Substitute, Open Approach—AHA CC: 2Q, 2015, 23-24

02UG3JH Supplement Mitral Valve with Synthetic Substitute, Transapical, Percutaneous Approach—AHA CC: 4Q, 2020, 52

02UM08Z Supplement Ventricular Septum with Zooplastic Tissue, Open Approach—AHA CC: 4Q, 2015, 25

02UM0JZ Supplement Ventricular Septum with Synthetic Substitute, Open Approach—AHA CC: 3Q, 2014, 16-17; 4Q, 2015, 22-23

02UP07Z Supplement Pulmonary Trunk with Autologous Tissue Substitute, Open Approach—AHA CC: 2Q, 2016, 23-24

02UP08Z Supplement Pulmonary Trunk with Zooplastic Tissue, Open Approach—AHA CC: 1Q, 2020, 24-25

02UQ0KZ Supplement Right Pulmonary Artery with Nonautologous Tissue Substitute, Open Approach—AHA CC: 3Q, 2015, 16-17

02UR07Z Supplement Left Pulmonary Artery with Autologous Tissue Substitute, Open Approach—AHA CC: 2Q, 2016, 23-24

02UR0KZ Supplement Left Pulmonary Artery with Nonautologous Tissue Substitute, Open Approach—AHA CC: 3Q, 2015, 16-17

02UW07Z Supplement Thoracic Aorta, Descending with Autologous Tissue Substitute, Open Approach—AHA CC: 4Q, 2015, 23-24

02UW0JZ Supplement Thoracic Aorta, Descending with Synthetic Substitute, Open Approach—AHA CC: 2Q, 2016, 26-27

02UX0KZ Supplement Thoracic Aorta, Ascending/Arch with Nonautologous Tissue Substitute, Open Approach—AHA CC: 1Q, 2017, 19-20

02VG0ZZ Restriction of Mitral Valve, Open Approach—AHA CC: 4Q, 2017, 36

02VW0DZ Restriction of Thoracic Aorta, Descending with Intraluminal Device, Open Approach—AHA CC: 1Q, 2020, 25-26

02VW3DZ Restriction of Thoracic Aorta, Descending with Intraluminal Device, Percutaneous Approach—AHA CC: 4Q, 2016, 92-93

02WA3JZ Revision of Synthetic Substitute in Heart, Percutaneous Approach—AHA CC: 3Q, 2014, 31-32

02WA3MZ Revision of Cardiac Lead in Heart, Percutaneous Approach—AHA CC: 3Q, 2015, 32

02WA3NZ Revision of Intracardiac Pacemaker in Heart, Percutaneous Approach—AHA CC: 4Q, 2016, 96

02WAXRZ Revision of Short-term External Heart Assist System in Heart, External Approach—AHA CC: 1Q, 2018, 17

02WY33Z Revision of Infusion Device in Great Vessel, Percutaneous Approach—AHA CC: 3Q, 2018, 9-10

02YA0Z0 Transplantation of Heart, Allogeneic, Open Approach—AHA CC: 3Q, 2013, 18-19

Arteries

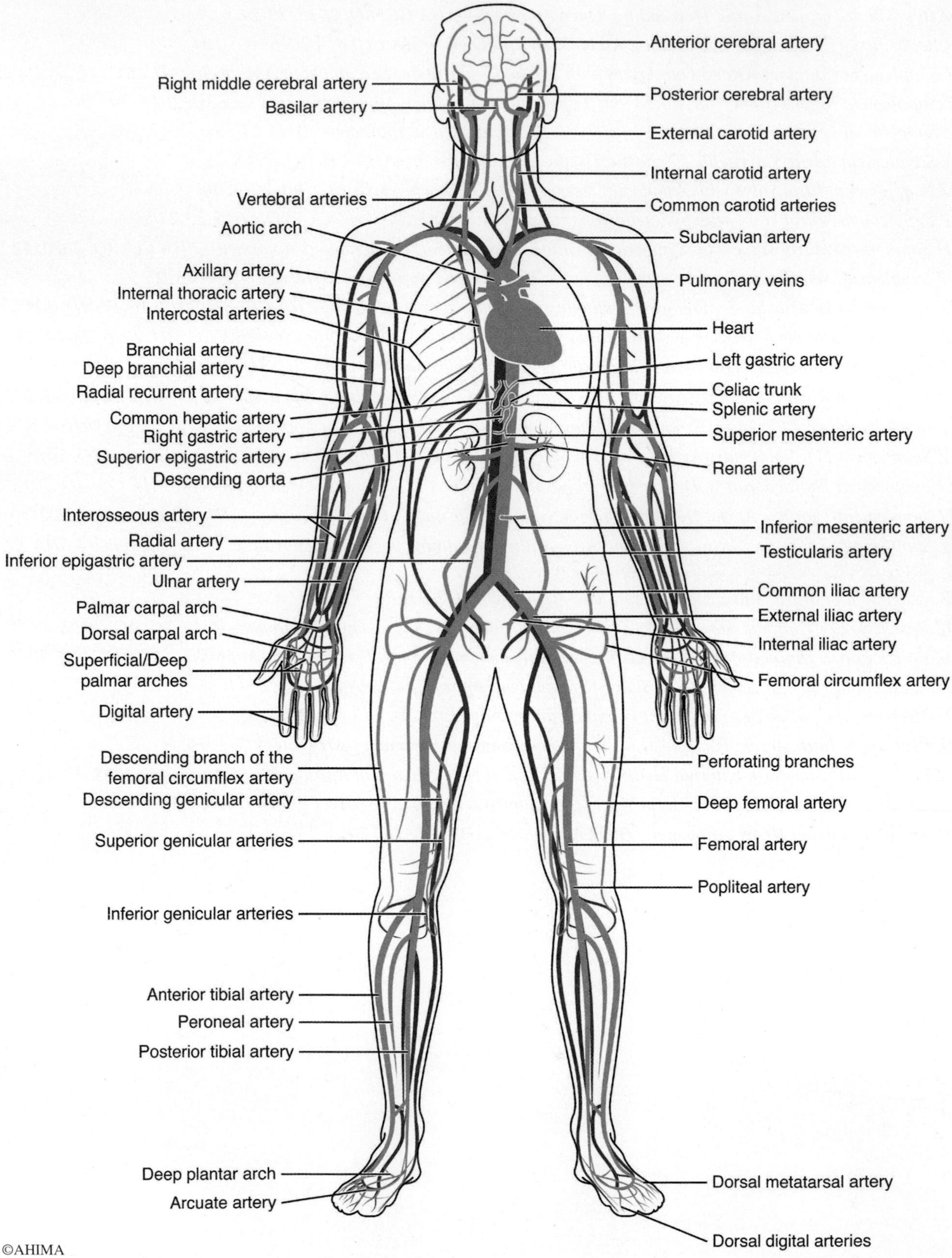
Anterior cerebral artery
Right middle cerebral artery
Posterior cerebral artery
Basilar artery
External carotid artery
Internal carotid artery
Vertebral arteries
Common carotid arteries
Aortic arch
Subclavian artery
Axillary artery
Pulmonary veins
Internal thoracic artery
Intercostal arteries
Heart
Branchial artery
Deep branchial artery
Left gastric artery
Radial recurrent artery
Celiac trunk
Splenic artery
Common hepatic artery
Right gastric artery
Superior mesenteric artery
Superior epigastric artery
Renal artery
Descending aorta
Interosseous artery
Inferior mesenteric artery
Radial artery
Testicularis artery
Inferior epigastric artery
Ulnar artery
Common iliac artery
Palmar carpal arch
External iliac artery
Dorsal carpal arch
Internal iliac artery
Superficial/Deep palmar arches
Femoral circumflex artery
Digital artery
Descending branch of the femoral circumflex artery
Perforating branches
Descending genicular artery
Deep femoral artery
Superior genicular arteries
Femoral artery
Popliteal artery
Inferior genicular arteries
Anterior tibial artery
Peroneal artery
Posterior tibial artery
Deep plantar arch
Dorsal metatarsal artery
Arcuate artery
Dorsal digital arteries

Arterial Anastomosis Around Elbow

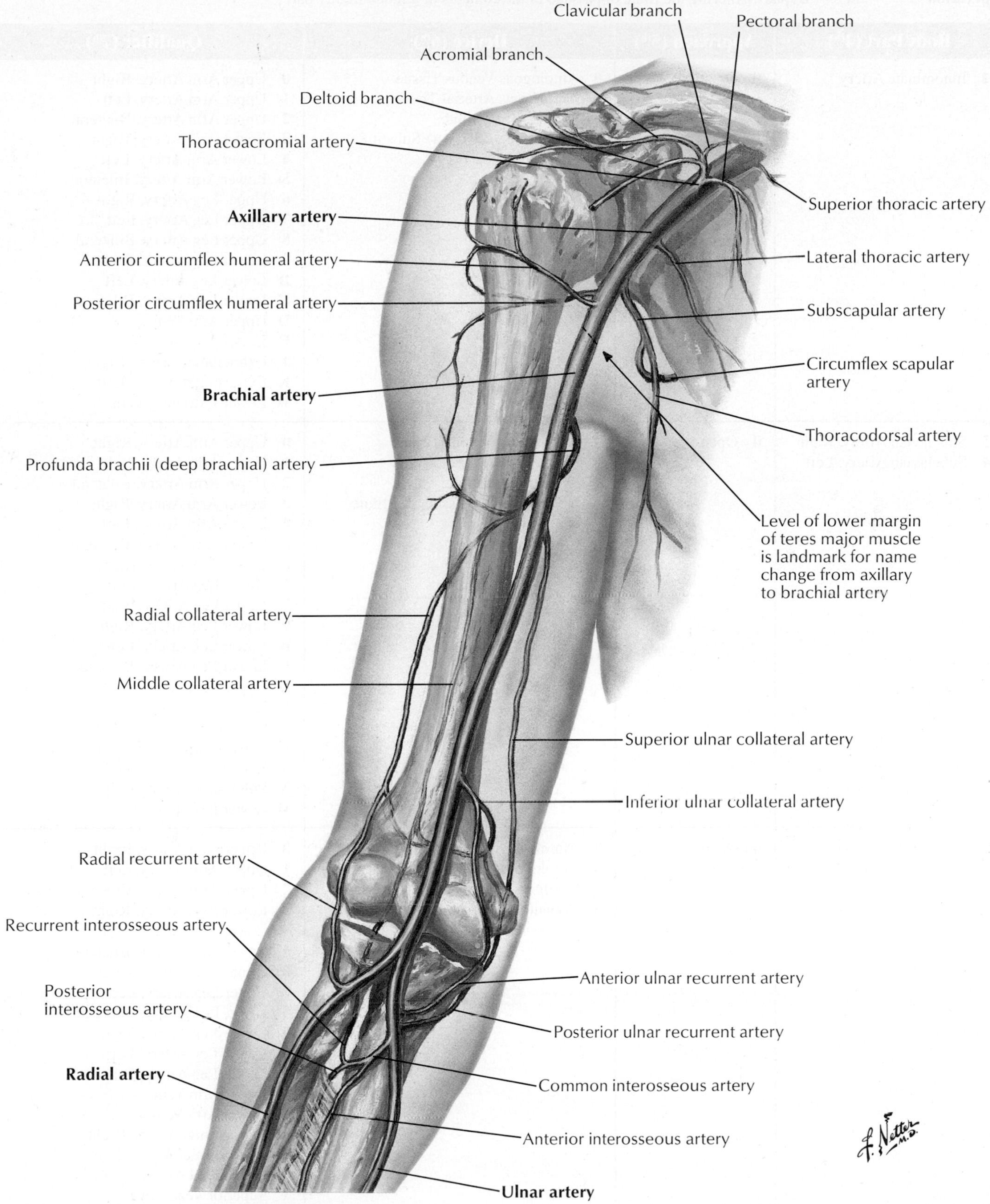
Clavicular branch
Pectoral branch
Acromial branch
Deltoid branch
Thoracoacromial artery
Superior thoracic artery
Axillary artery
Lateral thoracic artery
Anterior circumflex humeral artery
Posterior circumflex humeral artery
Subscapular artery
Circumflex scapular artery
Brachial artery
Thoracodorsal artery
Profunda brachii (deep brachial) artery
Level of lower margin of teres major muscle is landmark for name change from axillary to brachial artery
Radial collateral artery
Middle collateral artery
Superior ulnar collateral artery
Inferior ulnar collateral artery
Radial recurrent artery
Recurrent interosseous artery
Anterior ulnar recurrent artery
Posterior interosseous artery
Posterior ulnar recurrent artery
Radial artery
Common interosseous artery
Anterior interosseous artery
Ulnar artery

Section 0 **Medical and Surgical**
Body System 3 **Upper Arteries**
Operation 1 **Bypass:** Altering the route of passage of the contents of a tubular body part

Body Part (4th)	Approach (5th)	Device (6th)	Qualifier (7th)
2 Innominate Artery	0 Open	9 Autologous Venous Tissue A Autologous Arterial Tissue J Synthetic Substitute K Nonautologous Tissue Substitute Z No Device	0 Upper Arm Artery, Right 1 Upper Arm Artery, Left 2 Upper Arm Artery, Bilateral 3 Lower Arm Artery, Right 4 Lower Arm Artery, Left 5 Lower Arm Artery, Bilateral 6 Upper Leg Artery, Right 7 Upper Leg Artery, Left 8 Upper Leg Artery, Bilateral 9 Lower Leg Artery, Right B Lower Leg Artery, Left C Lower Leg Artery, Bilateral D Upper Arm Vein F Lower Arm Vein J Extracranial Artery, Right K Extracranial Artery, Left W Lower Extremity Vein
3 Subclavian Artery, Right 4 Subclavian Artery, Left	0 Open	9 Autologous Venous Tissue A Autologous Arterial Tissue J Synthetic Substitute K Nonautologous Tissue Substitute Z No Device	0 Upper Arm Artery, Right 1 Upper Arm Artery, Left 2 Upper Arm Artery, Bilateral 3 Lower Arm Artery, Right 4 Lower Arm Artery, Left 5 Lower Arm Artery, Bilateral 6 Upper Leg Artery, Right 7 Upper Leg Artery, Left 8 Upper Leg Artery, Bilateral 9 Lower Leg Artery, Right B Lower Leg Artery, Left C Lower Leg Artery, Bilateral D Upper Arm Vein F Lower Arm Vein J Extracranial Artery, Right K Extracranial Artery, Left M Pulmonary Artery, Right N Pulmonary Artery, Left W Lower Extremity Vein
5 Axillary Artery, Right 6 Axillary Artery, Left	0 Open	9 Autologous Venous Tissue A Autologous Arterial Tissue J Synthetic Substitute K Nonautologous Tissue Substitute Z No Device	0 Upper Arm Artery, Right 1 Upper Arm Artery, Left 2 Upper Arm Artery, Bilateral 3 Lower Arm Artery, Right 4 Lower Arm Artery, Left 5 Lower Arm Artery, Bilateral 6 Upper Leg Artery, Right 7 Upper Leg Artery, Left 8 Upper Leg Artery, Bilateral 9 Lower Leg Artery, Right B Lower Leg Artery, Left C Lower Leg Artery, Bilateral D Upper Arm Vein F Lower Arm Vein J Extracranial Artery, Right K Extracranial Artery, Left T Abdominal Artery V Superior Vena Cava W Lower Extremity Vein

Continued →

Section 0 **Medical and Surgical**
Body System 3 **Upper Arteries**
Operation 1 **Bypass:** Altering the route of passage of the contents of a tubular body part

Body Part (4th)	Approach (5th)	Device (6th)	Qualifier (7th)
7 Brachial Artery, Right	**0** Open	**9** Autologous Venous Tissue **A** Autologous Arterial Tissue **J** Synthetic Substitute **K** Nonautologous Tissue Substitute **Z** No Device	**0** Upper Arm Artery, Right **3** Lower Arm Artery, Right **D** Upper Arm Vein **F** Lower Arm Vein **V** Superior Vena Cava **W** Lower Extremity Vein
7 Brachial Artery, Right	**3** Percutaneous	**Z** No Device	**F** Lower Arm Vein
8 Brachial Artery, Left	**0** Open	**9** Autologous Venous Tissue **A** Autologous Arterial Tissue **J** Synthetic Substitute **K** Nonautologous Tissue Substitute **Z** No Device	**1** Upper Arm Artery, Left **4** Lower Arm Artery, Left **D** Upper Arm Vein **F** Lower Arm Vein **V** Superior Vena Cava **W** Lower Extremity Vein
8 Brachial Artery, Left	**3** Percutaneous	**Z** No Device	**F** Lower Arm Vein
9 Ulnar Artery, Right **B** Radial Artery, Right	**0** Open	**9** Autologous Venous Tissue **A** Autologous Arterial Tissue **J** Synthetic Substitute **K** Nonautologous Tissue Substitute **Z** No Device	**3** Lower Arm Artery, Right **F** Lower Arm Vein
9 Ulnar Artery, Right **B** Radial Artery, Right	**3** Percutaneous	**Z** No Device	**F** Lower Arm Vein
A Ulnar Artery, Left **C** Radial Artery, Left	**0** Open	**9** Autologous Venous Tissue **A** Autologous Arterial Tissue **J** Synthetic Substitute **K** Nonautologous Tissue Substitute **Z** No Device	**4** Lower Arm Artery, Left **F** Lower Arm Vein
A Ulnar Artery, Left **C** Radial Artery, Left	**3** Percutaneous	**Z** No Device	**F** Lower Arm Vein
G Intracranial Artery **S** Temporal Artery, Right **T** Temporal Artery, Left	**0** Open	**9** Autologous Venous Tissue **A** Autologous Arterial Tissue **J** Synthetic Substitute **K** Nonautologous Tissue Substitute **Z** No Device	**G** Intracranial Artery
H Common Carotid Artery, Right **J** Common Carotid Artery, Left	**0** Open	**9** Autologous Venous Tissue **A** Autologous Arterial Tissue **J** Synthetic Substitute **K** Nonautologous Tissue Substitute **Z** No Device	**G** Intracranial Artery **J** Extracranial Artery, Right **K** Extracranial Artery, Left **Y** Upper Artery
K Internal Carotid Artery, Right **L** Internal Carotid Artery, Left **M** External Carotid Artery, Right **N** External Carotid Artery, Left	**0** Open	**9** Autologous Venous Tissue **A** Autologous Arterial Tissue **J** Synthetic Substitute **K** Nonautologous Tissue Substitute **Z** No Device	**J** Extracranial Artery, Right **K** Extracranial Artery, Left

Section	**0**	**Medical and Surgical**
Body System	**3**	**Upper Arteries**
Operation	**5**	**Destruction:** Physical eradication of all or a portion of a body part by the direct use of energy, force, or a destructive agent

Body Part (4th)	Approach (5th)	Device (6th)	Qualifier (7th)
0 Internal Mammary Artery, Right **1** Internal Mammary Artery, Left **2** Innominate Artery **3** Subclavian Artery, Right **4** Subclavian Artery, Left **5** Axillary Artery, Right **6** Axillary Artery, Left **7** Brachial Artery, Right **8** Brachial Artery, Left **9** Ulnar Artery, Right **A** Ulnar Artery, Left **B** Radial Artery, Right **C** Radial Artery, Left **D** Hand Artery, Right **F** Hand Artery, Left **G** Intracranial Artery **H** Common Carotid Artery, Right **J** Common Carotid Artery, Left **K** Internal Carotid Artery, Right **L** Internal Carotid Artery, Left **M** External Carotid Artery, Right **N** External Carotid Artery, Left **P** Vertebral Artery, Right **Q** Vertebral Artery, Left **R** Face Artery **S** Temporal Artery, Right **T** Temporal Artery, Left **U** Thyroid Artery, Right **V** Thyroid Artery, Left **Y** Upper Artery	**0** Open **3** Percutaneous **4** Percutaneous Endoscopic	**Z** No Device	**Z** No Qualifier

Section 0 **Medical and Surgical**
Body System 3 **Upper Arteries**
Operation 7 **Dilation:** Expanding an orifice or the lumen of a tubular body part

Body Part (4th)	Approach (5th)	Device (6th)	Qualifier (7th)
0 Internal Mammary Artery, Right **1** Internal Mammary Artery, Left **2** Innominate Artery **3** Subclavian Artery, Right **4** Subclavian Artery, Left **5** Axillary Artery, Right **6** Axillary Artery, Left **7** Brachial Artery, Right **8** Brachial Artery, Left **9** Ulnar Artery, Right **A** Ulnar Artery, Left **B** Radial Artery, Right **C** Radial Artery, Left	**0** Open **3** Percutaneous **4** Percutaneous Endoscopic	**4** Intraluminal Device, Drug-eluting **5** Intraluminal Device, Drug-eluting, Two **6** Intraluminal Device, Drug-eluting, Three **7** Intraluminal Device, Drug-eluting, Four or More **E** Intraluminal Devices, Two **F** Intraluminal Devices, Three **G** Intraluminal Devices, Four or More	**Z** No Qualifier
0 Internal Mammary Artery, Right **1** Internal Mammary Artery, Left **2** Innominate Artery **3** Subclavian Artery, Right **4** Subclavian Artery, Left **5** Axillary Artery, Right **6** Axillary Artery, Left **7** Brachial Artery, Right **8** Brachial Artery, Left **9** Ulnar Artery, Right **A** Ulnar Artery, Left **B** Radial Artery, Right **C** Radial Artery, Left	**0** Open **3** Percutaneous **4** Percutaneous Endoscopic	**D** Intraluminal Device **Z** No Device	**1** Drug-Coated Balloon **Z** No Qualifier
D Hand Artery, Right **F** Hand Artery, Left **G** Intracranial Artery **H** Common Carotid Artery, Right **J** Common Carotid Artery, Left **K** Internal Carotid Artery, Right **L** Internal Carotid Artery, Left **M** External Carotid Artery, Right **N** External Carotid Artery, Left **P** Vertebral Artery, Right **Q** Vertebral Artery, Left **R** Face Artery **S** Temporal Artery, Right **T** Temporal Artery, Left **U** Thyroid Artery, Right **V** Thyroid Artery, Left **Y** Upper Artery	**0** Open **3** Percutaneous **4** Percutaneous Endoscopic	**4** Intraluminal Device, Drug-eluting **5** Intraluminal Device, Drug-eluting, Two **6** Intraluminal Device, Drug-eluting, Three **7** Intraluminal Device, Drug-eluting, Four or More **D** Intraluminal Device **E** Intraluminal Device, Two **F** Intraluminal Device, Three **G** Intraluminal Device, Four or More **Z** No Device	**Z** No Qualifier

Section **0** **Medical and Surgical**
Body System **3** **Upper Arteries**
Operation **9** **Drainage:** Taking or letting out fluids and/or gases from a body part

Body Part (4th)	Approach (5th)	Device (6th)	Qualifier (7th)
0 Internal Mammary Artery, Right **1** Internal Mammary Artery, Left **2** Innominate Artery **3** Subclavian Artery, Right **4** Subclavian Artery, Left **5** Axillary Artery, Right **6** Axillary Artery, Left **7** Brachial Artery, Right **8** Brachial Artery, Left **9** Ulnar Artery, Right **A** Ulnar Artery, Left **B** Radial Artery, Right **C** Radial Artery, Left **D** Hand Artery, Right **F** Hand Artery, Left **G** Intracranial Artery **H** Common Carotid Artery, Right **J** Common Carotid Artery, Left **K** Internal Carotid Artery, Right **L** Internal Carotid Artery, Left **M** External Carotid Artery, Right **N** External Carotid Artery, Left **P** Vertebral Artery, Right **Q** Vertebral Artery, Left **R** Face Artery **S** Temporal Artery, Right **T** Temporal Artery, Left **U** Thyroid Artery, Right **V** Thyroid Artery, Left **Y** Upper Artery	**0** Open **3** Percutaneous **4** Percutaneous Endoscopic	**0** Drainage Device	**Z** No Qualifier
0 Internal Mammary Artery, Right **1** Internal Mammary Artery, Left **2** Innominate Artery **3** Subclavian Artery, Right **4** Subclavian Artery, Left **5** Axillary Artery, Right **6** Axillary Artery, Left **7** Brachial Artery, Right **8** Brachial Artery, Left **9** Ulnar Artery, Right **A** Ulnar Artery, Left **B** Radial Artery, Right **C** Radial Artery, Left **D** Hand Artery, Right **F** Hand Artery, Left **G** Intracranial Artery **H** Common Carotid Artery, Right **J** Common Carotid Artery, Left **K** Internal Carotid Artery, Right **L** Internal Carotid Artery, Left **M** External Carotid Artery, Right **N** External Carotid Artery, Left **P** Vertebral Artery, Right **Q** Vertebral Artery, Left **R** Face Artery **S** Temporal Artery, Right **T** Temporal Artery, Left **U** Thyroid Artery, Right **V** Thyroid Artery, Left **Y** Upper Artery	**0** Open **3** Percutaneous **4** Percutaneous Endoscopic	**Z** No Device	**X** Diagnostic **Z** No Qualifier

Section 0 Medical and Surgical
Body System 3 Upper Arteries
Operation B **Excision:** Cutting out or off, without replacement, a portion of a body part

Body Part (4th)	Approach (5th)	Device (6th)	Qualifier (7th)
0 Internal Mammary Artery, Right **1** Internal Mammary Artery, Left **2** Innominate Artery **3** Subclavian Artery, Right **4** Subclavian Artery, Left **5** Axillary Artery, Right **6** Axillary Artery, Left **7** Brachial Artery, Right **8** Brachial Artery, Left **9** Ulnar Artery, Right **A** Ulnar Artery, Left **B** Radial Artery, Right **C** Radial Artery, Left **D** Hand Artery, Right **F** Hand Artery, Left **G** Intracranial Artery **H** Common Carotid Artery, Right **J** Common Carotid Artery, Left **K** Internal Carotid Artery, Right **L** Internal Carotid Artery, Left **M** External Carotid Artery, Right **N** External Carotid Artery, Left **P** Vertebral Artery, Right **Q** Vertebral Artery, Left **R** Face Artery **S** Temporal Artery, Right **T** Temporal Artery, Left **U** Thyroid Artery, Right **V** Thyroid Artery, Left **Y** Upper Artery	**0** Open **3** Percutaneous **4** Percutaneous Endoscopic	**Z** No Device	**X** Diagnostic **Z** No Qualifier

Section 0 Medical and Surgical
Body System 3 Upper Arteries
Operation C **Extirpation:** Taking or cutting out solid matter from a body part

Body Part (4th)	Approach (5th)	Device (6th)	Qualifier (7th)
0 Internal Mammary Artery, Right **1** Internal Mammary Artery, Left **2** Innominate Artery **3** Subclavian Artery, Right **4** Subclavian Artery, Left **5** Axillary Artery, Right **6** Axillary Artery, Left **7** Brachial Artery, Right **8** Brachial Artery, Left **9** Ulnar Artery, Right **A** Ulnar Artery, Left **B** Radial Artery, Right **C** Radial Artery, Left **D** Hand Artery, Right **F** Hand Artery, Left **R** Face Artery **S** Temporal Artery, Right **T** Temporal Artery, Left **U** Thyroid Artery, Right **V** Thyroid Artery, Left **Y** Upper Artery	**0** Open **3** Percutaneous **4** Percutaneous Endoscopic	**Z** No Device	**Z** No Qualifier

Continued →

Section 0 **Medical and Surgical**
Body System 3 **Upper Arteries**
Operation C **Extirpation:** Taking or cutting out solid matter from a body part

Body Part (4th)	Approach (5th)	Device (6th)	Qualifier (7th)
G Intracranial Artery H Common Carotid Artery, Right J Common Carotid Artery, Left K Internal Carotid Artery, Right L Internal Carotid Artery, Left M External Carotid Artery, Right N External Carotid Artery, Left P Vertebral Artery, Right Q Vertebral Artery, Left	0 Open 4 Percutaneous Endoscopic	Z No Device	Z No Qualifier
G Intracranial Artery H Common Carotid Artery, Right J Common Carotid Artery, Left K Internal Carotid Artery, Right L Internal Carotid Artery, Left M External Carotid Artery, Right N External Carotid Artery, Left P Vertebral Artery, Right Q Vertebral Artery, Left	3 Percutaneous	Z No Device	**7** Stent Retriever **Z** No Qualifier

Section 0 **Medical and Surgical**
Body System 3 **Upper Arteries**
Operation F **Fragmentation:** Breaking solid matter in a body part into pieces

Body Part (4th)	Approach (5th)	Device (6th)	Qualifier (7th)
2 Innominate Artery **3** Subclavian Artery, Right **4** Subclavian Artery, Left **5** Axillary Artery, Right **6** Axillary Artery, Left **7** Brachial Artery, Right **8** Brachial Artery, Left **9** Ulnar Artery, Right **A** Ulnar Artery, Left **B** Radial Artery, Right **C** Radial Artery, Left **G** Intracranial Artery **Y** Upper Artery	**3** Percutaneous	**Z** No Device	**0** Ultrasonic **Z** No Qualifier

Section 0 **Medical and Surgical**
Body System 3 **Upper Arteries**
Operation H **Insertion:** Putting in a nonbiological appliance that monitors, assists, performs, or prevents a physiological function but does not physically take the place of a body part

Body Part (4th)	Approach (5th)	Device (6th)	Qualifier (7th)
0 Internal Mammary Artery, Right **1** Internal Mammary Artery, Left **2** Innominate Artery **3** Subclavian Artery, Right **4** Subclavian Artery, Left **5** Axillary Artery, Right **6** Axillary Artery, Left **7** Brachial Artery, Right **8** Brachial Artery, Left **9** Ulnar Artery, Right **A** Ulnar Artery, Left **B** Radial Artery, Right **C** Radial Artery, Left **D** Hand Artery, Right **F** Hand Artery, Left **G** Intracranial Artery **H** Common Carotid Artery, Right **J** Common Carotid Artery, Left **M** External Carotid Artery, Right **N** External Carotid Artery, Left **P** Vertebral Artery, Right **Q** Vertebral Artery, Left **R** Face Artery **S** Temporal Artery, Right **T** Temporal Artery, Left **U** Thyroid Artery, Right **V** Thyroid Artery, Left	**0** Open **3** Percutaneous **4** Percutaneous Endoscopic	**3** Infusion Device **D** Intraluminal Device	**Z** No Qualifier
K Internal Carotid Artery, Right **L** Internal Carotid Artery, Left	**0** Open **3** Percutaneous **4** Percutaneous Endoscopic	**3** Infusion Device **D** Intraluminal Device **M** Stimulator Lead	**Z** No Qualifier
Y Upper Artery	**0** Open **3** Percutaneous **4** Percutaneous Endoscopic	**2** Monitoring Device **3** Infusion Device **D** Intraluminal Device **Y** Other Device	**Z** No Qualifier

Section 0 **Medical and Surgical**
Body System 3 **Upper Arteries**
Operation J **Inspection:** Visually and/or manually exploring a body part

Body Part (4th)	Approach (5th)	Device (6th)	Qualifier (7th)
Y Upper Artery	**0** Open **3** Percutaneous **4** Percutaneous Endoscopic **X** External	**Z** No Device	**Z** No Qualifier

Section 0 **Medical and Surgical**
Body System 3 **Upper Arteries**
Operation L **Occlusion:** Completely closing an orifice or the lumen of a tubular body part

Body Part (4th)	Approach (5th)	Device (6th)	Qualifier (7th)
0 Internal Mammary Artery, Right **1** Internal Mammary Artery, Left **2** Innominate Artery **3** Subclavian Artery, Right **4** Subclavian Artery, Left **5** Axillary Artery, Right **6** Axillary Artery, Left **7** Brachial Artery, Right **8** Brachial Artery, Left **9** Ulnar Artery, Right **A** Ulnar Artery, Left **B** Radial Artery, Right **C** Radial Artery, Left **D** Hand Artery, Right **F** Hand Artery, Left **R** Face Artery **S** Temporal Artery, Right **T** Temporal Artery, Left **U** Thyroid Artery, Right **V** Thyroid Artery, Left **Y** Upper Artery	**0** Open **3** Percutaneous **4** Percutaneous Endoscopic	**C** Extraluminal Device **D** Intraluminal Device **Z** No Device	**Z** No Qualifier
G Intracranial Artery **H** Common Carotid Artery, Right **J** Common Carotid Artery, Left **K** Internal Carotid Artery, Right **L** Internal Carotid Artery, Left **M** External Carotid Artery, Right **N** External Carotid Artery, Left **P** Vertebral Artery, Right **Q** Vertebral Artery, Left	**0** Open **3** Percutaneous **4** Percutaneous Endoscopic	**B** Intraluminal Device, Bioactive **C** Extraluminal Device **D** Intraluminal Device **Z** No Device	**Z** No Qualifier

Section 0 **Medical and Surgical**
Body System 3 **Upper Arteries**
Operation N **Release:** Freeing a body part from an abnormal physical constraint by cutting or by the use of force

Body Part (4th)	Approach (5th)	Device (6th)	Qualifier (7th)
0 Internal Mammary Artery, Right **1** Internal Mammary Artery, Left **2** Innominate Artery **3** Subclavian Artery, Right **4** Subclavian Artery, Left **5** Axillary Artery, Right **6** Axillary Artery, Left **7** Brachial Artery, Right **8** Brachial Artery, Left **9** Ulnar Artery, Right **A** Ulnar Artery, Left **B** Radial Artery, Right **C** Radial Artery, Left **D** Hand Artery, Right **F** Hand Artery, Left **G** Intracranial Artery **H** Common Carotid Artery, Right **J** Common Carotid Artery, Left **K** Internal Carotid Artery, Right **L** Internal Carotid Artery, Left **M** External Carotid Artery, Right **N** External Carotid Artery, Left **P** Vertebral Artery, Right **Q** Vertebral Artery, Left **R** Face Artery **S** Temporal Artery, Right **T** Temporal Artery, Left **U** Thyroid Artery, Right **V** Thyroid Artery, Left **Y** Upper Artery	**0** Open **3** Percutaneous **4** Percutaneous Endoscopic	**Z** No Device	**Z** No Qualifier

Section 0 **Medical and Surgical**
Body System 3 **Upper Arteries**
Operation P **Removal:** Taking out or off a device from a body part

Body Part (4th)	Approach (5th)	Device (6th)	Qualifier (7th)
Y Upper Artery	**0** Open **3** Percutaneous **4** Percutaneous Endoscopic	**0** Drainage Device **2** Monitoring Device **3** Infusion Device **7** Autologous Tissue Substitute **C** Extraluminal Device **D** Intraluminal Device **J** Synthetic Substitute **K** Nonautologous Tissue Substitute **M** Stimulator Lead **Y** Other Device	**Z** No Qualifier
Y Upper Artery	**X** External	**0** Drainage Device **2** Monitoring Device **3** Infusion Device **D** Intraluminal Device **M** Stimulator Lead	**Z** No Qualifier

Section 0 **Medical and Surgical**
Body System 3 **Upper Arteries**
Operation Q **Repair:** Restoring, to the extent possible, a body part to its normal anatomic structure and function

Body Part (4th)	Approach (5th)	Device (6th)	Qualifier (7th)
0 Internal Mammary Artery, Right **1** Internal Mammary Artery, Left **2** Innominate Artery **3** Subclavian Artery, Right **4** Subclavian Artery, Left **5** Axillary Artery, Right **6** Axillary Artery, Left **7** Brachial Artery, Right **8** Brachial Artery, Left **9** Ulnar Artery, Right **A** Ulnar Artery, Left **B** Radial Artery, Right **C** Radial Artery, Left **D** Hand Artery, Right **F** Hand Artery, Left **G** Intracranial Artery **H** Common Carotid Artery, Right **J** Common Carotid Artery, Left **K** Internal Carotid Artery, Right **L** Internal Carotid Artery, Left **M** External Carotid Artery, Right **N** External Carotid Artery, Left **P** Vertebral Artery, Right **Q** Vertebral Artery, Left **R** Face Artery **S** Temporal Artery, Right **T** Temporal Artery, Left **U** Thyroid Artery, Right **V** Thyroid Artery, Left **Y** Upper Artery	**0** Open **3** Percutaneous **4** Percutaneous Endoscopic	**Z** No Device	**Z** No Qualifier

Section 0 **Medical and Surgical**
Body System 3 **Upper Arteries**
Operation R **Replacement:** Putting in or on biological or synthetic material that physically takes the place and/or function of all or a portion of a body part

Body Part (4th)	Approach (5th)	Device (6th)	Qualifier (7th)
0 Internal Mammary Artery, Right **1** Internal Mammary Artery, Left **2** Innominate Artery **3** Subclavian Artery, Right **4** Subclavian Artery, Left **5** Axillary Artery, Right **6** Axillary Artery, Left **7** Brachial Artery, Right **8** Brachial Artery, Left **9** Ulnar Artery, Right **A** Ulnar Artery, Left **B** Radial Artery, Right **C** Radial Artery, Left **D** Hand Artery, Right **F** Hand Artery, Left **G** Intracranial Artery **H** Common Carotid Artery, Right **J** Common Carotid Artery, Left **K** Internal Carotid Artery, Right **L** Internal Carotid Artery, Left **M** External Carotid Artery, Right **N** External Carotid Artery, Left **P** Vertebral Artery, Right **Q** Vertebral Artery, Left **R** Face Artery **S** Temporal Artery, Right **T** Temporal Artery, Left **U** Thyroid Artery, Right **V** Thyroid Artery, Left **Y** Upper Artery	**0** Open **4** Percutaneous Endoscopic	**7** Autologous Tissue Substitute **J** Synthetic Substitute **K** Nonautologous Tissue Substitute	**Z** No Qualifier

Section 0 **Medical and Surgical**
Body System 3 **Upper Arteries**
Operation S **Reposition:** Moving to its normal location, or other suitable location, all or a portion of a body part

Body Part (4th)	Approach (5th)	Device (6th)	Qualifier (7th)
0 Internal Mammary Artery, Right **1** Internal Mammary Artery, Left **2** Innominate Artery **3** Subclavian Artery, Right **4** Subclavian Artery, Left **5** Axillary Artery, Right **6** Axillary Artery, Left **7** Brachial Artery, Right **8** Brachial Artery, Left **9** Ulnar Artery, Right **A** Ulnar Artery, Left **B** Radial Artery, Right **C** Radial Artery, Left **D** Hand Artery, Right **F** Hand Artery, Left **G** Intracranial Artery **H** Common Carotid Artery, Right **J** Common Carotid Artery, Left **K** Internal Carotid Artery, Right **L** Internal Carotid Artery, Left **M** External Carotid Artery, Right **N** External Carotid Artery, Left **P** Vertebral Artery, Right **Q** Vertebral Artery, Left **R** Face Artery **S** Temporal Artery, Right **T** Temporal Artery, Left **U** Thyroid Artery, Right **V** Thyroid Artery, Left **Y** Upper Artery	**0** Open **3** Percutaneous **4** Percutaneous Endoscopic	**Z** No Device	**Z** No Qualifier

Section 0 **Medical and Surgical**
Body System 3 **Upper Arteries**
Operation U **Supplement:** Putting in or on biological or synthetic material that physically reinforces and/or augments the function of a portion of a body part

Body Part (4th)	Approach (5th)	Device (6th)	Qualifier (7th)
0 Internal Mammary Artery, Right **1** Internal Mammary Artery, Left **2** Innominate Artery **3** Subclavian Artery, Right **4** Subclavian Artery, Left **5** Axillary Artery, Right **6** Axillary Artery, Left **7** Brachial Artery, Right **8** Brachial Artery, Left **9** Ulnar Artery, Right **A** Ulnar Artery, Left **B** Radial Artery, Right **C** Radial Artery, Left **D** Hand Artery, Right **F** Hand Artery, Left **G** Intracranial Artery **H** Common Carotid Artery, Right **J** Common Carotid Artery, Left **K** Internal Carotid Artery, Right **L** Internal Carotid Artery, Left **M** External Carotid Artery, Right **N** External Carotid Artery, Left **P** Vertebral Artery, Right **Q** Vertebral Artery, Left **R** Face Artery **S** Temporal Artery, Right **T** Temporal Artery, Left **U** Thyroid Artery, Right **V** Thyroid Artery, Left **Y** Upper Artery	**0** Open **3** Percutaneous **4** Percutaneous Endoscopic	**7** Autologous Tissue Substitute **J** Synthetic Substitute **K** Nonautologous Tissue Substitute	**Z** No Qualifier

Section 0 **Medical and Surgical**
Body System 3 **Upper Arteries**
Operation V **Restriction:** Partially closing an orifice or the lumen of a tubular body part

Body Part (4th)	Approach (5th)	Device (6th)	Qualifier (7th)
0 Internal Mammary Artery, Right **1** Internal Mammary Artery, Left **2** Innominate Artery **3** Subclavian Artery, Right **4** Subclavian Artery, Left **5** Axillary Artery, Right **6** Axillary Artery, Left **7** Brachial Artery, Right **8** Brachial Artery, Left **9** Ulnar Artery, Right **A** Ulnar Artery, Left **B** Radial Artery, Right **C** Radial Artery, Left **D** Hand Artery, Right **F** Hand Artery, Left **R** Face Artery **S** Temporal Artery, Right **T** Temporal Artery, Left **U** Thyroid Artery, Right **V** Thyroid Artery, Left **Y** Upper Artery	**0** Open **3** Percutaneous **4** Percutaneous Endoscopic	**C** Extraluminal Device **D** Intraluminal Device **Z** No Device	**Z** No Qualifier
G Intracranial Artery **H** Common Carotid Artery, Right **J** Common Carotid Artery, Left **K** Internal Carotid Artery, Right **L** Internal Carotid Artery, Left **M** External Carotid Artery, Right **N** External Carotid Artery, Left **P** Vertebral Artery, Right **Q** Vertebral Artery, Left	**0** Open **3** Percutaneous **4** Percutaneous Endoscopic	**B** Intraluminal Device, Bioactive **C** Extraluminal Device **D** Intraluminal Device **H** Intraluminal Device, Flow Diverter **Z** No Device	**Z** No Qualifier

Section 0 **Medical and Surgical**
Body System 3 **Upper Arteries**
Operation W **Revision:** Correcting, to the extent possible, a portion of a malfunctioning device or the position of a displaced device

Body Part (4th)	Approach (5th)	Device (6th)	Qualifier (7th)
Y Upper Artery	**0** Open **3** Percutaneous **4** Percutaneous Endoscopic	**0** Drainage Device **2** Monitoring Device **3** Infusion Device **7** Autologous Tissue Substitute **C** Extraluminal Device **D** Intraluminal Device **J** Synthetic Substitute **K** Nonautologous Tissue Substitute **M** Stimulator Lead **Y** Other Device	**Z** No Qualifier
Y Upper Artery	**X** External	**0** Drainage Device **2** Monitoring Device **3** Infusion Device **7** Autologous Tissue Substitute **C** Extraluminal Device **D** Intraluminal Device **J** Synthetic Substitute **K** Nonautologous Tissue Substitute **M** Neurostimulator Lead	**Z** No Qualifier

AHA Coding Clinic

03170ZD Bypass Right Brachial Artery to Upper Arm Vein, Open Approach—AHA CC: 4Q, 2013, 125-126

03180JD Bypass Left Brachial Artery to Upper Arm Vein with Synthetic Substitute, Open Approach—AHA CC: 3Q, 2016, 37-38

031C0ZF Bypass Left Radial Artery to Lower Arm Vein, Open Approach—AHA CC: 1Q, 2013, 27-28

031J0JJ Bypass Left Common Carotid Artery to Right Extracranial Artery with Synthetic Substitute, Open Approach—AHA CC: 4Q, 2017, 65

031J0ZK Bypass Left Common Carotid Artery to Left Extracranial Artery, Open Approach—AHA CC: 2Q, 2017, 22

037K3DZ Dilation of Right Internal Carotid Artery with Intraluminal Device, Percutaneous Approach—AHA CC: 3Q, 2019, 29-30

03BN0ZZ Excision of Left External Carotid Artery, Open Approach—AHA CC: 2Q, 2016, 12-14

03C70ZZ Extirpation of Matter from Right Brachial Artery, Open Approach—AHA CC: 3Q, 2020, 38-40

03CK0ZZ Extirpation of Matter from Right Internal Carotid Artery, Open Approach—AHA CC: 2Q, 2016, 11-12

03CL0ZZ Extirpation of Matter from Left Internal Carotid Artery, Open Approach—AHA CC: 2Q, 2021, 13

03CN0ZZ Extirpation of Matter from Left External Carotid Artery, Open Approach—AHA CC: 4Q, 2017, 65

03H40DZ Insertion of Intraluminal Device into Left Subclavian Artery, Open Approach—AHA CC: 1Q, 2020, 25-27

03HY32Z Insertion of Monitoring Device into Upper Artery, Percutaneous Approach—AHA CC: 2Q, 2016, 32-33

03JY0ZZ Inspection of Upper Artery, Open Approach—AHA CC: 1Q, 2015, 29

03JY3ZZ Inspection of Upper Artery, Percutaneous Approach—AHA CC: 1Q, 2021, 16-17

03LG0CZ Occlusion of Intracranial Artery with Extraluminal Device, Open Approach—AHA CC: 2Q, 2016, 30

03LG3DZ Occlusion of Intracranial Artery with Intraluminal Device, Percutaneous Approach—AHA CC: 4Q, 2014, 37

03LL0ZZ Occlusion of Left Internal Carotid Artery, Open Approach—AHA CC: 2Q, 2021, 13

03QH0ZZ Repair Right Common Carotid Artery, Open Approach—AHA CC: 1Q, 2017, 31-32

03SS0ZZ Reposition Right Temporal Artery, Open Approach—AHA CC: 3Q, 2015, 27-28

03UK0JZ Supplement Right Internal Carotid Artery with Synthetic Substitute, Open Approach—AHA CC: 2Q, 2016, 11-12

03VG0CZ Restriction of Intracranial Artery with Extraluminal Device, Open Approach—AHA CC: 1Q, 2019, 22

03VG3DZ Restriction of Intracranial Artery with Intraluminal Device, Percutaneous Approach—AHA CC: 1Q, 2016, 19-20

03VM3DZ Restriction of Right External Carotid Artery with Intraluminal Device, Percutaneous Approach—AHA CC: 4Q, 2016, 26

03WY0JZ Revision of Synthetic Substitute in Upper Artery, Open Approach—AHA CC: 3Q, 2016, 39-40

03WY3DZ Revision of Intraluminal Device in Upper Artery, Percutaneous Approach—AHA CC: 1Q, 2015, 32-33

Arteries

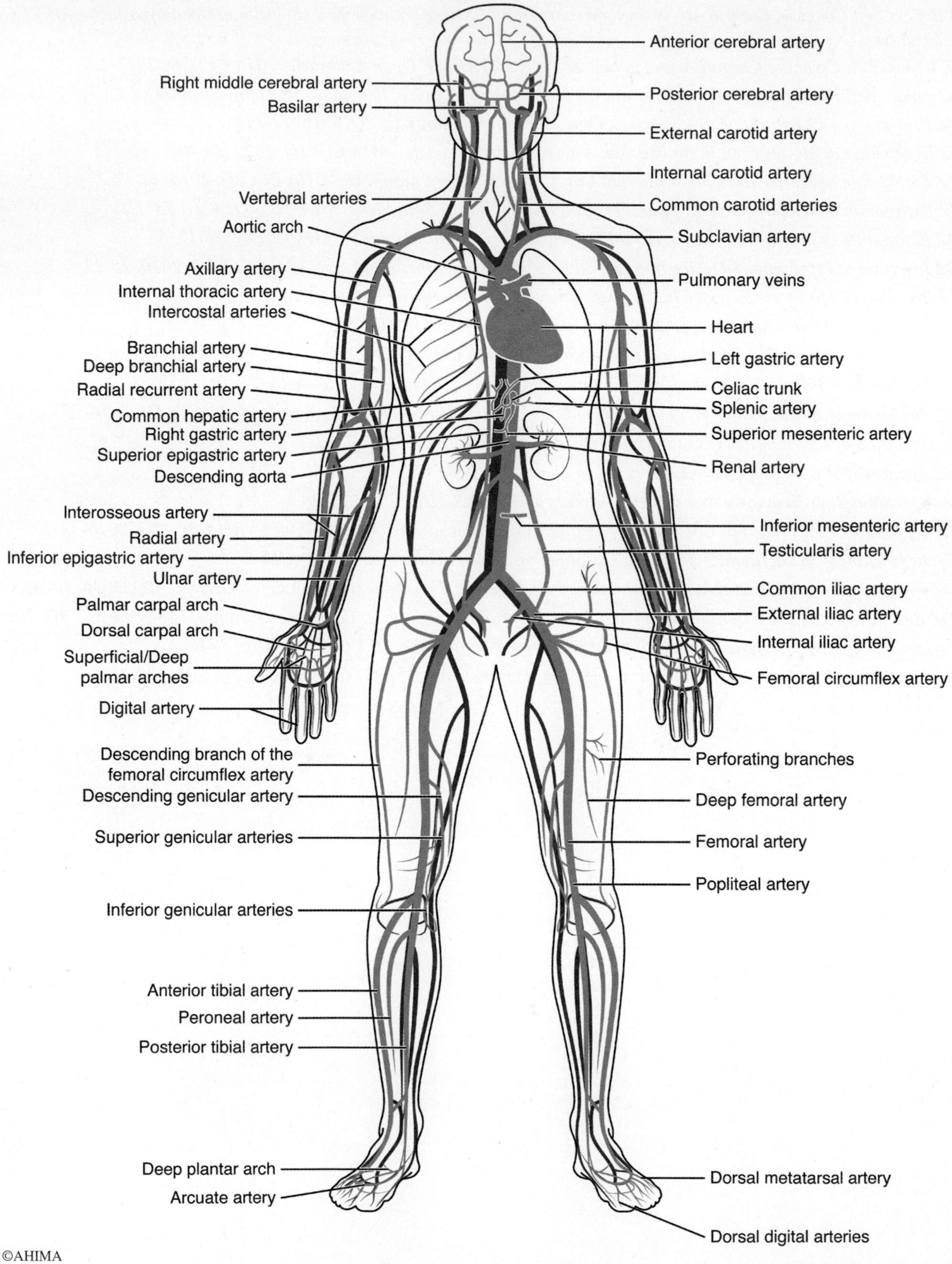
Anterior cerebral artery
Right middle cerebral artery
Posterior cerebral artery
Basilar artery
External carotid artery
Internal carotid artery
Vertebral arteries
Common carotid arteries
Aortic arch
Subclavian artery
Axillary artery
Pulmonary veins
Internal thoracic artery
Intercostal arteries
Heart
Branchial artery
Left gastric artery
Deep branchial artery
Radial recurrent artery
Celiac trunk
Splenic artery
Common hepatic artery
Superior mesenteric artery
Right gastric artery
Superior epigastric artery
Renal artery
Descending aorta
Interosseous artery
Inferior mesenteric artery
Radial artery
Testicularis artery
Inferior epigastric artery
Ulnar artery
Common iliac artery
Palmar carpal arch
External iliac artery
Dorsal carpal arch
Internal iliac artery
Superficial/Deep palmar arches
Femoral circumflex artery
Digital artery
Descending branch of the femoral circumflex artery
Perforating branches
Descending genicular artery
Deep femoral artery
Superior genicular arteries
Femoral artery
Popliteal artery
Inferior genicular arteries
Anterior tibial artery
Peroneal artery
Posterior tibial artery
Deep plantar arch
Dorsal metatarsal artery
Arcuate artery
Dorsal digital arteries

Lower Arteries Tables 041–04W

Section 0 **Medical and Surgical**
Body System 4 **Lower Arteries**
Operation 1 **Bypass:** Altering the route of passage of the contents of a tubular body part

Body Part (4th)	Approach (5th)	Device (6th)	Qualifier (7th)
0 Abdominal Aorta **C** Common Iliac Artery, Right **D** Common Iliac Artery, Left	**0** Open **4** Percutaneous Endoscopic	**9** Autologous Venous Tissue **A** Autologous Arterial Tissue **J** Synthetic Substitute **K** Nonautologous Tissue Substitute **Z** No Device	**0** Abdominal Aorta **1** Celiac Artery **2** Mesenteric Artery **3** Renal Artery, Right **4** Renal Artery, Left **5** Renal Artery, Bilateral **6** Common Iliac Artery, Right **7** Common Iliac Artery, Left **8** Common Iliac Arteries, Bilateral **9** Internal Iliac Artery, Right **B** Internal Iliac Artery, Left **C** Internal Iliac Arteries, Bilateral **D** External Iliac Artery, Right **F** External Iliac Artery, Left **G** External Iliac Arteries, Bilateral **H** Femoral Artery, Right **J** Femoral Artery, Left **K** Femoral Arteries, Bilateral **Q** Lower Extremity Artery **R** Lower Artery
3 Hepatic Artery **4** Splenic Artery	**0** Open **4** Percutaneous Endoscopic	**9** Autologous Venous Tissue **A** Autologous Arterial Tissue **J** Synthetic Substitute **K** Nonautologous Tissue Substitute **Z** No Device	**3** Renal Artery, Right **4** Renal Artery, Left **5** Renal Artery, Bilateral
E Internal Iliac Artery, Right **F** Internal Iliac Artery, Left **H** External Iliac Artery, Right **J** External Iliac Artery, Left	**0** Open **4** Percutaneous Endoscopic	**9** Autologous Venous Tissue **A** Autologous Arterial Tissue **J** Synthetic Substitute **K** Nonautologous Tissue Substitute **Z** No Device	**9** Internal Iliac Artery, Right **B** Internal Iliac Artery, Left **C** Internal Iliac Arteries, Bilateral **D** External Iliac Artery, Right **F** External Iliac Artery, Left **G** External Iliac Arteries, Bilateral **H** Femoral Artery, Right **J** Femoral Artery, Left **K** Femoral Arteries, Bilateral **P** Foot Artery **Q** Lower Extremity Artery
K Femoral Artery, Right **L** Femoral Artery, Left	**0** Open **4** Percutaneous Endoscopic	**9** Autologous Venous Tissue **A** Autologous Arterial Tissue **J** Synthetic Substitute **K** Nonautologous Tissue Substitute **Z** No Device	**H** Femoral Artery, Right **J** Femoral Artery, Left **K** Femoral Arteries, Bilateral **L** Popliteal Artery **M** Peroneal Artery **N** Posterior Tibial Artery **P** Foot Artery **Q** Lower Extremity Artery **S** Lower Extremity Vein
K Femoral Artery, Right **L** Femoral Artery, Left	**3** Percutaneous	**J** Synthetic Substitute	**Q** Lower Extremity Artery **S** Lower Extremity Vein
M Popliteal Artery, Right **N** Popliteal Artery, Left	**0** Open **4** Percutaneous Endoscopic	**9** Autologous Venous Tissue **A** Autologous Arterial Tissue **J** Synthetic Substitute **K** Nonautologous Tissue Substitute **Z** No Device	**L** Popliteal Artery **M** Peroneal Artery **P** Foot Artery **Q** Lower Extremity Artery **S** Lower Extremity Vein

Continued →

Section 0 Medical and Surgical
Body System 4 Lower Arteries
Operation 1 **Bypass:** Altering the route of passage of the contents of a tubular body part

Body Part (4th)	Approach (5th)	Device (6th)	Qualifier (7th)
M Popliteal Artery, Right **N** Popliteal Artery, Left	**3** Percutaneous	**J** Synthetic Substitute	**Q** Lower Extremity Artery **S** Lower Extremity Vein
P Anterior Tibial Artery, Right **Q** Anterior Tibial Artery, Left **R** Posterior Tibial Artery, Right **S** Posterior Tibial Artery, Left	**0** Open **3** Percutaneou **4** Percutaneous Endoscopic	**J** Synthetic Substitute	**Q** Lower Extremity Artery **S** Lower Extremity Vein
T Peroneal Artery, Right **U** Peroneal Artery, Left **V** Foot Artery, Right **W** Foot Artery, Left	**0** Open **4** Percutaneous Endoscopic	**9** Autologous Venous Tissue **A** Autologous Arterial Tissue **J** Synthetic Substitute **K** Nonautologous Tissue Substitute **Z** No Device	**P** Foot Artery **Q** Lower Extremity Artery **S** Lower Extremity Vein
T Peroneal Artery, Right **U** Peroneal Artery, Left **V** Foot Artery, Right **W** Foot Artery, Left	**3** Percutaneous	**J** Synthetic Substitute	**Q** Lower Extremity Artery **S** Lower Extremity Vein

Section 0 Medical and Surgical
Body System 4 Lower Arteries
Operation 5 **Destruction:** Physical eradication of all or a portion of a body part by the direct use of energy, force, or a destructive agent

Body Part (4th)	Approach (5th)	Device (6th)	Qualifier (7th)
0 Abdominal Aorta **1** Celiac Artery **2** Gastric Artery **3** Hepatic Artery **4** Splenic Artery **5** Superior Mesenteric Artery **6** Colic Artery, Right **7** Colic Artery, Left **8** Colic Artery, Middle **9** Renal Artery, Right **A** Renal Artery, Left **B** Inferior Mesenteric Artery **C** Common Iliac Artery, Right **D** Common Iliac Artery, Left **E** Internal Iliac Artery, Right **F** Internal Iliac Artery, Left **H** External Iliac Artery, Right **J** External Iliac Artery, Left **K** Femoral Artery, Right **L** Femoral Artery, Left **M** Popliteal Artery, Right **N** Popliteal Artery, Left **P** Anterior Tibial Artery, Right **Q** Anterior Tibial Artery, Left **R** Posterior Tibial Artery, Right **S** Posterior Tibial Artery, Left **T** Peroneal Artery, Right **U** Peroneal Artery, Left **V** Foot Artery, Right **W** Foot Artery, Left **Y** Lower Artery	**0** Open **3** Percutaneous **4** Percutaneous Endoscopic	**Z** No Device	**Z** No Qualifier

Section 0 **Medical and Surgical**
Body System 4 **Lower Arteries**
Operation 7 **Dilation:** Expanding an orifice or the lumen of a tubular body part

Body Part (4th)	Approach (5th)	Device (6th)	Qualifier (7th)
0 Abdominal Aorta **1** Celiac Artery **2** Gastric Artery **3** Hepatic Artery **4** Splenic Artery **5** Superior Mesenteric Artery **6** Colic Artery, Right **7** Colic Artery, Left **8** Colic Artery, Middle **9** Renal Artery, Right **A** Renal Artery, Left **B** Inferior Mesenteric Artery **C** Common Iliac Artery, Right **D** Common Iliac Artery, Left **E** Internal Iliac Artery, Right **F** Internal Iliac Artery, Left **H** External Iliac Artery, Right **J** External Iliac Artery, Left **K** Femoral Artery, Right **L** Femoral Artery, Left **M** Popliteal Artery, Right **N** Popliteal Artery, Left **P** Anterior Tibial Artery, Right **Q** Anterior Tibial Artery, Left **R** Posterior Tibial Artery, Right **S** Posterior Tibial Artery, Left **T** Peroneal Artery, Right **U** Peroneal Artery, Left **V** Foot Artery, Right **W** Foot Artery, Left **Y** Lower Artery	**0** Open **3** Percutaneous **4** Percutaneous Endoscopic	**4** Intraluminal Device, Drug-eluting **D** Intraluminal Device **Z** No Device	**1** Drug-Coated Balloon **Z** No Qualifier
0 Abdominal Aorta **1** Celiac Artery **2** Gastric Artery **3** Hepatic Artery **4** Splenic Artery **5** Superior Mesenteric Artery **6** Colic Artery, Right **7** Colic Artery, Left **8** Colic Artery, Middle **9** Renal Artery, Right **A** Renal Artery, Left **B** Inferior Mesenteric Artery **C** Common Iliac Artery, Right **D** Common Iliac Artery, Left **E** Internal Iliac Artery, Right **F** Internal Iliac Artery, Left **H** External Iliac Artery, Right **J** External Iliac Artery, Left **K** Femoral Artery, Right **L** Femoral Artery, Left **M** Popliteal Artery, Right **N** Popliteal Artery, Left **P** Anterior Tibial Artery, Right **Q** Anterior Tibial Artery, Left **R** Posterior Tibial Artery, Right **S** Posterior Tibial Artery, Left **T** Peroneal Artery, Right **U** Peroneal Artery, Left **V** Foot Artery, Right **W** Foot Artery, Left **Y** Lower Artery	**0** Open **3** Percutaneous **4** Percutaneous Endoscopic	**5** Intraluminal Device, Drug-eluting, Two **6** Intraluminal Device, Drug-eluting, Three **7** Intraluminal Device, Drug-eluting, Four or More **E** Intraluminal Devices, Two **F** Intraluminal Devices, Three **G** Intraluminal Devices, Four or More	**Z** No Qualifier

Section **0** **Medical and Surgical**
Body System **4** **Lower Arteries**
Operation **9** **Drainage:** Taking or letting out fluids and/or gases from a body part

Body Part (4th)	Approach (5th)	Device (6th)	Qualifier (7th)
0 Abdominal Aorta **1** Celiac Artery **2** Gastric Artery **3** Hepatic Artery **4** Splenic Artery **5** Superior Mesenteric Artery **6** Colic Artery, Right **7** Colic Artery, Left **8** Colic Artery, Middle **9** Renal Artery, Right **A** Renal Artery, Left **B** Inferior Mesenteric Artery **C** Common Iliac Artery, Right **D** Common Iliac Artery, Left **E** Internal Iliac Artery, Right **F** Internal Iliac Artery, Left **H** External Iliac Artery, Right **J** External Iliac Artery, Left **K** Femoral Artery, Right **L** Femoral Artery, Left **M** Popliteal Artery, Right **N** Popliteal Artery, Left **P** Anterior Tibial Artery, Right **Q** Anterior Tibial Artery, Left **R** Posterior Tibial Artery, Right **S** Posterior Tibial Artery, Left **T** Peroneal Artery, Right **U** Peroneal Artery, Left **V** Foot Artery, Right **W** Foot Artery, Left **Y** Lower Artery	**0** Open **3** Percutaneous **4** Percutaneous Endoscopic	**0** Drainage Device	**Z** No Qualifier
0 Abdominal Aorta **1** Celiac Artery **2** Gastric Artery **3** Hepatic Artery **4** Splenic Artery **5** Superior Mesenteric Artery **6** Colic Artery, Right **7** Colic Artery, Left **8** Colic Artery, Middle **9** Renal Artery, Right **A** Renal Artery, Left **B** Inferior Mesenteric Artery **C** Common Iliac Artery, Right **D** Common Iliac Artery, Left **E** Internal Iliac Artery, Right **F** Internal Iliac Artery, Left **H** External Iliac Artery, Right **J** External Iliac Artery, Left **K** Femoral Artery, Right **L** Femoral Artery, Left **M** Popliteal Artery, Right **N** Popliteal Artery, Left **P** Anterior Tibial Artery, Right **Q** Anterior Tibial Artery, Left **R** Posterior Tibial Artery, Right **S** Posterior Tibial Artery, Left **T** Peroneal Artery, Right **U** Peroneal Artery, Left **V** Foot Artery, Right **W** Foot Artery, Left **Y** Lower Artery	**0** Open **3** Percutaneous **4** Percutaneous Endoscopic	**Z** No Device	**X** Diagnostic **Z** No Qualifier

Section 0 **Medical and Surgical**
Body System 4 **Lower Arteries**
Operation B **Excision:** Cutting out or off, without replacement, a portion of a body part

Body Part (4th)	Approach (5th)	Device (6th)	Qualifier (7th)
0 Abdominal Aorta **1** Celiac Artery **2** Gastric Artery **3** Hepatic Artery **4** Splenic Artery **5** Superior Mesenteric Artery **6** Colic Artery, Right **7** Colic Artery, Left **8** Colic Artery, Middle **9** Renal Artery, Right **A** Renal Artery, Left **B** Inferior Mesenteric Artery **C** Common Iliac Artery, Right **D** Common Iliac Artery, Left **E** Internal Iliac Artery, Right **F** Internal Iliac Artery, Left **H** External Iliac Artery, Right **J** External Iliac Artery, Left **K** Femoral Artery, Right **L** Femoral Artery, Left **M** Popliteal Artery, Right **N** Popliteal Artery, Left **P** Anterior Tibial Artery, Right **Q** Anterior Tibial Artery, Left **R** Posterior Tibial Artery, Right **S** Posterior Tibial Artery, Left **T** Peroneal Artery, Right **U** Peroneal Artery, Left **V** Foot Artery, Right **W** Foot Artery, Left **Y** Lower Artery	**0** Open **3** Percutaneous **4** Percutaneous Endoscopic	**Z** No Device	**X** Diagnostic **Z** No Qualifier

Section 0 **Medical and Surgical**
Body System 4 **Lower Arteries**
Operation C **Extirpation:** Taking or cutting out solid matter from a body part

Body Part (4th)	Approach (5th)	Device (6th)	Qualifier (7th)
0 Abdominal Aorta **1** Celiac Artery **2** Gastric Artery **3** Hepatic Artery **4** Splenic Artery **5** Superior Mesenteric Artery **6** Colic Artery, Right **7** Colic Artery, Left **8** Colic Artery, Middle **9** Renal Artery, Right **A** Renal Artery, Left **B** Inferior Mesenteric Artery **C** Common Iliac Artery, Right **D** Common Iliac Artery, Left **E** Internal Iliac Artery, Right **F** Internal Iliac Artery, Left **H** External Iliac Artery, Right **J** External Iliac Artery, Left **K** Femoral Artery, Right **L** Femoral Artery, Left **M** Popliteal Artery, Right **N** Popliteal Artery, Left **P** Anterior Tibial Artery, Right **Q** Anterior Tibial Artery, Left **R** Posterior Tibial Artery, Right **S** Posterior Tibial Artery, Left **T** Peroneal Artery, Right **U** Peroneal Artery, Left **V** Foot Artery, Right **W** Foot Artery, Left **Y** Lower Artery	**0** Open **3** Percutaneous **4** Percutaneous Endoscopic	**Z** No Device	**Z** No Qualifier

Section 0 **Medical and Surgical**
Body System 4 **Lower Arteries**
Operation F **Fragmentation:** Breaking solid matter in a body part into pieces

Body Part (4th)	Approach (5th)	Device (6th)	Qualifier (7th)
C Common Iliac Artery, Right **D** Common Iliac Artery, Left **E** Internal Iliac Artery, Right **F** Internal Iliac Artery, Left **H** External Iliac Artery, Right **J** External Iliac Artery, Left **K** Femoral Artery, Right **L** Femoral Artery, Left **M** Popliteal Artery, Right **N** Popliteal Artery, Left **P** Anterior Tibial Artery, Right **Q** Anterior Tibial Artery, Left **R** Posterior Tibial Artery, Right **S** Posterior Tibial Artery, Left **T** Peroneal Artery, Right **U** Peroneal Artery, Left **Y** Lower Artery	**3** Percutaneous	**Z** No Device	**0** Ultrasonic **Z** No Qualifier

Section 0 **Medical and Surgical**
Body System 4 **Lower Arteries**
Operation H **Insertion:** Putting in a nonbiological appliance that monitors, assists, performs, or prevents a physiological function but does not physically take the place of a body part

Body Part (4th)	Approach (5th)	Device (6th)	Qualifier (7th)
0 Abdominal Aorta	**0** Open **3** Percutaneous **4** Percutaneous Endoscopic	**2** Monitoring Device **3** Infusion Device **D** Intraluminal Device	**Z** No Qualifier
1 Celiac Artery **2** Gastric Artery **3** Hepatic Artery **4** Splenic Artery **5** Superior Mesenteric Artery **6** Colic Artery, Right **7** Colic Artery, Left **8** Colic Artery, Middle **9** Renal Artery, Right **A** Renal Artery, Left **B** Inferior Mesenteric Artery **C** Common Iliac Artery, Right **D** Common Iliac Artery, Left **E** Internal Iliac Artery, Right **F** Internal Iliac Artery, Left **H** External Iliac Artery, Right **J** External Iliac Artery, Left **K** Femoral Artery, Right **L** Femoral Artery, Left **M** Popliteal Artery, Right **N** Popliteal Artery, Left **P** Anterior Tibial Artery, Right **Q** Anterior Tibial Artery, Left **R** Posterior Tibial Artery, Right **S** Posterior Tibial Artery, Left **T** Peroneal Artery, Right **U** Peroneal Artery, Left **V** Foot Artery, Right **W** Foot Artery, Left	**0** Open **3** Percutaneous **4** Percutaneous Endoscopic	**3** Infusion Device **D** Intraluminal Device	**Z** No Qualifier
Y Lower Artery	**0** Open **3** Percutaneous **4** Percutaneous Endoscopic	**2** Monitoring Device **3** Infusion Device **D** Intraluminal Device **Y** Other Device	**Z** No Qualifier

Section 0 **Medical and Surgical**
Body System 4 **Lower Arteries**
Operation J **Inspection:** Visually and/or manually exploring a body part

Body Part (4th)	Approach (5th)	Device (6th)	Qualifier (7th)
Y Lower Artery	**0** Open **3** Percutaneous **4** Percutaneous Endoscopic **X** External	**Z** No Device	**Z** No Qualifier

Section 0 **Medical and Surgical**
Body System 4 **Lower Arteries**
Operation L **Occlusion:** Completely closing an orifice or the lumen of a tubular body part

Body Part (4th)	Approach (5th)	Device (6th)	Qualifier (7th)
0 Abdominal Aorta	**0** Open **4** Percutaneous Endoscopic	**C** Extraluminal Device **D** Intraluminal Device **Z** No Device	**Z** No Qualifier
0 Abdominal Aorta	**3** Percutaneous	**C** Extraluminal Device **Z** No Device	**Z** No Qualifier
0 Abdominal Aorta	**3** Percutaneous	**D** Intraluminal Device	**J** Temporary **Z** No Qualifier
1 Celiac Artery **2** Gastric Artery **3** Hepatic Artery **4** Splenic Artery **5** Superior Mesenteric Artery **6** Colic Artery, Right **7** Colic Artery, Left **8** Colic Artery, Middle **9** Renal Artery, Right **A** Renal Artery, Left **B** Inferior Mesenteric Artery **C** Common Iliac Artery, Right **D** Common Iliac Artery, Left **H** External Iliac Artery, Right **J** External Iliac Artery, Left **K** Femoral Artery, Right **L** Femoral Artery, Left **M** Popliteal Artery, Right **N** Popliteal Artery, Left **P** Anterior Tibial Artery, Right **Q** Anterior Tibial Artery, Left **R** Posterior Tibial Artery, Right **S** Posterior Tibial Artery, Left **T** Peroneal Artery, Right **U** Peroneal Artery, Left **V** Foot Artery, Right **W** Foot Artery, Left **Y** Lower Artery	**0** Open **3** Percutaneous **4** Percutaneous Endoscopic	**C** Extraluminal Device **D** Intraluminal Device **Z** No Device	**Z** No Qualifier
E Internal Iliac Artery, Right	**0** Open **3** Percutaneous **4** Percutaneous Endoscopic	**C** Extraluminal Device **D** Intraluminal Device **Z** No Device	**T** Uterine Artery, Right **Z** No Qualifier
F Internal Iliac Artery, Left	**0** Open **3** Percutaneous **4** Percutaneous Endoscopic	**C** Extraluminal Device **D** Intraluminal Device **Z** No Device	**U** Uterine Artery, Left **Z** No Qualifier

Section 0 **Medical and Surgical**
Body System 4 **Lower Arteries**
Operation N **Release:** Freeing a body part from an abnormal physical constraint by cutting or by the use of force

Body Part (4th)	Approach (5th)	Device (6th)	Qualifier (7th)
0 Abdominal Aorta **1** Celiac Artery **2** Gastric Artery **3** Hepatic Artery **4** Splenic Artery **5** Superior Mesenteric Artery **6** Colic Artery, Right **7** Colic Artery, Left **8** Colic Artery, Middle **9** Renal Artery, Right **A** Renal Artery, Left **B** Inferior Mesenteric Artery **C** Common Iliac Artery, Right **D** Common Iliac Artery, Left **E** Internal Iliac Artery, Right **F** Internal Iliac Artery, Left **H** External Iliac Artery, Right **J** External Iliac Artery, Left **K** Femoral Artery, Right **L** Femoral Artery, Left **M** Popliteal Artery, Right **N** Popliteal Artery, Left **P** Anterior Tibial Artery, Right **Q** Anterior Tibial Artery, Left **R** Posterior Tibial Artery, Right **S** Posterior Tibial Artery, Left **T** Peroneal Artery, Right **U** Peroneal Artery, Left **V** Foot Artery, Right **W** Foot Artery, Left **Y** Lower Artery	**0** Open **3** Percutaneous **4** Percutaneous Endoscopic	**Z** No Device	**Z** No Qualifier

Section 0 **Medical and Surgical**
Body System 4 **Lower Arteries**
Operation P **Removal:** Taking out or off a device from a body part

Body Part (4th)	Approach (5th)	Device (6th)	Qualifier (7th)
Y Lower Artery	**0** Open **3** Percutaneous **4** Percutaneous Endoscopic	**0** Drainage Device **2** Monitoring Device **3** Infusion Device **7** Autologous Tissue Substitute **C** Extraluminal Device **D** Intraluminal Device **J** Synthetic Substitute **K** Nonautologous Tissue Substitute **Y** Other Device	**Z** No Qualifier
Y Lower Artery	**X** External	**0** Drainage Device **1** Radioactive Element **2** Monitoring Device **3** Infusion Device **D** Intraluminal Device	**Z** No Qualifier

Section 0 **Medical and Surgical**
Body System 4 **Lower Arteries**
Operation Q **Repair:** Restoring, to the extent possible, a body part to its normal anatomic structure and function

Body Part (4th)	Approach (5th)	Device (6th)	Qualifier (7th)
0 Abdominal Aorta **1** Celiac Artery **2** Gastric Artery **3** Hepatic Artery **4** Splenic Artery **5** Superior Mesenteric Artery **6** Colic Artery, Right **7** Colic Artery, Left **8** Colic Artery, Middle **9** Renal Artery, Right **A** Renal Artery, Left **B** Inferior Mesenteric Artery **C** Common Iliac Artery, Right **D** Common Iliac Artery, Left **E** Internal Iliac Artery, Right **F** Internal Iliac Artery, Left **H** External Iliac Artery, Right **J** External Iliac Artery, Left **K** Femoral Artery, Right **L** Femoral Artery, Left **M** Popliteal Artery, Right **N** Popliteal Artery, Left **P** Anterior Tibial Artery, Right **Q** Anterior Tibial Artery, Left **R** Posterior Tibial Artery, Right **S** Posterior Tibial Artery, Left **T** Peroneal Artery, Right **U** Peroneal Artery, Left **V** Foot Artery, Right **W** Foot Artery, Left **Y** Lower Artery	**0** Open **3** Percutaneous **4** Percutaneous Endoscopic	**Z** No Device	**Z** No Qualifier

Section 0 **Medical and Surgical**
Body System 4 **Lower Arteries**
Operation R **Replacement:** Putting in or on biological or synthetic material that physically takes the place and/or function of all or a portion of a body part

Body Part (4th)	Approach (5th)	Device (6th)	Qualifier (7th)
0 Abdominal Aorta **1** Celiac Artery **2** Gastric Artery **3** Hepatic Artery **4** Splenic Artery **5** Superior Mesenteric Artery **6** Colic Artery, Right **7** Colic Artery, Left **8** Colic Artery, Middle **9** Renal Artery, Right **A** Renal Artery, Left **B** Inferior Mesenteric Artery **C** Common Iliac Artery, Right **D** Common Iliac Artery, Left **E** Internal Iliac Artery, Right **F** Internal Iliac Artery, Left **H** External Iliac Artery, Right **J** External Iliac Artery, Left **K** Femoral Artery, Right **L** Femoral Artery, Left **M** Popliteal Artery, Right **N** Popliteal Artery, Left **P** Anterior Tibial Artery, Right **Q** Anterior Tibial Artery, Left **R** Posterior Tibial Artery, Right **S** Posterior Tibial Artery, Left **T** Peroneal Artery, Right **U** Peroneal Artery, Left **V** Foot Artery, Right **W** Foot Artery, Left **Y** Lower Artery	**0** Open **4** Percutaneous Endoscopic	**7** Autologous Tissue Substitute **J** Synthetic Substitute **K** Nonautologous Tissue Substitute	**Z** No Qualifier

Section **0** **Medical and Surgical**
Body System **4** **Lower Arteries**
Operation **S** **Reposition:** Moving to its normal location, or other suitable location, all or a portion of a body part

Body Part (4th)	Approach (5th)	Device (6th)	Qualifier (7th)
0 Abdominal Aorta **1** Celiac Artery **2** Gastric Artery **3** Hepatic Artery **4** Splenic Artery **5** Superior Mesenteric Artery **6** Colic Artery, Right **7** Colic Artery, Left **8** Colic Artery, Middle **9** Renal Artery, Right **A** Renal Artery, Left **B** Inferior Mesenteric Artery **C** Common Iliac Artery, Right **D** Common Iliac Artery, Left **E** Internal Iliac Artery, Right **F** Internal Iliac Artery, Left **H** External Iliac Artery, Right **J** External Iliac Artery, Left **K** Femoral Artery, Right **L** Femoral Artery, Left **M** Popliteal Artery, Right **N** Popliteal Artery, Left **P** Anterior Tibial Artery, Right **Q** Anterior Tibial Artery, Left **R** Posterior Tibial Artery, Right **S** Posterior Tibial Artery, Left **T** Peroneal Artery, Right **U** Peroneal Artery, Left **V** Foot Artery, Right **W** Foot Artery, Left **Y** Lower Artery	**0** Open **3** Percutaneous **4** Percutaneous Endoscopic	**Z** No Device	**Z** No Qualifier

Section 0 **Medical and Surgical**
Body System 4 **Lower Arteries**
Operation U **Supplement:** Putting in or on biological or synthetic material that physically reinforces and/or augments the function of a portion of a body part

Body Part (4th)	Approach (5th)	Device (6th)	Qualifier (7th)
0 Abdominal Aorta **1** Celiac Artery **2** Gastric Artery **3** Hepatic Artery **4** Splenic Artery **5** Superior Mesenteric Artery **6** Colic Artery, Right **7** Colic Artery, Left **8** Colic Artery, Middle **9** Renal Artery, Right **A** Renal Artery, Left **B** Inferior Mesenteric Artery **C** Common Iliac Artery, Right **D** Common Iliac Artery, Left **E** Internal Iliac Artery, Right **F** Internal Iliac Artery, Left **H** External Iliac Artery, Right **J** External Iliac Artery, Left **K** Femoral Artery, Right **L** Femoral Artery, Left **M** Popliteal Artery, Right **N** Popliteal Artery, Left **P** Anterior Tibial Artery, Right **Q** Anterior Tibial Artery, Left **R** Posterior Tibial Artery, Right **S** Posterior Tibial Artery, Left **T** Peroneal Artery, Right **U** Peroneal Artery, Left **V** Foot Artery, Right **W** Foot Artery, Left **Y** Lower Artery	**0** Open **3** Percutaneous **4** Percutaneous Endoscopic	**7** Autologous Tissue Substitute **J** Synthetic Substitute **K** Nonautologous Tissue Substitute	**Z** No Qualifier

Section 0 **Medical and Surgical**
Body System 4 **Lower Arteries**
Operation V **Restriction:** Partially closing an orifice or the lumen of a tubular body part

Body Part (4th)	Approach (5th)	Device (6th)	Qualifier (7th)
0 Abdominal Aorta	**0** Open **3** Percutaneous **4** Percutaneous Endoscopic	**C** Extraluminal Device **E** Intraluminal Device, Branched or Fenestrated, One or Two Arteries **F** Intraluminal Device, Branched or Fenestrated, Three or More Arteries **Z** No Device	**Z** No Qualifier
0 Abdominal Aorta	**0** Open **3** Percutaneous **4** Percutaneous Endoscopic	**D** Intraluminal Device	**J** Temporary **Z** No Qualifier

Continued →

Section 0 **Medical and Surgical**
Body System 4 **Lower Arteries**
Operation V **Restriction:** Partially closing an orifice or the lumen of a tubular body part

04V Continued

Body Part (4th)	Approach (5th)	Device (6th)	Qualifier (7th)
1 Celiac Artery **2** Gastric Artery **3** Hepatic Artery **4** Splenic Artery **5** Superior Mesenteric Artery **6** Colic Artery, Right **7** Colic Artery, Left **8** Colic Artery, Middle **9** Renal Artery, Right **A** Renal Artery, Left **B** Inferior Mesenteric Artery **E** Internal Iliac Artery, Right **F** Internal Iliac Artery, Left **H** External Iliac Artery, Right **J** External Iliac Artery, Left **K** Femoral Artery, Right **L** Femoral Artery, Left **M** Popliteal Artery, Right **N** Popliteal Artery, Left **P** Anterior Tibial Artery, Right **Q** Anterior Tibial Artery, Left **R** Posterior Tibial Artery, Right **S** Posterior Tibial Artery, Left **T** Peroneal Artery, Right **U** Peroneal Artery, Left **V** Foot Artery, Right **W** Foot Artery, Left **Y** Lower Artery	**0** Open **3** Percutaneous **4** Percutaneous Endoscopic	**C** Extraluminal Device **D** Intraluminal Device **Z** No Device	**Z** No Qualifier
C Common Iliac Artery, Right **D** Common Iliac Artery, Left	**0** Open **3** Percutaneous **4** Percutaneous Endoscopic	**C** Extraluminal Device **D** Intraluminal Device **E** Intraluminal Device, Branched or Fenestrated, One or Two Arteries **Z** No Device	**Z** No Qualifier

Section 0 **Medical and Surgical**
Body System 4 **Lower Arteries**
Operation W **Revision:** Correcting, to the extent possible, a portion of a malfunctioning device or the position of a displaced device

Body Part (4th)	Approach (5th)	Device (6th)	Qualifier (7th)
Y Lower Artery	**0** Open **3** Percutaneous **4** Percutaneous Endoscopic	**0** Drainage Device **2** Monitoring Device **3** Infusion Device **7** Autologous Tissue Substitute **C** Extraluminal Device **D** Intraluminal Device **J** Synthetic Substitute **K** Nonautologous Tissue Substitute **Y** Other Device	**Z** No Qualifier
Y Lower Artery	**X** External	**0** Drainage Device **2** Monitoring Device **3** Infusion Device **7** Autologous Tissue Substitute **C** Extraluminal Device **D** Intraluminal Device **J** Synthetic Substitute **K** Nonautologus Tissue Substitute	**Z** No Qualifier

AHA Coding Clinic

04100Z3 Bypass Abdominal Aorta to Right Renal Artery, Open Approach—AHA CC: 3Q, 2015, 28

04130Z3 Bypass Hepatic Artery to Right Renal Artery, Open Approach—AHA CC: 4Q, 2017, 47

04140Z4 Bypass Splenic Artery to Left Renal Artery, Open Approach—AHA CC: 3Q, 2015, 28; 4Q, 2017, 47

041C0J2 Bypass Right Common Iliac Artery to Mesenteric Artery with Synthetic Substitute, Open Approach—AHA CC: 3Q, 2017, 16

041C0J5 Bypass Right Common Iliac Artery to Bilateral Renal Artery with Synthetic Substitute, Open Approach—AHA CC: 3Q, 2017, 16

041K09N Bypass Right Femoral Artery to Posterior Tibial Artery with Autologous Venous Tissue, Open Approach—AHA CC: 3Q, 2017, 5-6

041K0JL Bypass Right Femoral Artery to Popliteal Artery with Synthetic Substitute, Open Approach—AHA CC: 3Q, 2018, 25

041K0JN Bypass Right Femoral Artery to Posterior Tibial Artery with Synthetic Substitute, Open Approach—AHA CC: 2Q, 2016, 18-19; 3Q, 2017, 5-6

041M09P Bypass Right Popliteal Artery to Foot Artery with Autologous Venous Tissue, Open Approach—AHA CC: 1Q, 2017, 32-33

047H3Z1 Dilation of Right External Iliac Artery using Drug-Coated Balloon, Percutaneous Approach—AHA CC: 4Q, 2020, 50-51

047K3D1 Dilation of Right Femoral Artery with Intraluminal Device, using Drug-Coated Balloon, Percutaneous Approach—AHA CC: 4Q, 2015, 7,15

047K3Z1 Dilation of Right Femoral Artery using Drug-Coated Balloon, Percutaneous Approach—AHA CC: 4Q, 2020, 50-51

047K3Z6 Dilation of Right Femoral Artery, Bifurcation, Percutaneous Approach—AHA CC: 4Q, 2016, 88-89

047L3Z1 Dilation of Left Femoral Artery using Drug-Coated Balloon, Percutaneous Approach—AHA CC: 4Q, 2015, 15

04CH0ZZ Extirpation of Matter from Right External Iliac Artery, Open Approach—AHA CC: 1Q, 2021, 15-16

04CJ0ZZ Extirpation of Matter from Left External Iliac Artery, Open Approach—AHA CC: 1Q, 2016, 31; 1Q, 2021, 15-16

04CK3Z6 Extirpation of Matter from Right Femoral Artery, Bifurcation, Percutaneous Approach—AHA CC: 4Q, 2016, 88-89

04CL3ZZ Extirpation of Matter from Left Femoral Artery, Percutaneous Approach—AHA CC: 1Q, 2015, 36

04FC3ZZ Fragmentation of Right Common Iliac Artery, Percutaneous Approach—AHA CC: 4Q, 2020, 51-52

04FH3ZZ Fragmentation of Right External Iliac Artery, Percutaneous Approach—AHA CC: 4Q, 2020, 50-52

04FK3ZZ Fragmentation of Right Femoral Artery, Percutaneous Approach—AHA CC: 4Q, 2020, 50-51

04H13DZ Insertion of Intraluminal Device into Celiac Artery, Percutaneous Approach—AHA CC: 1Q, 2019, 23

04H53DZ Insertion of Intraluminal Device into Superior Mesenteric Artery, Percutaneous Approach—AHA CC: 1Q, 2019, 23

04H93DZ Insertion of Intraluminal Device into Right Renal Artery, Percutaneous Approach—AHA CC: 1Q, 2019, 23

04HA3DZ Insertion of Intraluminal Device into Left Renal Artery, Percutaneous Approach—AHA CC: 1Q, 2019, 23

04HY32Z Insertion of Monitoring Device into Lower Artery, Percutaneous Approach—AHA CC: 1Q, 2017, 30

04HY33Z Insertion of Infusion Device into Lower Artery, Percutaneous Approach—AHA CC: 3Q, 2019, 20-21

04L24ZZ Occlusion of Gastric Artery, Percutaneous Endoscopic Approach—AHA CC: 3Q, 2020, 43

04L33DZ Occlusion of Hepatic Artery with Intraluminal Device, Percutaneous Approach—AHA CC: 3Q, 2014, 26-27

04L73DZ Occlusion of Left Colic Artery with Intraluminal Device, Percutaneous Approach—AHA CC: 1Q, 2014, 24

04LB3DZ Occlusion of Inferior Mesenteric Artery with Intraluminal Device, Percutaneous Approach—AHA CC: 1Q, 2014, 24

04LE3DT Occlusion of Right Uterine Artery with Intraluminal Device, Percutaneous Approach—AHA CC: 2Q, 2015, 27

04LH0CZ Occlusion of Right External Iliac Artery with Extraluminal Device, Open Approach—AHA CC: 2Q, 2018, 18-19

04LJ0CZ Occlusion of Left External Iliac Artery with Extraluminal Device, Open Approach—AHA CC: 2Q, 2018, 18-19

04N10ZZ Release Celiac Artery, Open Approach—AHA CC: 2Q, 2015, 28

04PY33Z Removal of Infusion Device from Lower Artery, Percutaneous Approach—AHA CC: 3Q, 2019, 20-21

04QK0ZZ Repair Right Femoral Artery, Open Approach—AHA CC: 1Q, 2014, 21-22

04R10JZ Replacement of Celiac Artery with Synthetic Substitute, Open Approach—AHA CC: 2Q, 2015, 28

04UJ0KZ Supplement Left External Iliac Artery with Nonautologous Tissue Substitute, Open Approach—AHA CC: 1Q, 2016, 31

04UK0KZ Supplement Right Femoral Artery with Nonautologous Tissue Substitute, Open Approach—AHA CC: 4Q, 2014, 37-38

04UK3JZ Supplement Right Femoral Artery with Synthetic Substitute, Percutaneous Approach—AHA CC: 1Q, 2014, 22-23

04UR07Z Supplement Right Posterior Tibial Artery with Autologous Tissue Substitute, Open Approach—AHA CC: 2Q, 2016, 18-19

04V00DZ Restriction of Abdominal Aorta with Intraluminal Device, Open Approach—AHA CC: 1Q, 2019, 22

04V03DZ Restriction of Abdominal Aorta with Intraluminal Device, Percutaneous Approach—AHA CC: 1Q, 2014, 9; 3Q, 2016, 39

04V03E6 Restriction of Abdominal Aorta, Bifurcation, with Branched or Fenestrated Intraluminal Device, One or Two Arteries, Percutaneous Approach—AHA CC: 4Q, 2016, 91-92

04V03F6 Restriction of Abdominal Aorta, Bifurcation, with Branched or Fenestrated Intraluminal Device, Three or More Arteries, Percutaneous Approach—AHA CC: 4Q, 2016, 92-94

04VC3EZ Restriction of Right Common Iliac Artery with Branched or Fenestrated Intraluminal Device, One or Two Arteries, Percutaneous Approach—AHA CC: 4Q, 2016, 93-94

04VD3EZ Restriction of Left Common Iliac Artery with Branched or Fenestrated Intraluminal Device, One or Two Arteries, Percutaneous Approach—AHA CC: 4Q, 2016, 93-94

04WY07Z Revision of Autologous Tissue Substitute in Lower Artery, Open Approach—AHA CC: 1Q, 2015, 36-37

04WY0JZ Revision of Synthetic Substitute in Lower Artery, Open Approach—AHA CC: 2Q, 2019, 14-15

04WY37Z Revision of Autologous Tissue Substitute in Lower Artery, Percutaneous Approach—AHA CC: 1Q, 2014, 22

04WY3DZ Revision of Intraluminal Device in Lower Artery, Percutaneous Approach—AHA CC: 1Q, 2014, 9-10; 3Q, 2020, 6

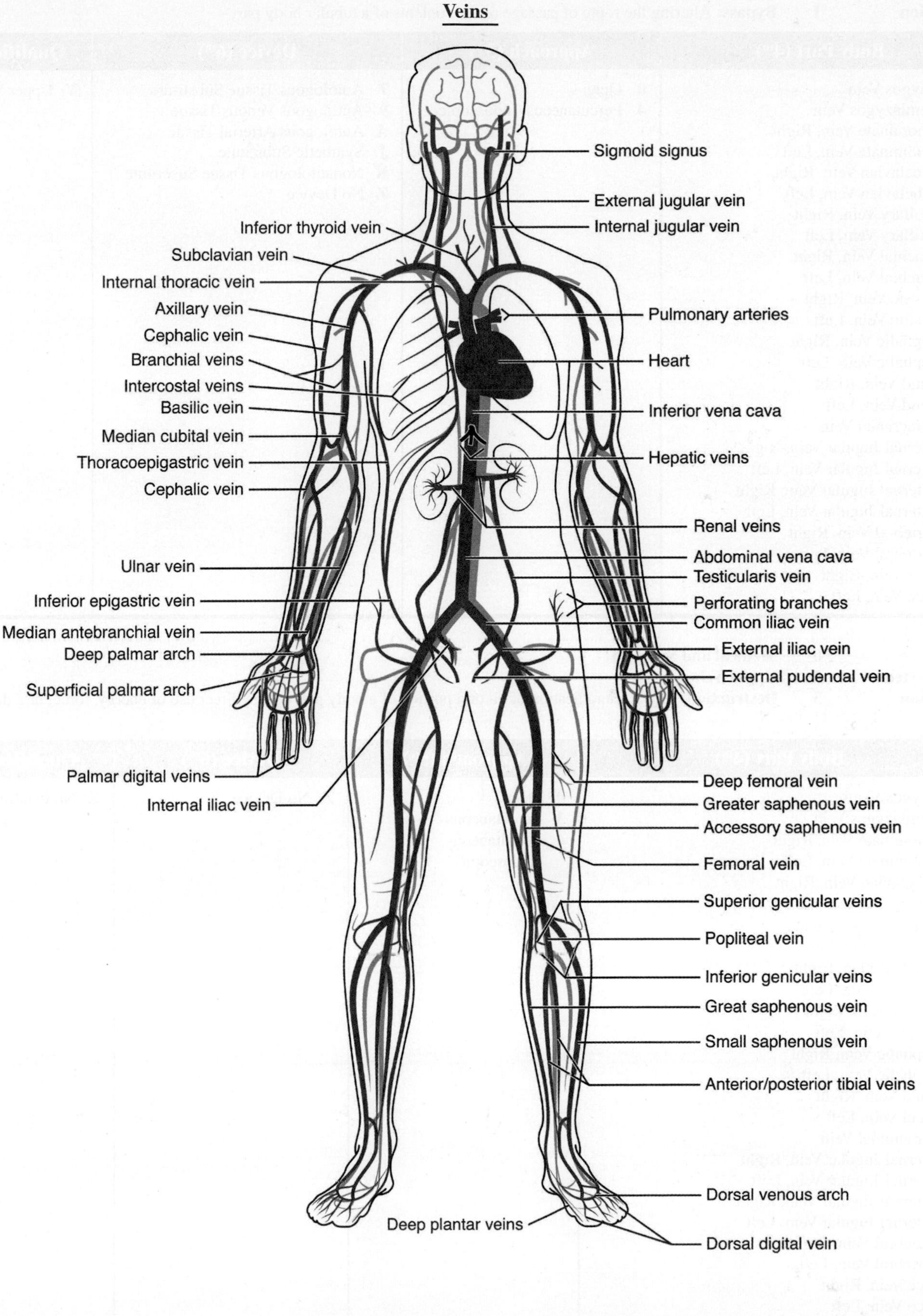
Veins
Sigmoid signus
External jugular vein
Internal jugular vein
Inferior thyroid vein
Subclavian vein
Internal thoracic vein
Axillary vein
Cephalic vein
Branchial veins
Intercostal veins
Basilic vein
Median cubital vein
Thoracoepigastric vein
Cephalic vein
Pulmonary arteries
Heart
Inferior vena cava
Hepatic veins
Renal veins
Abdominal vena cava
Testicularis vein
Perforating branches
Common iliac vein
External iliac vein
External pudendal vein
Ulnar vein
Inferior epigastric vein
Median antebranchial vein
Deep palmar arch
Superficial palmar arch
Palmar digital veins
Internal iliac vein
Deep femoral vein
Greater saphenous vein
Accessory saphenous vein
Femoral vein
Superior genicular veins
Popliteal vein
Inferior genicular veins
Great saphenous vein
Small saphenous vein
Anterior/posterior tibial veins
Dorsal venous arch
Deep plantar veins
Dorsal digital vein

Upper Veins Tables 051–05W

Section 0 **Medical and Surgical**
Body System 5 **Upper Veins**
Operation 1 **Bypass:** Altering the route of passage of the contents of a tubular body part

Body Part (4th)	Approach (5th)	Device (6th)	Qualifier (7th)
0 Azygos Vein	**0** Open	**7** Autologous Tissue Substitute	**Y** Upper Vein
1 Hemiazygos Vein	**4** Percutaneous Endoscopic	**9** Autologous Venous Tissue	
3 Innominate Vein, Right		**A** Autologous Arterial Tissue	
4 Innominate Vein, Left		**J** Synthetic Substitute	
5 Subclavian Vein, Right		**K** Nonautologous Tissue Substitute	
6 Subclavian Vein, Left		**Z** No Device	
7 Axillary Vein, Right			
8 Axillary Vein, Left			
9 Brachial Vein, Right			
A Brachial Vein, Left			
B Basilic Vein, Right			
C Basilic Vein, Left			
D Cephalic Vein, Right			
F Cephalic Vein, Left			
G Hand Vein, Right			
H Hand Vein, Left			
L Intracranial Vein			
M Internal Jugular Vein, Right			
N Internal Jugular Vein, Left			
P External Jugular Vein, Right			
Q External Jugular Vein, Left			
R Vertebral Vein, Right			
S Vertebral Vein, Left			
T Face Vein, Right			
V Face Vein, Left			

Section 0 **Medical and Surgical**
Body System 5 **Upper Veins**
Operation 5 **Destruction:** Physical eradication of all or a portion of a body part by the direct use of energy, force, or a destructive agent

Body Part (4th)	Approach (5th)	Device (6th)	Qualifier (7th)
0 Azygos Vein	**0** Open	**Z** No Device	**Z** No Qualifier
1 Hemiazygos Vein	**3** Percutaneous		
3 Innominate Vein, Right	**4** Percutaneous Endoscopic		
4 Innominate Vein, Left			
5 Subclavian Vein, Right			
6 Subclavian Vein, Left			
7 Axillary Vein, Right			
8 Axillary Vein, Left			
9 Brachial Vein, Right			
A Brachial Vein, Left			
B Basilic Vein, Right			
C Basilic Vein, Left			
D Cephalic Vein, Right			
F Cephalic Vein, Left			
G Hand Vein, Right			
H Hand Vein, Left			
L Intracranial Vein			
M Internal Jugular Vein, Right			
N Internal Jugular Vein, Left			
P External Jugular Vein, Right			
Q External Jugular Vein, Left			
R Vertebral Vein, Right			
S Vertebral Vein, Left			
T Face Vein, Right			
V Face Vein, Left			
Y Upper Vein			

Section 0 Medical and Surgical
Body System 5 Upper Veins
Operation 7 **Dilation:** Expanding an orifice or the lumen of a tubular body part

Body Part (4th)	Approach (5th)	Device (6th)	Qualifier (7th)
0 Azygos Vein **1** Hemiazygos Vein **G** Hand Vein, Right **H** Hand Vein, Left **L** Intracranial Vein **M** Internal Jugular Vein, Right **N** Internal Jugular Vein, Left **P** External Jugular Vein, Right **Q** External Jugular Vein, Left **R** Vertebral Vein, Right **S** Vertebral Vein, Left **T** Face Vein, Right **V** Face Vein, Left **Y** Upper Vein	**0** Open **3** Percutaneous **4** Percutaneous Endoscopic	**D** Intraluminal Device **Z** No Device	**Z** No Qualifier
3 Innominate Vein, Right **4** Innominate Vein, Left **5** Subclavian Vein, Right **6** Subclavian Vein, Left **7** Axillary Vein, Right **8** Axillary Vein, Left **9** Brachial Vein, Right **A** Brachial Vein, Left **B** Basilic Vein, Right **C** Basilic Vein, Left **D** Cephalic Vein, Right **F** Cephalic Vein, Left	**0** Open **3** Percutaneous **4** Percutaneous Endoscopic	**D** Intraluminal Device **Z** No Device	**1** Drug-Coated Balloon **Z** No Qualifier

Section 0 Medical and Surgical
Body System 5 Upper Veins
Operation 9 **Drainage:** Taking or letting out fluids and/or gases from a body part

Body Part (4th)	Approach (5th)	Device (6th)	Qualifier (7th)
0 Azygos Vein **1** Hemiazygos Vein **3** Innominate Vein, Right **4** Innominate Vein, Left **5** Subclavian Vein, Right **6** Subclavian Vein, Left **7** Axillary Vein, Right **8** Axillary Vein, Left **9** Brachial Vein, Right **A** Brachial Vein, Left **B** Basilic Vein, Right **C** Basilic Vein, Left **D** Cephalic Vein, Right **F** Cephalic Vein, Left **G** Hand Vein, Right **H** Hand Vein, Left **L** Intracranial Vein **M** Internal Jugular Vein, Right **N** Internal Jugular Vein, Left **P** External Jugular Vein, Right **Q** External Jugular Vein, Left **R** Vertebral Vein, Right **S** Vertebral Vein, Left **T** Face Vein, Right **V** Face Vein, Left **Y** Upper Vein	**0** Open **3** Percutaneous **4** Percutaneous Endoscopic	**0** Drainage Device	**Z** No Qualifier

Continued →

Section 0 **Medical and Surgical**
Body System 5 **Upper Veins**
Operation 9 **Drainage:** Taking or letting out fluids and/or gases from a body part

Body Part (4th)	Approach (5th)	Device (6th)	Qualifier (7th)
0 Azygos Vein 1 Hemiazygos Vein 3 Innominate Vein, Right 4 Innominate Vein, Left 5 Subclavian Vein, Right 6 Subclavian Vein, Left 7 Axillary Vein, Right 8 Axillary Vein, Left 9 Brachial Vein, Right A Brachial Vein, Left B Basilic Vein, Right C Basilic Vein, Left D Cephalic Vein, Right F Cephalic Vein, Left G Hand Vein, Right H Hand Vein, Left L Intracranial Vein M Internal Jugular Vein, Right N Internal Jugular Vein, Left P External Jugular Vein, Right Q External Jugular Vein, Left R Vertebral Vein, Right S Vertebral Vein, Left T Face Vein, Right V Face Vein, Left Y Upper Vein	0 Open 3 Percutaneous 4 Percutaneous Endoscopic	Z No Device	X Diagnostic Z No Qualifier

Section 0 **Medical and Surgical**
Body System 5 **Upper Veins**
Operation B **Excision:** Cutting out or off, without replacement, a portion of a body part

Body Part (4th)	Approach (5th)	Device (6th)	Qualifier (7th)
0 Azygos Vein 1 Hemiazygos Vein 3 Innominate Vein, Right 4 Innominate Vein, Left 5 Subclavian Vein, Right 6 Subclavian Vein, Left 7 Axillary Vein, Right 8 Axillary Vein, Left 9 Brachial Vein, Right A Brachial Vein, Left B Basilic Vein, Right C Basilic Vein, Left D Cephalic Vein, Right F Cephalic Vein, Left G Hand Vein, Right H Hand Vein, Left L Intracranial Vein M Internal Jugular Vein, Right N Internal Jugular Vein, Left P External Jugular Vein, Right Q External Jugular Vein, Left R Vertebral Vein, Right S Vertebral Vein, Left T Face Vein, Right V Face Vein, Left Y Upper Vein	0 Open 3 Percutaneous 4 Percutaneous Endoscopic	Z No Device	X Diagnostic Z No Qualifier

Section 0 Medical and Surgical
Body System 5 Upper Veins
Operation C **Extirpation:** Taking or cutting out solid matter from a body part

Body Part (4th)	Approach (5th)	Device (6th)	Qualifier (7th)
0 Azygos Vein **1** Hemiazygos Vein **3** Innominate Vein, Right **4** Innominate Vein, Left **5** Subclavian Vein, Right **6** Subclavian Vein, Left **7** Axillary Vein, Right **8** Axillary Vein, Left **9** Brachial Vein, Right **A** Brachial Vein, Left **B** Basilic Vein, Right **C** Basilic Vein, Left **D** Cephalic Vein, Right **F** Cephalic Vein, Left **G** Hand Vein, Right **H** Hand Vein, Left **L** Intracranial Vein **M** Internal Jugular Vein, Right **N** Internal Jugular Vein, Left **P** External Jugular Vein, Right **Q** External Jugular Vein, Left **R** Vertebral Vein, Right **S** Vertebral Vein, Left **T** Face Vein, Right **V** Face Vein, Left **Y** Upper Vein	**0** Open **3** Percutaneous **4** Percutaneous Endoscopic	**Z** No Device	**Z** No Qualifier

Section 0 Medical and Surgical
Body System 5 Upper Veins
Operation D **Extraction:** Pulling or stripping out or off all or a portion of a body part by the use of force

Body Part (4th)	Approach (5th)	Device (6th)	Qualifier (7th)
9 Brachial Vein, Right **A** Brachial Vein, Left **B** Basilic Vein, Right **C** Basilic Vein, Left **D** Cephalic Vein, Right **F** Cephalic Vein, Left **G** Hand Vein, Right **H** Hand Vein, Left **Y** Upper Vein	**0** Open **3** Percutaneous	**Z** No Device	**Z** No Qualifier

Section 0 Medical and Surgical
Body System 5 Upper Veins
Operation F **Fragmentation:** Breaking solid matter in a body part into pieces

Body Part (4th)	Approach (5th)	Device (6th)	Qualifier (7th)
3 Innominate Vein, Right **4** Innominate Vein, Left **5** Subclavian Vein, Right **6** Subclavian Vein, Left **7** Axillary Vein, Right **8** Axillary Vein, Left **9** Brachial Vein, Right **A** Brachial Vein, Left **B** Basilic Vein, Right **C** Basilic Vein, Left **D** Cephalic Vein, Right **F** Cephalic Vein, Left **Y** Upper Vein	**3** Percutaneous	**Z** No Device	**0** Ultrasonic **Z** No Qualifier

Section 0 **Medical and Surgical**
Body System 5 **Upper Veins**
Operation H **Insertion:** Putting in a nonbiological appliance that monitors, assists, performs, or prevents a physiological function but does not physically take the place of a body part

Body Part (4th)	Approach (5th)	Device (6th)	Qualifier (7th)
0 Azygos Vein	**0** Open **3** Percutaneous **4** Percutaneous Endoscopic	**2** Monitoring Device **3** Infusion Device **D** Intraluminal Device **M** Neurostimulator Lead	**Z** No Qualifier
1 Hemiazygos Vein **5** Subclavian Vein, Right **6** Subclavian Vein, Left **7** Axillary Vein, Right **8** Axillary Vein, Left **9** Brachial Vein, Right **A** Brachial Vein, Left **B** Basilic Vein, Right **C** Basilic Vein, Left **D** Cephalic Vein, Right **F** Cephalic Vein, Left **G** Hand Vein, Right **H** Hand Vein, Left **L** Intracranial Vein **M** Internal Jugular Vein, Right **N** Internal Jugular Vein, Left **P** External Jugular Vein, Right **Q** External Jugular Vein, Left **R** Vertebral Vein, Right **S** Vertebral Vein, Left **T** Face Vein, Right **V** Face Vein, Left	**0** Open **3** Percutaneous **4** Percutaneous Endoscopic	**3** Infusion Device **D** Intraluminal Device	**Z** No Qualifier
3 Innominate Vein, Right **4** Innominate Vein, Left	**0** Open **3** Percutaneous **4** Percutaneous Endoscopic	**3** Infusion Device **D** Intraluminal Device **M** Neurostimulator Lead	**Z** No Qualifier
Y Upper Vein	**0** Open **3** Percutaneous **4** Percutaneous Endoscopic	**2** Monitoring Device **3** Infusion Device **D** Intraluminal Device **Y** Other Device	**Z** No Qualifier

Section 0 **Medical and Surgical**
Body System 5 **Upper Veins**
Operation J **Inspection:** Visually and/or manually exploring a body part

Body Part (4th)	Approach (5th)	Device (6th)	Qualifier (7th)
Y Upper Vein	**0** Open **3** Percutaneous **4** Percutaneous Endoscopic **X** External	**Z** No Device	**Z** No Qualifier

Section 0 **Medical and Surgical**
Body System 5 **Upper Veins**
Operation L **Occlusion:** Completely closing an orifice or the lumen of a tubular body part

Body Part (4th)	Approach (5th)	Device (6th)	Qualifier (7th)
0 Azygos Vein **1** Hemiazygos Vein **3** Innominate Vein, Right **4** Innominate Vein, Left **5** Subclavian Vein, Right **6** Subclavian Vein, Left **7** Axillary Vein, Right **8** Axillary Vein, Left **9** Brachial Vein, Right **A** Brachial Vein, Left **B** Basilic Vein, Right **C** Basilic Vein, Left **D** Cephalic Vein, Right **F** Cephalic Vein, Left **G** Hand Vein, Right **H** Hand Vein, Left **L** Intracranial Vein **M** Internal Jugular Vein, Right **N** Internal Jugular Vein, Left **P** External Jugular Vein, Right **Q** External Jugular Vein, Left **R** Vertebral Vein, Right **S** Vertebral Vein, Left **T** Face Vein, Right **V** Face Vein, Left **Y** Upper Vein	**0** Open **3** Percutaneous **4** Percutaneous Endoscopic	**C** Extraluminal Device **D** Intraluminal Device **Z** No Device	**Z** No Qualifier

Section 0 **Medical and Surgical**
Body System 5 **Upper Veins**
Operation N **Release:** Freeing a body part from an abnormal physical constraint by cutting or by the use of force

Body Part (4th)	Approach (5th)	Device (6th)	Qualifier (7th)
0 Azygos Vein **1** Hemiazygos Vein **3** Innominate Vein, Right **4** Innominate Vein, Left **5** Subclavian Vein, Right **6** Subclavian Vein, Left **7** Axillary Vein, Right **8** Axillary Vein, Left **9** Brachial Vein, Right **A** Brachial Vein, Left **B** Basilic Vein, Right **C** Basilic Vein, Left **D** Cephalic Vein, Right **F** Cephalic Vein, Left **G** Hand Vein, Right **H** Hand Vein, Left **L** Intracranial Vein **M** Internal Jugular Vein, Right **N** Internal Jugular Vein, Left **P** External Jugular Vein, Right **Q** External Jugular Vein, Left **R** Vertebral Vein, Right **S** Vertebral Vein, Left **T** Face Vein, Right **V** Face Vein, Left **Y** Upper Vein	**0** Open **3** Percutaneous **4** Percutaneous Endoscopic	**Z** No Device	**Z** No Qualifier

Section 0 Medical and Surgical
Body System 5 Upper Veins
Operation P **Removal:** Taking out or off a device from a body part

Body Part (4th)	Approach (5th)	Device (6th)	Qualifier (7th)
0 Azygos Vein	0 Open 3 Percutaneous 4 Percutaneous Endoscopic X External	2 Monitoring Device M Neurostimulator Lead	Z No Qualifier
3 Innominate Vein, Right 4 Innominate Vein, Left	0 Open 3 Percutaneous 4 Percutaneous Endoscopic X External	M Neurostimulator Lead	Z No Qualifier
Y Upper Vein	0 Open 3 Percutaneous 4 Percutaneous Endoscopic	0 Drainage Device 2 Monitoring Device 3 Infusion Device 7 Autologous Tissue Substitute C Extraluminal Device D Intraluminal Device J Synthetic Substitute K Nonautologous Tissue Substitute Y Other Device	Z No Qualifier
Y Upper Vein	X External	0 Drainage Device 2 Monitoring Device 3 Infusion Device D Intraluminal Device	Z No Qualifier

Section 0 Medical and Surgical
Body System 5 Upper Veins
Operation Q **Repair:** Restoring, to the extent possible, a body part to its normal anatomic structure and function

Body Part (4th)	Approach (5th)	Device (6th)	Qualifier (7th)
0 Azygos Vein 1 Hemiazygos Vein 3 Innominate Vein, Right 4 Innominate Vein, Left 5 Subclavian Vein, Right 6 Subclavian Vein, Left 7 Axillary Vein, Right 8 Axillary Vein, Left 9 Brachial Vein, Right A Brachial Vein, Left B Basilic Vein, Right C Basilic Vein, Left D Cephalic Vein, Right F Cephalic Vein, Left G Hand Vein, Right H Hand Vein, Left L Intracranial Vein M Internal Jugular Vein, Right N Internal Jugular Vein, Left P External Jugular Vein, Right Q External Jugular Vein, Left R Vertebral Vein, Right S Vertebral Vein, Left T Face Vein, Right V Face Vein, Left Y Upper Vein	0 Open 3 Percutaneous 4 Percutaneous Endoscopic	Z No Device	Z No Qualifier

Section 0 **Medical and Surgical**
Body System 5 **Upper Veins**
Operation R **Replacement:** Putting in or on biological or synthetic material that physically takes the place and/or function of all or a portion of a body part

Body Part (4th)	Approach (5th)	Device (6th)	Qualifier (7th)
0 Azygos Vein **1** Hemiazygos Vein **3** Innominate Vein, Right **4** Innominate Vein, Left **5** Subclavian Vein, Right **6** Subclavian Vein, Left **7** Axillary Vein, Right **8** Axillary Vein, Left **9** Brachial Vein, Right **A** Brachial Vein, Left **B** Basilic Vein, Right **C** Basilic Vein, Left **D** Cephalic Vein, Right **F** Cephalic Vein, Left **G** Hand Vein, Right **H** Hand Vein, Left **L** Intracranial Vein **M** Internal Jugular Vein, Right **N** Internal Jugular Vein, Left **P** External Jugular Vein, Right **Q** External Jugular Vein, Left **R** Vertebral Vein, Right **S** Vertebral Vein, Left **T** Face Vein, Right **V** Face Vein, Left **Y** Upper Vein	**0** Open **4** Percutaneous Endoscopic	**7** Autologous Tissue Substitute **J** Synthetic Substitute **K** Nonautologous Tissue Substitute	**Z** No Qualifier

Section 0 **Medical and Surgical**
Body System 5 **Upper Veins**
Operation S **Reposition:** Moving to its normal location, or other suitable location, all or a portion of a body part

Body Part (4th)	Approach (5th)	Device (6th)	Qualifier (7th)
0 Azygos Vein **1** Hemiazygos Vein **3** Innominate Vein, Right **4** Innominate Vein, Left **5** Subclavian Vein, Right **6** Subclavian Vein, Left **7** Axillary Vein, Right **8** Axillary Vein, Left **9** Brachial Vein, Right **A** Brachial Vein, Left **B** Basilic Vein, Right **C** Basilic Vein, Left **D** Cephalic Vein, Right **F** Cephalic Vein, Left **G** Hand Vein, Right **H** Hand Vein, Left **L** Intracranial Vein **M** Internal Jugular Vein, Right **N** Internal Jugular Vein, Left **P** External Jugular Vein, Right **Q** External Jugular Vein, Left **R** Vertebral Vein, Right **S** Vertebral Vein, Left **T** Face Vein, Right **V** Face Vein, Left **Y** Upper Vein	**0** Open **3** Percutaneous **4** Percutaneous Endoscopic	**Z** No Device	**Z** No Qualifier

Section 0 **Medical and Surgical**
Body System 5 **Upper Veins**
Operation U **Supplement:** Putting in or on biological or synthetic material that physically reinforces and/or augments the function of a portion of a body part

Body Part (4th)	Approach (5th)	Device (6th)	Qualifier (7th)
0 Azygos Vein 1 Hemiazygos Vein 3 Innominate Vein, Right 4 Innominate Vein, Left 5 Subclavian Vein, Right 6 Subclavian Vein, Left 7 Axillary Vein, Right 8 Axillary Vein, Left 9 Brachial Vein, Right A Brachial Vein, Left B Basilic Vein, Right C Basilic Vein, Left D Cephalic Vein, Right F Cephalic Vein, Left G Hand Vein, Right H Hand Vein, Left L Intracranial Vein M Internal Jugular Vein, Right N Internal Jugular Vein, Left P External Jugular Vein, Right Q External Jugular Vein, Left R Vertebral Vein, Right S Vertebral Vein, Left T Face Vein, Right V Face Vein, Left Y Upper Vein	0 Open 3 Percutaneous 4 Percutaneous Endoscopic	7 Autologous Tissue Substitute J Synthetic Substitute K Nonautologous Tissue Substitute	Z No Qualifier

Section 0 **Medical and Surgical**
Body System 5 **Upper Veins**
Operation V **Restriction:** Partially closing an orifice or the lumen of a tubular body part

Body Part (4th)	Approach (5th)	Device (6th)	Qualifier (7th)
0 Azygos Vein 1 Hemiazygos Vein 3 Innominate Vein, Right 4 Innominate Vein, Left 5 Subclavian Vein, Right 6 Subclavian Vein, Left 7 Axillary Vein, Right 8 Axillary Vein, Left 9 Brachial Vein, Right A Brachial Vein, Left B Basilic Vein, Right C Basilic Vein, Left D Cephalic Vein, Right F Cephalic Vein, Left G Hand Vein, Right H Hand Vein, Left L Intracranial Vein M Internal Jugular Vein, Right N Internal Jugular Vein, Left P External Jugular Vein, Right Q External Jugular Vein, Left R Vertebral Vein, Right S Vertebral Vein, Left T Face Vein, Right V Face Vein, Left Y Upper Vein	0 Open 3 Percutaneous 4 Percutaneous Endoscopic	C Extraluminal Device D Intraluminal Device Z No Device	Z No Qualifier

Section 0 **Medical and Surgical**
Body System 5 **Upper Veins**
Operation W **Revision:** Correcting, to the extent possible, a portion of a malfunctioning device or the position of a displaced device

Body Part (4th)	Approach (5th)	Device (6th)	Qualifier (7th)
0 Azygos Vein	**0** Open **3** Percutaneous **4** Percutaneous Endoscopic **X** External	**2** Monitoring Device **M** Neurostimulator Lead	**Z** No Qualifier
3 Innominate Vein, Right **4** Innominate Vein, Left	**0** Open **3** Percutaneous **4** Percutaneous Endoscopic **X** External	**M** Neurostimulator Lead	**Z** No Qualifier
Y Upper Vein	**0** Open **3** Percutaneous **4** Percutaneous Endoscopic	**0** Drainage Device **2** Monitoring Device **3** Infusion Device **7** Autologous Tissue Substitute **C** Extraluminal Device **D** Intraluminal Device **J** Synthetic Substitute **K** Nonautologous Tissue Substitute **Y** Other Device	**Z** No Qualifier
Y Upper Vein	**X** External	**0** Drainage Device **2** Monitoring Device **3** Infusion Device **7** Autologous Tissue Substitute **C** Extraluminal Device **D** Intraluminal Device **J** Synthetic Substitute **K** Nonautologous Tissue Substitute	**Z** No Qualifier

AHA Coding Clinic

051Q49Y Bypass Left External Jugular Vein to Upper Vein with Autologous Venous Tissue, Percutaneous Endoscopic Approach—AHA CC: 1Q, 2020, 28-29
05733DZ Dilation of Right Innominate Vein with Intraluminal Device, Percutaneous Approach—AHA CC: 3Q, 2020, 38-40
059430Z Drainage of Left Innominate Vein with Drainage Device, Percutaneous Approach—AHA CC: 3Q, 2018, 7
05BD0ZZ Excision of Right Cephalic Vein, Open Approach—AHA CC: 3Q, 2020, 40
05BL0ZZ Excision of Intracranial Vein, Open Approach—AHA CC: 1Q, 2020, 24; 2Q, 2021, 15-16
05BN0ZZ Excision of Left Internal Jugular Vein, Open Approach—AHA CC: 2Q, 2016, 12-14
05BQ0ZZ Excision of Left External Jugular Vein, Open Approach—AHA CC: 2Q, 2016, 12-14
05CD0ZZ Extirpation of Matter from Right Cephalic Vein, Open Approach—AHA CC: 3Q, 2020, 37-40
05H032Z Insertion of Monitoring Device into Azygos Vein, Percutaneous Approach—AHA CC: 4Q, 2016, 98-99
05H43MZ Insertion of Neurostimulator Lead into Left Innominate Vein, Percutaneous Approach—AHA CC: 4Q, 2016, 98-99
05Q40ZZ Repair Left Innominate Vein, Open Approach—AHA CC: 3Q, 2017, 15-16
05SD0ZZ Reposition Right Cephalic Vein, Open Approach—AHA CC: 4Q, 2013, 125-126
05VD0ZZ Restriction of Right Cephalic Vein, Open Approach—AHA CC: 3Q, 2020, 37-38

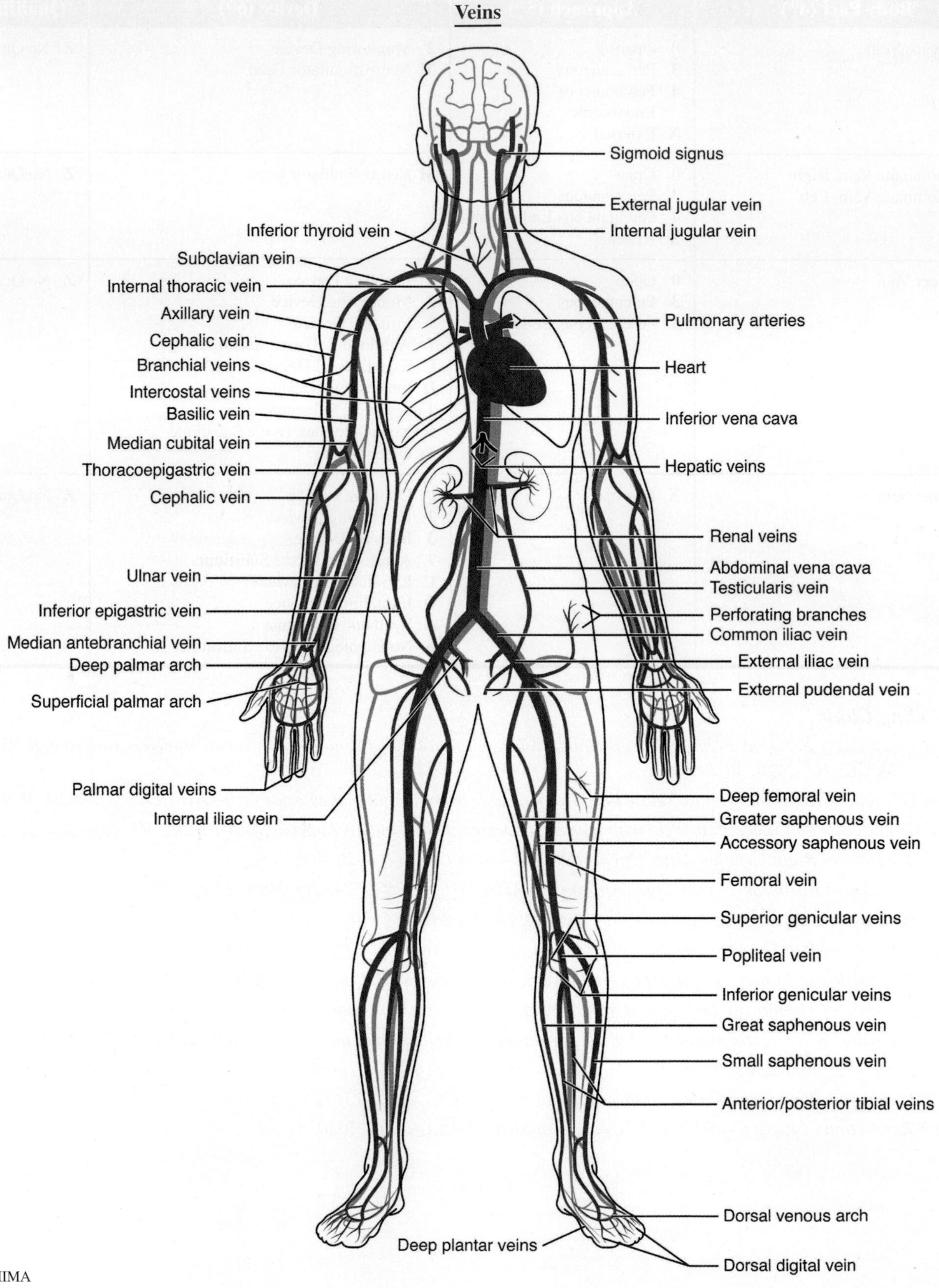
Veins
Sigmoid signus
External jugular vein
Inferior thyroid vein
Internal jugular vein
Subclavian vein
Internal thoracic vein
Axillary vein
Pulmonary arteries
Cephalic vein
Branchial veins
Heart
Intercostal veins
Basilic vein
Inferior vena cava
Median cubital vein
Thoracoepigastric vein
Hepatic veins
Cephalic vein
Renal veins
Ulnar vein
Abdominal vena cava
Testicularis vein
Inferior epigastric vein
Perforating branches
Median antebranchial vein
Common iliac vein
Deep palmar arch
External iliac vein
Superficial palmar arch
External pudendal vein
Palmar digital veins
Deep femoral vein
Internal iliac vein
Greater saphenous vein
Accessory saphenous vein
Femoral vein
Superior genicular veins
Popliteal vein
Inferior genicular veins
Great saphenous vein
Small saphenous vein
Anterior/posterior tibial veins
Dorsal venous arch
Deep plantar veins
Dorsal digital vein

Lower Veins Tables 061–06W

Section	**0**	**Medical and Surgical**
Body System	**6**	**Lower Veins**
Operation	**1**	**Bypass:** Altering the route of passage of the contents of a tubular body part

Body Part (4th)	Approach (5th)	Device (6th)	Qualifier (7th)
0 Inferior Vena Cava	**0** Open **4** Percutaneous Endoscopic	**7** Autologous Tissue Substitute **9** Autologous Venous Tissue **A** Autologous Arterial Tissue **J** Synthetic Substitute **K** Nonautologous Tissue Substitute **Z** No Device	**5** Superior Mesenteric Vein **6** Inferior Mesenteric Vein **P** Pulmonary Trunk **Q** Pulmonary Artery, Right **R** Pulmonary Artery, Left **Y** Lower Vein
1 Splenic Vein	**0** Open **4** Percutaneous Endoscopic	**7** Autologous Tissue Substitute **9** Autologous Venous Tissue **A** Autologous Arterial Tissue **J** Synthetic Substitute **K** Nonautologous Tissue Substitute **Z** No Device	**9** Renal Vein, Right **B** Renal Vein, Left **Y** Lower Vein
2 Gastric Vein **3** Esophageal Vein **4** Hepatic Vein **5** Superior Mesenteric Vein **6** Inferior Mesenteric Vein **7** Colic Vein **9** Renal Vein, Right **B** Renal Vein, Left **C** Common Iliac Vein, Right **D** Common Iliac Vein, Left **F** External Iliac Vein, Right **G** External Iliac Vein, Left **H** Hypogastric Vein, Right **J** Hypogastric Vein, Left **M** Femoral Vein, Right **N** Femoral Vein, Left **P** Saphenous Vein, Right **Q** Saphenous Vein, Left **T** Foot Vein, Right **V** Foot Vein, Left	**0** Open **4** Percutaneous Endoscopic	**7** Autologous Tissue Substitute **9** Autologous Venous Tissue **A** Autologous Arterial Tissue **J** Synthetic Substitute **K** Nonautologous Tissue Substitute **Z** No Device	**Y** Lower Vein
8 Portal Vein	**0** Open	**7** Autologous Tissue Substitute **9** Autologous Venous Tissue **A** Autologous Arterial Tissue **J** Synthetic Substitute **K** Nonautologous Tissue Substitute **Z** No Device	**9** Renal Vein, Right **B** Renal Vein, Left **Y** Lower Vein
8 Portal Vein	**3** Percutaneous	**J** Synthetic Substitute	**4** Hepatic Vein **Y** Lower Vein
8 Portal Vein	**4** Percutaneous Endoscopic	**7** Autologous Tissue Substitute **9** Autologous Venous Tissue **A** Autologous Arterial Tissue **K** Nonautologous Tissue Substitute **Z** No Device	**9** Renal Vein, Right **B** Renal Vein, Left **Y** Lower Vein
8 Portal Vein	**4** Percutaneous Endoscopic	**J** Synthetic Substitute	**4** Hepatic Vein **9** Renal Vein, Right **B** Renal Vein, Left **Y** Lower Vein

Section	**0**	**Medical and Surgical**
Body System	**6**	**Lower Veins**
Operation	**5**	**Destruction:** Physical eradication of all or a portion of a body part by the direct use of energy, force, or a destructive agent

Body Part (4th)	Approach (5th)	Device (6th)	Qualifier (7th)
0 Inferior Vena Cava **1** Splenic Vein **2** Gastric Vein **3** Esophageal Vein **4** Hepatic Vein **5** Superior Mesenteric Vein **6** Inferior Mesenteric Vein **7** Colic Vein **8** Portal Vein **9** Renal Vein, Right **B** Renal Vein, Left **C** Common Iliac Vein, Right **D** Common Iliac Vein, Left **F** External Iliac Vein, Right **G** External Iliac Vein, Left **H** Hypogastric Vein, Right **J** Hypogastric Vein, Left **M** Femoral Vein, Right **N** Femoral Vein, Left **P** Saphenous Vein, Right **Q** Saphenous Vein, Left **T** Foot Vein, Right **V** Foot Vein, Left	**0** Open **3** Percutaneous **4** Percutaneous Endoscopic	**Z** No Device	**Z** No Qualifier
Y Lower Vein	**0** Open **3** Percutaneous **4** Percutaneous Endoscopic	**Z** No Device	**C** Hemorrhoidal Plexus **Z** No Qualifier

Section	**0**	**Medical and Surgical**
Body System	**6**	**Lower Veins**
Operation	**7**	**Dilation:** Expanding an orifice or the lumen of a tubular body part

Body Part (4th)	Approach (5th)	Device (6th)	Qualifier (7th)
0 Inferior Vena Cava **1** Splenic Vein **2** Gastric Vein **3** Esophageal Vein **4** Hepatic Vein **5** Superior Mesenteric Vein **6** Inferior Mesenteric Vein **7** Colic Vein **8** Portal Vein **9** Renal Vein, Right **B** Renal Vein, Left **C** Common Iliac Vein, Right **D** Common Iliac Vein, Left **F** External Iliac Vein, Right **G** External Iliac Vein, Left **H** Hypogastric Vein, Right **J** Hypogastric Vein, Left **M** Femoral Vein, Right **N** Femoral Vein, Left **P** Saphenous Vein, Right **Q** Saphenous Vein, Left **T** Foot Vein, Right **V** Foot Vein, Left **Y** Lower Vein	**0** Open **3** Percutaneous **4** Percutaneous Endoscopic	**D** Intraluminal Device **Z** No Device	**Z** No Qualifier

Section 0 **Medical and Surgical**
Body System 6 **Lower Veins**
Operation 9 **Drainage:** Taking or letting out fluids and/or gases from a body part

Body Part (4th)	Approach (5th)	Device (6th)	Qualifier (7th)
0 Inferior Vena Cava **1** Splenic Vein **2** Gastric Vein **3** Esophageal Vein **4** Hepatic Vein **5** Superior Mesenteric Vein **6** Inferior Mesenteric Vein **7** Colic Vein **8** Portal Vein **9** Renal Vein, Right **B** Renal Vein, Left **C** Common Iliac Vein, Right **D** Common Iliac Vein, Left **F** External Iliac Vein, Right **G** External Iliac Vein, Left **H** Hypogastric Vein, Right **J** Hypogastric Vein, Left **M** Femoral Vein, Right **N** Femoral Vein, Left **P** Saphenous Vein, Right **Q** Saphenous Vein, Left **T** Foot Vein, Right **V** Foot Vein, Left **Y** Lower Vein	**0** Open **3** Percutaneous **4** Percutaneous Endoscopic	**0** Drainage Device	**Z** No Qualifier
0 Inferior Vena Cava **1** Splenic Vein **2** Gastric Vein **3** Esophageal Vein **4** Hepatic Vein **5** Superior Mesenteric Vein **6** Inferior Mesenteric Vein **7** Colic Vein **8** Portal Vein **9** Renal Vein, Right **B** Renal Vein, Left **C** Common Iliac Vein, Right **D** Common Iliac Vein, Left **F** External Iliac Vein, Right **G** External Iliac Vein, Left **H** Hypogastric Vein, Right **J** Hypogastric Vein, Left **M** Femoral Vein, Right **N** Femoral Vein, Left **P** Saphenous Vein, Right **Q** Saphenous Vein, Left **T** Foot Vein, Right **V** Foot Vein, Left **Y** Lower Vein	**0** Open **3** Percutaneous **4** Percutaneous Endoscopic	**Z** No Device	**X** Diagnostic **Z** No Qualifier

Section 0 **Medical and Surgical**
Body System 6 **Lower Veins**
Operation B **Excision:** Cutting out or off, without replacement, a portion of a body part

Body Part (4th)	Approach (5th)	Device (6th)	Qualifier (7th)
0 Inferior Vena Cava **1** Splenic Vein **2** Gastric Vein **3** Esophageal Vein **4** Hepatic Vein **5** Superior Mesenteric Vein **6** Inferior Mesenteric Vein **7** Colic Vein **8** Portal Vein **9** Renal Vein, Right **B** Renal Vein, Left **C** Common Iliac Vein, Right **D** Common Iliac Vein, Left **F** External Iliac Vein, Right **G** External Iliac Vein, Left **H** Hypogastric Vein, Right **J** Hypogastric Vein, Left **M** Femoral Vein, Right **N** Femoral Vein, Left **P** Saphenous Vein, Right **Q** Saphenous Vein, Left **T** Foot Vein, Right **V** Foot Vein, Left	**0** Open **3** Percutaneous **4** Percutaneous Endoscopic	**Z** No Device	**X** Diagnostic **Z** No Qualifier
Y Lower Vein	**0** Open **3** Percutaneous **4** Percutaneous Endoscopic	**Z** No Device	**C** Hemorrhoidal Plexus **X** Diagnostic **Z** No Qualifier

Section 0 **Medical and Surgical**
Body System 6 **Lower Veins**
Operation C **Extirpation:** Taking or cutting out solid matter from a body part

Body Part (4th)	Approach (5th)	Device (6th)	Qualifier (7th)
0 Inferior Vena Cava **1** Splenic Vein **2** Gastric Vein **3** Esophageal Vein **4** Hepatic Vein **5** Superior Mesenteric Vein **6** Inferior Mesenteric Vein **7** Colic Vein **8** Portal Vein **9** Renal Vein, Right **B** Renal Vein, Left **C** Common Iliac Vein, Right **D** Common Iliac Vein, Left **F** External Iliac Vein, Right **G** External Iliac Vein, Left **H** Hypogastric Vein, Right **J** Hypogastric Vein, Left **M** Femoral Vein, Right **N** Femoral Vein, Left **P** Saphenous Vein, Right **Q** Saphenous Vein, Left **T** Foot Vein, Right **V** Foot Vein, Left **Y** Lower Vein	**0** Open **3** Percutaneous **4** Percutaneous Endoscopic	**Z** No Device	**Z** No Qualifier

Section 0 **Medical and Surgical**
Body System 6 **Lower Veins**
Operation D **Extraction:** Pulling or stripping out or off all or a portion of a body part by the use of force

Body Part (4th)	Approach (5th)	Device (6th)	Qualifier (7th)
M Femoral Vein, Right **N** Femoral Vein, Left **P** Saphenous Vein, Right **Q** Saphenous Vein, Left **T** Foot Vein, Right **V** Foot Vein, Left **Y** Lower Vein	**0** Open **3** Percutaneous **4** Percutaneous Endoscopic	**Z** No Device	**Z** No Qualifier

Section 0 **Medical and Surgical**
Body System 6 **Lower Veins**
Operation F **Fragmentation:** Breaking solid matter in a body part into pieces

Body Part (4th)	Approach (5th)	Device (6th)	Qualifier (7th)
C Common Iliac Vein, Right **D** Common Iliac Vein, Left **F** External Iliac Vein, Right **G** External Iliac Vein, Left **H** Hypogastric Vein, Right **J** Hypogastric Vein, Left **M** Femoral Vein, Right **N** Femoral Vein, Left **P** Saphenous Vein, Right **Q** Saphenous Vein, Left **Y** Lower Vein	**3** Percutaneous	**Z** No Device	**0** Ultrasonic **Z** No Qualifier

Section 0 **Medical and Surgical**
Body System 6 **Lower Veins**
Operation H **Insertion:** Putting in a nonbiological appliance that monitors, assists, performs, or prevents a physiological function but does not physically take the place of a body part

Body Part (4th)	Approach (5th)	Device (6th)	Qualifier (7th)
0 Inferior Vena Cava	**0** Open **3** Percutaneous	**3** Infusion Device	**T** Via Umbilical Vein **Z** No Qualifier
0 Inferior Vena Cava	**0** Open **3** Percutaneous	**D** Intraluminal Device	**Z** No Qualifier
0 Inferior Vena Cava	**4** Percutaneous Endoscopic	**3** Infusion Device **D** Intraluminal Device	**Z** No Qualifier

Continued →

Section 0 **Medical and Surgical**
Body System 6 **Lower Veins**
Operation H **Insertion:** Putting in a nonbiological appliance that monitors, assists, performs, or prevents a physiological function but does not physically take the place of a body part

Body Part (4th)	Approach (5th)	Device (6th)	Qualifier (7th)
1 Splenic Vein **2** Gastric Vein **3** Esophageal Vein **4** Hepatic Vein **5** Superior Mesenteric Vein **6** Inferior Mesenteric Vein **7** Colic Vein **8** Portal Vein **9** Renal Vein, Right **B** Renal Vein, Left **C** Common Iliac Vein, Right **D** Common Iliac Vein, Left **F** External Iliac Vein, Right **G** External Iliac Vein, Left **H** Hypogastric Vein, Right **J** Hypogastric Vein, Left **M** Femoral Vein, Right **N** Femoral Vein, Left **P** Saphenous Vein, Right **Q** Saphenous Vein, Left **T** Foot Vein, Right **V** Foot Vein, Left	**0** Open **3** Percutaneous **4** Percutaneous Endoscopic	**3** Infusion Device **D** Intraluminal Device	**Z** No Qualifier
Y Lower Vein	**0** Open **3** Percutaneous **4** Percutaneous Endoscopic	**2** Monitoring Device **3** Infusion Device **D** Intraluminal Device **Y** Other Device	**Z** No Qualifier

Section 0 **Medical and Surgical**
Body System 6 **Lower Veins**
Operation J **Inspection:** Visually and/or manually exploring a body part

Body Part (4th)	Approach (5th)	Device (6th)	Qualifier (7th)
Y Lower Vein	**0** Open **3** Percutaneous **4** Percutaneous Endoscopic **X** External	**Z** No Device	**Z** No Qualifier

Section 0 **Medical and Surgical**
Body System 6 **Lower Veins**
Operation L **Occlusion:** Completely closing an orifice or the lumen of a tubular body part

Body Part (4th)	Approach (5th)	Device (6th)	Qualifier (7th)
0 Inferior Vena Cava **1** Splenic Vein **4** Hepatic Vein **5** Superior Mesenteric Vein **6** Inferior Mesenteric Vein **7** Colic Vein **8** Portal Vein **9** Renal Vein, Right **B** Renal Vein, Left **C** Common Iliac Vein, Right **D** Common Iliac Vein, Left **F** External Iliac Vein, Right **G** External Iliac Vein, Left **H** Hypogastric Vein, Right **J** Hypogastric Vein, Left **M** Femoral Vein, Right **N** Femoral Vein, Left **P** Saphenous Vein, Right **Q** Saphenous Vein, Left **T** Foot Vein, Right **V** Foot Vein, Left	**0** Open **3** Percutaneous **4** Percutaneous Endoscopic	**C** Extraluminal Device **D** Intraluminal Device **Z** No Device	**Z** No Qualifier
2 Gastric Vein **3** Esophageal Vein	**0** Open **3** Percutaneous **4** Percutaneous Endoscopic **7** Via Natural or Artificial Opening **8** Via Natural or Artificial Opening Endoscopic	**C** Extraluminal Device **D** Intraluminal Device **Z** No Device	**Z** No Qualifier
Y Lower Vein	**0** Open **3** Percutaneous **4** Percutaneous Endoscopic **7** Via Natural or Artificial Opening **8** Via Natural or Artificial Opening Endoscopic	**C** Extraluminal Device **D** Intraluminal Device **Z** No Device	**C** Hemorrhoidal Plexus **Z** No Qualifier

Section 0 **Medical and Surgical**
Body System 6 **Lower Veins**
Operation N **Release:** Freeing a body part from an abnormal physical constraint by cutting or by the use of force

Body Part (4th)	Approach (5th)	Device (6th)	Qualifier (7th)
0 Inferior Vena Cava **1** Splenic Vein **2** Gastric Vein **3** Esophageal Vein **4** Hepatic Vein **5** Superior Mesenteric Vein **6** Inferior Mesenteric Vein **7** Colic Vein **8** Portal Vein **9** Renal Vein, Right **B** Renal Vein, Left **C** Common Iliac Vein, Right **D** Common Iliac Vein, Left **F** External Iliac Vein, Right **G** External Iliac Vein, Left **H** Hypogastric Vein, Right **J** Hypogastric Vein, Left **M** Femoral Vein, Right **N** Femoral Vein, Left **P** Saphenous Vein, Right **Q** Saphenous Vein, Left **T** Foot Vein, Right **V** Foot Vein, Left **Y** Lower Vein	**0** Open **3** Percutaneous **4** Percutaneous Endoscopic	**Z** No Device	**Z** No Qualifier

Section 0 **Medical and Surgical**
Body System 6 **Lower Veins**
Operation P **Removal:** Taking out or off a device from a body part

Body Part (4th)	Approach (5th)	Device (6th)	Qualifier (7th)
Y Lower Vein	0 Open 3 Percutaneous 4 Percutaneous Endoscopic	0 Drainage Device 2 Monitoring Device 3 Infusion Device 7 Autologous Tissue Substitute C Extraluminal Device D Intraluminal Device J Synthetic Substitute K Nonautologous Tissue Substitute Y Other Device	Z No Qualifier
Y Lower Vein	X External	0 Drainage Device 2 Monitoring Device 3 Infusion Device D Intraluminal Device	Z No Qualifier

Section 0 **Medical and Surgical**
Body System 6 **Lower Veins**
Operation Q **Repair:** Restoring, to the extent possible, a body part to its normal anatomic structure and function

Body Part (4th)	Approach (5th)	Device (6th)	Qualifier (7th)
0 Inferior Vena Cava 1 Splenic Vein 2 Gastric Vein 3 Esophageal Vein 4 Hepatic Vein 5 Superior Mesenteric Vein 6 Inferior Mesenteric Vein 7 Colic Vein 8 Portal Vein 9 Renal Vein, Right B Renal Vein, Left C Common Iliac Vein, Right D Common Iliac Vein, Left F External Iliac Vein, Right G External Iliac Vein, Left H Hypogastric Vein, Right J Hypogastric Vein, Left M Femoral Vein, Right N Femoral Vein, Left P Saphenous Vein, Right Q Saphenous Vein, Left T Foot Vein, Right V Foot Vein, Left Y Lower Vein	0 Open 3 Percutaneous 4 Percutaneous Endoscopic	Z No Device	Z No Qualifier

Section 0 Medical and Surgical
Body System 6 Lower Veins
Operation R Replacement: Putting in or on biological or synthetic material that physically takes the place and/or function of all or a portion of a body part

Body Part (4th)	Approach (5th)	Device (6th)	Qualifier (7th)
0 Inferior Vena Cava 1 Splenic Vein 2 Gastric Vein 3 Esophageal Vein 4 Hepatic Vein 5 Superior Mesenteric Vein 6 Inferior Mesenteric Vein 7 Colic Vein 8 Portal Vein 9 Renal Vein, Right B Renal Vein, Left C Common Iliac Vein, Right D Common Iliac Vein, Left F External Iliac Vein, Right G External Iliac Vein, Left H Hypogastric Vein, Right J Hypogastric Vein, Left M Femoral Vein, Right N Femoral Vein, Left P Saphenous Vein, Right Q Saphenous Vein, Left T Foot Vein, Right V Foot Vein, Left Y Lower Vein	0 Open 4 Percutaneous Endoscopic	7 Autologous Tissue Substitute J Synthetic Substitute K Nonautologous Tissue Substitute	Z No Qualifier

Section 0 Medical and Surgical
Body System 6 Lower Veins
Operation S Reposition: Moving to its normal location, or other suitable location, all or a portion of a body part

Body Part (4th)	Approach (5th)	Device (6th)	Qualifier (7th)
0 Inferior Vena Cava 1 Splenic Vein 2 Gastric Vein 3 Esophageal Vein 4 Hepatic Vein 5 Superior Mesenteric Vein 6 Inferior Mesenteric Vein 7 Colic Vein 8 Portal Vein 9 Renal Vein, Right B Renal Vein, Left C Common Iliac Vein, Right D Common Iliac Vein, Left F External Iliac Vein, Right G External Iliac Vein, Left H Hypogastric Vein, Right J Hypogastric Vein, Left M Femoral Vein, Right N Femoral Vein, Left P Saphenous Vein, Right Q Saphenous Vein, Left T Foot Vein, Right V Foot Vein, Left Y Lower Vein	0 Open 3 Percutaneous 4 Percutaneous Endoscopic	Z No Device	Z No Qualifier

Section 0 **Medical and Surgical**
Body System 6 **Lower Veins**
Operation U **Supplement:** Putting in or on biological or synthetic material that physically reinforces and/or augments the function of a portion of a body part

Body Part (4th)	Approach (5th)	Device (6th)	Qualifier (7th)
0 Inferior Vena Cava **1** Splenic Vein **2** Gastric Vein **3** Esophageal Vein **4** Hepatic Vein **5** Superior Mesenteric Vein **6** Inferior Mesenteric Vein **7** Colic Vein **8** Portal Vein **9** Renal Vein, Right **B** Renal Vein, Left **C** Common Iliac Vein, Right **D** Common Iliac Vein, Left **F** External Iliac Vein, Right **G** External Iliac Vein, Left **H** Hypogastric Vein, Right **J** Hypogastric Vein, Left **M** Femoral Vein, Right **N** Femoral Vein, Left **P** Saphenous Vein, Right **Q** Saphenous Vein, Left **T** Foot Vein, Right **V** Foot Vein, Left **Y** Lower Vein	**0** Open **3** Percutaneous **4** Percutaneous Endoscopic	**7** Autologous Tissue Substitute **J** Synthetic Substitute **K** Nonautologous Tissue Substitute	**Z** No Qualifier

Section 0 **Medical and Surgical**
Body System 6 **Lower Veins**
Operation V **Restriction:** Partially closing an orifice or the lumen of a tubular body part

Body Part (4th)	Approach (5th)	Device (6th)	Qualifier (7th)
0 Inferior Vena Cava **1** Splenic Vein **2** Gastric Vein **3** Esophageal Vein **4** Hepatic Vein **5** Superior Mesenteric Vein **6** Inferior Mesenteric Vein **7** Colic Vein **8** Portal Vein **9** Renal Vein, Right **B** Renal Vein, Left **C** Common Iliac Vein, Right **D** Common Iliac Vein, Left **F** External Iliac Vein, Right **G** External Iliac Vein, Left **H** Hypogastric Vein, Right **J** Hypogastric Vein, Left **M** Femoral Vein, Right **N** Femoral Vein, Left **P** Saphenous Vein, Right **Q** Saphenous Vein, Left **T** Foot Vein, Right **V** Foot Vein, Left **Y** Lower Vein	**0** Open **3** Percutaneous **4** Percutaneous Endoscopic	**C** Extraluminal Device **D** Intraluminal Device **Z** No Device	**Z** No Qualifier

Section 0 **Medical and Surgical**
Body System 6 **Lower Veins**
Operation W **Revision:** Correcting, to the extent possible, a portion of a malfunctioning device or the position of a displaced device

Body Part (4th)	Approach (5th)	Device (6th)	Qualifier (7th)
Y Lower Vein	**0** Open **3** Percutaneous **4** Percutaneous Endoscopic **X** External	**0** Drainage Device **2** Monitoring Device **3** Infusion Device **7** Autologous Tissue Substitute **C** Extraluminal Device **D** Intraluminal Device **J** Synthetic Substitute **K** Nonautologous Tissue Substitute **Y** Other Device	**Z** No Qualifier
Y Lower Vein	**X** External	**0** Drainage Device **2** Monitoring Device **3** Infusion Device **7** Autologous Tissue Substitute **C** Extraluminal Device **D** Intraluminal Device **J** Synthetic Substitute **K** Nonautologus Tissue Substitute	**Z** No Qualifier

AHA Coding Clinic

06100JP Bypass Inferior Vena Cava to Pulmonary Trunk with Synthetic Substitute, Open Approach—AHA CC: 4Q, 2017, 37-38

06BP0ZZ Excision of Right Saphenous Vein, Open Approach—AHA CC: 1Q, 2014, 10-11; 2Q, 2016, 18-19; 1Q, 2017, 31-32; 3Q. 2017, 5-6

06BP4ZZ Excision of Right Saphenous Vein, Percutaneous Endoscopic Approach—AHA CC: 3Q, 2014, 20-21

06BQ0ZZ Excision of Left Saphenous Vein, Open Approach—AHA CC: 1Q, 2017, 32-33; 1Q, 2020, 28-29

06BQ4ZZ Excision of Left Saphenous Vein, Percutaneous Endoscopic Approach—AHA CC: 3Q, 2014, 20-21; 1Q, 2016, 27-28

06H033T Insertion of Infusion Device, Via Umbilical Vein, into Inferior Vena Cava, Percutaneous Approach—AHA CC: 1Q, 2017, 31

06H033Z Insertion of Infusion Device into Inferior Vena Cava, Percutaneous Approach—AHA CC: 3Q, 2013, 18-19

06HY33Z Insertion of Infusion Device into Lower Vein, Percutaneous Approach—AHA CC: 1Q, 2017, 31

06L34CZ Occlusion of Esophageal Vein with Extraluminal Device, Percutaneous Endoscopic Approach—AHA CC: 4Q, 2013, 112-113

06L38CZ Occlusion of Esophageal Vein with Extraluminal Device, Via Natural or Artificial Opening Endoscopic—AHA CC: 4Q, 2017, 57-58

06LF0CZ Occlusion of Right External Iliac Vein with Extraluminal Device, Open Approach—AHA CC: 2Q, 2018, 18-19

06LG0CZ Occlusion of Left External Iliac Vein with Extraluminal Device, Open Approach—AHA CC: 2Q, 2018, 18-19

06LY3DZ Occlusion of Lower Vein with Intraluminal Device, Percutaneous Approach—AHA CC: 3Q, 2020, 44-45

06V03DZ Restriction of Inferior Vena Cava with Intraluminal Device, Percutaneous Approach—AHA CC: 3Q, 2018, 11

06WY3DZ Revision of Intraluminal Device in Lower Vein, Percutaneous Approach—AHA CC: 3Q, 2014, 25-26

06WY3JZ Revision of Synthetic Substitute in Lower Vein, Percutaneous Approach—AHA CC: 1Q, 2018, 10; 2Q, 2019, 39

Lymph Vessels and Nodes of Head and Neck; Lymphatic Drainage of Mouth and Pharynx

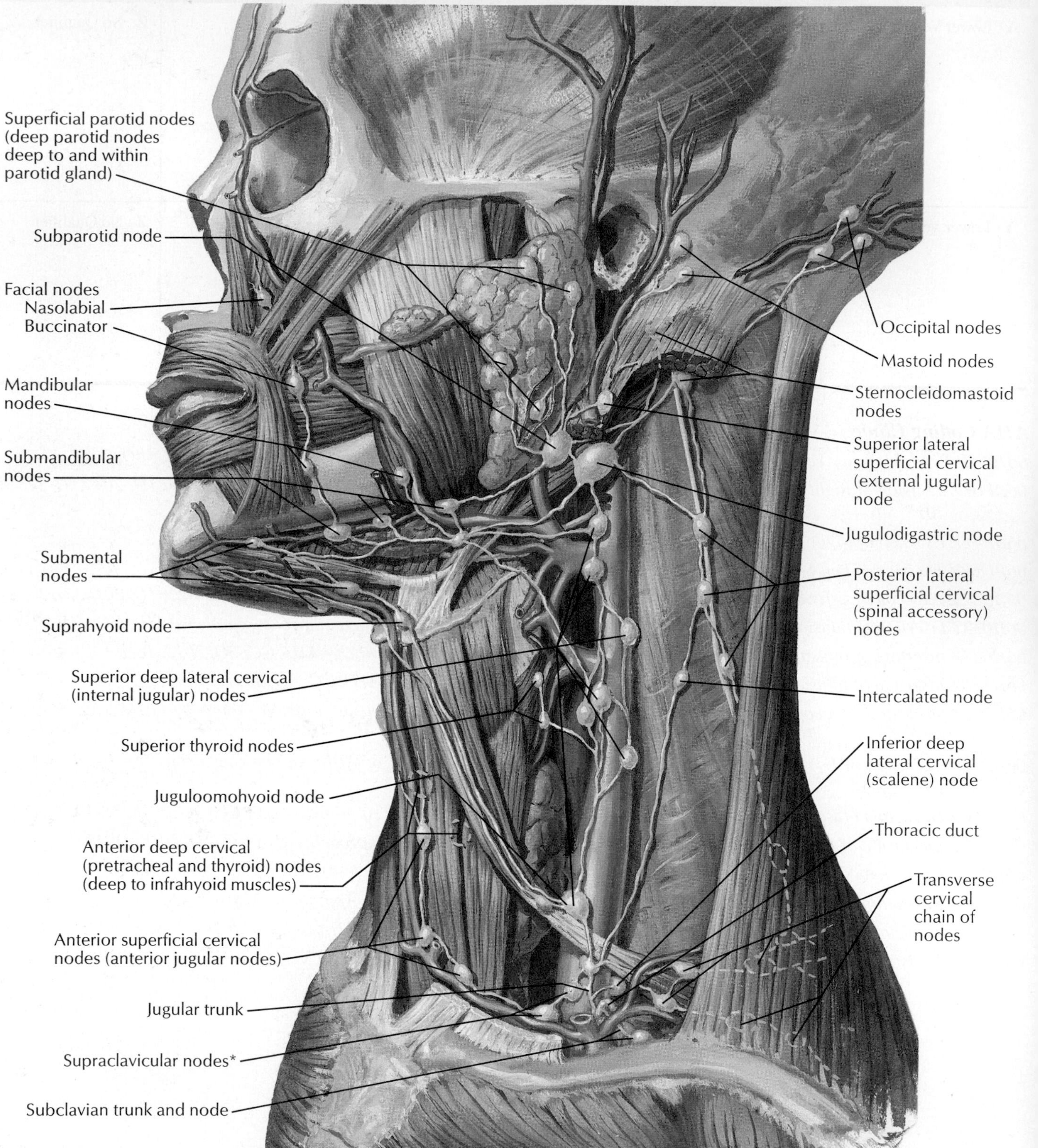
Superficial parotid nodes (deep parotid nodes deep to and within parotid gland)
Subparotid node
Facial nodes
Nasolabial
Buccinator
Mandibular nodes
Submandibular nodes
Submental nodes
Suprahyoid node
Superior deep lateral cervical (internal jugular) nodes
Superior thyroid nodes
Juguloomohyoid node
Anterior deep cervical (pretracheal and thyroid) nodes (deep to infrahyoid muscles)
Anterior superficial cervical nodes (anterior jugular nodes)
Jugular trunk
Supraclavicular nodes*
Subclavian trunk and node
Occipital nodes
Mastoid nodes
Sternocleidomastoid nodes
Superior lateral superficial cervical (external jugular) node
Jugulodigastric node
Posterior lateral superficial cervical (spinal accessory) nodes
Intercalated node
Inferior deep lateral cervical (scalene) node
Thoracic duct
Transverse cervical chain of nodes
F. Netter M.D.

*The supraclavicular group of nodes (also known as the lower deep cervical group), especially on the left, are also sometimes referred to as the signal or sentinel lymph nodes of Virchow or Troisier, especially when sufficiently enlarged and palpable. These nodes (or a single node) are so termed because they may be the first recognized presumptive evidence of malignant disease in the viscera.

Lymph Vessels and Nodes of Mammary Gland Lymphatic Drainage

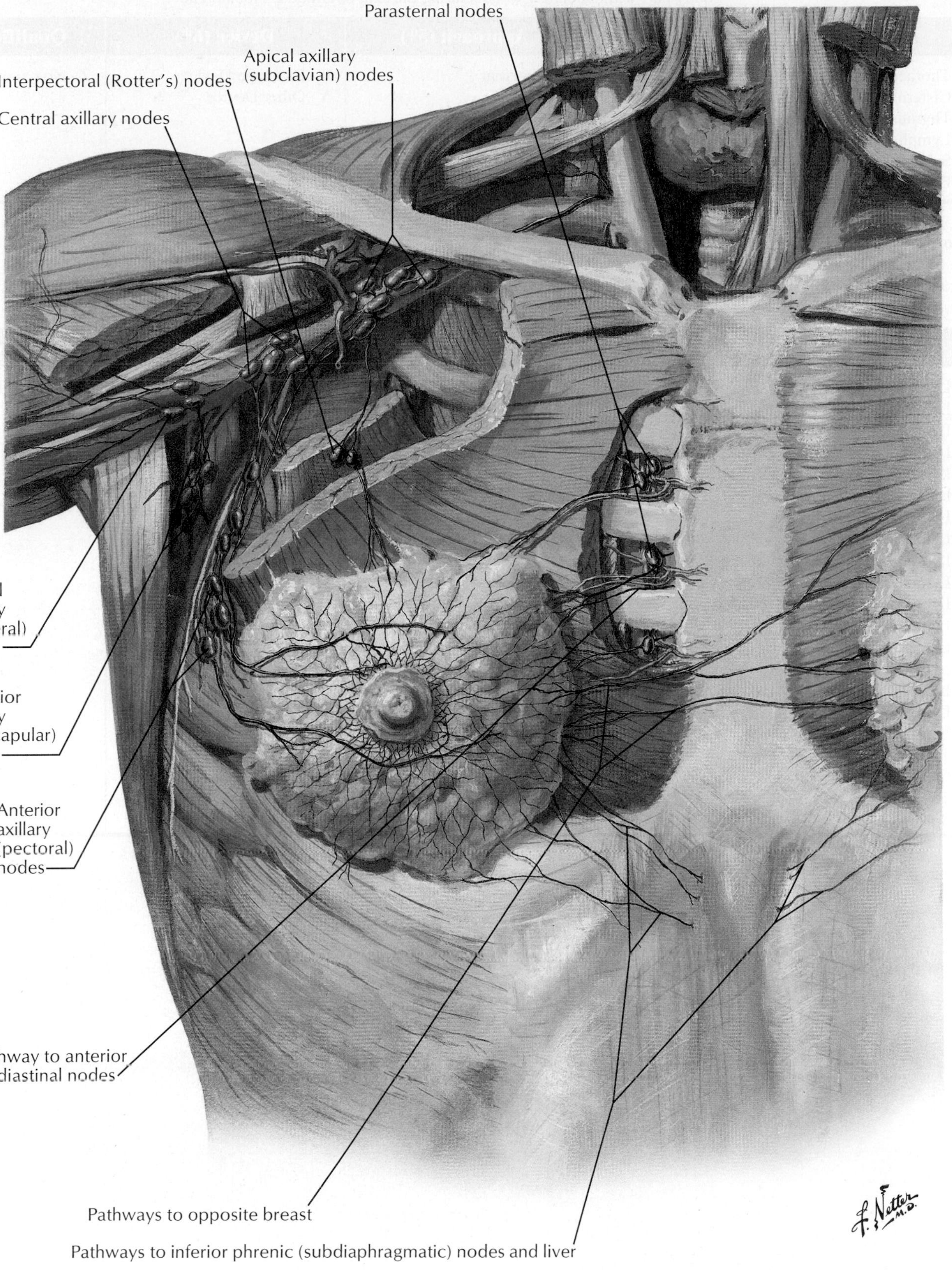
Parasternal nodes
Apical axillary (subclavian) nodes
Interpectoral (Rotter's) nodes
Central axillary nodes
Lateral axillary (humeral) nodes
Posterior axillary (subscapular) nodes
Anterior axillary (pectoral) nodes
Pathway to anterior mediastinal nodes
Pathways to opposite breast
Pathways to inferior phrenic (subdiaphragmatic) nodes and liver
F. Netter M.D.

Section 0 **Medical and Surgical**
Body System 7 **Lymphatic and Hemic Systems**
Operation 2 **Change:** Taking out or off a device from a body part and putting back an identical or similar device in or on the same body part without cutting or puncturing the skin or a mucous membrane

Body Part (4th)	Approach (5th)	Device (6th)	Qualifier (7th)
K Thoracic Duct **L** Cisterna Chyli **M** Thymus **N** Lymphatic **P** Spleen **T** Bone Marrow	**X** External	**0** Drainage Device **Y** Other Device	**Z** No Qualifier

Section 0 **Medical and Surgical**
Body System 7 **Lymphatic and Hemic Systems**
Operation 5 **Destruction:** Physical eradication of all or a portion of a body part by the direct use of energy, force, or a destructive agent

Body Part (4th)	Approach (5th)	Device (6th)	Qualifier (7th)
0 Lymphatic, Head **1** Lymphatic, Right Neck **2** Lymphatic, Left Neck **3** Lymphatic, Right Upper Extremity **4** Lymphatic, Left Upper Extremity **5** Lymphatic, Right Axillary **6** Lymphatic, Left Axillary **7** Lymphatic, Thorax **8** Lymphatic, Internal Mammary, Right **9** Lymphatic, Internal Mammary, Left **B** Lymphatic, Mesenteric **C** Lymphatic, Pelvis **D** Lymphatic, Aortic **F** Lymphatic, Right Lower Extremity **G** Lymphatic, Left Lower Extremity **H** Lymphatic, Right Inguinal **J** Lymphatic, Left Inguinal **K** Thoracic Duct **L** Cisterna Chyli **M** Thymus **P** Spleen	**0** Open **3** Percutaneous **4** Percutaneous Endoscopic	**Z** No Device	**Z** No Qualifier

Section 0 **Medical and Surgical**
Body System 7 **Lymphatic and Hemic Systems**
Operation 9 **Drainage:** Taking or letting out fluids and/or gases from a body part

Body Part (4th)	Approach (5th)	Device (6th)	Qualifier (7th)
0 Lymphatic, Head **1** Lymphatic, Right Neck **2** Lymphatic, Left Neck **3** Lymphatic, Right Upper Extremity **4** Lymphatic, Left Upper Extremity **5** Lymphatic, Right Axillary **6** Lymphatic, Left Axillary **7** Lymphatic, Thorax **8** Lymphatic, Internal Mammary, Right **9** Lymphatic, Internal Mammary, Left **B** Lymphatic, Mesenteric **C** Lymphatic, Pelvis **D** Lymphatic, Aortic **F** Lymphatic, Right Lower Extremity **G** Lymphatic, Left Lower Extremity **H** Lymphatic, Right Inguinal **J** Lymphatic, Left Inguinal **K** Thoracic Duct **L** Cisterna Chyli	**0** Open **3** Percutaneous **4** Percutaneous Endoscopic **8** Via Natural or Artificial Opening Endoscopic	**0** Drainage Device	**Z** No Qualifier
0 Lymphatic, Head **1** Lymphatic, Right Neck **2** Lymphatic, Left Neck **3** Lymphatic, Right Upper Extremity **4** Lymphatic, Left Upper Extremity **5** Lymphatic, Right Axillary **6** Lymphatic, Left Axillary **7** Lymphatic, Thorax **8** Lymphatic, Internal Mammary, Right **9** Lymphatic, Internal Mammary, Left **B** Lymphatic, Mesenteric **C** Lymphatic, Pelvis **D** Lymphatic, Aortic **F** Lymphatic, Right Lower Extremity **G** Lymphatic, Left Lower Extremity **H** Lymphatic, Right Inguinal **J** Lymphatic, Left Inguinal **K** Thoracic Duct **L** Cisterna Chyli	**0** Open **3** Percutaneous **4** Percutaneous Endoscopic **8** Via Natural or Artificial Opening Endoscopic	**Z** No Device	**X** Diagnostic **Z** No Qualifier
M Thymus **P** Spleen **T** Bone Marrow	**0** Open **3** Percutaneous **4** Percutaneous Endoscopic	**0** Drainage Device	**Z** No Qualifier
M Thymus **P** Spleen **T** Bone Marrow	**0** Open **3** Percutaneous **4** Percutaneous Endoscopic	**Z** No Device	**X** No Diagnostic **Z** No Qualifier

Section 0 **Medical and Surgical**
Body System 7 **Lymphatic and Hemic Systems**
Operation B **Excision:** Cutting out or off, without replacement, a portion of a body part

Body Part (4th)	Approach (5th)	Device (6th)	Qualifier (7th)
0 Lymphatic, Head **1** Lymphatic, Right Neck **2** Lymphatic, Left Neck **3** Lymphatic, Right Upper Extremity **4** Lymphatic, Left Upper Extremity **5** Lymphatic, Right Axillary **6** Lymphatic, Left Axillary **7** Lymphatic, Thorax **8** Lymphatic, Internal Mammary, Right **9** Lymphatic, Internal Mammary, Left **B** Lymphatic, Mesenteric **C** Lymphatic, Pelvis **D** Lymphatic, Aortic **F** Lymphatic, Right Lower Extremity **G** Lymphatic, Left Lower Extremity **H** Lymphatic, Right Inguinal **J** Lymphatic, Left Inguinal **K** Thoracic Duct **L** Cisterna Chyli **M** Thymus **P** Spleen	**0** Open **3** Percutaneous **4** Percutaneous Endoscopic	**Z** No Device	**X** Diagnostic **Z** No Qualifier

Section 0 **Medical and Surgical**
Body System 7 **Lymphatic and Hemic Systems**
Operation C **Extirpation:** Taking or cutting out solid matter from a body part

Body Part (4th)	Approach (5th)	Device (6th)	Qualifier (7th)
0 Lymphatic, Head **1** Lymphatic, Right Neck **2** Lymphatic, Left Neck **3** Lymphatic, Right Upper Extremity **4** Lymphatic, Left Upper Extremity **5** Lymphatic, Right Axillary **6** Lymphatic, Left Axillary **7** Lymphatic, Thorax **8** Lymphatic, Internal Mammary, Right **9** Lymphatic, Internal Mammary, Left **B** Lymphatic, Mesenteric **C** Lymphatic, Pelvis **D** Lymphatic, Aortic **F** Lymphatic, Right Lower Extremity **G** Lymphatic, Left Lower Extremity **H** Lymphatic, Right Inguinal **J** Lymphatic, Left Inguinal **K** Thoracic Duct **L** Cisterna Chyli **M** Thymus **P** Spleen	**0** Open **3** Percutaneous **4** Percutaneous Endoscopic	**Z** No Device	**Z** No Qualifier

Section 0 **Medical and Surgical**
Body System 7 **Lymphatic and Hemic Systems**
Operation D **Extraction:** Pulling or stripping out or off all or a portion of a body part by the use of force

Body Part (4th)	Approach (5th)	Device (6th)	Qualifier (7th)
0 Lymphatic, Head **1** Lymphatic, Right Neck **2** Lymphatic, Left Neck **3** Lymphatic, Right Upper Extremity **4** Lymphatic, Left Upper Extremity **5** Lymphatic, Right Axillary **6** Lymphatic, Left Axillary **7** Lymphatic, Thorax **8** Lymphatic, Internal Mammary, Right **9** Lymphatic, Internal Mammary, Left **B** Lymphatic, Mesenteric **C** Lymphatic, Pelvis **D** Lymphatic, Aortic **F** Lymphatic, Right Lower Extremity **G** Lymphatic, Left Lower Extremity **H** Lymphatic, Right Inguinal **J** Lymphatic, Left Inguinal **K** Thoracic Duct **L** Cisterna Chyli	**3** Percutaneous **4** Percutaneous Endoscopic **8** Via Natural or Artificial Opening Endoscopic	**Z** No Device	**X** Diagnostic
M Thymus **P** Spleen	**3** Percutaneous **4** Percutaneous Endoscopic	**Z** No Device	**X** No Diagnostic
Q Bone Marrow, Sternum **R** Bone Marrow, Iliac **S** Bone Marrow, Vertebral **T** Bone Marrow	**0** Open **3** Percutaneous	**Z** No Device	**X** Diagnostic **Z** No Qualifier

Section 0 **Medical and Surgical**
Body System 7 **Lymphatic and Hemic Systems**
Operation H **Insertion:** Putting in a nonbiological appliance that monitors, assists, performs, or prevents a physiological function but does not physically take the place of a body part

Body Part (4th)	Approach (5th)	Device (6th)	Qualifier (7th)
K Thoracic Duct **L** Cisterna Chyli **M** Thymus **N** Lymphatic **P** Spleen **T** Bone Marrow	**0** Open **3** Percutaneous **4** Percutaneous Endoscopic	**1** Radioactive Element **3** Infusion Device **Y** Other Device	**Z** No Qualifier

Section 0 **Medical and Surgical**
Body System 7 **Lymphatic and Hemic Systems**
Operation J **Inspection:** Visually and/or manually exploring a body part

Body Part (4th)	Approach (5th)	Device (6th)	Qualifier (7th)
K Thoracic Duct **L** Cisterna Chyli **M** Thymus **T** Bone Marrow	**0** Open **3** Percutaneous **4** Percutaneous Endoscopic	**Z** No Device	**Z** No Qualifier
N Lymphatic	**0** Open **3** Percutaneous **4** Percutaneous Endoscopic **8** Via Natural or Artificial Opening Endoscopic **X** External	**Z** No Device	**Z** No Qualifier
P Spleen	**0** Open **3** Percutaneous **4** Percutaneous Endoscopic **X** External	**Z** No Device	**Z** No Qualifier

Section 0 **Medical and Surgical**
Body System 7 **Lymphatic and Hemic Systems**
Operation L **Occlusion:** Completely closing an orifice or the lumen of a tubular body part

Body Part (4th)	Approach (5th)	Device (6th)	Qualifier (7th)
0 Lymphatic, Head **1** Lymphatic, Right Neck **2** Lymphatic, Left Neck **3** Lymphatic, Right Upper Extremity **4** Lymphatic, Left Upper Extremity **5** Lymphatic, Right Axillary **6** Lymphatic, Left Axillary **7** Lymphatic, Thorax **8** Lymphatic, Internal Mammary, Right **9** Lymphatic, Internal Mammary, Left **B** Lymphatic, Mesenteric **C** Lymphatic, Pelvis **D** Lymphatic, Aortic **F** Lymphatic, Right Lower Extremity **G** Lymphatic, Left Lower Extremity **H** Lymphatic, Right Inguinal **J** Lymphatic, Left Inguinal **K** Thoracic Duct **L** Cisterna Chyli	**0** Open **3** Percutaneous **4** Percutaneous Endoscopic	**C** Extraluminal Device **D** Intraluminal Device **Z** No Device	**Z** No Qualifier

Section 0 **Medical and Surgical**
Body System 7 **Lymphatic and Hemic Systems**
Operation N **Release:** Freeing a body part from an abnormal physical constraint by cutting or by the use of force

Body Part (4th)	Approach (5th)	Device (6th)	Qualifier (7th)
0 Lymphatic, Head **1** Lymphatic, Right Neck **2** Lymphatic, Left Neck **3** Lymphatic, Right Upper Extremity **4** Lymphatic, Left Upper Extremity **5** Lymphatic, Right Axillary **6** Lymphatic, Left Axillary **7** Lymphatic, Thorax **8** Lymphatic, Internal Mammary, Right **9** Lymphatic, Internal Mammary, Left **B** Lymphatic, Mesenteric **C** Lymphatic, Pelvis **D** Lymphatic, Aortic **F** Lymphatic, Right Lower Extremity **G** Lymphatic, Left Lower Extremity **H** Lymphatic, Right Inguinal **J** Lymphatic, Left Inguinal **K** Thoracic Duct **L** Cisterna Chyli **M** Thymus **P** Spleen	**0** Open **3** Percutaneous **4** Percutaneous Endoscopic	**Z** No Device	**Z** No Qualifier

Section 0 Medical and Surgical
Body System 7 Lymphatic and Hemic Systems
Operation P **Removal:** Taking out or off a device from a body part

Body Part (4th)	Approach (5th)	Device (6th)	Qualifier (7th)
K Thoracic Duct **L** Cisterna Chyli **N** Lymphatic	**0** Open **3** Percutaneous **4** Percutaneous Endoscopic	**0** Drainage Device **3** Infusion Device **7** Autologous Tissue Substitute **C** Extraluminal Device **D** Intraluminal Device **J** Synthetic Substitute **K** Nonautologous Tissue Substitute **Y** Other Device	**Z** No Qualifier
K Thoracic Duct **L** Cisterna Chyli **N** Lymphatic	**X** External	**0** Drainage Device **3** Infusion Device **D** Intraluminal Device	**Z** No Qualifier
M Thymus **P** Spleen	**0** Open **3** Percutaneous **4** Percutaneous Endoscopic	**0** Drainage Device **3** Infusion Device **Y** Other Device	**Z** No Qualifier
M Thymus **P** Spleen	**X** External	**0** Drainage Device **3** Infusion Device	**Z** No Qualifier
T Bone Marrow	**0** Open **3** Percutaneous **4** Percutaneous Endoscopic **X** External	**0** Drainage Device	**Z** No Qualifier

Section 0 Medical and Surgical
Body System 7 Lymphatic and Hemic Systems
Operation Q **Repair:** Restoring, to the extent possible, a body part to its normal anatomic structure and function

Body Part (4th)	Approach (5th)	Device (6th)	Qualifier (7th)
0 Lymphatic, Head **1** Lymphatic, Right Neck **2** Lymphatic, Left Neck **3** Lymphatic, Right Upper Extremity **4** Lymphatic, Left Upper Extremity **5** Lymphatic, Right Axillary **6** Lymphatic, Left Axillary **7** Lymphatic, Thorax **8** Lymphatic, Internal Mammary, Right **9** Lymphatic, Internal Mammary, Left **B** Lymphatic, Mesenteric **C** Lymphatic, Pelvis **D** Lymphatic, Aortic **F** Lymphatic, Right Lower Extremity **G** Lymphatic, Left Lower Extremity **H** Lymphatic, Right Inguinal **J** Lymphatic, Left Inguinal **K** Thoracic Duct **L** Cisterna Chyli	**0** Open **3** Percutaneous **4** Percutaneous Endoscopic **8** Via Natural or Artificial Opening Endoscopic	**Z** No Device	**Z** No Qualifier
M Thymus **P** Spleen	**0** Open **3** Percutaneous **4** Percutaneous Endoscopic	**Z** No Device	**Z** No Qualifier

Section 0 **Medical and Surgical**
Body System 7 **Lymphatic and Hemic Systems**
Operation S **Reposition:** Moving to its normal location, or other suitable location, all or a portion of a body part

Body Part (4th)	Approach (5th)	Device (6th)	Qualifier (7th)
M Thymus **P** Spleen	**0** Open	**Z** No Device	**Z** No Qualifier

Section 0 **Medical and Surgical**
Body System 7 **Lymphatic and Hemic Systems**
Operation T **Resection:** Cutting out or off, without replacement, all of a body part

Body Part (4th)	Approach (5th)	Device (6th)	Qualifier (7th)
0 Lymphatic, Head **1** Lymphatic, Right Neck **2** Lymphatic, Left Neck **3** Lymphatic, Right Upper Extremity **4** Lymphatic, Left Upper Extremity **5** Lymphatic, Right Axillary **6** Lymphatic, Left Axillary **7** Lymphatic, Thorax **8** Lymphatic, Internal Mammary, Right **9** Lymphatic, Internal Mammary, Left **B** Lymphatic, Mesenteric **C** Lymphatic, Pelvis **D** Lymphatic, Aortic **F** Lymphatic, Right Lower Extremity **G** Lymphatic, Left Lower Extremity **H** Lymphatic, Right Inguinal **J** Lymphatic, Left Inguinal **K** Thoracic Duct **L** Cisterna Chyli **M** Thymus **P** Spleen	**0** Open **4** Percutaneous Endoscopic	**Z** No Device	**Z** No Qualifier

Section 0 **Medical and Surgical**
Body System 7 **Lymphatic and Hemic Systems**
Operation U **Supplement:** Putting in or on biological or synthetic material that physically reinforces and/or augments the function of a portion of a body part

Body Part (4th)	Approach (5th)	Device (6th)	Qualifier (7th)
0 Lymphatic, Head **1** Lymphatic, Right Neck **2** Lymphatic, Left Neck **3** Lymphatic, Right Upper Extremity **4** Lymphatic, Left Upper Extremity **5** Lymphatic, Right Axillary **6** Lymphatic, Left Axillary **7** Lymphatic, Thorax **8** Lymphatic, Internal Mammary, Right **9** Lymphatic, Internal Mammary, Left **B** Lymphatic, Mesenteric **C** Lymphatic, Pelvis **D** Lymphatic, Aortic **F** Lymphatic, Right Lower Extremity **G** Lymphatic, Left Lower Extremity **H** Lymphatic, Right Inguinal **J** Lymphatic, Left Inguinal **K** Thoracic Duct **L** Cisterna Chyli	**0** Open **4** Percutaneous Endoscopic	**7** Autologous Tissue Substitute **J** Synthetic Substitute **K** Nonautologous Tissue Substitute	**Z** No Qualifier

Section 0 **Medical and Surgical**
Body System 7 **Lymphatic and Hemic Systems**
Operation V **Restriction:** Partially closing an orifice or the lumen of a tubular body part

Body Part (4th)	Approach (5th)	Device (6th)	Qualifier (7th)
0 Lymphatic, Head **1** Lymphatic, Right Neck **2** Lymphatic, Left Neck **3** Lymphatic, Right Upper Extremity **4** Lymphatic, Left Upper Extremity **5** Lymphatic, Right Axillary **6** Lymphatic, Left Axillary **7** Lymphatic, Thorax **8** Lymphatic, Internal Mammary, Right **9** Lymphatic, Internal Mammary, Left **B** Lymphatic, Mesenteric **C** Lymphatic, Pelvis **D** Lymphatic, Aortic **F** Lymphatic, Right Lower Extremity **G** Lymphatic, Left Lower Extremity **H** Lymphatic, Right Inguinal **J** Lymphatic, Left Inguinal **K** Thoracic Duct **L** Cisterna Chyli	**0** Open **3** Percutaneous **4** Percutaneous Endoscopic	**C** Extraluminal Device **D** Intraluminal Device **Z** No Device	**Z** No Qualifier

Section 0 **Medical and Surgical**
Body System 7 **Lymphatic and Hemic Systems**
Operation W **Revision:** Correcting, to the extent possible, a portion of a malfunctioning device or the position of a displaced device

Body Part (4th)	Approach (5th)	Device (6th)	Qualifier (7th)
K Thoracic Duct **L** Cisterna Chyli **N** Lymphatic	**0** Open **3** Percutaneous **4** Percutaneous Endoscopic	**0** Drainage Device **3** Infusion Device **7** Autologous Tissue Substitute **C** Extraluminal Device **D** Intraluminal Device **J** Synthetic Substitute **K** Nonautologous Tissue Substitute **Y** Other Device	**Z** No Qualifier
K Thoracic Duct **L** Cisterna Chyli **N** Lymphatic	**X** External	**0** Drainage Device **3** Infusion Device **7** Autologous Tissue Substitute **C** Extraluminal Device **D** Intraluminal Device **J** Synthetic Substitute **K** Nonautologous Tissue Substitute	**Z** No Qualifier
M Thymus **P** Spleen	**0** Open **3** Percutaneous **4** Percutaneous Endoscopic	**0** Drainage Device **3** Infusion Device **Y** Other Device	**Z** No Qualifier
M Thymus **P** Spleen	**X** External	**0** Drainage Device **3** Infusion Device	**Z** No Qualifier
T Bone Marrow	**0** Open **3** Percutaneous **4** Percutaneous Endoscopic **X** External	**0** Drainage Device	**Z** No Qualifier

Section 0 **Medical and Surgical**
Body System 7 **Lymphatic and Hemic Systems**
Operation Y **Transplantation:** Putting in or on all or a portion of a living body part taken from another individual or animal to physically take the place and/or function of all or a portion of a similar body part

Body Part (4th)	Approach (5th)	Device (6th)	Qualifier (7th)
M Thymus **P** Spleen	**0** Open	**Z** No Device	**0** Allogeneic **1** Syngeneic **2** Zooplastic

AHA Coding Clinic

07B74ZX Excision of Thorax Lymphatic, Percutaneous Endoscopic Approach, Diagnostic—AHA CC: 1Q, 2014, 20-21, 26; 3Q, 2014, 10-11

07BB0ZZ Excision of Mesenteric Lymphatic, Open Approach—AHA CC: 1Q, 2019, 6-7

07BD0ZZ Excision of Aortic Lymphatic, Open Approach—AHA CC: 1Q, 2019, 6-7

07Q60ZZ Repair Left Axillary Lymphatic, Open Approach—AHA CC: 1Q, 2017, 34

07T10ZZ Resection of Right Neck Lymphatic, Open Approach—AHA CC: 3Q, 2014, 9-10

07T20ZZ Resection of Left Neck Lymphatic, Open Approach—AHA CC: 3Q, 2014, 9-10; 2Q, 2016, 12-14

07T50ZZ Resection of Right Axillary Lymphatic, Open Approach—AHA CC: 1Q, 2016, 30

07TM0ZZ Resection of Thymus, Open Approach—AHA CC: 3Q, 2014, 16-17

07TP0ZZ Resection of Spleen, Open Approach—AHA CC: 4Q, 2015, 13

07YM0Z0 Transplantation of Thymus, Allogeneic, Open Approach—AHA CC: 3Q, 2019, 29

Anatomy of the Eyeball

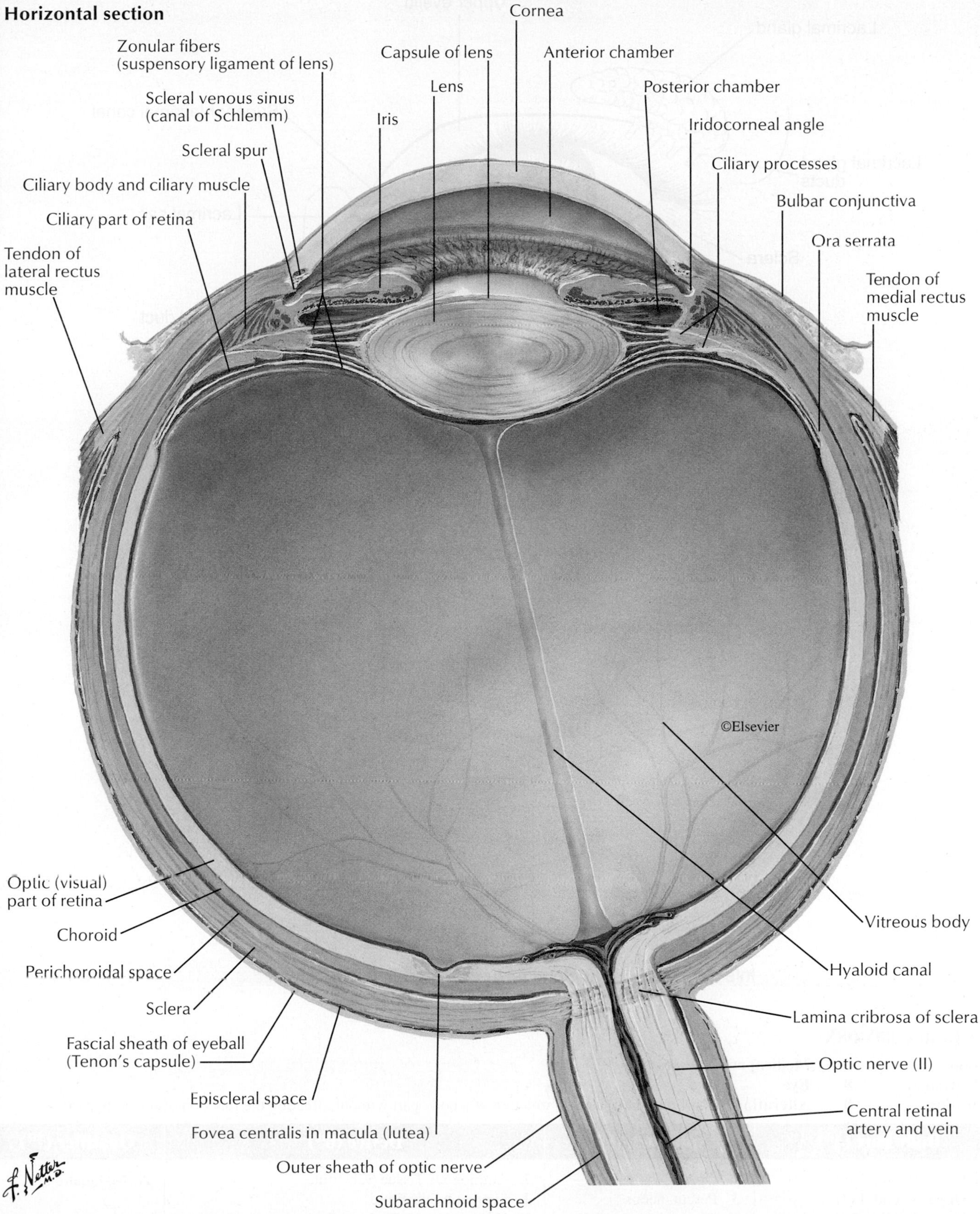

Horizontal section
Cornea
Zonular fibers
(suspensory ligament of lens)
Capsule of lens
Anterior chamber
Lens
Posterior chamber
Scleral venous sinus
(canal of Schlemm)
Iris
Iridocorneal angle
Scleral spur
Ciliary processes
Ciliary body and ciliary muscle
Bulbar conjunctiva
Ciliary part of retina
Ora serrata
Tendon of
lateral rectus
muscle
Tendon of
medial rectus
muscle
©Elsevier
Optic (visual)
part of retina
Choroid
Vitreous body
Perichoroidal space
Hyaloid canal
Sclera
Lamina cribrosa of sclera
Fascial sheath of eyeball
(Tenon's capsule)
Optic nerve (II)
Episcleral space
Central retinal
artery and vein
Fovea centralis in macula (lutea)
Outer sheath of optic nerve
Subarachnoid space

Eyelid

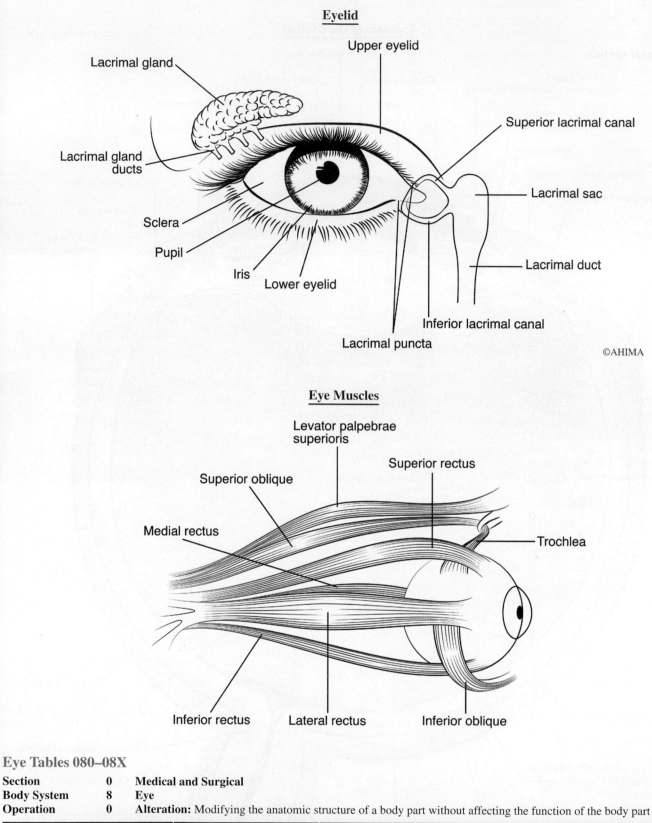

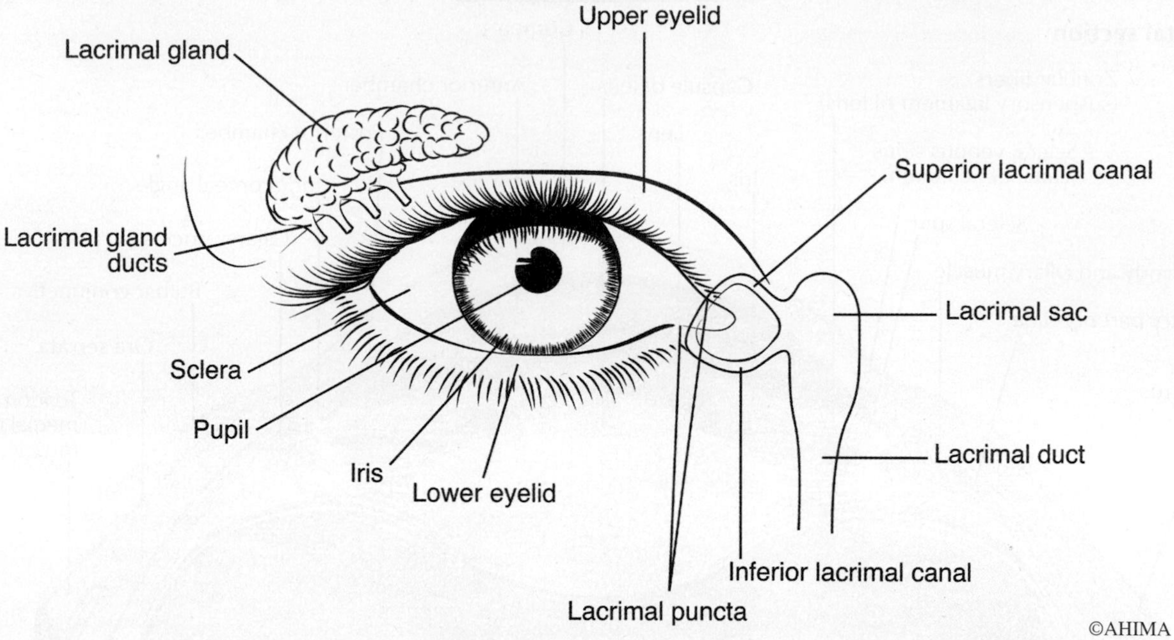
Upper eyelid
Lacrimal gland
Superior lacrimal canal
Lacrimal gland ducts
Lacrimal sac
Sclera
Pupil
Lacrimal duct
Iris
Lower eyelid
Inferior lacrimal canal
Lacrimal puncta

Eye Muscles

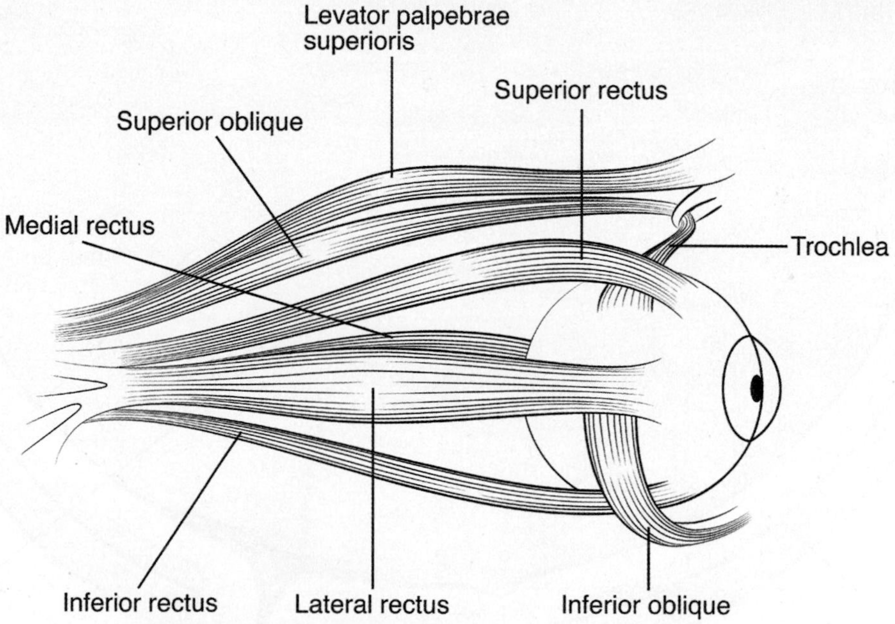
Levator palpebrae superioris
Superior rectus
Superior oblique
Medial rectus
Trochlea
Inferior rectus
Lateral rectus
Inferior oblique

Eye Tables 080–08X

Section	**0**	**Medical and Surgical**
Body System	**8**	**Eye**
Operation	**0**	**Alteration:** Modifying the anatomic structure of a body part without affecting the function of the body part

Body Part (4th)	Approach (5th)	Device (6th)	Qualifier (7th)
N Upper Eyelid, Right **P** Upper Eyelid, Left **Q** Lower Eyelid, Right **R** Lower Eyelid, Left	**0** Open **3** Percutaneous **X** External	**7** Autologous Tissue Substitute **J** Synthetic Substitute **K** Nonautologous Tissue Substitute **Z** No Device	**Z** No Qualifier

Section **0** **Medical and Surgical**
Body System **8** **Eye**
Operation **1** **Bypass:** Altering the route of passage of the contents of a tubular body part

Body Part (4th)	Approach (5th)	Device (6th)	Qualifier (7th)
2 Anterior Chamber, Right **3** Anterior Chamber, Left	**3** Percutaneous	**J** Synthetic Substitute **K** Nonautologous Tissue Substitute **Z** No Device	**4** Sclera
X Lacrimal Duct, Right **Y** Lacrimal Duct, Left	**0** Open **3** Percutaneous	**J** Synthetic Substitute **K** Nonautologous Tissue Substitute **Z** No Device	**3** Nasal Cavity

Section **0** **Medical and Surgical**
Body System **8** **Eye**
Operation **2** **Change:** Taking out or off a device from a body part and putting back an identical or similar device in or on the same body part without cutting or puncturing the skin or a mucous membrane

Body Part (4th)	Approach (5th)	Device (6th)	Qualifier (7th)
0 Eye, Right **1** Eye, Left	**X** External	**0** Drainage Device **Y** Other Device	**Z** No Qualifier

Section **0** **Medical and Surgical**
Body System **8** **Eye**
Operation **5** **Destruction:** Physical eradication of all or a portion of a body part by the direct use of energy, force, or a destructive agent

Body Part (4th)	Approach (5th)	Device (6th)	Qualifier (7th)
0 Eye, Right **1** Eye, Left **6** Sclera, Right **7** Sclera, Left **8** Cornea, Right **9** Cornea, Left **S** Conjunctiva, Right **T** Conjunctiva, Left	**X** External	**Z** No Device	**Z** No Qualifier
2 Anterior Chamber, Right **3** Anterior Chamber, Left **4** Vitreous, Right **5** Vitreous, Left **C** Iris, Right **D** Iris, Left **E** Retina, Right **F** Retina, Left **G** Retinal Vessel, Right **H** Retinal Vessel, Left **J** Lens, Right **K** Lens, Left	**3** Percutaneous	**Z** No Device	**Z** No Qualifier
A Choroid, Right **B** Choroid, Left **L** Extraocular Muscle, Right **M** Extraocular Muscle, Left **V** Lacrimal Gland, Right **W** Lacrimal Gland, Left	**0** Open **3** Percutaneous	**Z** No Device	**Z** No Qualifier
N Upper Eyelid, Right **P** Upper Eyelid, Left **Q** Lower Eyelid, Right **R** Lower Eyelid, Left	**0** Open **3** Percutaneous **X** External	**Z** No Device	**Z** No Qualifier
X Lacrimal Duct, Right **Y** Lacrimal Duct, Left	**0** Open **3** Percutaneous **7** Via Natural or Artificial Opening **8** Via Natural or Artificial Opening Endoscopic	**Z** No Device	**Z** No Qualifier

Section 0 **Medical and Surgical**
Body System 8 **Eye**
Operation 7 **Dilation:** Expanding an orifice or the lumen of a tubular body part

Body Part (4th)	Approach (5th)	Device (6th)	Qualifier (7th)
X Lacrimal Duct, Right **Y** Lacrimal Duct, Left	**0** Open **3** Percutaneous **7** Via Natural or Artificial Opening **8** Via Natural or Artificial Opening Endoscopic	**D** Intraluminal Device **Z** No Device	**Z** No Qualifier

Section 0 **Medical and Surgical**
Body System 8 **Eye**
Operation 9 **Drainage:** Taking or letting out fluids and/or gases from a body part

Body Part (4th)	Approach (5th)	Device (6th)	Qualifier (7th)
0 Eye, Right **1** Eye, Left **6** Sclera, Right **7** Sclera, Left **8** Cornea, Right **9** Cornea, Left **S** Conjunctiva, Right **T** Conjunctiva, Left	**X** External	**0** Drainage Device	**Z** No Qualifier
0 Eye, Right **1** Eye, Left **6** Sclera, Right **7** Sclera, Left **8** Cornea, Right **9** Cornea, Left **S** Conjunctiva, Right **T** Conjunctiva, Left	**X** External	**Z** No Device	**X** Diagnostic **Z** No Qualifier
2 Anterior Chamber, Right **3** Anterior Chamber, Left **4** Vitreous, Right **5** Vitreous, Left **C** Iris, Right **D** Iris, Left **E** Retina, Right **F** Retina, Left **G** Retinal Vessel, Right **H** Retinal Vessel, Left **J** Lens, Right **K** Lens, Left	**3** Percutaneous	**0** Drainage Device	**Z** No Qualifier
2 Anterior Chamber, Right **3** Anterior Chamber, Left **4** Vitreous, Right **5** Vitreous, Left **C** Iris, Right **D** Iris, Left **E** Retina, Right **F** Retina, Left **G** Retinal Vessel, Right **H** Retinal Vessel, Left **J** Lens, Right **K** Lens, Left	**3** Percutaneous	**Z** No Device	**X** Diagnostic **Z** No Qualifier
A Choroid, Right **B** Choroid, Left **L** Extraocular Muscle, Right **M** Extraocular Muscle, Left **V** Lacrimal Gland, Right **W** Lacrimal Gland, Left	**0** Open **3** Percutaneous	**0** Drainage Device	**Z** No Qualifier

Continued →

Section 0 **Medical and Surgical**
Body System 8 **Eye**
Operation 9 **Drainage:** Taking or letting out fluids and/or gases from a body part

Body Part (4th)	Approach (5th)	Device (6th)	Qualifier (7th)
A Choroid, Right **B** Choroid, Left **L** Extraocular Muscle, Right **M** Extraocular Muscle, Left **V** Lacrimal Gland, Right **W** Lacrimal Gland, Left	**0** Open **3** Percutaneous	**Z** No Device	**X** Diagnostic **Z** No Qualifier
N Upper Eyelid, Right **P** Upper Eyelid, Left **Q** Lower Eyelid, Right **R** Lower Eyelid, Left	**0** Open **3** Percutaneous **X** External	**0** Drainage Device	**Z** No Qualifier
N Upper Eyelid, Right **P** Upper Eyelid, Left **Q** Lower Eyelid, Right **R** Lower Eyelid, Left	**0** Open **3** Percutaneous **X** External	**Z** No Device	**X** Diagnostic **Z** No Qualifier
X Lacrimal Duct, Right **Y** Lacrimal Duct, Left	**0** Open **3** Percutaneous **7** Via Natural or Artificial Opening **8** Via Natural or Artificial Opening Endoscopic	**0** Drainage Device	**Z** No Qualifier
X Lacrimal Duct, Right **Y** Lacrimal Duct, Left	**0** Open **3** Percutaneous **7** Via Natural or Artificial Opening **8** Via Natural or Artificial Opening Endoscopic	**Z** No Device	**X** Diagnostic **Z** No Qualifier

Section 0 **Medical and Surgical**
Body System 8 **Eye**
Operation B **Excision:** Cutting out or off, without replacement, a portion of a body part

Body Part (4th)	Approach (5th)	Device (6th)	Qualifier (7th)
0 Eye, Right **1** Eye, Left **N** Upper Eyelid, Right **P** Upper Eyelid, Left **Q** Lower Eyelid, Right **R** Lower Eyelid, Left	**0** Open **3** Percutaneous **X** External	**Z** No Device	**X** Diagnostic **Z** No Qualifier
4 Vitreous, Right **5** Vitreous, Left **C** Iris, Right **D** Iris, Left **E** Retina, Right **F** Retina, Left **J** Lens, Right **K** Lens, Left	**3** Percutaneous	**Z** No Device	**X** Diagnostic **Z** No Qualifier
6 Sclera, Right **7** Sclera, Left **8** Cornea, Right **9** Cornea, Left **S** Conjunctiva, Right **T** Conjunctiva, Left	**X** External	**Z** No Device	**X** Diagnostic **Z** No Qualifier

Continued →

Section 0 **Medical and Surgical**
Body System 8 **Eye**
Operation B **Excision:** Cutting out or off, without replacement, a portion of a body part

Body Part (4th)	Approach (5th)	Device (6th)	Qualifier (7th)
A Choroid, Right **B** Choroid, Left **L** Extraocular Muscle, Right **M** Extraocular Muscle, Left **V** Lacrimal Gland, Right **W** Lacrimal Gland, Left	**0** Open **3** Percutaneous	**Z** No Device	**X** Diagnostic **Z** No Qualifier
X Lacrimal Duct, Right **Y** Lacrimal Duct, Left	**0** Open **3** Percutaneous **7** Via Natural or Artificial Opening **8** Via Natural or Artificial Opening Endoscopic	**Z** No Device	**X** Diagnostic **Z** No Qualifier

Section 0 **Medical and Surgical**
Body System 8 **Eye**
Operation C **Extirpation:** Taking or cutting out solid matter from a body part

Body Part (4th)	Approach (5th)	Device (6th)	Qualifier (7th)
0 Eye, Right **1** Eye, Left **6** Sclera, Right **7** Sclera, Left **8** Cornea, Right **9** Cornea, Left **S** Conjunctiva, Right **T** Conjunctiva, Left	**X** External	**Z** No Device	**Z** No Qualifier
2 Anterior Chamber, Right **3** Anterior Chamber, Left **4** Vitreous, Right **5** Vitreous, Left **C** Iris, Right **D** Iris, Left **E** Retina, Right **F** Retina, Left **G** Retinal Vessel, Right **H** Retinal Vessel, Left **J** Lens, Right **K** Lens, Left	**3** Percutaneous **X** External	**Z** No Device	**Z** No Qualifier
A Choroid, Right **B** Choroid, Left **L** Extraocular Muscle, Right **M** Extraocular Muscle, Left **N** Upper Eyelid, Right **P** Upper Eyelid, Left **Q** Lower Eyelid, Right **R** Lower Eyelid, Left **V** Lacrimal Gland, Right **W** Lacrimal Gland, Left	**0** Open **3** Percutaneous **X** External	**Z** No Device	**Z** No Qualifier
X Lacrimal Duct, Right **Y** Lacrimal Duct, Left	**0** Open **3** Percutaneous **7** Via Natural or Artificial Opening **8** Via Natural or Artificial Opening Endoscopic	**Z** No Device	**Z** No Qualifier

Section 0 Medical and Surgical
Body System 8 Eye
Operation D **Extraction:** Pulling or stripping out or off all or a portion of a body part by the use of force

Body Part (4th)	Approach (5th)	Device (6th)	Qualifier (7th)
8 Cornea, Right **9** Cornea, Left	**X** External	**Z** No Device	**X** Diagnostic **Z** No Qualifier
J Lens, Right **K** Lens, Left	**3** Percutaneous	**Z** No Device	**Z** No Qualifier

Section 0 Medical and Surgical
Body System 8 Eye
Operation F **Fragmentation:** Breaking solid matter in a body part into pieces

Body Part (4th)	Approach (5th)	Device (6th)	Qualifier (7th)
4 Vitreous, Right **5** Vitreous, Left	**3** Percutaneous **X** External	**Z** No Device	**Z** No Qualifier

Section 0 Medical and Surgical
Body System 8 Eye
Operation H **Insertion:** Putting in a nonbiological appliance that monitors, assists, performs, or prevents a physiological function but does not physically take the place of a body part

Body Part (4th)	Approach (5th)	Device (6th)	Qualifier (7th)
0 Eye, Right **1** Eye, Left	**0** Open	**5** Epiretinal Visual Prosthesis **Y** Other Device	**Z** No Qualifier
0 Eye, Right **1** Eye, Left	**3** Percutaneous	**1** Radioactive Element **3** Infusion Device **Y** Other Device	**Z** No Qualifier
0 Eye, Right **1** Eye, Left	**7** Via Natural or Artificial Opening **8** Via Natural or Artificial Opening Endoscopic	**Y** Other Device	**Z** No Qualifier
0 Eye, Right **1** Eye, Left	**X** External	**1** Radioactive Element **3** Infusion Device	**Z** No Qualifier

Section 0 Medical and Surgical
Body System 8 Eye
Operation J **Inspection:** Visually and/or manually exploring a body part

Body Part (4th)	Approach (5th)	Device (6th)	Qualifier (7th)
0 Eye, Right **1** Eye, Left **J** Lens, Right **K** Lens, Left	**X** External	**Z** No Device	**Z** No Qualifier
L Extraocular Muscle, Right **M** Extraocular Muscle, Left	**0** Open **X** External	**Z** No Device	**Z** No Qualifier

Section 0 **Medical and Surgical**
Body System 8 **Eye**
Operation L **Occlusion:** Completely closing an orifice or the lumen of a tubular body part

Body Part (4th)	Approach (5th)	Device (6th)	Qualifier (7th)
X Lacrimal Duct, Right **Y** Lacrimal Duct, Left	**0** Open **3** Percutaneous	**C** Extraluminal Device **D** Intraluminal Device **Z** No Device	**Z** No Qualifier
X Lacrimal Duct, Right **Y** Lacrimal Duct, Left	**7** Via Natural or Artificial Opening **8** Via Natural or Artificial Opening Endoscopic	**D** Intraluminal Device **Z** No Device	**Z** No Qualifier

Section 0 **Medical and Surgical**
Body System 8 **Eye**
Operation M **Reattachment:** Putting back in or on all or a portion of a separated body part to its normal location or other suitable location

Body Part (4th)	Approach (5th)	Device (6th)	Qualifier (7th)
N Upper Eyelid, Right **P** Upper Eyelid, Left **Q** Lower Eyelid, Right **R** Lower Eyelid, Left	**X** External	**Z** No Device	**Z** No Qualifier

Section 0 **Medical and Surgical**
Body System 8 **Eye**
Operation N **Release:** Freeing a body part from an abnormal physical constraint by cutting or by the use of force

Body Part (4th)	Approach (5th)	Device (6th)	Qualifier (7th)
0 Eye, Right **1** Eye, Left **6** Sclera, Right **7** Sclera, Left **8** Cornea, Right **9** Cornea, Left **S** Conjunctiva, Right **T** Conjunctiva, Left	**X** External	**Z** No Device	**Z** No Qualifier
2 Anterior Chamber, Right **3** Anterior Chamber, Left **4** Vitreous, Right **5** Vitreous, Left **C** Iris, Right **D** Iris, Left **E** Retina, Right **F** Retina, Left **G** Retinal Vessel, Right **H** Retinal Vessel, Left **J** Lens, Right **K** Lens, Left	**3** Percutaneous	**Z** No Device	**Z** No Qualifier
A Choroid, Right **B** Choroid, Left **L** Extraocular Muscle, Right **M** Extraocular Muscle, Left **V** Lacrimal Gland, Right **W** Lacrimal Gland, Left	**0** Open **3** Percutaneous	**Z** No Device	**Z** No Qualifier
N Upper Eyelid, Right **P** Upper Eyelid, Left **Q** Lower Eyelid, Right **R** Lower Eyelid, Left	**0** Open **3** Percutaneous **X** External	**Z** No Device	**Z** No Qualifier
X Lacrimal Duct, Right **Y** Lacrimal Duct, Left	**0** Open **3** Percutaneous **7** Via Natural or Artificial Opening **8** Via Natural or Artificial Opening Endoscopic	**Z** No Device	**Z** No Qualifier

Section 0 **Medical and Surgical**
Body System 8 **Eye**
Operation P **Removal:** Taking out or off a device from a body part

Body Part (4th)	Approach (5th)	Device (6th)	Qualifier (7th)
0 Eye, Right **1** Eye, Left	**0** Open **3** Percutaneous **7** Via Natural or Artificial Opening **8** Via Natural or Artificial Opening Endoscopic	**0** Drainage Device **1** Radioactive Element **3** Infusion Device **7** Autologous Tissue Substitute **C** Extraluminal Device **D** Intraluminal Device **J** Synthetic Substitute **K** Nonautologous Tissue Substitute **Y** Other Device	**Z** No Qualifier
0 Eye, Right **1** Eye, Left	**X** External	**0** Drainage Device **1** Radioactive Element **3** Infusion Device **7** Autologous Tissue Substitute **C** Extraluminal Device **D** Intraluminal Device **J** Synthetic Substitute **K** Nonautologous Tissue Substitute	**Z** No Qualifier
J Lens, Right **K** Lens, Left	**3** Percutaneous	**J** Synthetic Substitute **Y** Other Device	**Z** No Qualifier
L Extraocular Muscle, Right **M** Extraocular Muscle, Left	**0** Open **3** Percutaneous	**0** Drainage Device **7** Autologous Tissue Substitute **J** Synthetic Substitute **K** Nonautologous Tissue Substitute **Y** Other Device	**Z** No Qualifier

Section 0 **Medical and Surgical**
Body System 8 **Eye**
Operation Q **Repair:** Restoring, to the extent possible, a body part to its normal anatomic structure and function

Body Part (4th)	Approach (5th)	Device (6th)	Qualifier (7th)
0 Eye, Right **1** Eye, Left **6** Sclera, Right **7** Sclera, Left **8** Cornea, Right **9** Cornea, Left **S** Conjunctiva, Right **T** Conjunctiva, Left	**X** External	**Z** No Device	**Z** No Qualifier
2 Anterior Chamber, Right **3** Anterior Chamber, Left **4** Vitreous, Right **5** Vitreous, Left **C** Iris, Right **D** Iris, Left **E** Retina, Right **F** Retina, Left **G** Retinal Vessel, Right **H** Retinal Vessel, Left **J** Lens, Right **K** Lens, Left	**3** Percutaneous	**Z** No Device	**Z** No Qualifier

Continued →

Section	**0**	**Medical and Surgical**
Body System	**8**	**Eye**
Operation	**Q**	**Repair:** Restoring, to the extent possible, a body part to its normal anatomic structure and function

Body Part (4th)	Approach (5th)	Device (6th)	Qualifier (7th)
A Choroid, Right **B** Choroid, Left **L** Extraocular Muscle, Right **M** Extraocular Muscle, Left **V** Lacrimal Gland, Right **W** Lacrimal Gland, Left	**0** Open **3** Percutaneous	**Z** No Device	**Z** No Qualifier
N Upper Eyelid, Right **P** Upper Eyelid, Left **Q** Lower Eyelid, Right **R** Lower Eyelid, Left	**0** Open **3** Percutaneous **X** External	**Z** No Device	**Z** No Qualifier
X Lacrimal Duct, Right **Y** Lacrimal Duct, Left	**0** Open **3** Percutaneous **7** Via Natural or Artificial Opening **8** Via Natural or Artificial Opening Endoscopic	**Z** No Device	**Z** No Qualifier

Section	**0**	**Medical and Surgical**
Body System	**8**	**Eye**
Operation	**R**	**Replacement:** Putting in or on biological or synthetic material that physically takes the place and/or function of all or a portion of a body part

Body Part (4th)	Approach (5th)	Device (6th)	Qualifier (7th)
0 Eye, Right **1** Eye, Left **A** Choroid, Right **B** Choroid, Left	**0** Open **3** Percutaneous	**7** Autologous Tissue Substitute **J** Synthetic Substitute **K** Nonautologous Tissue Substitute	**Z** No Qualifier
4 Vitreous, Right **5** Vitreous, Left **C** Iris, Right **D** Iris, Left **G** Retinal Vessel, Right **H** Retinal Vessel, Left	**3** Percutaneous	**7** Autologous Tissue Substitute **J** Synthetic Substitute **K** Nonautologous Tissue Substitute	**Z** No Qualifier
6 Sclera, Right **7** Sclera, Left **S** Conjunctiva, Right **T** Conjunctiva, Left	**X** External	**7** Autologous Tissue Substitute **J** Synthetic Substitute **K** Nonautologous Tissue Substitute	**Z** No Qualifier
8 Cornea, Right **9** Cornea, Left	**3** Percutaneous **X** External	**7** Autologous Tissue Substitute **J** Synthetic Substitute **K** Nonautologous Tissue Substitute	**Z** No Qualifier
J Lens, Right **K** Lens, Left	**3** Percutaneous	**0** Synthetic Substitute, Intraocular Telescope **7** Autologous Tissue Substitute **J** Synthetic Substitute **K** Nonautologous Tissue Substitute	**Z** No Qualifier
N Upper Eyelid, Right **P** Upper Eyelid, Left **Q** Lower Eyelid, Right **R** Lower Eyelid, Left	**0** Open **3** Percutaneous **X** External	**7** Autologous Tissue Substitute **J** Synthetic Substitute **K** Nonautologous Tissue Substitute	**Z** No Qualifier
X Lacrimal Duct, Right **Y** Lacrimal Duct, Left	**0** Open **3** Percutaneous **7** Via Natural or Artificial Opening **8** Via Natural or Artificial Opening Endoscopic	**7** Autologous Tissue Substitute **J** Synthetic Substitute **K** Nonautologous Tissue Substitute	**Z** No Qualifier

Section	**0**	**Medical and Surgical**
Body System	**8**	**Eye**
Operation	**S**	**Reposition:** Moving to its normal location, or other suitable location, all or a portion of a body part

Body Part (4th)	Approach (5th)	Device (6th)	Qualifier (7th)
C Iris, Right **D** Iris, Left **G** Retinal Vessel, Right **H** Retinal Vessel, Left **J** Lens, Right **K** Lens, Left	**3** Percutaneous	**Z** No Device	**Z** No Qualifier
L Extraocular Muscle, Right **M** Extraocular Muscle, Left **V** Lacrimal Gland, Right **W** Lacrimal Gland, Left	**0** Open **3** Percutaneous	**Z** No Device	**Z** No Qualifier
N Upper Eyelid, Right **P** Upper Eyelid, Left **Q** Lower Eyelid, Right **R** Lower Eyelid, Left	**0** Open **3** Percutaneous **X** External	**Z** No Device	**Z** No Qualifier
X Lacrimal Duct, Right **Y** Lacrimal Duct, Left	**0** Open **3** Percutaneous **7** Via Natural or Artificial Opening **8** Via Natural or Artificial Opening Endoscopic	**Z** No Device	**Z** No Qualifier

Section	**0**	**Medical and Surgical**
Body System	**8**	**Eye**
Operation	**T**	**Resection:** Cutting out or off, without replacement, all of a body part

Body Part (4th)	Approach (5th)	Device (6th)	Qualifier (7th)
0 Eye, Right **1** Eye, Left **8** Cornea, Right **9** Cornea, Left	**X** External	**Z** No Device	**Z** No Qualifier
4 Vitreous, Right **5** Vitreous, Left **C** Iris, Right **D** Iris, Left **J** Lens, Right **K** Lens, Left	**3** Percutaneous	**Z** No Device	**Z** No Qualifier
L Extraocular Muscle, Right **M** Extraocular Muscle, Left **V** Lacrimal Gland, Right **W** Lacrimal Gland, Left	**0** Open **3** Percutaneous	**Z** No Device	**Z** No Qualifier
N Upper Eyelid, Right **P** Upper Eyelid, Left **Q** Lower Eyelid, Right **R** Lower Eyelid, Left	**0** Open **X** External	**Z** No Device	**Z** No Qualifier
X Lacrimal Duct, Right **Y** Lacrimal Duct, Left	**0** Open **3** Percutaneous **7** Via Natural or Artificial Opening **8** Via Natural or Artificial Opening Endoscopic	**Z** No Device	**Z** No Qualifier

Section 0 Medical and Surgical
Body System 8 Eye
Operation U **Supplement:** Putting in or on biological or synthetic material that physically reinforces and/or augments the function of a portion of a body part

Body Part (4th)	Approach (5th)	Device (6th)	Qualifier (7th)
0 Eye, Right **1** Eye, Left **C** Iris, Right **D** Iris, Left **E** Retina, Right **F** Retina, Left **G** Retinal Vessel, Right **H** Retinal Vessel, Left **L** Extraocular Muscle, Right **M** Extraocular Muscle, Left	**0** Open **3** Percutaneous	**7** Autologous Tissue Substitute **J** Synthetic Substitute **K** Nonautologous Tissue Substitute	**Z** No Qualifier
8 Cornea, Right **9** Cornea, Left **N** Upper Eyelid, Right **P** Upper Eyelid, Left **Q** Lower Eyelid, Right **R** Lower Eyelid, Left	**0** Open **3** Percutaneous **X** External	**7** Autologous Tissue Substitute **J** Synthetic Substitute **K** Nonautologous Tissue Substitute	**Z** No Qualifier
X Lacrimal Duct, Right **Y** Lacrimal Duct, Left	**0** Open **3** Percutaneous **7** Via Natural or Artificial Opening **8** Via Natural or Artificial Opening Endoscopic	**7** Autologous Tissue Substitute **J** Synthetic Substitute **K** Nonautologous Tissue Substitute	**Z** No Qualifier

Section 0 Medical and Surgical
Body System 8 Eye
Operation V **Restriction:** Partially closing an orifice or the lumen of a tubular body part

Body Part (4th)	Approach (5th)	Device (6th)	Qualifier (7th)
X Lacrimal Duct, Right **Y** Lacrimal Duct, Left	**0** Open **3** Percutaneous	**C** Extraluminal Device **D** Intraluminal Device **Z** No Device	**Z** No Qualifier
X Lacrimal Duct, Right **Y** Lacrimal Duct, Left	**7** Via Natural or Artificial Opening **8** Via Natural or Artificial Opening Endoscopic	**D** Intraluminal Device **Z** No Device	**Z** No Qualifier

Section 0 Medical and Surgical
Body System 8 Eye
Operation W **Revision:** Correcting, to the extent possible, a portion of a malfunctioning device or the position of a displaced device

Body Part (4th)	Approach (5th)	Device (6th)	Qualifier (7th)
0 Eye, Right **1** Eye, Left	**0** Open **3** Percutaneous **7** Via Natural or Artificial Opening **8** Via Natural or Artificial Opening Endoscopic	**0** Drainage Device **3** Infusion Device **7** Autologous Tissue Substitute **C** Extraluminal Device **D** Intraluminal Device **J** Synthetic Substitute **K** Nonautologous Tissue Substitute **Y** Other Device	**Z** No Qualifier
0 Eye, Right **1** Eye, Left	**X** External	**0** Drainage Device **3** Infusion Device **7** Autologous Tissue Substitute **C** Extraluminal Device **D** Intraluminal Device **J** Synthetic Substitute **K** Nonautologous Tissue Substitute	**Z** No Qualifier

Continued →

Section 0 Medical and Surgical
Body System 8 Eye
Operation W **Revision:** Correcting, to the extent possible, a portion of a malfunctioning device or the position of a displaced device

Body Part (4th)	Approach (5th)	Device (6th)	Qualifier (7th)
J Lens, Right K Lens, Left	3 Percutaneous	J Synthetic Substitute Y Other Device	Z No Qualifier
J Lens, Right K Lens, Left	X External	J Synthetic Substitute	Z No Qualifier
L Extraocular Muscle, Right M Extraocular Muscle, Left	0 Open 3 Percutaneous	0 Drainage Device 7 Autologous Tissue Substitute J Synthetic Substitute K Nonautologous Tissue Substitute Y Other Device	Z No Qualifier

Section 0 Medical and Surgical
Body System 8 Eye
Operation X **Transfer:** Moving, without taking out, all or a portion of a body part to another location to take over the function of all or a portion of a body part

Body Part (4th)	Approach (5th)	Device (6th)	Qualifier (7th)
L Extraocular Muscle, Right M Extraocular Muscle, Left	0 Open 3 Percutaneous	Z No Device	Z No Qualifier

AHA Coding Clinic

08133J4 Bypass Left Anterior Chamber to Sclera with Synthetic Substitute, Percutaneous Approach—AHA CC: 1Q, 2019, 27-28
08923ZZ Drainage of Right Anterior Chamber, Percutaneous Approach—AHA CC: 2Q, 2016, 21-22
08B43ZZ Excision of Right Vitreous, Percutaneous Approach—AHA CC: 4Q, 2014, 36-37
08B53ZZ Excision of Left Vitreous, Percutaneous Approach—AHA CC: 4Q, 2014, 35-36
08J0XZZ Inspection of Right Eye, External Approach—AHA CC: 1Q, 2015, 35-36
08NC3ZZ Release Right Iris, Percutaneous Approach—AHA CC: 2Q, 2015, 24-25
08Q7XZZ Repair Left Sclera, External Approach—AHA CC: 3Q, 2018, 13
08Q9XZZ Repair Left Cornea, External Approach—AHA CC: 3Q, 2018, 13
08R8XKZ Replacement of Right Cornea with Nonautologous Tissue Substitute, External Approach—AHA CC: 2Q, 2015, 24-26
08T1XZZ Resection of Left Eye, External Approach—AHA CC: 2Q, 2015, 12-13
08TM0ZZ Resection of Left Extraocular Muscle, Open Approach—AHA CC: 2Q, 2015, 12-13
08TR0ZZ Resection of Left Lower Eyelid, Open Approach—AHA CC: 2Q, 2015, 12-13
08U9XKZ Supplement Left Cornea with Nonautologous Tissue Substitute, External Approach—AHA CC: 3Q, 2014, 31

Nose and Sinuses

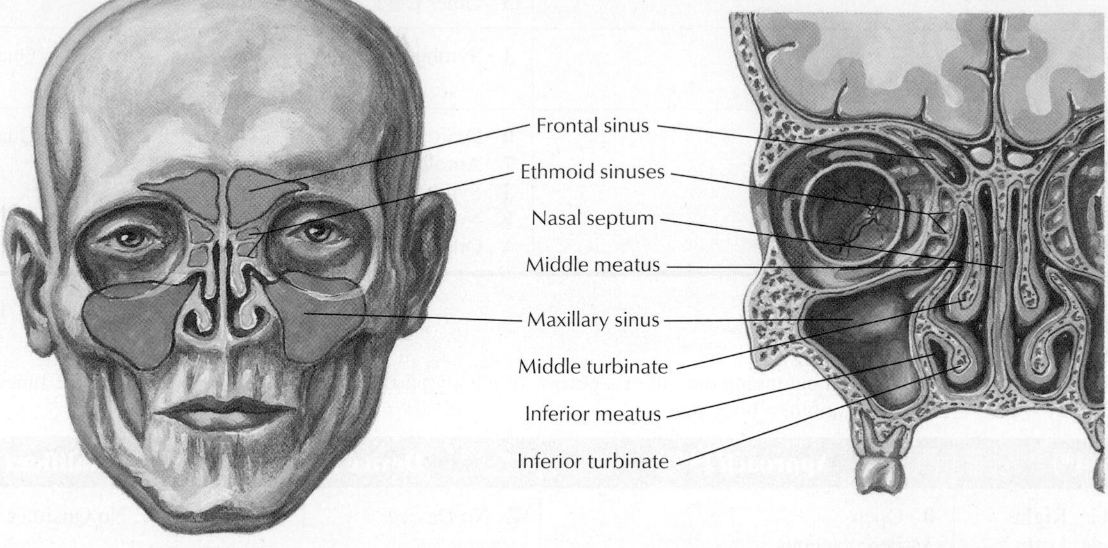
Frontal sinus
Ethmoid sinuses
Nasal septum
Middle meatus
Maxillary sinus
Middle turbinate
Inferior meatus
Inferior turbinate

Frontal view **Coronal section**

Anatomy of nasal cavity and sinuses

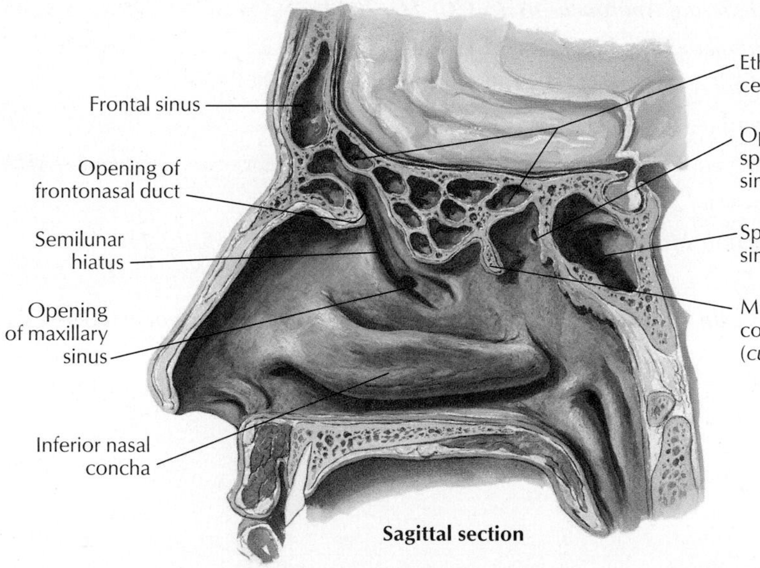
Frontal sinus
Opening of frontonasal duct
Semilunar hiatus
Opening of maxillary sinus
Inferior nasal concha
Ethmoidal cells
Opening of sphenoidal sinus
Sphenoidal sinus
Middle nasal concha (*cut away*)

Sagittal section

Paranasal sinuses

JOHN A.CRAIG—AD

Lateral Wall of Nasal Cavity

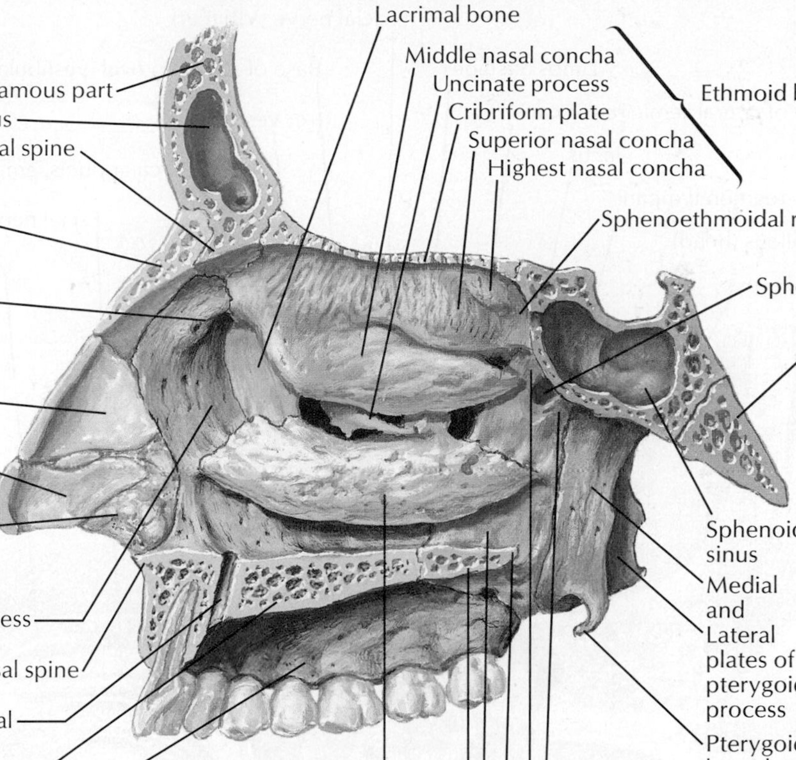

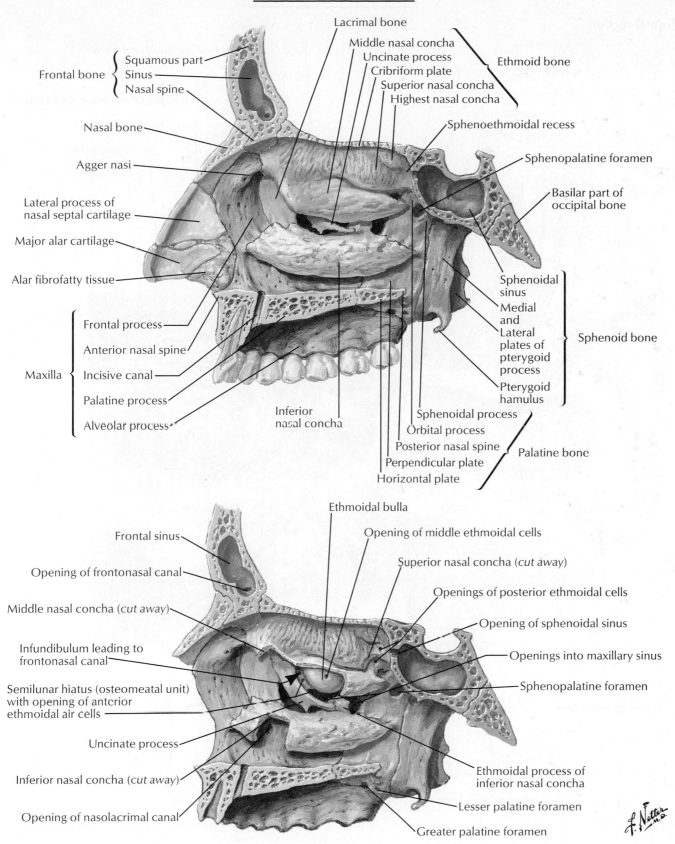

Lacrimal bone
Middle nasal concha
Uncinate process
Cribriform plate
Superior nasal concha
Highest nasal concha
Ethmoid bone
Frontal bone
Squamous part
Sinus
Nasal spine
Nasal bone
Sphenoethmoidal recess
Agger nasi
Sphenopalatine foramen
Basilar part of
occipital bone
Lateral process of
nasal septal cartilage
Major alar cartilage
Alar fibrofatty tissue
Sphenoidal
sinus
Medial
and
Lateral
plates of
pterygoid
process
Pterygoid
hamulus
Sphenoid bone
Maxilla
Frontal process
Anterior nasal spine
Incisive canal
Palatine process
Alveolar process
Inferior
nasal concha
Sphenoidal process
Orbital process
Posterior nasal spine
Perpendicular plate
Horizontal plate
Palatine bone

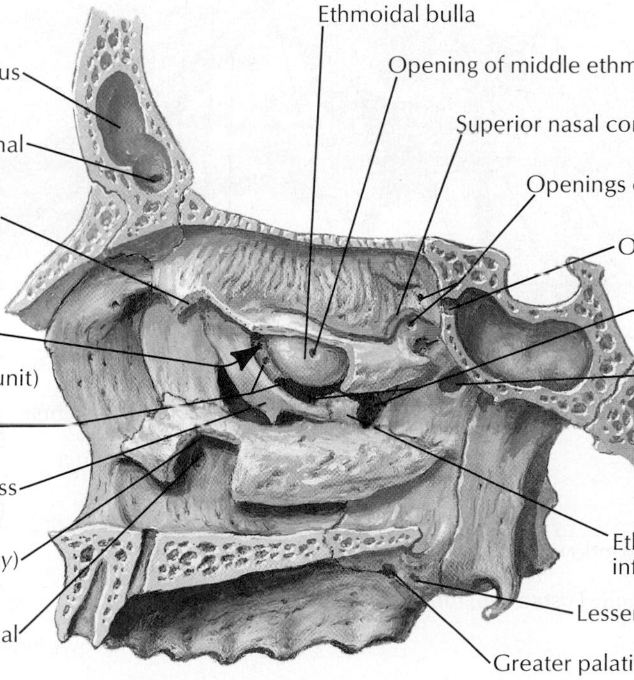

Ethmoidal bulla
Frontal sinus
Opening of middle ethmoidal cells
Superior nasal concha (cut away)
Opening of frontonasal canal
Openings of posterior ethmoidal cells
Middle nasal concha (cut away)
Opening of sphenoidal sinus
Infundibulum leading to
frontonasal canal
Openings into maxillary sinus
Sphenopalatine foramen
Semilunar hiatus (osteomeatal unit)
with opening of anterior
ethmoidal air cells
Uncinate process
Ethmoidal process of
inferior nasal concha
Inferior nasal concha (cut away)
Lesser palatine foramen
Opening of nasolacrimal canal
Greater palatine foramen

Pathway of Sound Reception

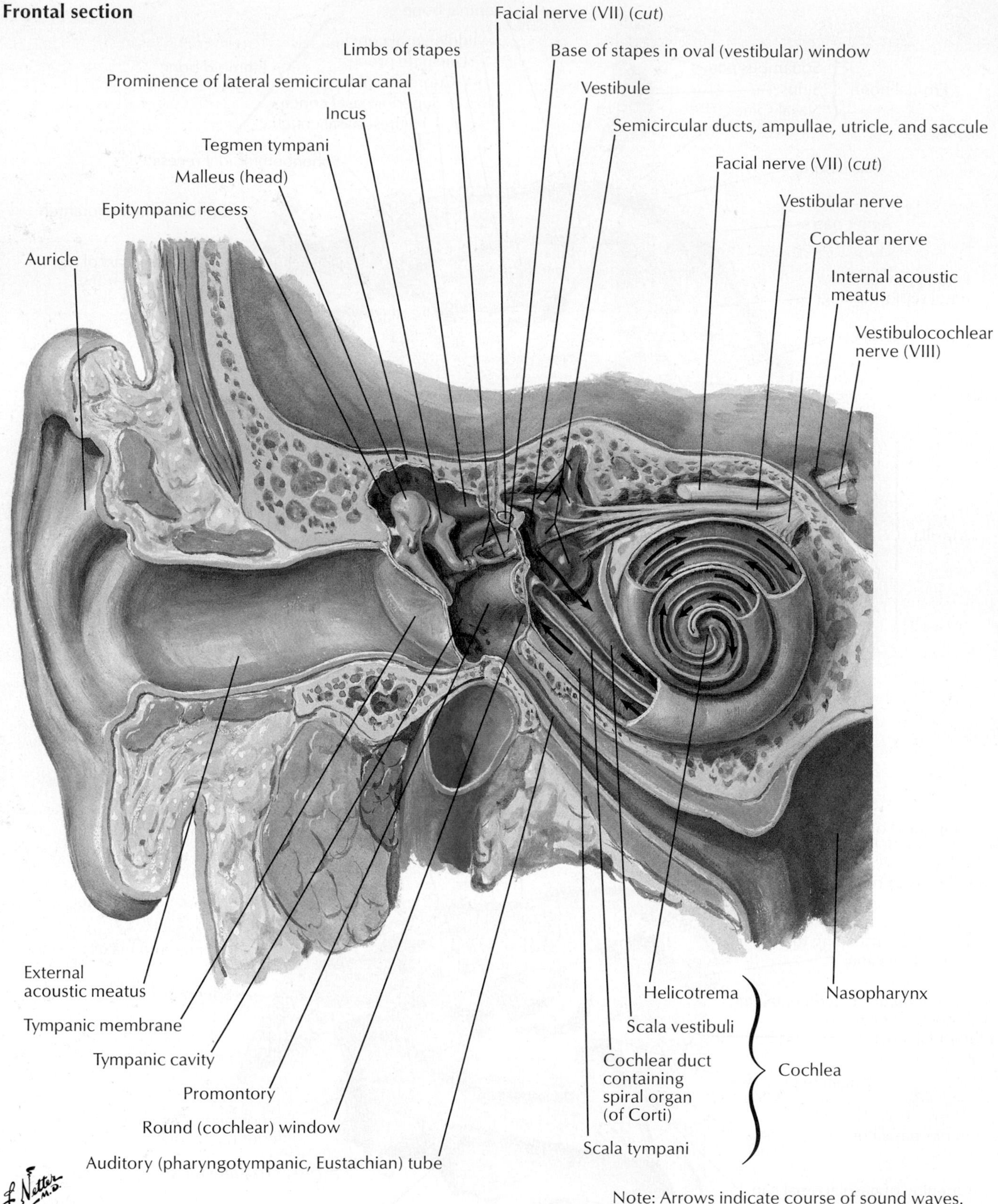
Frontal section
Facial nerve (VII) (cut)
Limbs of stapes
Base of stapes in oval (vestibular) window
Prominence of lateral semicircular canal
Vestibule
Incus
Semicircular ducts, ampullae, utricle, and saccule
Tegmen tympani
Facial nerve (VII) (cut)
Malleus (head)
Vestibular nerve
Epitympanic recess
Cochlear nerve
Auricle
Internal acoustic meatus
Vestibulocochlear nerve (VIII)
External acoustic meatus
Helicotrema
Nasopharynx
Tympanic membrane
Scala vestibuli
Tympanic cavity
Cochlear duct containing spiral organ (of Corti)
Cochlea
Promontory
Round (cochlear) window
Scala tympani
Auditory (pharyngotympanic, Eustachian) tube
F. Netter M.D.

Note: Arrows indicate course of sound waves.

Ear, Nose, Sinus Tables 090–09W

Section 0 **Medical and Surgical**
Body System 9 **Ear, Nose, Sinus**
Operation 0 **Alteration:** Modifying the anatomic structure of a body part without affecting the function of the body part

Body Part (4th)	Approach (5th)	Device (6th)	Qualifier (7th)
0 External Ear, Right **1** External Ear, Left **2** External Ear, Bilateral **K** Nasal Mucosa and Soft Tissue	**0** Open **3** Percutaneous **4** Percutaneous Endoscopic **X** External	**7** Autologous Tissue Substitute **J** Synthetic Substitute **K** Nonautologous Tissue Substitute **Z** No Device	**Z** No Qualifier

Section 0 **Medical and Surgical**
Body System 9 **Ear, Nose, Sinus**
Operation 1 **Bypass:** Altering the route of passage of the contents of a tubular body part

Body Part (4th)	Approach (5th)	Device (6th)	Qualifier (7th)
D Inner Ear, Right **E** Inner Ear, Left	**0** Open	**7** Autologous Tissue Substitute **J** Synthetic Substitute **K** Nonautologous Tissue Substitute **Z** No Device	**0** Endolymphatic

Section 0 **Medical and Surgical**
Body System 9 **Ear, Nose, Sinus**
Operation 2 **Change:** Taking out or off a device from a body part and putting back an identical or similar device in or on the same body part without cutting or puncturing the skin or a mucous membrane

Body Part (4th)	Approach (5th)	Device (6th)	Qualifier (7th)
H Ear, Right **J** Ear, Left **K** Nasal Mucosa and Soft Tissue **Y** Sinus	**X** External	**0** Drainage Device **Y** Other Device	**Z** No Qualifier

Section 0 **Medical and Surgical**
Body System 9 **Ear, Nose, Sinus**
Operation 3 **Control:** Stopping, or attempting to stop, postprocedural or other acute bleeding

Body Part (4th)	Approach (5th)	Device (6th)	Qualifier (7th)
K Nasal Mucosa and Soft Tissue	**7** Via Natural or Artificial Opening **8** Via Natural or Artificial Opening Endoscopic	**Z** No Device	**Z** No Qualifier

Section 0 **Medical and Surgical**
Body System 9 **Ear, Nose, Sinus**
Operation 5 **Destruction:** Physical eradication of all or a portion of a body part by the direct use of energy, force, or a destructive agent

Body Part (4th)	Approach (5th)	Device (6th)	Qualifier (7th)
0 External Ear, Right **1** External Ear, Left	**0** Open **3** Percutaneous **4** Percutaneous Endoscopic **X** External	**Z** No Device	**Z** No Qualifier
3 External Auditory Canal, Right **4** External Auditory Canal, Left	**0** Open **3** Percutaneous **4** Percutaneous Endoscopic **7** Via Natural or Artificial Opening **8** Via Natural or Artificial Opening Endoscopic **X** External	**Z** No Device	**Z** No Qualifier
5 Middle Ear, Right **6** Middle Ear, Left **9** Auditory Ossicle, Right **A** Auditory Ossicle, Left **D** Inner Ear, Right **E** Inner Ear, Left	**0** Open **8** Via Natural or Artificial Opening Endoscopic	**Z** No Device	**Z** No Qualifier

Continued →

Section 0 **Medical and Surgical**
Body System 9 **Ear, Nose, Sinus**
Operation 5 **Destruction:** Physical eradication of all or a portion of a body part by the direct use of energy, force, or a destructive agent

Body Part (4th)	Approach (5th)	Device (6th)	Qualifier (7th)
7 Tympanic Membrane, Right **8** Tympanic Membrane, Left **F** Eustachian Tube, Right **G** Eustachian Tube, Left **L** Nasal Turbinate **N** Nasopharynx	**0** Open **3** Percutaneous **4** Percutaneous Endoscopic **7** Via Natural or Artificial Opening **8** Via Natural or Artificial Opening Endoscopic	**Z** No Device	**Z** No Qualifier
B Mastoid Sinus, Right **C** Mastoid Sinus, Left **M** Nasal Septum **P** Accessory Sinus **Q** Maxillary Sinus, Right **R** Maxillary Sinus, Left **S** Frontal Sinus, Right **T** Frontal Sinus, Left **U** Ethmoid Sinus, Right **V** Ethmoid Sinus, Left **W** Sphenoid Sinus, Right **X** Sphenoid Sinus, Left	**0** Open **3** Percutaneous **4** Percutaneous Endoscopic **8** Via Natural or Artificial Opening Endoscopic	**Z** No Device	**Z** No Qualifier
K Nasal Mucosa and Soft Tissue	**0** Open **3** Percutaneous **4** Percutaneous Endoscopic **8** Via Natural or Artificial Opening Endoscopic **X** External	**Z** No Device	**Z** No Qualifier

Section 0 **Medical and Surgical**
Body System 9 **Ear, Nose, Sinus**
Operation 7 **Dilation:** Expanding an orifice or the lumen of a tubular body part

Body Part (4th)	Approach (5th)	Device (6th)	Qualifier (7th)
F Eustachian Tube, Right **G** Eustachian Tube, Left	**0** Open **7** Via Natural or Artificial Opening **8** Via Natural or Artificial Opening Endoscopic	**D** Intraluminal Device **Z** No Device	**Z** No Qualifier
F Eustachian Tube, Right **G** Eustachian Tube, Left	**3** Percutaneous **4** Percutaneous Endoscopic	**Z** No Device	**Z** No Qualifier

Section 0 **Medical and Surgical**
Body System 9 **Ear, Nose, Sinus**
Operation 8 **Division:** Cutting into a body part, without draining fluids and/or gases from the body part, in order to separate or transect a body part

Body Part (4th)	Approach (5th)	Device (6th)	Qualifier (7th)
L Nasal Turbinate	**0** Open **3** Percutaneous **4** Percutaneous Endoscopic **7** Via Natural or Artificial Opening **8** Via Natural or Artificial Opening Endoscopic	**Z** No Device	**Z** No Qualifier

Section 0 **Medical and Surgical**
Body System 9 **Ear, Nose, Sinus**
Operation 9 **Drainage:** Taking or letting out fluids and/or gases from a body part

Body Part (4th)	Approach (5th)	Device (6th)	Qualifier (7th)
0 External Ear, Right **1** External Ear, Left	**0** Open **3** Percutaneous **4** Percutaneous Endoscopic **X** External	**0** Drainage Device	**Z** No Qualifier
0 External Ear, Right **1** External Ear, Left	**0** Open **3** Percutaneous **4** Percutaneous Endoscopic **X** External	**Z** No Device	**X** Diagnostic **Z** No Qualifier
3 External Auditory Canal, Right **4** External Auditory Canal, Left **K** Nasal Mucosa and Soft Tissue	**0** Open **3** Percutaneous **4** Percutaneous Endoscopic **7** Via Natural or Artificial Opening **8** Via Natural or Artificial Opening Endoscopic **X** External	**0** Drainage Device	**Z** No Qualifier
3 External Auditory Canal, Right **4** External Auditory Canal, Left **K** Nasal Mucosa and Soft Tissue	**0** Open **3** Percutaneous **4** Percutaneous Endoscopic **7** Via Natural or Artificial Opening **8** Via Natural or Artificial Opening Endoscopic **X** External	**Z** No Device	**X** Diagnostic **Z** No Qualifier
5 Middle Ear, Right **6** Middle Ear, Left **9** Auditory Ossicle, Right **A** Auditory Ossicle, Left **D** Inner Ear, Right **E** Inner Ear, Left	**0** Open **7** Via Natural or Artificial Opening **8** Via Natural or Artificial Opening Endoscopic	**0** Drainage Device	**Z** No Qualifier
5 Middle Ear, Right **6** Middle Ear, Left **9** Auditory Ossicle, Right **A** Auditory Ossicle, Left **D** Inner Ear, Right **E** Inner Ear, Left	**0** Open **7** Via Natural or Artificial Opening **8** Via Natural or Artificial Opening Endoscopic	**Z** No Device	**X** Diagnostic **Z** No Qualifier
7 Tympanic Membrane, Right **8** Tympanic Membrane, Left **B** Mastoid Sinus, Right **C** Mastoid Sinus, Left **F** Eustachian Tube, Right **G** Eustachian Tube, Left **L** Nasal Turbinate **M** Nasal Septum **N** Nasopharynx **P** Accessory Sinus **Q** Maxillary Sinus, Right **R** Maxillary Sinus, Left **S** Frontal Sinus, Right **T** Frontal Sinus, Left **U** Ethmoid Sinus, Right **V** Ethmoid Sinus, Left **W** Sphenoid Sinus, Right **X** Sphenoid Sinus, Left	**0** Open **3** Percutaneous **4** Percutaneous Endoscopic **7** Via Natural or Artificial Opening **8** Via Natural or Artificial Opening Endoscopic	**0** Drainage Device	**Z** No Qualifier

Continued →

Section 0 Medical and Surgical
Body System 9 Ear, Nose, Sinus
Operation 9 **Drainage:** Taking or letting out fluids and/or gases from a body part

Body Part (4th)	Approach (5th)	Device (6th)	Qualifier (7th)
7 Tympanic Membrane, Right 8 Tympanic Membrane, Left B Mastoid Sinus, Right C Mastoid Sinus, Left F Eustachian Tube, Right G Eustachian Tube, Left L Nasal Turbinate M Nasal Septum N Nasopharynx P Accessory Sinus Q Maxillary Sinus, Right R Maxillary Sinus, Left S Frontal Sinus, Right T Frontal Sinus, Left U Ethmoid Sinus, Right V Ethmoid Sinus, Left W Sphenoid Sinus, Right X Sphenoid Sinus, Left	0 Open 3 Percutaneous 4 Percutaneous Endoscopic 7 Via Natural or Artificial Opening 8 Via Natural or Artificial Opening Endoscopic	Z No Device	X Diagnostic Z No Qualifier

Section 0 Medical and Surgical
Body System 9 Ear, Nose, Sinus
Operation B **Excision:** Cutting out or off, without replacement, a portion of a body part

Body Part (4th)	Approach (5th)	Device (6th)	Qualifier (7th)
0 External Ear, Right 1 External Ear, Left	0 Open 3 Percutaneous 4 Percutaneous Endoscopic X External	Z No Device	X Diagnostic Z No Qualifier
3 External Auditory Canal, Right 4 External Auditory Canal, Left	0 Open 3 Percutaneous 4 Percutaneous Endoscopic 7 Via Natural or Artificial Opening 8 Via Natural or Artificial Opening Endoscopic X External	Z No Device	X Diagnostic Z No Qualifier
5 Middle Ear, Right 6 Middle Ear, Left 9 Auditory Ossicle, Right A Auditory Ossicle, Left D Inner Ear, Right E Inner Ear, Left	0 Open 8 Via Natural or Artificial Opening Endoscopic	Z No Device	X Diagnostic Z No Qualifier
7 Tympanic Membrane, Right 8 Tympanic Membrane, Left F Eustachian Tube, Right G Eustachian Tube, Left L Nasal Turbinate N Nasopharynx	0 Open 3 Percutaneous 4 Percutaneous Endoscopic 7 Via Natural or Artificial Opening 8 Via Natural or Artificial Opening Endoscopic	Z No Device	X Diagnostic Z No Qualifier
B Mastoid Sinus, Right C Mastoid Sinus, Left M Nasal Septum P Accessory Sinus Q Maxillary Sinus, Right R Maxillary Sinus, Left S Frontal Sinus, Right T Frontal Sinus, Left U Ethmoid Sinus, Right V Ethmoid Sinus, Left W Sphenoid Sinus, Right X Sphenoid Sinus, Left	0 Open 3 Percutaneous 4 Percutaneous Endoscopic 8 Via Natural or Artificial Opening Endoscopic	Z No Device	X Diagnostic Z No Qualifier

Continued →

Section 0 **Medical and Surgical**
Body System 9 **Ear, Nose, Sinus**
Operation B **Excision:** Cutting out or off, without replacement, a portion of a body part

Body Part (4th)	Approach (5th)	Device (6th)	Qualifier (7th)
K Nasal Mucosa and Soft Tissue	**0** Open **3** Percutaneous **4** Percutaneous Endoscopic **8** Via Natural or Artificial Opening Endoscopic **X** External	**Z** No Device	**X** Diagnostic **Z** No Qualifier

Section 0 **Medical and Surgical**
Body System 9 **Ear, Nose, Sinus**
Operation C **Extirpation:** Taking or cutting out solid matter from a body part

Body Part (4th)	Approach (5th)	Device (6th)	Qualifier (7th)
0 External Ear, Right **1** External Ear, Left	**0** Open **3** Percutaneous **4** Percutaneous Endoscopic **X** External	**Z** No Device	**Z** No Qualifier
3 External Auditory Canal, Right **4** External Auditory Canal, Left	**0** Open **3** Percutaneous **4** Percutaneous Endoscopic **7** Via Natural or Artificial Opening **8** Via Natural or Artificial Opening Endoscopic **X** External	**Z** No Device	**Z** No Qualifier
5 Middle Ear, Right **6** Middle Ear, Left **9** Auditory Ossicle, Right **A** Auditory Ossicle, Left **D** Inner Ear, Right **E** Inner Ear, Left	**0** Open **8** Via Natural or Artificial Opening Endoscopic	**Z** No Device	**Z** No Qualifier
7 Tympanic Membrane, Right **8** Tympanic Membrane, Left **F** Eustachian Tube, Right **G** Eustachian Tube, Left **L** Nasal Turbinate **N** Nasopharynx	**0** Open **3** Percutaneous **4** Percutaneous Endoscopic **7** Via Natural or Artificial Opening **8** Via Natural or Artificial Opening Endoscopic	**Z** No Device	**Z** No Qualifier
B Mastoid Sinus, Right **C** Mastoid Sinus, Left **M** Nasal Septum **P** Accessory Sinus **Q** Maxillary Sinus, Right **R** Maxillary Sinus, Left **S** Frontal Sinus, Right **T** Frontal Sinus, Left **U** Ethmoid Sinus, Right **V** Ethmoid Sinus, Left **W** Sphenoid Sinus, Right **X** Sphenoid Sinus, Left	**0** Open **3** Percutaneous **4** Percutaneous Endoscopic **8** Via Natural or Artificial Opening Endoscopic	**Z** No Device	**Z** No Qualifier
K Nasal Mucosa and Soft Tissue	**0** Open **3** Percutaneous **4** Percutaneous Endoscopic **8** Via Natural or Artificial Opening Endoscopic **X** External	**Z** No Device	**Z** No Qualifier

Section 0 **Medical and Surgical**
Body System 9 **Ear, Nose, Sinus**
Operation D **Extraction:** Pulling or stripping out or off all or a portion of a body part by the use of force

Body Part (4th)	Approach (5th)	Device (6th)	Qualifier (7th)
7 Tympanic Membrane, Right **8** Tympanic Membrane, Left **L** Nasal Turbinate	**0** Open **3** Percutaneous **4** Percutaneous Endoscopic **7** Via Natural or Artificial Opening **8** Via Natural or Artificial Opening Endoscopic	**Z** No Device	**Z** No Qualifier
9 Auditory Ossicle, Right **A** Auditory Ossicle, Left	**0** Open	**Z** No Device	**Z** No Qualifier
B Mastoid Sinus, Right **C** Mastoid Sinus, Left **M** Nasal Septum **P** Accessory Sinus **Q** Maxillary Sinus, Right **R** Maxillary Sinus, Left **S** Frontal Sinus, Right **T** Frontal Sinus, Left **U** Ethmoid Sinus, Right **V** Ethmoid Sinus, Left **W** Sphenoid Sinus, Right **X** Sphenoid Sinus, Left	**0** Open **3** Percutaneous **4** Percutaneous Endoscopic	**Z** No Device	**Z** No Qualifier

Section 0 **Medical and Surgical**
Body System 9 **Ear, Nose, Sinus**
Operation H **Insertion:** Putting in a nonbiological appliance that monitors, assists, performs, or prevents a physiological function but does not physically take the place of a body part

Body Part (4th)	Approach (5th)	Device (6th)	Qualifier (7th)
D Inner Ear, Right **E** Inner Ear, Left	**0** Open **3** Percutaneous **4** Percutaneous Endoscopic	**1** Radioactive Element **4** Hearing Device, Bone Conduction **5** Hearing Device, Single Channel Cochlear Prosthesis **6** Hearing Device, Multiple Channel Cochlear Prosthesis **S** Hearing Device	**Z** No Qualifier
H Ear, Right **J** Ear, Left **K** Nasal Mucosa and Soft Tissue **Y** Sinus	**0** Open **3** Percutaneous **4** Percutaneous Endoscopic **7** Via Natural or Artificial Opening **8** Via Natural or Artificial Opening Endoscopic	**1** Radioactive Element **Y** Other Device	**Z** No Qualifier
N Nasopharynx	**7** Via Natural or Artificial Opening **8** Via Natural or Artificial Opening Endoscopic	**1** Radioactive Element **B** Intraluminal Device, Airway	**Z** No Qualifier

Section 0 **Medical and Surgical**
Body System 9 **Ear, Nose, Sinus**
Operation J **Inspection:** Visually and/or manually exploring a body part

Body Part (4th)	Approach (5th)	Device (6th)	Qualifier (7th)
7 Tympanic Membrane, Right **8** Tympanic Membrane, Left **H** Ear, Right **J** Ear, Left	**0** Open **3** Percutaneous **4** Percutaneous Endoscopic **7** Via Natural or Artificial Opening **8** Via Natural or Artificial Opening Endoscopic **X** External	**Z** No Device	**Z** No Qualifier
D Inner Ear, Right **E** Inner Ear, Left **K** Nose **Y** Sinus	**0** Open **3** Percutaneous **4** Percutaneous Endoscopic **8** Via Natural or Artificial Opening Endoscopic **X** External	**Z** No Device	**Z** No Qualifier

Section 0 **Medical and Surgical**
Body System 9 **Ear, Nose, Sinus**
Operation M **Reattachment:** Putting back in or on all or a portion of a separated body part to its normal location or other suitable location

Body Part (4th)	Approach (5th)	Device (6th)	Qualifier (7th)
0 External Ear, Right **1** External Ear, Left **K** Nasal Mucosa and Soft Tissue	**X** External	**Z** No Device	**Z** No Qualifier

Section 0 **Medical and Surgical**
Body System 9 **Ear, Nose, Sinus**
Operation N **Release:** Freeing a body part from an abnormal physical constraint by cutting or by the use of force

Body Part (4th)	Approach (5th)	Device (6th)	Qualifier (7th)
0 External Ear, Right **1** External Ear, Left	**0** Open **3** Percutaneous **4** Percutaneous Endoscopic **X** External	**Z** No Device	**Z** No Qualifier
3 External Auditory Canal, Right **4** External Auditory Canal, Left	**0** Open **3** Percutaneous **4** Percutaneous Endoscopic **7** Via Natural or Artificial Opening **8** Via Natural or Artificial Opening Endoscopic **X** External	**Z** No Device	**Z** No Qualifier
5 Middle Ear, Right **6** Middle Ear, Left **9** Auditory Ossicle, Right **A** Auditory Ossicle, Left **D** Inner Ear, Right **E** Inner Ear, Left	**0** Open **8** Via Natural or Artificial Opening Endoscopic	**Z** No Device	**Z** No Qualifier
7 Tympanic Membrane, Right **8** Tympanic Membrane, Left **F** Eustachian Tube, Right **G** Eustachian Tube, Left **L** Nasal Turbinate **N** Nasopharynx	**0** Open **3** Percutaneous **4** Percutaneous Endoscopic **7** Via Natural or Artificial Opening **8** Via Natural or Artificial Opening Endoscopic	**Z** No Device	**Z** No Qualifier
B Mastoid Sinus, Right **C** Mastoid Sinus, Left **M** Nasal Septum **P** Accessory Sinus **Q** Maxillary Sinus, Right **R** Maxillary Sinus, Left **S** Frontal Sinus, Right **T** Frontal Sinus, Left **U** Ethmoid Sinus, Right **V** Ethmoid Sinus, Left **W** Sphenoid Sinus, Right **X** Sphenoid Sinus, Left	**0** Open **3** Percutaneous **4** Percutaneous Endoscopic **8** Via Natural or Artificial Opening Endoscopic	**Z** No Device	**Z** No Qualifier
K Nasal Mucosa and Soft Tissue	**0** Open **3** Percutaneous **4** Percutaneous Endoscopic **8** Via Natural or Artificial Opening Endoscopic **X** External	**Z** No Device	**Z** No Qualifier

Section 0 Medical and Surgical
Body System 9 Ear, Nose, Sinus
Operation P **Removal:** Taking out or off a device from a body part

Body Part (4th)	Approach (5th)	Device (6th)	Qualifier (7th)
7 Tympanic Membrane, Right 8 Tympanic Membrane, Left	0 Open 7 Via Natural or Artificial Opening 8 Via Natural or Artificial Opening Endoscopic X External	0 Drainage Device	Z No Qualifier
D Inner Ear, Right E Inner Ear, Left	0 Open 7 Via Natural or Artificial Opening 8 Via Natural or Artificial Opening Endoscopic	S Hearing Device	Z No Qualifier
H Ear, Right J Ear, Left K Nasal Mucosa and Soft Tissue	0 Open 3 Percutaneous 4 Percutaneous Endoscopic 7 Via Natural or Artificial Opening 8 Via Natural or Artificial Opening Endoscopic	0 Drainage Device 7 Autologous Tissue Substitute D Intraluminal Device J Synthetic Substitute K Nonautologous Tissue Substitute Y Other Device	Z No Qualifier
H Ear, Right J Ear, Left K Nasal Mucosa and Soft Tissue	X External	0 Drainage Device 7 Autologous Tissue Substitute D Intraluminal Device J Synthetic Substitute K Nonautologous Tissue Substitute	Z No Qualifier
Y Sinus	0 Open 3 Percutaneous 4 Percutaneous Endoscopic	0 Drainage Device Y Other Device	Z No Qualifier
Y Sinus	7 Via Natural or Artificial Opening 8 Via Natural or Artificial Opening Endoscopic	Y Other Device	Z No Qualifier
Y Sinus	X External	0 Drainage Device	Z No Qualifier

Section 0 Medical and Surgical
Body System 9 Ear, Nose, Sinus
Operation Q **Repair:** Restoring, to the extent possible, a body part to its normal anatomic structure and function

Body Part (4th)	Approach (5th)	Device (6th)	Qualifier (7th)
0 External Ear, Right 1 External Ear, Left 2 External Ear, Bilateral	0 Open 3 Percutaneous 4 Percutaneous Endoscopic X External	Z No Device	Z No Qualifier
3 External Auditory Canal, Right 4 External Auditory Canal, Left F Eustachian Tube, Right G Eustachian Tube, Left	0 Open 3 Percutaneous 4 Percutaneous Endoscopic 7 Via Natural or Artificial Opening 8 Via Natural or Artificial Opening Endoscopic X External	Z No Device	Z No Qualifier
5 Middle Ear, Right 6 Middle Ear, Left 9 Auditory Ossicle, Right A Auditory Ossicle, Left D Inner Ear, Right E Inner Ear, Left	0 Open 8 Via Natural or Artificial Opening Endoscopic	Z No Device	Z No Qualifier
7 Tympanic Membrane, Right 8 Tympanic Membrane, Left L Nasal Turbinate N Nasopharynx	0 Open 3 Percutaneous 4 Percutaneous Endoscopic 7 Via Natural or Artificial Opening 8 Via Natural or Artificial Opening Endoscopic	Z No Device	Z No Qualifier

Continued →

Section 0 **Medical and Surgical**
Body System 9 **Ear, Nose, Sinus**
Operation Q **Repair:** Restoring, to the extent possible, a body part to its normal anatomic structure and function

Body Part (4th)	Approach (5th)	Device (6th)	Qualifier (7th)
B Mastoid Sinus, Right **C** Mastoid Sinus, Left **M** Nasal Septum **P** Accessory Sinus **Q** Maxillary Sinus, Right **R** Maxillary Sinus, Left **S** Frontal Sinus, Right **T** Frontal Sinus, Left **U** Ethmoid Sinus, Right **V** Ethmoid Sinus, Left **W** Sphenoid Sinus, Right **X** Sphenoid Sinus, Left	**0** Open **3** Percutaneous **4** Percutaneous Endoscopic **8** Via Natural or Artificial Opening Endoscopic	**Z** No Device	**Z** No Qualifier
K Nasal Mucosa and Soft Tissue	**0** Open **3** Percutaneous **4** Percutaneous Endoscopic **8** Via Natural or Artificial Opening Endoscopic **X** External	**Z** No Device	**Z** No Qualifier

Section 0 **Medical and Surgical**
Body System 9 **Ear, Nose, Sinus**
Operation R **Replacement:** Putting in or on biological or synthetic material that physically takes the place and/or function of all or a portion of a body part

Body Part (4th)	Approach (5th)	Device (6th)	Qualifier (7th)
0 External Ear, Right **1** External Ear, Left **2** External Ear, Bilateral **K** Nasal Mucosa and Soft Tissue	**0** Open **X** External	**7** Autologous Tissue Substitute **J** Synthetic Substitute **K** Nonautologous Tissue Substitute	**Z** No Qualifier
5 Middle Ear, Right **6** Middle Ear, Left **9** Auditory Ossicle, Right **A** Auditory Ossicle, Left **D** Inner Ear, Right **E** Inner Ear, Left	**0** Open	**7** Autologous Tissue Substitute **J** Synthetic Substitute **K** Nonautologous Tissue Substitute	**Z** No Qualifier
7 Tympanic Membrane, Right **8** Tympanic Membrane, Left **N** Nasopharynx	**0** Open **7** Via Natural or Artificial Opening **8** Via Natural or Artificial Opening Endoscopic	**7** Autologous Tissue Substitute **J** Synthetic Substitute **K** Nonautologous Tissue Substitute	**Z** No Qualifier
L Nasal Turbinate	**0** Open **3** Percutaneous **4** Percutaneous Endoscopic **7** Via Natural or Artificial Opening **8** Via Natural or Artificial Opening Endoscopic	**7** Autologous Tissue Substitute **J** Synthetic Substitute **K** Nonautologous Tissue Substitute	**Z** No Qualifier
M Nasal Septum	**0** Open **3** Percutaneous **4** Percutaneous Endoscopic	**7** Autologous Tissue Substitute **J** Synthetic Substitute **K** Nonautologous Tissue Substitute	**Z** No Qualifier

Section 0 **Medical and Surgical**
Body System 9 **Ear, Nose, Sinus**
Operation S **Reposition:** Moving to its normal location, or other suitable location, all or a portion of a body part

Body Part (4th)	Approach (5th)	Device (6th)	Qualifier (7th)
0 External Ear, Right **1** External Ear, Left **2** External Ear, Bilateral **K** Nasal Mucosa and Soft Tissue	**0** Open **4** Percutaneous Endoscopic **X** External	**Z** No Device	**Z** No Qualifier
7 Tympanic Membrane, Right **8** Tympanic Membrane, Left **F** Eustachian Tube, Right **G** Eustachian Tube, Left **L** Nasal Turbinate	**0** Open **4** Percutaneous Endoscopic **7** Via Natural or Artificial Opening **8** Via Natural or Artificial Opening Endoscopic	**Z** No Device	**Z** No Qualifier
9 Auditory Ossicle, Right **A** Auditory Ossicle, Left **M** Nasal Septum	**0** Open **4** Percutaneous Endoscopic	**Z** No Device	**Z** No Qualifier

Section 0 **Medical and Surgical**
Body System 9 **Ear, Nose, Sinus**
Operation T **Resection:** Cutting out or off, without replacement, all of a body part

Body Part (4th)	Approach (5th)	Device (6th)	Qualifier (7th)
0 External Ear, Right **1** External Ear, Left	**0** Open **4** Percutaneous Endoscopic **X** External	**Z** No Device	**Z** No Qualifier
5 Middle Ear, Right **6** Middle Ear, Left **9** Auditory Ossicle, Right **A** Auditory Ossicle, Left **D** Inner Ear, Right **E** Inner Ear, Left	**0** Open **8** Via Natural or Artificial Opening Endoscopic	**Z** No Device	**Z** No Qualifier
7 Tympanic Membrane, Right **8** Tympanic Membrane, Left **F** Eustachian Tube, Right **G** Eustachian Tube, Left **L** Nasal Turbinate **N** Nasopharynx	**0** Open **4** Percutaneous Endoscopic **7** Via Natural or Artificial Opening **8** Via Natural or Artificial Opening Endoscopic	**Z** No Device	**Z** No Qualifier
B Mastoid Sinus, Right **C** Mastoid Sinus, Left **M** Nasal Septum **P** Accessory Sinus **Q** Maxillary Sinus, Right **R** Maxillary Sinus, Left **S** Frontal Sinus, Right **T** Frontal Sinus, Left **U** Ethmoid Sinus, Right **V** Ethmoid Sinus, Left **W** Sphenoid Sinus, Right **X** Sphenoid Sinus, Left	**0** Open **4** Percutaneous Endoscopic **8** Via Natural or Artificial Opening Endoscopic	**Z** No Device	**Z** No Qualifier
K Nasal Mucosa and Soft Tissue	**0** Open **4** Percutaneous Endoscopic **8** Via Natural or Artificial Opening Endoscopic **X** External	**Z** No Device	**Z** No Qualifier

Section 0 **Medical and Surgical**
Body System 9 **Ear, Nose, Sinus**
Operation U **Supplement:** Putting in or on biological or synthetic material that physically reinforces and/or augments the function of a portion of a body part

Body Part (4th)	Approach (5th)	Device (6th)	Qualifier (7th)
0 External Ear, Right **1** External Ear, Left **2** External Ear, Bilateral	**0** Open **X** External	**7** Autologous Tissue Substitute **J** Synthetic Substitute **K** Nonautologous Tissue Substitute	**Z** No Qualifier
5 Middle Ear, Right **6** Middle Ear, Left **9** Auditory Ossicle, Right **A** Auditory Ossicle, Left **D** Inner Ear, Right **E** Inner Ear, Left	**0** Open **8** Via Natural or Artificial Opening Endoscopic	**7** Autologous Tissue Substitute **J** Synthetic Substitute **K** Nonautologous Tissue Substitute	**Z** No Qualifier
7 Tympanic Membrane, Right **8** Tympanic Membrane, Left **N** Nasopharynx	**0** Open **7** Via Natural or Artificial Opening **8** Via Natural or Artificial Opening Endoscopic	**7** Autologous Tissue Substitute **J** Synthetic Substitute **K** Nonautologous Tissue Substitute	**Z** No Qualifier
B Mastoid Sinus, Right **C** Mastoid Sinus, Left **L** Nasal Turbinate **P** Accessory Sinus **Q** Maxillary Sinus, Right **R** Maxillary Sinus, Left **S** Frontal Sinus, Right **T** Frontal Sinus, Left **U** Ethmoid Sinus, Right **V** Ethmoid Sinus, Left **W** Sphenoid Sinus, Right **X** Sphenoid Sinus, Left	**0** Open **3** Percutaneous **4** Percutaneous Endoscopic **7** Via Natural or Artificial Opening **8** Via Natural or Artificial Opening Endoscopic	**7** Autologous Tissue Substitute **J** Synthetic Substitute **K** Nonautologous Tissue Substitute	**Z** No Qualifier
K Nasal Mucosa and Soft Tissue	**0** Open **8** Via Natural or Artificial Opening Endoscopic **X** External	**7** Autologous Tissue Substitute **J** Synthetic Substitute **K** Nonautologous Tissue Substitute	**Z** No Qualifier
M Nasal Septum	**0** Open **3** Percutaneous **4** Percutaneous Endoscopic **8** Via Natural or Artificial Opening Endoscopic	**7** Autologous Tissue Substitute **J** Synthetic Substitute **K** Nonautologous Tissue Substitute	**Z** No Qualifier

Section 0 **Medical and Surgical**
Body System 9 **Ear, Nose, Sinus**
Operation W **Revision:** Correcting, to the extent possible, a portion of a malfunctioning device or the position of a displaced device

Body Part (4th)	Approach (5th)	Device (6th)	Qualifier (7th)
7 Tympanic Membrane, Right **8** Tympanic Membrane, Left **9** Auditory Ossicle, Right **A** Auditory Ossicle, Left	**0** Open **7** Via Natural or Artificial Opening **8** Via Natural or Artificial Opening Endoscopic	**7** Autologous Tissue Substitute **J** Synthetic Substitute **K** Nonautologous Tissue Substitute	**Z** No Qualifier
D Inner Ear, Right **E** Inner Ear, Left	**0** Open **7** Via Natural or Artificial Opening **8** Via Natural or Artificial Opening Endoscopic	**S** Hearing Device	**Z** No Qualifier
H Ear, Right **J** Ear, Left **K** Nasal Mucosa and Soft Tissue	**0** Open **3** Percutaneous **4** Percutaneous Endoscopic **7** Via Natural or Artificial Opening **8** Via Natural or Artificial Opening Endoscopic	**0** Drainage Device **7** Autologous Tissue Substitute **D** Intraluminal Device **J** Synthetic Substitute **K** Nonautologous Tissue Substitute **Y** Other Device	**Z** No Qualifier

Continued →

Section 0 **Medical and Surgical**
Body System 9 **Ear, Nose, Sinus**
Operation W **Revision:** Correcting, to the extent possible, a portion of a malfunctioning device or the position of a displaced device

Body Part (4th)	Approach (5th)	Device (6th)	Qualifier (7th)
H Ear, Right **J** Ear, Left **K** Nasal Mucosa and Soft Tissue	**X** External	**0** Drainage Device **7** Autologous Tissue Substitute **D** Intraluminal Device **J** Synthetic Substitute **K** Nonautologous Tissue Substitute	**Z** No Qualifier
Y Sinus	**0** Open **3** Percutaneous **4** Percutaneous Endoscopic	**0** Drainage Device **Y** Other Device	**Z** No Qualifier
Y Sinus	**7** Via Natural or Artificial Opening **8** Via Natural or Artificial Opening Endoscopic	**Y** Other Device	**Z** No Qualifier
Y Sinus	**X** External	**0** Drainage Device	**Z** No Qualifier

AHA Coding Clinic

093K8ZZ Control Bleeding in Nasal Mucosa and Soft Tissue, Via Natural or Artificial Opening Endoscopic—AHA CC: 4Q, 2018, 38
09QKXZZ Repair Nasal Mucosa and Soft Tissue, External Approach—AHA CC: 4Q, 2014, 20-21
09QT4ZZ Repair Left Frontal Sinus, Percutaneous Endoscopic Approach—AHA CC: 4Q, 2013, 114
09QW0ZZ Repair Right Sphenoid Sinus, Open Approach—AHA CC: 3Q, 2014, 22-23
09QX0ZZ Repair Left Sphenoid Sinus, Open Approach—AHA CC: 3Q, 2014, 22-23

Topography of Lungs: Anterior View

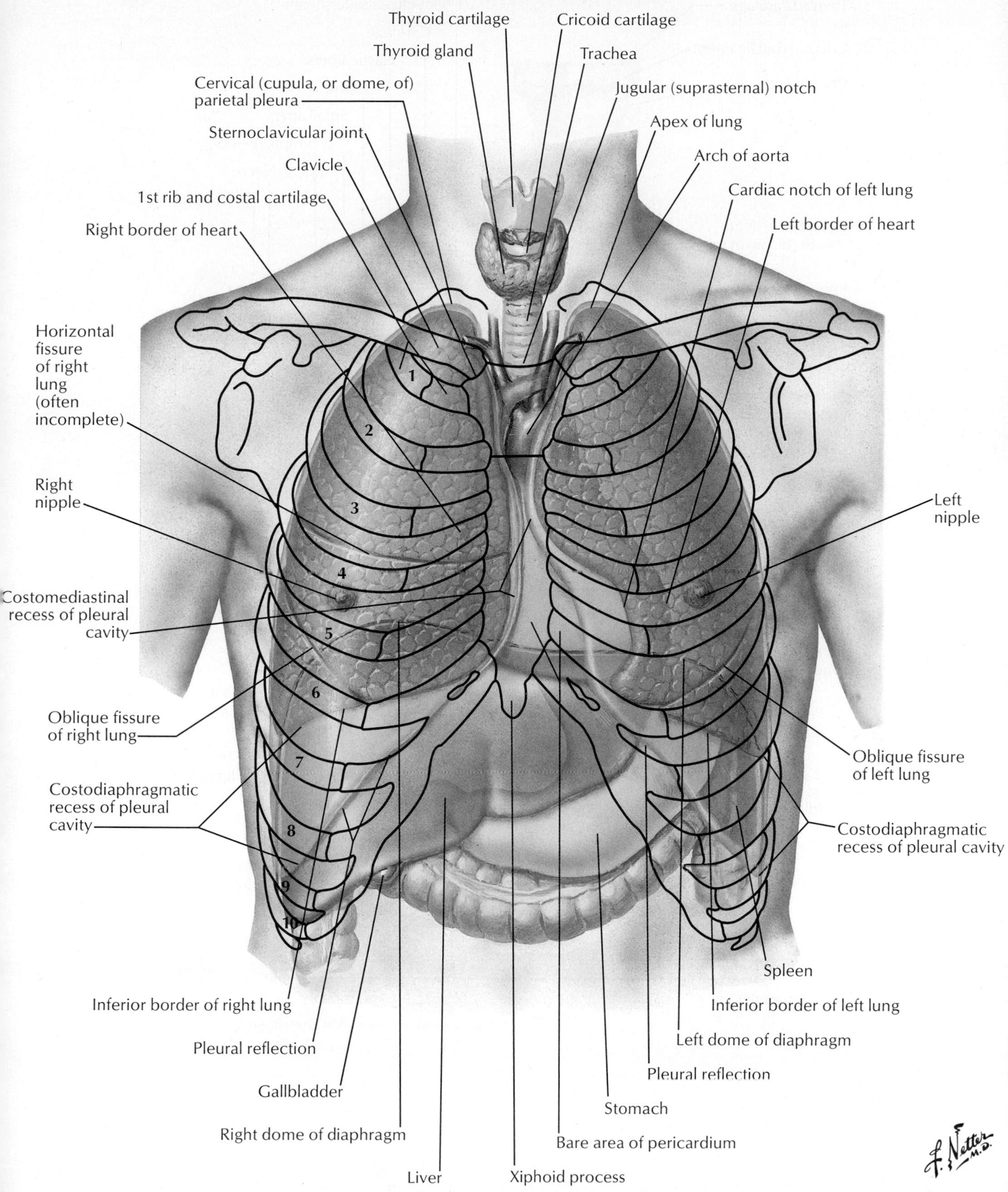
Thyroid cartilage
Cricoid cartilage
Thyroid gland
Trachea
Cervical (cupula, or dome, of) parietal pleura
Jugular (suprasternal) notch
Apex of lung
Sternoclavicular joint
Clavicle
Arch of aorta
1st rib and costal cartilage
Cardiac notch of left lung
Right border of heart
Left border of heart
Horizontal fissure of right lung (often incomplete)
1
2
3
4
5
6
7
8
9
10
Right nipple
Left nipple
Costomediastinal recess of pleural cavity
Oblique fissure of right lung
Oblique fissure of left lung
Costodiaphragmatic recess of pleural cavity
Costodiaphragmatic recess of pleural cavity
Spleen
Inferior border of right lung
Inferior border of left lung
Left dome of diaphragm
Pleural reflection
Pleural reflection
Gallbladder
Stomach
Right dome of diaphragm
Bare area of pericardium
Liver
Xiphoid process
F. Netter M.D.

Structure of the Trachea and Major Bronchi

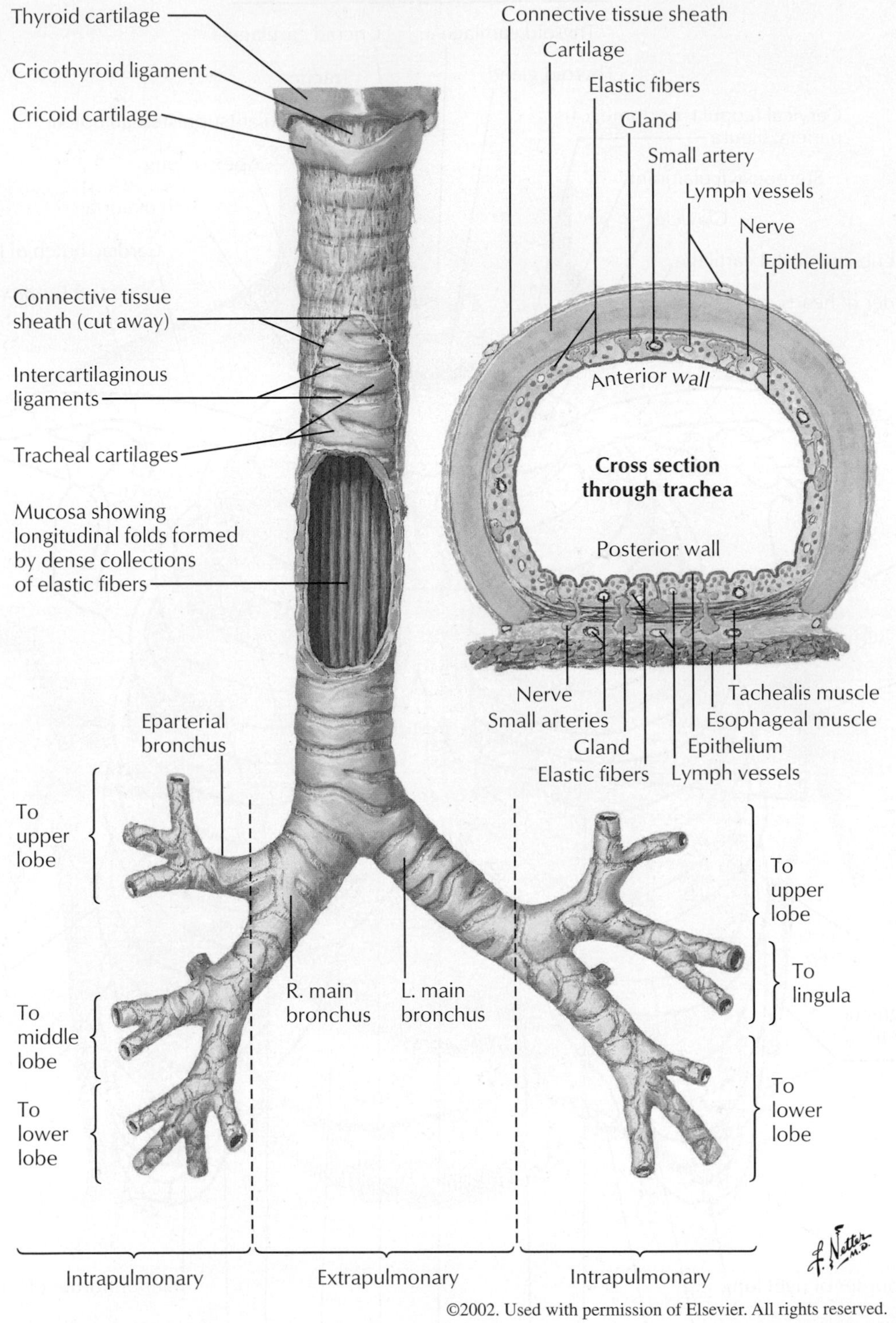

Thyroid cartilage
Cricothyroid ligament
Cricoid cartilage
Connective tissue sheath (cut away)
Intercartilaginous ligaments
Tracheal cartilages
Mucosa showing longitudinal folds formed by dense collections of elastic fibers
Connective tissue sheath
Cartilage
Elastic fibers
Gland
Small artery
Lymph vessels
Nerve
Epithelium
Anterior wall
Cross section through trachea
Posterior wall
Nerve
Small arteries
Gland
Elastic fibers
Tachealis muscle
Esophageal muscle
Epithelium
Lymph vessels
Eparterial bronchus
To upper lobe
To middle lobe
To lower lobe
R. main bronchus
L. main bronchus
To upper lobe
To lingula
To lower lobe
Intrapulmonary
Extrapulmonary
Intrapulmonary

Sublobar Resection and Surgical Lung Biopsy

Segmental resection

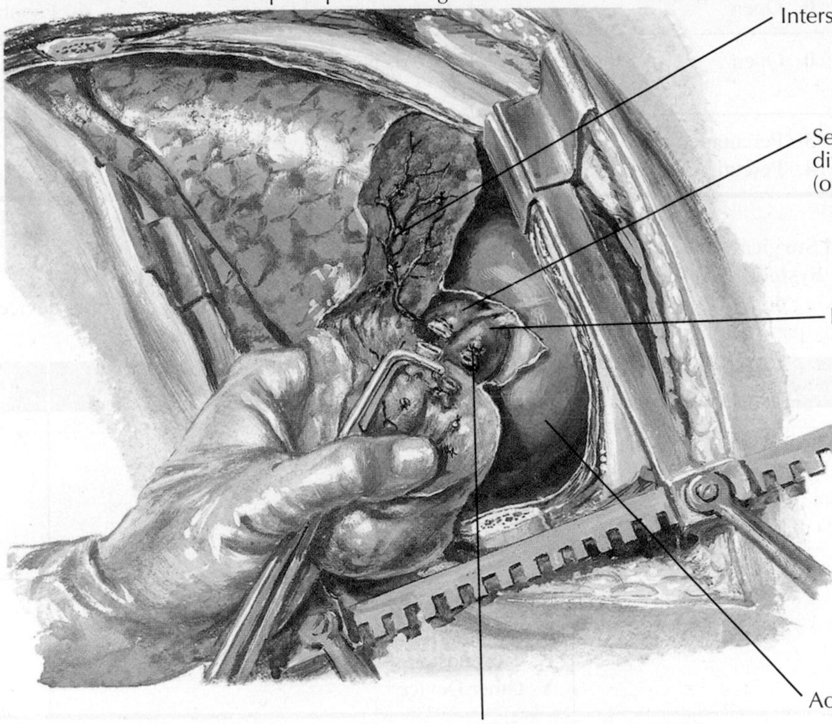

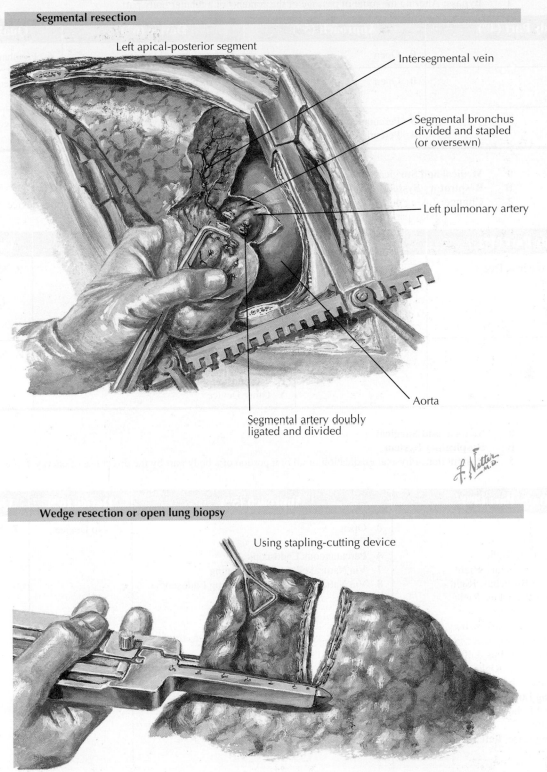

Left apical-posterior segment
Intersegmental vein
Segmental bronchus divided and stapled (or oversewn)
Left pulmonary artery
Aorta
Segmental artery doubly ligated and divided
F. Netter M.D.

Wedge resection or open lung biopsy

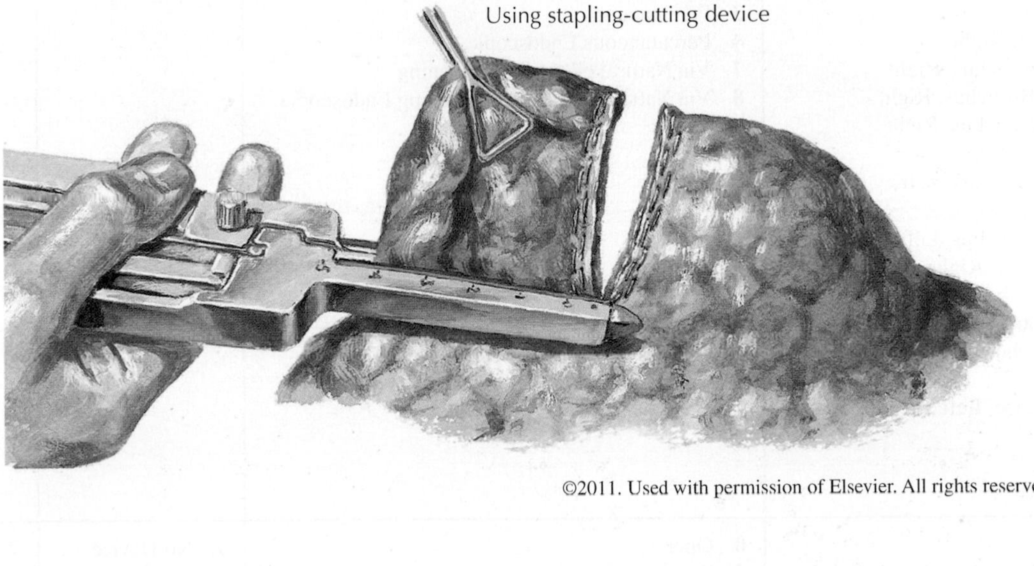

Using stapling-cutting device

Respiratory System Tables 0B1–0BY

Section 0 **Medical and Surgical**
Body System B **Respiratory System**
Operation 1 **Bypass:** Altering the route of passage of the contents of a tubular body part

Body Part (4th)	Approach (5th)	Device (6th)	Qualifier (7th)
1 Trachea	0 Open	D Intraluminal Device	6 Esophagus
1 Trachea	0 Open	F Tracheostomy Device Z No Device	4 Cutaneous
1 Trachea	3 Percutaneous 4 Percutaneous Endoscopic	F Tracheostomy Device Z No Device	4 Cutaneous

Section 0 **Medical and Surgical**
Body System B **Respiratory System**
Operation 2 **Change:** Taking out or off a device from a body part and putting back an identical or similar device in or on the same body part without cutting or puncturing the skin or a mucous membrane

Body Part (4th)	Approach (5th)	Device (6th)	Qualifier (7th)
0 Tracheobronchial Tree K Lung, Right L Lung, Left Q Pleura T Diaphragm	X External	0 Drainage Device Y Other Device	Z No Qualifier
1 Trachea	X External	0 Drainage Device E Intraluminal Device, Endotracheal Airway F Tracheostomy Device Y Other Device	Z No Qualifier

Section 0 **Medical and Surgical**
Body System B **Respiratory System**
Operation 5 **Destruction:** Physical eradication of all or a portion of a body part by the direct use of energy, force, or a destructive agent

Body Part (4th)	Approach (5th)	Device (6th)	Qualifier (7th)
1 Trachea 2 Carina 3 Main Bronchus, Right 4 Upper Lobe Bronchus, Right 5 Middle Lobe Bronchus, Right 6 Lower Lobe Bronchus, Right 7 Main Bronchus, Left 8 Upper Lobe Bronchus, Left 9 Lingula Bronchus B Lower Lobe Bronchus, Left C Upper Lung Lobe, Right D Middle Lung Lobe, Right F Lower Lung Lobe, Right G Upper Lung Lobe, Left H Lung Lingula J Lower Lung Lobe, Left K Lung, Right L Lung, Left M Lungs, Bilateral	0 Open 3 Percutaneous 4 Percutaneous Endoscopic 7 Via Natural or Artificial Opening 8 Via Natural or Artificial Opening Endoscopic	Z No Device	Z No Qualifier
N Pleura, Right P Pleura, Left T Diaphragm	0 Open 3 Percutaneous 4 Percutaneous Endoscopic	Z No Device	Z No Qualifier

Section 0 **Medical and Surgical**
Body System B **Respiratory System**
Operation 7 **Dilation:** Expanding an orifice or the lumen of a tubular body part

Body Part (4th)	Approach (5th)	Device (6th)	Qualifier (7th)
1 Trachea **2** Carina **3** Main Bronchus, Right **4** Upper Lobe Bronchus, Right **5** Middle Lobe Bronchus, Right **6** Lower Lobe Bronchus, Right **7** Main Bronchus, Left **8** Upper Lobe Bronchus, Left **9** Lingula Bronchus **B** Lower Lobe Bronchus, Left	**0** Open **3** Percutaneous **4** Percutaneous Endoscopic **7** Via Natural or Artificial Opening **8** Via Natural or Artificial Opening Endoscopic	**D** Intraluminal Device **Z** No Device	**Z** No Qualifier

Section 0 **Medical and Surgical**
Body System B **Respiratory System**
Operation 9 **Drainage:** Taking or letting out fluids and/or gases from a body part

Body Part (4th)	Approach (5th)	Device (6th)	Qualifier (7th)
1 Trachea **2** Carina **3** Main Bronchus, Right **4** Upper Lobe Bronchus, Right **5** Middle Lobe Bronchus, Right **6** Lower Lobe Bronchus, Right **7** Main Bronchus, Left **8** Upper Lobe Bronchus, Left **9** Lingula Bronchus **B** Lower Lobe Bronchus, Left **C** Upper Lung Lobe, Right **D** Middle Lung Lobe, Right **F** Lower Lung Lobe, Right **G** Upper Lung Lobe, Left **H** Lung Lingula **J** Lower Lung Lobe, Left **K** Lung, Right **L** Lung, Left **M** Lungs, Bilateral	**0** Open **3** Percutaneous **4** Percutaneous Endoscopic **7** Via Natural or Artificial Opening **8** Via Natural or Artificial Opening Endoscopic	**0** Drainage Device	**Z** No Qualifier
1 Trachea **2** Carina **3** Main Bronchus, Right **4** Upper Lobe Bronchus, Right **5** Middle Lobe Bronchus, Right **6** Lower Lobe Bronchus, Right **7** Main Bronchus, Left **8** Upper Lobe Bronchus, Left **9** Lingula Bronchus **B** Lower Lobe Bronchus, Left **C** Upper Lung Lobe, Right **D** Middle Lung Lobe, Right **F** Lower Lung Lobe, Right **G** Upper Lung Lobe, Left **H** Lung Lingula **J** Lower Lung Lobe, Left **K** Lung, Right **L** Lung, Left **M** Lungs, Bilateral	**0** Open **3** Percutaneous **4** Percutaneous Endoscopic **7** Via Natural or Artificial Opening **8** Via Natural or Artificial Opening Endoscopic	**Z** No Device	**X** Diagnostic **Z** No Qualifier
N Pleura, Right **P** Pleura, Left	**0** Open **3** Percutaneous **4** Percutaneous Endoscopic **8** Via Natural or Artificial Opening Endoscopic	**0** Drainage Device	**Z** No Qualifier

Continued →

Section 0 **Medical and Surgical**
Body System B **Respiratory System**
Operation 9 **Drainage:** Taking or letting out fluids and/or gases from a body part

Body Part (4th)	Approach (5th)	Device (6th)	Qualifier (7th)
N Pleura, Right **P** Pleura, Left	**0** Open **3** Percutaneous **4** Percutaneous Endoscopic **8** Via Natural or Artificial Opening Endoscopic	**Z** No Device	**X** Diagnostic **Z** No Qualifier
T Diaphragm	**0** Open **3** Percutaneous **4** Percutaneous Endoscopic	**0** Drainage Device	**Z** No Qualifier
T Diaphragm	**0** Open **3** Percutaneous **4** Percutaneous Endoscopic	**Z** No Device	**X** Diagnostic **Z** No Qualifier

Section 0 **Medical and Surgical**
Body System B **Respiratory System**
Operation B **Excision:** Cutting out or off, without replacement, a portion of a body part

Body Part (4th)	Approach (5th)	Device (6th)	Qualifier (7th)
1 Trachea **2** Carina **3** Main Bronchus, Right **4** Upper Lobe Bronchus, Right **5** Middle Lobe Bronchus, Right **6** Lower Lobe Bronchus, Right **7** Main Bronchus, Left **8** Upper Lobe Bronchus, Left **9** Lingula Bronchus **B** Lower Lobe Bronchus, Left **C** Upper Lung Lobe, Right **D** Middle Lung Lobe, Right **F** Lower Lung Lobe, Right **G** Upper Lung Lobe, Left **H** Lung Lingula **J** Lower Lung Lobe, Left **K** Lung, Right **L** Lung, Left **M** Lungs, Bilateral	**0** Open **3** Percutaneous **4** Percutaneous Endoscopic **7** Via Natural or Artificial Opening **8** Via Natural or Artificial Opening Endoscopic	**Z** No Device	**X** Diagnostic **Z** No Qualifier
N Pleura, Right **P** Pleura, Left	**0** Open **3** Percutaneous **4** Percutaneous Endoscopic **8** Via Natural or Artificial Opening Endoscopic	**Z** No Device	**X** Diagnostic **Z** No Qualifier
T Diaphragm	**0** Open **3** Percutaneous **4** Percutaneous Endoscopic	**Z** No Device	**X** Diagnostic **Z** No Qualifier

Section 0 **Medical and Surgical**
Body System B **Respiratory System**
Operation C **Extirpation:** Taking or cutting out solid matter from a body part

Body Part (4th)	Approach (5th)	Device (6th)	Qualifier (7th)
1 Trachea 2 Carina 3 Main Bronchus, Right 4 Upper Lobe Bronchus, Right 5 Middle Lobe Bronchus, Right 6 Lower Lobe Bronchus, Right 7 Main Bronchus, Left 8 Upper Lobe Bronchus, Left 9 Lingula Bronchus B Lower Lobe Bronchus, Left C Upper Lung Lobe, Right D Middle Lung Lobe, Right F Lower Lung Lobe, Right G Upper Lung Lobe, Left H Lung Lingula J Lower Lung Lobe, Left K Lung, Right L Lung, Left M Lungs, Bilateral	0 Open 3 Percutaneous 4 Percutaneous Endoscopic 7 Via Natural or Artificial Opening 8 Via Natural or Artificial Opening Endoscopic	Z No Device	Z No Qualifier
N Pleura, Right P Pleura, Left T Diaphragm	0 Open 3 Percutaneous 4 Percutaneous Endoscopic	Z No Device	Z No Qualifier

Section 0 **Medical and Surgical**
Body System B **Respiratory System**
Operation D **Extraction:** Pulling or stripping out or off all or a portion of a body part by the use of force

Body Part (4th)	Approach (5th)	Device (6th)	Qualifier (7th)
1 Trachea 2 Carina 3 Main Bronchus, Right 4 Upper Lobe Bronchus, Right 5 Middle Lobe Bronchus, Right 6 Lower Lobe Bronchus, Right 7 Main Bronchus, Left 8 Upper Lobe Bronchus, Left 9 Lingula Bronchus B Lower Lobe Bronchus, Left C Upper Lung Lobe, Right D Middle Lung Lobe, Right F Lower Lung Lobe, Right G Upper Lung Lobe, Left H Lung Lingula J Lower Lung Lobe, Left K Lung, Right L Lung, Left M Lung, Bilateral	4 Percutaneous Endoscopic 8 Via Natural or Artificial Opening Endoscopic	Z No Device	X Diagnostic
N Pleura, Right P Pleura, Left	0 Open 3 Percutaneous 4 Percutaneous Endoscopic	Z No Device	X Diagnostic Z No Qualifier

Section 0 **Medical and Surgical**
Body System B **Respiratory System**
Operation F **Fragmentation:** Breaking solid matter in a body part into pieces

Body Part (4th)	Approach (5th)	Device (6th)	Qualifier (7th)
1 Trachea **2** Carina **3** Main Bronchus, Right **4** Upper Lobe Bronchus, Right **5** Middle Lobe Bronchus, Right **6** Lower Lobe Bronchus, Right **7** Main Bronchus, Left **8** Upper Lobe Bronchus, Left **9** Lingula Bronchus **B** Lower Lobe Bronchus, Left	**0** Open **3** Percutaneous **4** Percutaneous Endoscopic **7** Via Natural or Artificial Opening **8** Via Natural or Artificial Opening Endoscopic **X** External	**Z** No Device	**Z** No Qualifier

Section 0 **Medical and Surgical**
Body System B **Respiratory System**
Operation H **Insertion:** Putting in a nonbiological appliance that monitors, assists, performs, or prevents a physiological function but does not physically take the place of a body part

Body Part (4th)	Approach (5th)	Device (6th)	Qualifier (7th)
0 Tracheobronchial Tree	**0** Open **3** Percutaneous **4** Percutaneous Endoscopic **7** Via Natural or Artificial Opening **8** Via Natural or Artificial Opening Endoscopic	**1** Radioactive Element **2** Monitoring Device **3** Infusion Device **D** Intraluminal Device **Y** Other Device	**Z** No Qualifier
1 Trachea	**0** Open	**2** Monitoring Device **D** Intraluminal Device **Y** Other Device	**Z** No Qualifier
1 Trachea	**3** Percutaneous	**D** Intraluminal Device **E** Intraluminal Device, Endotracheal Airway **Y** Other Device	**Z** No Qualifier
1 Trachea	**4** Percutaneous Endoscopic	**D** Intraluminal Device **Y** Other Device	**Z** No Qualifier
1 Trachea	**7** Via Natural or Artificial Opening **8** Via Natural or Artificial Opening Endoscopic	**2** Monitoring Device **D** Intraluminal Device **E** Intraluminal Device, Endotracheal Airway **Y** Other Device	**Z** No Qualifier
3 Main Bronchus, Right **4** Upper Lobe Bronchus, Right **5** Middle Lobe Bronchus, Right **6** Lower Lobe Bronchus, Right **7** Main Bronchus, Left **8** Upper Lobe Bronchus, Left **9** Lingula Bronchus **B** Lower Lobe Bronchus, Left	**0** Open **3** Percutaneous **4** Percutaneous Endoscopic **7** Via Natural or Artificial Opening **8** Via Natural or Artificial Opening Endoscopic	**G** Intraluminal Device, Endobronchial Valve	**Z** No Qualifier
K Lung, Right **L** Lung, Left	**0** Open **3** Percutaneous **4** Percutaneous Endoscopic **7** Via Natural or Artificial Opening **8** Via Natural or Artificial Opening Endoscopic	**1** Radioactive Element **2** Monitoring Device **3** Infusion Device **Y** Other Device	**Z** No Qualifier
Q Pleura	**0** Open **3** Percutaneous **4** Percutaneous Endoscopic **7** Via Natural or Artificial Opening **8** Via Natural or Artificial Opening Endoscopic	**Y** Other Device	**Z** No Qualifier

Continued →

Section 0 **Medical and Surgical**
Body System B **Respiratory System**
Operation H **Insertion:** Putting in a nonbiological appliance that monitors, assists, performs, or prevents a physiological function but does not physically take the place of a body part

Body Part (4th)	Approach (5th)	Device (6th)	Qualifier (7th)
T Diaphragm	**0** Open **3** Percutaneous **4** Percutaneous Endoscopic	**2** Monitoring Device **M** Diaphragmatic Pacemaker Lead **Y** Other Device	**Z** No Qualifier
T Diaphragm	**7** Via Natural or Artificial Opening **8** Via Natural or Artificial Opening Endoscopic	**Y** Other Device	**Z** No Qualifier

Section 0 **Medical and Surgical**
Body System B **Respiratory System**
Operation J **Inspection:** Visually and/or manually exploring a body part

Body Part (4th)	Approach (5th)	Device (6th)	Qualifier (7th)
0 Tracheobronchial Tree **1** Trachea **K** Lung, Right **L** Lung, Left **Q** Pleura **T** Diaphragm	**0** Open **3** Percutaneous **4** Percutaneous Endoscopic **7** Via Natural or Artificial Opening **8** Via Natural or Artificial Opening Endoscopic **X** External	**Z** No Device	**Z** No Qualifier

Section 0 **Medical and Surgical**
Body System B **Respiratory System**
Operation L **Occlusion:** Completely closing an orifice or the lumen of a tubular body part

Body Part (4th)	Approach (5th)	Device (6th)	Qualifier (7th)
1 Trachea **2** Carina **3** Main Bronchus, Right **4** Upper Lobe Bronchus, Right **5** Middle Lobe Bronchus, Right **6** Lower Lobe Bronchus, Right **7** Main Bronchus, Left **8** Upper Lobe Bronchus, Left **9** Lingula Bronchus **B** Lower Lobe Bronchus, Left	**0** Open **3** Percutaneous **4** Percutaneous Endoscopic	**C** Extraluminal Device **D** Intraluminal Device **Z** No Device	**Z** No Qualifier
1 Trachea **2** Carina **3** Main Bronchus, Right **4** Upper Lobe Bronchus, Right **5** Middle Lobe Bronchus, Right **6** Lower Lobe Bronchus, Right **7** Main Bronchus, Left **8** Upper Lobe Bronchus, Left **9** Lingula Bronchus **B** Lower Lobe Bronchus, Left	**7** Via Natural or Artificial Opening **8** Via Natural or Artificial Opening Endoscopic	**D** Intraluminal Device **Z** No Device	**Z** No Qualifier

Section 0 **Medical and Surgical**
Body System B **Respiratory System**
Operation M **Reattachment:** Putting back in or on all or a portion of a separated body part to its normal location or other suitable location

Body Part (4th)	Approach (5th)	Device (6th)	Qualifier (7th)
1 Trachea **2** Carina **3** Main Bronchus, Right **4** Upper Lobe Bronchus, Right **5** Middle Lobe Bronchus, Right **6** Lower Lobe Bronchus, Right **7** Main Bronchus, Left **8** Upper Lobe Bronchus, Left **9** Lingula Bronchus **B** Lower Lobe Bronchus, Left **C** Upper Lung Lobe, Right **D** Middle Lung Lobe, Right **F** Lower Lung Lobe, Right **G** Upper Lung Lobe, Left **H** Lung Lingula **J** Lower Lung Lobe, Left **K** Lung, Right **L** Lung, Left **T** Diaphragm	**0** Open	**Z** No Device	**Z** No Qualifier

Section 0 **Medical and Surgical**
Body System B **Respiratory System**
Operation N **Release:** Freeing a body part from an abnormal physical constraint by cutting or by the use of force

Body Part (4th)	Approach (5th)	Device (6th)	Qualifier (7th)
1 Trachea **2** Carina **3** Main Bronchus, Right **4** Upper Lobe Bronchus, Right **5** Middle Lobe Bronchus, Right **6** Lower Lobe Bronchus, Right **7** Main Bronchus, Left **8** Upper Lobe Bronchus, Left **9** Lingula Bronchus **B** Lower Lobe Bronchus, Left **C** Upper Lung Lobe, Right **D** Middle Lung Lobe, Right **F** Lower Lung Lobe, Right **G** Upper Lung Lobe, Left **H** Lung Lingula **J** Lower Lung Lobe, Left **K** Lung, Right **L** Lung, Left **M** Lungs, Bilateral	**0** Open **3** Percutaneous **4** Percutaneous Endoscopic **7** Via Natural or Artificial Opening **8** Via Natural or Artificial Opening Endoscopic	**Z** No Device	**Z** No Qualifier
N Pleura, Right **P** Pleura, Left **T** Diaphragm	**0** Open **3** Percutaneous **4** Percutaneous Endoscopic	**Z** No Device	**Z** No Qualifier

Section **0** **Medical and Surgical**
Body System **B** **Respiratory System**
Operation **P** **Removal:** Taking out or off a device from a body part

Body Part (4th)	Approach (5th)	Device (6th)	Qualifier (7th)
0 Tracheobronchial Tree	**0** Open **3** Percutaneous **4** Percutaneous Endoscopic **7** Via Natural or Artificial Opening **8** Via Natural or Artificial Opening Endoscopic	**0** Drainage Device **1** Radioactive Element **2** Monitoring Device **3** Infusion Device **7** Autologous Tissue Substitute **C** Extraluminal Device **D** Intraluminal Device **J** Synthetic Substitute **K** Nonautologous Tissue Substitute **Y** Other Device	**Z** No Qualifier
0 Tracheobronchial Tree	**X** External	**0** Drainage Device **1** Radioactive Element **2** Monitoring Device **3** Infusion Device **D** Intraluminal Device	**Z** No Qualifier
1 Trachea	**0** Open **3** Percutaneous **4** Percutaneous Endoscopic **7** Via Natural or Artificial Opening **8** Via Natural or Artificial Opening Endoscopic	**0** Drainage Device **2** Monitoring Device **7** Autologous Tissue Substitute **C** Extraluminal Device **D** Intraluminal Device **F** Tracheostomy Device **J** Synthetic Substitute **K** Nonautologous Tissue Substitute	**Z** No Qualifier
1 Trachea	**X** External	**0** Drainage Device **2** Monitoring Device **D** Intraluminal Device **F** Tracheostomy Device	**Z** No Qualifier
K Lung, Right **L** Lung, Left	**0** Open **3** Percutaneous **4** Percutaneous Endoscopic **7** Via Natural or Artificial Opening **8** Via Natural or Artificial Opening Endoscopic	**0** Drainage Device **1** Radioactive Element **2** Monitoring Device **3** Infusion Device **Y** Other Device	**Z** No Qualifier
K Lung, Right **L** Lung, Left	**X** External	**0** Drainage Device **1** Radioactive Element **2** Monitoring Device **3** Infusion Device	**Z** No Qualifier
Q Pleura	**0** Open **3** Percutaneous **4** Percutaneous Endoscopic **7** Via Natural or Artificial Opening **8** Via Natural or Artificial Opening Endoscopic	**0** Drainage Device **1** Radioactive Element **2** Monitoring Device **Y** Other Device	**Z** No Qualifier
Q Pleura	**X** External	**0** Drainage Device **1** Radioactive Element **2** Monitoring Device	**Z** No Qualifier
T Diaphragm	**0** Open **3** Percutaneous **4** Percutaneous Endoscopic **7** Via Natural or Artificial Opening **8** Via Natural or Artificial Opening Endoscopic	**0** Drainage Device **2** Monitoring Device **7** Autologous Tissue Substitute **J** Synthetic Substitute **K** Nonautologous Tissue Substitute **M** Diaphragmatic Pacemaker Lead **Y** Other Device	**Z** No Qualifier
T Diaphragm	**X** External	**0** Drainage Device **2** Monitoring Device **M** Diaphragmatic Pacemaker Lead	**Z** No Qualifier

Section 0 **Medical and Surgical**
Body System B **Respiratory System**
Operation Q **Repair:** Restoring, to the extent possible, a body part to its normal anatomic structure and function

Body Part (4th)	Approach (5th)	Device (6th)	Qualifier (7th)
1 Trachea **2** Carina **3** Main Bronchus, Right **4** Upper Lobe Bronchus, Right **5** Middle Lobe Bronchus, Right **6** Lower Lobe Bronchus, Right **7** Main Bronchus, Left **8** Upper Lobe Bronchus, Left **9** Lingula Bronchus **B** Lower Lobe Bronchus, Left **C** Upper Lung Lobe, Right **D** Middle Lung Lobe, Right **F** Lower Lung Lobe, Right **G** Upper Lung Lobe, Left **H** Lung Lingula **J** Lower Lung Lobe, Left **K** Lung, Right **L** Lung, Left **M** Lungs, Bilateral	**0** Open **3** Percutaneous **4** Percutaneous Endoscopic **7** Via Natural or Artificial Opening **8** Via Natural or Artificial Opening Endoscopic	**Z** No Device	**Z** No Qualifier
N Pleura, Right **P** Pleura, Left **T** Diaphragm	**0** Open **3** Percutaneous **4** Percutaneous Endoscopic	**Z** No Device	**Z** No Qualifier

Section 0 **Medical and Surgical**
Body System B **Respiratory**
Operation R **Replacement:** Putting in or on biological or synthetic material that physically takes the place and/or function of all or a portion of a body part

Body Part (4th)	Approach (5th)	Device (6th)	Qualifier (7th)
1 Trachea **2** Carina **3** Main Bronchus, Right **4** Upper Lobe Bronchus, Right **5** Middle Lobe Bronchus, Right **6** Lower Lobe Bronchus, Right **7** Main Bronchus, Left **8** Upper Lobe Bronchus, Left **9** Lingula Bronchus **B** Lower Lobe Bronchus, Left **T** Diaphragm	**0** Open **4** Percutaneous Endoscopic	**7** Autologous Tissue Substitute **J** Synthetic Substitute **K** Nonautologous Tissue Substitute	**Z** No Qualifier

Section 0 **Medical and Surgical**
Body System B **Respiratory System**
Operation S **Reposition:** Moving to its normal location, or other suitable location, all or a portion of a body part

Body Part (4th)	Approach (5th)	Device (6th)	Qualifier (7th)
1 Trachea 2 Carina 3 Main Bronchus, Right 4 Upper Lobe Bronchus, Right 5 Middle Lobe Bronchus, Right 6 Lower Lobe Bronchus, Right 7 Main Bronchus, Left 8 Upper Lobe Bronchus, Left 9 Lingula Bronchus B Lower Lobe Bronchus, Left C Upper Lung Lobe, Right D Middle Lung Lobe, Right F Lower Lung Lobe, Right G Upper Lung Lobe, Left H Lung Lingula J Lower Lung Lobe, Left K Lung, Right L Lung, Left T Diaphragm	0 Open	Z No Device	Z No Qualifier

Section 0 **Medical and Surgical**
Body System B **Respiratory System**
Operation T **Resection:** Cutting out or off, without replacement, all of a body part

Body Part (4th)	Approach (5th)	Device (6th)	Qualifier (7th)
1 Trachea 2 Carina 3 Main Bronchus, Right 4 Upper Lobe Bronchus, Right 5 Middle Lobe Bronchus, Right 6 Lower Lobe Bronchus, Right 7 Main Bronchus, Left 8 Upper Lobe Bronchus, Left 9 Lingula Bronchus B Lower Lobe Bronchus, Left C Upper Lung Lobe, Right D Middle Lung Lobe, Right F Lower Lung Lobe, Right G Upper Lung Lobe, Left H Lung Lingula J Lower Lung Lobe, Left K Lung, Right L Lung, Left M Lungs, Bilateral T Diaphragm	0 Open 4 Percutaneous Endoscopic	Z No Device	Z No Qualifier

Section 0 **Medical and Surgical**
Body System B **Respiratory System**
Operation U **Supplement:** Putting in or on biological or synthetic material that physically reinforces and/or augments the function of a portion of a body part

Body Part (4th)	Approach (5th)	Device (6th)	Qualifier (7th)
1 Trachea **2** Carina **3** Main Bronchus, Right **4** Upper Lobe Bronchus, Right **5** Middle Lobe Bronchus, Right **6** Lower Lobe Bronchus, Right **7** Main Bronchus, Left **8** Upper Lobe Bronchus, Left **9** Lingula Bronchus **B** Lower Lobe Bronchus, Left	**0** Open **4** Percutaneous Endoscopic **8** Via Natural or Artificial Opening Endoscopic	**7** Autologous Tissue Substitute **J** Synthetic Substitute **K** Nonautologous Tissue Substitute	**Z** No Qualifier
T Diaphragm	**0** Open **4** Percutaneous Endoscopic	**7** Autologous Tissue Substitute **J** Synthetic Substitute **K** Nonautologous Tissue Substitute	**Z** No Qualifier

Section 0 **Medical and Surgical**
Body System B **Respiratory System**
Operation V **Restriction:** Partially closing an orifice or the lumen of a tubular body part

Body Part (4th)	Approach (5th)	Device (6th)	Qualifier (7th)
1 Trachea **2** Carina **3** Main Bronchus, Right **4** Upper Lobe Bronchus, Right **5** Middle Lobe Bronchus, Right **6** Lower Lobe Bronchus, Right **7** Main Bronchus, Left **8** Upper Lobe Bronchus, Left **9** Lingula Bronchus **B** Lower Lobe Bronchus, Left	**0** Open **3** Percutaneous **4** Percutaneous Endoscopic	**C** Extraluminal Device **D** Intraluminal Device **Z** No Device	**Z** No Qualifier
1 Trachea **2** Carina **3** Main Bronchus, Right **4** Upper Lobe Bronchus, Right **5** Middle Lobe Bronchus, Right **6** Lower Lobe Bronchus, Right **7** Main Bronchus, Left **8** Upper Lobe Bronchus, Left **9** Lingula Bronchus **B** Lower Lobe Bronchus, Left	**7** Via Natural or Artificial Opening **8** Via Natural or Artificial Opening Endoscopic	**D** Intraluminal Device **Z** No Device	**Z** No Qualifier

Section 0 **Medical and Surgical**
Body System B **Respiratory System**
Operation W **Revision:** Correcting, to the extent possible, a portion of a malfunctioning device or the position of a displaced device

Body Part (4th)	Approach (5th)	Device (6th)	Qualifier (7th)
0 Tracheobronchial Tree	**0** Open **3** Percutaneous **4** Percutaneous Endoscopic **7** Via Natural or Artificial Opening **8** Via Natural or Artificial Opening Endoscopic	**0** Drainage Device **2** Monitoring Device **3** Infusion Device **7** Autologous Tissue Substitute **C** Extraluminal Device **D** Intraluminal Device **J** Synthetic Substitute **K** Nonautologous Tissue Substitute **Y** Other Device	**Z** No Qualifier

Continued →

Section 0 Medical and Surgical
Body System B Respiratory System
Operation W **Revision:** Correcting, to the extent possible, a portion of a malfunctioning device or the position of a displaced device

Body Part (4th)	Approach (5th)	Device (6th)	Qualifier (7th)
0 Tracheobronchial Tree	**X** External	**0** Drainage Device **2** Monitoring Device **3** Infusion Device **7** Autologous Tissue Substitute **C** Extraluminal Device **D** Intraluminal Device **J** Synthetic Substitute **K** Nonautologous Tissue Substitute	**Z** No Qualifier
1 Trachea	**0** Open **3** Percutaneous **4** Percutaneous Endoscopic **7** Via Natural or Artificial Opening **8** Via Natural or Artificial Opening Endoscopic **X** External	**0** Drainage Device **2** Monitoring Device **7** Autologous Tissue Substitute **C** Extraluminal Device **D** Intraluminal Device **F** Tracheostomy Device **J** Synthetic Substitute **K** Nonautologous Tissue Substitute	**Z** No Qualifier
K Lung, Right **L** Lung, Left	**0** Open **3** Percutaneous **4** Percutaneous Endoscopic **7** Via Natural or Artificial Opening **8** Via Natural or Artificial Opening Endoscopic	**0** Drainage Device **2** Monitoring Device **3** Infusion Device **Y** Other Device	**Z** No Qualifier
K Lung, Right **L** Lung, Left	**X** External	**0** Drainage Device **2** Monitoring Device **3** Infusion Device	**Z** No Qualifier
Q Pleura	**0** Open **3** Percutaneous **4** Percutaneous Endoscopic **7** Via Natural or Artificial Opening **8** Via Natural or Artificial Opening Endoscopic	**0** Drainage Device **2** Monitoring Device **Y** Other Device	**Z** No Qualifier
Q Pleura	**X** External	**0** Drainage Device **2** Monitoring Device	**Z** No Qualifier
T Diaphragm	**0** Open **3** Percutaneous **4** Percutaneous Endoscopic **7** Via Natural or Artificial Opening **8** Via Natural or Artificial Opening Endoscopic	**0** Drainage Device **2** Monitoring Device **7** Autologous Tissue Substitute **J** Synthetic Substitute **K** Nonautologous Tissue Substitute **M** Diaphragmatic Pacemaker Lead **Y** Other Device	**Z** No Qualifier
T Diaphragm	**X** External	**0** Drainage Device **2** Monitoring Device **7** Autologous Tissue Substitute **J** Synthetic Substitute **K** Nonautologous Tissue Substitute **M** Diaphragmatic Pacemaker Lead	**Z** No Qualifier

Section **0** **Medical and Surgical**
Body System **B** **Respiratory System**
Operation **Y** **Transplantation:** Putting in or on all or a portion of a living body part taken from another individual or animal to physically take the place and/or function of all or a portion of a similar body part

Body Part (4th)	Approach (5th)	Device (6th)	Qualifier (7th)
C Upper Lung Lobe, Right **D** Middle Lung Lobe, Right **F** Lower Lung Lobe, Right **G** Upper Lung Lobe, Left **H** Lung Lingula **J** Lower Lung Lobe, Left **K** Lung, Right **L** Lung, Left **M** Lungs, Bilateral	**0** Open	**Z** No Device	**0** Allogeneic **1** Syngeneic **2** Zooplastic

AHA Coding Clinic

0B5P0ZZ Destruction of Left Pleura, Open Approach—AHA CC: 2Q, 2016, 17-18

0B948ZX Drainage of Right Upper Lobe Bronchus, Via Natural or Artificial Opening Endoscopic, Diagnostic—AHA CC: 1Q, 2016, 26-27

0B988ZX Drainage of Left Upper Lobe Bronchus, Via Natural or Artificial Opening Endoscopic, Diagnostic—AHA CC: 1Q, 2016, 27

0B9J8ZX Drainage of Left Lower Lung Lobe, Via Natural or Artificial Opening Endoscopic, Diagnostic—AHA CC: 1Q, 2016, 26-27; 1Q, 2017, 51

0B9M8ZZ Drainage of Bilateral Lungs, Via Natural or Artificial Opening Endoscopic—AHA CC: 3Q, 2017, 15

0BB10ZZ Excision of Trachea, Open Approach—AHA CC: 1Q, 2015, 15-16

0BB48ZX Excision of Right Upper Lobe Bronchus, Via Natural or Artificial Opening Endoscopic, Diagnostic—AHA CC: 1Q, 2016, 26-27

0BB88ZX Excision of Left Upper Lobe Bronchus, Via Natural or Artificial Opening Endoscopic, Diagnostic—AHA CC: 1Q, 2016, 27

0BBC8ZX Excision of Right Upper Lung Lobe, Via Natural or Artificial Opening Endoscopic, Diagnostic—AHA CC: 1Q, 2016, 26-27

0BBK8ZX Excision of Right Lung, Via Natural or Artificial Opening Endoscopic, Diagnostic—AHA CC: 1Q, 2014, 20-21

0BC58ZZ Extirpation of Matter from Right Middle Lobe Bronchus, Via Natural or Artificial Opening Endoscopic—AHA CC: 3Q, 2017, 14-15

0BDC8ZX Extraction of Right Upper Lung Lobe, Via Natural or Artificial Opening Endoscopic, Diagnostic—AHA CC: 3Q, 2020, 40-41

0BDD8ZX Extraction of Right Middle Lung Lobe, Via Natural or Artificial Opening Endoscopic, Diagnostic—AHA CC: 3Q, 2020, 40-41

0BDF8ZX Extraction of Right Lower Lung Lobe, Via Natural or Artificial Opening Endoscopic, Diagnostic—AHA CC: 3Q, 2020, 40-41

0BH17EZ Insertion of Endotracheal Airway into Trachea, Via Natural or Artificial Opening—AHA CC: 4Q, 2014, 3-15

0BH18EZ Insertion of Endotracheal Airway into Trachea, Via Natural or Artificial Opening Endoscopic—AHA CC: 4Q, 2014, 3-15

0BHB8GZ Insertion of Endobronchial Valve into Left Lower Lobe Bronchus, Via Natural or Artificial Opening Endoscopic—AHA CC: 3Q, 2019, 33-34

0BJL8ZZ Inspection of Left Lung, Via Natural or Artificial Opening Endoscopic—AHA CC: 1Q, 2014, 20

0BJQ4ZZ Inspection of Pleura, Percutaneous Endoscopic Approach—AHA CC: 2Q, 2015, 31

0BN10ZZ Release Trachea, Open Approach—AHA CC: 3Q, 2015, 15-16

0BNL0ZZ Release Left Lung, Open Approach—AHA CC: 3Q, 2018, 28

0BNN0ZZ Release Right Pleura, Open Approach—AHA CC: 2Q, 2019, 20-21

0BQT4ZZ Repair Diaphragm, Percutaneous Endoscopic Approach—AHA CC: 3Q, 2020, 41-42

0BU18JZ Supplement Trachea with Synthetic Substitute, Via Natural or Artificial Opening Endoscopic—AHA CC: 3Q, 2020, 43-44

0BU307Z Supplement Right Main Bronchus with Autologous Tissue Substitute, Open Approach—AHA CC: 1Q, 2015, 28-29

Oral Cavity

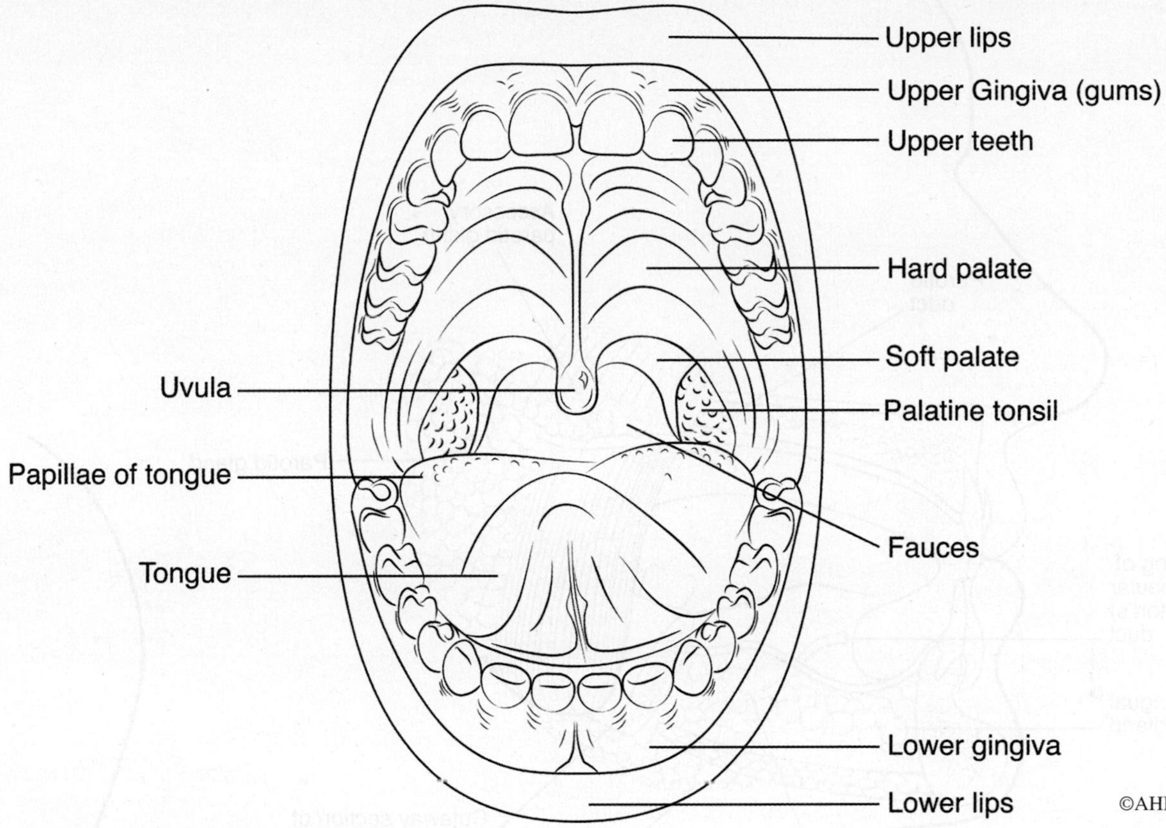
Upper lips
Upper Gingiva (gums)
Upper teeth
Hard palate
Soft palate
Uvula
Palatine tonsil
Papillae of tongue
Fauces
Tongue
Lower gingiva
Lower lips

Glands of the Oral Cavity

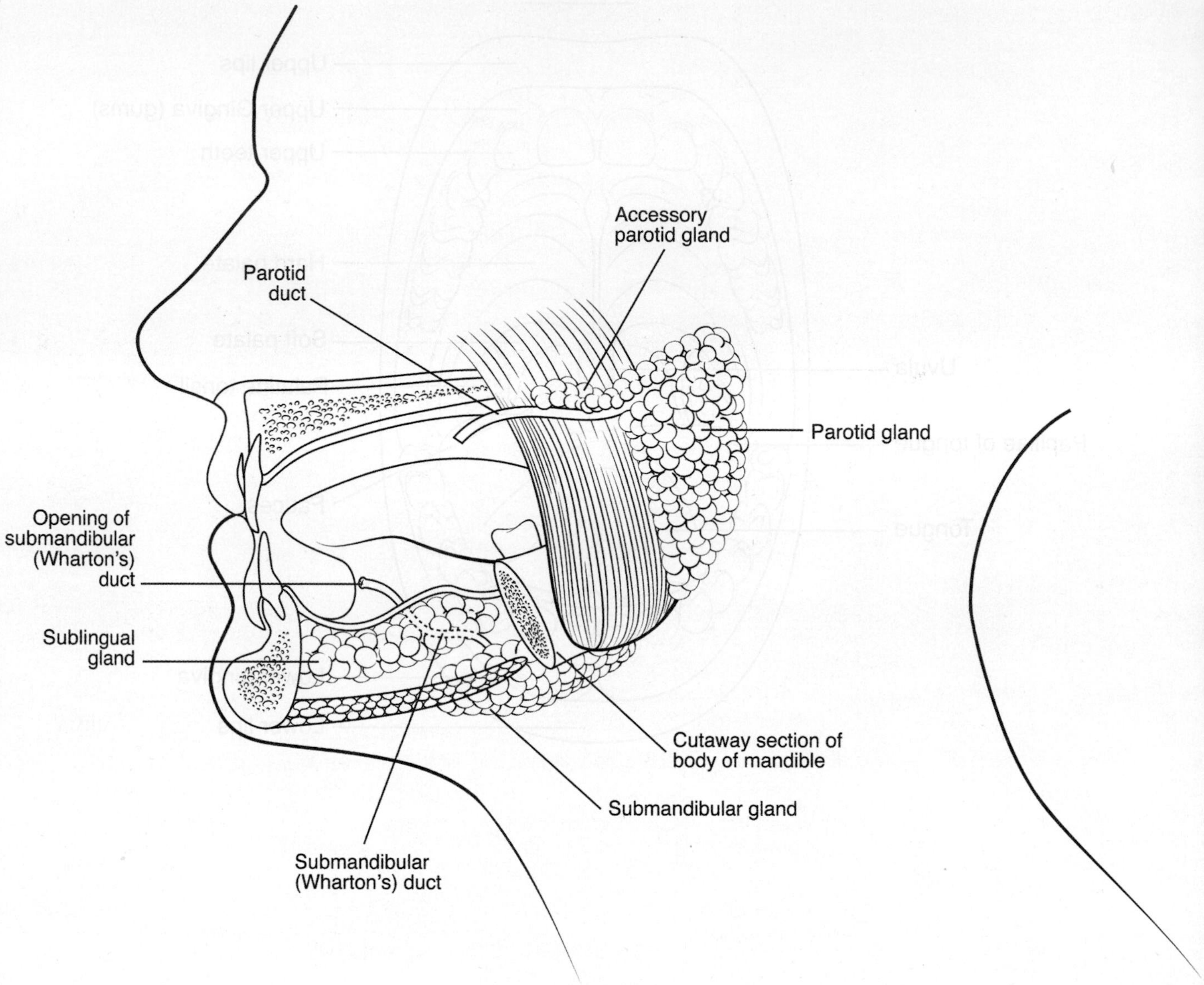

Accessory parotid gland
Parotid duct
Parotid gland
Opening of submandibular (Wharton's) duct
Sublingual gland
Cutaway section of body of mandible
Submandibular gland
Submandibular (Wharton's) duct

Throat

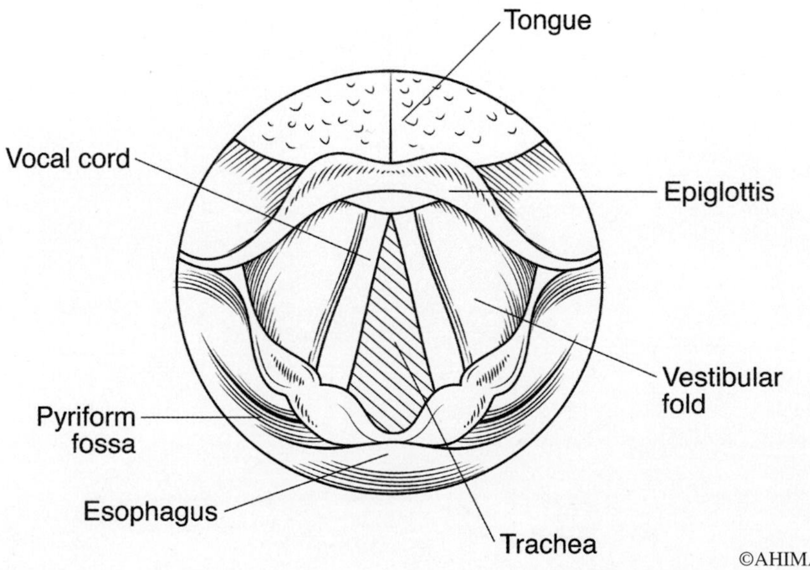

Tongue
Vocal cord
Epiglottis
Vestibular fold
Pyriform fossa
Esophagus
Trachea

Section 0 **Medical and Surgical**
Body System C **Mouth and Throat**
Operation 0 **Alteration:** Modifying the anatomic structure of a body part without affecting the function of the body part

Body Part (4th)	Approach (5th)	Device (6th)	Qualifier (7th)
0 Upper Lip **1** Lower Lip	**X** External	**7** Autologous Tissue Substitute **J** Synthetic Substitute **K** Nonautologous Tissue Substitute **Z** No Device	**Z** No Qualifier

Section 0 **Medical and Surgical**
Body System C **Mouth and Throat**
Operation 2 **Change:** Taking out or off a device from a body part and putting back an identical or similar device in or on the same body part without cutting or puncturing the skin or a mucous membrane

Body Part (4th)	Approach (5th)	Device (6th)	Qualifier (7th)
A Salivary Gland **S** Larynx **Y** Mouth and Throat	**X** External	**0** Drainage Device **Y** Other Device	**Z** No Qualifier

Section 0 **Medical and Surgical**
Body System C **Mouth and Throat**
Operation 5 **Destruction:** Physical eradication of all or a portion of a body part by the direct use of energy, force, or a destructive agent

Body Part (4th)	Approach (5th)	Device (6th)	Qualifier (7th)
0 Upper Lip **1** Lower Lip **2** Hard Palate **3** Soft Palate **4** Buccal Mucosa **5** Upper Gingiva **6** Lower Gingiva **7** Tongue **N** Uvula **P** Tonsils **Q** Adenoids	**0** Open **3** Percutaneous **X** External	**Z** No Device	**Z** No Qualifier
8 Parotid Gland, Right **9** Parotid Gland, Left **B** Parotid Duct, Right **C** Parotid Duct, Left **D** Sublingual Gland, Right **F** Sublingual Gland, Left **G** Submaxillary Gland, Right **H** Submaxillary Gland, Left **J** Minor Salivary Gland	**0** Open **3** Percutaneous	**Z** No Device	**Z** No Qualifier
M Pharynx **R** Epiglottis **S** Larynx **T** Vocal Cord, Right **V** Vocal Cord, Left	**0** Open **3** Percutaneous **4** Percutaneous Endoscopic **7** Via Natural or Artificial Opening **8** Via Natural or Artificial Opening Endoscopic	**Z** No Device	**Z** No Qualifier
W Upper Tooth **X** Lower Tooth	**0** Open **X** External	**Z** No Device	**0** Single **1** Multiple **2** All

Section 0 **Medical and Surgical**
Body System C **Mouth and Throat**
Operation 7 **Dilation:** Expanding an orifice or the lumen of a tubular body part

Body Part (4th)	Approach (5th)	Device (6th)	Qualifier (7th)
B Parotid Duct, Right **C** Parotid Duct, Left	**0** Open **3** Percutaneous **7** Via Natural or Artificial Opening	**D** Intraluminal Device **Z** No Device	**Z** No Qualifier
M Pharynx	**7** Via Natural or Artificial Opening **8** Via Natural or Artificial Opening Endoscopic	**D** Intraluminal Device **Z** No Device	**Z** No Qualifier
S Larynx	**0** Open **3** Percutaneous **4** Percutaneous Endoscopic **7** Via Natural or Artificial Opening **8** Via Natural or Artificial Opening Endoscopic	**D** Intraluminal Device **Z** No Device	**Z** No Qualifier

Section 0 **Medical and Surgical**
Body System C **Mouth and Throat**
Operation 9 **Drainage:** Taking or letting out fluids and/or gases from a body part

Body Part (4th)	Approach (5th)	Device (6th)	Qualifier (7th)
0 Upper Lip **1** Lower Lip **2** Hard Palate **3** Soft Palate **4** Buccal Mucosa **5** Upper Gingiva **6** Lower Gingiva **7** Tongue **N** Uvula **P** Tonsils **Q** Adenoids	**0** Open **3** Percutaneous **X** External	**0** Drainage Device	**Z** No Qualifier
0 Upper Lip **1** Lower Lip **2** Hard Palate **3** Soft Palate **4** Buccal Mucosa **5** Upper Gingiva **6** Lower Gingiva **7** Tongue **N** Uvula **P** Tonsils **Q** Adenoids	**0** Open **3** Percutaneous **X** External	**Z** No Device	**X** Diagnostic **Z** No Qualifier
8 Parotid Gland, Right **9** Parotid Gland, Left **B** Parotid Duct, Right **C** Parotid Duct, Left **D** Sublingual Gland, Right **F** Sublingual Gland, Left **G** Submaxillary Gland, Right **H** Submaxillary Gland, Left **J** Minor Salivary Gland	**0** Open **3** Percutaneous	**0** Drainage Device	**Z** No Qualifier
8 Parotid Gland, Right **9** Parotid Gland, Left **B** Parotid Duct, Right **C** Parotid Duct, Left **D** Sublingual Gland, Right **F** Sublingual Gland, Left **G** Submaxillary Gland, Right **H** Submaxillary Gland, Left **J** Minor Salivary Gland	**0** Open **3** Percutaneous	**Z** No Device	**X** Diagnostic **Z** No Qualifier

Continued →

Section 0 **Medical and Surgical**
Body System C **Mouth and Throat**
Operation 9 **Drainage:** Taking or letting out fluids and/or gases from a body part

Body Part (4th)	Approach (5th)	Device (6th)	Qualifier (7th)
M Pharynx **R** Epiglottis **S** Larynx **T** Vocal Cord, Right **V** Vocal Cord, Left	**0** Open **3** Percutaneous **4** Percutaneous Endoscopic **7** Via Natural or Artificial Opening **8** Via Natural or Artificial Opening Endoscopic	**0** Drainage Device	**Z** No Qualifier
M Pharynx **R** Epiglottis **S** Larynx **T** Vocal Cord, Right **V** Vocal Cord, Left	**0** Open **3** Percutaneous **4** Percutaneous Endoscopic **7** Via Natural or Artificial Opening **8** Via Natural or Artificial Opening Endoscopic	**Z** No Device	**X** Diagnostic **Z** No Qualifier
W Upper Tooth **X** Lower Tooth	**0** Open **X** External	**0** Drainage Device **Z** No Device	**0** Single **1** Multiple **2** All

Section 0 **Medical and Surgical**
Body System C **Mouth and Throat**
Operation B **Excision:** Cutting out or off, without replacement, a portion of a body part

Body Part (4th)	Approach (5th)	Device (6th)	Qualifier (7th)
0 Upper Lip **1** Lower Lip **2** Hard Palate **3** Soft Palate **4** Buccal Mucosa **5** Upper Gingiva **6** Lower Gingiva **7** Tongue **N** Uvula **P** Tonsils **Q** Adenoids	**0** Open **3** Percutaneous **X** External	**Z** No Device	**X** Diagnostic **Z** No Qualifier
8 Parotid Gland, Right **9** Parotid Gland, Left **B** Parotid Duct, Right **C** Parotid Duct, Left **D** Sublingual Gland, Right **F** Sublingual Gland, Left **G** Submaxillary Gland, Right **H** Submaxillary Gland, Left **J** Minor Salivary Gland	**0** Open **3** Percutaneous	**Z** No Device	**X** Diagnostic **Z** No Qualifier
M Pharynx **R** Epiglottis **S** Larynx **T** Vocal Cord, Right **V** Vocal Cord, Left	**0** Open **3** Percutaneous **4** Percutaneous Endoscopic **7** Via Natural or Artificial Opening **8** Via Natural or Artificial Opening Endoscopic	**Z** No Device	**X** Diagnostic **Z** No Qualifier
W Upper Tooth **X** Lower Tooth	**0** Open **X** External	**Z** No Device	**0** Single **1** Multiple **2** All

Section 0 **Medical and Surgical**
Body System C **Mouth and Throat**
Operation C **Extirpation:** Taking or cutting out solid matter from a body part

Body Part (4th)	Approach (5th)	Device (6th)	Qualifier (7th)
0 Upper Lip **1** Lower Lip **2** Hard Palate **3** Soft Palate **4** Buccal Mucosa **5** Upper Gingiva **6** Lower Gingiva **7** Tongue **N** Uvula **P** Tonsils **Q** Adenoids	**0** Open **3** Percutaneous **X** External	**Z** No Device	**Z** No Qualifier
8 Parotid Gland, Right **9** Parotid Gland, Left **B** Parotid Duct, Right **C** Parotid Duct, Left **D** Sublingual Gland, Right **F** Sublingual Gland, Left **G** Submaxillary Gland, Right **H** Submaxillary Gland, Left **J** Minor Salivary Gland	**0** Open **3** Percutaneous	**Z** No Device	**Z** No Qualifier
M Pharynx **R** Epiglottis **S** Larynx **T** Vocal Cord, Right **V** Vocal Cord, Left	**0** Open **3** Percutaneous **4** Percutaneous Endoscopic **7** Via Natural or Artificial Opening **8** Via Natural or Artificial Opening Endoscopic	**Z** No Device	**Z** No Qualifier
W Upper Tooth **X** Lower Tooth	**0** Open **X** External	**Z** No Device	**0** Single **1** Multiple **2** All

Section 0 **Medical and Surgical**
Body System C **Mouth and Throat**
Operation D **Extraction:** Pulling or stripping out or off all or a portion of a body part by the use of force

Body Part (4th)	Approach (5th)	Device (6th)	Qualifier (7th)
T Vocal Cord, Right **V** Vocal Cord, Left	**0** Open **3** Percutaneous **4** Percutaneous Endoscopic **7** Via Natural or Artificial Opening **8** Via Natural or Artificial Opening Endoscopic	**Z** No Device	**Z** No Qualifier
W Upper Tooth **X** Lower Tooth	**X** External	**Z** No Device	**0** Single **1** Multiple **2** All

Section 0 **Medical and Surgical**
Body System C **Mouth and Throat**
Operation F **Fragmentation:** Breaking solid matter in a body part into pieces

Body Part (4th)	Approach (5th)	Device (6th)	Qualifier (7th)
B Parotid Duct, Right **C** Parotid Duct, Left	**0** Open **3** Percutaneous **7** Via Natural or Artificial Opening **X** External	**Z** No Device	**Z** No Qualifier

Section	**0**	**Medical and Surgical**
Body System	**C**	**Mouth and Throat**
Operation	**H**	**Insertion:** Putting in a nonbiological appliance that monitors, assists, performs, or prevents a physiological function but does not physically take the place of a body part

Body Part (4th)	Approach (5th)	Device (6th)	Qualifier (7th)
7 Tongue	**0** Open **3** Percutaneous **X** External	**1** Radioactive Element	**Z** No Qualifier
A Salivary Gland **S** Larynx	**0** Open **3** Percutaneous **7** Via Natural or Artificial Opening **8** Via Natural or Artificial Opening Endoscopic	**1** Radioactive Element **Y** Other Device	**Z** No Qualifier
Y Mouth and Throat	**0** Open **3** Percutaneous	**1** Radioactive Element **Y** Other Device	**Z** No Qualifier
Y Mouth and Throat	**7** Via Natural or Artificial Opening **8** Via Natural or Artificial Opening Endoscopic	**1** Radioactive Element **B** Intraluminal Device, Airway **Y** Other Device	**Z** No Qualifier

Section	**0**	**Medical and Surgical**
Body System	**C**	**Mouth and Throat**
Operation	**J**	**Inspection:** Visually and/or manually exploring a body part

Body Part (4th)	Approach (5th)	Device (6th)	Qualifier (7th)
A SalivaryGland	**0** Open **3** Percutaneous **X** External	**Z** No Device	**Z** No Qualifier
S Larynx **Y** Mouth and Throat	**0** Open **3** Percutaneous **4** Percutaneous Endoscopic **7** Via Natural or Artificial Opening **8** Via Natural or Artificial Opening Endoscopic **X** External	**Z** No Device	**Z** No Qualifier

Section	**0**	**Medical and Surgical**
Body System	**C**	**Mouth and Throat**
Operation	**L**	**Occlusion:** Completely closing an orifice or the lumen of a tubular body part

Body Part (4th)	Approach (5th)	Device (6th)	Qualifier (7th)
B Parotid Duct, Right **C** Parotid Duct, Left	**0** Open **3** Percutaneous **4** Percutaneous Endoscopic	**C** Extraluminal Device **D** Intraluminal Device **Z** No Device	**Z** No Qualifier
B Parotid Duct, Right **C** Parotid Duct, Left	**7** Via Natural or Artificial Opening **8** Via Natural or Artificial Opening Endoscopic	**D** Intraluminal Device **Z** No Device	**Z** No Qualifier

Section	**0**	**Medical and Surgical**
Body System	**C**	**Mouth and Throat**
Operation	**M**	**Reattachment:** Putting back in or on all or a portion of a separated body part to its normal location or other suitable location

Body Part (4th)	Approach (5th)	Device (6th)	Qualifier (7th)
0 Upper Lip **1** Lower Lip **3** Soft Palate **7** Tongue **N** Uvula	**0** Open	**Z** No Device	**Z** No Qualifier
W Upper Tooth **X** Lower Tooth	**0** Open **X** External	**Z** No Device	**0** Single **1** Multiple **2** All

Section 0 **Medical and Surgical**
Body System C **Mouth and Throat**
Operation N **Release:** Freeing a body part from an abnormal physical constraint by cutting or by the use of force

Body Part (4th)	Approach (5th)	Device (6th)	Qualifier (7th)
0 Upper Lip **1** Lower Lip **2** Hard Palate **3** Soft Palate **4** Buccal Mucosa **5** Upper Gingiva **6** Lower Gingiva **7** Tongue **N** Uvula **P** Tonsils **Q** Adenoids	**0** Open **3** Percutaneous **X** External	**Z** No Device	**Z** No Qualifier
8 Parotid Gland, Right **9** Parotid Gland, Left **B** Parotid Duct, Right **C** Parotid Duct, Left **D** Sublingual Gland, Right **F** Sublingual Gland, Left **G** Submaxillary Gland, Right **H** Submaxillary Gland, Left **J** Minor Salivary Gland	**0** Open **3** Percutaneous	**Z** No Device	**Z** No Qualifier
M Pharynx **R** Epiglottis **S** Larynx **T** Vocal Cord, Right **V** Vocal Cord, Left	**0** Open **3** Percutaneous **4** Percutaneous Endoscopic **7** Via Natural or Artificial Opening **8** Via Natural or Artificial Opening Endoscopic	**Z** No Device	**Z** No Qualifier
W Upper Tooth **X** Lower Tooth	**0** Open **X** External	**Z** No Device	**0** Single **1** Multiple **2** All

Section 0 **Medical and Surgical**
Body System C **Mouth and Throat**
Operation P **Removal:** Taking out or off a device from a body part

Body Part (4th)	Approach (5th)	Device (6th)	Qualifier (7th)
A Salivary Gland	**0** Open **3** Percutaneous	**0** Drainage Device **C** Extraluminal Device **Y** Other Device	**Z** No Qualifier
A Salivary Gland	**7** Via Natural or Artificial Opening **8** Via Natural or Artificial Opening Endoscopic	**Y** Other Device	**Z** No Qualifier
S Larynx	**0** Open **3** Percutaneous **7** Via Natural or Artificial Opening **8** Via Natural or Artificial Opening Endoscopic	**0** Drainage Device **7** Autologous Tissue Substitute **D** Intraluminal Device **J** Synthetic Substitute **K** Nonautologous Tissue Substitute **Y** Other Device	**Z** No Qualifier
S Larynx	**X** External	**0** Drainage Device **7** Autologous Tissue Substitute **D** Intraluminal Device **J** Synthetic Substitute **K** Nonautologous Tissue Substitute	**Z** No Qualifier

Continued →

Section 0 **Medical and Surgical**
Body System C **Mouth and Throat**
Operation P **Removal:** Taking out or off a device from a body part

Body Part (4th)	Approach (5th)	Device (6th)	Qualifier (7th)
Y Mouth and Throat	**0** Open **3** Percutaneous **7** Via Natural or Artificial Opening **8** Via Natural or Artificial Opening Endoscopic	**0** Drainage Device **1** Radioactive Element **7** Autologous Tissue Substitute **D** Intraluminal Device **J** Synthetic Substitute **K** Nonautologous Tissue Substitute **Y** Other Device	**Z** No Qualifier
Y Mouth and Throat	**X** External	**0** Drainage Device **1** Radioactive Element **7** Autologous Tissue Substitute **D** Intraluminal Device **J** Synthetic Substitute **K** Nonautologous Tissue Substitute	**Z** No Qualifier

Section 0 **Medical and Surgical**
Body System C **Mouth and Throat**
Operation Q **Repair:** Restoring, to the extent possible, a body part to its normal anatomic structure and function

Body Part (4th)	Approach (5th)	Device (6th)	Qualifier (7th)
0 Upper Lip **1** Lower Lip **2** Hard Palate **3** Soft Palate **4** Buccal Mucosa **5** Upper Gingiva **6** Lower Gingiva **7** Tongue **N** Uvula **P** Tonsils **Q** Adenoids	**0** Open **3** Percutaneous **X** External	**Z** No Device	**Z** No Qualifier
8 Parotid Gland, Right **9** Parotid Gland, Left **B** Parotid Duct, Right **C** Parotid Duct, Left **D** Sublingual Gland, Right **F** Sublingual Gland, Left **G** Submaxillary Gland, Right **H** Submaxillary Gland, Left **J** Minor Salivary Gland	**0** Open **3** Percutaneous	**Z** No Device	**Z** No Qualifier
M Pharynx **R** Epiglottis **S** Larynx **T** Vocal Cord, Right **V** Vocal Cord, Left	**0** Open **3** Percutaneous **4** Percutaneous Endoscopic **7** Via Natural or Artificial Opening **8** Via Natural or Artificial Opening Endoscopic	**Z** No Device	**Z** No Qualifier
W Upper Tooth **X** Lower Tooth	**0** Open **X** External	**Z** No Device	**0** Single **1** Multiple **2** All

Section 0 **Medical and Surgical**
Body System C **Mouth and Throat**
Operation R **Replacement:** Putting in or on biological or synthetic material that physically takes the place and/or function of all or a portion of a body part

Body Part (4th)	Approach (5th)	Device (6th)	Qualifier (7th)
0 Upper Lip **1** Lower Lip **2** Hard Palate **3** Soft Palate **4** Buccal Mucosa **5** Upper Gingiva **6** Lower Gingiva **7** Tongue **N** Uvula	**0** Open **3** Percutaneous **X** External	**7** Autologous Tissue Substitute **J** Synthetic Substitute **K** Nonautologous Tissue Substitute	**Z** No Qualifier
B Parotid Duct, Right **C** Parotid Duct, Left	**0** Open **3** Percutaneous	**7** Autologous Tissue Substitute **J** Synthetic Substitute **K** Nonautologous Tissue Substitute	**Z** No Qualifier
M Pharynx **R** Epiglottis **S** Larynx **T** Vocal Cord, Right **V** Vocal Cord, Left	**0** Open **7** Via Natural or Artificial Opening **8** Via Natural or Artificial Opening Endoscopic	**7** Autologous Tissue Substitute **J** Synthetic Substitute **K** Nonautologous Tissue Substitute	**Z** No Qualifier
W Upper Tooth **X** Lower Tooth	**0** Open **X** External	**7** Autologous Tissue Substitute **J** Synthetic Substitute **K** Nonautologous Tissue Substitute	**0** Single **1** Multiple **2** All

Section 0 **Medical and Surgical**
Body System C **Mouth and Throat**
Operation S **Reposition:** Moving to its normal location, or other suitable location, all or a portion of a body part

Body Part (4th)	Approach (5th)	Device (6th)	Qualifier (7th)
0 Upper Lip **1** Lower Lip **2** Hard Palate **3** Soft Palate **7** Tongue **N** Uvula	**0** Open **X** External	**Z** No Device	**Z** No Qualifier
B Parotid Duct, Right **C** Parotid Duct, Left	**0** Open **3** Percutaneous	**Z** No Device	**Z** No Qualifier
R Epiglottis **T** Vocal Cord, Right **V** Vocal Cord, Left	**0** Open **7** Via Natural or Artificial Opening **8** Via Natural or Artificial Opening Endoscopic	**Z** No Device	**Z** No Qualifier
W Upper Tooth **X** Lower Tooth	**0** Open **X** External	**5** External Fixation Device **Z** No Device	**0** Single **1** Multiple **2** All

Section 0 **Medical and Surgical**
Body System C **Mouth and Throat**
Operation T **Resection:** Cutting out or off, without replacement, all of a body part

Body Part (4th)	Approach (5th)	Device (6th)	Qualifier (7th)
0 Upper Lip **1** Lower Lip **2** Hard Palate **3** Soft Palate **7** Tongue **N** Uvula **P** Tonsils **Q** Adenoids	**0** Open **X** External	**Z** No Device	**Z** No Qualifier
8 Parotid Gland, Right **9** Parotid Gland, Left **B** Parotid Duct, Right **C** Parotid Duct, Left **D** Sublingual Gland, Right **F** Sublingual Gland, Left **G** Submaxillary Gland, Right **H** Submaxillary Gland, Left **J** Minor Salivary Gland	**0** Open	**Z** No Device	**Z** No Qualifier
M Pharynx **R** Epiglottis **S** Larynx **T** Vocal Cord, Right **V** Vocal Cord, Left	**0** Open **4** Percutaneous Endoscopic **7** Via Natural or Artificial Opening **8** Via Natural or Artificial Opening Endoscopic	**Z** No Device	**Z** No Qualifier
W Upper Tooth **X** Lower Tooth	**0** Open	**Z** No Device	**0** Single **1** Multiple **2** All

Section 0 **Medical and Surgical**
Body System C **Mouth and Throat**
Operation U **Supplement:** Putting in or on biological or synthetic material that physically reinforces and/or augments the function of a portion of a body part

Body Part (4th)	Approach (5th)	Device (6th)	Qualifier (7th)
0 Upper Lip **1** Lower Lip **2** Hard Palate **3** Soft Palate **4** Buccal Mucosa **5** Upper Gingiva **6** Lower Gingiva **7** Tongue **N** Uvula	**0** Open **3** Percutaneous **X** External	**7** Autologous Tissue Substitute **J** Synthetic Substitute **K** Nonautologous Tissue Substitute	**Z** No Qualifier
M Pharynx **R** Epiglottis **S** Larynx **T** Vocal Cord, Right **V** Vocal Cord, Left	**0** Open **7** Via Natural or Artificial Opening **8** Via Natural or Artificial Opening Endoscopic	**7** Autologous Tissue Substitute **J** Synthetic Substitute **K** Nonautologous Tissue Substitute	**Z** No Qualifier

Section 0 **Medical and Surgical**
Body System C **Mouth and Throat**
Operation V **Restriction:** Partially closing an orifice or the lumen of a tubular body part

Body Part (4th)	Approach (5th)	Device (6th)	Qualifier (7th)
B Parotid Duct, Right **C** Parotid Duct, Left	**0** Open **3** Percutaneous	**C** Extraluminal Device **D** Intraluminal Device **Z** No Device	**Z** No Qualifier
B Parotid Duct, Right **C** Parotid Duct, Left	**7** Via Natural or Artificial Opening **8** Via Natural or Artificial Opening Endoscopic	**D** Intraluminal Device **Z** No Device	**Z** No Qualifier

Section 0 **Medical and Surgical**
Body System C **Mouth and Throat**
Operation W **Revision:** Correcting, to the extent possible, a portion of a malfunctioning device or the position of a displaced device

Body Part (4th)	Approach (5th)	Device (6th)	Qualifier (7th)
A Salivary Gland	**0** Open **3** Percutaneous	**0** Drainage Device **C** Extraluminal Device **Y** Other Device	**Z** No Qualifier
A Salivary Gland	**7** Via Natural or Artificial Opening **8** Via Natural or Artificial Opening Endoscopic	**Y** Other Device	**Z** No Qualifier
A Salivary Gland	**X** External	**0** Drainage Device **C** Extraluminal Device	**Z** No Qualifier
S Larynx	**0** Open **3** Percutaneous **7** Via Natural or Artificial Opening **8** Via Natural or Artificial Opening Endoscopic	**0** Drainage Device **7** Autologous Tissue Substitute **D** Intraluminal Device **J** Synthetic Substitute **K** Nonautologous Tissue Substitute **Y** Other Device	**Z** No Qualifier
S Larynx	**X** External	**0** Drainage Device **7** Autologous Tissue Substitute **D** Intraluminal Device **J** Synthetic Substitute **K** Nonautologous Tissue Substitute	**Z** No Qualifier
Y Mouth and Throat	**0** Open **3** Percutaneous **7** Via Natural or Artificial Opening **8** Via Natural or Artificial Opening Endoscopic	**0** Drainage Device **1** Radioactive Element **7** Autologous Tissue Substitute **D** Intraluminal Device **J** Synthetic Substitute **K** Nonautologous Tissue Substitute **Y** Other Device	**Z** No Qualifier
Y Mouth and Throat	**X** External	**0** Drainage Device **1** Radioactive Element **7** Autologous Tissue Substitute **D** Intraluminal Device **J** Synthetic Substitute **K** Nonautologous Tissue Substitute	**Z** No Qualifier

Section 0 **Medical and Surgical**
Body System C **Mouth and Throat**
Operation X **Transfer:** Moving, without taking out, all or a portion of a body part to another location to take over the function of all or a portion of a body part

Body Part (4th)	Approach (5th)	Device (6th)	Qualifier (7th)
0 Upper Lip **1** Lower Lip **3** Soft Palate **4** Buccal Mucosa **5** Upper Gingiva **6** Lower Gingiva **7** Tongue	**0** Open **X** External	**Z** No Device	**Z** No Qualifier

AHA Coding Clinic

0CB80ZZ Excision of Right Parotid Gland, Open Approach—AHA CC: 3Q, 2014, 21-22
0CBM8ZX Excision of Pharynx, Via Natural or Artificial Opening Endoscopic, Diagnostic—AHA CC: 2Q, 2016, 20
0CBM8ZZ Excision of Pharynx, Via Natural or Artificial Opening Endoscopic—AHA CC: 3Q, 2016, 28-29
0CCH3ZZ Extirpation of Matter from Left Submaxillary Gland, Percutaneous Approach—AHA CC: 2Q, 2016, 20
0CQ50ZZ Repair Upper Gingiva, Open Approach—AHA CC: 1Q, 2017, 20-21
0CR3XJZ Replacement of Soft Palate with Synthetic Substitute, External Approach—AHA CC: 3Q, 2014, 25
0CR4XKZ Replacement of Buccal Mucosa with Nonautologous Tissue Substitute, External Approach—AHA CC: 2Q, 2014, 5-6
0CSR8ZZ Reposition Epiglottis, Via Natural or Artificial Opening Endoscopic—AHA CC: 3Q, 2016, 28-29
0CT90ZZ Resection of Left Parotid Gland, Open Approach—AHA CC: 2Q, 2016, 12-14
0CTW0Z1 Resection of Upper Tooth, Multiple, Open Approach—AHA CC: 3Q, 2014, 23-24
0CTX0Z1 Resection of Lower Tooth, Multiple, Open Approach—AHA CC: 3Q, 2014, 23-24

Gastrointestinal System: Organization

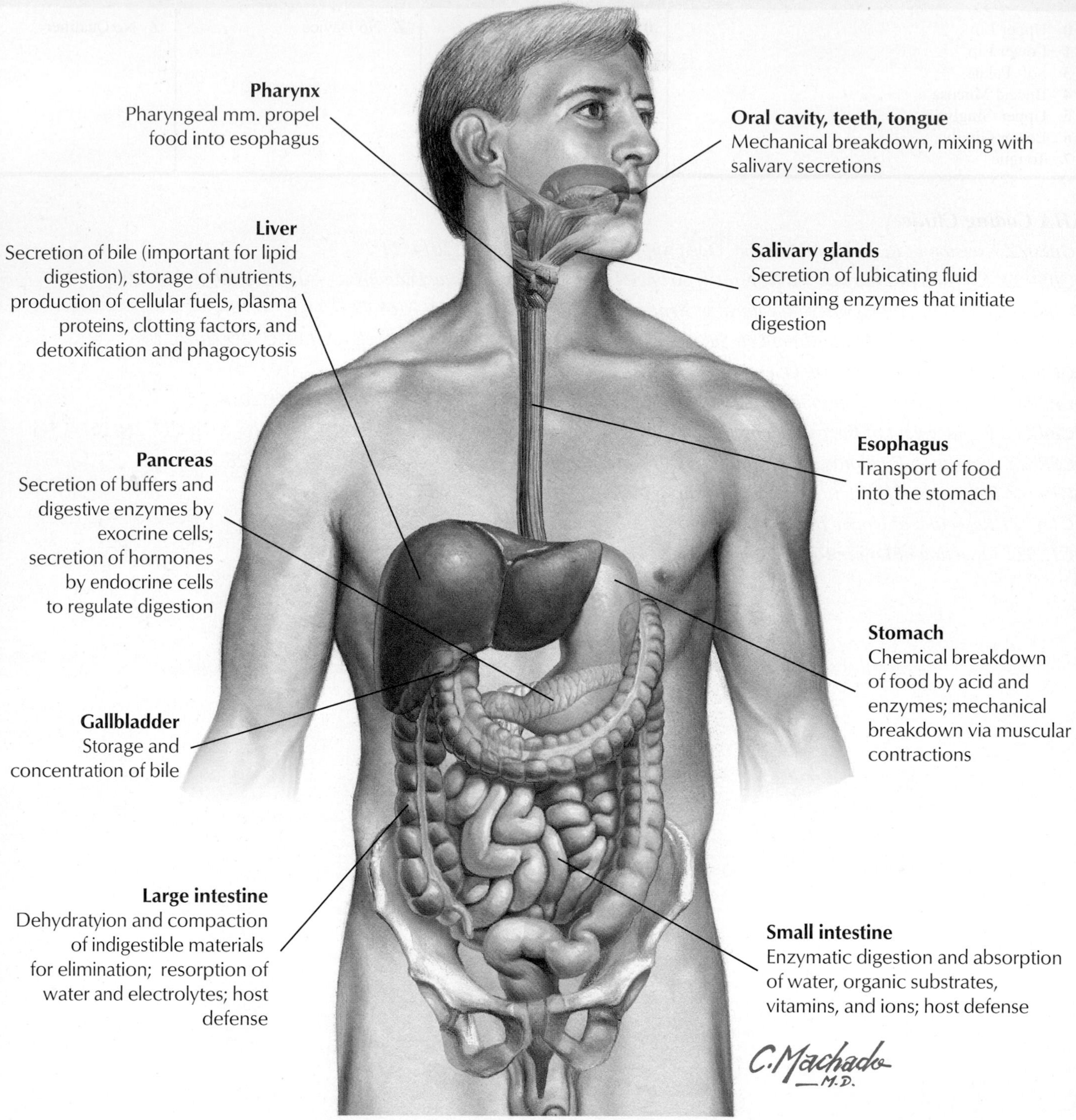
Pharynx
Pharyngeal mm. propel food into esophagus
Oral cavity, teeth, tongue
Mechanical breakdown, mixing with salivary secretions
Liver
Secretion of bile (important for lipid digestion), storage of nutrients, production of cellular fuels, plasma proteins, clotting factors, and detoxification and phagocytosis
Salivary glands
Secretion of lubicating fluid containing enzymes that initiate digestion
Esophagus
Transport of food into the stomach
Pancreas
Secretion of buffers and digestive enzymes by exocrine cells; secretion of hormones by endocrine cells to regulate digestion
Stomach
Chemical breakdown of food by acid and enzymes; mechanical breakdown via muscular contractions
Gallbladder
Storage and concentration of bile
Large intestine
Dehydratyion and compaction of indigestible materials for elimination; resorption of water and electrolytes; host defense
Small intestine
Enzymatic digestion and absorption of water, organic substrates, vitamins, and ions; host defense
C. Machado M.D.

Stomach, Liver, Gallbladder

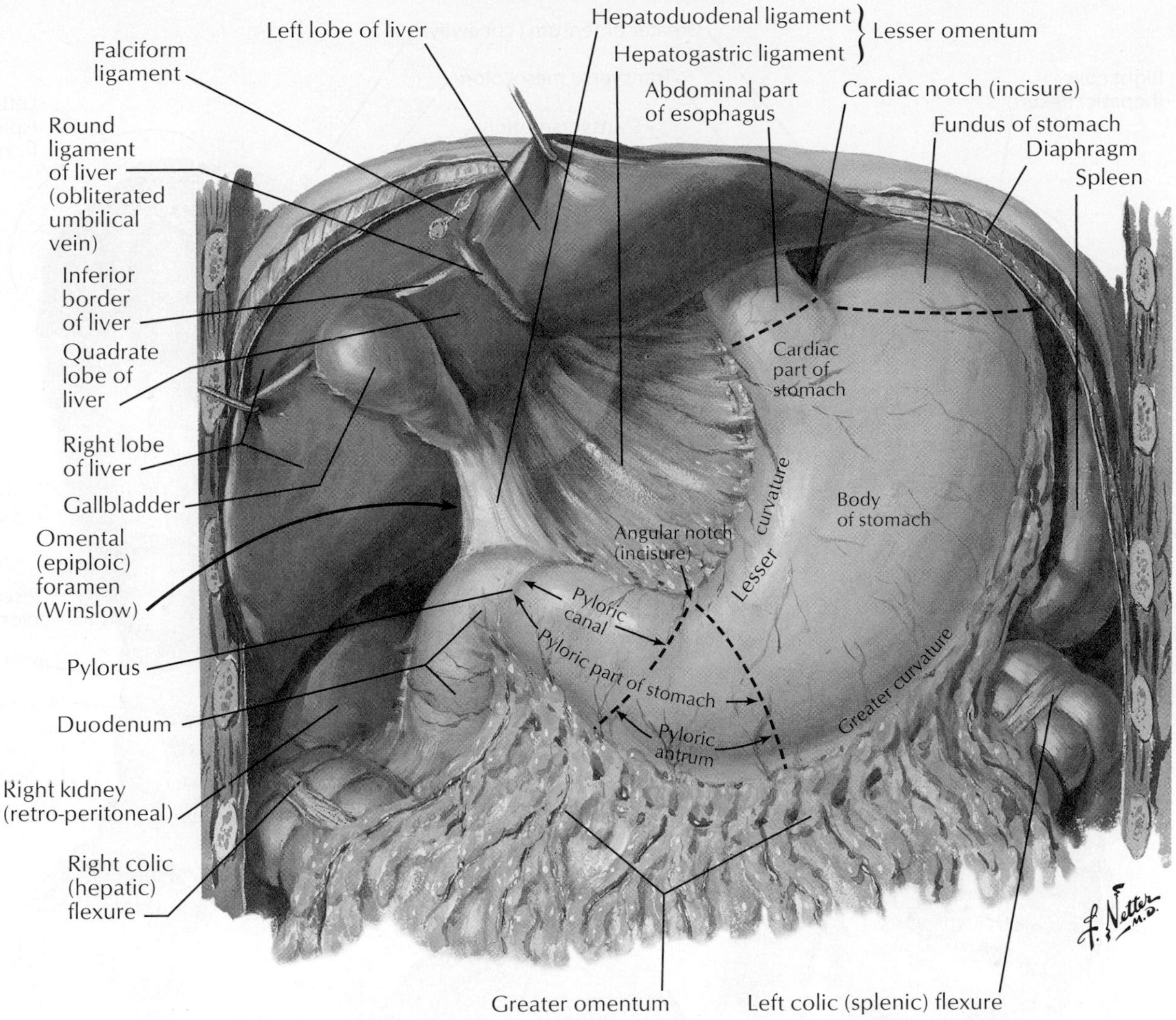

Left lobe of liver
Hepatoduodenal ligament
Hepatogastric ligament
Lesser omentum
Falciform ligament
Round ligament of liver (obliterated umbilical vein)
Abdominal part of esophagus
Cardiac notch (incisure)
Fundus of stomach
Diaphragm
Spleen
Inferior border of liver
Quadrate lobe of liver
Cardiac part of stomach
Right lobe of liver
Gallbladder
Lesser curvature
Body of stomach
Omental (epiploic) foramen (Winslow)
Angular notch (incisure)
Pyloric canal
Pylorus
Pyloric part of stomach
Greater curvature
Duodenum
Pyloric antrum
Right kidney (retro-peritoneal)
Right colic (hepatic) flexure
F. Netter M.D.
Greater omentum
Left colic (splenic) flexure

Large Intestine Structure of Colon

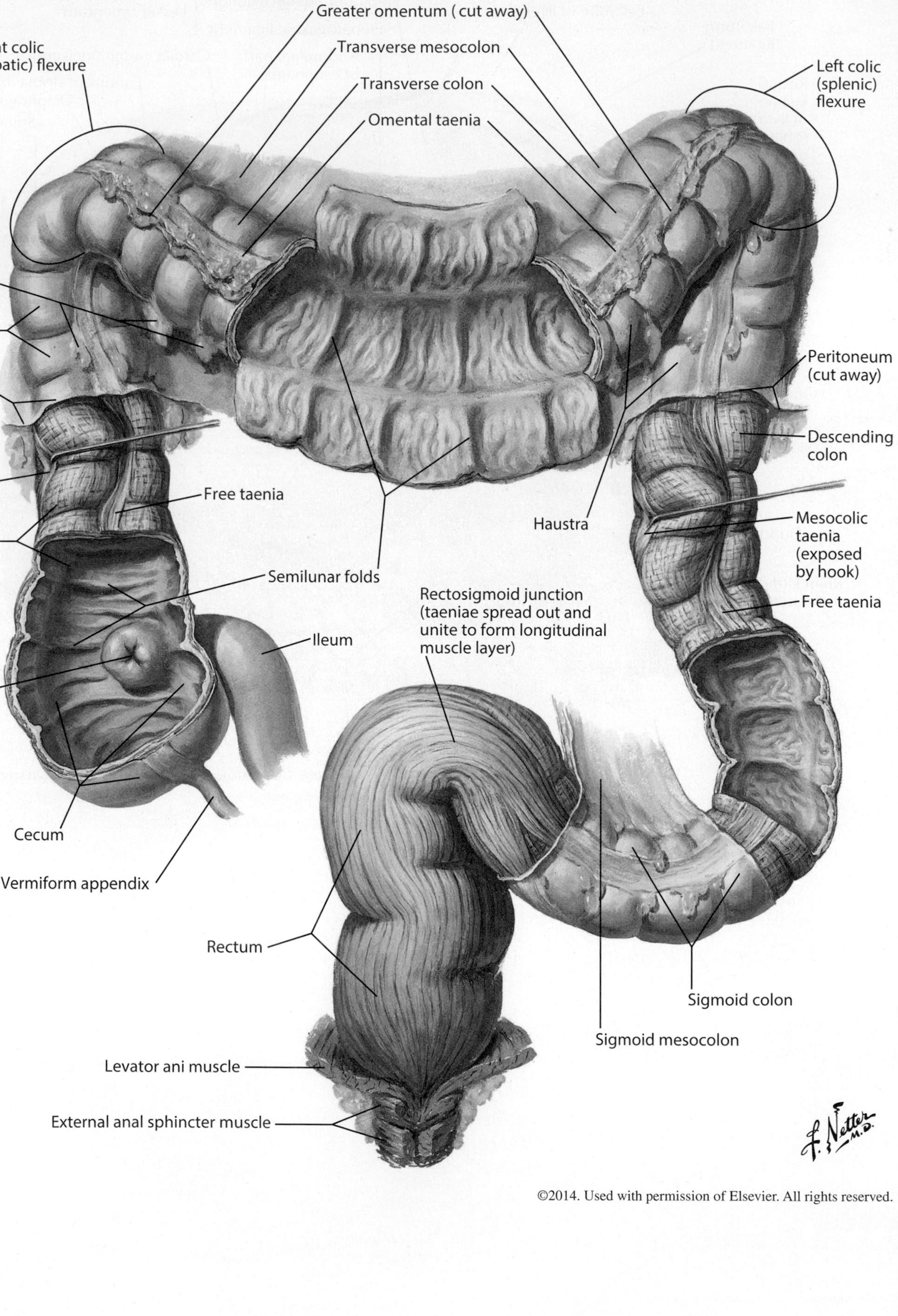

Greater omentum (cut away)
Transverse mesocolon
Transverse colon
Omental taenia
Right colic (hepatic) flexure
Left colic (splenic) flexure
Omental (epiploic) appendices
Haustra
Peritoneum (cut away)
Omental taenia (exposed by hook)
Free taenia
Ascending colon
Semilunar folds
Haustra
Peritoneum (cut away)
Descending colon
Mesocolic taenia (exposed by hook)
Free taenia
Rectosigmoid junction (taeniae spread out and unite to form longitudinal muscle layer)
Ileum
Ileal orifice
Cecum
Vermiform appendix
Rectum
Sigmoid colon
Sigmoid mesocolon
Levator ani muscle
External anal sphincter muscle
F. Netter M.D.

Treatment of Morbid Obesity

Gastric stapling (vertical banded gastroplasty)

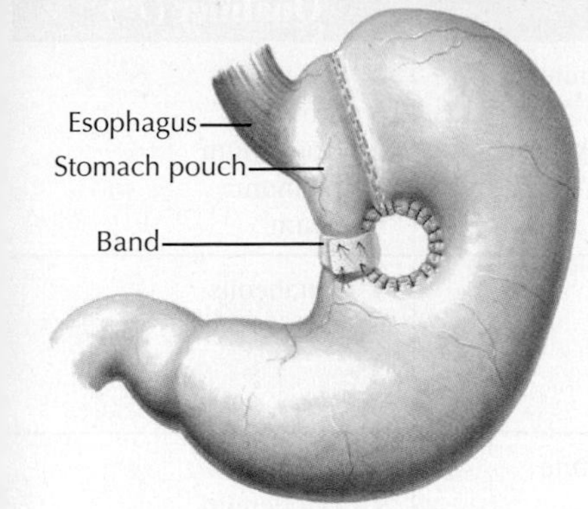
Esophagus
Stomach pouch
Band

Gastric bypass (Roux-en-Y)

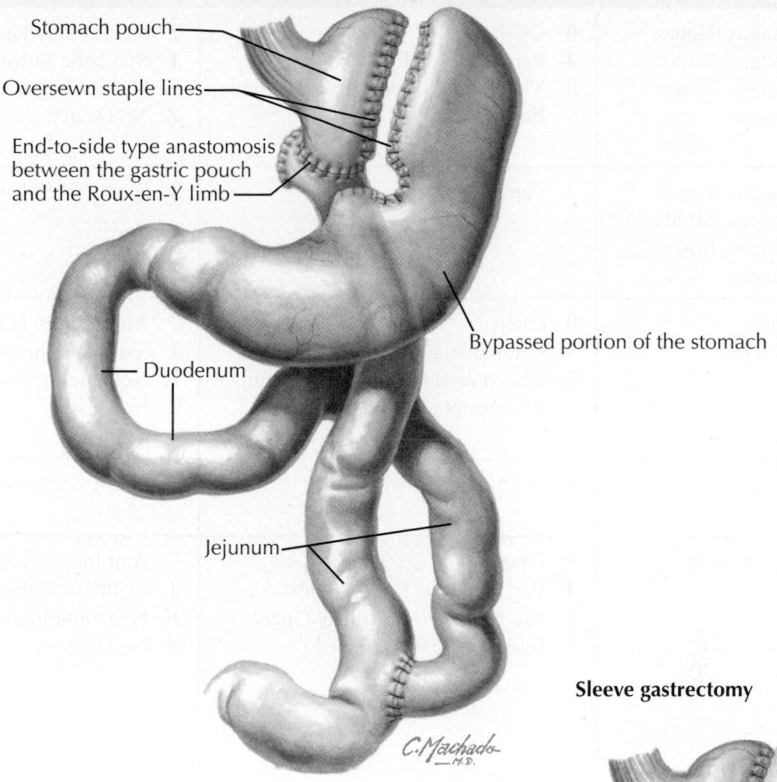
Stomach pouch
Oversewn staple lines
End-to-side type anastomosis between the gastric pouch and the Roux-en-Y limb
Bypassed portion of the stomach
Duodenum
Jejunum
C. Machado M.D.

Laparoscopic adjustable gastric banding

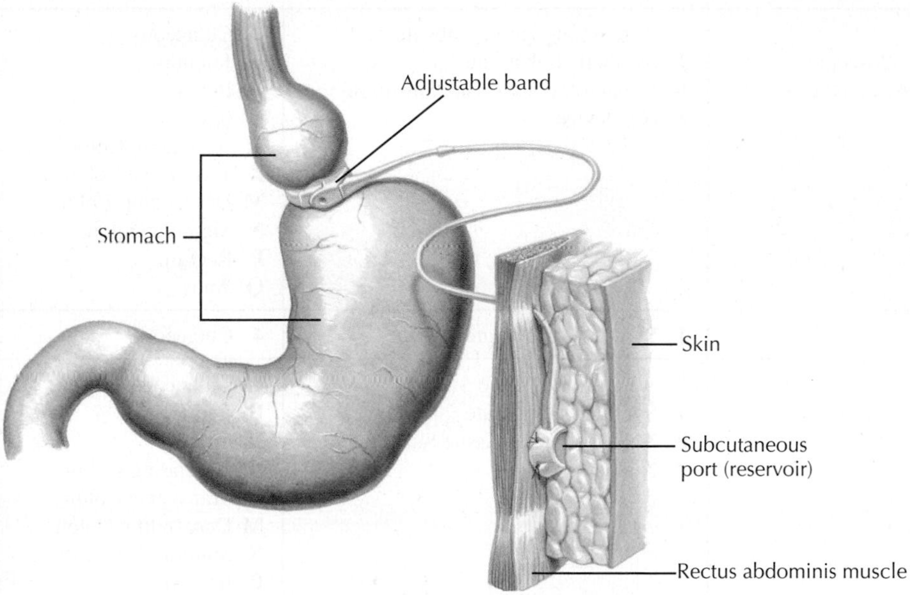
Adjustable band
Stomach
Skin
Subcutaneous port (reservoir)
Rectus abdominis muscle

Sleeve gastrectomy

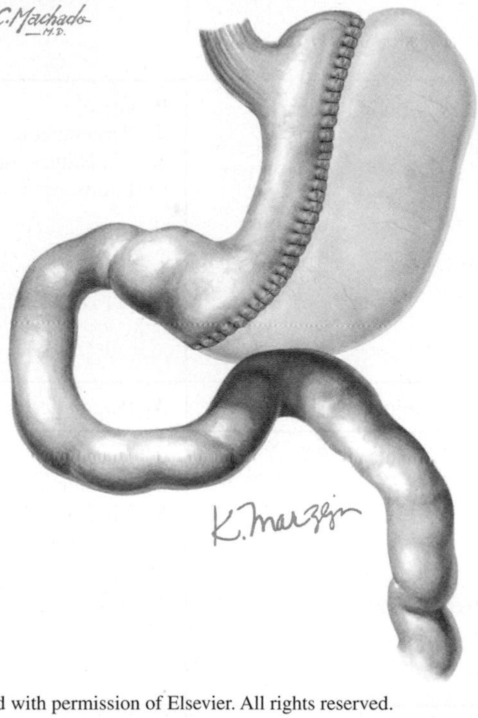
K. Marzejon

Gastrointestinal System Tables 0D1–0DY

Section	0	**Medical and Surgical**
Body System	D	**Gastrointestinal System**
Operation	1	**Bypass:** Altering the route of passage of the contents of a tubular body part

Body Part (4th)	Approach (5th)	Device (6th)	Qualifier (7th)
1 Esophagus, Upper **2** Esophagus, Middle **3** Esophagus, Lower **5** Esophagus	**0** Open **4** Percutaneous Endoscopic **8** Via Natural or Artificial Opening Endoscopic	**7** Autologous Tissue Substitute **J** Synthetic Substitute **K** Nonautologous Tissue Substitute **Z** No Device	**4** Cutaneous **6** Stomach **9** Duodenum **A** Jejunum **B** Ileum
1 Esophagus, Upper **2** Esophagus, Middle **3** Esophagus, Lower **5** Esophagus	**3** Percutaneous	**J** Synthetic Substitute	**4** Cutaneous
6 Stomach **9** Duodenum	**0** Open **4** Percutaneous Endoscopic **8** Via Natural or Artificial Opening Endoscopic	**7** Autologous Tissue Substitute **J** Synthetic Substitute **K** Nonautologous Tissue Substitute **Z** No Device	**4** Cutaneous **9** Duodenum **A** Jejunum **B** Ileum **L** Transverse Colon
6 Stomach **9** Duodenum	**3** Percutaneous	**J** Synthetic Substitute	**4** Cutaneous
8 Small Intestine	**0** Open **4** Percutaneous Endoscopic **8** Via Natural or Artificial Opening Endoscopic	**7** Autologous Tissue Substitute **J** Synthetic Substitute **K** Nonautologous Tissue **Z** No Device	**4** Cutaneous **8** Small Intestine **H** Cecum **K** Ascending Colon **L** Transverse Colon **M** Descending Colon **N** Sigmoid Colon **P** Rectum **Q** Anus
A Jejunum	**0** Open **4** Percutaneous Endoscopic **8** Via Natural or Artificial Opening Endoscopic	**7** Autologous Tissue Substitute **J** Synthetic Substitute **K** Nonautologous Tissue Substitute **Z** No Device	**4** Cutaneous **A** Jejunum **B** Ileum **H** Cecum **K** Ascending Colon **L** Transverse Colon **M** Descending Colon **N** Sigmoid Colon **P** Rectum **Q** Anus
A Jejunum	**3** Percutaneous	**J** Synthetic Substitute	**4** Cutaneous
B Ileum	**0** Open **4** Percutaneous Endoscopic **8** Via Natural or Artificial Opening Endoscopic	**7** Autologous Tissue Substitute **J** Synthetic Substitute **K** Nonautologous Tissue Substitute **Z** No Device	**4** Cutaneous **B** Ileum **H** Cecum **K** Ascending Colon **L** Transverse Colon **M** Descending Colon **N** Sigmoid Colon **P** Rectum **Q** Anus
B Ileum	**3** Percutaneous	**J** Synthetic Substitute	**4** Cutaneous
E Large Intestine	**0** Open **4** Percutaneous Endoscopic **8** Via Natural or Artificial Opening Endoscopic	**7** Autologous Tissue Substitute **J** Synthetic Substitute **K** Nonautologous Tissue **Z** No Device	**4** Cutaneous **E** Large Intestine **P** Rectum

Continued →

Section 0 **Medical and Surgical**
Body System D **Gastrointestinal System**
Operation 1 **Bypass:** Altering the route of passage of the contents of a tubular body part

Body Part (4th)	Approach (5th)	Device (6th)	Qualifier (7th)
H Cecum	**0** Open **4** Percutaneous Endoscopic **8** Via Natural or Artificial Opening Endoscopic	**7** Autologous Tissue Substitute **J** Synthetic Substitute **K** Nonautologous Tissue Substitute **Z** No Device	**4** Cutaneous **H** Cecum **K** Ascending Colon **L** Transverse Colon **M** Descending Colon **N** Sigmoid Colon **P** Rectum
H Cecum	**3** Percutaneous	**J** Synthetic Substitute	**4** Cutaneous
K Ascending Colon	**0** Open **4** Percutaneous Endoscopic **8** Via Natural or Artificial Opening Endoscopic	**7** Autologous Tissue Substitute **J** Synthetic Substitute **K** Nonautologous Tissue Substitute **Z** No Device	**4** Cutaneous **K** Ascending Colon **L** Transverse Colon **M** Descending Colon **N** Sigmoid Colon **P** Rectum
K Ascending Colon	**3** Percutaneous	**J** Synthetic Substitute	**4** Cutaneous
L Transverse Colon	**0** Open **4** Percutaneous Endoscopic **8** Via Natural or Artificial Opening Endoscopic	**7** Autologous Tissue Substitute **J** Synthetic Substitute **K** Nonautologous Tissue Substitute **Z** No Device	**4** Cutaneous **L** Transverse Colon **M** Descending Colon **N** Sigmoid Colon **P** Rectum
L Transverse Colon	**3** Percutaneous	**J** Synthetic Substitute	**4** Cutaneous
M Descending Colon	**0** Open **4** Percutaneous Endoscopic **8** Via Natural or Artificial Opening Endoscopic	**7** Autologous Tissue Substitute **J** Synthetic Substitute **K** Nonautologous Tissue Substitute **Z** No Device	**4** Cutaneous **M** Descending Colon **N** Sigmoid Colon **P** Rectum
M Descending Colon	**3** Percutaneous	**J** Synthetic Substitute	**4** Cutaneous
N Sigmoid Colon	**0** Open **4** Percutaneous Endoscopic **8** Via Natural or Artificial Opening Endoscopic	**7** Autologous Tissue Substitute **J** Synthetic Substitute **K** Nonautologous Tissue Substitute **Z** No Device	**4** Cutaneous **N** Sigmoid Colon **P** Rectum
N Sigmoid Colon	**3** Percutaneous	**J** Synthetic Substitute	**4** Cutaneous

Section 0 **Medical and Surgical**
Body System D **Gastrointestinal System**
Operation 2 **Change:** Taking out or off a device from a body part and putting back an identical or similar device in or on the same body part without cutting or puncturing the skin or a mucous membrane

Body Part (4th)	Approach (5th)	Device (6th)	Qualifier (7th)
0 Upper Intestinal Tract **D** Lower Intestinal Tract	**X** External	**0** Drainage Device **U** Feeding Device **Y** Other Device	**Z** No Qualifier
U Omentum **V** Mesentery **W** Peritoneum	**X** External	**0** Drainage Device **Y** Other Device	**Z** No Qualifier

Section 0 **Medical and Surgical**
Body System D **Gastrointestinal System**
Operation 5 **Destruction:** Physical eradication of all or a portion of a body part by the direct use of energy, force, or a destructive agent

Body Part (4th)	Approach (5th)	Device (6th)	Qualifier (7th)
1 Esophagus, Upper **2** Esophagus, Middle **3** Esophagus, Lower **4** Esophagogastric Junction **5** Esophagus **6** Stomach **7** Stomach, Pylorus **8** Small Intestine **9** Duodenum **A** Jejunum **B** Ileum **C** Ileocecal Valve **E** Large Intestine **F** Large Intestine, Right **G** Large Intestine, Left **H** Cecum **J** Appendix **K** Ascending Colon **L** Transverse Colon **M** Descending Colon **N** Sigmoid Colon **P** Rectum	**0** Open **3** Percutaneous **4** Percutaneous Endoscopic **7** Via Natural or Artificial Opening **8** Via Natural or Artificial Opening Endoscopic	**Z** No Device	**Z** No Qualifier
Q Anus	**0** Open **3** Percutaneous **4** Percutaneous Endoscopic **7** Via Natural or Artificial Opening **8** Via Natural or Artificial Opening Endoscopic **X** External	**Z** No Device	**Z** No Qualifier
R Anal Sphincter **U** Omentum **V** Mesentery **W** Peritoneum	**0** Open **3** Percutaneous **4** Percutaneous Endoscopic	**Z** No Device	**Z** No Qualifier

Section 0 **Medical and Surgical**
Body System D **Gastrointestinal System**
Operation 7 **Dilation:** Expanding an orifice or the lumen of a tubular body part

Body Part (4th)	Approach (5th)	Device (6th)	Qualifier (7th)
1 Esophagus, Upper **2** Esophagus, Middle **3** Esophagus, Lower **4** Esophagogastric Junction **5** Esophagus **6** Stomach **7** Stomach, Pylorus **8** Small Intestine **9** Duodenum **A** Jejunum **B** Ileum **C** Ileocecal Valve **E** Large Intestine **F** Large Intestine, Right **G** Large Intestine, Left **H** Cecum **K** Ascending Colon **L** Transverse Colon **M** Descending Colon **N** Sigmoid Colon **P** Rectum **Q** Anus	**0** Open **3** Percutaneous **4** Percutaneous Endoscopic **7** Via Natural or Artificial Opening **8** Via Natural or Artificial Opening Endoscopic	**D** Intraluminal Device **Z** No Device	**Z** No Qualifier

Section 0 **Medical and Surgical**
Body System D **Gastrointestinal System**
Operation 8 **Division:** Cutting into a body part, without draining fluids and/or gases from the body part, in order to separate or transect a body part

Body Part (4th)	Approach (5th)	Device (6th)	Qualifier (7th)
4 Esophagogastric Junction 7 Stomach, Pylorus	0 Open 3 Percutaneous 4 Percutaneous Endoscopic 7 Via Natural or Artificial Opening 8 Via Natural or Artificial Opening Endoscopic	Z No Device	Z No Qualifier
R Anal Sphincter	0 Open 3 Percutaneous	Z No Device	Z No Qualifier

Section 0 **Medical and Surgical**
Body System D **Gastrointestinal System**
Operation 9 **Drainage:** Taking or letting out fluids and/or gases from a body part

Body Part (4th)	Approach (5th)	Device (6th)	Qualifier (7th)
1 Esophagus, Upper 2 Esophagus, Middle 3 Esophagus, Lower 4 Esophagogastric Junction 5 Esophagus 6 Stomach 7 Stomach, Pylorus 8 Small Intestine 9 Duodenum A Jejunum B Ileum C Ileocecal Valve E Large Intestine F Large Intestine, Right G Large Intestine, Left H Cecum J Appendix K Ascending Colon L Transverse Colon M Descending Colon N Sigmoid Colon P Rectum	0 Open 3 Percutaneous 4 Percutaneous Endoscopic 7 Via Natural or Artificial Opening 8 Via Natural or Artificial Opening Endoscopic	0 Drainage Device	Z No Qualifier
1 Esophagus, Upper 2 Esophagus, Middle 3 Esophagus, Lower 4 Esophagogastric Junction 5 Esophagus 6 Stomach 7 Stomach, Pylorus 8 Small Intestine 9 Duodenum A Jejunum B Ileum C Ileocecal Valve E Large Intestine F Large Intestine, Right G Large Intestine, Left H Cecum J Appendix K Ascending Colon L Transverse Colon M Descending Colon N Sigmoid Colon P Rectum	0 Open 3 Percutaneous 4 Percutaneous Endoscopic 7 Via Natural or Artificial Opening 8 Via Natural or Artificial Opening Endoscopic	Z No Device	X Diagnostic Z No Qualifier

Continued →

0D9 Continued

Section 0 **Medical and Surgical**
Body System D **Gastrointestinal System**
Operation 9 **Drainage:** Taking or letting out fluids and/or gases from a body part

Body Part (4th)	Approach (5th)	Device (6th)	Qualifier (7th)
Q Anus	**0** Open **3** Percutaneous **4** Percutaneous Endoscopic **7** Via Natural or Artificial Opening **8** Via Natural or Artificial Opening Endoscopic **X** External	**0** Drainage Device	**Z** No Qualifier
Q Anus	**0** Open **3** Percutaneous **4** Percutaneous Endoscopic **7** Via Natural or Artificial Opening **8** Via Natural or Artificial Opening Endoscopic **X** External	**Z** No Device	**X** Diagnostic **Z** No Qualifier
R Anal Sphincter **U** Omentum **V** Mesentery **W** Peritoneum	**0** Open **3** Percutaneous **4** Percutaneous Endoscopic	**0** Drainage Device	**Z** No Qualifier
R Anal Sphincter **U** Omentum **V** Mesentery **W** Peritoneum	**0** Open **3** Percutaneous **4** Percutaneous Endoscopic	**Z** No Device	**X** Diagnostic **Z** No Qualifier

Section 0 **Medical and Surgical**
Body System D **Gastrointestinal System**
Operation B **Excision:** Cutting out or off, without replacement, a portion of a body part

Body Part (4th)	Approach (5th)	Device (6th)	Qualifier (7th)
1 Esophagus, Upper **2** Esophagus, Middle **3** Esophagus, Lower **4** Esophagogastric Junction **5** Esophagus **7** Stomach, Pylorus **8** Small Intestine **9** Duodenum **A** Jejunum **B** Ileum **C** Ileocecal Valve **E** Large Intestine **F** Large Intestine, Right **H** Cecum **J** Appendix **K** Ascending Colon **P** Rectum	**0** Open **3** Percutaneous **4** Percutaneous Endoscopic **7** Via Natural or Artificial Opening **8** Via Natural or Artificial Opening Endoscopic	**Z** No Device	**X** Diagnostic **Z** No Qualifier
6 Stomach	**0** Open **3** Percutaneous **4** Percutaneous Endoscopic **7** Via Natural or Artificial Opening **8** Via Natural or Artificial Opening Endoscopic	**Z** No Device	**3** Vertical **X** Diagnostic **Z** No Qualifier
G Large Intestine, Left **L** Transverse Colon **M** Descending Colon **N** Sigmoid Colon	**0** Open **3** Percutaneous **4** Percutaneous Endoscopic **7** Via Natural or Artificial Opening **8** Via Natural or Artificial Opening Endoscopic	**Z** No Device	**X** Diagnostic **Z** No Qualifier

Continued →

Section **0** **Medical and Surgical**
Body System **D** **Gastrointestinal System**
Operation **B** **Excision:** Cutting out or off, without replacement, a portion of a body part

Body Part (4th)	Approach (5th)	Device (6th)	Qualifier (7th)
G Large Intestine, Left **L** Transverse Colon **M** Descending Colon **N** Sigmoid Colon	**F** Via Natural or Artificial Opening With Percutaneous Endoscopic Assistance	**Z** No Device	**Z** No Qualifier
Q Anus	**0** Open **3** Percutaneous **4** Percutaneous Endoscopic **7** Via Natural or Artificial Opening **8** Via Natural or Artificial Opening Endoscopic **X** External	**Z** No Device	**X** Diagnostic **Z** No Qualifier
R Anal Sphincter **U** Omentum **V** Mesentery **W** Peritoneum	**0** Open **3** Percutaneous **4** Percutaneous Endoscopic	**Z** No Device	**X** Diagnostic **Z** No Qualifier

Section **0** **Medical and Surgical**
Body System **D** **Gastrointestinal System**
Operation **C** **Extirpation:** Taking or cutting out solid matter from a body part

Body Part (4th)	Approach (5th)	Device (6th)	Qualifier (7th)
1 Esophagus, Upper **2** Esophagus, Middle **3** Esophagus, Lower **4** Esophagogastric Junction **5** Esophagus **6** Stomach **7** Stomach, Pylorus **8** Small Intestine **9** Duodenum **A** Jejunum **B** Ileum **C** Ileocecal Valve **E** Large Intestine **F** Large Intestine, Right **G** Large Intestine, Left **H** Cecum **J** Appendix **K** Ascending Colon **L** Transverse Colon **M** Descending Colon **N** Sigmoid Colon **P** Rectum	**0** Open **3** Percutaneous **4** Percutaneous Endoscopic **7** Via Natural or Artificial Opening **8** Via Natural or Artificial Opening Endoscopic	**Z** No Device	**Z** No Qualifier
Q Anus	**0** Open **3** Percutaneous **4** Percutaneous Endoscopic **7** Via Natural or Artificial Opening **8** Via Natural or Artificial Opening Endoscopic **X** External	**Z** No Device	**Z** No Qualifier
R Anal Sphincter **U** Omentum **V** Mesentery **W** Peritoneum	**0** Open **3** Percutaneous **4** Percutaneous Endoscopic	**Z** No Device	**Z** No Qualifier

Section 0 **Medical and Surgical**
Body System D **Gastrointestinal System**
Operation D **Extraction:** Pulling or stripping out or off all or a portion of a body part by the use of force

Body Part (4th)	Approach (5th)	Device (6th)	Qualifier (7th)
1 Esophagus, Upper **2** Esophagus, Middle **3** Esophagus, Lower **4** Esophagogastric Junction **5** Esophagus **6** Stomach **7** Stomach, Pylorus **8** Small Intestine **9** Duodenum **A** Jejunum **B** Ileum **C** Ileocecal Valve **E** Large Intestine **F** Large Intestine, Right **G** Large Intestine, Left **H** Cecum **J** Appendix **K** Ascending Colon **L** Transverse Colon **M** Descending Colon **N** Sigmoid Colon **P** Rectum	**3** Percutaneous **4** Percutaneous Endoscopic **8** Via Natural or Artificial Opening Endoscopic	**Z** No Device	**X** Diagnostic
Q Anus	**3** Percutaneous **4** Percutaneous Endoscopic **8** Via Natural or Artificial Opening Endoscopic **X** External	**Z** No Device	**X** Diagnostic

Section 0 **Medical and Surgical**
Body System D **Gastrointestinal System**
Operation F **Fragmentation:** Breaking solid matter in a body part into pieces

Body Part (4th)	Approach (5th)	Device (6th)	Qualifier (7th)
5 Esophagus **6** Stomach **8** Small Intestine **9** Duodenum **A** Jejunum **B** Ileum **E** Large Intestine **F** Large Intestine, Right **G** Large Intestine, Left **H** Cecum **J** Appendix **K** Ascending Colon **L** Transverse Colon **M** Descending Colon **N** Sigmoid Colon **P** Rectum **Q** Anus	**0** Open **3** Percutaneous **4** Percutaneous Endoscopic **7** Via Natural or Artificial Opening **8** Via Natural or Artificial Opening Endoscopic **X** External	**Z** No Device	**Z** No Qualifier

Section 0 **Medical and Surgical**
Body System D **Gastrointestinal System**
Operation H **Insertion:** Putting in a nonbiological appliance that monitors, assists, performs, or prevents a physiological function but does not physically take the place of a body part

Body Part (4th)	Approach (5th)	Device (6th)	Qualifier (7th)
0 Upper Intestinal Tract **D** Lower Intestinal Tract	**0** Open **3** Percutaneous **4** Percutaneous Endoscopic **7** Via Natural or Artificial Opening **8** Via Natural or Artificial Opening Endoscopic	**Y** Other Device	**Z** No Qualifier
5 Esophagus	**0** Open **3** Percutaneous **4** Percutaneous Endoscopic	**1** Radioactive Element **2** Monitoring Device **3** Infusion Device **D** Intraluminal Device **U** Feeding Device **Y** Other Device	**Z** No Qualifier
5 Esophagus	**7** Via Natural or Artificial Opening **8** Via Natural or Artificial Opening Endoscopic	**1** Radioactive Element **2** Monitoring Device **3** Infusion Device **B** Intraluminal Device, Airway **D** Intraluminal Device **U** Feeding Device **Y** Other Device	**Z** No Qualifier
6 Stomach	**0** Open **3** Percutaneous **4** Percutaneous Endoscopic	**1** Radioactive Element **2** Monitoring Device **3** Infusion Device **D** Intraluminal Device **M** Stimulator Lead **U** Feeding Device **Y** Other Device	**Z** No Qualifier
6 Stomach	**7** Via Natural or Artificial Opening **8** Via Natural or Artificial Opening Endoscopic	**1** Radioactive Element **2** Monitoring Device **3** Infusion Device **D** Intraluminal Device **U** Feeding Device **Y** Other Device	**Z** No Qualifier
8 Small Intestine **9** Duodenum **A** Jejunum **B** Ileum	**0** Open **3** Percutaneous **4** Percutaneous Endoscopic **7** Via Natural or Artificial Opening **8** Via Natural or Artificial Opening Endoscopic	**1** Radioactive Element **2** Monitoring Device **3** Infusion Device **D** Intraluminal Device **U** Feeding Device	**Z** No Qualifier
E Large Intestine **P** Rectum	**0** Open **3** Percutaneous **4** Percutaneous Endoscopic **7** Via Natural or Artificial Opening **8** Via Natural or Artificial Opening Endoscopic	**1** Radioactive Element **D** Intraluminal Device	**Z** No Qualifier
Q Anus	**0** Open **3** Percutaneous **4** Percutaneous Endoscopic	**D** Intraluminal Device **L** Artificial Sphincter	**Z** No Qualifier
Q Anus	**7** Via Natural or Artificial Opening **8** Via Natural or Artificial Opening Endoscopic	**D** Intraluminal Device	**Z** No Qualifier
R Anal Sphincter	**0** Open **3** Percutaneous **4** Percutaneous Endoscopic	**M** Stimulator Lead	**Z** No Qualifier

Section 0 **Medical and Surgical**
Body System D **Gastrointestinal System**
Operation J **Inspection:** Visually and/or manually exploring a body part

Body Part (4th)	Approach (5th)	Device (6th)	Qualifier (7th)
0 Upper Intestinal Tract **6** Stomach **D** Lower Intestinal Tract	**0** Open **3** Percutaneous **4** Percutaneous Endoscopic **7** Via Natural or Artificial Opening **8** Via Natural or Artificial Opening Endoscopic **X** External	**Z** No Device	**Z** No Qualifier
U Omentum **V** Mesentery **W** Peritoneum	**0** Open **3** Percutaneous **4** Percutaneous Endoscopic **X** External	**Z** No Device	**Z** No Qualifier

Section 0 **Medical and Surgical**
Body System D **Gastrointestinal System**
Operation L **Occlusion:** Completely closing an orifice or the lumen of a tubular body part

Body Part (4th)	Approach (5th)	Device (6th)	Qualifier (7th)
1 Esophagus, Upper **2** Esophagus, Middle **3** Esophagus, Lower **4** Esophagogastric Junction **5** Esophagus **6** Stomach **7** Stomach, Pylorus **8** Small Intestine **9** Duodenum **A** Jejunum **B** Ileum **C** Ileocecal Valve **E** Large Intestine **F** Large Intestine, Right **G** Large Intestine, Left **H** Cecum **K** Ascending Colon **L** Transverse Colon **M** Descending Colon **N** Sigmoid Colon **P** Rectum	**0** Open **3** Percutaneous **4** Percutaneous Endoscopic	**C** Extraluminal Device **D** Intraluminal Device **Z** No Device	**Z** No Qualifier
1 Esophagus, Upper **2** Esophagus, Middle **3** Esophagus, Lower **4** Esophagogastric Junction **5** Esophagus **6** Stomach **7** Stomach, Pylorus **8** Small Intestine **9** Duodenum **A** Jejunum **B** Ileum **C** Ileocecal Valve **E** Large Intestine **F** Large Intestine, Right **G** Large Intestine, Left **H** Cecum **K** Ascending Colon **L** Transverse Colon **M** Descending Colon **N** Sigmoid Colon **P** Rectum	**7** Via Natural or Artificial Opening **8** Via Natural or Artificial Opening Endoscopic	**D** Intraluminal Device **Z** No Device	**Z** No Qualifier

Continued →

Section **0** **Medical and Surgical**
Body System **D** **Gastrointestinal System**
Operation **L** **Occlusion:** Completely closing an orifice or the lumen of a tubular body part

Body Part (4th)	Approach (5th)	Device (6th)	Qualifier (7th)
Q Anus	**0** Open **3** Percutaneous **4** Percutaneous Endoscopic **X** External	**C** Extraluminal Device **D** Intraluminal Device **Z** No Device	**Z** No Qualifier
Q Anus	**7** Via Natural or Artificial Opening **8** Via Natural or Artificial Opening Endoscopic	**D** Intraluminal Device **Z** No Device	**Z** No Qualifier

Section **0** **Medical and Surgical**
Body System **D** **Gastrointestinal System**
Operation **M** **Reattachment:** Putting back in or on all or a portion of a separated body part to its normal location or other suitable location

Body Part (4th)	Approach (5th)	Device (6th)	Qualifier (7th)
5 Esophagus **6** Stomach **8** Small Intestine **9** Duodenum **A** Jejunum **B** Ileum **E** Large Intestine **F** Large Intestine, Right **G** Large Intestine, Left **H** Cecum **K** Ascending Colon **L** Transverse Colon **M** Descending Colon **N** Sigmoid Colon **P** Rectum	**0** Open **4** Percutaneous Endoscopic	**Z** No Device	**Z** No Qualifier

Section **0** **Medical and Surgical**
Body System **D** **Gastrointestinal System**
Operation **N** **Release:** Freeing a body part from an abnormal physical constraint by cutting or by the use of force

Body Part (4th)	Approach (5th)	Device (6th)	Qualifier (7th)
1 Esophagus, Upper **2** Esophagus, Middle **3** Esophagus, Lower **4** Esophagogastric Junction **5** Esophagus **6** Stomach **7** Stomach, Pylorus **8** Small Intestine **9** Duodenum **A** Jejunum **B** Ileum **C** Ileocecal Valve **E** Large Intestine **F** Large Intestine, Right **G** Large Intestine, Left **H** Cecum **J** Appendix **K** Ascending Colon **L** Transverse Colon **M** Descending Colon **N** Sigmoid Colon **P** Rectum	**0** Open **3** Percutaneous **4** Percutaneous Endoscopic **7** Via Natural or Artificial Opening **8** Via Natural or Artificial Opening Endoscopic	**Z** No Device	**Z** No Qualifier

Continued →

Section 0 **Medical and Surgical**
Body System D **Gastrointestinal System**
Operation N **Release:** Freeing a body part from an abnormal physical constraint by cutting or by the use of force

Body Part (4th)	Approach (5th)	Device (6th)	Qualifier (7th)
Q Anus	**0** Open **3** Percutaneous **4** Percutaneous Endoscopic **7** Via Natural or Artificial Opening **8** Via Natural or Artificial Opening Endoscopic **X** External	**Z** No Device	**Z** No Qualifier
R Anal Sphincter **U** Omentum **V** Mesentery **W** Peritoneum	**0** Open **3** Percutaneous **4** Percutaneous Endoscopic	**Z** No Device	**Z** No Qualifier

Section 0 **Medical and Surgical**
Body System D **Gastrointestinal System**
Operation P **Removal:** Taking out or off a device from a body part

Body Part (4th)	Approach (5th)	Device (6th)	Qualifier (7th)
0 Upper Intestinal Tract **D** Lower Intestinal Tract	**0** Open **3** Percutaneous **4** Percutaneous Endoscopic **7** Via Natural or Artificial Opening **8** Via Natural or Artificial Opening Endoscopic	**0** Drainage Device **2** Monitoring Device **3** Infusion Device **7** Autologous Tissue Substitute **C** Extraluminal Device **D** Intraluminal Device **J** Synthetic Substitute **K** Nonautologous Tissue Substitute **U** Feeding Device **Y** Other Device	**Z** No Qualifier
0 Upper Intestinal Tract **D** Lower Intestinal Tract	**X** External	**0** Drainage Device **2** Monitoring Device **3** Infusion Device **D** Intraluminal Device **U** Feeding Device	**Z** No Qualifier
5 Esophagus	**0** Open **3** Percutaneous **4** Percutaneous Endoscopic	**1** Radioactive Element **2** Monitoring Device **3** Infusion Device **U** Feeding Device **Y** Other Device	**Z** No Qualifier
5 Esophagus	**7** Via Natural or Artificial Opening **8** Via Natural or Artificial Opening Endoscopic	**1** Radioactive Element **D** Intraluminal Device **Y** Other Device	**Z** No Qualifier
5 Esophagus	**X** External	**1** Radioactive Element **2** Monitoring Device **3** Infusion Device **D** Intraluminal Device **U** Feeding Device	**Z** No Qualifier

Continued →

Body Part (4th)	Approach (5th)	Device (6th)	Qualifier (7th)
6 Stomach	**0** Open **3** Percutaneous **4** Percutaneous Endoscopic	**0** Drainage Device **2** Monitoring Device **3** Infusion Device **7** Autologous Tissue Substitute **C** Extraluminal Device **D** Intraluminal Device **J** Synthetic Substitute **K** Nonautologous Tissue Substitute **M** Stimulator Lead **U** Feeding Device **Y** Other Device	**Z** No Qualifier
6 Stomach	**7** Via Natural or Artificial Opening **8** Via Natural or Artificial Opening Endoscopic	**0** Drainage Device **2** Monitoring Device **3** Infusion Device **7** Autologous Tissue Substitute **C** Extraluminal Device **D** Intraluminal Device **J** Synthetic Substitute **K** Nonautologous Tissue Substitute **U** Feeding Device **Y** Other Device	**Z** No Qualifier
6 Stomach	**X** External	**0** Drainage Device **2** Monitoring Device **3** Infusion Device **D** Intraluminal Device **U** Feeding Device	**Z** No Qualifier
P Rectum	**0** Open **3** Percutaneous **4** Percutaneous Endoscopic **7** Via Natural or Artificial Opening **8** Via Natural or Artificial Opening Endoscopic **X** External	**1** Radioactive Element	**Z** No Qualifier
Q Anus	**0** Open **3** Percutaneous **4** Percutaneous Endoscopic **7** Via Natural or Artificial Opening **8** Via Natural or Artificial Opening Endoscopic	**L** Artificial Sphincter	**Z** No Qualifier
R Anal Sphincter	**0** Open **3** Percutaneous **4** Percutaneous Endoscopic	**M** Stimulator Lead	**Z** No Qualifier
U Omentum **V** Mesentery **W** Peritoneum	**0** Open **3** Percutaneous **4** Percutaneous Endoscopic	**0** Drainage Device **1** Radioactive Element **7** Autologous Tissue Substitute **J** Synthetic Substitute **K** Nonautologous Tissue Substitute	**Z** No Qualifier

Section **0** **Medical and Surgical**
Body System **D** **Gastrointestinal System**
Operation **Q** **Repair:** Restoring, to the extent possible, a body part to its normal anatomic structure and function

Body Part (4th)	Approach (5th)	Device (6th)	Qualifier (7th)
1 Esophagus, Upper **2** Esophagus, Middle **3** Esophagus, Lower **4** Esophagogastric Junction **5** Esophagus **6** Stomach **7** Stomach, Pylorus **8** Small Intestine **9** Duodenum **A** Jejunum **B** Ileum **C** Ileocecal Valve **E** Large Intestine **F** Large Intestine, Right **G** Large Intestine, Left **H** Cecum **J** Appendix **K** Ascending Colon **L** Transverse Colon **M** Descending Colon **N** Sigmoid Colon **P** Rectum	**0** Open **3** Percutaneous **4** Percutaneous Endoscopic **7** Via Natural or Artificial Opening **8** Via Natural or Artificial Opening Endoscopic	**Z** No Device	**Z** No Qualifier
Q Anus	**0** Open **3** Percutaneous **4** Percutaneous Endoscopic **7** Via Natural or Artificial Opening **8** Via Natural or Artificial Opening Endoscopic **X** External	**Z** No Device	**Z** No Qualifier
R Anal Sphincter **U** Omentum **V** Mesentery **W** Peritoneum	**0** Open **3** Percutaneous **4** Percutaneous Endoscopic	**Z** No Device	**Z** No Qualifier

Section **0** **Medical and Surgical**
Body System **D** **Gastrointestinal System**
Operation **R** **Replacement:** Putting in or on biological or synthetic material that physically takes the place and/or function of all or a portion of a body part

Body Part (4th)	Approach (5th)	Device (6th)	Qualifier (7th)
5 Esophagus	**0** Open **4** Percutaneous Endoscopic **7** Via Natural or Artificial Opening **8** Via Natural or Artificial Opening Endoscopic	**7** Autologous Tissue Substitute **J** Synthetic Substitute **K** Nonautologous Tissue Substitute	**Z** No Qualifier
R Anal Sphincter **U** Omentum **V** Mesentery **W** Peritoneum	**0** Open **4** Percutaneous Endoscopic	**7** Autologous Tissue Substitute **J** Synthetic Substitute **K** Nonautologous Tissue Substitute	**Z** No Qualifier

Section **0** **Medical and Surgical**
Body System **D** **Gastrointestinal System**
Operation **S** **Reposition:** Moving to its normal location, or other suitable location, all or a portion of a body part

Body Part (4th)	Approach (5th)	Device (6th)	Qualifier (7th)
5 Esophagus **6** Stomach **9** Duodenum **A** Jejunum **B** Ileum **H** Cecum **K** Ascending Colon **L** Transverse Colon **M** Descending Colon **N** Sigmoid Colon **P** Rectum **Q** Anus	**0** Open **4** Percutaneous Endoscopic **7** Via Natural or Artificial Opening **8** Via Natural or Artificial Opening Endoscopic **X** External	**Z** No Device	**Z** No Qualifier
8 Small Intestine **E** Large Intestine	**0** Open **4** Percutaneous Endoscopic **7** Via Natural or Artificial Opening **8** Via Natural or Artificial Opening Endoscopic	**Z** No Device	**Z** No Qualifier

Section **0** **Medical and Surgical**
Body System **D** **Gastrointestinal System**
Operation **T** **Resection:** Cutting out or off, without replacement, all of a body part

Body Part (4th)	Approach (5th)	Device (6th)	Qualifier (7th)
1 Esophagus, Upper **2** Esophagus, Middle **3** Esophagus, Lower **4** Esophagogastric Junction **5** Esophagus **6** Stomach **7** Stomach, Pylorus **8** Small Intestine **9** Duodenum **A** Jejunum **B** Ileum **C** Ileocecal Valve **E** Large Intestine **F** Large Intestine, Right **H** Cecum **J** Appendix **K** Ascending Colon **P** Rectum **Q** Anus	**0** Open **4** Percutaneous Endoscopic **7** Via Natural or Artificial Opening **8** Via Natural or Artificial Opening Endoscopic	**Z** No Device	**Z** No Qualifier
G Large Intestine, Left **L** Transverse Colon **M** Descending Colon **N** Sigmoid Colon	**0** Open **4** Percutaneous Endoscopic **7** Via Natural or Artificial Opening **8** Via Natural or Artificial Opening Endoscopic **F** Via Natural or Artificial Opening With Percutaneous Endoscopic Assistance	**Z** No Device	**Z** No Qualifier
R Anal Sphincter **U** Omentum	**0** Open **4** Percutaneous Endoscopic	**Z** No Device	**Z** No Qualifier

Section 0 **Medical and Surgical**
Body System D **Gastrointestinal System**
Operation U **Supplement:** Putting in or on biological or synthetic material that physically reinforces and/or augments the function of a portion of a body part

Body Part (4th)	Approach (5th)	Device (6th)	Qualifier (7th)
1 Esophagus, Upper 2 Esophagus, Middle 3 Esophagus, Lower 4 Esophagogastric Junction 5 Esophagus 6 Stomach 7 Stomach, Pylorus 8 Small Intestine 9 Duodenum A Jejunum B Ileum C Ileocecal Valve E Large Intestine F Large Intestine, Right G Large Intestine, Left H Cecum K Ascending Colon L Transverse Colon M Descending Colon N Sigmoid Colon P Rectum	0 Open 4 Percutaneous Endoscopic 7 Via Natural or Artificial Opening 8 Via Natural or Artificial Opening Endoscopic	7 Autologous Tissue Substitute J Synthetic Substitute K Nonautologous Tissue Substitute	Z No Qualifier
Q Anus	0 Open 4 Percutaneous Endoscopic 7 Via Natural or Artificial Opening 8 Via Natural or Artificial Opening Endoscopic X External	7 Autologous Tissue Substitute J Synthetic Substitute K Nonautologous Tissue Substitute	Z No Qualifier
R Anal Sphincter U Omentum V Mesentery W Peritoneum	0 Open 4 Percutaneous Endoscopic	7 Autologous Tissue Substitute J Synthetic Substitute K Nonautologous Tissue Substitute	Z No Qualifier

Section 0 **Medical and Surgical**
Body System D **Gastrointestinal System**
Operation V **Restriction:** Partially closing an orifice or the lumen of a tubular body part

Body Part (4th)	Approach (5th)	Device (6th)	Qualifier (7th)
1 Esophagus, Upper 2 Esophagus, Middle 3 Esophagus, Lower 4 Esophagogastric Junction 5 Esophagus 6 Stomach 7 Stomach, Pylorus 8 Small Intestine 9 Duodenum A Jejunum B Ileum C Ileocecal Valve E Large Intestine F Large Intestine, Right G Large Intestine, Left H Cecum K Ascending Colon L Transverse Colon M Descending Colon N Sigmoid Colon P Rectum	0 Open 3 Percutaneous 4 Percutaneous Endoscopic	C Extraluminal Device D Intraluminal Device Z No Device	Z No Qualifier

Continued →

Section 0 **Medical and Surgical**
Body System D **Gastrointestinal System**
Operation V **Restriction:** Partially closing an orifice or the lumen of a tubular body part

Body Part (4th)	Approach (5th)	Device (6th)	Qualifier (7th)
1 Esophagus, Upper **2** Esophagus, Middle **3** Esophagus, Lower **4** Esophagogastric Junction **5** Esophagus **6** Stomach **7** Stomach, Pylorus **8** Small Intestine **9** Duodenum **A** Jejunum **B** Ileum **C** Ileocecal Valve **E** Large Intestine **F** Large Intestine, Right **G** Large Intestine, Left **H** Cecum **K** Ascending Colon **L** Transverse Colon **M** Descending Colon **N** Sigmoid Colon **P** Rectum	**7** Via Natural or Artificial Opening **8** Via Natural or Artificial Opening Endoscopic	**D** Intraluminal Device **Z** No Device	**Z** No Qualifier
Q Anus	**0** Open **3** Percutaneous **4** Percutaneous Endoscopic **X** External	**C** Extraluminal Device **D** Intraluminal Device **Z** No Device	**Z** No Qualifier
Q Anus	**7** Via Natural or Artificial Opening **8** Via Natural or Artificial Opening Endoscopic	**D** Intraluminal Device **Z** No Device	**Z** No Qualifier

Section 0 **Medical and Surgical**
Body System D **Gastrointestinal System**
Operation W **Revision:** Correcting, to the extent possible, a portion of a malfunctioning device or the position of a displaced device

Body Part (4th)	Approach (5th)	Device (6th)	Qualifier (7th)
0 Upper Intestinal Tract **D** Lower Intestinal Tract	**0** Open **3** Percutaneous **4** Percutaneous Endoscopic **7** Via Natural or Artificial Opening **8** Via Natural or Artificial Opening Endoscopic	**0** Drainage Device **2** Monitoring Device **3** Infusion Device **7** Autologous Tissue Substitute **C** Extraluminal Device **D** Intraluminal Device **J** Synthetic Substitute **K** Nonautologous Tissue Substitute **U** Feeding Device **Y** Other Device	**Z** No Qualifier
0 Upper Intestinal Tract **D** Lower Intestinal Tract	**X** External	**0** Drainage Device **2** Monitoring Device **3** Infusion Device **7** Autologous Tissue Substitute **C** Extraluminal Device **D** Intraluminal Device **J** Synthetic Substitute **K** Nonautologous Tissue Substitute **U** Feeding Device	**Z** No Qualifier

Continued →

Section 0 **Medical and Surgical**
Body System D **Gastrointestinal System**
Operation W **Revision:** Correcting, to the extent possible, a portion of a malfunctioning device or the position of a displaced device

Body Part (4th)	Approach (5th)	Device (6th)	Qualifier (7th)
5 Esophagus	**0** Open **3** Percutaneous **4** Percutaneous Endoscopic	**Y** Other Device	**Z** No Qualifier
5 Esophagus	**7** Via Natural or Artificial Opening **8** Via Natural or Artificial Opening Endoscopic	**D** Intraluminal Device **Y** Other Device	**Z** No Qualifier
5 Esophagus	**X** External	**D** Intraluminal Device	**Z** No Qualifier
6 Stomach	**0** Open **3** Percutaneous **4** Percutaneous Endoscopic	**0** Drainage Device **2** Monitoring Device **3** Infusion Device **7** Autologous Tissue Substitute **C** Extraluminal Device **D** Intraluminal Device **J** Synthetic Substitute **K** Nonautologous Tissue Substitute **M** Stimulator Lead **U** Feeding Device **Y** Other Device	**Z** No Qualifier
6 Stomach	**7** Via Natural or Artificial Opening **8** Via Natural or Artificial Opening Endoscopic	**0** Drainage Device **2** Monitoring Device **3** Infusion Device **7** Autologous Tissue Substitute **C** Extraluminal Device **D** Intraluminal Device **J** Synthetic Substitute **K** Nonautologous Tissue Substitute **U** Feeding Device **Y** Other Device	**Z** No Qualifier
6 Stomach	**X** External	**0** Drainage Device **2** Monitoring Device **3** Infusion Device **7** Autologous Tissue Substitute **C** Extraluminal Device **D** Intraluminal Device **J** Synthetic Substitute **K** Nonautologous Tissue Substitute **U** Feeding Device	**Z** No Qualifier
8 Small Intestine **E** Large Intestine	**0** Open **4** Percutaneous Endoscopic **7** Via Natural or Artificial Opening **8** Via Natural or Artificial Opening Endoscopic	**7** Autologous Tissue Substitute **J** Synthetic Substitute **K** Nonautologous Tissue Substitute	**Z** No Qualifier
Q Anus	**0** Open **3** Percutaneous **4** Percutaneous Endoscopic **7** Via Natural or Artificial Opening **8** Via Natural or Artificial Opening Endoscopic	**L** Artificial Sphincter	**Z** No Qualifier
R Anal Sphincter	**0** Open **3** Percutaneous **4** Percutaneous Endoscopic	**M** Stimulator Lead	**Z** No Qualifier
U Omentum **V** Mesentery **W** Peritoneum	**0** Open **3** Percutaneous **4** Percutaneous Endoscopic	**0** Drainage Device **7** Autologous Tissue Substitute **J** Synthetic Substitute **K** Nonautologous Tissue Substitute	**Z** No Qualifier

Section 0 **Medical and Surgical**
Body System D **Gastrointestinal System**
Operation X **Transfer:** Moving, without taking out, all or a portion of a body part to another location to take over the function of all or a portion of a body part

Body Part (4th)	Approach (5th)	Device (6th)	Qualifier (7th)
6 Stomach 8 Small Intestine	0 Open 4 Percutaneous Endoscopic	Z No Device	5 Esophagus
E Large Intestine	0 Open 4 Percutaneous Endoscopic	Z No Device	5 Esophagus 7 Vagina

Section 0 **Medical and Surgical**
Body System D **Gastrointestinal System**
Operation Y **Transplantation:** Putting in or on all or a portion of a living body part taken from another individual or animal to physically take the place and/or function of all or a portion of a similar body part

Body Part (4th)	Approach (5th)	Device (6th)	Qualifier (7th)
5 Esophagus 6 Stomach 8 Small Intestine E Large Intestine	0 Open	Z No Device	0 Allogeneic 1 Syngeneic 2 Zooplastic

AHA Coding Clinic

0D160ZA Bypass Stomach to Jejunum, Open Approach—AHA CC: 2Q, 2017, 17-18
0D194ZB Bypass Duodenum to Ileum, Percutaneous Endoscopic Approach—AHA CC: 2Q, 2016, 31
0D1N0Z4 Bypass Sigmoid Colon to Cutaneous, Open Approach—AHA CC: 4Q, 2014, 41-42
0D2DXUZ Change Feeding Device in Lower Intestinal Tract, External Approach—AHA CC: 1Q, 2019, 26-27
0D5W0ZZ Destruction of Peritoneum, Open Approach—AHA CC: 1Q, 2017, 34-35
0D768ZZ Dilation of Stomach, Via Natural or Artificial Opening Endoscopic—AHA CC: 4Q, 2014, 40
0D7A8ZZ Dilation of Jejunum, Via Natural or Artificial Opening Endoscopic—AHA CC: 4Q, 2014, 40
0D844ZZ Division of Esophagogastric Junction, Percutaneous Endoscopic Approach—AHA CC: 3Q, 2017, 22-23
0D874ZZ Division of Stomach, Pylorus, Percutaneous Endoscopic Approach—AHA CC: 3Q, 2017, 23-24; 2Q, 2019, 15-16
0D9670Z Drainage of Stomach with Drainage Device, Via Natural or Artificial Opening—AHA CC: 2Q, 2015, 29
0DB28ZX Excision of Middle Esophagus, Via Natural or Artificial Opening Endoscopic, Diagnostic—AHA CC: 1Q, 2016, 24-25
0DB60ZZ Excision of Stomach, Open Approach—AHA CC: 2Q, 2017, 17-18; 1Q, 2019, 4-7
0DB64Z3 Excision of Stomach, Percutaneous Endoscopic Approach, Vertical—AHA CC: 2Q, 2016, 31
0DB80ZZ Excision of Small Intestine, Open Approach—AHA CC: 2Q, 2021, 11-12
0DB90ZZ Excision of Duodenum, Open Approach—AHA CC: 3Q, 2014, 32-33; 1Q, 2019, 4-7
0DBA0ZZ Excision of Jejunum, Open Approach—AHA CC: 1Q, 2019 4-5
0DBA4ZZ Excision of Jejunum, Percutaneous Endoscopic Approach—AHA CC: 2Q, 2019, 15-16
0DBB0ZZ Excision of Ileum, Open Approach—AHA CC: 3Q, 2014, 28-29; 3Q, 2016, 5-6
0DBK8ZZ Excision of Ascending Colon, Via Natural or Artificial Opening Endoscopic—AHA CC: 1Q, 2017, 16
0DBN0ZZ Excision of Sigmoid Colon, Open Approach—AHA CC: 4Q, 2014, 40-41; 1Q, 2019, 27
0DBP0ZZ Excision of Rectum, Open Approach—AHA CC: 1Q, 2019, 27
0DBP7ZZ Excision of Rectum, Via Natural or Artificial Opening—AHA CC: 1Q, 2016, 22
0DD68ZX Extraction of Stomach, Via Natural or Artificial Opening Endoscopic, Diagnostic—AHA CC: 4Q, 2017, 42
0DDP8ZX Extraction of Rectum, Via Natural or Artificial Opening Endoscopic, Diagnostic—AHA CC: 1Q, 2021, 20-21
0DH63UZ Insertion of Feeding Device into Stomach, Percutaneous Approach—AHA CC: 4Q, 2013, 117
0DH67UZ Insertion of Feeding Device into Stomach, Via Natural or Artificial Opening—AHA CC: 3Q, 2016, 26-27
0DH68YZ Insertion of Monitoring Device into Stomach, Via Natural or Artificial Opening Endoscopic—AHA CC: 2Q, 2019, 18
0DHA3UZ Insertion of Feeding Device into Jejunum, Percutaneous Approach—AHA CC: 3Q, 2020, 43
0DJ07ZZ Inspection of Upper Intestinal Tract, Via Natural or Artificial Opening—AHA CC: 2Q, 2016, 20-21

0DJ08ZZ Inspection of Upper Intestinal Tract, Via Natural or Artificial Opening Endoscopic—AHA CC: 3Q, 2015, 24-25
0DJD0ZZ Inspection of Lower Intestinal Tract, Open Approach—AHA CC: 1Q, 2019, 25-26
0DJD8ZZ Inspection of Lower Intestinal Tract, Via Natural or Artificial Opening Endoscopic—AHA CC: 2Q, 2017, 15-16
0DN50ZZ Release Esophagus, Open Approach—AHA CC: 3Q, 2015, 15-16
0DN80ZZ Release Small Intestine, Open Approach—AHA CC: 4Q, 2017, 49-50
0DNW0ZZ Release Peritoneum, Open Approach—AHA CC: 1Q, 2017, 35
0DP68YZ Removal of Other Device from Stomach, Via Natural or Artificial Opening Endoscopic—AHA CC: 2Q, 2019, 18-19
0DQ64ZZ Repair Stomach, Percutaneous Endoscopic Approach—AHA CC: 2Q, 2019, 15-16
0DQ98ZZ Repair Duodenum, Via Natural or Artificial Opening Endoscopic—AHA CC: 4Q, 2014, 20
0DQP0ZZ Repair Rectum, Open Approach—AHA CC: 1Q, 2016, 7-8
0DQR0ZZ Repair Anal Sphincter, Open Approach—AHA CC: 1Q, 2016, 7-8
0DQV4ZZ Repair Mesentery, Percutaneous Endoscopic Approach— AHA CC: 1Q, 2018, 11-12
0DS80ZZ Reposition Small Intestine, Open Approach—AHA CC: 4Q, 2017, 49-50
0DSB7ZZ Reposition Ileum, Via Natural or Artificial Opening—AHA CC: 3Q, 2017, 9-10
0DSE0ZZ Reposition Large Intestine, Open Approach—AHA CC: 4Q, 2017, 49-50
0DSK7ZZ Reposition Ascending Colon, Via Natural or Artificial Opening—AHA CC: 3Q, 2017, 9-10
0DSM4ZZ Reposition Descending Colon, Percutaneous Endoscopic Approach—AHA CC: 3Q, 2016, 5-6
0DSP0ZZ Reposition Rectum, Open Approach—AHA CC: 3Q, 2017, 17-18; 1Q, 2019, 30-31
0DT30ZZ Resection of Lower Esophagus, Open Approach—AHA CC: 1Q, 2019, 14-15
0DT90ZZ Resection of Duodenum, Open Approach—AHA CC: 1Q, 2019, 4-7
0DTF0ZZ Resection of Right Large Intestine, Open Approach—AHA CC: 3Q, 2014, 6-7; 4Q, 2014, 42-43
0DTH0ZZ Resection of Cecum, Open Approach—AHA CC: 3Q, 2014, 6
0DTJ0ZZ Resection of Appendix, Open Approach—AHA CC: 4Q, 2017, 49-50
0DTP0ZZ Resection of Rectum, Open Approach—AHA CC: 4Q, 2014, 40-41
0DTQ0ZZ Resection of Anus, Open Approach—AHA CC: 4Q, 2014, 40-41
0DUE07Z Supplement Large Intestine with Autologous Tissue Substitute, Open Approach—AHA CC: 2Q, 2021, 20-21
0DUP0JZ Supplement Rectum with Synthetic Substitute, Open Approach—AHA CC: 1Q, 2019, 30-31
0DUP47Z Supplement Rectum with Autologous Tissue Substitute, Percutaneous Endoscopic Approach—AHA CC: 1Q, 2021, 22-23
0DV40ZZ Restriction of Esophagogastric Junction, Open Approach—AHA CC: 2Q, 2016, 22-23
0DV44ZZ Restriction of Esophagogastric Junction, Percutaneous Endoscopic Approach—AHA CC: 3Q, 2014, 28; 3Q, 2017, 22-23
0DW63CZ Revision of Extraluminal Device in Stomach, Percutaneous Approach—AHA CC: 1Q, 2018, 20
0DW807Z Revision of Autologous Tissue Substitute in Small Intestine, Open Approach—AHA CC: 1Q, 2021, 19-20
0DX60Z5 Transfer Stomach to Esophagus, Open Approach—AHA CC: 2Q, 2016, 22-23; 2Q, 2017, 18
0DXE0Z5 Transfer Large Intestine to Esophagus, Open Approach—AHA CC: 1Q, 2019, 14-15
0DXE0Z7 Transfer Large Intestine to Vagina, Open Approach—AHA CC: 4Q, 2019, 30

Surfaces and Bed of Liver

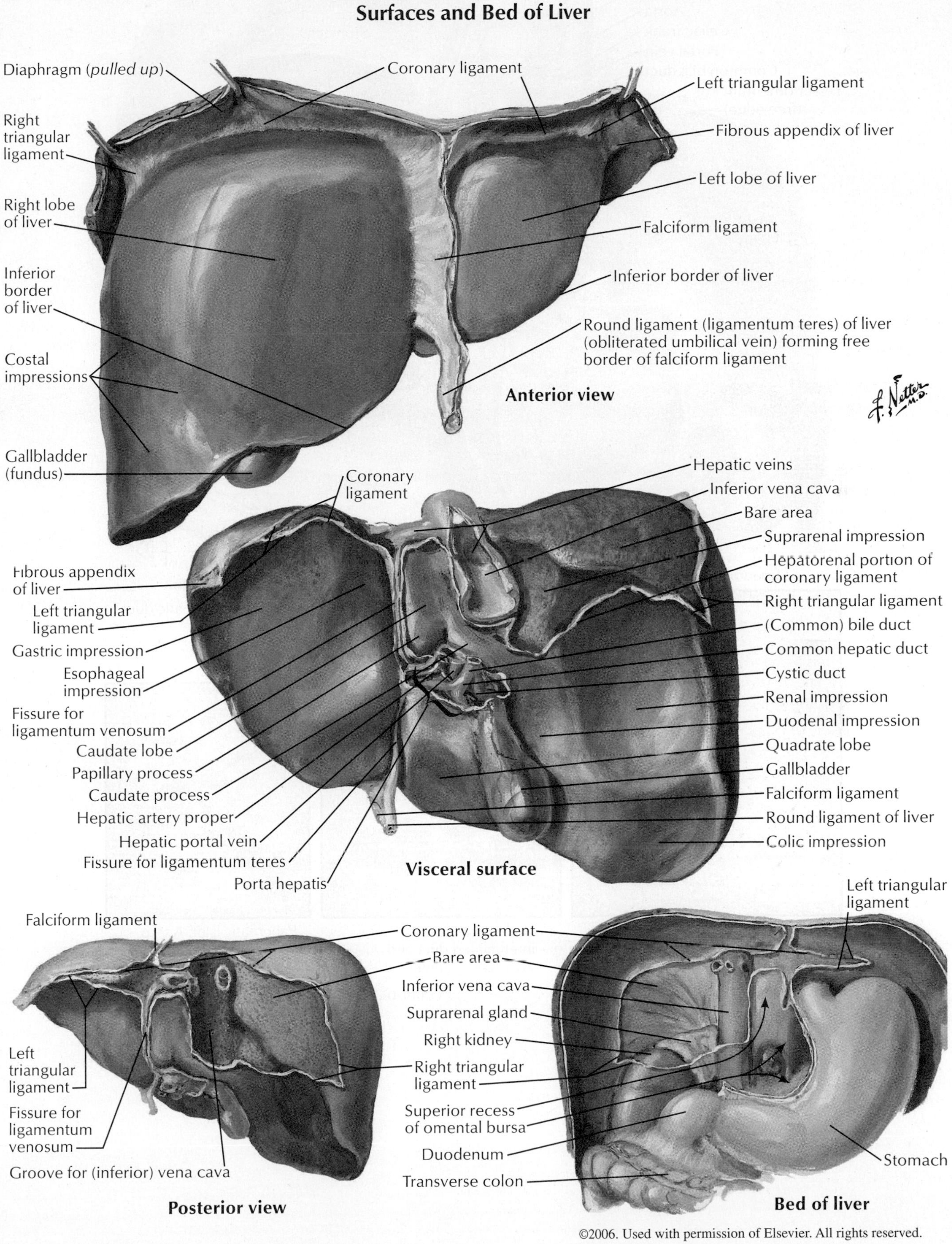
Surfaces and Bed of Liver
Diaphragm (pulled up)
Coronary ligament
Left triangular ligament
Right triangular ligament
Fibrous appendix of liver
Left lobe of liver
Right lobe of liver
Falciform ligament
Inferior border of liver
Inferior border of liver
Round ligament (ligamentum teres) of liver (obliterated umbilical vein) forming free border of falciform ligament
Costal impressions
Anterior view
Gallbladder (fundus)
Coronary ligament
Hepatic veins
Inferior vena cava
Bare area
Suprarenal impression
Hepatorenal portion of coronary ligament
Fibrous appendix of liver
Left triangular ligament
Right triangular ligament
Gastric impression
(Common) bile duct
Common hepatic duct
Esophageal impression
Cystic duct
Fissure for ligamentum venosum
Renal impression
Duodenal impression
Caudate lobe
Quadrate lobe
Papillary process
Gallbladder
Caudate process
Falciform ligament
Hepatic artery proper
Round ligament of liver
Hepatic portal vein
Colic impression
Fissure for ligamentum teres
Visceral surface
Porta hepatis
Left triangular ligament
Falciform ligament
Coronary ligament
Bare area
Inferior vena cava
Suprarenal gland
Right kidney
Left triangular ligament
Right triangular ligament
Superior recess of omental bursa
Fissure for ligamentum venosum
Duodenum
Stomach
Groove for (inferior) vena cava
Transverse colon
Posterior view
Bed of liver

Pancreas: Anatomy and Histology

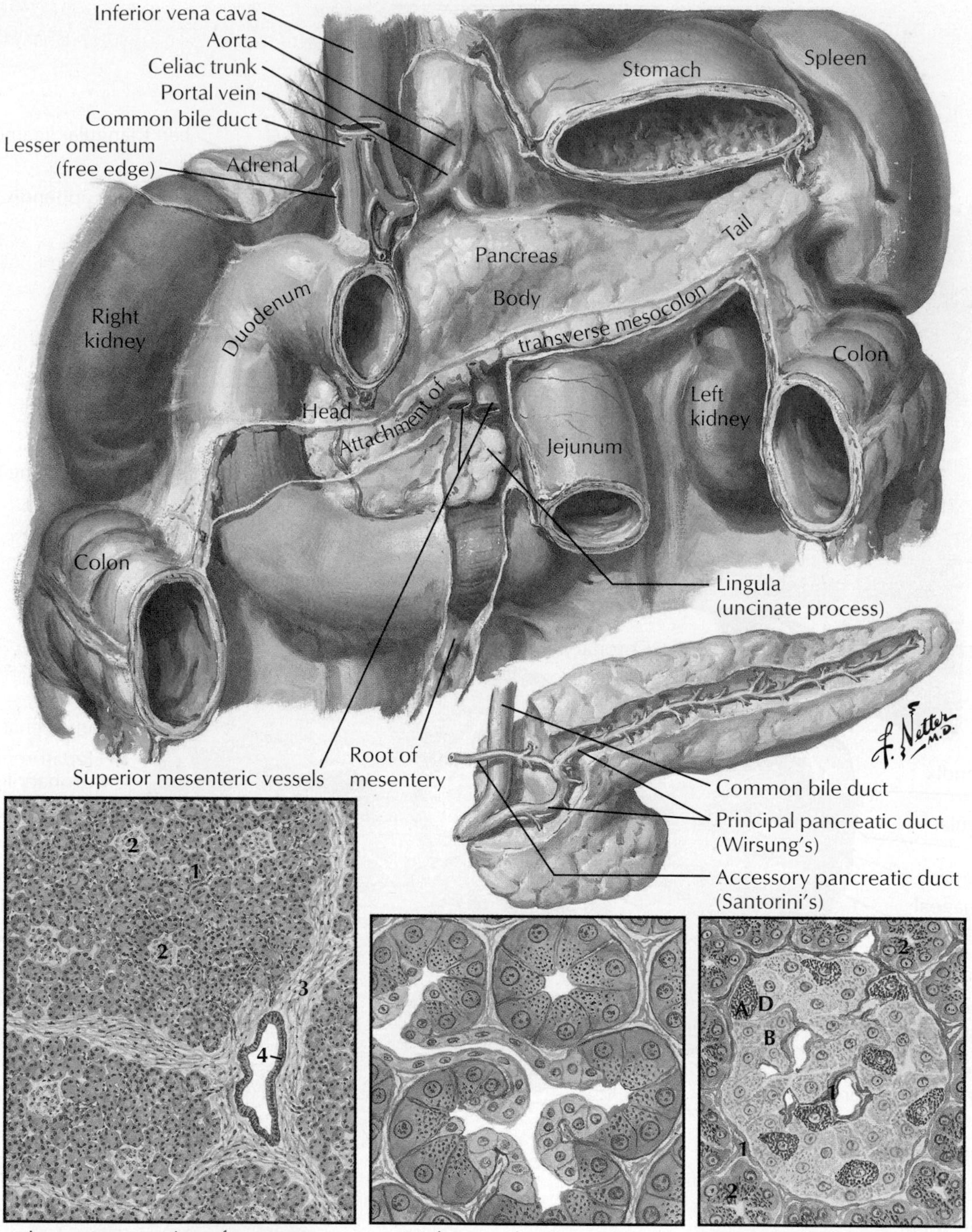
Inferior vena cava
Aorta
Celiac trunk
Portal vein
Common bile duct
Lesser omentum
(free edge)
Adrenal
Stomach
Spleen
Pancreas
Tail
Body
Duodenum
Right
kidney
transverse mesocolon
Attachment of
Head
Colon
Left
kidney
Jejunum
Colon
Lingula
(uncinate process)
Superior mesenteric vessels
Root of
mesentery
Common bile duct
Principal pancreatic duct
(Wirsung's)
Accessory pancreatic duct
(Santorini's)
F. Netter M.D.
2
1
2
3
4
A
D
B
1
1
2
2

Low-power section of pancreas
1. Acini, **2.** islet, **3.** interlobular septum, **4.** interlobular duct

High magnification: acini, intercalated duct and zymogen granules

Pancreatic islet: **A** (=α−), **B** (=β−), and **D** (=δ−) cells.
1. Reticulum, **2.** acini

Section 0 Medical and Surgical
Body System F Hepatobiliary System and Pancreas
Operation 1 **Bypass:** Altering the route of passage of the contents of a tubular body part

Body Part (4th)	Approach (5th)	Device (6th)	Qualifier (7th)
4 Gallbladder 5 Hepatic Duct, Right 6 Hepatic Duct, Left 7 Hepatic Duct, Common 8 Cystic Duct 9 Common Bile Duct	0 Open 4 Percutaneous Endoscopic	D Intraluminal Device Z No Device	3 Duodenum 4 Stomach 5 Hepatic Duct, Right 6 Hepatic Duct, Left 7 Hepatic Duct, Caudate 8 Cystic Duct 9 Common Bile Duct B Small Intestine
D Pancreatic Duct	0 Open 4 Percutaneous Endoscopic	D Intraluminal Device Z No Device	3 Duodenum 4 Stomach B Small Intestine C Large Intestine
F Pancreatic Duct, Accessory G Pancreas	0 Open 4 Percutaneous Endoscopic	D Intraluminal Device Z No Device	3 Duodenum B Small Intestine C Large Intestine

Section 0 Medical and Surgical
Body System F Hepatobiliary System and Pancreas
Operation 2 **Change:** Taking out or off a device from a body part and putting back an identical or similar device in or on the same body part without cutting or puncturing the skin or a mucous membrane

Body Part (4th)	Approach (5th)	Device (6th)	Qualifier (7th)
0 Liver 4 Gallbladder B Hepatobiliary Duct D Pancreatic Duct G Pancreas	X External	0 Drainage Device Y Other Device	Z No Qualifier

Section 0 Medical and Surgical
Body System F Hepatobiliary System and Pancreas
Operation 5 **Destruction:** Physical eradication of all or a portion of a body part by the direct use of energy, force, or a destructive agent

Body Part (4th)	Approach (5th)	Device (6th)	Qualifier (7th)
0 Liver 1 Liver, Right Lobe 2 Liver, Left Lobe	0 Open 3 Percutaneous 4 Percutaneous Endoscopic	Z No Device	F Irreversible Electroporation Z No Qualifier
4 Gallbladder	0 Open 3 Percutaneous 4 Percutaneous Endoscopic 8 Via Natural or Artificial Opening Endoscopic	Z No Device	Z No Qualifier
5 Hepatic Duct, Right 6 Hepatic Duct, Left 7 Hepatic Duct, Common 8 Cystic Duct 9 Common Bile Duct C Ampulla of Vater D Pancreatic Duct F Pancreatic Duct, Accessory	0 Open 3 Percutaneous 4 Percutaneous Endoscopic 7 Via Natural or Artificial Opening 8 Via Natural or Artificial Opening Endoscopic	Z No Device	Z No Qualifier
G Pancreas	0 Open 3 Percutaneous 4 Percutaneous Endoscopic	Z No Device	F Irreversible Electroporation Z No Qualifier
G Pancreas	8 Via Natural or Artificial Opening Endoscopic	Z No Device	Z No Qualifier

Section 0 **Medical and Surgical**
Body System F **Hepatobiliary System and Pancreas**
Operation 7 **Dilation:** Expanding an orifice or the lumen of a tubular body part

Body Part (4th)	Approach (5th)	Device (6th)	Qualifier (7th)
5 Hepatic Duct, Right 6 Hepatic Duct, Left 7 Hepatic Duct, Common 8 Cystic Duct 9 Common Bile Duct C Ampulla of Vater D Pancreatic Duct F Pancreatic Duct, Accessory	0 Open 3 Percutaneous 4 Percutaneous Endoscopic 7 Via Natural or Artificial Opening 8 Via Natural or Artificial Opening Endoscopic	D Intraluminal Device Z No Device	Z No Qualifier

Section 0 **Medical and Surgical**
Body System F **Hepatobiliary System and Pancreas**
Operation 8 **Division:** Cutting into a body part, without draining fluids and/or gases from the body part, in order to separate or transect a body part

Body Part (4th)	Approach (5th)	Device (6th)	Qualifier (7th)
0 Liver 1 Liver, Right Lobe 2 Liver, Left Lobe G Pancreas	0 Open 3 Percutaneous 4 Percutaneous Endoscopic	Z No Device	Z No Qualifier

Section 0 **Medical and Surgical**
Body System F **Hepatobiliary System and Pancreas**
Operation 9 **Drainage:** Taking or letting out fluids and/or gases from a body part

Body Part (4th)	Approach (5th)	Device (6th)	Qualifier (7th)
0 Liver 1 Liver, Right Lobe 2 Liver, Left Lobe	0 Open 3 Percutaneous 4 Percutaneous Endoscopic	0 Drainage Device	Z No Qualifier
0 Liver 1 Liver, Right Lobe 2 Liver, Left Lobe	0 Open 3 Percutaneous 4 Percutaneous Endoscopic	Z No Device	X Diagnostic Z No Qualifier
4 Gallbladder G Pancreas	0 Open 3 Percutaneous 4 Percutaneous Endoscopic 8 Via Natural or Artificial Opening Endoscopic	0 Drainage Device	Z No Qualifier
4 Gallbladder G Pancreas	0 Open 3 Percutaneous 4 Percutaneous Endoscopic 8 Via Natural or Artificial Opening Endoscopic	Z No Device	X Diagnostic Z No Qualifier
5 Hepatic Duct, Right 6 Hepatic Duct, Left 7 Hepatic Duct, Common 8 Cystic Duct 9 Common Bile Duct C Ampulla of Vater D Pancreatic Duct F Pancreatic Duct, Accessory	0 Open 3 Percutaneous 4 Percutaneous Endoscopic 7 Via Natural or Artificial Opening 8 Via Natural or Artificial Opening Endoscopic	0 Drainage Device	Z No Qualifier
5 Hepatic Duct, Right 6 Hepatic Duct, Left 7 Hepatic Duct, Common 8 Cystic Duct 9 Common Bile Duct C Ampulla of Vater D Pancreatic Duct F Pancreatic Duct, Accessory	0 Open 3 Percutaneous 4 Percutaneous Endoscopic 7 Via Natural or Artificial Opening 8 Via Natural or Artificial Opening Endoscopic	Z No Device	X Diagnostic Z No Qualifier

Section	**0**	**Medical and Surgical**
Body System	**F**	**Hepatobiliary System and Pancreas**
Operation	**B**	**Excision:** Cutting out or off, without replacement, a portion of a body part

Body Part (4th)	Approach (5th)	Device (6th)	Qualifier (7th)
0 Liver **1** Liver, Right Lobe **2** Liver, Left Lobe	**0** Open **3** Percutaneous **4** Percutaneous Endoscopic	**Z** No Device	**X** Diagnostic **Z** No Qualifier
4 Gallbladder **G** Pancreas	**0** Open **3** Percutaneous **4** Percutaneous Endoscopic **8** Via Natural or Artificial Opening Endoscopic	**Z** No Device	**X** Diagnostic **Z** No Qualifier
5 Hepatic Duct, Right **6** Hepatic Duct, Left **7** Hepatic Duct, Common **8** Cystic Duct **9** Common Bile Duct **C** Ampulla of Vater **D** Pancreatic Duct **F** Pancreatic Duct, Accessory	**0** Open **3** Percutaneous **4** Percutaneous Endoscopic **7** Via Natural or Artificial Opening **8** Via Natural or Artificial Opening Endoscopic	**Z** No Device	**X** Diagnostic **Z** No Qualifier

Section	**0**	**Medical and Surgical**
Body System	**F**	**Hepatobiliary System and Pancreas**
Operation	**C**	**Extirpation:** Taking or cutting out solid matter from a body part

Body Part (4th)	Approach (5th)	Device (6th)	Qualifier (7th)
0 Liver **1** Liver, Right Lobe **2** Liver, Left Lobe	**0** Open **3** Percutaneous **4** Percutaneous Endoscopic	**Z** No Device	**Z** No Qualifier
4 Gallbladder **G** Pancreas	**0** Open **3** Percutaneous **4** Percutaneous Endoscopic **8** Via Natural or Artificial Opening Endoscopic	**Z** No Device	**Z** No Qualifier
5 Hepatic Duct, Right **6** Hepatic Duct, Left **7** Hepatic Duct, Common **8** Cystic Duct **9** Common Bile Duct **C** Ampulla of Vater **D** Pancreatic Duct **F** Pancreatic Duct, Accessory	**0** Open **3** Percutaneous **4** Percutaneous Endoscopic **7** Via Natural or Artificial Opening **8** Via Natural or Artificial Opening Endoscopic	**Z** No Device	**Z** No Qualifier

Section	**0**	**Medical and Surgical**
Body System	**F**	**Hepatobiliary System and Pancreas**
Operation	**D**	**Extraction:** Pulling or stripping out or off all or a portion of a body part by the use of force

Body Part (4th)	Approach (5th)	Device (6th)	Qualifier (7th)
0 Liver **1** Liver, Right Lobe **2** Liver, Left Lobe	**3** Percutaneous **4** Percutaneous Endoscopic	**Z** No Device	**X** Diagnostic
4 Gallbladder **5** Hepatic Duct, Right **6** Hepatic Duct, Left **7** Hepatic Duct, Common **8** Cystic Duct **9** Common Bile Duct **C** Ampulla of Vater **D** Pancreatic Duct **F** Pancreatic Duct, Accessory **G** Pancreas	**3** Percutaneous **4** Percutaneous Endoscopic **8** Via Natural or Artificial Opening Endoscopic	**Z** No Device	**X** Diagnostic

Section 0 **Medical and Surgical**
Body System F **Hepatobiliary System and Pancreas**
Operation F **Fragmentation:** Breaking solid matter in a body part into pieces

Body Part (4th)	Approach (5th)	Device (6th)	Qualifier (7th)
4 Gallbladder **5** Hepatic Duct, Right **6** Hepatic Duct, Left **7** Hepatic Duct, Common **8** Cystic Duct **9** Common Bile Duct **C** Ampulla of Vater **D** Pancreatic Duct **F** Pancreatic Duct, Accessory	**0** Open **3** Percutaneous **4** Percutaneous Endoscopic **7** Via Natural or Artificial Opening **8** Via Natural or Artificial Opening Endoscopic **X** External	**Z** No Device	**Z** No Qualifier

Section 0 **Medical and Surgical**
Body System F **Hepatobiliary System and Pancreas**
Operation H **Insertion:** Putting in a nonbiological appliance that monitors, assists, performs, or prevents a physiological function but does not physically take the place of a body part

Body Part (4th)	Approach (5th)	Device (6th)	Qualifier (7th)
0 Liver **4** Gallbladder **G** Pancreas	**0** Open **3** Percutaneous **4** Percutaneous Endoscopic	**1** Radioactive Element **2** Monitoring Device **3** Infusion Device **Y** Other Device	**Z** No Qualifier
1 Liver, Right Lobe **2** Liver, Left Lobe	**0** Open **3** Percutaneous **4** Percutaneous Endoscopic	**2** Monitoring Device **3** Infusion Device	**Z** No Qualifier
B Hepatobiliary Duct **D** Pancreatic Duct	**0** Open **3** Percutaneous **4** Percutaneous Endoscopic **7** Via Natural or Artificial Opening **8** Via Natural or Artificial Opening Endoscopic	**1** Radioactive Element **2** Monitoring Device **3** Infusion Device **D** Intraluminal Device **Y** Other Device	**Z** No Qualifier

Section 0 **Medical and Surgical**
Body System F **Hepatobiliary System and Pancreas**
Operation J **Inspection:** Visually and/or manually exploring a body part

Body Part (4th)	Approach (5th)	Device (6th)	Qualifier (7th)
0 Liver	**0** Open **3** Percutaneous **4** Percutaneous Endoscopic **X** External	**Z** No Device	**Z** No Qualifier
4 Gallbladder **G** Pancreas	**0** Open **3** Percutaneous **4** Percutaneous Endoscopic **8** Via Natural or Artificial Opening Endoscopic **X** External	**Z** No Device	**Z** No Qualifier
B Hepatobiliary Duct **D** Pancreatic Duct	**0** Open **3** Percutaneous **4** Percutaneous Endoscopic **7** Via Natural or Artificial Opening **8** Via Natural or Artificial Opening Endoscopic	**Z** No Device	**Z** No Qualifier

Section 0 **Medical and Surgical**
Body System F **Hepatobiliary System and Pancreas**
Operation L **Occlusion:** Completely closing an orifice or the lumen of a tubular body part

Body Part (4th)	Approach (5th)	Device (6th)	Qualifier (7th)
5 Hepatic Duct, Right **6** Hepatic Duct, Left **7** Hepatic Duct, Common **8** Cystic Duct **9** Common Bile Duct **C** Ampulla of Vater **D** Pancreatic Duct **F** Pancreatic Duct, Accessory	**0** Open **3** Percutaneous **4** Percutaneous Endoscopic	**C** Extraluminal Device **D** Intraluminal Device **Z** No Device	**Z** No Qualifier
5 Hepatic Duct, Right **6** Hepatic Duct, Left **7** Hepatic Duct, Common **8** Cystic Duct **9** Common Bile Duct **C** Ampulla of Vater **D** Pancreatic Duct **F** Pancreatic Duct, Accessory	**7** Via Natural or Artificial Opening **8** Via Natural or Artificial Opening Endoscopic	**D** Intraluminal Device **Z** No Device	**Z** No Qualifier

Section 0 **Medical and Surgical**
Body System F **Hepatobiliary System and Pancreas**
Operation M **Reattachment:** Putting back in or on all or a portion of a separated body part to its normal location or other suitable location

Body Part (4th)	Approach (5th)	Device (6th)	Qualifier (7th)
0 Liver **1** Liver, Right Lobe **2** Liver, Left Lobe **4** Gallbladder **5** Hepatic Duct, Right **6** Hepatic Duct, Left **7** Hepatic Duct, Common **8** Cystic Duct **9** Common Bile Duct **C** Ampulla of Vater **D** Pancreatic Duct **F** Pancreatic Duct, Accessory **G** Pancreas	**0** Open **4** Percutaneous Endoscopic	**Z** No Device	**Z** No Qualifier

Section 0 **Medical and Surgical**
Body System F **Hepatobiliary System and Pancreas**
Operation N **Release:** Freeing a body part from an abnormal physical constraint by cutting or by the use of force

Body Part (4th)	Approach (5th)	Device (6th)	Qualifier (7th)
0 Liver **1** Liver, Right Lobe **2** Liver, Left Lobe	**0** Open **3** Percutaneous **4** Percutaneous Endoscopic	**Z** No Device	**Z** No Qualifier
4 Gallbladder **G** Pancreas	**0** Open **3** Percutaneous **4** Percutaneous Endoscopic **8** Via Natural or Artificial Opening Endoscopic	**Z** No Device	**Z** No Qualifier
5 Hepatic Duct, Right **6** Hepatic Duct, Left **7** Hepatic Duct, Common **8** Cystic Duct **9** Common Bile Duct **C** Ampulla of Vater **D** Pancreatic Duct **F** Pancreatic Duct, Accessory	**0** Open **3** Percutaneous **4** Percutaneous Endoscopic **7** Via Natural or Artificial Opening **8** Via Natural or Artificial Opening Endoscopic	**Z** No Device	**Z** No Qualifier

Section 0 **Medical and Surgical**
Body System F **Hepatobiliary System and Pancreas**
Operation P **Removal:** Taking out or off a device from a body part

Body Part (4th)	Approach (5th)	Device (6th)	Qualifier (7th)
0 Liver	**0** Open **3** Percutaneous **4** Percutaneous Endoscopic	**0** Drainage Device **2** Monitoring Device **3** Infusion Device **Y** Other Device	**Z** No Qualifier
0 Liver	**X** External	**0** Drainage Device **2** Monitoring Device **3** Infusion Device	**Z** No Qualifier
4 Gallbladder **G** Pancreas	**0** Open **3** Percutaneous **4** Percutaneous Endoscopic **X** External	**0** Drainage Device **2** Monitoring Device **3** Infusion Device **D** Intraluminal Device **Y** Other Device	**Z** No Qualifier
4 Gallbladder **G** Pancreas	**X** External	**0** Drainage Device **2** Monitoring Device **3** Infusion Device **D** Intraluminal Device	**Z** No Qualifier
B Hepatobiliary Duct **D** Pancreatic Duct	**0** Open **3** Percutaneous **4** Percutaneous Endoscopic **7** Via Natural or Artificial Opening **8** Via Natural or Artificial Opening Endoscopic	**0** Drainage Device **1** Radioactive Element **2** Monitoring Device **3** Infusion Device **7** Autologous Tissue Substitute **C** Extraluminal Device **D** Intraluminal Device **J** Synthetic Substitute **K** Nonautologous Tissue Substitute **Y** Other Device	**Z** No Qualifier
B Hepatobiliary Duct **D** Pancreatic Duct	**X** External	**0** Drainage Device **1** Radioactive Element **2** Monitoring Device **3** Infusion Device **D** Intraluminal Device	**Z** No Qualifier

Section 0 **Medical and Surgical**
Body System F **Hepatobiliary System and Pancreas**
Operation Q **Repair:** Restoring, to the extent possible, a body part to its normal anatomic structure and function

Body Part (4th)	Approach (5th)	Device (6th)	Qualifier (7th)
0 Liver **1** Liver, Right Lobe **2** Liver, Left Lobe	**0** Open **3** Percutaneous **4** Percutaneous Endoscopic	**Z** No Device	**Z** No Qualifier
4 Gallbladder **G** Pancreas	**0** Open **3** Percutaneous **4** Percutaneous Endoscopic **8** Via Natural or Artificial Opening Endoscopic	**Z** No Device	**Z** No Qualifier
5 Hepatic Duct, Right **6** Hepatic Duct, Left **7** Hepatic Duct, Common **8** Cystic Duct **9** Common Bile Duct **C** Ampulla of Vater **D** Pancreatic Duct **F** Pancreatic Duct, Accessory	**0** Open **3** Percutaneous **4** Percutaneous Endoscopic **7** Via Natural or Artificial Opening **8** Via Natural or Artificial Opening Endoscopic	**Z** No Device	**Z** No Qualifier

Section 0 **Medical and Surgical**
Body System F **Hepatobiliary System and Pancreas**
Operation R **Replacement:** Putting in or on biological or synthetic material that physically takes the place and/or function of all or a portion of a body part

Body Part (4th)	Approach (5th)	Device (6th)	Qualifier (7th)
5 Hepatic Duct, Right **6** Hepatic Duct, Left **7** Hepatic Duct, Common **8** Cystic Duct **9** Common Bile Duct **C** Ampulla of Vater **D** Pancreatic Duct **F** Pancreatic Duct, Accessory	**0** Open **4** Percutaneous Endoscopic **8** Via Natural or Artificial Opening Endoscopic	**7** Autologous Tissue Substitute **J** Synthetic Substitute **K** Nonautologous Tissue Substitute	**Z** No Qualifier

Section 0 **Medical and Surgical**
Body System F **Hepatobiliary System and Pancreas**
Operation S **Reposition:** Moving to its normal location, or other suitable location, all or a portion of a body part

Body Part (4th)	Approach (5th)	Device (6th)	Qualifier (7th)
0 Liver **4** Gallbladder **5** Hepatic Duct, Right **6** Hepatic Duct, Left **7** Hepatic Duct, Common **8** Cystic Duct **9** Common Bile Duct **C** Ampulla of Vater **D** Pancreatic Duct **F** Pancreatic Duct, Accessory **G** Pancreas	**0** Open **4** Percutaneous Endoscopic	**Z** No Device	**Z** No Qualifier

Section 0 **Medical and Surgical**
Body System F **Hepatobiliary System and Pancreas**
Operation T **Resection:** Cutting out or off, without replacement, all of a body part

Body Part (4th)	Approach (5th)	Device (6th)	Qualifier (7th)
0 Liver **1** Liver, Right Lobe **2** Liver, Left Lobe **4** Gallbladder **G** Pancreas	**0** Open **4** Percutaneous Endoscopic	**Z** No Device	**Z** No Qualifier
5 Hepatic Duct, Right **6** Hepatic Duct, Left **7** Hepatic Duct, Common **8** Cystic Duct **9** Common Bile Duct **C** Ampulla of Vater **D** Pancreatic Duct **F** Pancreatic Duct, Accessory	**0** Open **4** Percutaneous Endoscopic **7** Via Natural or Artificial Opening **8** Via Natural or Artificial Opening Endoscopic	**Z** No Device	**Z** No Qualifier

Section 0 **Medical and Surgical**
Body System F **Hepatobiliary System and Pancreas**
Operation U **Supplement:** Putting in or on biological or synthetic material that physically reinforces and/or augments the function of a portion of a body part

Body Part (4th)	Approach (5th)	Device (6th)	Qualifier (7th)
5 Hepatic Duct, Right **6** Hepatic Duct, Left **7** Hepatic Duct, Common **8** Cystic Duct **9** Common Bile Duct **C** Ampulla of Vater **D** Pancreatic Duct **F** Pancreatic Duct, Accessory	**0** Open **3** Percutaneous **4** Percutaneous Endoscopic **8** Via Natural or Artificial Opening Endoscopic	**7** Autologous Tissue Substitute **J** Synthetic Substitute **K** Nonautologous Tissue Substitute	**Z** No Qualifier

Section 0 **Medical and Surgical**
Body System F **Hepatobiliary System and Pancreas**
Operation V **Restriction:** Partially closing an orifice or the lumen of a tubular body part

Body Part (4th)	Approach (5th)	Device (6th)	Qualifier (7th)
5 Hepatic Duct, Right **6** Hepatic Duct, Left **7** Hepatic Duct, Common **8** Cystic Duct **9** Common Bile Duct **C** Ampulla of Vater **D** Pancreatic Duct **F** Pancreatic Duct, Accessory	**0** Open **3** Percutaneous **4** Percutaneous Endoscopic	**C** Extraluminal Device **D** Intraluminal Device **Z** No Device	**Z** No Qualifier
5 Hepatic Duct, Right **6** Hepatic Duct, Left **7** Hepatic Duct, Common **8** Cystic Duct **9** Common Bile Duct **C** Ampulla of Vater **D** Pancreatic Duct **F** Pancreatic Duct, Accessory	**7** Via Natural or Artificial Opening **8** Via Natural or Artificial Opening Endoscopic	**D** Intraluminal Device **Z** No Device	**Z** No Qualifier

Section 0 **Medical and Surgical**
Body System F **Hepatobiliary System and Pancreas**
Operation W **Revision:** Correcting, to the extent possible, a portion of a malfunctioning device or the position of a displaced device

Body Part (4th)	Approach (5th)	Device (6th)	Qualifier (7th)
0 Liver	**0** Open **3** Percutaneous **4** Percutaneous Endoscopic	**0** Drainage Device **2** Monitoring Device **3** Infusion Device **Y** Other Device	**Z** No Qualifier
0 Liver	**X** External	**0** Drainage Device **2** Monitoring Device **3** Infusion Device	**Z** No Qualifier
4 Gallbladder **G** Pancreas	**0** Open **3** Percutaneous **4** Percutaneous Endoscopic	**0** Drainage Device **2** Monitoring Device **3** Infusion Device **D** Intraluminal Device **Y** Other Device	**Z** No Qualifier
4 Gallbladder **G** Pancreas	**X** External	**0** Drainage Device **2** Monitoring Device **3** Infusion Device **D** Intraluminal Device	**Z** No Qualifier

Continued

Section 0 Medical and Surgical
Body System F Hepatobiliary System and Pancreas
Operation W **Revision:** Correcting, to the extent possible, a portion of a malfunctioning device or the position of a displaced device

Body Part (4th)	Approach (5th)	Device (6th)	Qualifier (7th)
B Hepatobiliary Duct **D** Pancreatic Duct	**0** Open **3** Percutaneous **4** Percutaneous Endoscopic **7** Via Natural or Artificial Opening **8** Via Natural or Artificial Opening Endoscopic	**0** Drainage Device **2** Monitoring Device **3** Infusion Device **7** Autologous Tissue Substitute **C** Extraluminal Device **D** Intraluminal Device **J** Synthetic Substitute **K** Nonautologous Tissue Substitute **Y** Other Device	**Z** No Qualifier
B Hepatobiliary Duct **D** Pancreatic Duct	**X** External	**0** Drainage Device **2** Monitoring Device **3** Infusion Device **7** Autologous Tissue Substitute **C** Extraluminal Device **D** Intraluminal Device **J** Synthetic Substitute **K** Nonautologous Tissue Substitute	**Z** No Qualifier

Section 0 Medical and Surgical
Body System F Hepatobiliary System and Pancreas
Operation Y **Transplantation:** Putting in or on all or a portion of a living body part taken from another individual or animal to physically take the place and/or function of all or a portion of a similar body part

Body Part (4th)	Approach (5th)	Device (6th)	Qualifier (7th)
0 Liver **G** Pancreas	**0** Open	**Z** No Device	**0** Allogeneic **1** Syngeneic **2** Zooplastic

AHA Coding Clinic

0F1D4Z4 Bypass Pancreatic Duct to Stomach, Percutaneous Endoscopic Approach—AHA CC: 4Q, 2020, 53-54

0F5G4ZF Destruction of Pancreas using Irreversible Electroporation, Percutaneous Endoscopic Approach—AHA CC: 4Q, 2018, 39-40

0F798DZ Dilation of Common Bile Duct with Intraluminal Device, Via Natural or Artificial Opening Endoscopic—AHA CC: 3Q, 2014, 15-16; 1Q, 2016, 25

0F7D8DZ Dilation of Pancreatic Duct with Intraluminal Device, Via Natural or Artificial Opening Endoscopic—AHA CC: 1Q, 2016, 25; 3Q, 2016, 27-28

0F9630Z Drainage of Left Hepatic Duct with Drainage Device, Percutaneous Approach—AHA CC: 1Q, 2015, 32

0F9G40Z Drainage of Pancreas with Drainage Device, Percutaneous Endoscopic Approach AHA CC: 3Q, 2014, 15-16

0F9G80Z Drainage of Pancreas with Drainage Device, Via Natural or Artificial Opening Endoscopic—AHA CC: 3Q, 2020 34-35

0FB00ZX Excision of Liver, Open Approach, Diagnostic—AHA CC: 3Q, 2016, 41

0FB90ZZ Excision of Common Bile Duct, Open Approach—AHA CC: 1Q, 2019, 4-7

0FB98ZX Excision of Common Bile Duct, Via Natural or Artificial Opening Endoscopic, Diagnostic—AHA CC: 1Q, 2016, 23-25

0FBD8ZX Excision of Pancreatic Duct, Via Natural or Artificial Opening Endoscopic, Diagnostic—AHA CC: 1Q, 2016, 25

0FBG0ZZ Excision of Pancreas, Open Approach—AHA CC: 3Q, 2014, 32-33; 1Q, 2019, 4-8

0FQ00ZZ Repair Liver, Open Approach—AHA CC: 4Q, 2013, 109-111

0FQ90ZZ Repair Common Bile Duct, Open Approach—AHA CC: 3Q, 2016, 27

0FT00ZZ Resection of Liver, Open Approach—AHA CC: 4Q, 2012, 99-101

0FT40ZZ Resection of Gallbladder, Open Approach—AHA CC: 1Q, 2019, 4-5

0FY00Z0 Transplantation of Liver, Allogeneic, Open Approach—AHA CC: 4Q, 2012, 99-101; 3Q, 2014, 13-14

Endocrine System

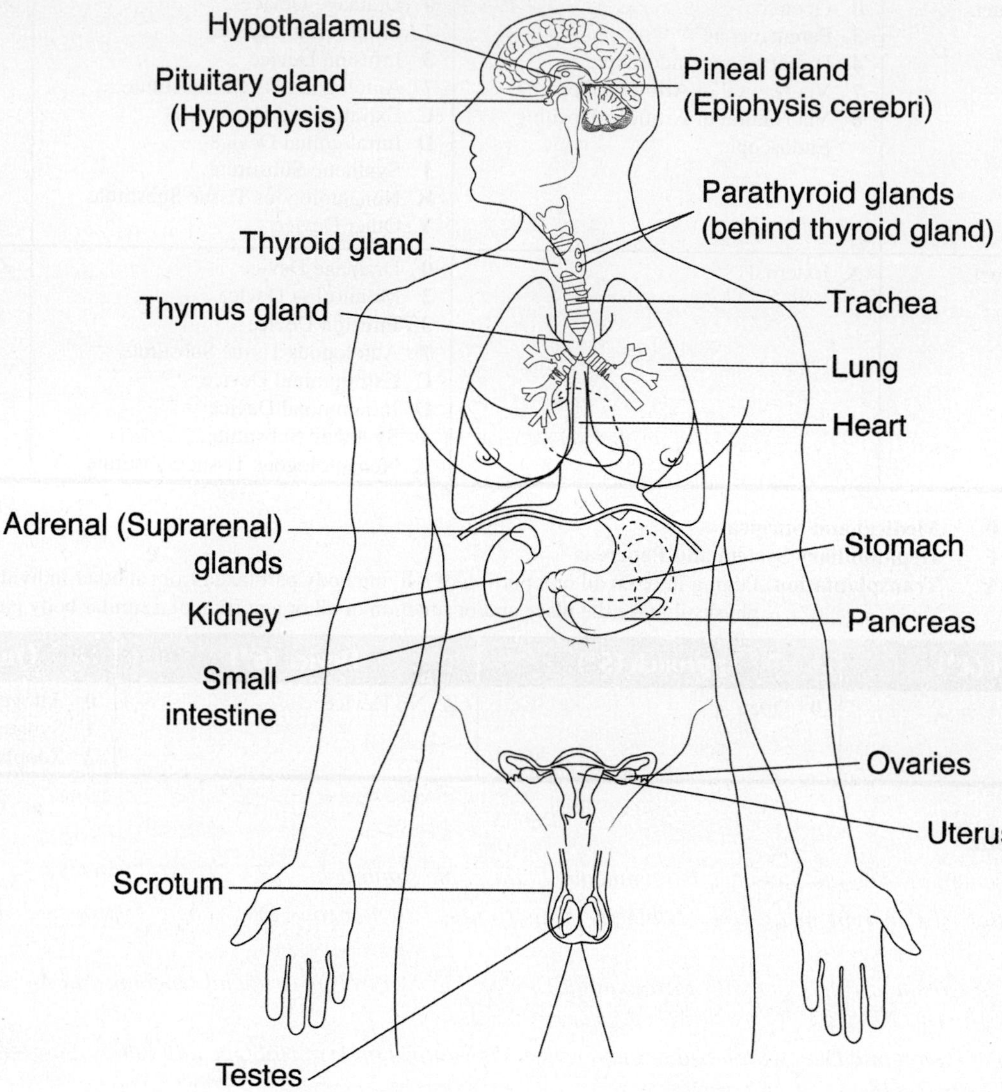
Hypothalamus
Pituitary gland
(Hypophysis)
Pineal gland
(Epiphysis cerebri)
Parathyroid glands
(behind thyroid gland)
Thyroid gland
Thymus gland
Trachea
Lung
Heart
Adrenal (Suprarenal)
glands
Stomach
Kidney
Pancreas
Small
intestine
Ovaries
Uterus
Scrotum
Testes

Endocrine System Tables 0G2–0GW

Section 0 **Medical and Surgical**
Body System G **Endocrine System**
Operation 2 **Change:** Taking out or off a device from a body part and putting back an identical or similar device in or on the same body part without cutting or puncturing the skin or a mucous membrane

Body Part (4th)	Approach (5th)	Device (6th)	Qualifier (7th)
0 Pituitary Gland **1** Pineal Body **5** Adrenal Gland **K** Thyroid Gland **R** Parathyroid Gland **S** Endocrine Gland	**X** External	**0** Drainage Device **Y** Other Device	**Z** No Qualifier

Section 0 **Medical and Surgical**
Body System G **Endocrine System**
Operation 5 **Destruction:** Physical eradication of all or a portion of a body part by the direct use of energy, force, or a destructive agent

Body Part (4th)	Approach (5th)	Device (6th)	Qualifier (7th)
0 Pituitary Gland **1** Pineal Body **2** Adrenal Gland, Left **3** Adrenal Gland, Right **4** Adrenal Glands, Bilateral **6** Carotid Body, Left **7** Carotid Body, Right **8** Carotid Bodies, Bilateral **9** Para-aortic Body **B** Coccygeal Glomus **C** Glomus Jugulare **D** Aortic Body **F** Paraganglion Extremity **G** Thyroid Gland Lobe, Left **H** Thyroid Gland Lobe, Right **K** Thyroid Gland **L** Superior Parathyroid Gland, Right **M** Superior Parathyroid Gland, Left **N** Inferior Parathyroid Gland, Right **P** Inferior Parathyroid Gland, Left **Q** Parathyroid Glands, Multiple **R** Parathyroid Gland	**0** Open **3** Percutaneous **4** Percutaneous Endoscopic	**Z** No Device	**Z** No Qualifier

Section 0 **Medical and Surgical**
Body System G **Endocrine System**
Operation 8 **Division:** Cutting into a body part, without draining fluids and/or gases from the body part, in order to separate or transect a body part

Body Part (4th)	Approach (5th)	Device (6th)	Qualifier (7th)
0 Pituitary Gland **J** Thyroid Gland Isthmus	**0** Open **3** Percutaneous **4** Percutaneous Endoscopic	**Z** No Device	**Z** No Qualifier

Section 0 **Medical and Surgical**
Body System G **Endocrine System**
Operation 9 **Drainage:** Taking or letting out fluids and/or gases from a body part

Body Part (4th)	Approach (5th)	Device (6th)	Qualifier (7th)
0 Pituitary Gland **1** Pineal Body **2** Adrenal Gland, Left **3** Adrenal Gland, Right **4** Adrenal Glands, Bilateral **6** Carotid Body, Left **7** Carotid Body, Right **8** Carotid Bodies, Bilateral **9** Para-aortic Body **B** Coccygeal Glomus **C** Glomus Jugulare **D** Aortic Body **F** Paraganglion Extremity **G** Thyroid Gland Lobe, Left **H** Thyroid Gland Lobe, Right **K** Thyroid Gland **L** Superior Parathyroid Gland, Right **M** Superior Parathyroid Gland, Left **N** Inferior Parathyroid Gland, Right **P** Inferior Parathyroid Gland, Left **Q** Parathyroid Glands, Multiple **R** Parathyroid Gland	**0** Open **3** Percutaneous **4** Percutaneous Endoscopic	**0** Drainage Device	**Z** No Qualifier
0 Pituitary Gland **1** Pineal Body **2** Adrenal Gland, Left **3** Adrenal Gland, Right **4** Adrenal Glands, Bilateral **6** Carotid Body, Left **7** Carotid Body, Right **8** Carotid Bodies, Bilateral **9** Para-aortic Body **B** Coccygeal Glomus **C** Glomus Jugulare **D** Aortic Body **F** Paraganglion Extremity **G** Thyroid Gland Lobe, Left **H** Thyroid Gland Lobe, Right **K** Thyroid Gland **L** Superior Parathyroid Gland, Right **M** Superior Parathyroid Gland, Left **N** Inferior Parathyroid Gland, Right **P** Inferior Parathyroid Gland, Left **Q** Parathyroid Glands, Multiple **R** Parathyroid Gland	**0** Open **3** Percutaneous **4** Percutaneous Endoscopic	**Z** No Device	**X** Diagnostic **Z** No Qualifier

Section **0 Medical and Surgical**
Body System **G Endocrine System**
Operation **B Excision:** Cutting out or off, without replacement, a portion of a body part

Body Part (4th)	Approach (5th)	Device (6th)	Qualifier (7th)
0 Pituitary Gland 1 Pineal Body 2 Adrenal Gland, Left 3 Adrenal Gland, Right 4 Adrenal Glands, Bilateral 6 Carotid Body, Left 7 Carotid Body, Right 8 Carotid Bodies, Bilateral 9 Para-aortic Body B Coccygeal Glomus C Glomus Jugulare D Aortic Body F Paraganglion Extremity G Thyroid Gland Lobe, Left H Thyroid Gland Lobe, Right J Thyroid Gland Isthmus L Superior Parathyroid Gland, Right M Superior Parathyroid Gland, Left N Inferior Parathyroid Gland, Right P Inferior Parathyroid Gland, Left Q Parathyroid Glands, Multiple R Parathyroid Gland	0 Open 3 Percutaneous 4 Percutaneous Endoscopic	Z No Device	X Diagnostic Z No Qualifier

Section **0 Medical and Surgical**
Body System **G Endocrine System**
Operation **C Extirpation:** Taking or cutting out solid matter from a body part

Body Part (4th)	Approach (5th)	Device (6th)	Qualifier (7th)
0 Pituitary Gland 1 Pineal Body 2 Adrenal Gland, Left 3 Adrenal Gland, Right 4 Adrenal Glands, Bilateral 6 Carotid Body, Left 7 Carotid Body, Right 8 Carotid Bodies, Bilateral 9 Para-aortic Body B Coccygeal Glomus C Glomus Jugulare D Aortic Body F Paraganglion Extremity G Thyroid Gland Lobe, Left H Thyroid Gland Lobe, Right K Thyroid Gland L Superior Parathyroid Gland, Right M Superior Parathyroid Gland, Left N Inferior Parathyroid Gland, Right P Inferior Parathyroid Gland, Left Q Parathyroid Glands, Multiple R Parathyroid Gland	0 Open 3 Percutaneous 4 Percutaneous Endoscopic	Z No Device	Z No Qualifier

Section **0 Medical and Surgical**
Body System **G Endocrine System**
Operation **H Insertion:** Putting in a nonbiological appliance that monitors, assists, performs, or prevents a physiological function but does not physically take the place of a body part

Body Part (4th)	Approach (5th)	Device (6th)	Qualifier (7th)
S Endocrine Gland	0 Open 3 Percutaneous 4 Percutaneous Endoscopic	1 Radioactive Element 2 Monitoring Device 3 Infusion Device Y Other Device	Z No Qualifier

Section 0 **Medical and Surgical**
Body System G **Endocrine System**
Operation J **Inspection:** Visually and/or manually exploring a body part

Body Part (4th)	Approach (5th)	Device (6th)	Qualifier (7th)
0 Pituitary Gland **1** Pineal Body **5** Adrenal Gland **K** Thyroid Gland **R** Parathyroid Gland **S** Endocrine Gland	**0** Open **3** Percutaneous **4** Percutaneous Endoscopic	**Z** No Device	**Z** No Qualifier

Section 0 **Medical and Surgical**
Body System G **Endocrine System**
Operation M **Reattachment:** Putting back in or on all or a portion of a separated body part to its normal location or other suitable location

Body Part (4th)	Approach (5th)	Device (6th)	Qualifier (7th)
2 Adrenal Gland, Left **3** Adrenal Gland, Right **G** Thyroid Gland Lobe, Left **H** Thyroid Gland Lobe, Right **L** Superior Parathyroid Gland, Right **M** Superior Parathyroid Gland, Left **N** Inferior Parathyroid Gland, Right **P** Inferior Parathyroid Gland, Left **Q** Parathyroid Glands, Multiple **R** Parathyroid Gland	**0** Open **4** Percutaneous Endoscopic	**Z** No Device	**Z** No Qualifier

Section 0 **Medical and Surgical**
Body System G **Endocrine System**
Operation N **Release:** Freeing a body part from an abnormal physical constraint by cutting or by the use of force

Body Part (4th)	Approach (5th)	Device (6th)	Qualifier (7th)
0 Pituitary Gland **1** Pineal Body **2** Adrenal Gland, Left **3** Adrenal Gland, Right **4** Adrenal Glands, Bilateral **6** Carotid Body, Left **7** Carotid Body, Right **8** Carotid Bodies, Bilateral **9** Para-aortic Body **B** Coccygeal Glomus **C** Glomus Jugulare **D** Aortic Body **F** Paraganglion Extremity **G** Thyroid Gland Lobe, Left **H** Thyroid Gland Lobe, Right **K** Thyroid Gland **L** Superior Parathyroid Gland, Right **M** Superior Parathyroid Gland, Left **N** Inferior Parathyroid Gland, Right **P** Inferior Parathyroid Gland, Left **Q** Parathyroid Glands, Multiple **R** Parathyroid Gland	**0** Open **3** Percutaneous **4** Percutaneous Endoscopic	**Z** No Device	**Z** No Qualifier

Section 0 **Medical and Surgical**
Body System G **Endocrine System**
Operation P **Removal:** Taking out or off a device from a body part

Body Part (4th)	Approach (5th)	Device (6th)	Qualifier (7th)
0 Pituitary Gland **1** Pineal Body **5** Adrenal Gland **K** Thyroid Gland **R** Parathyroid Gland	**0** Open **3** Percutaneous **4** Percutaneous Endoscopic **X** External	**0** Drainage Device	**Z** No Qualifier
S Endocrine Gland	**0** Open **3** Percutaneous **4** Percutaneous Endoscopic	**0** Drainage Device **2** Monitoring Device **3** Infusion Device **Y** Other Device	**Z** No Qualifier
S Endocrine Gland	**X** External	**0** Drainage Device **2** Monitoring Device **3** Infusion Device	**Z** No Qualifier

Section 0 **Medical and Surgical**
Body System G **Endocrine System**
Operation Q **Repair:** Restoring, to the extent possible, a body part to its normal anatomic structure and function

Body Part (4th)	Approach (5th)	Device (6th)	Qualifier (7th)
0 Pituitary Gland **1** Pineal Body **2** Adrenal Gland, Left **3** Adrenal Gland, Right **4** Adrenal Glands, Bilateral **6** Carotid Body, Left **7** Carotid Body, Right **8** Carotid Bodies, Bilateral **9** Para-aortic Body **B** Coccygeal Glomus **C** Glomus Jugulare **D** Aortic Body **F** Paraganglion Extremity **G** Thyroid Gland Lobe, Left **H** Thyroid Gland Lobe, Right **J** Thyroid Gland Isthmus **K** Thyroid Gland **L** Superior Parathyroid Gland, Right **M** Superior Parathyroid Gland, Left **N** Inferior Parathyroid Gland, Right **P** Inferior Parathyroid Gland, Left **Q** Parathyroid Glands, Multiple **R** Parathyroid Gland	**0** Open **3** Percutaneous **4** Percutaneous Endoscopic	**Z** No Device	**Z** No Qualifier

Section 0 **Medical and Surgical**
Body System G **Endocrine System**
Operation S **Reposition:** Moving to its normal location, or other suitable location, all or a portion of a body part

Body Part (4th)	Approach (5th)	Device (6th)	Qualifier (7th)
2 Adrenal Gland, Left **3** Adrenal Gland, Right **G** Thyroid Gland Lobe, Left **H** Thyroid Gland Lobe, Right **L** Superior Parathyroid Gland, Right **M** Superior Parathyroid Gland, Left **N** Inferior Parathyroid Gland, Right **P** Inferior Parathyroid Gland, Left **Q** Parathyroid Glands, Multiple **R** Parathyroid Gland	**0** Open **4** Percutaneous Endoscopic	**Z** No Device	**Z** No Qualifier

Section 0 **Medical and Surgical**
Body System G **Endocrine System**
Operation T **Resection:** Cutting out or off, without replacement, all of a body part

Body Part (4th)	Approach (5th)	Device (6th)	Qualifier (7th)
0 Pituitary Gland **1** Pineal Body **2** Adrenal Gland, Left **3** Adrenal Gland, Right **4** Adrenal Glands, Bilateral **6** Carotid Body, Left **7** Carotid Body, Right **8** Carotid Bodies, Bilateral **9** Para-aortic Body **B** Coccygeal Glomus **C** Glomus Jugulare **D** Aortic Body **F** Paraganglion Extremity **G** Thyroid Gland Lobe, Left **H** Thyroid Gland Lobe, Right **J** Thyroid Gland Isthmus **K** Thyroid Gland **L** Superior Parathyroid Gland, Right **M** Superior Parathyroid Gland, Left **N** Inferior Parathyroid Gland, Right **P** Inferior Parathyroid Gland, Left **Q** Parathyroid Glands, Multiple **R** Parathyroid Gland	**0** Open **4** Percutaneous Endoscopic	**Z** No Device	**Z** No Qualifier

Section 0 **Medical and Surgical**
Body System G **Endocrine System**
Operation W **Revision:** Correcting, to the extent possible, a portion of a malfunctioning device or the position of a displaced device

Body Part (4th)	Approach (5th)	Device (6th)	Qualifier (7th)
0 Pituitary Gland **1** Pineal Body **5** Adrenal Gland **K** Thyroid Gland **R** Parathyroid Gland	**0** Open **3** Percutaneous **4** Percutaneous Endoscopic **X** External	**0** Drainage Device	**Z** No Qualifier
S Endocrine Gland	**0** Open **3** Percutaneous **4** Percutaneous Endoscopic	**0** Drainage Device **2** Monitoring Device **3** Infusion Device **Y** Other Device	**Z** No Qualifier
S Endocrine Gland	**X** External	**0** Drainage Device **2** Monitoring Device **3** Infusion Device	**Z** No Qualifier

AHA Coding Clinic

0GB00ZZ Excision of Pituitary Gland, Open Approach—AHA CC: 3Q, 2014, 22-23

0GB90ZZ Excision of Para-aortic Body, Open Approach—AHA CC: 2Q, 2021, 7

0GBG0ZZ Excision of Left Thyroid Gland Lobe, Open Approach—AHA CC: 2Q, 2017, 20

0GBH0ZZ Excision of Right Thyroid Gland Lobe, Open Approach—AHA CC: 2Q, 2017, 20

Cross-Section of the Skin Showing Layers and Types of Infections

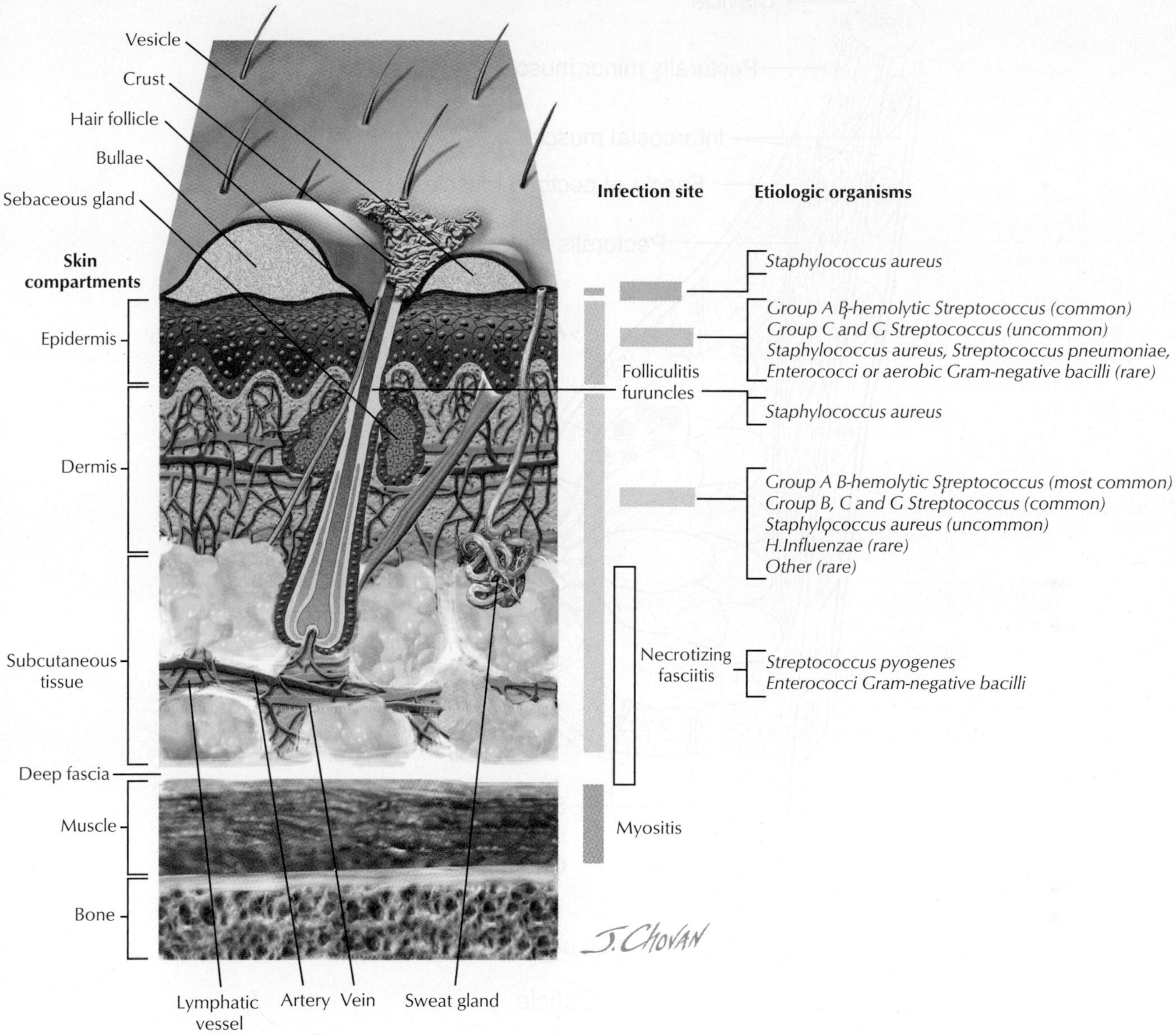
Vesicle
Crust
Hair follicle
Bullae
Sebaceous gland
Skin compartments
Epidermis
Dermis
Subcutaneous tissue
Deep fascia
Muscle
Bone
Lymphatic vessel
Artery
Vein
Sweat gland
Infection site
Etiologic organisms
Staphylococcus aureus
Group A β-hemolytic Streptococcus (common)
Group C and G Streptococcus (uncommon)
Staphylococcus aureus, Streptococcus pneumoniae,
Enterococci or aerobic Gram-negative bacilli (rare)
Folliculitis furuncles
Staphylococcus aureus
Group A B-hemolytic Streptococcus (most common)
Group B, C and G Streptococcus (common)
Staphylococcus aureus (uncommon)
H.Influenzae (rare)
Other (rare)
Necrotizing fasciitis
Streptococcus pyogenes
Enterococci Gram-negative bacilli
Myositis
J. Chovan

Breast

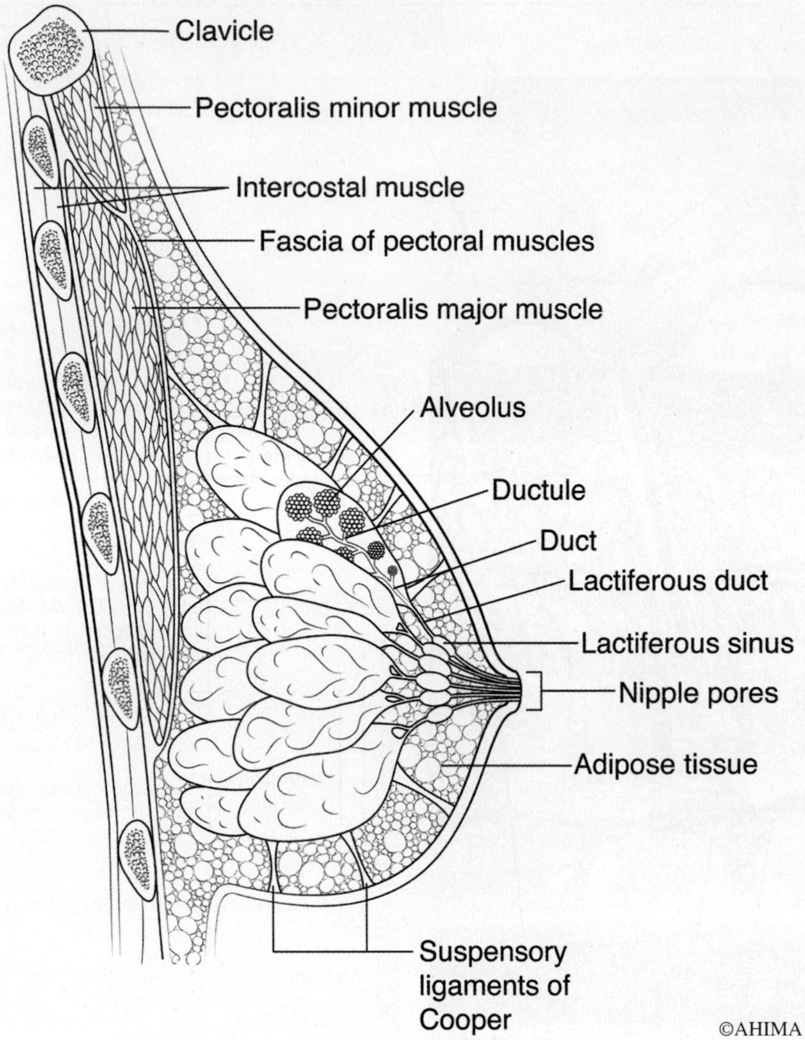

Clavicle
Pectoralis minor muscle
Intercostal muscle
Fascia of pectoral muscles
Pectoralis major muscle
Alveolus
Ductule
Duct
Lactiferous duct
Lactiferous sinus
Nipple pores
Adipose tissue
Suspensory ligaments of Cooper

©AHIMA

Nail Bed

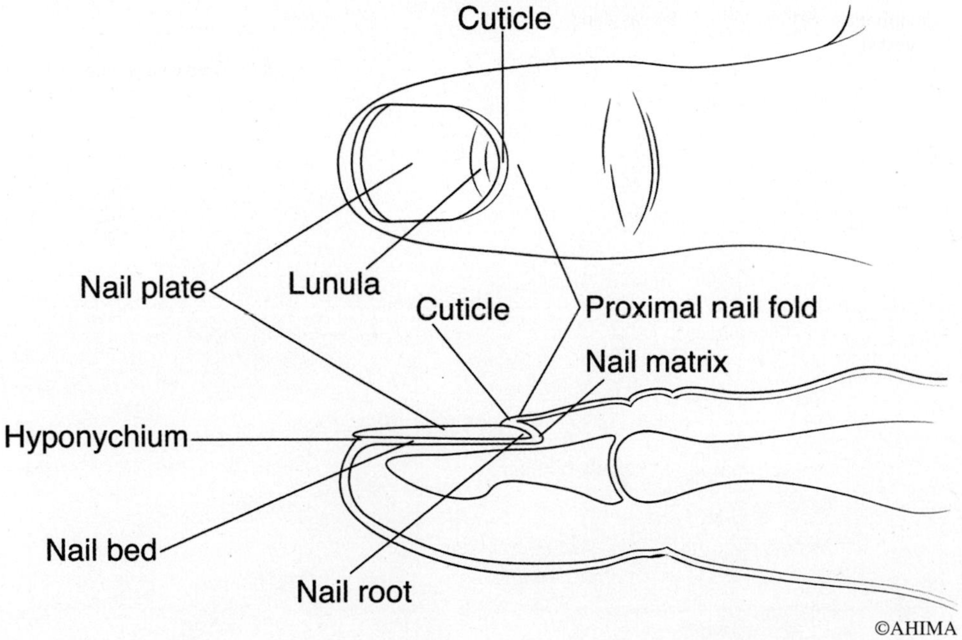

Cuticle
Nail plate
Lunula
Cuticle
Proximal nail fold
Nail matrix
Hyponychium
Nail bed
Nail root

©AHIMA

Section 0 **Medical and Surgical**
Body System H **Skin and Breast**
Operation 0 **Alteration:** Modifying the anatomic structure of a body part without affecting the function of the body part

Body Part (4th)	Approach (5th)	Device (6th)	Qualifier (7th)
T Breast, Right **U** Breast, Left **V** Breast, Bilateral	**0** Open **3** Percutaneous	**7** Autologous Tissue Substitute **J** Synthetic Substitute **K** Nonautologous Tissue Substitute **Z** No Device	**Z** No Qualifier

Section 0 **Medical and Surgical**
Body System H **Skin and Breast**
Operation 2 **Change:** Taking out or off a device from a body part and putting back an identical or similar device in or on the same body part without cutting or puncturing the skin or a mucous membrane

Body Part (4th)	Approach (5th)	Device (6th)	Qualifier (7th)
P Skin **T** Breast, Right **U** Breast, Left	**X** External	**0** Drainage Device **Y** Other Device	**Z** No Qualifier

Section 0 **Medical and Surgical**
Body System H **Skin and Breast**
Operation 5 **Destruction:** Physical eradication of all or a portion of a body part by the direct use of energy, force, or a destructive agent

Body Part (4th)	Approach (5th)	Device (6th)	Qualifier (7th)
0 Skin, Scalp **1** Skin, Face **2** Skin, Right Ear **3** Skin, Left Ear **4** Skin, Neck **5** Skin, Chest **6** Skin, Back **7** Skin, Abdomen **8** Skin, Buttock **9** Skin, Perineum **A** Skin, Inguinal **B** Skin, Right Upper Arm **C** Skin, Left Upper Arm **D** Skin, Right Lower Arm **E** Skin, Left Lower Arm **F** Skin, Right Hand **G** Skin, Left Hand **H** Skin, Right Upper Leg **J** Skin, Left Upper Leg **K** Skin, Right Lower Leg **L** Skin, Left Lower Leg **M** Skin, Right Foot **N** Skin, Left Foot	**X** External	**Z** No Device	**D** Multiple **Z** No Qualifier
Q Finger Nail **R** Toe Nail	**X** External	**Z** No Device	**Z** No Qualifier
T Breast, Right **U** Breast, Left **V** Breast, Bilateral	**0** Open **3** Percutaneous **7** Via Natural or Artificial Opening **8** Via Natural or Artificial Opening Endoscopic	**Z** No Device	**Z** No Qualifier
W Nipple, Right **X** Nipple, Left	**0** Open **3** Percutaneous **7** Via Natural or Artificial Opening **8** Via Natural or Artificial Opening Endoscopic **X** External	**Z** No Device	**Z** No Qualifier

Section 0 Medical and Surgical
Body System H Skin and Breast
Operation 8 **Division:** Cutting into a body part, without draining fluids and/or gases from the body part, in order to separate or transect a body part

Body Part (4th)	Approach (5th)	Device (6th)	Qualifier (7th)
0 Skin, Scalp 1 Skin, Face 2 Skin, Right Ear 3 Skin, Left Ear 4 Skin, Neck 5 Skin, Chest 6 Skin, Back 7 Skin, Abdomen 8 Skin, Buttock 9 Skin, Perineum A Skin, Inguinal B Skin, Right Upper Arm C Skin, Left Upper Arm D Skin, Right Lower Arm E Skin, Left Lower Arm F Skin, Right Hand G Skin, Left Hand H Skin, Right Upper Leg J Skin, Left Upper Leg K Skin, Right Lower Leg L Skin, Left Lower Leg M Skin, Right Foot N Skin, Left Foot	X External	Z No Device	Z No Qualifier

Section 0 Medical and Surgical
Body System H Skin and Breast
Operation 9 **Drainage:** Taking or letting out fluids and/or gases from a body part

Body Part (4th)	Approach (5th)	Device (6th)	Qualifier (7th)
0 Skin, Scalp 1 Skin, Face 2 Skin, Right Ear 3 Skin, Left Ear 4 Skin, Neck 5 Skin, Chest 6 Skin, Back 7 Skin, Abdomen 8 Skin, Buttock 9 Skin, Perineum A Skin, Inguinal B Skin, Right Upper Arm C Skin, Left Upper Arm D Skin, Right Lower Arm E Skin, Left Lower Arm F Skin, Right Hand G Skin, Left Hand H Skin, Right Upper Leg J Skin, Left Upper Leg K Skin, Right Lower Leg L Skin, Left Lower Leg M Skin, Right Foot N Skin, Left Foot Q Finger Nail R Toe Nail	X External	0 Drainage Device	Z No Qualifier

Continued →

Section 0 **Medical and Surgical**
Body System H **Skin and Breast**
Operation 9 **Drainage:** Taking or letting out fluids and/or gases from a body part

Body Part (4th)	Approach (5th)	Device (6th)	Qualifier (7th)
0 Skin, Scalp **1** Skin, Face **2** Skin, Right Ear **3** Skin, Left Ear **4** Skin, Neck **5** Skin, Chest **6** Skin, Back **7** Skin, Abdomen **8** Skin, Buttock **9** Skin, Perineum **A** Skin, Inguinal **B** Skin, Right Upper Arm **C** Skin, Left Upper Arm **D** Skin, Right Lower Arm **E** Skin, Left Lower Arm **F** Skin, Right Hand **G** Skin, Left Hand **H** Skin, Right Upper Leg **J** Skin, Left Upper Leg **K** Skin, Right Lower Leg **L** Skin, Left Lower Leg **M** Skin, Right Foot **N** Skin, Left Foot **Q** Finger Nail **R** Toe Nail	**X** External	**Z** No Device	**X** Diagnostic **Z** No Qualifier
T Breast, Right **U** Breast, Left **V** Breast, Bilateral	**0** Open **3** Percutaneous **7** Via Natural or Artificial Opening **8** Via Natural or Artificial Opening Endoscopic	**0** Drainage Device	**Z** No Qualifier
T Breast, Right **U** Breast, Left **V** Breast, Bilateral	**0** Open **3** Percutaneous **7** Via Natural or Artificial Opening **8** Via Natural or Artificial Opening Endoscopic	**Z** No Device	**X** Diagnostic **Z** No Qualifier
W Nipple, Right **X** Nipple, Left	**0** Open **3** Percutaneous **7** Via Natural or Artificial Opening **8** Via Natural or Artificial Opening Endoscopic **X** External	**0** Drainage Device	**Z** No Qualifier
W Nipple, Right **X** Nipple, Left	**0** Open **3** Percutaneous **7** Via Natural or Artificial Opening **8** Via Natural or Artificial Opening Endoscopic **X** External	**Z** No Device	**X** Diagnostic **Z** No Qualifier

Section 0 **Medical and Surgical**
Body System H **Skin and Breast**
Operation B **Excision:** Cutting out or off, without replacement, a portion of a body part

Body Part (4th)	Approach (5th)	Device (6th)	Qualifier (7th)
0 Skin, Scalp **1** Skin, Face **2** Skin, Right Ear **3** Skin, Left Ear **4** Skin, Neck **5** Skin, Chest **6** Skin, Back **7** Skin, Abdomen **8** Skin, Buttock **9** Skin, Perineum **A** Skin, Inguinal **B** Skin, Right Upper Arm **C** Skin, Left Upper Arm **D** Skin, Right Lower Arm **E** Skin, Left Lower Arm **F** Skin, Right Hand **G** Skin, Left Hand **H** Skin, Right Upper Leg **J** Skin, Left Upper Leg **K** Skin, Right Lower Leg **L** Skin, Left Lower Leg **M** Skin, Right Foot **N** Skin, Left Foot **Q** Finger Nail **R** Toe Nail	**X** External	**Z** No Device	**X** Diagnostic **Z** No Qualifier
T Breast, Right **U** Breast, Left **V** Breast, Bilateral **Y** Supernumerary Breast	**0** Open **3** Percutaneous **7** Via Natural or Artificial Opening **8** Via Natural or Artificial Opening Endoscopic	**Z** No Device	**X** Diagnostic **Z** No Qualifier
W Nipple, Right **X** Nipple, Left	**0** Open **3** Percutaneous **7** Via Natural or Artificial Opening **8** Via Natural or Artificial Opening Endoscopic **X** External	**Z** No Device	**X** Diagnostic **Z** No Qualifier

Section 0 **Medical and Surgical**
Body System H **Skin and Breast**
Operation C **Extirpation:** Taking or cutting out solid matter from a body part

Body Part (4th)	Approach (5th)	Device (6th)	Qualifier (7th)
0 Skin, Scalp **1** Skin, Face **2** Skin, Right Ear **3** Skin, Left Ear **4** Skin, Neck **5** Skin, Chest **6** Skin, Back **7** Skin, Abdomen **8** Skin, Buttock **9** Skin, Perineum **A** Skin, Inguinal **B** Skin, Right Upper Arm **C** Skin, Left Upper Arm **D** Skin, Right Lower Arm **E** Skin, Left Lower Arm **F** Skin, Right Hand **G** Skin, Left Hand **H** Skin, Right Upper Leg **J** Skin, Left Upper Leg **K** Skin, Right Lower Leg **L** Skin, Left Lower Leg **M** Skin, Right Foot **N** Skin, Left Foot **Q** Finger Nail **R** Toe Nail	**X** External	**Z** No Device	**Z** No Qualifier
T Breast, Right **U** Breast, Left **V** Breast, Bilateral	**0** Open **3** Percutaneous **7** Via Natural or Artificial Opening **8** Via Natural or Artificial Opening Endoscopic	**Z** No Device	**Z** No Qualifier
W Nipple, Right **X** Nipple, Left	**0** Open **3** Percutaneous **7** Via Natural or Artificial Opening **8** Via Natural or Artificial Opening Endoscopic **X** External	**Z** No Device	**Z** No Qualifier

Section 0 **Medical and Surgical**
Body System H **Skin and Breast**
Operation D **Extraction:** Pulling or stripping out or off all or a portion of a body part by the use of force

Body Part (4th)	Approach (5th)	Device (6th)	Qualifier (7th)
0 Skin, Scalp **1** Skin, Face **2** Skin, Right Ear **3** Skin, Left Ear **4** Skin, Neck **5** Skin, Chest **6** Skin, Back **7** Skin, Abdomen **8** Skin, Buttock **9** Skin, Perineum **A** Skin, Inguinal **B** Skin, Right Upper Arm **C** Skin, Left Upper Arm **D** Skin, Right Lower Arm **E** Skin, Left Lower Arm **F** Skin, Right Hand **G** Skin, Left Hand **H** Skin, Right Upper Leg **J** Skin, Left Upper Leg **K** Skin, Right Lower Leg **L** Skin, Left Lower Leg **M** Skin, Right Foot **N** Skin, Left Foot **Q** Finger Nail **R** Toe Nail **S** Hair	**X** External	**Z** No Device	**Z** No Qualifier
T Breast, Right **U** Breast, Left **V** Breast, Bilateral **Y** Supernumerary Breast	**0** Open	**Z** No Device	**Z** No Qualifier

Section 0 **Medical and Surgical**
Body System H **Skin and Breast**
Operation H **Insertion:** Putting in a nonbiological appliance that monitors, assists, performs, or prevents a physiological function but does not physically take the place of a body part

Body Part (4th)	Approach (5th)	Device (6th)	Qualifier (7th)
P Skin	**X** External	**Y** Other Device	**Z** No Qualifier
T Breast, Right **U** Breast, Left	**0** Open **3** Percutaneous **7** Via Natural or Artificial Opening **8** Via Natural or Artificial Opening Endoscopic	**1** Radioactive Element **N** Tissue Expander **Y** Other Device	**Z** No Qualifier
V Breast, Bilateral	**0** Open **3** Percutaneous **7** Via Natural or Artificial Opening **8** Via Natural or Artificial Opening Endoscopic	**1** Radioactive Element **N** Tissue Expander	**Z** No Qualifier
W Nipple, Right **X** Nipple, Left	**0** Open **3** Percutaneous **7** Via Natural or Artificial Opening **8** Via Natural or Artificial Opening Endoscopic	**1** Radioactive Element **N** Tissue Expander	**Z** No Qualifier
W Nipple, Right **X** Nipple, Left	**X** External	**1** Radioactive Element	**Z** No Qualifier

Section 0 **Medical and Surgical**
Body System H **Skin and Breast**
Operation J **Inspection:** Visually and/or manually exploring a body part

Body Part (4th)	Approach (5th)	Device (6th)	Qualifier (7th)
P Skin **Q** Finger Nail **R** Toe Nail	**X** External	**Z** No Device	**Z** No Qualifier
T Breast, Right **U** Breast, Left	**0** Open **3** Percutaneous **7** Via Natural or Artificial Opening **8** Via Natural or Artificial Opening Endoscopic	**Z** No Device	**Z** No Qualifier

Section 0 **Medical and Surgical**
Body System H **Skin and Breast**
Operation M **Reattachment:** Putting back in or on all or a portion of a separated body part to its normal location or other suitable location

Body Part (4th)	Approach (5th)	Device (6th)	Qualifier (7th)
0 Skin, Scalp **1** Skin, Face **2** Skin, Right Ear **3** Skin, Left Ear **4** Skin, Neck **5** Skin, Chest **6** Skin, Back **7** Skin, Abdomen **8** Skin, Buttock **9** Skin, Perineum **A** Skin, Inguinal **B** Skin, Right Upper Arm **C** Skin, Left Upper Arm **D** Skin, Right Lower Arm **E** Skin, Left Lower Arm **F** Skin, Right Hand **G** Skin, Left Hand **H** Skin, Right Upper Leg **J** Skin, Left Upper Leg **K** Skin, Right Lower Leg **L** Skin, Left Lower Leg **M** Skin, Right Foot **N** Skin, Left Foot **T** Breast, Right **U** Breast, Left **V** Breast, Bilateral **W** Nipple, Right **X** Nipple, Left	**X** External	**Z** No Device	**Z** No Qualifier

Section 0 **Medical and Surgical**
Body System H **Skin and Breast**
Operation N **Release:** Freeing a body part from an abnormal physical constraint by cutting or by the use of force

Body Part (4th)	Approach (5th)	Device (6th)	Qualifier (7th)
0 Skin, Scalp **1** Skin, Face **2** Skin, Right Ear **3** Skin, Left Ear **4** Skin, Neck **5** Skin, Chest **6** Skin, Back **7** Skin, Abdomen **8** Skin, Buttock **9** Skin, Perineum **A** Skin, Inguinal **B** Skin, Right Upper Arm **C** Skin, Left Upper Arm **D** Skin, Right Lower Arm **E** Skin, Left Lower Arm **F** Skin, Right Hand **G** Skin, Left Hand **H** Skin, Right Upper Leg **J** Skin, Left Upper Leg **K** Skin, Right Lower Leg **L** Skin, Left Lower Leg **M** Skin, Right Foot **N** Skin, Left Foot **Q** Finger Nail **R** Toe Nail	**X** External	**Z** No Device	**Z** No Qualifier
T Breast, Right **U** Breast, Left **V** Breast, Bilateral	**0** Open **3** Percutaneous **7** Via Natural or Artificial Opening **8** Via Natural or Artificial Opening Endoscopic	**Z** No Device	**Z** No Qualifier
W Nipple, Right **X** Nipple, Left	**0** Open **3** Percutaneous **7** Via Natural or Artificial Opening **8** Via Natural or Artificial Opening Endoscopic **X** External	**Z** No Device	**Z** No Qualifier

Section 0 **Medical and Surgical**
Body System H **Skin and Breast**
Operation P **Removal:** Taking out or off a device from a body part

Body Part (4th)	Approach (5th)	Device (6th)	Qualifier (7th)
P Skin	**X** External	**0** Drainage Device **7** Autologous Tissue Substitute **J** Synthetic Substitute **K** Nonautologous Tissue Substitute **Y** Other Device	**Z** No Qualifier
Q Finger Nail **R** Toe Nail	**X** External	**0** Drainage Device **7** Autologous Tissue Substitute **J** Synthetic Substitute **K** Nonautologous Tissue Substitute	**Z** No Qualifier
S Hair	**X** External	**7** Autologous Tissue Substitute **J** Synthetic Substitute **K** Nonautologous Tissue Substitute	**Z** No Qualifier
T Breast, Right **U** Breast, Left	**0** Open **3** Percutaneous **7** Via Natural or Artificial Opening **8** Via Natural or Artificial Opening Endoscopic	**0** Drainage Device **1** Radioactive Element **7** Autologous Tissue Substitute **J** Synthetic Substitute **K** Nonautologous Tissue Substitute **N** Tissue Expander **Y** Other Device	**Z** No Qualifier

Section 0 **Medical and Surgical**
Body System H **Skin and Breast**
Operation Q **Repair:** Restoring, to the extent possible, a body part to its normal anatomic structure and function

Body Part (4th)	Approach (5th)	Device (6th)	Qualifier (7th)
0 Skin, Scalp **1** Skin, Face **2** Skin, Right Ear **3** Skin, Left Ear **4** Skin, Neck **5** Skin, Chest **6** Skin, Back **7** Skin, Abdomen **8** Skin, Buttock **9** Skin, Perineum **A** Skin, Inguinal **B** Skin, Right Upper Arm **C** Skin, Left Upper Arm **D** Skin, Right Lower Arm **E** Skin, Left Lower Arm **F** Skin, Right Hand **G** Skin, Left Hand **H** Skin, Right Upper Leg **J** Skin, Left Upper Leg **K** Skin, Right Lower Leg **L** Skin, Left Lower Leg **M** Skin, Right Foot **N** Skin, Left Foot **Q** Finger Nail **R** Toe Nail	**X** External	**Z** No Device	**Z** No Qualifier
T Breast, Right **U** Breast, Left **V** Breast, Bilateral **Y** Supernumerary Breast	**0** Open **3** Percutaneous **7** Via Natural or Artificial Opening **8** Via Natural or Artificial Opening Endoscopic	**Z** No Device	**Z** No Qualifier

Continued →

Section 0 **Medical and Surgical**
Body System H **Skin and Breast**
Operation Q **Repair:** Restoring, to the extent possible, a body part to its normal anatomic structure and function

Body Part (4th)	Approach (5th)	Device (6th)	Qualifier (7th)
W Nipple, Right **X** Nipple, Left	**0** Open **3** Percutaneous **7** Via Natural or Artificial Opening **8** Via Natural or Artificial Opening Endoscopic **X** External	**Z** No Device	**Z** No Qualifier

Section 0 **Medical and Surgical**
Body System H **Skin and Breast**
Operation R **Replacement:** Putting in or on biological or synthetic material that physically takes the place and/or function of all or a portion of a body part

Body Part (4th)	Approach (5th)	Device (6th)	Qualifier (7th)
0 Skin, Scalp **1** Skin, Face **2** Skin, Right Ear **3** Skin, Left Ear **4** Skin, Neck **5** Skin, Chest **6** Skin, Back **7** Skin, Abdomen **8** Skin, Buttock **9** Skin, Perineum **A** Skin, Inguinal **B** Skin, Right Upper Arm **C** Skin, Left Upper Arm **D** Skin, Right Lower Arm **E** Skin, Left Lower Arm **F** Skin, Right Hand **G** Skin, Left Hand **H** Skin, Right Upper Leg **J** Skin, Left Upper Leg **K** Skin, Right Lower Leg **L** Skin, Left Lower Leg **M** Skin, Right Foot **N** Skin, Left Foot	**X** External	**7** Autologous Tissue Substitute	**2** Cell Suspension Technique **3** Full Thickness **4** Partial Thickness
0 Skin, Scalp **1** Skin, Face **2** Skin, Right Ear **3** Skin, Left Ear **4** Skin, Neck **5** Skin, Chest **6** Skin, Back **7** Skin, Abdomen **8** Skin, Buttock **9** Skin, Perineum **A** Skin, Inguinal **B** Skin, Right Upper Arm **C** Skin, Left Upper Arm **D** Skin, Right Lower Arm **E** Skin, Left Lower Arm **F** Skin, Right Hand **G** Skin, Left Hand **H** Skin, Right Upper Leg **J** Skin, Left Upper Leg **K** Skin, Right Lower Leg **L** Skin, Left Lower Leg **M** Skin, Right Foot **N** Skin, Left Foot	**X** External	**J** Synthetic Substitute	**3** Full Thickness **4** Partial Thickness **Z** No Qualifier

Continued →

Section 0 Medical and Surgical
Body System H Skin and Breast
Operation R **Replacement:** Putting in or on biological or synthetic material that physically takes the place and/or function of all or a portion of a body part

Body Part (4th)	Approach (5th)	Device (6th)	Qualifier (7th)
0 Skin, Scalp **1** Skin, Face **2** Skin, Right Ear **3** Skin, Left Ear **4** Skin, Neck **5** Skin, Chest **6** Skin, Back **7** Skin, Abdomen **8** Skin, Buttock **9** Skin, Perineum **A** Skin, Inguinal **B** Skin, Right Upper Arm **C** Skin, Left Upper Arm **D** Skin, Right Lower Arm **E** Skin, Left Lower Arm **F** Skin, Right Hand **G** Skin, Left Hand **H** Skin, Right Upper Leg **J** Skin, Left Upper Leg **K** Skin, Right Lower Leg **L** Skin, Left Lower Leg **M** Skin, Right Foot **N** Skin, Left Foot	**X** External	**K** Nonautologous Tissue Substitute	**3** Full Thickness **4** Partial Thickness
Q Finger Nail **R** Toe Nail **S** Hair	**X** External	**7** Autologous Tissue Substitute **J** Synthetic Substitute **K** Nonautologous Tissue Substitute	**Z** No Qualifier
T Breast, Right **U** Breast, Left **V** Breast, Bilateral	**0** Open	**7** Autologous Tissue Substitute	**5** Latissimus Dorsi Myocutaneous Flap **6** Transverse Rectus Abdominis Myocutaneous Flap **7** Deep Inferior Epigastric Artery Perforator Flap **8** Superficial Inferior Epigastric Artery Flap **9** Gluteal Artery Perforator Flap **Z** No Qualifier
T Breast, Right **U** Breast, Left **V** Breast, Bilateral	**0** Open	**J** Synthetic Substitute **K** Nonautologous Tissue Substitute	**Z** No Qualifier
T Breast, Right **U** Breast, Left **V** Breast, Bilateral	**3** Percutaneous	**7** Autologous Tissue Substitute **J** Synthetic Substitute **K** Nonautologous Tissue Substitute	**Z** No Qualifier
W Nipple, Right **X** Nipple, Left	**0** Open **3** Percutaneous **X** External	**7** Autologous Tissue Substitute **J** Synthetic Substitute **K** Nonautologous Tissue Substitute	**Z** No Qualifier

Section 0 Medical and Surgical
Body System H Skin and Breast
Operation S **Reposition:** Moving to its normal location, or other suitable location, all or a portion of a body part

Body Part (4th)	Approach (5th)	Device (6th)	Qualifier (7th)
S Hair W Nipple, Right X Nipple, Left	X External	Z No Device	Z No Qualifier
T Breast, Right U Breast, Left V Breast, Bilateral	0 Open	Z No Device	Z No Qualifier

Section 0 Medical and Surgical
Body System H Skin and Breast
Operation T **Resection:** Cutting out or off, without replacement, all of a body part

Body Part (4th)	Approach (5th)	Device (6th)	Qualifier (7th)
Q Finger Nail R Toe Nail W Nipple, Right X Nipple, Left	X External	Z No Device	Z No Qualifier
T Breast, Right U Breast, Left V Breast, Bilateral Y Supernumerary Breast	0 Open	Z No Device	Z No Qualifier

Section 0 Medical and Surgical
Body System H Skin and Breast
Operation U **Supplement:** Putting in or on biological or synthetic material that physically reinforces and/or augments the function of a portion of a body part

Body Part (4th)	Approach (5th)	Device (6th)	Qualifier (7th)
T Breast, Right U Breast, Left V Breast, Bilateral	0 Open 3 Percutaneous 7 Via Natural or Artificial Opening 8 Via Natural or Artificial Opening Endoscopic	7 Autologous Tissue Substitute J Synthetic Substitute K Nonautologous Tissue Substitute	Z No Qualifier
W Nipple, Right X Nipple, Left	0 Open 3 Percutaneous 7 Via Natural or Artificial Opening 8 Via Natural or Artificial Opening Endoscopic X External	7 Autologous Tissue Substitute J Synthetic Substitute K Nonautologous Tissue Substitute	Z No Qualifier

Section **0** **Medical and Surgical**
Body System **H** **Skin and Breast**
Operation **W** **Revision:** Correcting, to the extent possible, a portion of a malfunctioning device or the position of a displaced device

Body Part (4th)	Approach (5th)	Device (6th)	Qualifier (7th)
P Skin	**X** External	**0** Drainage Device **7** Autologous Tissue Substitute **J** Synthetic Substitute **K** Nonautologous Tissue Substitute **Y** Other Device	**Z** No Qualifier
Q Finger Nail **R** Toe Nail	**X** External	**0** Drainage Device **7** Autologous Tissue Substitute **J** Synthetic Substitute **K** Nonautologous Tissue Substitute	**Z** No Qualifier
S Hair	**X** External	**7** Autologous Tissue Substitute **J** Synthetic Substitute **K** Nonautologous Tissue Substitute	**Z** No Qualifier
T Breast, Right **U** Breast, Left	**0** Open **3** Percutaneous **7** Via Natural or Artificial Opening **8** Via Natural or Artificial Opening Endoscopic	**0** Drainage Device **7** Autologous Tissue Substitute **J** Synthetic Substitute **K** Nonautologous Tissue Substitute **N** Tissue Expander **Y** Other Device	**Z** No Qualifier

Section **0** **Medical and Surgical**
Body System **H** **Skin and Breast**
Operation **X** **Transfer:** Moving, without taking out, all or a portion of a body part to another location to take over the function of all or a portion of a body part

Body Part (4th)	Approach (5th)	Device (6th)	Qualifier (7th)
0 Skin, Scalp **1** Skin, Face **2** Skin, Right Ear **3** Skin, Left Ear **4** Skin, Neck **5** Skin, Chest **6** Skin, Back **7** Skin, Abdomen **8** Skin, Buttock **9** Skin, Perineum **A** Skin, Inguinal **B** Skin, Right Upper Arm **C** Skin, Left Upper Arm **D** Skin, Right Lower Arm **E** Skin, Left Lower Arm **F** Skin, Right Hand **G** Skin, Left Hand **H** Skin, Right Upper Leg **J** Skin, Left Upper Leg **K** Skin, Right Lower Leg **L** Skin, Left Lower Leg **M** Skin, Right Foot **N** Skin, Left Foot	**X** External	**Z** No Device	**Z** No Qualifier

AHA Coding Clinic

0HB8XZZ Excision of Buttock Skin, External Approach—AHA CC: 3Q, 2015, 3
0HBHXZZ Excision of Right Upper Leg Skin, External Approach—AHA CC: 1Q, 2020, 31-32
0HBJXZZ Excision of Left Upper Leg Skin, External Approach—AHA CC: 3Q, 2016, 29-30
0HBT0ZZ Excision of Right Breast, Open Approach—AHA CC: 1Q, 2018, 14-15
0HD6XZZ Extraction of Back Skin, External Approach—AHA CC: 3Q, 2015, 5-6
0HDHXZZ Extraction of Right Upper Leg Skin, External Approach—AHA CC: 3Q, 2015, 5
0HHT0NZ Insertion of Tissue Expander into Right Breast, Open Approach—AHA CC: 4Q, 2017, 67

0HHU0YZ Insertion of Other Device into Left Breast, Open Approach—AHA CC: 4Q, 2013, 107

0HHV0NZ Insertion of Tissue Expander into Bilateral Breast, Open Approach—AHA CC: 2Q, 2014, 12

0HPT07Z Removal of Autologous Tissue Substitute from Right Breast, Open Approach—AHA CC: 2Q, 2016, 27

0HPT0NZ Removal of Tissue Expander from Right Breast, Open Approach—AHA CC: 3Q, 2018, 13-14

0HPU07Z Removal of Autologous Tissue Substitute from Left Breast, Open Approach—AHA CC: 2Q, 2016, 27

0HQ9XZZ Repair Perineum Skin, External Approach—AHA CC: 1Q, 2016, 7

0HQEXZZ Repair Left Lower Arm Skin, External Approach—AHA CC: 4Q, 2014, 31-32

0HRMXK3 Replacement of Right Foot Skin with Nonautologous Tissue Substitute, Full Thickness, External Approach—AHA CC: 1Q, 2017, 35-36

0HRNXK3 Replacement of Left Foot Skin with Nonautologous Tissue Substitute, Full Thickness, External Approach—AHA CC: 3Q, 2014, 14-15

0HRU07Z Replacement of Left Breast with Autologous Tissue Substitute, Open Approach—AHA CC: 1Q, 2020, 27-28

0HRV077 Replacement of Bilateral Breast using Deep Inferior Epigastric Artery Perforator Flap, Open Approach—AHA CC: 3Q, 2018, 13-14

0HTT0ZZ Resection of Right Breast, Open Approach—AHA CC: 4Q, 2014, 34

0HTU0ZZ Resection of Left Breast, Open Approach—AHA CC: 3Q, 2018, 13-14

0HTV0ZZ Resection of Bilateral Breast, Open Approach—AHA CC: 2Q, 2021, 16-17

Cross-Section of the Skin Showing Layer and Types of Infections

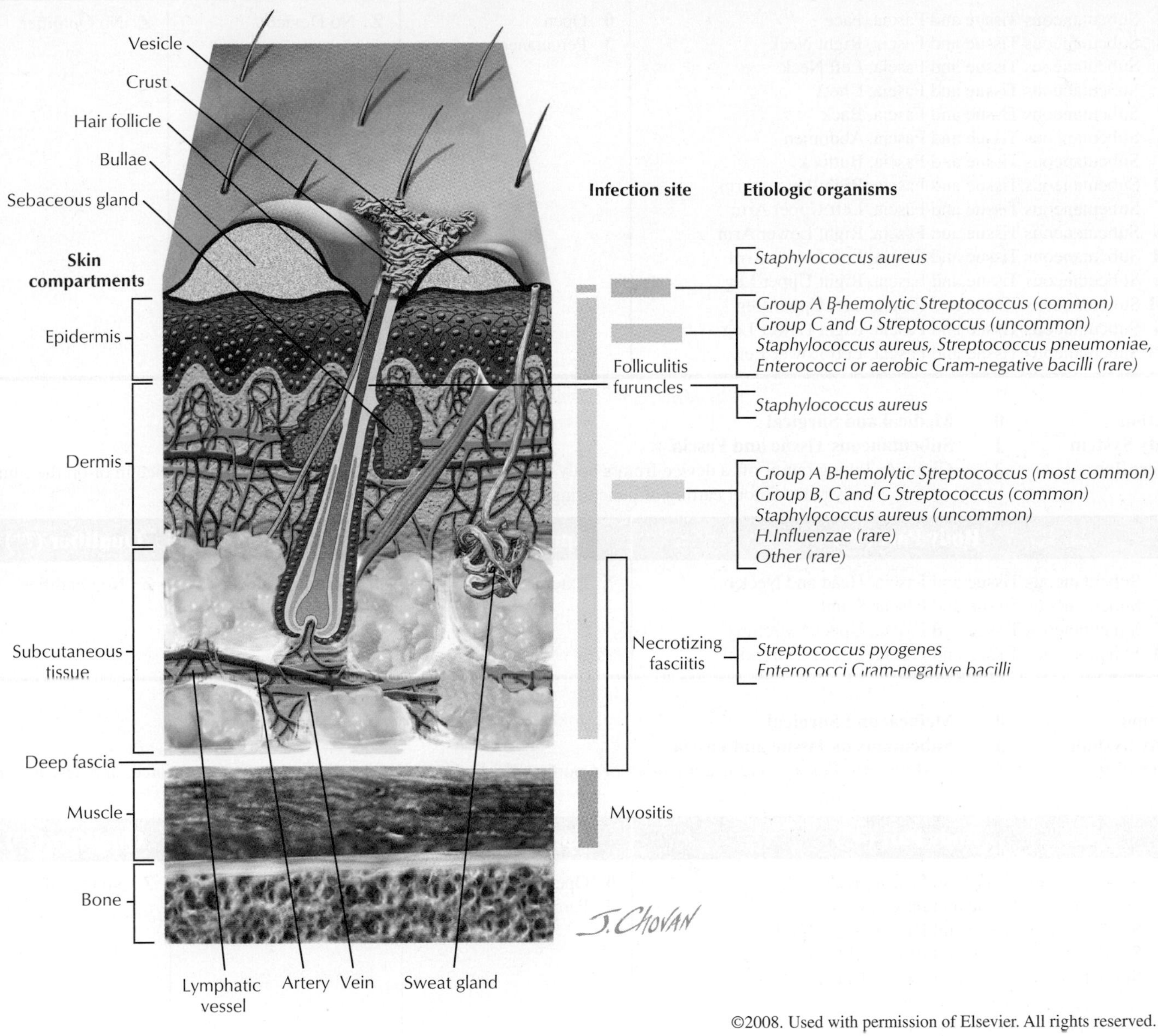
Vesicle
Crust
Hair follicle
Bullae
Sebaceous gland
Skin compartments
Epidermis
Dermis
Subcutaneous tissue
Deep fascia
Muscle
Bone
Lymphatic vessel
Artery
Vein
Sweat gland
J. CHOVAN
Infection site
Etiologic organisms
Staphylococcus aureus
Group A β-hemolytic Streptococcus (common)
Group C and G Streptococcus (uncommon)
Staphylococcus aureus, Streptococcus pneumoniae,
Enterococci or aerobic Gram-negative bacilli (rare)
Folliculitis furuncles
Staphylococcus aureus
Group A B-hemolytic Streptococcus (most common)
Group B, C and G Streptococcus (common)
Staphylococcus aureus (uncommon)
H.Influenzae (rare)
Other (rare)
Necrotizing fasciitis
Streptococcus pyogenes
Enterococci Gram-negative bacilli
Myositis

Subcutaneous Tissue and Fascia Tables 0J0–0JX

Section 0 **Medical and Surgical**
Body System J **Subcutaneous Tissue and Fascia**
Operation 0 **Alteration:** Modifying the anatomic structure of a body part without affecting the function of the body part

Body Part (4th)	Approach (5th)	Device (6th)	Qualifier (7th)
1 Subcutaneous Tissue and Fascia, Face **4** Subcutaneous Tissue and Fascia, Right Neck **5** Subcutaneous Tissue and Fascia, Left Neck **6** Subcutaneous Tissue and Fascia, Chest **7** Subcutaneous Tissue and Fascia, Back **8** Subcutaneous Tissue and Fascia, Abdomen **9** Subcutaneous Tissue and Fascia, Buttock **D** Subcutaneous Tissue and Fascia, Right Upper Arm **F** Subcutaneous Tissue and Fascia, Left Upper Arm **G** Subcutaneous Tissue and Fascia, Right Lower Arm **H** Subcutaneous Tissue and Fascia, Left Lower Arm **L** Subcutaneous Tissue and Fascia, Right Upper Leg **M** Subcutaneous Tissue and Fascia, Left Upper Leg **N** Subcutaneous Tissue and Fascia, Right Lower Leg **P** Subcutaneous Tissue and Fascia, Left Lower Leg	**0** Open **3** Percutaneous	**Z** No Device	**Z** No Qualifier

Section 0 **Medical and Surgical**
Body System J **Subcutaneous Tissue and Fascia**
Operation 2 **Change:** Taking out or off a device from a body part and putting back an identical or similar device in or on the same body part without cutting or puncturing the skin or a mucous membrane

Body Part (4th)	Approach (5th)	Device (6th)	Qualifier (7th)
S Subcutaneous Tissue and Fascia, Head and Neck **T** Subcutaneous Tissue and Fascia, Trunk **V** Subcutaneous Tissue and Fascia, Upper Extremity **W** Subcutaneous Tissue and Fascia, Lower Extremity	**X** External	**0** Drainage Device **Y** Other Device	**Z** No Qualifier

Section 0 **Medical and Surgical**
Body System J **Subcutaneous Tissue and Fascia**
Operation 5 **Destruction:** Physical eradication of all or a portion of a body part by the direct use of energy, force, or a destructive agent

Body Part (4th)	Approach (5th)	Device (6th)	Qualifier (7th)
0 Subcutaneous Tissue and Fascia, Scalp **1** Subcutaneous Tissue and Fascia, Face **4** Subcutaneous Tissue and Fascia, Right Neck **5** Subcutaneous Tissue and Fascia, Left Neck **6** Subcutaneous Tissue and Fascia, Chest **7** Subcutaneous Tissue and Fascia, Back **8** Subcutaneous Tissue and Fascia, Abdomen **9** Subcutaneous Tissue and Fascia, Buttock **B** Subcutaneous Tissue and Fascia, Perineum **C** Subcutaneous Tissue and Fascia, Pelvic Region **D** Subcutaneous Tissue and Fascia, Right Upper Arm **F** Subcutaneous Tissue and Fascia, Left Upper Arm **G** Subcutaneous Tissue and Fascia, Right Lower Arm **H** Subcutaneous Tissue and Fascia, Left Lower Arm **J** Subcutaneous Tissue and Fascia, Right Hand **K** Subcutaneous Tissue and Fascia, Left Hand **L** Subcutaneous Tissue and Fascia, Right Upper Leg **M** Subcutaneous Tissue and Fascia, Left Upper Leg **N** Subcutaneous Tissue and Fascia, Right Lower Leg **P** Subcutaneous Tissue and Fascia, Left Lower Leg **Q** Subcutaneous Tissue and Fascia, Right Foot **R** Subcutaneous Tissue and Fascia, Left Foot	**0** Open **3** Percutaneous	**Z** No Device	**Z** No Qualifier

Section 0 Medical and Surgical
Body System J Subcutaneous Tissue and Fascia
Operation 8 **Division:** Cutting into a body part, without draining fluids and/or gases from the body part, in order to separate or transect a body part

Body Part (4th)	Approach (5th)	Device (6th)	Qualifier (7th)
0 Subcutaneous Tissue and Fascia, Scalp 1 Subcutaneous Tissue and Fascia, Face 4 Subcutaneous Tissue and Fascia, Right Neck 5 Subcutaneous Tissue and Fascia, Left Neck 6 Subcutaneous Tissue and Fascia, Chest 7 Subcutaneous Tissue and Fascia, Back 8 Subcutaneous Tissue and Fascia, Abdomen 9 Subcutaneous Tissue and Fascia, Buttock B Subcutaneous Tissue and Fascia, Perineum C Subcutaneous Tissue and Fascia, Pelvic Region D Subcutaneous Tissue and Fascia, Right Upper Arm F Subcutaneous Tissue and Fascia, Left Upper Arm G Subcutaneous Tissue and Fascia, Right Lower Arm H Subcutaneous Tissue and Fascia, Left Lower Arm J Subcutaneous Tissue and Fascia, Right Hand K Subcutaneous Tissue and Fascia, Left Hand L Subcutaneous Tissue and Fascia, Right Upper Leg M Subcutaneous Tissue and Fascia, Left Upper Leg N Subcutaneous Tissue and Fascia, Right Lower Leg P Subcutaneous Tissue and Fascia, Left Lower Leg Q Subcutaneous Tissue and Fascia, Right Foot R Subcutaneous Tissue and Fascia, Left Foot S Subcutaneous Tissue and Fascia, Head and Neck T Subcutaneous Tissue and Fascia, Trunk V Subcutaneous Tissue and Fascia, Upper Extremity W Subcutaneous Tissue and Fascia, Lower Extremity	0 Open 3 Percutaneous	Z No Device	Z No Qualifier

Section 0 Medical and Surgical
Body System J Subcutaneous Tissue and Fascia
Operation 9 **Drainage:** Taking or letting out fluids and/or gases from a body part

Body Part (4th)	Approach (5th)	Device (6th)	Qualifier (7th)
0 Subcutaneous Tissue and Fascia, Scalp 1 Subcutaneous Tissue and Fascia, Face 4 Subcutaneous Tissue and Fascia, Right Neck 5 Subcutaneous Tissue and Fascia, Left Neck 6 Subcutaneous Tissue and Fascia, Chest 7 Subcutaneous Tissue and Fascia, Back 8 Subcutaneous Tissue and Fascia, Abdomen 9 Subcutaneous Tissue and Fascia, Buttock B Subcutaneous Tissue and Fascia, Perineum C Subcutaneous Tissue and Fascia, Pelvic Region D Subcutaneous Tissue and Fascia, Right Upper Arm F Subcutaneous Tissue and Fascia, Left Upper Arm G Subcutaneous Tissue and Fascia, Right Lower Arm H Subcutaneous Tissue and Fascia, Left Lower Arm J Subcutaneous Tissue and Fascia, Right Hand K Subcutaneous Tissue and Fascia, Left Hand L Subcutaneous Tissue and Fascia, Right Upper Leg M Subcutaneous Tissue and Fascia, Left Upper Leg N Subcutaneous Tissue and Fascia, Right Lower Leg P Subcutaneous Tissue and Fascia, Left Lower Leg Q Subcutaneous Tissue and Fascia, Right Foot R Subcutaneous Tissue and Fascia, Left Foot	0 Open 3 Percutaneous	0 Drainage Device	Z No Qualifier

Continued →

Section	**0**	**Medical and Surgical**
Body System	**J**	**Subcutaneous Tissue and Fascia**
Operation	**9**	**Drainage:** Taking or letting out fluids and/or gases from a body part

Body Part (4th)	Approach (5th)	Device (6th)	Qualifier (7th)
0 Subcutaneous Tissue and Fascia, Scalp **1** Subcutaneous Tissue and Fascia, Face **4** Subcutaneous Tissue and Fascia, Right Neck **5** Subcutaneous Tissue and Fascia, Left Neck **6** Subcutaneous Tissue and Fascia, Chest **7** Subcutaneous Tissue and Fascia, Back **8** Subcutaneous Tissue and Fascia, Abdomen **9** Subcutaneous Tissue and Fascia, Buttock **B** Subcutaneous Tissue and Fascia, Perineum **C** Subcutaneous Tissue and Fascia, Pelvic Region **D** Subcutaneous Tissue and Fascia, Right Upper Arm **F** Subcutaneous Tissue and Fascia, Left Upper Arm **G** Subcutaneous Tissue and Fascia, Right Lower Arm **H** Subcutaneous Tissue and Fascia, Left Lower Arm **J** Subcutaneous Tissue and Fascia, Right Hand **K** Subcutaneous Tissue and Fascia, Left Hand **L** Subcutaneous Tissue and Fascia, Right Upper Leg **M** Subcutaneous Tissue and Fascia, Left Upper Leg **N** Subcutaneous Tissue and Fascia, Right Lower Leg **P** Subcutaneous Tissue and Fascia, Left Lower Leg **Q** Subcutaneous Tissue and Fascia, Right Foot **R** Subcutaneous Tissue and Fascia, Left Foot	**0** Open **3** Percutaneous	**Z** No Device	**X** Diagnostic **Z** No Qualifier

Section	**0**	**Medical and Surgical**
Body System	**J**	**Subcutaneous Tissue and Fascia**
Operation	**B**	**Excision:** Cutting out or off, without replacement, a portion of a body part

Body Part (4th)	Approach (5th)	Device (6th)	Qualifier (7th)
0 Subcutaneous Tissue and Fascia, Scalp **1** Subcutaneous Tissue and Fascia, Face **4** Subcutaneous Tissue and Fascia, Right Neck **5** Subcutaneous Tissue and Fascia, Left Neck **6** Subcutaneous Tissue and Fascia, Chest **7** Subcutaneous Tissue and Fascia, Back **8** Subcutaneous Tissue and Fascia, Abdomen **9** Subcutaneous Tissue and Fascia, Buttock **B** Subcutaneous Tissue and Fascia, Perineum **C** Subcutaneous Tissue and Fascia, Pelvic Region **D** Subcutaneous Tissue and Fascia, Right Upper Arm **F** Subcutaneous Tissue and Fascia, Left Upper Arm **G** Subcutaneous Tissue and Fascia, Right Lower Arm **H** Subcutaneous Tissue and Fascia, Left Lower Arm **J** Subcutaneous Tissue and Fascia, Right Hand **K** Subcutaneous Tissue and Fascia, Left Hand **L** Subcutaneous Tissue and Fascia, Right Upper Leg **M** Subcutaneous Tissue and Fascia, Left Upper Leg **N** Subcutaneous Tissue and Fascia, Right Lower Leg **P** Subcutaneous Tissue and Fascia, Left Lower Leg **Q** Subcutaneous Tissue and Fascia, Right Foot **R** Subcutaneous Tissue and Fascia, Left Foot	**0** Open **3** Percutaneous	**Z** No Device	**X** Diagnostic **Z** No Qualifier

Section 0 Medical and Surgical
Body System J Subcutaneous Tissue and Fascia
Operation C **Extirpation:** Taking or cutting out solid matter from a body part

Body Part (4th)	Approach (5th)	Device (6th)	Qualifier (7th)
0 Subcutaneous Tissue and Fascia, Scalp 1 Subcutaneous Tissue and Fascia, Face 4 Subcutaneous Tissue and Fascia, Right Neck 5 Subcutaneous Tissue and Fascia, Left Neck 6 Subcutaneous Tissue and Fascia, Chest 7 Subcutaneous Tissue and Fascia, Back 8 Subcutaneous Tissue and Fascia, Abdomen 9 Subcutaneous Tissue and Fascia, Buttock B Subcutaneous Tissue and Fascia, Perineum C Subcutaneous Tissue and Fascia, Pelvic Region D Subcutaneous Tissue and Fascia, Right Upper Arm F Subcutaneous Tissue and Fascia, Left Upper Arm G Subcutaneous Tissue and Fascia, Right Lower Arm H Subcutaneous Tissue and Fascia, Left Lower Arm J Subcutaneous Tissue and Fascia, Right Hand K Subcutaneous Tissue and Fascia, Left Hand L Subcutaneous Tissue and Fascia, Right Upper Leg M Subcutaneous Tissue and Fascia, Left Upper Leg N Subcutaneous Tissue and Fascia, Right Lower Leg P Subcutaneous Tissue and Fascia, Left Lower Leg Q Subcutaneous Tissue and Fascia, Right Foot R Subcutaneous Tissue and Fascia, Left Foot	0 Open 3 Percutaneous	Z No Device	Z No Qualifier

Section 0 Medical and Surgical
Body System J Subcutaneous Tissue and Fascia
Operation D **Extraction:** Pulling or stripping out or off all or a portion of a body part by the use of force

Body Part (4th)	Approach (5th)	Device (6th)	Qualifier (7th)
0 Subcutaneous Tissue and Fascia, Scalp 1 Subcutaneous Tissue and Fascia, Face 4 Subcutaneous Tissue and Fascia, Right Neck 5 Subcutaneous Tissue and Fascia, Left Neck 6 Subcutaneous Tissue and Fascia, Chest 7 Subcutaneous Tissue and Fascia, Back 8 Subcutaneous Tissue and Fascia, Abdomen 9 Subcutaneous Tissue and Fascia, Buttock B Subcutaneous Tissue and Fascia, Perineum C Subcutaneous Tissue and Fascia, Pelvic Region D Subcutaneous Tissue and Fascia, Right Upper Arm F Subcutaneous Tissue and Fascia, Left Upper Arm G Subcutaneous Tissue and Fascia, Right Lower Arm H Subcutaneous Tissue and Fascia, Left Lower Arm J Subcutaneous Tissue and Fascia, Right Hand K Subcutaneous Tissue and Fascia, Left Hand L Subcutaneous Tissue and Fascia, Right Upper Leg M Subcutaneous Tissue and Fascia, Left Upper Leg N Subcutaneous Tissue and Fascia, Right Lower Leg P Subcutaneous Tissue and Fascia, Left Lower Leg Q Subcutaneous Tissue and Fascia, Right Foot R Subcutaneous Tissue and Fascia, Left Foot	0 Open 3 Percutaneous	Z No Device	Z No Qualifier

Section 0 **Medical and Surgical**
Body System J **Subcutaneous Tissue and Fascia**
Operation H **Insertion:** Putting in a nonbiological appliance that monitors, assists, performs, or prevents a physiological function but does not physically take the place of a body part

Body Part (4th)	Approach (5th)	Device (6th)	Qualifier (7th)
0 Subcutaneous Tissue and Fascia, Scalp **1** Subcutaneous Tissue and Fascia, Face **4** Subcutaneous Tissue and Fascia, Right Neck **5** Subcutaneous Tissue and Fascia, Left Neck **9** Subcutaneous Tissue and Fascia, Buttock **B** Subcutaneous Tissue and Fascia, Perineum **C** Subcutaneous Tissue and Fascia, Pelvic Region **J** Subcutaneous Tissue and Fascia, Right Hand **K** Subcutaneous Tissue and Fascia, Left Hand **Q** Subcutaneous Tissue and Fascia, Right Foot **R** Subcutaneous Tissue and Fascia, Left Foot	**0** Open **3** Percutaneous	**N** Tissue Expander	**Z** No Qualifier
6 Subcutaneous Tissue and Fascia, Chest	**0** Open **3** Percutaneous	**0** Monitoring Device, Hemodynamic **2** Monitoring Device **4** Pacemaker, Single Chamber **5** Pacemaker, Single Chamber Rate Responsive **6** Pacemaker, Dual Chamber **7** Cardiac Resynchronization Pacemaker Pulse Generator **8** Defibrillator Generator **9** Cardiac Resynchronization Defibrillator Pulse Generator **A** Contractility Modulation Device **B** Stimulator Generator, Single Array **C** Stimulator Generator, Single Array Rechargeable **D** Stimulator Generator, Multiple Array **E** Stimulator Generator, Multiple Array Rechargeable **F** Subcutaneous Defibrillator Lead **H** Contraceptive Device **M** Stimulator Generator **N** Tissue Expander **P** Cardiac Rhythm Related Device **V** Infusion Device, Pump **W** Vascular Access Device, Totally Implantable **X** Vascular Access Device, Tunneled **Y** Other Device	**Z** No Qualifier
7 Subcutaneous Tissue and Fascia, Back	**0** Open **3** Percutaneous	**B** Stimulator Generator, Single Array **C** Stimulator Generator, Single Array Rechargeable **D** Stimulator Generator, Multiple Array **E** Stimulator Generator, Multiple Array Rechargeable **M** Stimulator Generator **N** Tissue Expander **V** Infusion Device, Pump **Y** Other Device	**Z** No Qualifier

Continued →

Section 0 **Medical and Surgical**
Body System J **Subcutaneous Tissue and Fascia**
Operation H **Insertion:** Putting in a nonbiological appliance that monitors, assists, performs, or prevents a physiological function but does not physically take the place of a body part

Body Part (4th)	Approach (5th)	Device (6th)	Qualifier (7th)
8 Subcutaneous Tissue and Fascia, Abdomen	**0** Open **3** Percutaneous	**0** Monitoring Device, Hemodynamic **2** Monitoring Device **4** Pacemaker, Single Chamber **5** Pacemaker, Single Chamber Rate Responsive **6** Pacemaker, Dual Chamber **7** Cardiac Resynchronization Pacemaker Pulse Generator **8** Defibrillator Generator **9** Cardiac Resynchronization Defibrillator Pulse Generator **A** Contractility Modulation Device **B** Stimulator Generator, Single Array **C** Stimulator Generator, Single Array Rechargeable **D** Stimulator Generator, Multiple Array **E** Stimulator Generator, Multiple Array Rechargeable **H** Contraceptive Device **M** Stimulator Generator **N** Tissue Expander **P** Cardiac Rhythm Related Device **V** Infusion Device, Pump **W** Vascular Access Device Totally Implantable **X** Vascular Access Device, Tunneled **Y** Other Device	**Z** No Qualifier
D Subcutaneous Tissue and Fascia, Right Upper Arm **F** Subcutaneous Tissue and Fascia, Left Upper Arm **G** Subcutaneous Tissue and Fascia, Right Lower Arm **H** Subcutaneous Tissue and Fascia, Left Lower Arm **L** Subcutaneous Tissue and Fascia, Right Upper Leg **M** Subcutaneous Tissue and Fascia, Left Upper Leg **N** Subcutaneous Tissue and Fascia, Right Lower Leg **P** Subcutaneous Tissue and Fascia, Left Lower Leg	**0** Open **3** Percutaneous	**H** Contraceptive Device **N** Tissue Expander **V** Infusion Device, Pump **W** Vascular Access Device, Totally Implantable **X** Vascular Access Device, Tunneled	**Z** No Qualifier
S Subcutaneous Tissue and Fascia, Head and Neck **V** Subcutaneous Tissue and Fascia, Upper Extremity **W** Subcutaneous Tissue and Fascia, Lower Extremity	**0** Open **3** Percutaneous	**1** Radioactive Element **3** Infusion Device **Y** Other Device	**Z** No Qualifier
T Subcutaneous Tissue and Fascia, Trunk	**0** Open **3** Percutaneous	**1** Radioactive Element **3** Infusion Device **V** Infusion Device, Pump **Y** Other Device	**Z** No Qualifier

Section 0 **Medical and Surgical**
Body System J **Subcutaneous Tissue and Fascia**
Operation J **Inspection:** Visually and/or manually exploring a body part

Body Part (4th)	Approach (5th)	Device (6th)	Qualifier (7th)
S Subcutaneous Tissue and Fascia, Head and Neck **T** Subcutaneous Tissue and Fascia, Trunk **V** Subcutaneous Tissue and Fascia, Upper Extremity **W** Subcutaneous Tissue and Fascia, Lower Extremity	**0** Open **3** Percutaneous **X** External	**Z** No Device	**Z** No Qualifier

Section 0 **Medical and Surgical**
Body System J **Subcutaneous Tissue and Fascia**
Operation N **Release:** Freeing a body part from an abnormal physical constraint by cutting or by the use of force

Body Part (4th)	Approach (5th)	Device (6th)	Qualifier (7th)
0 Subcutaneous Tissue and Fascia, Scalp **1** Subcutaneous Tissue and Fascia, Face **4** Subcutaneous Tissue and Fascia, Right Neck **5** Subcutaneous Tissue and Fascia, Left Neck **6** Subcutaneous Tissue and Fascia, Chest **7** Subcutaneous Tissue and Fascia, Back **8** Subcutaneous Tissue and Fascia, Abdomen **9** Subcutaneous Tissue and Fascia, Buttock **B** Subcutaneous Tissue and Fascia, Perineum **C** Subcutaneous Tissue and Fascia, Pelvic Region **D** Subcutaneous Tissue and Fascia, Right Upper Arm **F** Subcutaneous Tissue and Fascia, Left Upper Arm **G** Subcutaneous Tissue and Fascia, Right Lower Arm **H** Subcutaneous Tissue and Fascia, Left Lower Arm **J** Subcutaneous Tissue and Fascia, Right Hand **K** Subcutaneous Tissue and Fascia, Left Hand **L** Subcutaneous Tissue and Fascia, Right Upper Leg **M** Subcutaneous Tissue and Fascia, Left Upper Leg **N** Subcutaneous Tissue and Fascia, Right Lower Leg **P** Subcutaneous Tissue and Fascia, Left Lower Leg **Q** Subcutaneous Tissue and Fascia, Right Foot **R** Subcutaneous Tissue and Fascia, Left Foot	**0** Open **3** Percutaneous **X** External	**Z** No Device	**Z** No Qualifier

Section 0 **Medical and Surgical**
Body System J **Subcutaneous Tissue and Fascia**
Operation P **Removal:** Taking out or off a device from a body part

Body Part (4th)	Approach (5th)	Device (6th)	Qualifier (7th)
S Subcutaneous Tissue and Fascia, Head and Neck	**0** Open **3** Percutaneous	**0** Drainage Device **1** Radioactive Element **3** Infusion Device **7** Autologous Tissue Substitute **J** Synthetic Substitute **K** Nonautologous Tissue Substitute **N** Tissue Expander **Y** Other Device	**Z** No Qualifier
S Subcutaneous Tissue and Fascia, Head and Neck	**X** External	**0** Drainage Device **1** Radioactive Element **3** Infusion Device	**Z** No Qualifier
T Subcutaneous Tissue and Fascia, Trunk	**0** Open **3** Percutaneous	**0** Drainage Device **1** Radioactive Element **2** Monitoring Device **3** Infusion Device **7** Autologous Tissue Substitute **F** Subcutaneous Defibrillator Lead **H** Contraceptive Device **J** Synthetic Substitute **K** Nonautologous Tissue Substitute **M** Stimulator Generator **N** Tissue Expander **P** Cardiac Rhythm Related Device **V** Infusion Device, Pump **W** Vascular Access Device, Totally Implantable **X** Vascular Access Device, Tunneled **Y** Other Device	**Z** No Qualifier

Continued →

Section 0 **Medical and Surgical**
Body System J **Subcutaneous Tissue and Fascia**
Operation P **Removal:** Taking out or off a device from a body part

Body Part (4th)	Approach (5th)	Device (6th)	Qualifier (7th)
T Subcutaneous Tissue and Fascia, Trunk	**X** External	**0** Drainage Device **1** Radioactive Element **2** Monitoring Device **3** Infusion Device **H** Contraceptive Device **V** Infusion Device, Pump **X** Vascular Access Device, Tunneled	**Z** No Qualifier
V Subcutaneous Tissue and Fascia, Upper Extremity **W** Subcutaneous Tissue and Fascia, Lower Extremity	**0** Open **3** Percutaneous	**0** Drainage Device **1** Radioactive Element **3** Infusion Device **7** Autologous Tissue Substitute **H** Contraceptive Device **J** Synthetic Substitute **K** Nonautologous Tissue Substitute **N** Tissue Expander **V** Infusion Device, Pump **W** Vascular Access Device, Totally Implantable **X** Vascular Access Device, Tunneled **Y** Other Device	**Z** No Qualifier
V Subcutaneous Tissue and Fascia, Upper Extremity **W** Subcutaneous Tissue and Fascia, Lower Extremity	**X** External	**0** Drainage Device **1** Radioactive Element **3** Infusion Device **H** Contraceptive Device **V** Infusion Device, Pump **X** Vascular Access Device, Tunneled	**Z** No Qualifier

Section 0 **Medical and Surgical**
Body System J **Subcutaneous Tissue and Fascia**
Operation Q **Repair:** Restoring, to the extent possible, a body part to its normal anatomic structure and function

Body Part (4th)	Approach (5th)	Device (6th)	Qualifier (7th)
0 Subcutaneous Tissue and Fascia, Scalp **1** Subcutaneous Tissue and Fascia, Face **4** Subcutaneous Tissue and Fascia, Right Neck **5** Subcutaneous Tissue and Fascia, Left Neck **6** Subcutaneous Tissue and Fascia, Chest **7** Subcutaneous Tissue and Fascia, Back **8** Subcutaneous Tissue and Fascia, Abdomen **9** Subcutaneous Tissue and Fascia, Buttock **B** Subcutaneous Tissue and Fascia, Perineum **C** Subcutaneous Tissue and Fascia, Pelvic Region **D** Subcutaneous Tissue and Fascia, Right Upper Arm **F** Subcutaneous Tissue and Fascia, Left Upper Arm **G** Subcutaneous Tissue and Fascia, Right Lower Arm **H** Subcutaneous Tissue and Fascia, Left Lower Arm **J** Subcutaneous Tissue and Fascia, Right Hand **K** Subcutaneous Tissue and Fascia, Left Hand **L** Subcutaneous Tissue and Fascia, Right Upper Leg **M** Subcutaneous Tissue and Fascia, Left Upper Leg **N** Subcutaneous Tissue and Fascia, Right Lower Leg **P** Subcutaneous Tissue and Fascia, Left Lower Leg **Q** Subcutaneous Tissue and Fascia, Right Foot **R** Subcutaneous Tissue and Fascia, Left Foot	**0** Open **3** Percutaneous	**Z** No Device	**Z** No Qualifier

Section 0 Medical and Surgical
Body System J Subcutaneous Tissue and Fascia
Operation R Replacement: Putting in or on biological or synthetic material that physically takes the place and/or function of all or a portion of a body part

Body Part (4th)	Approach (5th)	Device (6th)	Qualifier (7th)
0 Subcutaneous Tissue and Fascia, Scalp 1 Subcutaneous Tissue and Fascia, Face 4 Subcutaneous Tissue and Fascia, Right Neck 5 Subcutaneous Tissue and Fascia, Left Neck 6 Subcutaneous Tissue and Fascia, Chest 7 Subcutaneous Tissue and Fascia, Back 8 Subcutaneous Tissue and Fascia, Abdomen 9 Subcutaneous Tissue and Fascia, Buttock B Subcutaneous Tissue and Fascia, Perineum C Subcutaneous Tissue and Fascia, Pelvic Region D Subcutaneous Tissue and Fascia, Right Upper Arm F Subcutaneous Tissue and Fascia, Left Upper Arm G Subcutaneous Tissue and Fascia, Right Lower Arm H Subcutaneous Tissue and Fascia, Left Lower Arm J Subcutaneous Tissue and Fascia, Right Hand K Subcutaneous Tissue and Fascia, Left Hand L Subcutaneous Tissue and Fascia, Right Upper Leg M Subcutaneous Tissue and Fascia, Left Upper Leg N Subcutaneous Tissue and Fascia, Right Lower Leg P Subcutaneous Tissue and Fascia, Left Lower Leg Q Subcutaneous Tissue and Fascia, Right Foot R Subcutaneous Tissue and Fascia, Left Foot	0 Open 3 Percutaneous	7 Autologous Tissue Substitute J Synthetic Substitute K Nonautologous Tissue Substitute	Z No Qualifier

Section 0 Medical and Surgical
Body System J Subcutaneous Tissue and Fascia
Operation U Supplement: Putting in or on biological or synthetic material that physically reinforces and/or augments the function of a portion of a body part

Body Part (4th)	Approach (5th)	Device (6th)	Qualifier (7th)
0 Subcutaneous Tissue and Fascia, Scalp 1 Subcutaneous Tissue and Fascia, Face 4 Subcutaneous Tissue and Fascia, Right Neck 5 Subcutaneous Tissue and Fascia, Left Neck 6 Subcutaneous Tissue and Fascia, Chest 7 Subcutaneous Tissue and Fascia, Back 8 Subcutaneous Tissue and Fascia, Abdomen 9 Subcutaneous Tissue and Fascia, Buttock B Subcutaneous Tissue and Fascia, Perineum C Subcutaneous Tissue and Fascia, Pelvic Region D Subcutaneous Tissue and Fascia, Right Upper Arm F Subcutaneous Tissue and Fascia, Left Upper Arm G Subcutaneous Tissue and Fascia, Right Lower Arm H Subcutaneous Tissue and Fascia, Left Lower Arm J Subcutaneous Tissue and Fascia, Right Hand K Subcutaneous Tissue and Fascia, Left Hand L Subcutaneous Tissue and Fascia, Right Upper Leg M Subcutaneous Tissue and Fascia, Left Upper Leg N Subcutaneous Tissue and Fascia, Right Lower Leg P Subcutaneous Tissue and Fascia, Left Lower Leg Q Subcutaneous Tissue and Fascia, Right Foot R Subcutaneous Tissue and Fascia, Left Foot	0 Open 3 Percutaneous	7 Autologous Tissue Substitute J Synthetic Substitute K Nonautologous Tissue Substitute	Z No Qualifier

Section **0** **Medical and Surgical**
Body System **J** **Subcutaneous Tissue and Fascia**
Operation **W** **Revision:** Correcting, to the extent possible, a portion of a malfunctioning device or the position of a displaced device

Body Part (4th)	Approach (5th)	Device (6th)	Qualifier (7th)
S Subcutaneous Tissue and Fascia, Head and Neck	**0** Open **3** Percutaneous	**0** Drainage Device **3** Infusion Device **7** Autologous Tissue Substitute **J** Synthetic Substitute **K** Nonautologous Tissue Substitute **N** Tissue Expander **Y** Other Device	**Z** No Qualifier
S Subcutaneous Tissue and Fascia, Head and Neck	**X** External	**0** Drainage Device **3** Infusion Device **7** Autologous Tissue Substitute **J** Synthetic Substitute **K** Nonautologous Tissue Substitute **N** Tissue Expander	**Z** No Qualifier
T Subcutaneous Tissue and Fascia, Trunk	**0** Open **3** Percutaneous	**0** Drainage Device **2** Monitoring Device **3** Infusion Device **7** Autologous Tissue Substitute **F** Subcutaneous Defibrillator Lead **H** Contraceptive Device **J** Synthetic Substitute **K** Nonautologous Tissue Substitute **M** Stimulator Generator **N** Tissue Expander **P** Cardiac Rhythm Related Device **V** Infusion Device, Pump **W** Vascular Access Device, Totally Implantable **X** Vascular Access Device, Tunneled **Y** Other Device	**Z** No Qualifier
T Subcutaneous Tissue and Fascia, Trunk	**X** External	**0** Drainage Device **2** Monitoring Device **3** Infusion Device **7** Autologous Tissue Substitute **F** Subcutaneous Defibrillator Lead **H** Contraceptive Device **J** Synthetic Substitute **K** Nonautologous Tissue Substitute **M** Stimulator Generator **N** Tissue Expander **P** Cardiac Rhythm Related Device **V** Infusion Device, Pump **W** Vascular Access Device, Totally Implantable **X** Vascular Access Device, Tunneled	**Z** No Qualifier
V Subcutaneous Tissue and Fascia, Upper Extremity **W** Subcutaneous Tissue and Fascia, Lower Extremity	**0** Open **3** Percutaneous	**0** Drainage Device **3** Infusion Device **7** Autologous Tissue Substitute **H** Contraceptive Device **J** Synthetic Substitute **K** Nonautologous Tissue Substitute **N** Tissue Expander **V** Infusion Device, Pump **W** Vascular Access Device, Totally Implantable **X** Vascular Access Device, Tunneled **Y** Other Device	**Z** No Qualifier

Continued →

Section 0 **Medical and Surgical**
Body System J **Subcutaneous Tissue and Fascia**
Operation W **Revision:** Correcting, to the extent possible, a portion of a malfunctioning device or the position of a displaced device

Body Part (4th)	Approach (5th)	Device (6th)	Qualifier (7th)
V Subcutaneous Tissue and Fascia, Upper Extremity **W** Subcutaneous Tissue and Fascia, Lower Extremity	**X** External	**0** Drainage Device **3** Infusion Device **7** Autologous Tissue Substitute **H** Contraceptive Device **J** Synthetic Substitute **K** Nonautologous Tissue Substitute **N** Tissue Expander **V** Infusion Device, Pump **W** Vascular Access Device, Totally Implantable **X** Vascular Access Device, Tunneled	**Z** No Qualifier

Section 0 **Medical and Surgical**
Body System J **Subcutaneous Tissue and Fascia**
Operation X **Transfer:** Moving, without taking out, all or a portion of a body part to another location to take over the function of all or a portion of a body part

Body Part (4th)	Approach (5th)	Device (6th)	Qualifier (7th)
0 Subcutaneous Tissue and Fascia, Scalp **1** Subcutaneous Tissue and Fascia, Face **4** Subcutaneous Tissue and Fascia, Right Neck **5** Subcutaneous Tissue and Fascia, Left Neck **6** Subcutaneous Tissue and Fascia, Chest **7** Subcutaneous Tissue and Fascia, Back **8** Subcutaneous Tissue and Fascia, Abdomen **9** Subcutaneous Tissue and Fascia, Buttock **B** Subcutaneous Tissue and Fascia, Perineum **C** Subcutaneous Tissue and Fascia, Pelvic Region **D** Subcutaneous Tissue and Fascia, Right Upper Arm **F** Subcutaneous Tissue and Fascia, Left Upper Arm **G** Subcutaneous Tissue and Fascia, Right Lower Arm **H** Subcutaneous Tissue and Fascia, Left Lower Arm **J** Subcutaneous Tissue and Fascia, Right Hand **K** Subcutaneous Tissue and Fascia, Left Hand **L** Subcutaneous Tissue and Fascia, Right Upper Leg **M** Subcutaneous Tissue and Fascia, Left Upper Leg **N** Subcutaneous Tissue and Fascia, Right Lower Leg **P** Subcutaneous Tissue and Fascia, Left Lower Leg **Q** Subcutaneous Tissue and Fascia, Right Foot **R** Subcutaneous Tissue and Fascia, Left Foot	**0** Open **3** Percutaneous	**Z** No Device	**B** Skin and Subcutaneous Tissue **C** Skin, Subcutaneous Tissue and Fascia **Z** No Qualifier

AHA Coding Clinic

0J2TXYZ Change Other Device in Trunk Subcutaneous Tissue and Fascia, External Approach—AHA CC: 2Q, 2017, 26; 3Q, 2018, 10

0J910ZZ Drainage of Face Subcutaneous Tissue and Fascia, Open Approach—AHA CC: 3Q, 2018, 16

0J940ZZ Drainage of Right Neck Subcutaneous Tissue and Fascia, Open Approach—AHA CC: 3Q, 2018, 16-17

0J960ZZ Drainage of Chest Subcutaneous Tissue and Fascia, Open Approach—AHA CC: 3Q, 2015, 23-24

0J9C0ZZ Drainage of Pelvic Region Subcutaneous Tissue and Fascia, Open Approach—AHA CC: 3Q, 2015, 23-24

0J9D0ZZ Drainage of Right Upper Arm Subcutaneous Tissue and Fascia, Open Approach—AHA CC: 3Q, 2015, 23-24

0J9F0ZZ Drainage of Left Upper Arm Subcutaneous Tissue and Fascia, Open Approach—AHA CC: 3Q, 2015, 23-24

0J9L0ZZ Drainage of Right Upper Leg Subcutaneous Tissue and Fascia, Open Approach—AHA CC: 3Q, 2015, 23-24

0J9M0ZZ Drainage of Left Upper Leg Subcutaneous Tissue and Fascia, Open Approach—AHA CC: 3Q, 2015, 23-24

0JB70ZZ Excision of Back Subcutaneous Tissue and Fascia, Open Approach—AHA CC: 1Q, 2018, 7-8

0JB80ZZ Excision of Abdomen Subcutaneous Tissue and Fascia, Open Approach—AHA CC: 3Q, 2014, 22-23; 4Q, 2014, 39-40; 1Q, 2020, 31-32

0JB90ZZ Excision of Buttock Subcutaneous Tissue and Fascia, Open Approach—AHA CC: 3Q, 2015, 6-7

0JB93ZZ Excision of Buttock Subcutaneous Tissue and Fascia, Percutaneous Approach—AHA CC: 3Q, 2019, 25

0JBB0ZZ Excision of Perineum Subcutaneous Tissue and Fascia, Open Approach—AHA CC: 1Q, 2015, 29-30

0JBH0ZZ Excision of Left Lower Arm Subcutaneous Tissue and Fascia, Open Approach—AHA CC: 2Q, 2015, 13

0JC80ZZ Extirpation of Matter from Abdomen Subcutaneous Tissue and Fascia, Open Approach—AHA CC: 3Q, 2017, 22

0JD70ZZ Extraction of Back Subcutaneous Tissue and Fascia, Open Approach—AHA CC: 3Q, 2016, 21

0JDC0ZZ Extraction of Pelvic Region Subcutaneous Tissue and Fascia, Open Approach—AHA CC: 1Q, 2015, 23

0JDL0ZZ Extraction of Right Upper Leg Subcutaneous Tissue and Fascia, Open Approach—AHA CC: 1Q, 2016, 40

0JDN0ZZ Extraction of Right Lower Leg Subcutaneous Tissue and Fascia, Open Approach—AHA CC: 3Q, 2016, 20-21

0JDR0ZZ Extraction of Left Foot Subcutaneous Tissue and Fascia, Open Approach—AHA CC: 3Q, 2016, 22

0JH608Z Insertion of Defibrillator Generator into Chest Subcutaneous Tissue and Fascia, Open Approach—AHA CC: 4Q, 2012, 104-106

0JH60MZ Insertion of Stimulator Generator into Chest Subcutaneous Tissue and Fascia, Open Approach—AHA CC: 4Q, 2016, 98-99

0JH60PZ Insertion of Cardiac Rhythm Related Device into Chest Subcutaneous Tissue and Fascia, Open Approach—AHA CC: 4Q, 2012, 104-106

0JH60WZ Insertion of Totally Implantable Vascular Access Device into Chest Subcutaneous Tissue and Fascia, Open Approach—AHA CC: 4Q, 2017, 63-64

0JH60XZ Insertion of Tunneled Vascular Access Device into Chest Subcutaneous Tissue and Fascia, Open Approach—AHA CC: 2Q, 2015, 33-34

0JH63VZ Insertion of Infusion Pump into Chest Subcutaneous Tissue and Fascia, Percutaneous Approach—AHA CC: 4Q, 2015, 14-15

0JH63XZ Insertion of Tunneled Vascular Access Device into Chest Subcutaneous Tissue and Fascia, Percutaneous Approach—AHA CC: 4Q, 2015, 30-32; 2Q, 2016, 15-16; 2Q, 2017, 24-26

0JH80VZ Insertion of Infusion Pump into Abdomen Subcutaneous Tissue and Fascia, Open Approach—AHA CC: 3Q, 2014, 19-20

0JH80WZ Insertion of Totally Implantable Vascular Access Device into Abdomen Subcutaneous Tissue and Fascia, Open Approach—AHA CC: 2Q, 2016, 14

0JH80YZ Insertion of Other Device into Abdomen Subcutaneous Tissue and Fascia, Open Approach—AHA CC: 4Q, 2020, 55

0JHS33Z Insertion of Infusion Device into Head and Neck Subcutaneous Tissue and Fascia, Percutaneous Approach—AHA CC: 2Q, 2020, 15-16

0JHT03Z Insertion of Infusion Device into Trunk Subcutaneous Tissue and Fascia, Open Approach—AHA CC: 2Q, 2020, 16-17

0JHT0YZ Insertion of Other Device into Trunk Subcutaneous Tissue and Fascia, Open Approach—AHA CC: 4Q, 2018, 42-43

0JNL0ZZ Release Right Upper Leg Subcutaneous Tissue and Fascia, Open Approach—AHA CC: 3Q, 2017, 11-12

0JNM0ZZ Release Left Upper Leg Subcutaneous Tissue and Fascia, Open Approach—AHA CC: 3Q, 2017, 11-12

0JNN0ZZ Release Right Lower Leg Subcutaneous Tissue and Fascia, Open Approach—AHA CC: 3Q, 2017, 11-12

0JNP0ZZ Release Left Lower Leg Subcutaneous Tissue and Fascia, Open Approach—AHA CC: 3Q, 2017, 11-12

0JNQ0ZZ Release Right Foot Subcutaneous Tissue and Fascia, Open Approach—AHA CC: 3Q, 2017, 11-12

0JNR0ZZ Release Left Foot Subcutaneous Tissue and Fascia, Open Approach—AHA CC: 3Q, 2017, 11-12

0JPT0NZ Removal of Tissue Expander from Trunk Subcutaneous Tissue and Fascia, Open Approach—AHA CC: 4Q, 2013, 109-111

0JPT0PZ Removal of Cardiac Rhythm Related Device from Trunk Subcutaneous Tissue and Fascia, Open Approach—AHA CC: 4Q, 2012, 104-106

0JPT0VZ Removal of Infusion Pump from Trunk Subcutaneous Tissue and Fascia, Open Approach—AHA CC: 3Q, 2014, 19-20

0JPT0XZ Removal of Tunneled Vascular Access Device from Trunk Subcutaneous Tissue and Fascia, Open Approach—AHA CC: 4Q, 2015, 31-32; 2Q, 2016, 15-16

0JPT3JZ Removal of Synthetic Substitute from Trunk Subcutaneous Tissue and Fascia, Percutaneous Approach—AHA CC: 4Q, 2018, 86

0JPT3YZ Removal of Other Device from Trunk Subcutaneous Tissue and Fascia, Percutaneous Approach—AHA CC: 3Q, 2018, 29

0JQC0ZZ Repair Pelvic Region Subcutaneous Tissue and Fascia, Open Approach—AHA CC: 4Q, 2014, 44-45; 3Q, 2017, 19

0JR107Z Replacement of Face Subcutaneous Tissue and Fascia with Autologous Tissue Substitute, Open Approach—AHA CC: 2Q, 2015, 13

0JU707Z Supplement of Back Subcutaneous Tissue and Fascia with Autologous Tissue Substitute, Open Approach—AHA CC: 1Q, 2018, 7-8

0JUH0KZ Supplement of Left Lower Arm Subcutaneous Tissue and Fascia with Nonautologous Tissue Substitute, Open Approach—AHA CC: 2Q, 2018, 20

0JWS0JZ Revision of Synthetic Substitute in Head and Neck Subcutaneous Tissue and Fascia, Open Approach—AHA CC: 2Q, 2015, 9-10

0JWT0JZ Revision of Synthetic Substitute in Trunk Subcutaneous Tissue and Fascia, Open Approach— AHA CC: 1Q, 2018, 8-9

0JWT0PZ Revision of Cardiac Rhythm Related Device in Trunk Subcutaneous Tissue and Fascia, Open Approach—AHA CC: 4Q, 2012, 104-106

0JWT33Z Revision of Infusion Device in Trunk Subcutaneous Tissue and Fascia, Percutaneous Approach—AHA CC: 4Q, 2015, 33

0JX00ZC Transfer Scalp Subcutaneous Tissue and Fascia with Skin, Subcutaneous Tissue and Fascia, Open Approach—AHA CC: 1Q, 2018, 10

0JX60ZB Transfer Chest Subcutaneous Tissue and Fascia with Skin and Subcutaneous Tissue, Open Approach—AHA CC: 4Q, 2013, 109-111; 2Q, 2021, 16-17

0JX80ZB Transfer Abdomen Subcutaneous Tissue and Fascia with Skin and Subcutaneous Tissue, Open Approach—AHA CC: 4Q, 2013, 109-111

0JXN0ZC Transfer Right Lower Leg Subcutaneous Tissue and Fascia with Skin, Subcutaneous Tissue and Fascia, Open Approach—AHA CC: 3Q, 2014, 18-19

Muscles

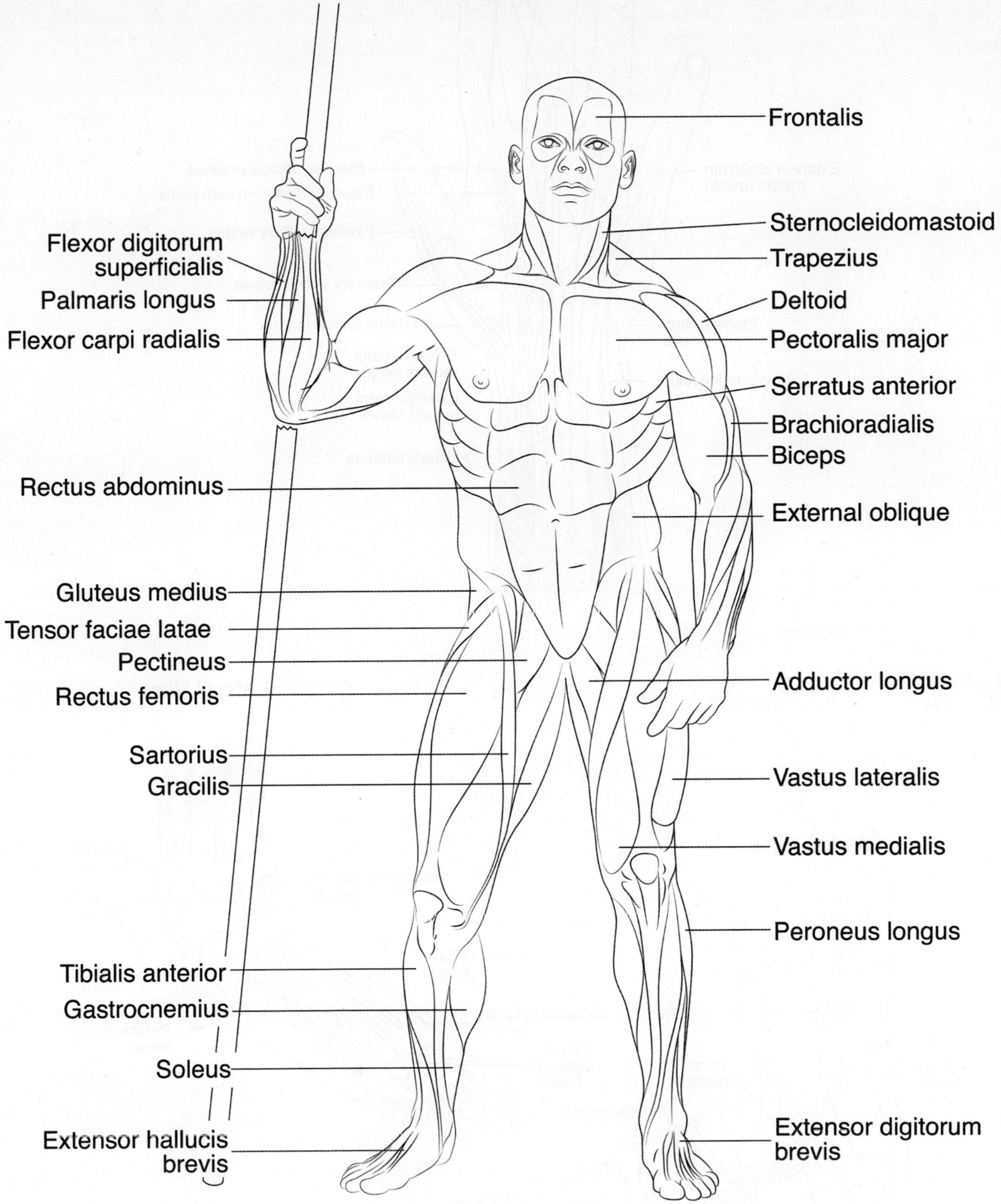
Frontalis
Sternocleidomastoid
Trapezius
Deltoid
Pectoralis major
Serratus anterior
Brachioradialis
Biceps
External oblique
Adductor longus
Vastus lateralis
Vastus medialis
Peroneus longus
Extensor digitorum brevis
Flexor digitorum superficialis
Palmaris longus
Flexor carpi radialis
Rectus abdominus
Gluteus medius
Tensor faciae latae
Pectineus
Rectus femoris
Sartorius
Gracilis
Tibialis anterior
Gastrocnemius
Soleus
Extensor hallucis brevis

Muscles of the Hand

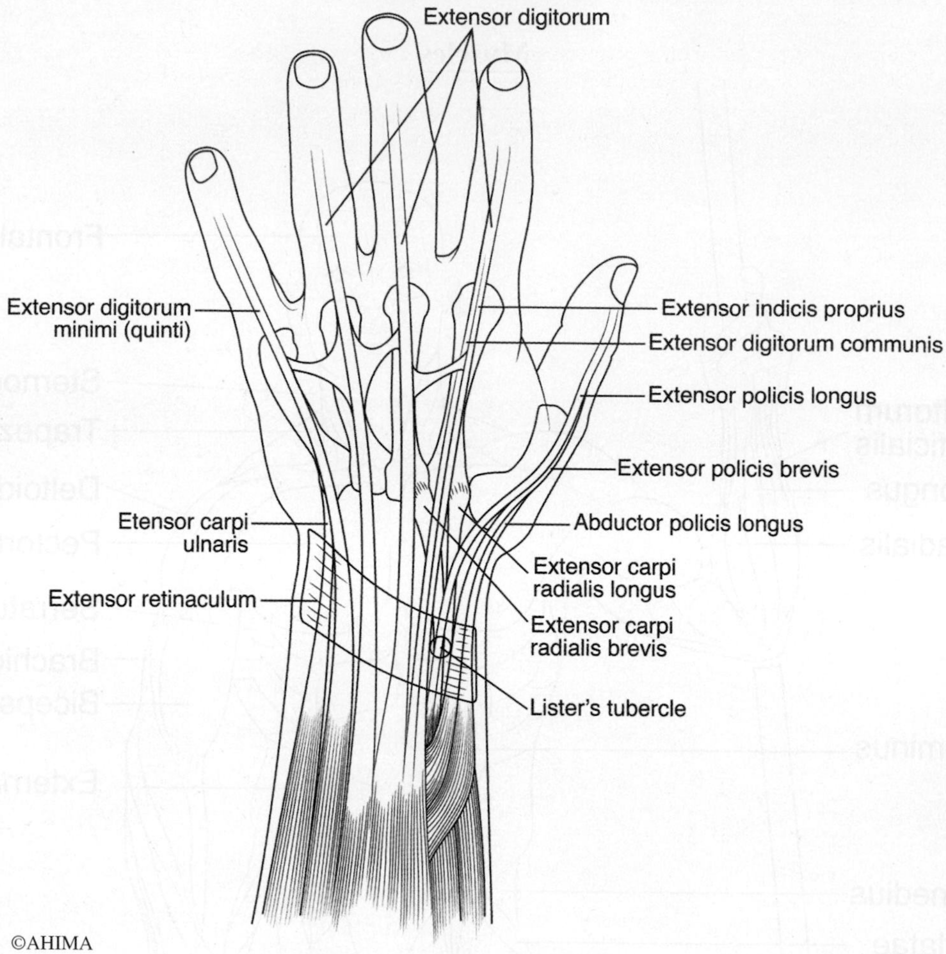
Extensor digitorum
Extensor digitorum minimi (quinti)
Extensor indicis proprius
Extensor digitorum communis
Extensor policis longus
Extensor policis brevis
Etensor carpi ulnaris
Abductor policis longus
Extensor carpi radialis longus
Extensor retinaculum
Extensor carpi radialis brevis
Lister's tubercle

Muscles of the Foot

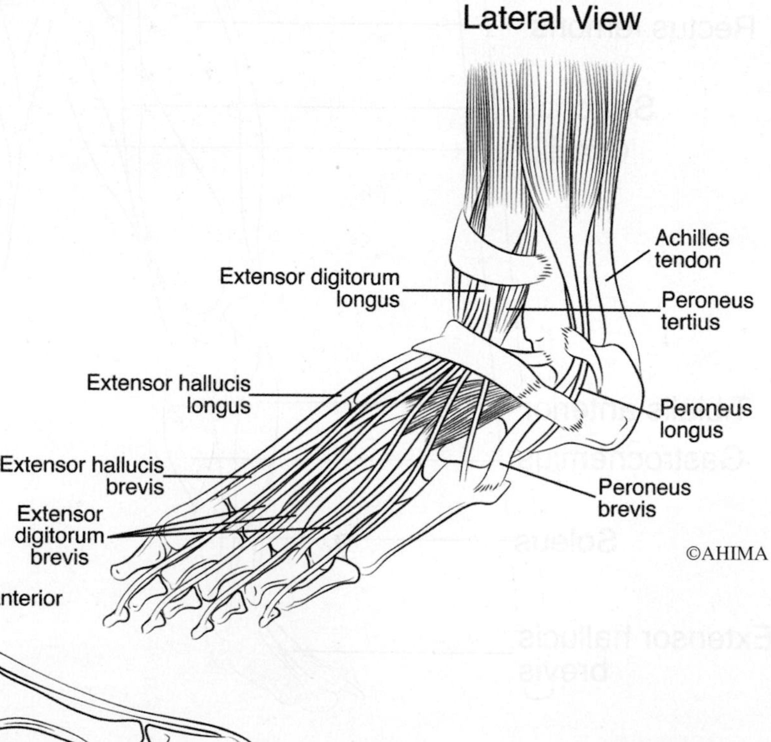
Lateral View
Achilles tendon
Extensor digitorum longus
Peroneus tertius
Extensor hallucis longus
Peroneus longus
Extensor hallucis brevis
Peroneus brevis
Extensor digitorum brevis

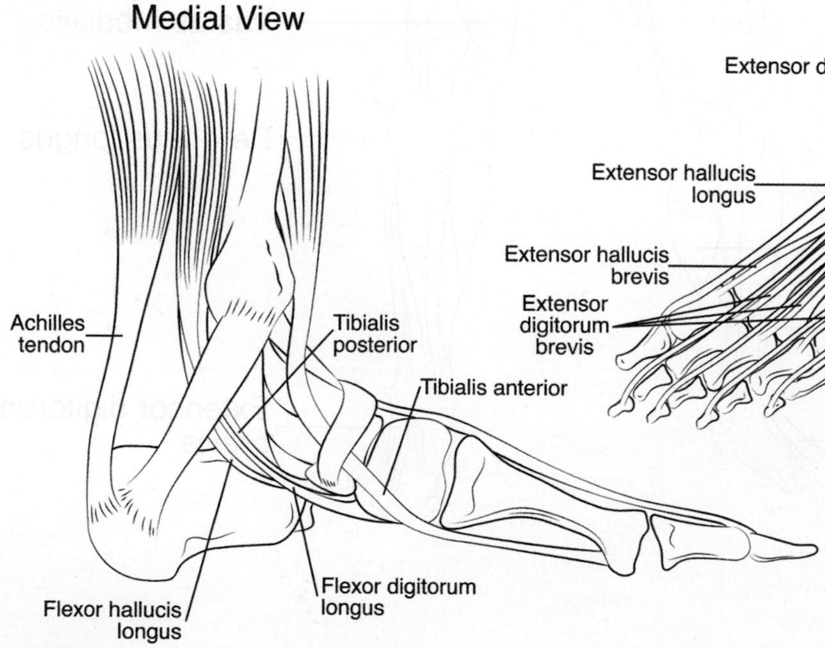
Medial View
Achilles tendon
Tibialis posterior
Tibialis anterior
Flexor digitorum longus
Flexor hallucis longus

Muscles Tables 0K2–0KX

Section 0 **Medical and Surgical**
Body System K **Muscles**
Operation 2 **Change:** Taking out or off a device from a body part and putting back an identical or similar device in or on the same body part without cutting or puncturing the skin or a mucous membrane

Body Part (4th)	Approach (5th)	Device (6th)	Qualifier (7th)
X Upper Muscle **Y** Lower Muscle	**X** External	**0** Drainage Device **Y** Other Device	**Z** No Qualifier

Section 0 **Medical and Surgical**
Body System K **Muscles**
Operation 5 **Destruction:** Physical eradication of all or a portion of a body part by the direct use of energy, force, or a destructive agent

Body Part (4th)	Approach (5th)	Device (6th)	Qualifier (7th)
0 Head Muscle **1** Facial Muscle **2** Neck Muscle, Right **3** Neck Muscle, Left **4** Tongue, Palate, Pharynx Muscle **5** Shoulder Muscle, Right **6** Shoulder Muscle, Left **7** Upper Arm Muscle, Right **8** Upper Arm Muscle, Left **9** Lower Arm and Wrist Muscle, Right **B** Lower Arm and Wrist Muscle, Left **C** Hand Muscle, Right **D** Hand Muscle, Left **F** Trunk Muscle, Right **G** Trunk Muscle, Left **H** Thorax Muscle, Right **J** Thorax Muscle, Left **K** Abdomen Muscle, Right **L** Abdomen Muscle, Left **M** Perineum Muscle **N** Hip Muscle, Right **P** Hip Muscle, Left **Q** Upper Leg Muscle, Right **R** Upper Leg Muscle, Left **S** Lower Leg Muscle, Right **T** Lower Leg Muscle, Left **V** Foot Muscle, Right **W** Foot Muscle, Left	**0** Open **3** Percutaneous **4** Percutaneous Endoscopic	**Z** No Device	**Z** No Qualifier

Section 0 **Medical and Surgical**
Body System K **Muscles**
Operation 8 **Division:** Cutting into a body part, without draining fluids and/or gases from the body part, in order to separate or transect a body part

Body Part (4th)	Approach (5th)	Device (6th)	Qualifier (7th)
0 Head Muscle **1** Facial Muscle **2** Neck Muscle, Right **3** Neck Muscle, Left **5** Shoulder Muscle, Right **6** Shoulder Muscle, Left **7** Upper Arm Muscle, Right **8** Upper Arm Muscle, Left **9** Lower Arm and Wrist Muscle, Right **B** Lower Arm and Wrist Muscle, Left **C** Hand Muscle, Right **D** Hand Muscle, Left **F** Trunk Muscle, Right **G** Trunk Muscle, Left **H** Thorax Muscle, Right **J** Thorax Muscle, Left **K** Abdomen Muscle, Right **L** Abdomen Muscle, Left **M** Perineum Muscle **N** Hip Muscle, Right **P** Hip Muscle, Left **Q** Upper Leg Muscle, Right **R** Upper Leg Muscle, Left **S** Lower Leg Muscle, Right **T** Lower Leg Muscle, Left **V** Foot Muscle, Right **W** Foot Muscle, Left	**0** Open **3** Percutaneous **4** Percutaneous Endoscopic	**Z** No Device	**Z** No Qualifier
4 Tongue, Palate, Pharynx Muscle	**0** Open **3** Percutaneous **4** Percutaneous Endoscopic **7** Via Natural or Artificial Opening **8** Via Natural or Artificial Opening Endoscopic	**Z** No Device	**Z** No Qualifier

Section 0 **Medical and Surgical**
Body System K **Muscles**
Operation 9 **Drainage:** Taking or letting out fluids and/or gases from a body part

Body Part (4th)	Approach (5th)	Device (6th)	Qualifier (7th)
0 Head Muscle **1** Facial Muscle **2** Neck Muscle, Right **3** Neck Muscle, Left **4** Tongue, Palate, Pharynx Muscle **5** Shoulder Muscle, Right **6** Shoulder Muscle, Left **7** Upper Arm Muscle, Right **8** Upper Arm Muscle, Left **9** Lower Arm and Wrist Muscle, Right **B** Lower Arm and Wrist Muscle, Left **C** Hand Muscle, Right **D** Hand Muscle, Left **F** Trunk Muscle, Right **G** Trunk Muscle, Left **H** Thorax Muscle, Right **J** Thorax Muscle, Left **K** Abdomen Muscle, Right **L** Abdomen Muscle, Left **M** Perineum Muscle **N** Hip Muscle, Right **P** Hip Muscle, Left **Q** Upper Leg Muscle, Right **R** Upper Leg Muscle, Left **S** Lower Leg Muscle, Right **T** Lower Leg Muscle, Left **V** Foot Muscle, Right **W** Foot Muscle, Left	**0** Open **3** Percutaneous **4** Percutaneous Endoscopic	**0** Drainage Device	**Z** No Qualifier
0 Head Muscle **1** Facial Muscle **2** Neck Muscle, Right **3** Neck Muscle, Left **4** Tongue, Palate, Pharynx Muscle **5** Shoulder Muscle, Right **6** Shoulder Muscle, Left **7** Upper Arm Muscle, Right **8** Upper Arm Muscle, Left **9** Lower Arm and Wrist Muscle, Right **B** Lower Arm and Wrist Muscle, Left **C** Hand Muscle, Right **D** Hand Muscle, Left **F** Trunk Muscle, Right **G** Trunk Muscle, Left **H** Thorax Muscle, Right **J** Thorax Muscle, Left **K** Abdomen Muscle, Right **L** Abdomen Muscle, Left **M** Perineum Muscle **N** Hip Muscle, Right **P** Hip Muscle, Left **Q** Upper Leg Muscle, Right **R** Upper Leg Muscle, Left **S** Lower Leg Muscle, Right **T** Lower Leg Muscle, Left **V** Foot Muscle, Right **W** Foot Muscle, Left	**0** Open **3** Percutaneous **4** Percutaneous Endoscopic	**Z** No Device	**X** Diagnostic **Z** No Qualifier

Section 0 **Medical and Surgical**
Body System K **Muscles**
Operation B **Excision:** Cutting out or off, without replacement, a portion of a body part

Body Part (4th)	Approach (5th)	Device (6th)	Qualifier (7th)
0 Head Muscle 1 Facial Muscle 2 Neck Muscle, Right 3 Neck Muscle, Left 4 Tongue, Palate, Pharynx Muscle 5 Shoulder Muscle, Right 6 Shoulder Muscle, Left 7 Upper Arm Muscle, Right 8 Upper Arm Muscle, Left 9 Lower Arm and Wrist Muscle, Right B Lower Arm and Wrist Muscle, Left C Hand Muscle, Right D Hand Muscle, Left F Trunk Muscle, Right G Trunk Muscle, Left H Thorax Muscle, Right J Thorax Muscle, Left K Abdomen Muscle, Right L Abdomen Muscle, Left M Perineum Muscle N Hip Muscle, Right P Hip Muscle, Left Q Upper Leg Muscle, Right R Upper Leg Muscle, Left S Lower Leg Muscle, Right T Lower Leg Muscle, Left V Foot Muscle, Right W Foot Muscle, Left	0 Open 3 Percutaneous 4 Percutaneous Endoscopic	Z No Device	X Diagnostic Z No Qualifier

Section 0 **Medical and Surgical**
Body System K **Muscles**
Operation C **Extirpation:** Taking or cutting out solid matter from a body part

Body Part (4th)	Approach (5th)	Device (6th)	Qualifier (7th)
0 Head Muscle 1 Facial Muscle 2 Neck Muscle, Right 3 Neck Muscle, Left 4 Tongue, Palate, Pharynx Muscle 5 Shoulder Muscle, Right 6 Shoulder Muscle, Left 7 Upper Arm Muscle, Right 8 Upper Arm Muscle, Left 9 Lower Arm and Wrist Muscle, Right B Lower Arm and Wrist Muscle, Left C Hand Muscle, Right D Hand Muscle, Left F Trunk Muscle, Right G Trunk Muscle, Left H Thorax Muscle, Right J Thorax Muscle, Left K Abdomen Muscle, Right L Abdomen Muscle, Left M Perineum Muscle N Hip Muscle, Right P Hip Muscle, Left Q Upper Leg Muscle, Right R Upper Leg Muscle, Left S Lower Leg Muscle, Right T Lower Leg Muscle, Left V Foot Muscle, Right W Foot Muscle, Left	0 Open 3 Percutaneous 4 Percutaneous Endoscopic	Z No Device	Z No Qualifier

Section	**0**	**Medical and Surgical**
Body System	**K**	**Muscles**
Operation	**D**	**Extraction:** Pulling or stripping out or off all or a portion of a body part by the use of force

Body Part (4th)	Approach (5th)	Device (6th)	Qualifier (7th)
0 Head Muscle **1** Facial Muscle **2** Neck Muscle, Right **3** Neck Muscle, Left **4** Tongue, Palate, Pharynx Muscle **5** Shoulder Muscle, Right **6** Shoulder Muscle, Left **7** Upper Arm Muscle, Right **8** Upper Arm Muscle, Left **9** Lower Arm and Wrist Muscle, Right **B** Lower Arm and Wrist Muscle, Left **C** Hand Muscle, Right **D** Hand Muscle, Left **F** Trunk Muscle, Right **G** Trunk Muscle, Left **H** Thorax Muscle, Right **J** Thorax Muscle, Left **K** Abdomen Muscle, Right **L** Abdomen Muscle, Left **M** Perineum **N** Hip Muscle, Right **P** Hip Muscle, Left **Q** Upper Leg Muscle, Right **R** Upper Leg Muscle, Left **S** Lower Leg Muscle, Right **T** Lower Leg Muscle, Left **V** Foot Muscle, Right **W** Foot Muscle, Left	**0** Open	**Z** No Device	**Z** No Qualifier

Section	**0**	**Medical and Surgical**
Body System	**K**	**Muscles**
Operation	**H**	**Insertion:** Putting in a nonbiological appliance that monitors, assists, performs, or prevents a physiological function but does not physically take the place of a body part

Body Part (4th)	Approach (5th)	Device (6th)	Qualifier (7th)
X Upper Muscle **Y** Lower Muscle	**0** Open **3** Percutaneous **4** Percutaneous Endoscopic	**M** Stimulator Lead **Y** Other Device	**Z** No Qualifier

Section	**0**	**Medical and Surgical**
Body System	**K**	**Muscles**
Operation	**J**	**Inspection:** Visually and/or manually exploring a body part

Body Part (4th)	Approach (5th)	Device (6th)	Qualifier (7th)
X Upper Muscle **Y** Lower Muscle	**0** Open **3** Percutaneous **4** Percutaneous Endoscopic **X** External	**Z** No Device	**Z** No Qualifier

Section 0 **Medical and Surgical**
Body System K **Muscles**
Operation M **Reattachment:** Putting back in or on all or a portion of a separated body part to its normal location or other suitable location

Body Part (4th)	Approach (5th)	Device (6th)	Qualifier (7th)
0 Head Muscle **1** Facial Muscle **2** Neck Muscle, Right **3** Neck Muscle, Left **4** Tongue, Palate, Pharynx Muscle **5** Shoulder Muscle, Right **6** Shoulder Muscle, Left **7** Upper Arm Muscle, Right **8** Upper Arm Muscle, Left **9** Lower Arm and Wrist Muscle, Right **B** Lower Arm and Wrist Muscle, Left **C** Hand Muscle, Right **D** Hand Muscle, Left **F** Trunk Muscle, Right **G** Trunk Muscle, Left **H** Thorax Muscle, Right **J** Thorax Muscle, Left **K** Abdomen Muscle, Right **L** Abdomen Muscle, Left **M** Perineum Muscle **N** Hip Muscle, Right **P** Hip Muscle, Left **Q** Upper Leg Muscle, Right **R** Upper Leg Muscle, Left **S** Lower Leg Muscle, Right **T** Lower Leg Muscle, Left **V** Foot Muscle, Right **W** Foot Muscle, Left	**0** Open **4** Percutaneous Endoscopic	**Z** No Device	**Z** No Qualifier

Section 0 **Medical and Surgical**
Body System K **Muscles**
Operation N **Release:** Freeing a body part from an abnormal physical constraint by cutting or by the use of force

Body Part (4th)	Approach (5th)	Device (6th)	Qualifier (7th)
0 Head Muscle **1** Facial Muscle **2** Neck Muscle, Right **3** Neck Muscle, Left **4** Tongue, Palate, Pharynx Muscle **5** Shoulder Muscle, Right **6** Shoulder Muscle, Left **7** Upper Arm Muscle, Right **8** Upper Arm Muscle, Left **9** Lower Arm and Wrist Muscle, Right **B** Lower Arm and Wrist Muscle, Left **C** Hand Muscle, Right **D** Hand Muscle, Left **F** Trunk Muscle, Right **G** Trunk Muscle, Left **H** Thorax Muscle, Right **J** Thorax Muscle, Left **K** Abdomen Muscle, Right **L** Abdomen Muscle, Left **M** Perineum Muscle **N** Hip Muscle, Right **P** Hip Muscle, Left **Q** Upper Leg Muscle, Right **R** Upper Leg Muscle, Left **S** Lower Leg Muscle, Right **T** Lower Leg Muscle, Left **V** Foot Muscle, Right **W** Foot Muscle, Left	**0** Open **3** Percutaneous **4** Percutaneous Endoscopic **X** External	**Z** No Device	**Z** No Qualifier

Section 0 Medical and Surgical
Body System K Muscles
Operation P **Removal:** Taking out or off a device from a body part

Body Part (4th)	Approach (5th)	Device (6th)	Qualifier (7th)
X Upper Muscle **Y** Lower Muscle	**0** Open **3** Percutaneous **4** Percutaneous Endoscopic	**0** Drainage Device **7** Autologous Tissue Substitute **J** Synthetic Substitute **K** Nonautologous Tissue Substitute **M** Stimulator Lead **Y** Other Device	**Z** No Qualifier
X Upper Muscle **Y** Lower Muscle	**X** External	**0** Drainage Device **M** Stimulator Lead	**Z** No Qualifier

Section 0 Medical and Surgical
Body System K Muscles
Operation Q **Repair:** Restoring, to the extent possible, a body part to its normal anatomic structure and function

Body Part (4th)	Approach (5th)	Device (6th)	Qualifier (7th)
0 Head Muscle **1** Facial Muscle **2** Neck Muscle, Right **3** Neck Muscle, Left **4** Tongue, Palate, Pharynx Muscle **5** Shoulder Muscle, Right **6** Shoulder Muscle, Left **7** Upper Arm Muscle, Right **8** Upper Arm Muscle, Left **9** Lower Arm and Wrist Muscle, Right **B** Lower Arm and Wrist Muscle, Left **C** Hand Muscle, Right **D** Hand Muscle, Left **F** Trunk Muscle, Right **G** Trunk Muscle, Left **H** Thorax Muscle, Right **J** Thorax Muscle, Left **K** Abdomen Muscle, Right **L** Abdomen Muscle, Left **M** Perineum Muscle **N** Hip Muscle, Right **P** Hip Muscle, Left **Q** Upper Leg Muscle, Right **R** Upper Leg Muscle, Left **S** Lower Leg Muscle, Right **T** Lower Leg Muscle, Left **V** Foot Muscle, Right **W** Foot Muscle, Left	**0** Open **3** Percutaneous **4** Percutaneous Endoscopic	**Z** No Device	**Z** No Qualifier

Section 0 **Medical and Surgical**
Body System K **Muscles**
Operation R **Replacement:** Putting in or on biological or synthetic material that physically takes the place and/or function of all or a portion of a body part

Body Part (4th)	Approach (5th)	Device (6th)	Qualifier (7th)
0 Head Muscle **1** Facial Muscle **2** Neck Muscle, Right **3** Neck Muscle, Left **4** Tongue, Palate, Pharynx Muscle **5** Shoulder Muscle, Right **6** Shoulder Muscle, Left **7** Upper Arm Muscle, Right **8** Upper Arm Muscle, Left **9** Lower Arm and Wrist Muscle, Right **B** Lower Arm and Wrist Muscle, Left **C** Hand Muscle, Right **D** Hand Muscle, Left **F** Trunk Muscle, Right **G** Trunk Muscle, Left **H** Thorax Muscle, Right **J** Thorax Muscle, Left **K** Abdomen Muscle, Right **L** Abdomen Muscle, Left **M** Perineum **N** Hip Muscle, Right **P** Hip Muscle, Left **Q** Upper Leg Muscle, Right **R** Upper Leg Muscle, Left **S** Lower Leg Muscle, Right **T** Lower Leg Muscle, Left **V** Foot Muscle, Right **W** Foot Muscle, Left	**0** Open **4** Percutaneous Endoscopic	**7** Autologous Tissue Substitute **J** Synthetic Substitute **K** Nonautologous Tissue Substitute	**Z** No Qualifier

Section 0 **Medical and Surgical**
Body System K **Muscles**
Operation S **Reposition:** Moving to its normal location, or other suitable location, all or a portion of a body part

Body Part (4th)	Approach (5th)	Device (6th)	Qualifier (7th)
0 Head Muscle **1** Facial Muscle **2** Neck Muscle, Right **3** Neck Muscle, Left **4** Tongue, Palate, Pharynx Muscle **5** Shoulder Muscle, Right **6** Shoulder Muscle, Left **7** Upper Arm Muscle, Right **8** Upper Arm Muscle, Left **9** Lower Arm and Wrist Muscle, Right **B** Lower Arm and Wrist Muscle, Left **C** Hand Muscle, Right **D** Hand Muscle, Left **F** Trunk Muscle, Right **G** Trunk Muscle, Left **H** Thorax Muscle, Right **J** Thorax Muscle, Left **K** Abdomen Muscle, Right **L** Abdomen Muscle, Left **M** Perineum Muscle **N** Hip Muscle, Right **P** Hip Muscle, Left **Q** Upper Leg Muscle, Right **R** Upper Leg Muscle, Left **S** Lower Leg Muscle, Right **T** Lower Leg Muscle, Left **V** Foot Muscle, Right **W** Foot Muscle, Left	**0** Open **4** Percutaneous Endoscopic	**Z** No Device	**Z** No Qualifier

Section 0 **Medical and Surgical**
Body System K **Muscles**
Operation T **Resection:** Cutting out or off, without replacement, all of a body part

Body Part (4th)	Approach (5th)	Device (6th)	Qualifier (7th)
0 Head Muscle	**0** Open	**Z** No Device	**Z** No Qualifier
1 Facial Muscle	**4** Percutaneous Endoscopic		
2 Neck Muscle, Right			
3 Neck Muscle, Left			
4 Tongue, Palate, Pharynx Muscle			
5 Shoulder Muscle, Right			
6 Shoulder Muscle, Left			
7 Upper Arm Muscle, Right			
8 Upper Arm Muscle, Left			
9 Lower Arm and Wrist Muscle, Right			
B Lower Arm and Wrist Muscle, Left			
C Hand Muscle, Right			
D Hand Muscle, Left			
F Trunk Muscle, Right			
G Trunk Muscle, Left			
H Thorax Muscle, Right			
J Thorax Muscle, Left			
K Abdomen Muscle, Right			
L Abdomen Muscle, Left			
M Perineum Muscle			
N Hip Muscle, Right			
P Hip Muscle, Left			
Q Upper Leg Muscle, Right			
R Upper Leg Muscle, Left			
S Lower Leg Muscle, Right			
T Lower Leg Muscle, Left			
V Foot Muscle, Right			
W Foot Muscle, Left			

Section 0 **Medical and Surgical**
Body System K **Muscles**
Operation U **Supplement:** Putting in or on biological or synthetic material that physically reinforces and/or augments the function of a portion of a body part

Body Part (4th)	Approach (5th)	Device (6th)	Qualifier (7th)
0 Head Muscle	**0** Open	**7** Autologous Tissue Substitute	**Z** No Qualifier
1 Facial Muscle	**4** Percutaneous Endoscopic	**J** Synthetic Substitute	
2 Neck Muscle, Right		**K** Nonautologous Tissue Substitute	
3 Neck Muscle, Left			
4 Tongue, Palate, Pharynx Muscle			
5 Shoulder Muscle, Right			
6 Shoulder Muscle, Left			
7 Upper Arm Muscle, Right			
8 Upper Arm Muscle, Left			
9 Lower Arm and Wrist Muscle, Right			
B Lower Arm and Wrist Muscle, Left			
C Hand Muscle, Right			
D Hand Muscle, Left			
F Trunk Muscle, Right			
G Trunk Muscle, Left			
H Thorax Muscle, Right			
J Thorax Muscle, Left			
K Abdomen Muscle, Right			
L Abdomen Muscle, Left			
M Perineum Muscle			
N Hip Muscle, Right			
P Hip Muscle, Left			
Q Upper Leg Muscle, Right			
R Upper Leg Muscle, Left			
S Lower Leg Muscle, Right			
T Lower Leg Muscle, Left			
V Foot Muscle, Right			
W Foot Muscle, Left			

Section 0 **Medical and Surgical**
Body System K **Muscles**
Operation W **Revision:** Correcting, to the extent possible, a portion of a malfunctioning device or the position of a displaced device

Body Part (4th)	Approach (5th)	Device (6th)	Qualifier (7th)
X Upper Muscle Y Lower Muscle	0 Open 3 Percutaneous 4 Percutaneous Endoscopic	0 Drainage Device 7 Autologous Tissue Substitute J Synthetic Substitute K Nonautologous Tissue Substitute M Stimulator Lead Y Other Device	Z No Qualifier
X Upper Muscle Y Lower Muscle	X External	0 Drainage Device 7 Autologous Tissue Substitute J Synthetic Substitute K Nonautologous Tissue Substitute M Stimulator Lead	Z No Qualifier

Section 0 **Medical and Surgical**
Body System K **Muscles**
Operation X **Transfer:** Moving, without taking out, all or a portion of a body part to another location to take over the function of all or a portion of a body part

Body Part (4th)	Approach (5th)	Device (6th)	Qualifier (7th)
0 Head Muscle 1 Facial Muscle 2 Neck Muscle, Right 3 Neck Muscle, Left 4 Tongue, Palate, Pharynx Muscle 5 Shoulder Muscle, Right 6 Shoulder Muscle, Left 7 Upper Arm Muscle, Right 8 Upper Arm Muscle, Left 9 Lower Arm and Wrist Muscle, Right B Lower Arm and Wrist Muscle, Left C Hand Muscle, Right D Hand Muscle, Left H Thorax Muscle, Right J Thorax Muscle, Left M Perineum Muscle N Hip Muscle, Right P Hip Muscle, Left Q Upper Leg Muscle, Right R Upper Leg Muscle, Left S Lower Leg Muscle, Right T Lower Leg Muscle, Left V Foot Muscle, Right W Foot Muscle, Left	0 Open 4 Percutaneous Endoscopic	Z No Device	0 Skin 1 Subcutaneous Tissue 2 Skin and Subcutaneous Tissue Z No Qualifier
F Trunk Muscle, Right G Trunk Muscle, Left	0 Open 4 Percutaneous Endoscopic	Z No Device	0 Skin 1 Subcutaneous Tissue 2 Skin and Subcutaneous Tissue 5 Latissimus Dorsi Myocutaneous Flap 7 Deep Inferior Epigastric Artery Perforator Flap 8 Superficial Inferior Epigastric Artery Flap 9 Gluteal Artery Perforator Flap Z No Qualifier
K Abdomen Muscle, Right L Abdomen Muscle, Left	0 Open 4 Percutaneous Endoscopic	Z No Device	0 Skin 1 Subcutaneous Tissue 2 Skin and Subcutaneous Tissue 6 Transverse Rectus Abdominis Myocutaneous Flap Z No Qualifier

AHA Coding Clinic

0K844ZZ Division of Tongue, Palate, Pharynx Muscle, Percutaneous Endoscopic Approach—AHA CC: 2Q, 2020, 25

0KBN0ZZ Excision of Right Hip Muscle, Open Approach—AHA CC: 3Q, 2016, 20

0KBP0ZZ Excision of Left Hip Muscle, Open Approach—AHA CC: 3Q, 2016, 20; 4Q, 2019, 43-44

0KBR0ZZ Excision of Left Upper Leg Muscle, Open Approach—AHA CC: 1Q, 2020, 27-28

0KDS0ZZ Extraction of Right Lower Leg Muscle, Open Approach—AHA CC: 4Q, 2017, 42

0KHY3YZ Insertion of Other Device into Lower Muscle, Percutaneous Approach—AHA CC: 4Q, 2020, 63-64

0KN84ZZ Release Left Upper Arm Muscle, Percutaneous Endoscopic Approach—AHA CC: 2Q, 2015, 22-23

0KNK0ZZ Release Right Abdomen Muscle, Open Approach—AHA CC: 4Q, 2014, 39-40

0KNL0ZZ Release Left Abdomen Muscle, Open Approach—AHA CC: 4Q, 2014, 39-40

0KNT0ZZ Release Left Lower Leg Muscle, Open Approach—AHA CC: 2Q, 2017, 12-14

0KNV0ZZ Release Right Foot Muscle, Open Approach—AHA CC: 2Q, 2017, 12-14

0KQM0ZZ Repair Perineum Muscle, Open Approach—AHA CC: 4Q, 2013, 120; 1Q, 2016, 7; 2Q, 2016, 34-35

0KT30ZZ Resection of Left Neck Muscle, Open Approach—AHA CC: 2Q, 2016, 12-14

0KTM0ZZ Resection of Perineum Muscle, Open Approach—AHA CC: 4Q, 2014, 40-41; 1Q, 2015, 38

0KX10Z2 Transfer Facial Muscle with Skin and Subcutaneous Tissue, Open Approach—AHA CC: 3Q, 2015, 33

0KX40Z2 Transfer Tongue, Palate, Pharynx Muscle with Skin and Subcutaneous Tissue, Open Approach—AHA CC: 2Q, 2015, 26

0KXF0Z2 Transfer Right Trunk Muscle with Skin and Subcutaneous Tissue, Open Approach—AHA CC: 2Q, 2014, 12

0KXF0Z5 Transfer Right Trunk Muscle, Latissimus Dorsi Myocutaneous Flap, Open Approach—AHA CC: 4Q, 2017, 67

0KXK0Z6 Transfer Right Abdomen Muscle, Transverse Rectus Abdominis Myocutaneous Flap, Open Approach—AHA CC: 4Q, 2014, 41

0KXL0Z6 Transfer Left Abdomen Muscle, Transverse Rectus Abdominis Myocutaneous Flap, Open Approach—AHA CC: 2Q, 2014, 10-11

0KXQ0ZZ Transfer Right Upper Leg Muscle, Open Approach—AHA CC: 3Q, 2016, 30-31

0KXR0ZZ Transfer Left Upper Leg Muscle, Open Approach—AHA CC: 3Q, 2016, 30-31

Shoulder Tendons and Ligaments

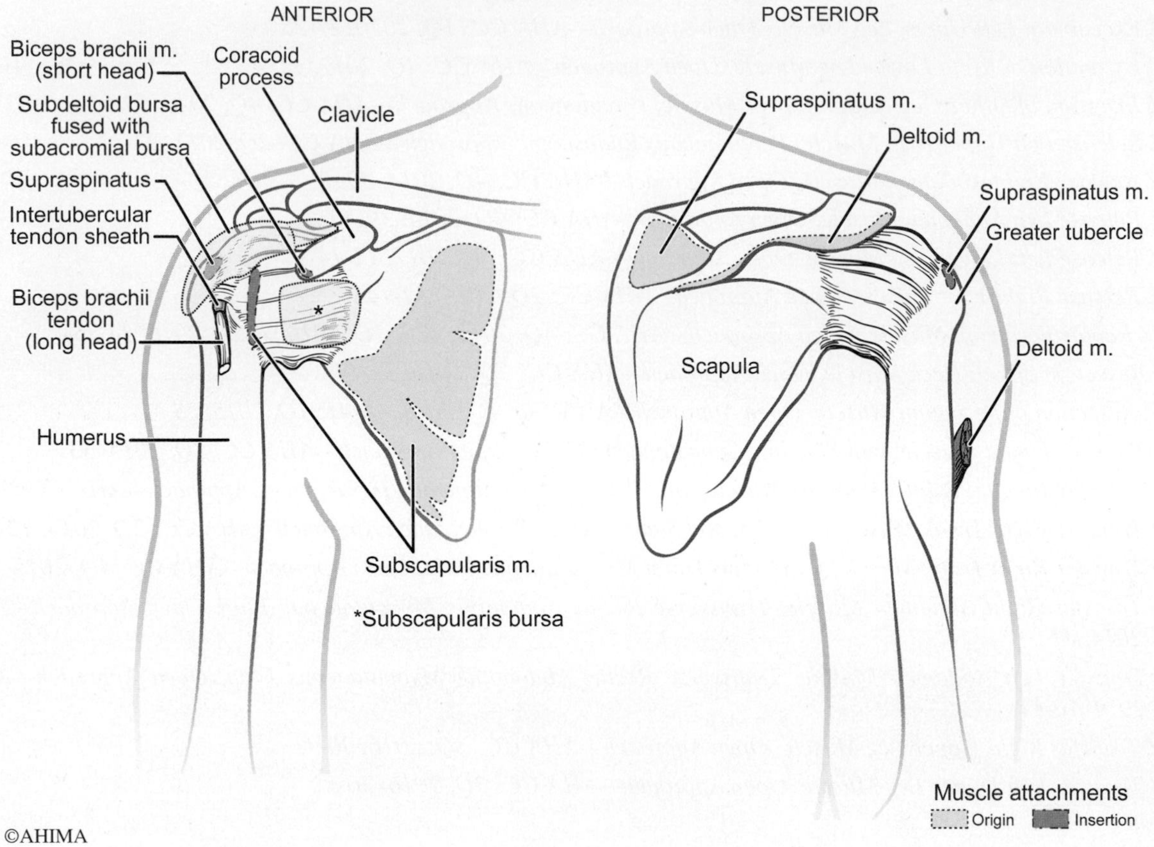
ANTERIOR
POSTERIOR
Biceps brachii m. (short head)
Coracoid process
Subdeltoid bursa fused with subacromial bursa
Clavicle
Supraspinatus
Intertubercular tendon sheath
Biceps brachii tendon (long head)
Humerus
Subscapularis m.
*Subscapularis bursa
Supraspinatus m.
Deltoid m.
Supraspinatus m.
Greater tubercle
Scapula
Deltoid m.
Muscle attachments
Origin
Insertion

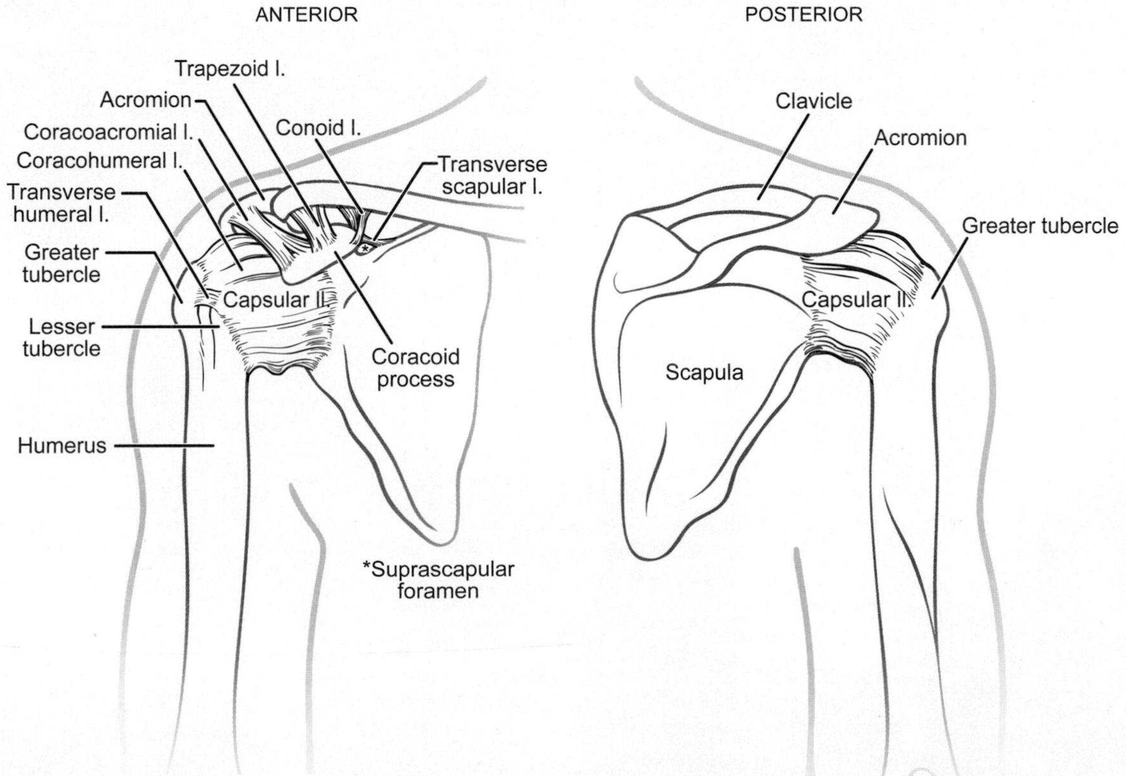
ANTERIOR
POSTERIOR
Trapezoid l.
Acromion
Coracoacromial l.
Conoid l.
Coracohumeral l.
Transverse scapular l.
Transverse humeral l.
Greater tubercle
Capsular ll.
Lesser tubercle
Coracoid process
Humerus
*Suprascapular foramen
Clavicle
Acromion
Greater tubercle
Capsular ll.
Scapula

Hip Tendons and Ligaments

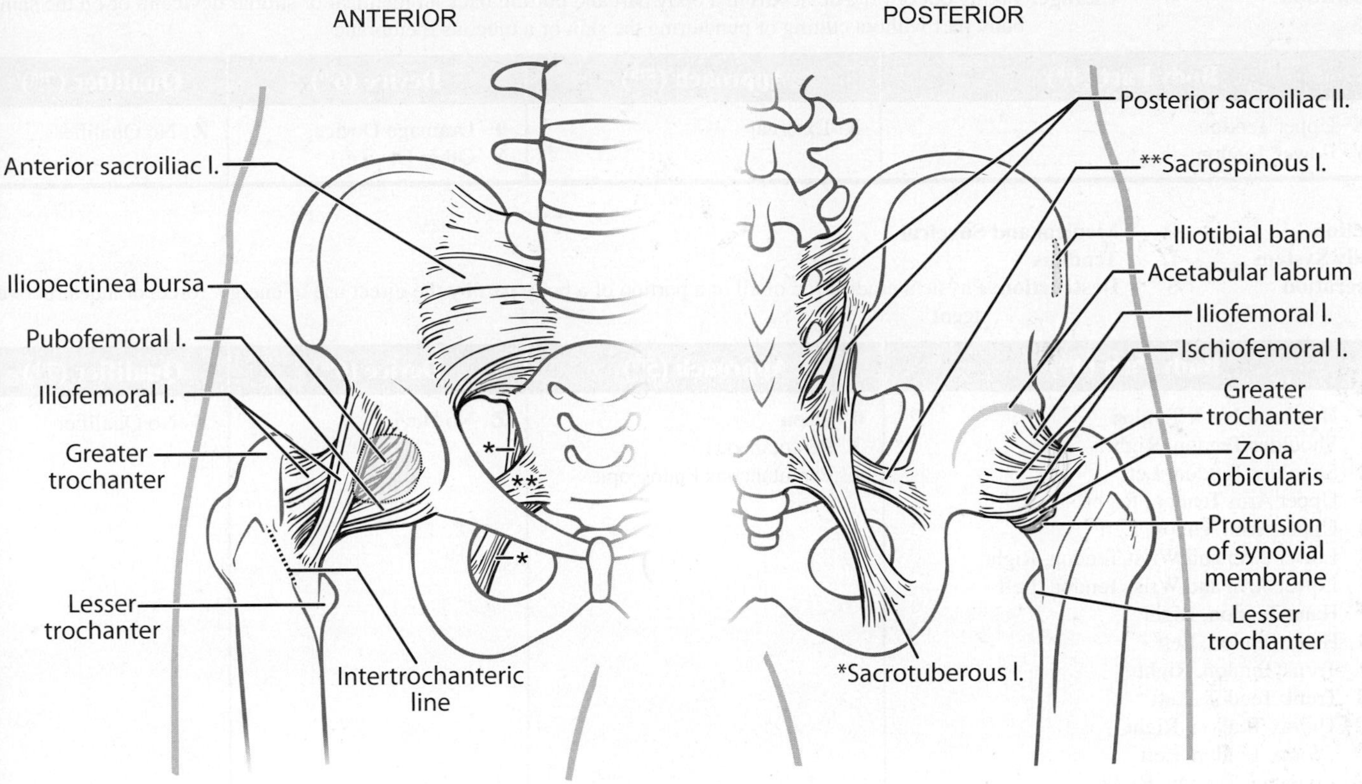
ANTERIOR
POSTERIOR
Anterior sacroiliac l.
Iliopectinea bursa
Pubofemoral l.
Iliofemoral l.
Greater trochanter
Lesser trochanter
Intertrochanteric line
*
**
*
Posterior sacroiliac ll.
**Sacrospinous l.
Iliotibial band
Acetabular labrum
Iliofemoral l.
Ischiofemoral l.
Greater trochanter
Zona orbicularis
Protrusion of synovial membrane
Lesser trochanter
*Sacrotuberous l.

Knee Tendons and Ligaments

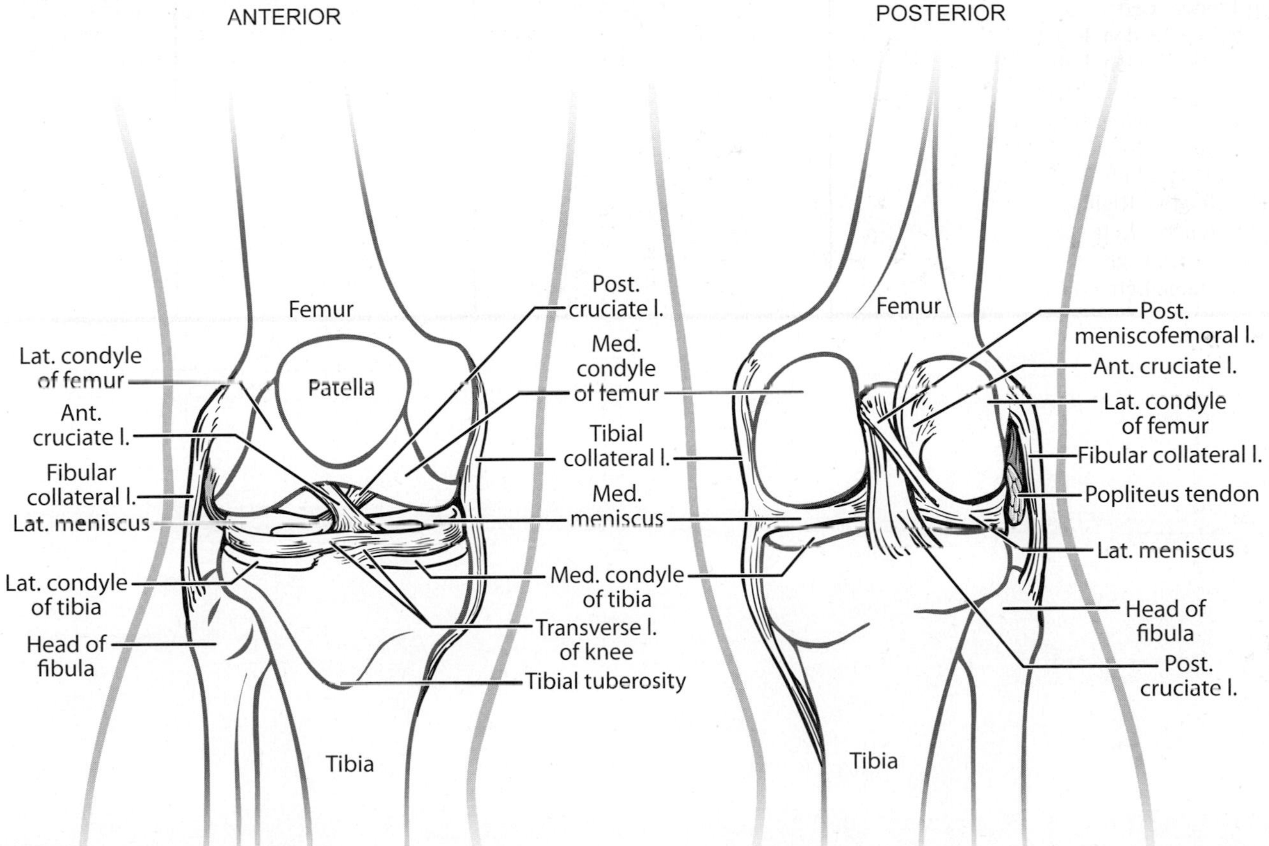
ANTERIOR
POSTERIOR
Femur
Patella
Lat. condyle of femur
Ant. cruciate l.
Fibular collateral l.
Lat. meniscus
Lat. condyle of tibia
Head of fibula
Tibia
Post. cruciate l.
Med. condyle of femur
Tibial collateral l.
Med. meniscus
Med. condyle of tibia
Transverse l. of knee
Tibial tuberosity
Femur
Post. meniscofemoral l.
Ant. cruciate l.
Lat. condyle of femur
Fibular collateral l.
Popliteus tendon
Lat. meniscus
Head of fibula
Post. cruciate l.
Tibia

Tendons Tables 0L2–0LX

Section 0 **Medical and Surgical**
Body System L **Tendons**
Operation 2 **Change:** Taking out or off a device from a body part and putting back an identical or similar device in or on the same body part without cutting or puncturing the skin or a mucous membrane

Body Part (4th)	Approach (5th)	Device (6th)	Qualifier (7th)
X Upper Tendon **Y** Lower Tendon	**X** External	**0** Drainage Device **Y** Other Device	**Z** No Qualifier

Section 0 **Medical and Surgical**
Body System L **Tendons**
Operation 5 **Destruction:** Physical eradication of all or a portion of a body part by the direct use of energy, force, or a destructive agent

Body Part (4th)	Approach (5th)	Device (6th)	Qualifier (7th)
0 Head and Neck Tendon **1** Shoulder Tendon, Right **2** Shoulder Tendon, Left **3** Upper Arm Tendon, Right **4** Upper Arm Tendon, Left **5** Lower Arm and Wrist Tendon, Right **6** Lower Arm and Wrist Tendon, Left **7** Hand Tendon, Right **8** Hand Tendon, Left **9** Trunk Tendon, Right **B** Trunk Tendon, Left **C** Thorax Tendon, Right **D** Thorax Tendon, Left **F** Abdomen Tendon, Right **G** Abdomen Tendon, Left **H** Perineum Tendon **J** Hip Tendon, Right **K** Hip Tendon, Left **L** Upper Leg Tendon, Right **M** Upper Leg Tendon, Left **N** Lower Leg Tendon, Right **P** Lower Leg Tendon, Left **Q** Knee Tendon, Right **R** Knee Tendon, Left **S** Ankle Tendon, Right **T** Ankle Tendon, Left **V** Foot Tendon, Right **W** Foot Tendon, Left	**0** Open **3** Percutaneous **4** Percutaneous Endoscopic	**Z** No Device	**Z** No Qualifier

Section 0 **Medical and Surgical**
Body System L **Tendons**
Operation 8 **Division:** Cutting into a body part, without draining fluids and/or gases from the body part, in order to separate or transect a body part

Body Part (4th)	Approach (5th)	Device (6th)	Qualifier (7th)
0 Head and Neck Tendon **1** Shoulder Tendon, Right **2** Shoulder Tendon, Left **3** Upper Arm Tendon, Right **4** Upper Arm Tendon, Left **5** Lower Arm and Wrist Tendon, Right **6** Lower Arm and Wrist Tendon, Left **7** Hand Tendon, Right **8** Hand Tendon, Left **9** Trunk Tendon, Right **B** Trunk Tendon, Left **C** Thorax Tendon, Right **D** Thorax Tendon, Left **F** Abdomen Tendon, Right **G** Abdomen Tendon, Left **H** Perineum Tendon **J** Hip Tendon, Right **K** Hip Tendon, Left **L** Upper Leg Tendon, Right **M** Upper Leg Tendon, Left **N** Lower Leg Tendon, Right **P** Lower Leg Tendon, Left **Q** Knee Tendon, Right **R** Knee Tendon, Left **S** Ankle Tendon, Right **T** Ankle Tendon, Left **V** Foot Tendon, Right **W** Foot Tendon, Left	**0** Open **3** Percutaneous **4** Percutaneous Endoscopic	**Z** No Device	**Z** No Qualifier

Section 0 **Medical and Surgical**
Body System L **Tendons**
Operation 9 **Drainage:** Taking or letting out fluids and/or gases from a body part

Body Part (4th)	Approach (5th)	Device (6th)	Qualifier (7th)
0 Head and Neck Tendon **1** Shoulder Tendon, Right **2** Shoulder Tendon, Left **3** Upper Arm Tendon, Right **4** Upper Arm Tendon, Left **5** Lower Arm and Wrist Tendon, Right **6** Lower Arm and Wrist Tendon, Left **7** Hand Tendon, Right **8** Hand Tendon, Left **9** Trunk Tendon, Right **B** Trunk Tendon, Left **C** Thorax Tendon, Right **D** Thorax Tendon, Left **F** Abdomen Tendon, Right **G** Abdomen Tendon, Left **H** Perineum Tendon **J** Hip Tendon, Right **K** Hip Tendon, Left **L** Upper Leg Tendon, Right **M** Upper Leg Tendon, Left **N** Lower Leg Tendon, Right **P** Lower Leg Tendon, Left **Q** Knee Tendon, Right **R** Knee Tendon, Left **S** Ankle Tendon, Right **T** Ankle Tendon, Left **V** Foot Tendon, Right **W** Foot Tendon, Left	**0** Open **3** Percutaneous **4** Percutaneous Endoscopic	**0** Drainage Device	**Z** No Qualifier

Continued →

Section **0** **Medical and Surgical**
Body System **L** **Tendons**
Operation **9** **Drainage:** Taking or letting out fluids and/or gases from a body part

Body Part (4th)	Approach (5th)	Device (6th)	Qualifier (7th)
0 Head and Neck Tendon **1** Shoulder Tendon, Right **2** Shoulder Tendon, Left **3** Upper Arm Tendon, Right **4** Upper Arm Tendon, Left **5** Lower Arm and Wrist Tendon, Right **6** Lower Arm and Wrist Tendon, Left **7** Hand Tendon, Right **8** Hand Tendon, Left **9** Trunk Tendon, Right **B** Trunk Tendon, Left **C** Thorax Tendon, Right **D** Thorax Tendon, Left **F** Abdomen Tendon, Right **G** Abdomen Tendon, Left **H** Perineum Tendon **J** Hip Tendon, Right **K** Hip Tendon, Left **L** Upper Leg Tendon, Right **M** Upper Leg Tendon, Left **N** Lower Leg Tendon, Right **P** Lower Leg Tendon, Left **Q** Knee Tendon, Right **R** Knee Tendon, Left **S** Ankle Tendon, Right **T** Ankle Tendon, Left **V** Foot Tendon, Right **W** Foot Tendon, Left	**0** Open **3** Percutaneous **4** Percutaneous Endoscopic	**Z** No Device	**X** Diagnostic **Z** No Qualifier

Section **0** **Medical and Surgical**
Body System **L** **Tendons**
Operation **B** **Excision:** Cutting out or off, without replacement, a portion of a body part

Body Part (4th)	Approach (5th)	Device (6th)	Qualifier (7th)
0 Head and Neck Tendon **1** Shoulder Tendon, Right **2** Shoulder Tendon, Left **3** Upper Arm Tendon, Right **4** Upper Arm Tendon, Left **5** Lower Arm and Wrist Tendon, Right **6** Lower Arm and Wrist Tendon, Left **7** Hand Tendon, Right **8** Hand Tendon, Left **9** Trunk Tendon, Right **B** Trunk Tendon, Left **C** Thorax Tendon, Right **D** Thorax Tendon, Left **F** Abdomen Tendon, Right **G** Abdomen Tendon, Left **H** Perineum Tendon **J** Hip Tendon, Right **K** Hip Tendon, Left **L** Upper Leg Tendon, Right **M** Upper Leg Tendon, Left **N** Lower Leg Tendon, Right **P** Lower Leg Tendon, Left **Q** Knee Tendon, Right **R** Knee Tendon, Left **S** Ankle Tendon, Right **T** Ankle Tendon, Left **V** Foot Tendon, Right **W** Foot Tendon, Left	**0** Open **3** Percutaneous **4** Percutaneous Endoscopic	**Z** No Device	**X** Diagnostic **Z** No Qualifier

Section 0 **Medical and Surgical**
Body System L **Tendons**
Operation C **Extirpation:** Taking or cutting out solid matter from a body part

Body Part (4th)	Approach (5th)	Device (6th)	Qualifier (7th)
0 Head and Neck Tendon **1** Shoulder Tendon, Right **2** Shoulder Tendon, Left **3** Upper Arm Tendon, Right **4** Upper Arm Tendon, Left **5** Lower Arm and Wrist Tendon, Right **6** Lower Arm and Wrist Tendon, Left **7** Hand Tendon, Right **8** Hand Tendon, Left **9** Trunk Tendon, Right **B** Trunk Tendon, Left **C** Thorax Tendon, Right **D** Thorax Tendon, Left **F** Abdomen Tendon, Right **G** Abdomen Tendon, Left **H** Perineum Tendon **J** Hip Tendon, Right **K** Hip Tendon, Left **L** Upper Leg Tendon, Right **M** Upper Leg Tendon, Left **N** Lower Leg Tendon, Right **P** Lower Leg Tendon, Left **Q** Knee Tendon, Right **R** Knee Tendon, Left **S** Ankle Tendon, Right **T** Ankle Tendon, Left **V** Foot Tendon, Right **W** Foot Tendon, Left	**0** Open **3** Percutaneous **4** Percutaneous Endoscopic	**Z** No Device	**Z** No Qualifier

Section 0 **Medical and Surgical**
Body System L **Tendons**
Operation D **Extraction:** Pulling or stripping out or off all or a portion of a body part by the use of force

Body Part (4th)	Approach (5th)	Device (6th)	Qualifier (7th)
0 Head and Neck Tendon **1** Shoulder Tendon, Right **2** Shoulder Tendon, Left **3** Upper Arm Tendon, Right **4** Upper Arm Tendon, Left **5** Lower Arm and Wrist Tendon, Right **6** Lower Arm and Wrist Tendon, Left **7** Hand Tendon, Right **8** Hand Tendon, Left **9** Trunk Tendon, Right **B** Trunk Tendon, Left **C** Thorax Tendon, Right **D** Thorax Tendon, Left **F** Abdomen Tendon, Right **G** Abdomen Tendon, Left **H** Perineum Tendon **J** Hip Tendon, Right **K** Hip Tendon, Left **L** Upper Leg Tendon, Right **M** Upper Leg Tendon, Left **N** Lower Leg Tendon, Right **P** Lower Leg Tendon, Left **Q** Knee Tendon, Right **R** Knee Tendon, Left **S** Ankle Tendon, Right **T** Ankle Tendon, Left **V** Foot Tendon, Right **W** Foot Tendon, Left	**0** Open	**Z** No Device	**Z** No Qualifier

Section 0 **Medical and Surgical**
Body System L **Tendons**
Operation H **Inspection:** Putting in a nonbiological appliance that monitors, assists, performs, or prevents a physiological function but does not physically take the place of a body part

Body Part (4th)	Approach (5th)	Device (6th)	Qualifier (7th)
X Upper Tendon **Y** Lower Tendon	**0** Open **3** Percutaneous **4** Percutaneous Endoscopic	**Y** Other Device	**Z** No Qualifier

Section 0 **Medical and Surgical**
Body System L **Tendons**
Operation J **Inspection:** Visually and/or manually exploring a body part

Body Part (4th)	Approach (5th)	Device (6th)	Qualifier (7th)
X Upper Tendon **Y** Lower Tendon	**0** Open **3** Percutaneous **4** Percutaneous Endoscopic **X** External	**Z** No Device	**Z** No Qualifier

Section 0 **Medical and Surgical**
Body System L **Tendons**
Operation M **Reattachment:** Putting back in or on all or a portion of a separated body part to its normal location or other suitable location

Body Part (4th)	Approach (5th)	Device (6th)	Qualifier (7th)
0 Head and Neck Tendon **1** Shoulder Tendon, Right **2** Shoulder Tendon, Left **3** Upper Arm Tendon, Right **4** Upper Arm Tendon, Left **5** Lower Arm and Wrist Tendon, Right **6** Lower Arm and Wrist Tendon, Left **7** Hand Tendon, Right **8** Hand Tendon, Left **9** Trunk Tendon, Right **B** Trunk Tendon, Left **C** Thorax Tendon, Right **D** Thorax Tendon, Left **F** Abdomen Tendon, Right **G** Abdomen Tendon, Left **H** Perineum Tendon **J** Hip Tendon, Right **K** Hip Tendon, Left **L** Upper Leg Tendon, Right **M** Upper Leg Tendon, Left **N** Lower Leg Tendon, Right **P** Lower Leg Tendon, Left **Q** Knee Tendon, Right **R** Knee Tendon, Left **S** Ankle Tendon, Right **T** Ankle Tendon, Left **V** Foot Tendon, Right **W** Foot Tendon, Left	**0** Open **4** Percutaneous Endoscopic	**Z** No Device	**Z** No Qualifier

ection 0 Medical and Surgical
ody System L Tendons
)peration N **Release:** Freeing a body part from an abnormal physical constraint by cutting or by the use of force

Body Part (4th)	Approach (5th)	Device (6th)	Qualifier (7th)
0 Head and Neck Tendon **1** Shoulder Tendon, Right **2** Shoulder Tendon, Left **3** Upper Arm Tendon, Right **4** Upper Arm Tendon, Left **5** Lower Arm and Wrist Tendon, Right **6** Lower Arm and Wrist Tendon, Left **7** Hand Tendon, Right **8** Hand Tendon, Left **9** Trunk Tendon, Right **B** Trunk Tendon, Left **C** Thorax Tendon, Right **D** Thorax Tendon, Left **F** Abdomen Tendon, Right **G** Abdomen Tendon, Left **H** Perineum Tendon **J** Hip Tendon, Right **K** Hip Tendon, Left **L** Upper Leg Tendon, Right **M** Upper Leg Tendon, Left **N** Lower Leg Tendon, Right **P** Lower Leg Tendon, Left **Q** Knee Tendon, Right **R** Knee Tendon, Left **S** Ankle Tendon, Right **T** Ankle Tendon, Left **V** Foot Tendon, Right **W** Foot Tendon, Left	**0** Open **3** Percutaneous **4** Percutaneous Endoscopic **X** External	**Z** No Device	**Z** No Qualifier

ection 0 Medical and Surgical
ody System L Tendons
)peration P **Removal:** Taking out or off a device from a body part

Body Part (4th)	Approach (5th)	Device (6th)	Qualifier (7th)
X Upper Tendon **Y** Lower Tendon	**0** Open **3** Percutaneous **4** Percutaneous Endoscopic	**0** Drainage Device **7** Autologous Tissue Substitute **J** Synthetic Substitute **K** Nonautologous Tissue Substitute **Y** Other Device	**Z** No Qualifier
X Upper Tendon **Y** Lower Tendon	**X** External	**0** Drainage Device	**Z** No Qualifier

Section 0 **Medical and Surgical**
Body System L **Tendons**
Operation Q **Repair:** Restoring, to the extent possible, a body part to its normal anatomic structure and function

Body Part (4th)	Approach (5th)	Device (6th)	Qualifier (7th)
0 Head and Neck Tendon **1** Shoulder Tendon, Right **2** Shoulder Tendon, Left **3** Upper Arm Tendon, Right **4** Upper Arm Tendon, Left **5** Lower Arm and Wrist Tendon, Right **6** Lower Arm and Wrist Tendon, Left **7** Hand Tendon, Right **8** Hand Tendon, Left **9** Trunk Tendon, Right **B** Trunk Tendon, Left **C** Thorax Tendon, Right **D** Thorax Tendon, Left **F** Abdomen Tendon, Right **G** Abdomen Tendon, Left **H** Perineum Tendon **J** Hip Tendon, Right **K** Hip Tendon, Left **L** Upper Leg Tendon, Right **M** Upper Leg Tendon, Left **N** Lower Leg Tendon, Right **P** Lower Leg Tendon, Left **Q** Knee Tendon, Right **R** Knee Tendon, Left **S** Ankle Tendon, Right **T** Ankle Tendon, Left **V** Foot Tendon, Right **W** Foot Tendon, Left	**0** Open **3** Percutaneous **4** Percutaneous Endoscopic	**Z** No Device	**Z** No Qualifier

Section 0 **Medical and Surgical**
Body System L **Tendons**
Operation R **Replacement:** Putting in or on biological or synthetic material that physically takes the place and/or function of all or a portion of a body part

Body Part (4th)	Approach (5th)	Device (6th)	Qualifier (7th)
0 Head and Neck Tendon **1** Shoulder Tendon, Right **2** Shoulder Tendon, Left **3** Upper Arm Tendon, Right **4** Upper Arm Tendon, Left **5** Lower Arm and Wrist Tendon, Right **6** Lower Arm and Wrist Tendon, Left **7** Hand Tendon, Right **8** Hand Tendon, Left **9** Trunk Tendon, Right **B** Trunk Tendon, Left **C** Thorax Tendon, Right **D** Thorax Tendon, Left **F** Abdomen Tendon, Right **G** Abdomen Tendon, Left **H** Perineum Tendon **J** Hip Tendon, Right **K** Hip Tendon, Left **L** Upper Leg Tendon, Right **M** Upper Leg Tendon, Left **N** Lower Leg Tendon, Right **P** Lower Leg Tendon, Left **Q** Knee Tendon, Right **R** Knee Tendon, Left **S** Ankle Tendon, Right **T** Ankle Tendon, Left **V** Foot Tendon, Right **W** Foot Tendon, Left	**0** Open **4** Percutaneous Endoscopic	**7** Autologous Tissue Substitute **J** Synthetic Substitute **K** Nonautologous Tissue Substitute	**Z** No Qualifier

Section 0 **Medical and Surgical**
Body System L **Tendons**
Operation S **Reposition:** Moving to its normal location, or other suitable location, all or a portion of a body part

Body Part (4th)	Approach (5th)	Device (6th)	Qualifier (7th)
0 Head and Neck Tendon **1** Shoulder Tendon, Right **2** Shoulder Tendon, Left **3** Upper Arm Tendon, Right **4** Upper Arm Tendon, Left **5** Lower Arm and Wrist Tendon, Right **6** Lower Arm and Wrist Tendon, Left **7** Hand Tendon, Right **8** Hand Tendon, Left **9** Trunk Tendon, Right **B** Trunk Tendon, Left **C** Thorax Tendon, Right **D** Thorax Tendon, Left **F** Abdomen Tendon, Right **G** Abdomen Tendon, Left **H** Perineum Tendon **J** Hip Tendon, Right **K** Hip Tendon, Left **L** Upper Leg Tendon, Right **M** Upper Leg Tendon, Left **N** Lower Leg Tendon, Right **P** Lower Leg Tendon, Left **Q** Knee Tendon, Right **R** Knee Tendon, Left **S** Ankle Tendon, Right **T** Ankle Tendon, Left **V** Foot Tendon, Right **W** Foot Tendon, Left	**0** Open **4** Percutaneous Endoscopic	**Z** No Device	**Z** No Qualifier

Section 0 **Medical and Surgical**
Body System L **Tendons**
Operation T **Resection:** Cutting out or off, without replacement, all of a body part

Body Part (4th)	Approach (5th)	Device (6th)	Qualifier (7th)
0 Head and Neck Tendon **1** Shoulder Tendon, Right **2** Shoulder Tendon, Left **3** Upper Arm Tendon, Right **4** Upper Arm Tendon, Left **5** Lower Arm and Wrist Tendon, Right **6** Lower Arm and Wrist Tendon, Left **7** Hand Tendon, Right **8** Hand Tendon, Left **9** Trunk Tendon, Right **B** Trunk Tendon, Left **C** Thorax Tendon, Right **D** Thorax Tendon, Left **F** Abdomen Tendon, Right **G** Abdomen Tendon, Left **H** Perineum Tendon **J** Hip Tendon, Right **K** Hip Tendon, Left **L** Upper Leg Tendon, Right **M** Upper Leg Tendon, Left **N** Lower Leg Tendon, Right **P** Lower Leg Tendon, Left **Q** Knee Tendon, Right **R** Knee Tendon, Left **S** Ankle Tendon, Right **T** Ankle Tendon, Left **V** Foot Tendon, Right **W** Foot Tendon, Left	**0** Open **4** Percutaneous Endoscopic	**Z** No Device	**Z** No Qualifier

Section 0 Medical and Surgical
Body System L Tendons
Operation U **Supplement:** Putting in or on biological or synthetic material that physically reinforces and/or augments the function of a portion of a body part

Body Part (4th)	Approach (5th)	Device (6th)	Qualifier (7th)
0 Head and Neck Tendon 1 Shoulder Tendon, Right 2 Shoulder Tendon, Left 3 Upper Arm Tendon, Right 4 Upper Arm Tendon, Left 5 Lower Arm and Wrist Tendon, Right 6 Lower Arm and Wrist Tendon, Left 7 Hand Tendon, Right 8 Hand Tendon, Left 9 Trunk Tendon, Right B Trunk Tendon, Left C Thorax Tendon, Right D Thorax Tendon, Left F Abdomen Tendon, Right G Abdomen Tendon, Left H Perineum Tendon J Hip Tendon, Right K Hip Tendon, Left L Upper Leg Tendon, Right M Upper Leg Tendon, Left N Lower Leg Tendon, Right P Lower Leg Tendon, Left Q Knee Tendon, Right R Knee Tendon, Left S Ankle Tendon, Right T Ankle Tendon, Left V Foot Tendon, Right W Foot Tendon, Left	0 Open 4 Percutaneous Endoscopic	7 Autologous Tissue Substitute J Synthetic Substitute K Nonautologous Tissue Substitute	Z No Qualifier

Section 0 Medical and Surgical
Body System L Tendons
Operation W **Revision:** Correcting, to the extent possible, a portion of a malfunctioning device or the position of a displaced device

Body Part (4th)	Approach (5th)	Device (6th)	Qualifier (7th)
X Upper Tendon Y Lower Tendon	0 Open 3 Percutaneous 4 Percutaneous Endoscopic	0 Drainage Device 7 Autologous Tissue Substitute J Synthetic Substitute K Nonautologous Tissue Substitute Y Other Device	Z No Qualifier
X Upper Tendon Y Lower Tendon	X External	0 Drainage Device 7 Autologous Tissue Substitute J Synthetic Substitute K Nonautologous Tissue Substitute	Z No Qualifier

Section 0 **Medical and Surgical**
Body System L **Tendons**
Operation X **Transfer:** Moving, without taking out, all or a portion of a body part to another location to take over the function of all or a portion of a body part

Body Part (4th)	Approach (5th)	Device (6th)	Qualifier (7th)
0 Head and Neck Tendon **1** Shoulder Tendon, Right **2** Shoulder Tendon, Left **3** Upper Arm Tendon, Right **4** Upper Arm Tendon, Left **5** Lower Arm and Wrist Tendon, Right **6** Lower Arm and Wrist Tendon, Left **7** Hand Tendon, Right **8** Hand Tendon, Left **9** Trunk Tendon, Right **B** Trunk Tendon, Left **C** Thorax Tendon, Right **D** Thorax Tendon, Left **F** Abdomen Tendon, Right **G** Abdomen Tendon, Left **H** Perineum Tendon **J** Hip Tendon, Right **K** Hip Tendon, Left **L** Upper Leg Tendon, Right **M** Upper Leg Tendon, Left **N** Lower Leg Tendon, Right **P** Lower Leg Tendon, Left **Q** Knee Tendon, Right **R** Knee Tendon, Left **S** Ankle Tendon, Right **T** Ankle Tendon, Left **V** Foot Tendon, Right **W** Foot Tendon, Left	**0** Open **4** Percutaneous Endoscopic	**Z** No Device	**Z** No Qualifier

AHA Coding Clinic

0L8J0ZZ Division of Right Hip Tendon, Open Approach—AHA CC: 3Q, 2016, 30-31
0LB60ZZ Excision of Left Lower Arm and Wrist Tendon, Open Approach—AHA CC: 3Q, 2015, 26-27
0LBL0ZZ Excision of Right Upper Leg Tendon, Open Approach—AHA CC: 2Q, 2017, 21-22
0LBP0ZZ Excision of Left Lower Leg Tendon, Open Approach—AHA CC: 3Q, 2014, 18-19
0LBT0ZZ Excision of Left Ankle Tendon, Open Approach—AHA CC: 3Q, 2014, 14-15
0LQ14ZZ Repair Right Shoulder Tendon, Percutaneous Endoscopic Approach—AHA CC: 3Q, 2013, 20-22; 3Q, 2016, 32-33
0LS30ZZ Reposition Right Upper Arm Tendon, Open Approach—AHA CC: 3Q, 2016, 32-33
0LS40ZZ Reposition Left Upper Arm Tendon, Open Approach—AHA CC: 3Q, 2015, 14-15
0LUM0KZ Supplement Left Upper Leg Tendon with Nonautologous Tissue Substitute, Open Approach—AHA CC: 2Q, 2015, 11
0LUQ0KZ Supplement Right Knee Tendon with Nonautologous Tissue Substitute, Open Approach—AHA CC: 2Q, 2015, 11

Bursa of the Knee

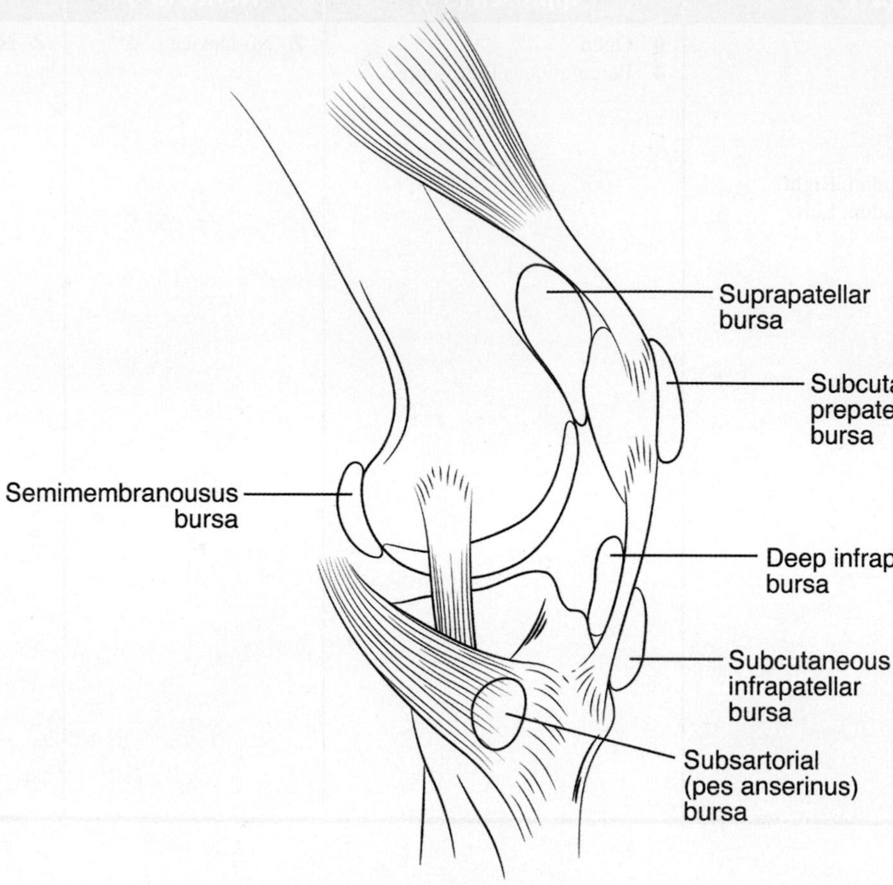
Suprapatellar bursa
Subcutaneous prepatellar bursa
Semimembranousus bursa
Deep infrapatellar bursa
Subcutaneous infrapatellar bursa
Subsartorial (pes anserinus) bursa

Ligaments of the Knee

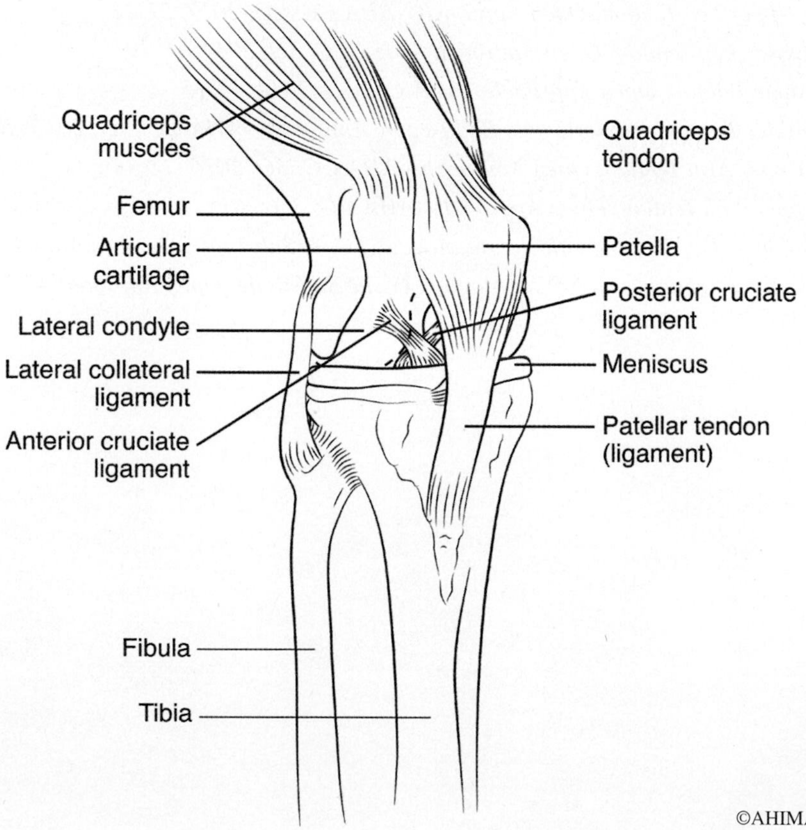
Quadriceps muscles
Femur
Articular cartilage
Lateral condyle
Lateral collateral ligament
Anterior cruciate ligament
Fibula
Tibia
Quadriceps tendon
Patella
Posterior cruciate ligament
Meniscus
Patellar tendon (ligament)

Shoulder Tendons and Ligaments

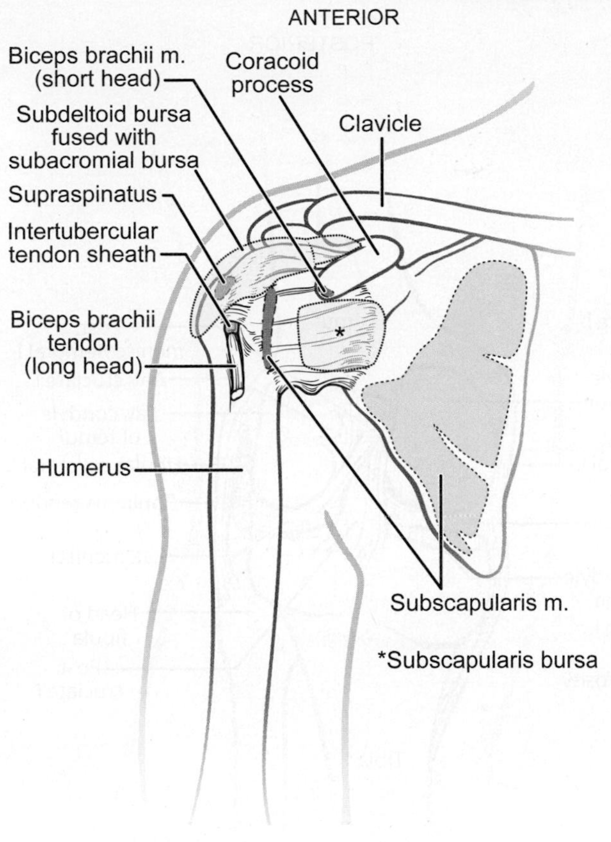
ANTERIOR
Biceps brachii m. (short head)
Coracoid process
Subdeltoid bursa fused with subacromial bursa
Clavicle
Supraspinatus
Intertubercular tendon sheath
Biceps brachii tendon (long head)
Humerus
Subscapularis m.
*Subscapularis bursa

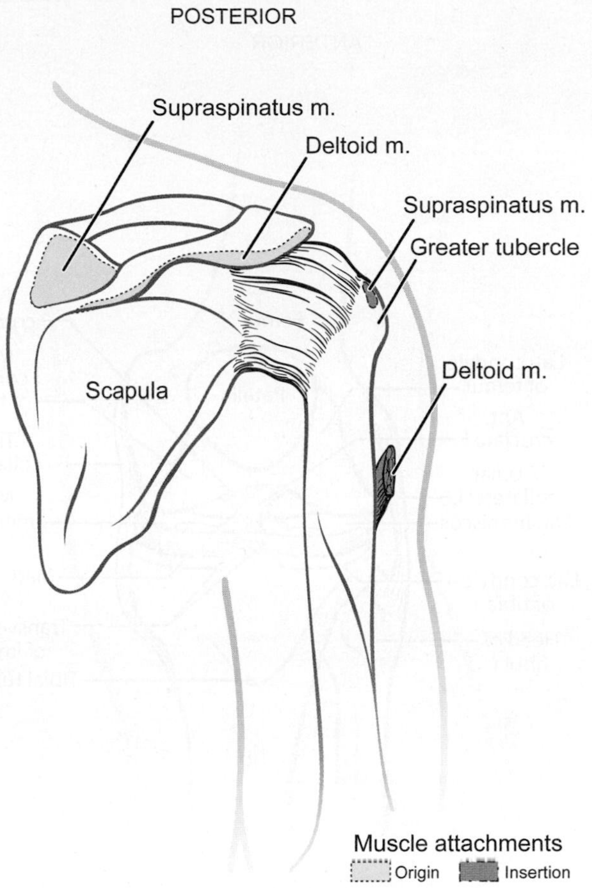
POSTERIOR
Supraspinatus m.
Deltoid m.
Supraspinatus m.
Greater tubercle
Scapula
Deltoid m.
Muscle attachments
Origin
Insertion

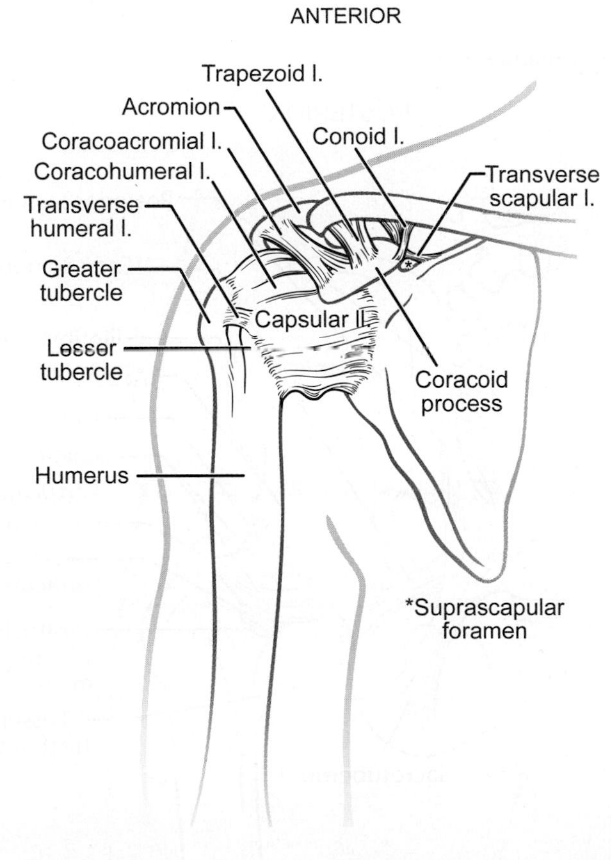
ANTERIOR
Trapezoid l.
Acromion
Coracoacromial l.
Conoid l.
Coracohumeral l.
Transverse scapular l.
Transverse humeral l.
Greater tubercle
Capsular ll.
Lesser tubercle
Coracoid process
Humerus
*Suprascapular foramen

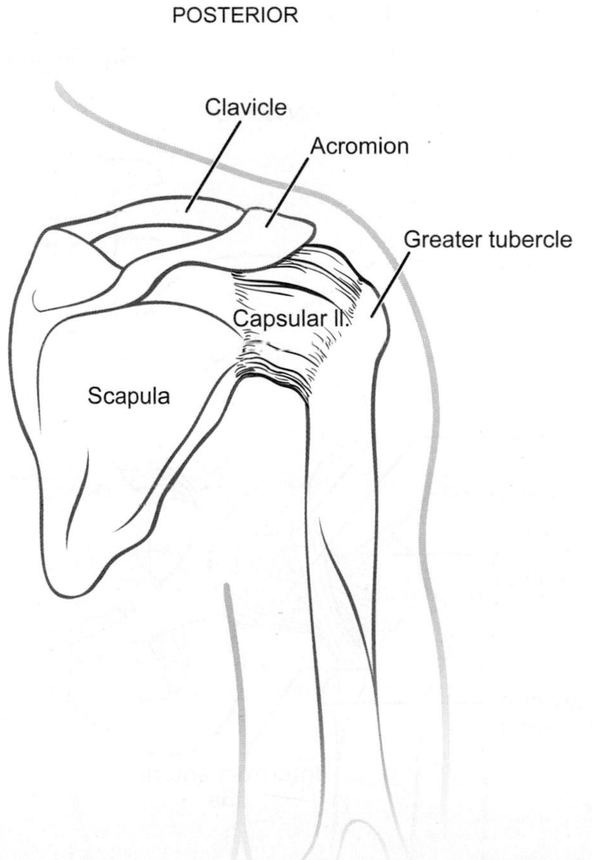
POSTERIOR
Clavicle
Acromion
Greater tubercle
Capsular ll.
Scapula

Knee Tendons and Ligaments

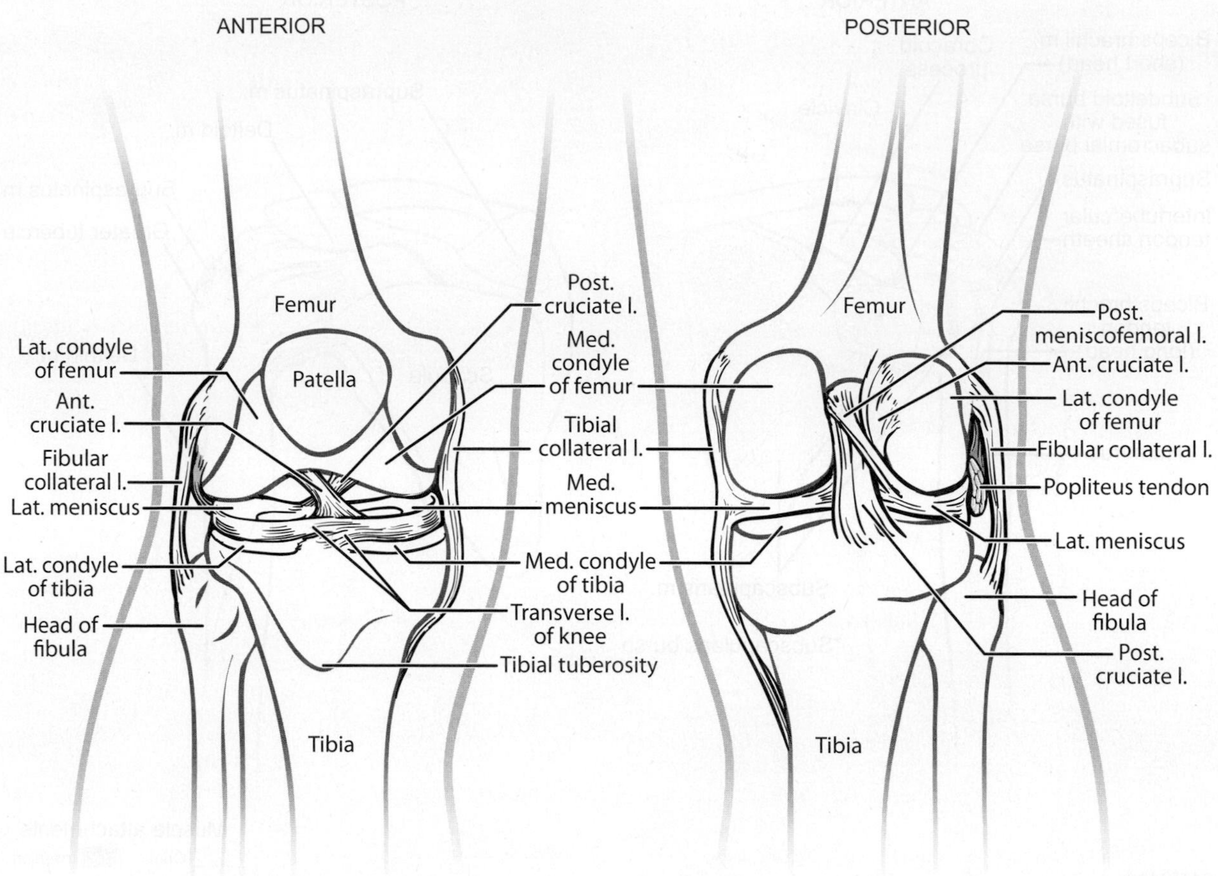

ANTERIOR
POSTERIOR
Femur
Patella
Lat. condyle of femur
Ant. cruciate l.
Fibular collateral l.
Lat. meniscus
Lat. condyle of tibia
Head of fibula
Post. cruciate l.
Med. condyle of femur
Tibial collateral l.
Med. meniscus
Med. condyle of tibia
Transverse l. of knee
Tibial tuberosity
Tibia
Femur
Post. meniscofemoral l.
Ant. cruciate l.
Lat. condyle of femur
Fibular collateral l.
Popliteus tendon
Lat. meniscus
Head of fibula
Post. cruciate l.
Tibia

Hip Tendons and Ligaments

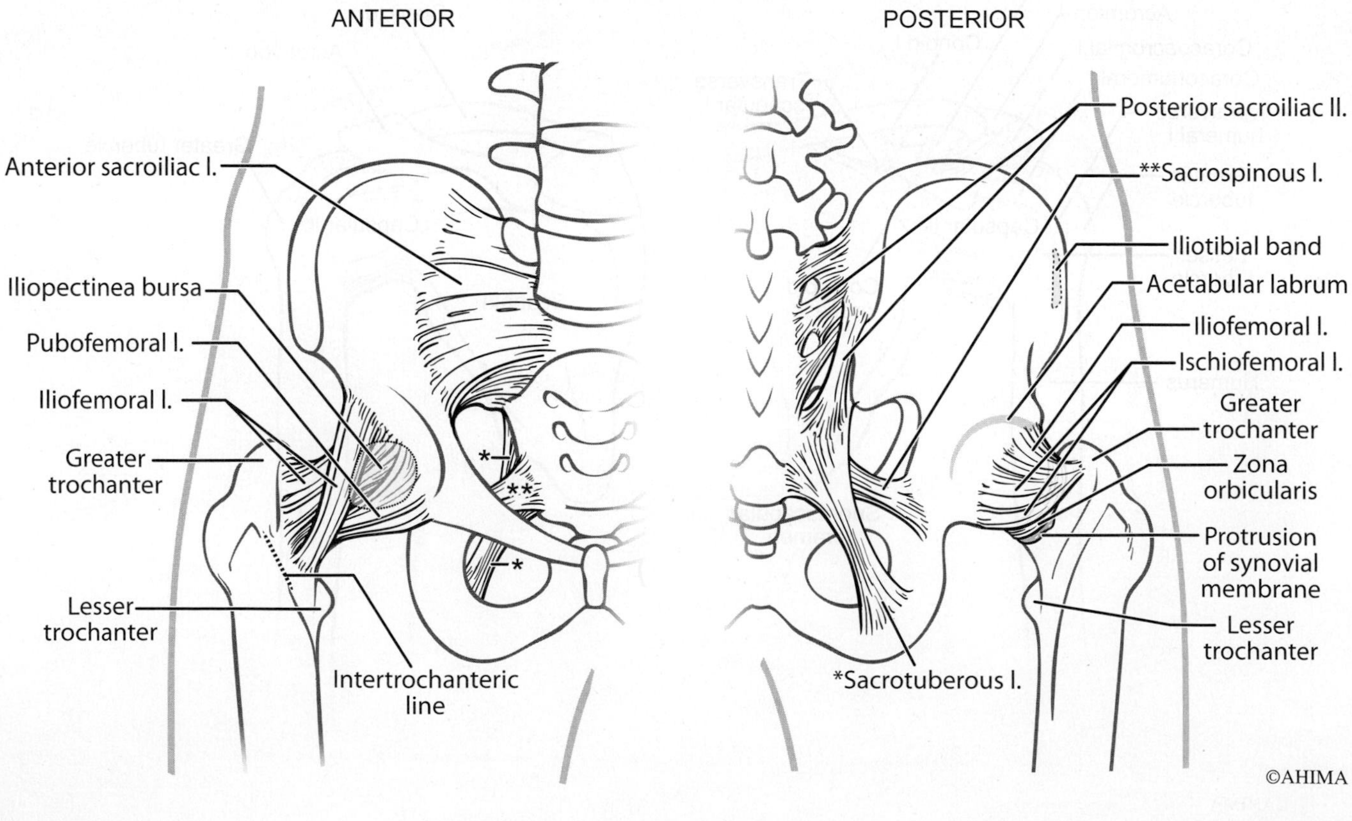

ANTERIOR
POSTERIOR
Anterior sacroiliac l.
Iliopectinea bursa
Pubofemoral l.
Iliofemoral l.
Greater trochanter
Lesser trochanter
Intertrochanteric line
*
**
*
Posterior sacroiliac ll.
**Sacrospinous l.
Iliotibial band
Acetabular labrum
Iliofemoral l.
Ischiofemoral l.
Greater trochanter
Zona orbicularis
Protrusion of synovial membrane
Lesser trochanter
*Sacrotuberous l.

Section 0 **Medical and Surgical**
Body System M **Bursae and Ligaments**
Operation 2 **Change:** Taking out or off a device from a body part and putting back an identical or similar device in or on the same body part without cutting or puncturing the skin or a mucous membrane

Body Part (4th)	Approach (5th)	Device (6th)	Qualifier (7th)
X Upper Bursa and Ligament **Y** Lower Bursa and Ligament	**X** External	**0** Drainage Device **Y** Other Device	**Z** No Qualifier

Section 0 **Medical and Surgical**
Body System M **Bursae and Ligaments**
Operation 5 **Destruction:** Physical eradication of all or a portion of a body part by the direct use of energy, force, or a destructive agent

Body Part (4th)	Approach (5th)	Device (6th)	Qualifier (7th)
0 Head and Neck Bursa and Ligament **1** Shoulder Bursa and Ligament, Right **2** Shoulder Bursa and Ligament, Left **3** Elbow Bursa and Ligament, Right **4** Elbow Bursa and Ligament, Left **5** Wrist Bursa and Ligament, Right **6** Wrist Bursa and Ligament, Left **7** Hand Bursa and Ligament, Right **8** Hand Bursa and Ligament, Left **9** Upper Extremity Bursa and Ligament, Right **B** Upper Extremity Bursa and Ligament, Left **C** Upper Spine Bursa and Ligament, Right **D** Lower Spine Bursa and Ligament, Left **F** Sternum Bursa and Ligament, Right **G** Rib(s) Bursa and Ligament, Left **H** Abdomen Bursa and Ligament, Right **J** Abdomen Bursa and Ligament, Left **K** Perineum Bursa and Ligament **L** Hip Bursa and Ligament, Right **M** Hip Bursa and Ligament, Left **N** Knee Bursa and Ligament, Right **P** Knee Bursa and Ligament, Left **Q** Ankle Bursa and Ligament, Right **R** Ankle Bursa and Ligament, Left **S** Foot Bursa and Ligament, Right **T** Foot Bursa and Ligament, Left **V** Lower Extremity Bursa and Ligament, Right **W** Lower Extremity Bursa and Ligament, Left	**0** Open **3** Percutaneous **4** Percutaneous Endoscopic	**Z** No Device	**Z** No Qualifier

Section 0 **Medical and Surgical**
Body System M **Bursae and Ligaments**
Operation 8 **Division:** Cutting into a body part, without draining fluids and/or gases from the body part, in order to separate or transect a body part

Body Part (4th)	Approach (5th)	Device (6th)	Qualifier (7th)
0 Head and Neck Bursa and Ligament **1** Shoulder Bursa and Ligament, Right **2** Shoulder Bursa and Ligament, Left **3** Elbow Bursa and Ligament, Right **4** Elbow Bursa and Ligament, Left **5** Wrist Bursa and Ligament, Right **6** Wrist Bursa and Ligament, Left **7** Hand Bursa and Ligament, Right **8** Hand Bursa and Ligament, Left **9** Upper Extremity Bursa and Ligament, Right **B** Upper Extremity Bursa and Ligament, Left **C** Upper Spine Bursa and Ligament, Right **D** Lower Spine Bursa and Ligament, Left **F** Sternum Bursa and Ligament, Right **G** Rib(s) Bursa and Ligament, Left **H** Abdomen Bursa and Ligament, Right **J** Abdomen Bursa and Ligament, Left **K** Perineum Bursa and Ligament **L** Hip Bursa and Ligament, Right **M** Hip Bursa and Ligament, Left **N** Knee Bursa and Ligament, Right **P** Knee Bursa and Ligament, Left **Q** Ankle Bursa and Ligament, Right **R** Ankle Bursa and Ligament, Left **S** Foot Bursa and Ligament, Right **T** Foot Bursa and Ligament, Left **V** Lower Extremity Bursa and Ligament, Right **W** Lower Extremity Bursa and Ligament, Left	**0** Open **3** Percutaneous **4** Percutaneous Endoscopic	**Z** No Device	**Z** No Qualifier

Section 0 **Medical and Surgical**
Body System M **Bursae and Ligaments**
Operation 9 **Drainage:** Taking or letting out fluids and/or gases from a body part

Body Part (4th)	Approach (5th)	Device (6th)	Qualifier (7th)
0 Head and Neck Bursa and Ligament **1** Shoulder Bursa and Ligament, Right **2** Shoulder Bursa and Ligament, Left **3** Elbow Bursa and Ligament, Right **4** Elbow Bursa and Ligament, Left **5** Wrist Bursa and Ligament, Right **6** Wrist Bursa and Ligament, Left **7** Hand Bursa and Ligament, Right **8** Hand Bursa and Ligament, Left **9** Upper Extremity Bursa and Ligament, Right **B** Upper Extremity Bursa and Ligament, Left **C** Upper Spine Bursa and Ligament, Right **D** Lower Spine Bursa and Ligament, Left **F** Sternum Bursa and Ligament, Right **G** Rib(s) Bursa and Ligament, Left **H** Abdomen Bursa and Ligament, Right **J** Abdomen Bursa and Ligament, Left **K** Perineum Bursa and Ligament **L** Hip Bursa and Ligament, Right **M** Hip Bursa and Ligament, Left **N** Knee Bursa and Ligament, Right **P** Knee Bursa and Ligament, Left **Q** Ankle Bursa and Ligament, Right **R** Ankle Bursa and Ligament, Left **S** Foot Bursa and Ligament, Right **T** Foot Bursa and Ligament, Left **V** Lower Extremity Bursa and Ligament, Right **W** Lower Extremity Bursa and Ligament, Left	**0** Open **3** Percutaneous **4** Percutaneous Endoscopic	**0** Drainage Device	**Z** No Qualifier

Continued →

Section 0 **Medical and Surgical**
Body System M **Bursae and Ligaments**
Operation 9 **Drainage:** Taking or letting out fluids and/or gases from a body part

Body Part (4th)	Approach (5th)	Device (6th)	Qualifier (7th)
0 Head and Neck Bursa and Ligament **1** Shoulder Bursa and Ligament, Right **2** Shoulder Bursa and Ligament, Left **3** Elbow Bursa and Ligament, Right **4** Elbow Bursa and Ligament, Left **5** Wrist Bursa and Ligament, Right **6** Wrist Bursa and Ligament, Left **7** Hand Bursa and Ligament, Right **8** Hand Bursa and Ligament, Left **9** Upper Extremity Bursa and Ligament, Right **B** Upper Extremity Bursa and Ligament, Left **C** Upper Spine Bursa and Ligament, Right **D** Lower Spine Bursa and Ligament, Left **F** Sternum Bursa and Ligament, Right **G** Rib(s) Bursa and Ligament, Left **H** Abdomen Bursa and Ligament, Right **J** Abdomen Bursa and Ligament, Left **K** Perineum Bursa and Ligament **L** Hip Bursa and Ligament, Right **M** Hip Bursa and Ligament, Left **N** Knee Bursa and Ligament, Right **P** Knee Bursa and Ligament, Left **Q** Ankle Bursa and Ligament, Right **R** Ankle Bursa and Ligament, Left **S** Foot Bursa and Ligament, Right **T** Foot Bursa and Ligament, Left **V** Lower Extremity Bursa and Ligament, Right **W** Lower Extremity Bursa and Ligament, Left	**0** Open **3** Percutaneous **4** Percutaneous Endoscopic	**Z** No Device	**X** Diagnostic **Z** No Qualifier

Section 0 **Medical and Surgical**
Body System M **Bursae and Ligaments**
Operation B **Excision:** Cutting out or off, without replacement, a portion of a body part

Body Part (4th)	Approach (5th)	Device (6th)	Qualifier (7th)
0 Head and Neck Bursa and Ligament **1** Shoulder Bursa and Ligament, Right **2** Shoulder Bursa and Ligament, Left **3** Elbow Bursa and Ligament, Right **4** Elbow Bursa and Ligament, Left **5** Wrist Bursa and Ligament, Right **6** Wrist Bursa and Ligament, Left **7** Hand Bursa and Ligament, Right **8** Hand Bursa and Ligament, Left **9** Upper Extremity Bursa and Ligament, Right **B** Upper Extremity Bursa and Ligament, Left **C** Upper Spine Bursa and Ligament, Right **D** Lower Spine Bursa and Ligament, Left **F** Sternum Bursa and Ligament, Right **G** Rib(s) Bursa and Ligament, Left **H** Abdomen Bursa and Ligament, Right **J** Abdomen Bursa and Ligament, Left **K** Perineum Bursa and Ligament **L** Hip Bursa and Ligament, Right **M** Hip Bursa and Ligament, Left **N** Knee Bursa and Ligament, Right **P** Knee Bursa and Ligament, Left **Q** Ankle Bursa and Ligament, Right **R** Ankle Bursa and Ligament, Left **S** Foot Bursa and Ligament, Right **T** Foot Bursa and Ligament, Left **V** Lower Extremity Bursa and Ligament, Right **W** Lower Extremity Bursa and Ligament, Left	**0** Open **3** Percutaneous **4** Percutaneous Endoscopic	**Z** No Device	**X** Diagnostic **Z** No Qualifier

Section **0** **Medical and Surgical**
Body System **M** **Bursae and Ligaments**
Operation **C** **Extirpation:** Taking or cutting out solid matter from a body part

Body Part (4th)	Approach (5th)	Device (6th)	Qualifier (7th)
0 Head and Neck Bursa and Ligament	**0** Open	**Z** No Device	**Z** No Qualifier
1 Shoulder Bursa and Ligament, Right	**3** Percutaneous		
2 Shoulder Bursa and Ligament, Left	**4** Percutaneous Endoscopic		
3 Elbow Bursa and Ligament, Right			
4 Elbow Bursa and Ligament, Left			
5 Wrist Bursa and Ligament, Right			
6 Wrist Bursa and Ligament, Left			
7 Hand Bursa and Ligament, Right			
8 Hand Bursa and Ligament, Left			
9 Upper Extremity Bursa and Ligament, Right			
B Upper Extremity Bursa and Ligament, Left			
C Upper Spine Bursa and Ligament, Right			
D Trunk Bursa and Ligament, Left			
F Sternum Bursa and Ligament, Right			
G Rib(s) Bursa and Ligament, Left			
H Abdomen Bursa and Ligament, Right			
J Abdomen Bursa and Ligament, Left			
K Perineum Bursa and Ligament			
L Hip Bursa and Ligament, Right			
M Hip Bursa and Ligament, Left			
N Knee Bursa and Ligament, Right			
P Knee Bursa and Ligament, Left			
Q Ankle Bursa and Ligament, Right			
R Ankle Bursa and Ligament, Left			
S Foot Bursa and Ligament, Right			
T Foot Bursa and Ligament, Left			
V Lower Extremity Bursa and Ligament, Right			
W Lower Extremity Bursa and Ligament, Left			

Section **0** **Medical and Surgical**
Body System **M** **Bursae and Ligaments**
Operation **D** **Extraction:** Pulling or stripping out or off all or a portion of a body part by the use of force

Body Part (4th)	Approach (5th)	Device (6th)	Qualifier (7th)
0 Head and Neck Bursa and Ligament	**0** Open	**Z** No Device	**Z** No Qualifier
1 Shoulder Bursa and Ligament, Right	**3** Percutaneous		
2 Shoulder Bursa and Ligament, Left	**4** Percutaneous Endoscopic		
3 Elbow Bursa and Ligament, Right			
4 Elbow Bursa and Ligament, Left			
5 Wrist Bursa and Ligament, Right			
6 Wrist Bursa and Ligament, Left			
7 Hand Bursa and Ligament, Right			
8 Hand Bursa and Ligament, Left			
9 Upper Extremity Bursa and Ligament, Right			
B Upper Extremity Bursa and Ligament, Left			
C Upper Spine Bursa and Ligament, Right			
D Lower Spine Bursa and Ligament, Left			
F Sternum Bursa and Ligament, Right			
G Rib(s) Bursa and Ligament, Left			
H Abdomen Bursa and Ligament, Right			
J Abdomen Bursa and Ligament, Left			
K Perineum Bursa and Ligament			
L Hip Bursa and Ligament, Right			
M Hip Bursa and Ligament, Left			
N Knee Bursa and Ligament, Right			
P Knee Bursa and Ligament, Left			
Q Ankle Bursa and Ligament, Right			
R Ankle Bursa and Ligament, Left			
S Foot Bursa and Ligament, Right			
T Foot Bursa and Ligament, Left			
V Lower Extremity Bursa and Ligament, Right			
W Lower Extremity Bursa and Ligament, Left			

Section 0 **Medical and Surgical**
Body System M **Bursae and Ligaments**
Operation H **Insertion:** Putting in a nonbiological appliance that monitors, assists, performs, or prevents a physiological function but does not physically take the place of a body part

Body Part (4th)	Approach (5th)	Device (6th)	Qualifier (7th)
X Upper Bursa and Ligament **Y** Lower Bursa and Ligament	**0** Open **3** Percutaneous **4** Percutaneous Endoscopic	**Y** Other Device	**Z** No Qualifier

Section 0 **Medical and Surgical**
Body System M **Bursae and Ligaments**
Operation J **Inspection:** Visually and/or manually exploring a body part

Body Part (4th)	Approach (5th)	Device (6th)	Qualifier (7th)
X Upper Bursa and Ligament **Y** Lower Bursa and Ligament	**0** Open **3** Percutaneous **4** Percutaneous Endoscopic **X** External	**Z** No Device	**Z** No Qualifier

Section 0 **Medical and Surgical**
Body System M **Bursae and Ligaments**
Operation M **Reattachment:** Putting back in or on all or a portion of a separated body part to its normal location or other suitable location

Body Part (4th)	Approach (5th)	Device (6th)	Qualifier (7th)
0 Head and Neck Bursa and Ligament **1** Shoulder Bursa and Ligament, Right **2** Shoulder Bursa and Ligament, Left **3** Elbow Bursa and Ligament, Right **4** Elbow Bursa and Ligament, Left **5** Wrist Bursa and Ligament, Right **6** Wrist Bursa and Ligament, Left **7** Hand Bursa and Ligament, Right **8** Hand Bursa and Ligament, Left **9** Upper Extremity Bursa and Ligament, Right **B** Upper Extremity Bursa and Ligament, Left **C** Upper Spine Bursa and Ligament, Right **D** Lower Spine Bursa and Ligament, Left **F** Sternum Bursa and Ligament, Right **G** Rib(s) Bursa and Ligament, Left **H** Abdomen Bursa and Ligament, Right **J** Abdomen Bursa and Ligament, Left **K** Perineum Bursa and Ligament **L** Hip Bursa and Ligament, Right **M** Hip Bursa and Ligament, Left **N** Knee Bursa and Ligament, Right **P** Knee Bursa and Ligament, Left **Q** Ankle Bursa and Ligament, Right **R** Ankle Bursa and Ligament, Left **S** Foot Bursa and Ligament, Right **T** Foot Bursa and Ligament, Left **V** Lower Extremity Bursa and Ligament, Right **W** Lower Extremity Bursa and Ligament, Left	**0** Open **4** Percutaneous Endoscopic	**Z** No Device	**Z** No Qualifier

Section 0 **Medical and Surgical**
Body System M **Bursae and Ligaments**
Operation N **Release:** Freeing a body part from an abnormal physical constraint by cutting or by the use of force

Body Part (4th)	Approach (5th)	Device (6th)	Qualifier (7th)
0 Head and Neck Bursa and Ligament **1** Shoulder Bursa and Ligament, Right **2** Shoulder Bursa and Ligament, Left **3** Elbow Bursa and Ligament, Right **4** Elbow Bursa and Ligament, Left **5** Wrist Bursa and Ligament, Right **6** Wrist Bursa and Ligament, Left **7** Hand Bursa and Ligament, Right **8** Hand Bursa and Ligament, Left **9** Upper Extremity Bursa and Ligament, Right **B** Upper Extremity Bursa and Ligament, Left **C** Upper Spine Bursa and Ligament, Right **D** Lower Spine Bursa and Ligament, Left **F** Sternum Bursa and Ligament, Right **G** Rib(s) Bursa and Ligament, Left **H** Abdomen Bursa and Ligament, Right **J** Abdomen Bursa and Ligament, Left **K** Perineum Bursa and Ligament **L** Hip Bursa and Ligament, Right **M** Hip Bursa and Ligament, Left **N** Knee Bursa and Ligament, Right **P** Knee Bursa and Ligament, Left **Q** Ankle Bursa and Ligament, Right **R** Ankle Bursa and Ligament, Left **S** Foot Bursa and Ligament, Right **T** Foot Bursa and Ligament, Left **V** Lower Extremity Bursa and Ligament, Right **W** Lower Extremity Bursa and Ligament, Left	**0** Open **3** Percutaneous **4** Percutaneous Endoscopic **X** External	**Z** No Device	**Z** No Qualifier

Section 0 **Medical and Surgical**
Body System M **Bursae and Ligaments**
Operation P **Removal:** Taking out or off a device from a body part

Body Part (4th)	Approach (5th)	Device (6th)	Qualifier (7th)
X Upper Bursa and Ligament **Y** Lower Bursa and Ligament	**0** Open **3** Percutaneous **4** Percutaneous Endoscopic	**0** Drainage Device **7** Autologous Tissue Substitute **J** Synthetic Substitute **K** Nonautologous Tissue Substitute **Y** Other Device	**Z** No Qualifier
X Upper Bursa and Ligament **Y** Lower Bursa and Ligament	**X** External	**0** Drainage Device	**Z** No Qualifier

Section	**0**	**Medical and Surgical**
Body System	**M**	**Bursae and Ligaments**
Operation	**Q**	**Repair:** Restoring, to the extent possible, a body part to its normal anatomic structure and function

Body Part (4th)	Approach (5th)	Device (6th)	Qualifier (7th)
0 Head and Neck Bursa and Ligament **1** Shoulder Bursa and Ligament, Right **2** Shoulder Bursa and Ligament, Left **3** Elbow Bursa and Ligament, Right **4** Elbow Bursa and Ligament, Left **5** Wrist Bursa and Ligament, Right **6** Wrist Bursa and Ligament, Left **7** Hand Bursa and Ligament, Right **8** Hand Bursa and Ligament, Left **9** Upper Extremity Bursa and Ligament, Right **B** Upper Extremity Bursa and Ligament, Left **C** Upper Spine Bursa and Ligament, Right **D** Lower Spine Bursa and Ligament, Left **F** Sternum Bursa and Ligament, Right **G** Rib(s) Bursa and Ligament, Left **H** Abdomen Bursa and Ligament, Right **J** Abdomen Bursa and Ligament, Left **K** Perineum Bursa and Ligament **L** Hip Bursa and Ligament, Right **M** Hip Bursa and Ligament, Left **N** Knee Bursa and Ligament, Right **P** Knee Bursa and Ligament, Left **Q** Ankle Bursa and Ligament, Right **R** Ankle Bursa and Ligament, Left **S** Foot Bursa and Ligament, Right **T** Foot Bursa and Ligament, Left **V** Lower Extremity Bursa and Ligament, Right **W** Lower Extremity Bursa and Ligament, Left	**0** Open **3** Percutaneous **4** Percutaneous Endoscopic	**Z** No Device	**Z** No Qualifier

Section	**0**	**Medical and Surgical**
Body System	**M**	**Bursae and Ligaments**
Operation	**R**	**Replacement:** Putting in or on biological or synthetic material that physically takes the place and/or function of all or a portion of a body part

Body Part (4th)	Approach (5th)	Device (6th)	Qualifier (7th)
0 Head and Neck Bursa and Ligament **1** Shoulder Bursa and Ligament, Right **2** Shoulder Bursa and Ligament, Left **3** Elbow Bursa and Ligament, Right **4** Elbow Bursa and Ligament, Left **5** Wrist Bursa and Ligament, Right **6** Wrist Bursa and Ligament, Left **7** Hand Bursa and Ligament, Right **8** Hand Bursa and Ligament, Left **9** Upper Extremity Bursa and Ligament, Right **B** Upper Extremity Bursa and Ligament, Left **C** Upper Spine Bursa and Ligament **D** Lower Spine Bursa and Ligament **F** Sternum Bursa and Ligament **G** Rib(s) Bursa and Ligament **H** Abdomen Bursa and Ligament, Right **J** Abdomen Bursa and Ligament, Left **K** Perineum Bursa and Ligament **L** Hip Bursa and Ligament, Right **M** Hip Bursa and Ligament, Left **N** Knee Bursa and Ligament, Right **P** Knee Bursa and Ligament, Left **Q** Ankle Bursa and Ligament, Right **R** Ankle Bursa and Ligament, Left **S** Foot Bursa and Ligament, Right **T** Foot Bursa and Ligament, Left **V** Lower Extremity Bursa and Ligament, Right **W** Lower Extremity Bursa and Ligament, Left	**0** Open **4** Percutaneous Endoscopic	**7** Autologous Tissue Substitute **J** Synthetic Substitute **K** Nonautologous Tissue Substitute	**Z** No Qualifier

Section 0 **Medical and Surgical**
Body System M **Bursae and Ligaments**
Operation S **Reposition:** Moving to its normal location, or other suitable location, all or a portion of a body part

Body Part (4th)	Approach (5th)	Device (6th)	Qualifier (7th)
0 Head and Neck Bursa and Ligament **1** Shoulder Bursa and Ligament, Right **2** Shoulder Bursa and Ligament, Left **3** Elbow Bursa and Ligament, Right **4** Elbow Bursa and Ligament, Left **5** Wrist Bursa and Ligament, Right **6** Wrist Bursa and Ligament, Left **7** Hand Bursa and Ligament, Right **8** Hand Bursa and Ligament, Left **9** Upper Extremity Bursa and Ligament, Right **B** Upper Extremity Bursa and Ligament, Left **C** Upper Spine Bursa and Ligament, Right **D** Lower Spine Bursa and Ligament, Left **F** Sternum Bursa and Ligament, Right **G** Rib(s) Bursa and Ligament, Left **H** Abdomen Bursa and Ligament, Right **J** Abdomen Bursa and Ligament, Left **K** Perineum Bursa and Ligament **L** Hip Bursa and Ligament, Right **M** Hip Bursa and Ligament, Left **N** Knee Bursa and Ligament, Right **P** Knee Bursa and Ligament, Left **Q** Ankle Bursa and Ligament, Right **R** Ankle Bursa and Ligament, Left **S** Foot Bursa and Ligament, Right **T** Foot Bursa and Ligament, Left **V** Lower Extremity Bursa and Ligament, Right **W** Lower Extremity Bursa and Ligament, Left	**0** Open **4** Percutaneous Endoscopic	**Z** No Device	**Z** No Qualifier

Section 0 **Medical and Surgical**
Body System M **Bursae and Ligaments**
Operation T **Resection:** Cutting out or off, without replacement, all of a body part

Body Part (4th)	Approach (5th)	Device (6th)	Qualifier (7th)
0 Head and Neck Bursa and Ligament **1** Shoulder Bursa and Ligament, Right **2** Shoulder Bursa and Ligament, Left **3** Elbow Bursa and Ligament, Right **4** Elbow Bursa and Ligament, Left **5** Wrist Bursa and Ligament, Right **6** Wrist Bursa and Ligament, Left **7** Hand Bursa and Ligament, Right **8** Hand Bursa and Ligament, Left **9** Upper Extremity Bursa and Ligament, Right **B** Upper Extremity Bursa and Ligament, Left **C** Upper Spine Bursa and Ligament, Right **D** Lower Spine Bursa and Ligament, Left **F** Sternum Bursa and Ligament, Right **G** Rib(s) Bursa and Ligament, Left **H** Abdomen Bursa and Ligament, Right **J** Abdomen Bursa and Ligament, Left **K** Perineum Bursa and Ligament **L** Hip Bursa and Ligament, Right **M** Hip Bursa and Ligament, Left **N** Knee Bursa and Ligament, Right **P** Knee Bursa and Ligament, Left **Q** Ankle Bursa and Ligament, Right **R** Ankle Bursa and Ligament, Left **S** Foot Bursa and Ligament, Right **T** Foot Bursa and Ligament, Left **V** Lower Extremity Bursa and Ligament, Right **W** Lower Extremity Bursa and Ligament, Left	**0** Open **4** Percutaneous Endoscopic	**Z** No Device	**Z** No Qualifier

Section 0 **Medical and Surgical**
Body System M **Bursae and Ligaments**
Operation U **Supplement:** Putting in or on biological or synthetic material that physically reinforces and/or augments the function of a portion of a body part

Body Part (4th)	Approach (5th)	Device (6th)	Qualifier (7th)
0 Head and Neck Bursa and Ligament **1** Shoulder Bursa and Ligament, Right **2** Shoulder Bursa and Ligament, Left **3** Elbow Bursa and Ligament, Right **4** Elbow Bursa and Ligament, Left **5** Wrist Bursa and Ligament, Right **6** Wrist Bursa and Ligament, Left **7** Hand Bursa and Ligament, Right **8** Hand Bursa and Ligament, Left **9** Upper Extremity Bursa and Ligament, Right **B** Upper Extremity Bursa and Ligament, Left **C** Upper Spine Bursa and Ligament, Right **D** Lower Spine Bursa and Ligament, Left **F** Sternum Bursa and Ligament, Right **G** Rib(s) Bursa and Ligament, Left **H** Abdomen Bursa and Ligament, Right **J** Abdomen Bursa and Ligament, Left **K** Perineum Bursa and Ligament **L** Hip Bursa and Ligament, Right **M** Hip Bursa and Ligament, Left **N** Knee Bursa and Ligament, Right **P** Knee Bursa and Ligament, Left **Q** Ankle Bursa and Ligament, Right **R** Ankle Bursa and Ligament, Left **S** Foot Bursa and Ligament, Right **T** Foot Bursa and Ligament, Left **V** Lower Extremity Bursa and Ligament, Right **W** Lower Extremity Bursa and Ligament, Left	**0** Open **4** Percutaneous Endoscopic	**7** Autologous Tissue Substitute **J** Synthetic Substitute **K** Nonautologous Tissue Substitute	**Z** No Qualifier

Section 0 **Medical and Surgical**
Body System M **Bursae and Ligaments**
Operation W **Revision:** Correcting, to the extent possible, a portion of a malfunctioning device or the position of a displaced device

Body Part (4th)	Approach (5th)	Device (6th)	Qualifier (7th)
X Upper Bursa and Ligament **Y** Lower Bursa and Ligament	**0** Open **3** Percutaneous **4** Percutaneous Endoscopic	**0** Drainage Device **7** Autologous Tissue Substitute **J** Synthetic Substitute **K** Nonautologous Tissue Substitute **Y** Other Device	**Z** No Qualifier
X Upper Bursa and Ligament **Y** Lower Bursa and Ligament	**X** External	**0** Drainage Device **7** Autologous Tissue Substitute **J** Synthetic Substitute **K** Nonautologous Tissue Substitute	**Z** No Qualifier

Section 0 **Medical and Surgical**
Body System M **Bursae and Ligaments**
Operation X **Transfer:** Moving, without taking out, all or a portion of a body part to another location to take over the function of all or a portion of a body part

Body Part (4th)	Approach (5th)	Device (6th)	Qualifier (7th)
0 Head and Neck Bursa and Ligament **1** Shoulder Bursa and Ligament, Right **2** Shoulder Bursa and Ligament, Left **3** Elbow Bursa and Ligament, Right **4** Elbow Bursa and Ligament, Left **5** Wrist Bursa and Ligament, Right **6** Wrist Bursa and Ligament, Left **7** Hand Bursa and Ligament, Right **8** Hand Bursa and Ligament, Left **9** Upper Extremity Bursa and Ligament, Right **B** Upper Extremity Bursa and Ligament, Left **C** Upper Spine Bursa and Ligament, Right **D** Lower Spine Bursa and Ligament, Left **F** Sternum Bursa and Ligament, Right **G** Rib(s) Bursa and Ligament, Left **H** Abdomen Bursa and Ligament, Right **J** Abdomen Bursa and Ligament, Left **K** Perineum Bursa and Ligament **L** Hip Bursa and Ligament, Right **M** Hip Bursa and Ligament, Left **N** Knee Bursa and Ligament, Right **P** Knee Bursa and Ligament, Left **Q** Ankle Bursa and Ligament, Right **R** Ankle Bursa and Ligament, Left **S** Foot Bursa and Ligament, Right **T** Foot Bursa and Ligament, Left **V** Lower Extremity Bursa and Ligament, Right **W** Lower Extremity Bursa and Ligament, Left	**0** Open **4** Percutaneous Endoscopic	**Z** No Device	**Z** No Qualifier

AHA Coding Clinic

0MM14ZZ Reattachment of Right Shoulder Bursa and Ligament, Percutaneous Endoscopic Approach—AHA CC: 3Q, 2013, 20-22

0MQ00ZZ Repair Head and Neck Bursa and Ligament, Open Approach—AHA CC: 3Q, 2014, 9

0MUN47Z Supplement Right Knee Bursa and Ligament with Autologous Tissue Substitute, Percutaneous Endoscopic Approach—AHA CC: 2Q, 2017, 21-22

Head and Facial Bones

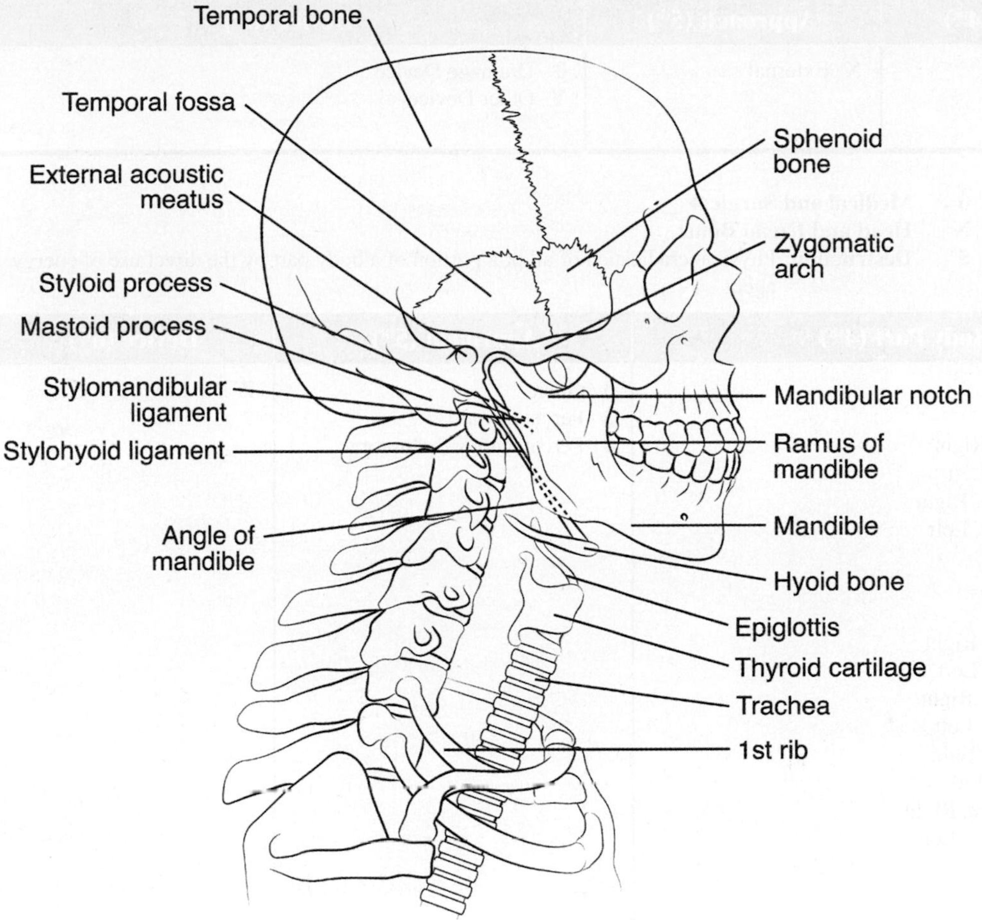
Temporal bone
Temporal fossa
External acoustic meatus
Styloid process
Mastoid process
Stylomandibular ligament
Stylohyoid ligament
Angle of mandible
Sphenoid bone
Zygomatic arch
Mandibular notch
Ramus of mandible
Mandible
Hyoid bone
Epiglottis
Thyroid cartilage
Trachea
1st rib

©AHIMA

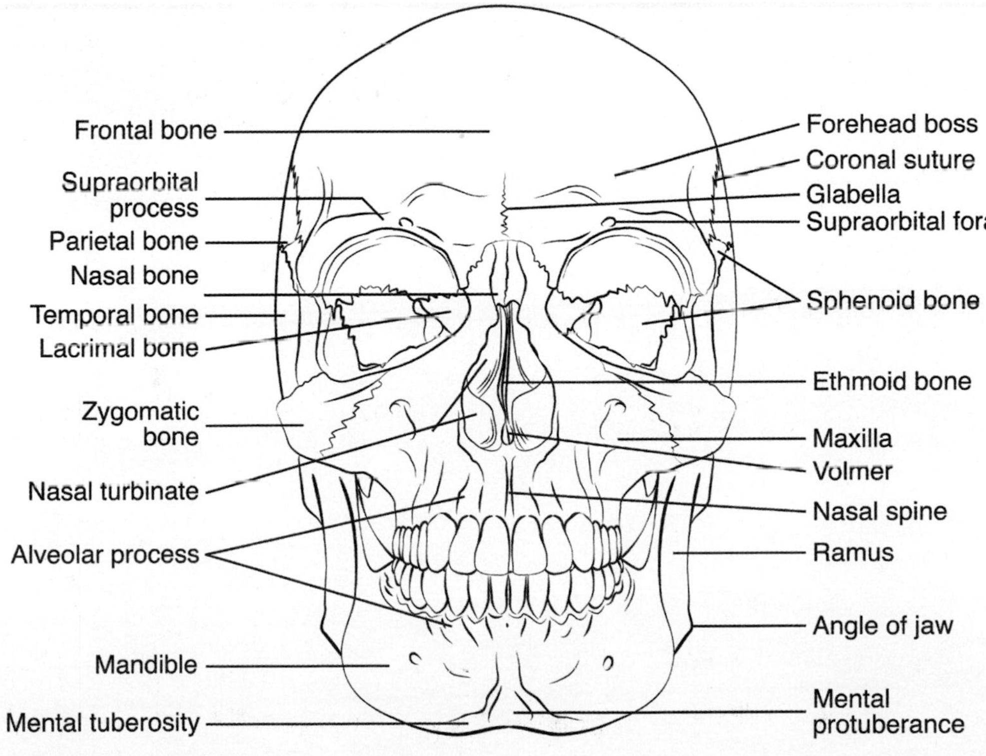
Frontal bone
Supraorbital process
Parietal bone
Nasal bone
Temporal bone
Lacrimal bone
Zygomatic bone
Nasal turbinate
Alveolar process
Mandible
Mental tuberosity
Forehead boss
Coronal suture
Glabella
Supraorbital foramen
Sphenoid bone
Ethmoid bone
Maxilla
Volmer
Nasal spine
Ramus
Angle of jaw
Mental protuberance

©AHIMA

Section 0 **Medical and Surgical**
Body System N **Head and Facial Bones**
Operation 2 **Change:** Taking out or off a device from a body part and putting back an identical or similar device in or on the same body part without cutting or puncturing the skin or a mucous membrane

Body Part (4th)	Approach (5th)	Device (6th)	Qualifier (7th)
0 Skull **B** Nasal Bone **W** Facial Bone	**X** External	**0** Drainage Device **Y** Other Device	**Z** No Qualifier

Section 0 **Medical and Surgical**
Body System N **Head and Facial Bones**
Operation 5 **Destruction:** Physical eradication of all or a portion of a body part by the direct use of energy, force, or a destructive agent

Body Part (4th)	Approach (5th)	Device (6th)	Qualifier (7th)
0 Skull **1** Frontal Bone **3** Parietal Bone, Right **4** Parietal Bone, Left **5** Temporal Bone, Right **6** Temporal Bone, Left **7** Occipital Bone **B** Nasal Bone **C** Sphenoid Bone **F** Ethmoid Bone, Right **G** Ethmoid Bone, Left **H** Lacrimal Bone, Right **J** Lacrimal Bone, Left **K** Palatine Bone, Right **L** Palatine Bone, Left **M** Zygomatic Bone, Right **N** Zygomatic Bone, Left **P** Orbit, Right **Q** Orbit, Left **R** Maxilla **T** Mandible, Right **V** Mandible, Left **X** Hyoid Bone	**0** Open **3** Percutaneous **4** Percutaneous Endoscopic	**Z** No Device	**Z** No Qualifier

Section 0 **Medical and Surgical**
Body System N **Head and Facial Bones**
Operation 8 **Division:** Cutting into a body part, without draining fluids and/or gases from the body part, in order to separate or transect a body part

Body Part (4th)	Approach (5th)	Device (6th)	Qualifier (7th)
0 Skull **1** Frontal Bone **3** Parietal Bone, Right **4** Parietal Bone, Left **5** Temporal Bone, Right **6** Temporal Bone, Left **7** Occipital Bone **B** Nasal Bone **C** Sphenoid Bone **F** Ethmoid Bone, Right **G** Ethmoid Bone, Left **H** Lacrimal Bone, Right **J** Lacrimal Bone, Left **K** Palatine Bone, Right **L** Palatine Bone, Left **M** Zygomatic Bone, Right **N** Zygomatic Bone, Left **P** Orbit, Right **Q** Orbit, Left **R** Maxilla **T** Mandible, Right **V** Mandible, Left **X** Hyoid Bone	**0** Open **3** Percutaneous **4** Percutaneous Endoscopic	**Z** No Device	**Z** No Qualifier

Section 0 **Medical and Surgical**
Body System N **Head and Facial Bones**
Operation 9 **Drainage:** Taking or letting out fluids and/or gases from a body part

Body Part (4th)	Approach (5th)	Device (6th)	Qualifier (7th)
0 Skull **1** Frontal Bone **3** Parietal Bone, Right **4** Parietal Bone, Left **5** Temporal Bone, Right **6** Temporal Bone, Left **7** Occipital Bone **B** Nasal Bone **C** Sphenoid Bone **F** Ethmoid Bone, Right **G** Ethmoid Bone, Left **H** Lacrimal Bone, Right **J** Lacrimal Bone, Left **K** Palatine Bone, Right **L** Palatine Bone, Left **M** Zygomatic Bone, Right **N** Zygomatic Bone, Left **P** Orbit, Right **Q** Orbit, Left **R** Maxilla **T** Mandible, Right **V** Mandible, Left **X** Hyoid Bone	**0** Open **3** Percutaneous **4** Percutaneous Endoscopic	**0** Drainage Device	**Z** No Qualifier

Continued →

Section 0 **Medical and Surgical**
Body System N **Head and Facial Bones**
Operation 9 **Drainage:** Taking or letting out fluids and/or gases from a body part

Body Part (4th)	Approach (5th)	Device (6th)	Qualifier (7th)
0 Skull **1** Frontal Bone **3** Parietal Bone, Right **4** Parietal Bone, Left **5** Temporal Bone, Right **6** Temporal Bone, Left **7** Occipital Bone **B** Nasal Bone **C** Sphenoid Bone **F** Ethmoid Bone, Right **G** Ethmoid Bone, Left **H** Lacrimal Bone, Right **J** Lacrimal Bone, Left **K** Palatine Bone, Right **L** Palatine Bone, Left **M** Zygomatic Bone, Right **N** Zygomatic Bone, Left **P** Orbit, Right **Q** Orbit, Left **R** Maxilla **T** Mandible, Right **V** Mandible, Left **X** Hyoid Bone	**0** Open **3** Percutaneous **4** Percutaneous Endoscopic	**Z** No Device	**X** Diagnostic **Z** No Qualifier

Section 0 **Medical and Surgical**
Body System N **Head and Facial Bones**
Operation B **Excision:** Cutting out or off, without replacement, a portion of a body part

Body Part (4th)	Approach (5th)	Device (6th)	Qualifier (7th)
0 Skull **1** Frontal Bone **3** Parietal Bone, Right **4** Parietal Bone, Left **5** Temporal Bone, Right **6** Temporal Bone, Left **7** Occipital Bone **B** Nasal Bone **C** Sphenoid Bone **F** Ethmoid Bone, Right **G** Ethmoid Bone, Left **H** Lacrimal Bone, Right **J** Lacrimal Bone, Left **K** Palatine Bone, Right **L** Palatine Bone, Left **M** Zygomatic Bone, Right **N** Zygomatic Bone, Left **P** Orbit, Right **Q** Orbit, Left **R** Maxilla **T** Mandible, Right **V** Mandible, Left **X** Hyoid Bone	**0** Open **3** Percutaneous **4** Percutaneous Endoscopic	**Z** No Device	**X** Diagnostic **Z** No Qualifier

Section 0 **Medical and Surgical**
Body System N **Head and Facial Bones**
Operation C **Extirpation: Taking or cutting out solid matter from a body part**

Body Part (4th)	Approach (5th)	Device (6th)	Qualifier (7th)
1 Frontal Bone 3 Parietal Bone, Right 4 Parietal Bone, Left 5 Temporal Bone, Right 6 Temporal Bone, Left 7 Occipital Bone B Nasal Bone C Sphenoid Bone F Ethmoid Bone, Right G Ethmoid Bone, Left H Lacrimal Bone, Right J Lacrimal Bone, Left K Palatine Bone, Right L Palatine Bone, Left M Zygomatic Bone, Right N Zygomatic Bone, Left P Orbit, Right Q Orbit, Left R Maxilla T Mandible, Right V Mandible, Left X Hyoid Bone	0 Open 3 Percutaneous 4 Percutaneous Endoscopic	Z No Device	Z No Qualifier

Section 0 **Medical and Surgical**
Body System N **Head and Facial Bones**
Operation D **Extraction:** Pulling or stripping out or off all or a portion of a body part by the use of force

Body Part (4th)	Approach (5th)	Device (6th)	Qualifier (7th)
0 Skull 1 Frontal Bone 3 Parietal Bone, Right 4 Parietal Bone, Left 5 Temporal Bone, Right 6 Temporal Bone, Left 7 Occipital Bone B Nasal Bone C Sphenoid Bone F Ethmoid Bone, Right G Ethmoid Bone, Left H Lacrimal Bone, Right J Lacrimal Bone, Left K Palatine Bone, Right L Palatine Bone, Left M Zygomatic Bone, Right N Zygomatic Bone, Left P Orbit, Right Q Orbit, Left R Maxilla T Mandible, Right V Mandible, Left X Hyoid Bone	0 Open	Z No Device	Z No Qualifier

Section 0 **Medical and Surgical**
Body System N **Head and Facial Bones**
Operation H **Insertion:** Putting in a nonbiological appliance that monitors, assists, performs, or prevents a physiological function but does not physically take the place of a body part

Body Part (4th)	Approach (5th)	Device (6th)	Qualifier (7th)
0 Skull	**0** Open	**3** Infusion Device **4** Internal Fixation Device **5** External Fixation Device **M** Bone Growth Stimulator **N** Neurostimulator Generator	**Z** No Qualifier
0 Skull	**3** Percutaneous **4** Percutaneous Endoscopic	**3** Infusion Device **4** Internal Fixation Device **5** External Fixation Device **M** Bone Growth Stimulator	**Z** No Qualifier
1 Frontal Bone **3** Parietal Bone, Right **4** Parietal Bone, Left **7** Occipital Bone **C** Sphenoid Bone **F** Ethmoid Bone, Right **G** Ethmoid Bone, Left **H** Lacrimal Bone, Right **J** Lacrimal Bone, Left **K** Palatine Bone, Right **L** Palatine Bone, Left **M** Zygomatic Bone, Right **N** Zygomatic Bone, Left **P** Orbit, Right **Q** Orbit, Left **X** Hyoid Bone	**0** Open **3** Percutaneous **4** Percutaneous Endoscopic	**4** Internal Fixation Device	**Z** No Qualifier
5 Temporal Bone, Right **6** Temporal Bone, Left	**0** Open **3** Percutaneous **4** Percutaneous Endoscopic	**4** Internal Fixation Device **S** Hearing Device	**Z** No Qualifier
B Nasal Bone	**0** Open **3** Percutaneous **4** Percutaneous Endoscopic	**4** Internal Fixation Device **M** Bone Growth Stimulator	**Z** No Qualifier
R Maxilla **T** Mandible, Right **V** Mandible, Left	**0** Open **3** Percutaneous **4** Percutaneous Endoscopic	**4** Internal Fixation Device **5** External Fixation Device	**Z** No Qualifier
W Facial Bone	**0** Open **3** Percutaneous **4** Percutaneous Endoscopic	**M** Bone Growth Stimulator	**Z** No Qualifier

Section 0 **Medical and Surgical**
Body System N **Head and Facial Bones**
Operation J **Inspection:** Visually and/or manually exploring a body part

Body Part (4th)	Approach (5th)	Device (6th)	Qualifier (7th)
0 Skull **B** Nasal Bone **W** Facial Bone	**0** Open **3** Percutaneous **4** Percutaneous Endoscopic **X** External	**Z** No Device	**Z** No Qualifier

Section	**0**	**Medical and Surgical**
Body System	**N**	**Head and Facial Bones**
Operation	**N**	**Release:** Freeing a body part from an abnormal physical constraint by cutting or by the use of force

Body Part (4th)	Approach (5th)	Device (6th)	Qualifier (7th)
1 Frontal Bone **3** Parietal Bone, Right **4** Parietal Bone, Left **5** Temporal Bone, Right **6** Temporal Bone, Left **7** Occipital Bone **B** Nasal Bone **C** Sphenoid Bone **F** Ethmoid Bone, Right **G** Ethmoid Bone, Left **H** Lacrimal Bone, Right **J** Lacrimal Bone, Left **K** Palatine Bone, Right **L** Palatine Bone, Left **M** Zygomatic Bone, Right **N** Zygomatic Bone, Left **P** Orbit, Right **Q** Orbit, Left **R** Maxilla **T** Mandible, Right **V** Mandible, Left **X** Hyoid Bone	**0** Open **3** Percutaneous **4** Percutaneous Endoscopic	**Z** No Device	**Z** No Qualifier

Section	**0**	**Medical and Surgical**
Body System	**N**	**Head and Facial Bones**
Operation	**P**	**Removal:** Taking out or off a device from a body part

Body Part (4th)	Approach (5th)	Device (6th)	Qualifier (7th)
0 Skull	**0** Open	**0** Drainage Device **4** Internal Fixation Device **5** External Fixation Device **7** Autologous Tissue Substitute **J** Synthetic Substitute **K** Nonautologous Tissue Substitute **M** Bone Growth Stimulator **N** Neurostimulator Generator **S** Hearing Device	**Z** No Qualifier
0 Skull	**3** Percutaneous **4** Percutaneous Endoscopic	**0** Drainage Device **4** Internal Fixation Device **5** External Fixation Device **7** Autologous Tissue Substitute **J** Synthetic Substitute **K** Nonautologous Tissue Substitute **M** Bone Growth Stimulator **S** Hearing Device	**Z** No Qualifier
0 Skull	**X** External	**0** Drainage Device **4** Internal Fixation Device **5** External Fixation Device **M** Bone Growth Stimulator **S** Hearing Device	**Z** No Qualifier
B Nasal Bone **W** Facial Bone	**0** Open **3** Percutaneous **4** Percutaneous Endoscopic	**0** Drainage Device **4** Internal Fixation Device **7** Autologous Tissue Substitute **J** Synthetic Substitute **K** Nonautologous Tissue Substitute **M** Bone Growth Stimulator	**Z** No Qualifier
B Nasal Bone **W** Facial Bone	**X** External	**0** Drainage Device **4** Internal Fixation Device **M** Bone Growth Stimulator	**Z** No Qualifier

Section 0 **Medical and Surgical**
Body System N **Head and Facial Bones**
Operation Q **Repair:** Restoring, to the extent possible, a body part to its normal anatomic structure and function

Body Part (4th)	Approach (5th)	Device (6th)	Qualifier (7th)
0 Skull **1** Frontal Bone **3** Parietal Bone, Right **4** Parietal Bone, Left **5** Temporal Bone, Right **6** Temporal Bone, Left **7** Occipital Bone **B** Nasal Bone **C** Sphenoid Bone **F** Ethmoid Bone, Right **G** Ethmoid Bone, Left **H** Lacrimal Bone, Right **J** Lacrimal Bone, Left **K** Palatine Bone, Right **L** Palatine Bone, Left **M** Zygomatic Bone, Right **N** Zygomatic Bone, Left **P** Orbit, Right **Q** Orbit, Left **R** Maxilla **T** Mandible, Right **V** Mandible, Left **X** Hyoid Bone	**0** Open **3** Percutaneous **4** Percutaneous Endoscopic **X** External	**Z** No Device	**Z** No Qualifier

Section 0 **Medical and Surgical**
Body System N **Head and Facial Bones**
Operation R **Replacement:** Putting in or on biological or synthetic material that physically takes the place and/or function of all or a portion of a body part

Body Part (4th)	Approach (5th)	Device (6th)	Qualifier (7th)
0 Skull **1** Frontal Bone **3** Parietal Bone, Right **4** Parietal Bone, Left **5** Temporal Bone, Right **6** Temporal Bone, Left **7** Occipital Bone **B** Nasal Bone **C** Sphenoid Bone **F** Ethmoid Bone, Right **G** Ethmoid Bone, Left **H** Lacrimal Bone, Right **J** Lacrimal Bone, Left **K** Palatine Bone, Right **L** Palatine Bone, Left **M** Zygomatic Bone, Right **N** Zygomatic Bone, Left **P** Orbit, Right **Q** Orbit, Left **R** Maxilla **T** Mandible, Right **V** Mandible, Left **X** Hyoid Bone	**0** Open **3** Percutaneous **4** Percutaneous Endoscopic	**7** Autologous Tissue Substitute **J** Synthetic Substitute **K** Nonautologous Tissue Substitute	**Z** No Qualifier

Section **0** **Medical and Surgical**
Body System **N** **Head and Facial Bones**
Operation **S** **Reposition:** Moving to its normal location, or other suitable location, all or a portion of a body part

Body Part (4th)	Approach (5th)	Device (6th)	Qualifier (7th)
0 Skull **R** Maxilla **T** Mandible, Right **V** Mandible, Left	**0** Open **3** Percutaneous **4** Percutaneous Endoscopic	**4** Internal Fixation Device **5** External Fixation Device **Z** No Device	**Z** No Qualifier
0 Skull **R** Maxilla **T** Mandible, Right **V** Mandible, Left	**X** External	**Z** No Device	**Z** No Qualifier
1 Frontal Bone **3** Parietal Bone, Right **4** Parietal Bone, Left **5** Temporal Bone, Right **6** Temporal Bone, Left **7** Occipital Bone **B** Nasal Bone **C** Sphenoid Bone **F** Ethmoid Bone, Right **G** Ethmoid Bone, Left **H** Lacrimal Bone, Right **J** Lacrimal Bone, Left **K** Palatine Bone, Right **L** Palatine Bone, Left **M** Zygomatic Bone, Right **N** Zygomatic Bone, Left **P** Orbit, Right **Q** Orbit, Left **X** Hyoid Bone	**0** Open **3** Percutaneous **4** Percutaneous Endoscopic	**4** Internal Fixation Device **Z** No Device	**Z** No Qualifier
1 Frontal Bone **3** Parietal Bone, Right **4** Parietal Bone, Left **5** Temporal Bone, Right **6** Temporal Bone, Left **7** Occipital Bone **B** Nasal Bone **C** Sphenoid Bone **F** Ethmoid Bone, Right **G** Ethmoid Bone, Left **H** Lacrimal Bone, Right **J** Lacrimal Bone, Left **K** Palatine Bone, Right **L** Palatine Bone, Left **M** Zygomatic Bone, Right **N** Zygomatic Bone, Left **P** Orbit, Right **Q** Orbit, Left **X** Hyoid Bone	**X** External	**Z** No Device	**Z** No Qualifier

Section 0 **Medical and Surgical**
Body System N **Head and Facial Bones**
Operation T **Resection:** Cutting out or off, without replacement, all of a body part

Body Part (4th)	Approach (5th)	Device (6th)	Qualifier (7th)
1 Frontal Bone **3** Parietal Bone, Right **4** Parietal Bone, Left **5** Temporal Bone, Right **6** Temporal Bone, Left **7** Occipital Bone **B** Nasal Bone **C** Sphenoid Bone **F** Ethmoid Bone, Right **G** Ethmoid Bone, Left **H** Lacrimal Bone, Right **J** Lacrimal Bone, Left **K** Palatine Bone, Right **L** Palatine Bone, Left **M** Zygomatic Bone, Right **N** Zygomatic Bone, Left **P** Orbit, Right **Q** Orbit, Left **R** Maxilla **T** Mandible, Right **V** Mandible, Left **X** Hyoid Bone	**0** Open	**Z** No Device	**Z** No Qualifier

Section 0 **Medical and Surgical**
Body System N **Head and Facial Bones**
Operation U **Supplement:** Putting in or on biological or synthetic material that physically reinforces and/or augments the function of a portion of a body part

Body Part (4th)	Approach (5th)	Device (6th)	Qualifier (7th)
0 Skull **1** Frontal Bone **3** Parietal Bone, Right **4** Parietal Bone, Left **5** Temporal Bone, Right **6** Temporal Bone, Left **7** Occipital Bone **B** Nasal Bone **C** Sphenoid Bone **F** Ethmoid Bone, Right **G** Ethmoid Bone, Left **H** Lacrimal Bone, Right **J** Lacrimal Bone, Left **K** Palatine Bone, Right **L** Palatine Bone, Left **M** Zygomatic Bone, Right **N** Zygomatic Bone, Left **P** Orbit, Right **Q** Orbit, Left **R** Maxilla **T** Mandible, Right **V** Mandible, Left **X** Hyoid Bone	**0** Open **3** Percutaneous **4** Percutaneous Endoscopic	**7** Autologous Tissue Substitute **J** Synthetic Substitute **K** Nonautologous Tissue Substitute	**Z** No Qualifier

Section	0	Medical and Surgical
Body System	N	Head and Facial Bones
Operation	W	**Revision:** Correcting, to the extent possible, a portion of a malfunctioning device or the position of a displaced device

Body Part (4th)	Approach (5th)	Device (6th)	Qualifier (7th)
0 Skull	**0** Open	**0** Drainage Device **4** Internal Fixation Device **5** External Fixation Device **7** Autologous Tissue Substitute **J** Synthetic Substitute **K** Nonautologous Tissue Substitute **M** Bone Growth Stimulator **N** Neurostimulator Generator **S** Hearing Device	**Z** No Qualifier
0 Skull	**3** Percutaneous **4** Percutaneous Endoscopic **X** External	**0** Drainage Device **4** Internal Fixation Device **5** External Fixation Device **7** Autologous Tissue Substitute **J** Synthetic Substitute **K** Nonautologous Tissue Substitute **M** Bone Growth Stimulator **S** Hearing Device	**Z** No Qualifier
B Nasal Bone **W** Facial Bone	**0** Open **3** Percutaneous **4** Percutaneous Endoscopic **X** External	**0** Drainage Device **4** Internal Fixation Device **7** Autologous Tissue Substitute **J** Synthetic Substitute **K** Nonautologous Tissue Substitute **M** Bone Growth Stimulator	**Z** No Qualifier

AHA Coding Clinic

0NBB0ZZ Excision of Nasal Bone, Open Approach—AHA CC: 1Q, 2017, 20-21
0NBQ0ZZ Excision of Left Orbit, Open Approach—AHA CC: 2Q, 2015, 12-13
0NBR0ZZ Excision of Maxilla, Open Approach—AHA CC: 1Q, 2021, 21-22
0NH004Z Insertion of Internal Fixation Device into Skull, Open Approach—AHA CC: 3Q, 2015, 13-14
0NP004Z Removal of Internal Fixation Device from Skull, Open Approach—AHA CC: 3Q, 2015, 13-14
0NR00JZ Replacement of Skull with Synthetic Substitute, Open Approach—AHA CC: 3Q, 2014, 7-8
0NR70JZ Replacement of Occipital Bone with Synthetic Substitute, Open Approach—AHA CC: 3Q, 2017, 17
0NRR0JZ Replacement of Maxilla with Synthetic Substitute, Open Approach—AHA CC: 1Q, 2021, 21-22
0NRV07Z Replacement of Left Mandible with Autologous Tissue Substitute, Open Approach—AHA CC: 1Q, 2017, 23-24
0NRV0JZ Replacement of Left Mandible with Synthetic Substitute, Open Approach—AHA CC: 1Q, 2017, 23-24
0NS004Z Reposition Skull with Internal Fixation Device, Open Approach—AHA CC: 3Q, 2017, 22
0NS005Z Reposition Skull with External Fixation Device, Open Approach—AHA CC: 3Q, 2013, 24-25
0NS00ZZ Reposition Skull, Open Approach—AHA CC: 3Q, 2015, 17-18; 2Q, 2016, 30
0NS104Z Reposition Frontal Bone with Internal Fixation Device, Open Approach—AHA CC: 3Q, 2013, 25
0NS504Z Reposition Right Temporal Bone with Internal Fixation Device, Open Approach—AHA CC: 3Q, 2015, 27-28
0NSR04Z Reposition Maxilla with Internal Fixation Device, Open Approach—AHA CC: 3Q, 2014, 23-24
0NSR0ZZ Reposition Maxilla, Open Approach—AHA CC: 1Q, 2017, 20-21
0NU00JZ Supplement Skull with Synthetic Substitute, Open Approach—AHA CC: 3Q, 2013, 24-25
0NUR07Z Supplement Maxilla with Autologous Tissue Substitute, Open Approach—AHA CC: 3Q, 2016, 29-30

Bones - Front and Back Views

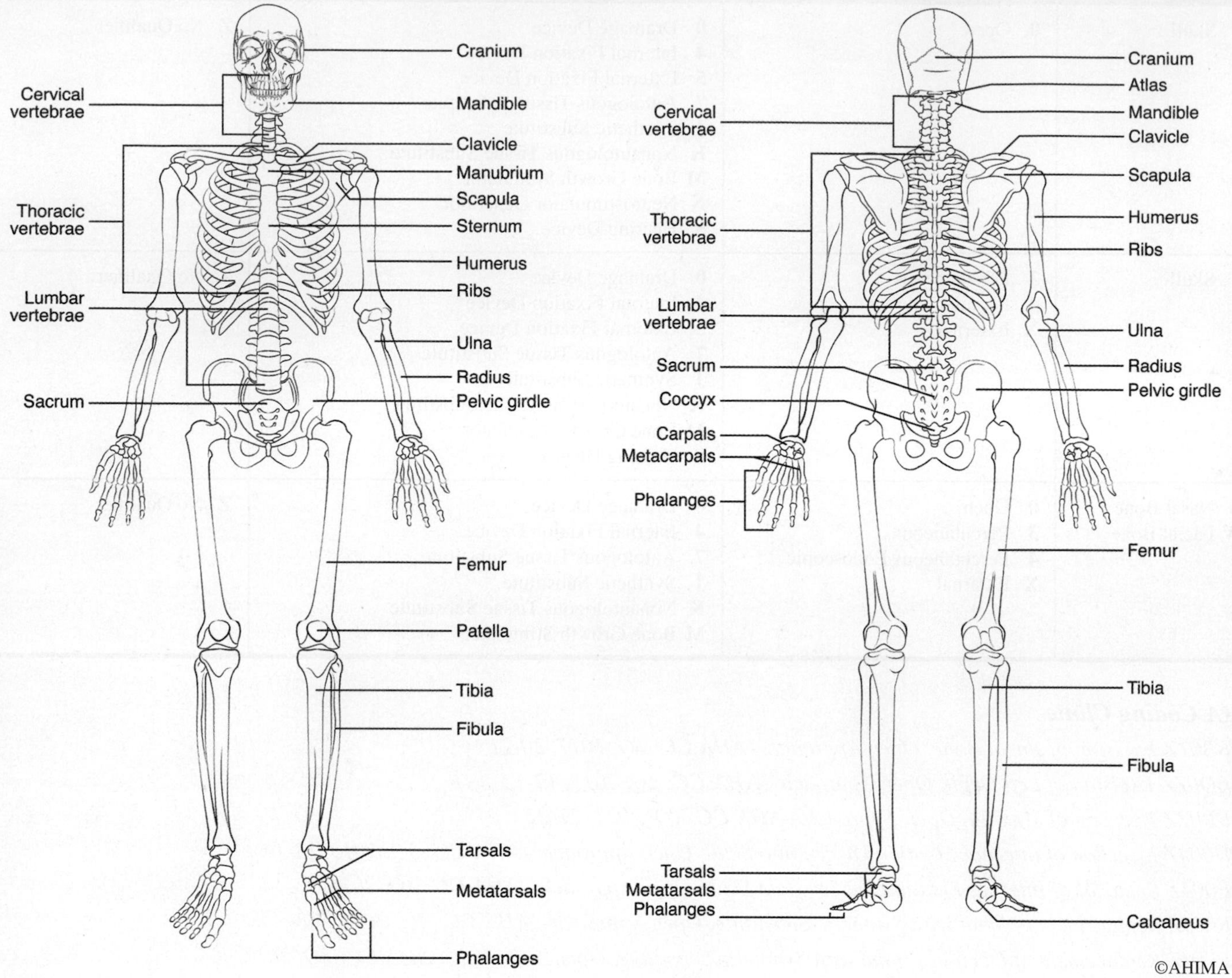

Vertebral Column

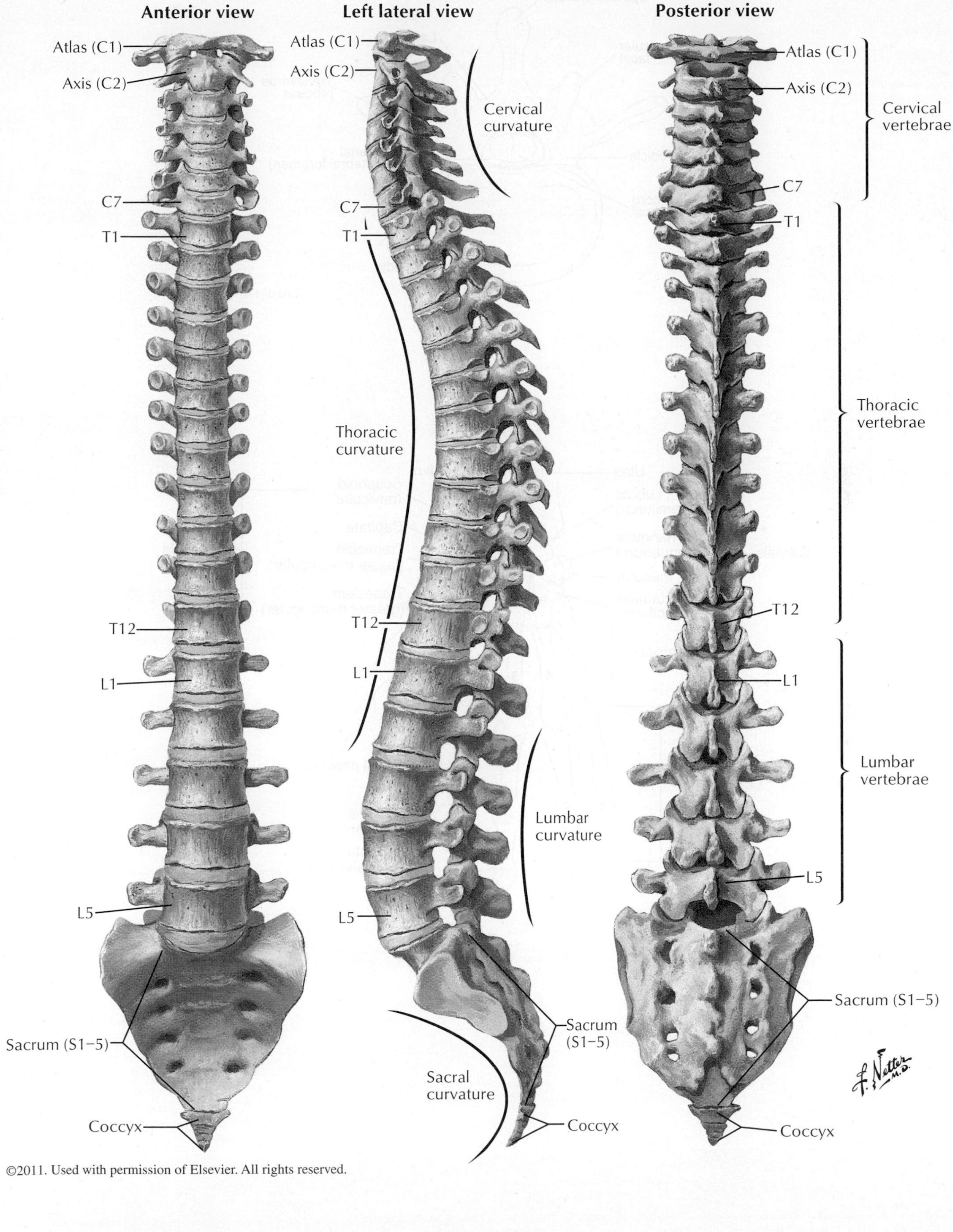
Anterior view
Left lateral view
Posterior view
Atlas (C1)
Axis (C2)
C7
T1
T12
L1
L5
Sacrum (S1–5)
Coccyx
Cervical curvature
Thoracic curvature
Lumbar curvature
Sacral curvature
Cervical vertebrae
Thoracic vertebrae
Lumbar vertebrae
F. Netter M.D.

Cross-section Spine

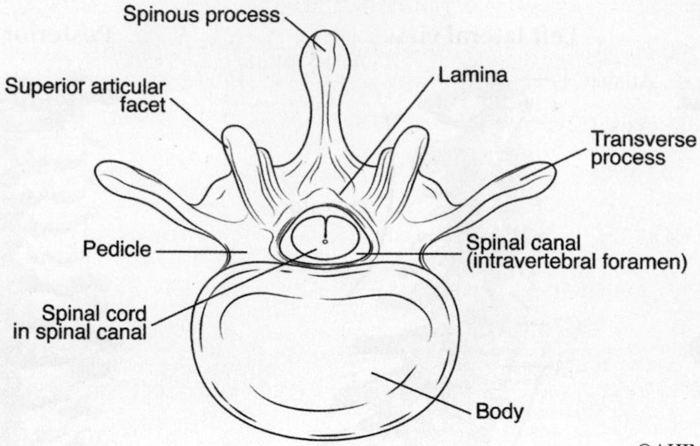
Spinous process
Superior articular facet
Lamina
Transverse process
Pedicle
Spinal canal (intravertebral foramen)
Spinal cord in spinal canal
Body

Hand Bones

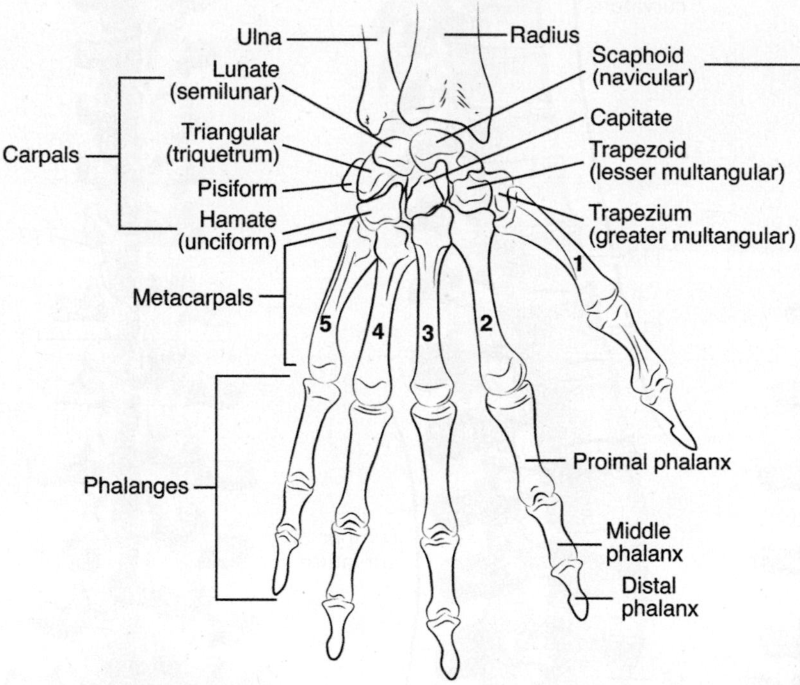
Ulna
Radius
Lunate (semilunar)
Scaphoid (navicular)
Carpals
Capitate
Triangular (triquetrum)
Trapezoid (lesser multangular)
Carpals
Pisiform
Hamate (unciform)
Trapezium (greater multangular)
1
Metacarpals
5
4
3
2
Phalanges
Proimal phalanx
Middle phalanx
Distal phalanx

Upper Bones Tables 0P2–0PW

Section 0 **Medical and Surgical**
Body System P **Upper Bones**
Operation 2 **Change:** Taking out or off a device from a body part and putting back an identical or similar device in or on the same body part without cutting or puncturing the skin or a mucous membrane

Body Part (4th)	Approach (5th)	Device (6th)	Qualifier (7th)
Y Upper Bone	**X** External	**0** Drainage Device **Y** Other Device	**Z** No Qualifier

Section 0 **Medical and Surgical**
Body System P **Upper Bones**
Operation 5 **Destruction:** Physical eradication of all or a portion of a body part by the direct use of energy, force, or a destructive agent

Body Part (4th)	Approach (5th)	Device (6th)	Qualifier (7th)
0 Sternum **1** Ribs, 1 to 2 **2** Ribs, 3 or More **3** Cervical Vertebra **4** Thoracic Vertebra **5** Scapula, Right **6** Scapula, Left **7** Glenoid Cavity, Right **8** Glenoid Cavity, Left **9** Clavicle, Right **B** Clavicle, Left **C** Humeral Head, Right **D** Humeral Head, Left **F** Humeral Shaft, Right **G** Humeral Shaft, Left **H** Radius, Right **J** Radius, Left **K** Ulna, Right **L** Ulna, Left **M** Carpal, Right **N** Carpal, Left **P** Metacarpal, Right **Q** Metacarpal, Left **R** Thumb Phalanx, Right **S** Thumb Phalanx, Left **T** Finger Phalanx, Right **V** Finger Phalanx, Left	**0** Open **3** Percutaneous **4** Percutaneous Endoscopic	**Z** No Device	**Z** No Qualifier

Section 0 **Medical and Surgical**
Body System P **Upper Bones**
Operation 8 **Division:** Cutting into a body part, without draining fluids and/or gases from the body part, in order to separate or transect a body part

Body Part (4th)	Approach (5th)	Device (6th)	Qualifier (7th)
0 Sternum **1** Ribs, 1 to 2 **2** Ribs, 3 or More **3** Cervical Vertebra **4** Thoracic Vertebra **5** Scapula, Right **6** Scapula, Left **7** Glenoid Cavity, Right **8** Glenoid Cavity, Left **9** Clavicle, Right **B** Clavicle, Left **C** Humeral Head, Right **D** Humeral Head, Left **F** Humeral Shaft, Right **G** Humeral Shaft, Left **H** Radius, Right **J** Radius, Left **K** Ulna, Right **L** Ulna, Left **M** Carpal, Right **N** Carpal, Left **P** Metacarpal, Right **Q** Metacarpal, Left **R** Thumb Phalanx, Right **S** Thumb Phalanx, Left **T** Finger Phalanx, Right **V** Finger Phalanx, Left	**0** Open **3** Percutaneous **4** Percutaneous Endoscopic	**Z** No Device	**Z** No Qualifier

Section 0 **Medical and Surgical**
Body System P **Upper Bones**
Operation 9 **Drainage:** Taking or letting out fluids and/or gases from a body part

Body Part (4th)	Approach (5th)	Device (6th)	Qualifier (7th)
0 Sternum **1** Ribs, 1 to 2 **2** Ribs, 3 or More **3** Cervical Vertebra **4** Thoracic Vertebra **5** Scapula, Right **6** Scapula, Left **7** Glenoid Cavity, Right **8** Glenoid Cavity, Left **9** Clavicle, Right **B** Clavicle, Left **C** Humeral Head, Right **D** Humeral Head, Left **F** Humeral Shaft, Right **G** Humeral Shaft, Left **H** Radius, Right **J** Radius, Left **K** Ulna, Right **L** Ulna, Left **M** Carpal, Right **N** Carpal, Left **P** Metacarpal, Right **Q** Metacarpal, Left **R** Thumb Phalanx, Right **S** Thumb Phalanx, Left **T** Finger Phalanx, Right **V** Finger Phalanx, Left	**0** Open **3** Percutaneous **4** Percutaneous Endoscopic	**0** Drainage Device	**Z** No Qualifier

Continued →

Section 0 **Medical and Surgical**
Body System P **Upper Bones**
Operation 9 **Drainage:** Taking or letting out fluids and/or gases from a body part

Body Part (4th)	Approach (5th)	Device (6th)	Qualifier (7th)
0 Sternum **1** Ribs, 1 to 2 **2** Ribs, 3 or More **3** Cervical Vertebra **4** Thoracic Vertebra **5** Scapula, Right **6** Scapula, Left **7** Glenoid Cavity, Right **8** Glenoid Cavity, Left **9** Clavicle, Right **B** Clavicle, Left **C** Humeral Head, Right **D** Humeral Head, Left **F** Humeral Shaft, Right **G** Humeral Shaft, Left **H** Radius, Right **J** Radius, Left **K** Ulna, Right **L** Ulna, Left **M** Carpal, Right **N** Carpal, Left **P** Metacarpal, Right **Q** Metacarpal, Left **R** Thumb Phalanx, Right **S** Thumb Phalanx, Left **T** Finger Phalanx, Right **V** Finger Phalanx, Left	**0** Open **3** Percutaneous **4** Percutaneous Endoscopic	**Z** No Device	**X** Diagnostic **Z** No Qualifier

Section 0 **Medical and Surgical**
Body System P **Upper Bones**
Operation B **Excision:** Cutting out or off, without replacement, a portion of a body part

Body Part (4th)	Approach (5th)	Device (6th)	Qualifier (7th)
0 Sternum **1** Ribs, 1 to 2 **2** Ribs, 3 or More **3** Cervical Vertebra **4** Thoracic Vertebra **5** Scapula, Right **6** Scapula, Left **7** Glenoid Cavity, Right **8** Glenoid Cavity, Left **9** Clavicle, Right **B** Clavicle, Left **C** Humeral Head, Right **D** Humeral Head, Left **F** Humeral Shaft, Right **G** Humeral Shaft, Left **H** Radius, Right **J** Radius, Left **K** Ulna, Right **L** Ulna, Left **M** Carpal, Right **N** Carpal, Left **P** Metacarpal, Right **Q** Metacarpal, Left **R** Thumb Phalanx, Right **S** Thumb Phalanx, Left **T** Finger Phalanx, Right **V** Finger Phalanx, Left	**0** Open **3** Percutaneous **4** Percutaneous Endoscopic	**Z** No Device	**X** Diagnostic **Z** No Qualifier

Section 0 **Medical and Surgical**
Body System P **Upper Bones**
Operation C **Extirpation:** Taking or cutting out solid matter from a body part

Body Part (4th)	Approach (5th)	Device (6th)	Qualifier (7th)
0 Sternum **1** Ribs, 1 to 2 **2** Ribs, 3 or More **3** Cervical Vertebra **4** Thoracic Vertebra **5** Scapula, Right **6** Scapula, Left **7** Glenoid Cavity, Right **8** Glenoid Cavity, Left **9** Clavicle, Right **B** Clavicle, Left **C** Humeral Head, Right **D** Humeral Head, Left **F** Humeral Shaft, Right **G** Humeral Shaft, Left **H** Radius, Right **J** Radius, Left **K** Ulna, Right **L** Ulna, Left **M** Carpal, Right **N** Carpal, Left **P** Metacarpal, Right **Q** Metacarpal, Left **R** Thumb Phalanx, Right **S** Thumb Phalanx, Left **T** Finger Phalanx, Right **V** Finger Phalanx, Left	**0** Open **3** Percutaneous **4** Percutaneous Endoscopic	**Z** No Device	**Z** No Qualifier

Section 0 **Medical and Surgical**
Body System P **Upper Bones**
Operation D **Extraction:** Pulling or stripping out or off all or a portion of a body part by the use of force

Body Part (4th)	Approach (5th)	Device (6th)	Qualifier (7th)
0 Sternum **1** Ribs, 1 to 2 **2** Ribs, 3 or More **3** Cervical Vertebra **4** Thoracic Vertebra **5** Scapula, Right **6** Scapula, Left **7** Glenoid Cavity, Right **8** Glenoid Cavity, Left **9** Clavical, Right **B** Clavical, Left **C** Humeral Head, Right **D** Humeral Head, Left **F** Humeral Shaft, Right **G** Humeral Shaft, Left **H** Radius, Right **J** Radius, Left **K** Ulna, Right **L** Ulna, Left **M** Carpal, Right **N** Carpal, Left **P** Metacarpal, Right **Q** Metacarpal, Left **R** Thumb Phalanx, Right **S** Thumb Phalanx, Left **T** Finger Phalanx, Right **V** Finger Phalanx, Left	**0** Open	**Z** No Device	**Z** No Qualifier

Section 0 **Medical and Surgical**
Body System P **Upper Bones**
Operation H **Insertion:** Putting in a nonbiological appliance that monitors, assists, performs, or prevents a physiological function but does not physically take the place of a body part

Body Part (4th)	Approach (5th)	Device (6th)	Qualifier (7th)
0 Sternum	**0** Open **3** Percutaneous **4** Percutaneous Endoscopic	**0** Internal Fixation Device, Rigid Plate **4** Internal Fixation Device	**Z** No Qualifier
1 Ribs, 1 to 2 **2** Ribs, 3 or More **3** Cervical Vertebra **4** Thoracic Vertebra **5** Scapula, Right **6** Scapula, Left **7** Glenoid Cavity, Right **8** Glenoid Cavity, Left **9** Clavicle, Right **B** Clavicle, Left	**0** Open **3** Percutaneous **4** Percutaneous Endoscopic	**4** Internal Fixation Device	**Z** No Qualifier
C Humeral Head, Right **D** Humeral Head, Left **H** Radius, Right **J** Radius, Left **K** Ulna, Right **L** Ulna, Left	**0** Open **3** Percutaneous **4** Percutaneous Endoscopic	**4** Internal Fixation Device **5** External Fixation Device **6** Internal Fixation Device, Intramedullary **8** External Fixation Device, Limb Lengthening **B** External Fixation Device, Monoplanar **C** External Fixation Device, Ring **D** External Fixation Device, Hybrid	**Z** No Qualifier
F Humeral Shaft, Right **G** Humeral Shaft, Left	**0** Open **3** Percutaneous **4** Percutaneous Endoscopic	**4** Internal Fixation Device **5** External Fixation Device **6** Internal Fixation Device, Intramedullary **7** Internal Fixation Device, Intramedullary Limb Lengthening **8** External Fixation Device, Limb Lengthening **B** External Fixation Device, Monoplanar **C** External Fixation Device, Ring **D** External Fixation Device, Hybrid	**Z** No Qualifier
M Carpal, Right **N** Carpal, Left **P** Metacarpal, Right **Q** Metacarpal, Left **R** Thumb Phalanx, Right **S** Thumb Phalanx, Left **T** Finger Phalanx, Right **V** Finger Phalanx, Left	**0** Open **3** Percutaneous **4** Percutaneous Endoscopic	**4** Internal Fixation Device **5** External Fixation Device	**Z** No Qualifier
Y Upper Bone	**0** Open **3** Percutaneous **4** Percutaneous Endoscopic	**M** Bone Growth Stimulator	**Z** No Qualifier

Section 0 **Medical and Surgical**
Body System P **Upper Bones**
Operation J **Inspection:** Visually and/or manually exploring a body part

Body Part (4th)	Approach (5th)	Device (6th)	Qualifier (7th)
Y Upper Bone	**0** Open **3** Percutaneous **4** Percutaneous Endoscopic **X** External	**Z** No Device	**Z** No Qualifier

Section 0 **Medical and Surgical**
Body System P **Upper Bones**
Operation N **Release:** Freeing a body part from an abnormal physical constraint by cutting or by the use of force

Body Part (4th)	Approach (5th)	Device (6th)	Qualifier (7th)
0 Sternum **1** Ribs, 1 to 2 **2** Ribs, 3 or More **3** Cervical Vertebra **4** Thoracic Vertebra **5** Scapula, Right **6** Scapula, Left **7** Glenoid Cavity, Right **8** Glenoid Cavity, Left **9** Clavicle, Right **B** Clavicle, Left **C** Humeral Head, Right **D** Humeral Head, Left **F** Humeral Shaft, Right **G** Humeral Shaft, Left **H** Radius, Right **J** Radius, Left **K** Ulna, Right **L** Ulna, Left **M** Carpal, Right **N** Carpal, Left **P** Metacarpal, Right **Q** Metacarpal, Left **R** Thumb Phalanx, Right **S** Thumb Phalanx, Left **T** Finger Phalanx, Right **V** Finger Phalanx, Left	**0** Open **3** Percutaneous **4** Percutaneous Endoscopic	**Z** No Device	**Z** No Qualifier

Section 0 **Medical and Surgical**
Body System P **Upper Bones**
Operation P **Removal:** Taking out or off a device from a body part

Body Part (4th)	Approach (5th)	Device (6th)	Qualifier (7th)
0 Sternum **1** Ribs, 1 to 2 **2** Ribs, 3 or More **3** Cervical Vertebra **4** Thoracic Vertebra **5** Scapula, Right **6** Scapula, Left **7** Glenoid Cavity, Right **8** Glenoid Cavity, Left **9** Clavicle, Right **B** Clavicle, Left	**0** Open **3** Percutaneous **4** Percutaneous Endoscopic	**4** Internal Fixation Device **7** Autologous Tissue Substitute **J** Synthetic Substitute **K** Nonautologous Tissue Substitute	**Z** No Qualifier
0 Sternum **1** Ribs, 1 to 2 **2** Ribs, 3 or More **3** Cervical Vertebra **4** Thoracic Vertebra **5** Scapula, Right **6** Scapula, Left **7** Glenoid Cavity, Right **8** Glenoid Cavity, Left **9** Clavicle, Right **B** Clavicle, Left	**X** External	**4** Internal Fixation Device	**Z** No Qualifier

Continued →

Section **0** **Medical and Surgical**
Body System **P** **Upper Bones**
Operation **P** **Removal:** Taking out or off a device from a body part

Body Part (4th)	Approach (5th)	Device (6th)	Qualifier (7th)
C Humeral Head, Right **D** Humeral Head, Left **F** Humeral Shaft, Right **G** Humeral Shaft, Left **H** Radius, Right **J** Radius, Left **K** Ulna, Right **L** Ulna, Left **M** Carpal, Right **N** Carpal, Left **P** Metacarpal, Right **Q** Metacarpal, Left **R** Thumb Phalanx, Right **S** Thumb Phalanx, Left **T** Finger Phalanx, Right **V** Finger Phalanx, Left	**0** Open **3** Percutaneous **4** Percutaneous Endoscopic	**4** Internal Fixation Device **5** External Fixation Device **7** Autologous Tissue Substitute **J** Synthetic Substitute **K** Nonautologous Tissue Substitute	**Z** No Qualifier
C Humeral Head, Right **D** Humeral Head, Left **F** Humeral Shaft, Right **G** Humeral Shaft, Left **H** Radius, Right **J** Radius, Left **K** Ulna, Right **L** Ulna, Left **M** Carpal, Right **N** Carpal, Left **P** Metacarpal, Right **Q** Metacarpal, Left **R** Thumb Phalanx, Right **S** Thumb Phalanx, Left **T** Finger Phalanx, Right **V** Finger Phalanx, Left	**X** External	**4** Internal Fixation Device **5** External Fixation Device	**Z** No Qualifier
Y Upper Bone	**0** Open **3** Percutaneous **4** Percutaneous Endoscopic **X** External	**0** Drainage Device **M** Bone Growth Stimulator	**Z** No Qualifier

Section 0 **Medical and Surgical**
Body System P **Upper Bones**
Operation Q **Repair:** Restoring, to the extent possible, a body part to its normal anatomic structure and function

Body Part (4th)	Approach (5th)	Device (6th)	Qualifier (7th)
0 Sternum **1** Ribs, 1 to 2 **2** Ribs, 3 or More **3** Cervical Vertebra **4** Thoracic Vertebra **5** Scapula, Right **6** Scapula, Left **7** Glenoid Cavity, Right **8** Glenoid Cavity, Left **9** Clavicle, Right **B** Clavicle, Left **C** Humeral Head, Right **D** Humeral Head, Left **F** Humeral Shaft, Right **G** Humeral Shaft, Left **H** Radius, Right **J** Radius, Left **K** Ulna, Right **L** Ulna, Left **M** Carpal, Right **N** Carpal, Left **P** Metacarpal, Right **Q** Metacarpal, Left **R** Thumb Phalanx, Right **S** Thumb Phalanx, Left **T** Finger Phalanx, Right **V** Finger Phalanx, Left	**0** Open **3** Percutaneous **4** Percutaneous Endoscopic **X** External	**Z** No Device	**Z** No Qualifier

Section 0 **Medical and Surgical**
Body System P **Upper Bones**
Operation R **Replacement:** Putting in or on biological or synthetic material that physically takes the place and/or function of all or a portion of a body part

Body Part (4th)	Approach (5th)	Device (6th)	Qualifier (7th)
0 Sternum **1** Ribs, 1 to 2 **2** Ribs, 3 or More **3** Cervical Vertebra **4** Thoracic Vertebra **5** Scapula, Right **6** Scapula, Left **7** Glenoid Cavity, Right **8** Glenoid Cavity, Left **9** Clavicle, Right **B** Clavicle, Left **C** Humeral Head, Right **D** Humeral Head, Left **F** Humeral Shaft, Right **G** Humeral Shaft, Left **H** Radius, Right **J** Radius, Left **K** Ulna, Right **L** Ulna, Left **M** Carpal, Right **N** Carpal, Left **P** Metacarpal, Right **Q** Metacarpal, Left **R** Thumb Phalanx, Right **S** Thumb Phalanx, Left **T** Finger Phalanx, Right **V** Finger Phalanx, Left	**0** Open **3** Percutaneous **4** Percutaneous Endoscopic	**7** Autologous Tissue Substitute **J** Synthetic Substitute **K** Nonautologous Tissue Substitute	**Z** No Qualifier

Section 0 **Medical and Surgical**
Body System P **Upper Bones**
Operation S **Reposition:** Moving to its normal location, or other suitable location, all or a portion of a body part

Body Part (4th)	Approach (5th)	Device (6th)	Qualifier (7th)
0 Sternum	**0** Open **3** Percutaneous **4** Percutaneous Endoscopic	**0** Internal Fixation Device, Rigid Plate **4** Internal Fixation Device **Z** No Device	**Z** No Qualifier
0 Sternum	**X** External	**Z** No Device	**Z** No Qualifier
1 Ribs, 1 to 2 **2** Ribs, 3 or More **3** Cervical Vertebra **5** Scapula, Right **6** Scapula, Left **7** Glenoid Cavity, Right **8** Glenoid Cavity, Left **9** Clavicle, Right **B** Clavicle, Left	**0** Open **3** Percutaneous **4** Percutaneous Endoscopic	**4** Internal Fixation Device **Z** No Device	**Z** No Qualifier
1 Ribs, 1 to 2 **2** Ribs, 3 or More **3** Cervical Vertebra **5** Scapula, Right **6** Scapula, Left **7** Glenoid Cavity, Right **8** Glenoid Cavity, Left **9** Clavicle, Right **B** Clavicle, Left	**X** External	**Z** No Device	**Z** No Qualifier
4 Thoracic Vertebra	**0** Open **4** Percutaneous Endoscopic	**3** Spinal Stabilization Device, Vertebral Body Tether **4** Internal Fixation Device **Z** No Device	**Z** No Qualifier
4 Thoracic Vertebra	**3** Percutaneous	**4** Internal Fixation Device **Z** No Device	**Z** No Qualifier
4 Thoracic Vertebra	**X** External	**Z** No Device	**Z** No Qualifier
C Humeral Head, Right **D** Humeral Head, Left **F** Humeral Shaft, Right **G** Humeral Shaft, Left **H** Radius, Right **J** Radius, Left **K** Ulna, Right **L** Ulna, Left	**0** Open **3** Percutaneous **4** Percutaneous Endoscopic	**4** Internal Fixation Device **5** External Fixation Device **6** Internal Fixation Device, Intramedullary **B** External Fixation Device, Monoplanar **C** External Fixation Device, Ring **D** External Fixation Device, Hybrid **Z** No Device	**Z** No Qualifier
C Humeral Head, Right **D** Humeral Head, Left **F** Humeral Shaft, Right **G** Humeral Shaft, Left **H** Radius, Right **J** Radius, Left **K** Ulna, Right **L** Ulna, Left	**X** External	**Z** No Device	**Z** No Qualifier
M Carpal, Right **N** Carpal, Left **P** Metacarpal, Right **Q** Metacarpal, Left **R** Thumb Phalanx, Right **S** Thumb Phalanx, Left **T** Finger Phalanx, Right **V** Finger Phalanx, Left	**0** Open **3** Percutaneous **4** Percutaneous Endoscopic	**4** Internal Fixation Device **5** External Fixation Device **Z** No Device	**Z** No Qualifier

Continued →

Section 0 Medical and Surgical
Body System P Upper Bones
Operation S **Reposition:** Moving to its normal location, or other suitable location, all or a portion of a body part

Body Part (4th)	Approach (5th)	Device (6th)	Qualifier (7th)
M Carpal, Right **N** Carpal, Left **P** Metacarpal, Right **Q** Metacarpal, Left **R** Thumb Phalanx, Right **S** Thumb Phalanx, Left **T** Finger Phalanx, Right **V** Finger Phalanx, Left	**X** External	**Z** No Device	**Z** No Qualifier

Section 0 Medical and Surgical
Body System P Upper Bones
Operation T **Resection:** Cutting out or off, without replacement, all of a body part

Body Part (4th)	Approach (5th)	Device (6th)	Qualifier (7th)
0 Sternum **1** Ribs, 1 to 2 **2** Ribs, 3 or More **5** Scapula, Right **6** Scapula, Left **7** Glenoid Cavity, Right **8** Glenoid Cavity, Left **9** Clavicle, Right **B** Clavicle, Left **C** Humeral Head, Right **D** Humeral Head, Left **F** Humeral Shaft, Right **G** Humeral Shaft, Left **H** Radius, Right **J** Radius, Left **K** Ulna, Right **L** Ulna, Left **M** Carpal, Right **N** Carpal, Left **P** Metacarpal, Right **Q** Metacarpal, Left **R** Thumb Phalanx, Right **S** Thumb Phalanx, Left **T** Finger Phalanx, Right **V** Finger Phalanx, Left	**0** Open	**Z** No Device	**Z** No Qualifier

Section 0 **Medical and Surgical**
Body System P **Upper Bones**
Operation U **Supplement:** Putting in or on biological or synthetic material that physically reinforces and/or augments the function of a portion of a body part

Body Part (4th)	Approach (5th)	Device (6th)	Qualifier (7th)
0 Sternum **1** Ribs, 1 to 2 **2** Ribs, 3 or More **3** Cervical Vertebra **4** Thoracic Vertebra **5** Scapula, Right **6** Scapula, Left **7** Glenoid Cavity, Right **8** Glenoid Cavity, Left **9** Clavicle, Right **B** Clavicle, Left **C** Humeral Head, Right **D** Humeral Head, Left **F** Humeral Shaft, Right **G** Humeral Shaft, Left **H** Radius, Right **J** Radius, Left **K** Ulna, Right **L** Ulna, Left **M** Carpal, Right **N** Carpal, Left **P** Metacarpal, Right **Q** Metacarpal, Left **R** Thumb Phalanx, Right **S** Thumb Phalanx, Left **T** Finger Phalanx, Right **V** Finger Phalanx, Left	**0** Open **3** Percutaneous **4** Percutaneous Endoscopic	**7** Autologous Tissue Substitute **J** Synthetic Substitute **K** Nonautologous Tissue Substitute	**Z** No Qualifier

Section 0 **Medical and Surgical**
Body System P **Upper Bones**
Operation W **Revision:** Correcting, to the extent possible, a portion of a malfunctioning device or the position of a displaced device

Body Part (4th)	Approach (5th)	Device (6th)	Qualifier (7th)
0 Sternum **1** Ribs, 1 to 2 **2** Ribs, 3 or More **3** Cervical Vertebra **4** Thoracic Vertebra **5** Scapula, Right **6** Scapula, Left **7** Glenoid Cavity, Right **8** Glenoid Cavity, Left **9** Clavicle, Right **B** Clavicle, Left	**0** Open **3** Percutaneous **4** Percutaneous Endoscopic **X** External	**4** Internal Fixation Device **7** Autologous Tissue Substitute **J** Synthetic Substitute **K** Nonautologous Tissue Substitute	**Z** No Qualifier

Continued →

Body Part (4th)	Approach (5th)	Device (6th)	Qualifier (7th)
C Humeral Head, Right **D** Humeral Head, Left **F** Humeral Shaft, Right **G** Humeral Shaft, Left **H** Radius, Right **J** Radius, Left **K** Ulna, Right **L** Ulna, Left **M** Carpal, Right **N** Carpal, Left **P** Metacarpal, Right **Q** Metacarpal, Left **R** Thumb Phalanx, Right **S** Thumb Phalanx, Left **T** Finger Phalanx, Right **V** Finger Phalanx, Left	**0** Open **3** Percutaneous **4** Percutaneous Endoscopic **X** External	**4** Internal Fixation Device **5** External Fixation Device **7** Autologous Tissue Substitute **J** Synthetic Substitute **K** Nonautologous Tissue Substitute	**Z** No Qualifier
Y Upper Bone	**0** Open **3** Percutaneous **4** Percutaneous Endoscopic **X** External	**0** Drainage Device **M** Bone Growth Stimulator	**Z** No Qualifier

AHA Coding Clinic

0PB10ZZ Excision of 1 to 2 Ribs, Open Approach—AHA CC: 4Q, 2012, 101-102; 4Q, 2013, 109-111
0PB20ZZ Excision of 3 or More Ribs, Open Approach—AHA CC: 4Q, 2013, 109-111
0PB54ZZ Excision of Right Scapula, Percutaneous Endoscopic Approach—AHA CC: 3Q, 2013, 20-22
0PC00ZZ Extirpation of Matter from Sternum, Open Approach—AHA CC: 3Q, 2019, 19
0PH000Z Insertion of Rigid Plate Internal Fixation Device into Sternum, Open Approach—AHA CC: 1Q, 2020, 29-30
0PH304Z Insertion of Internal Fixation Device into Cervical Vertebra, Open Approach—AHA CC: 2Q, 2017, 23-24; 2Q, 2019, 40
0PH404Z Insertion of Internal Fixation Device into Thoracic Vertebra, Open Approach—AHA CC: 4Q, 2014, 28-29
0PH504Z Insertion of Internal Fixation Device into Right Scapula, Open Approach—AHA CC: 4Q, 2018, 12-13
0PP404Z Removal of Internal Fixation Device from Thoracic Vertebra, Open Approach—AHA CC: 4Q, 2014, 28-29
0PRH0JZ Replacement of Right Radius with Synthetic Substitute, Open Approach—AHA CC: 4Q, 2018, 92-93
0PS00ZZ Reposition Sternum, Open Approach—AHA CC: 4Q, 2015, 34
0PS204Z Reposition 3 or More Ribs with Internal Fixation Device, Open Approach—AHA CC: 4Q, 2014, 26; 4Q, 2017, 53
0PS3XZZ Reposition Cervical Vertebra, External Approach—AHA CC: 2Q, 2015, 35
0PS404Z Reposition Thoracic Vertebra with Internal Fixation Device, Open Approach—AHA CC: 1Q, 2020, 33-34
0PS444Z Reposition Thoracic Vertebra with Internal Fixation Device, Percutaneous Endoscopic Approach—AHA CC: 3Q, 2018, 26-27
0PS4XZZ Reposition Thoracic Vertebra, External Approach—AHA CC: 1Q, 2016, 21
0PSJ04Z Reposition Left Radius with Internal Fixation Device, Open Approach—AHA CC: 3Q, 2014, 33-34; 4Q, 2014, 32-33
0PSL04Z Reposition Left Ulna with Internal Fixation Device, Open Approach—AHA CC: 4Q, 2014, 32-33
0PTN0ZZ Resection of Left Carpal, Open Approach—AHA CC: 3Q, 2015, 26-27
0PU00JZ Supplement Sternum with Synthetic Substitute, Open Approach—AHA CC: 4Q, 2013, 109-111
0PU30KZ Supplement Cervical Vertebra with Nonautologous Tissue Substitute, Open Approach—AHA CC: 2Q, 2015, 20-21
0PU507Z Supplement Right Scapula with Autologous Tissue Substitute, Open Approach—AHA CC: 4Q, 2018, 12-13
0PU50KZ Supplement Right Scapula with Nonautologous Tissue Substitute, Open Approach—AHA CC: 4Q, 2018, 12-13
0PW104Z Revision of Internal Fixation Device in 1 to 2 Ribs, Open Approach—AHA CC: 4Q, 2014, 26-27
0PW204Z Revision of Internal Fixation Device in 3 or More Ribs, Open Approach—AHA CC: 4Q, 2014, 26-27
0PW404Z Revision of Internal Fixation Device in Thoracic Vertebra, Open Approach—AHA CC: 4Q, 2014, 27-28

Bones - Front and Back Views

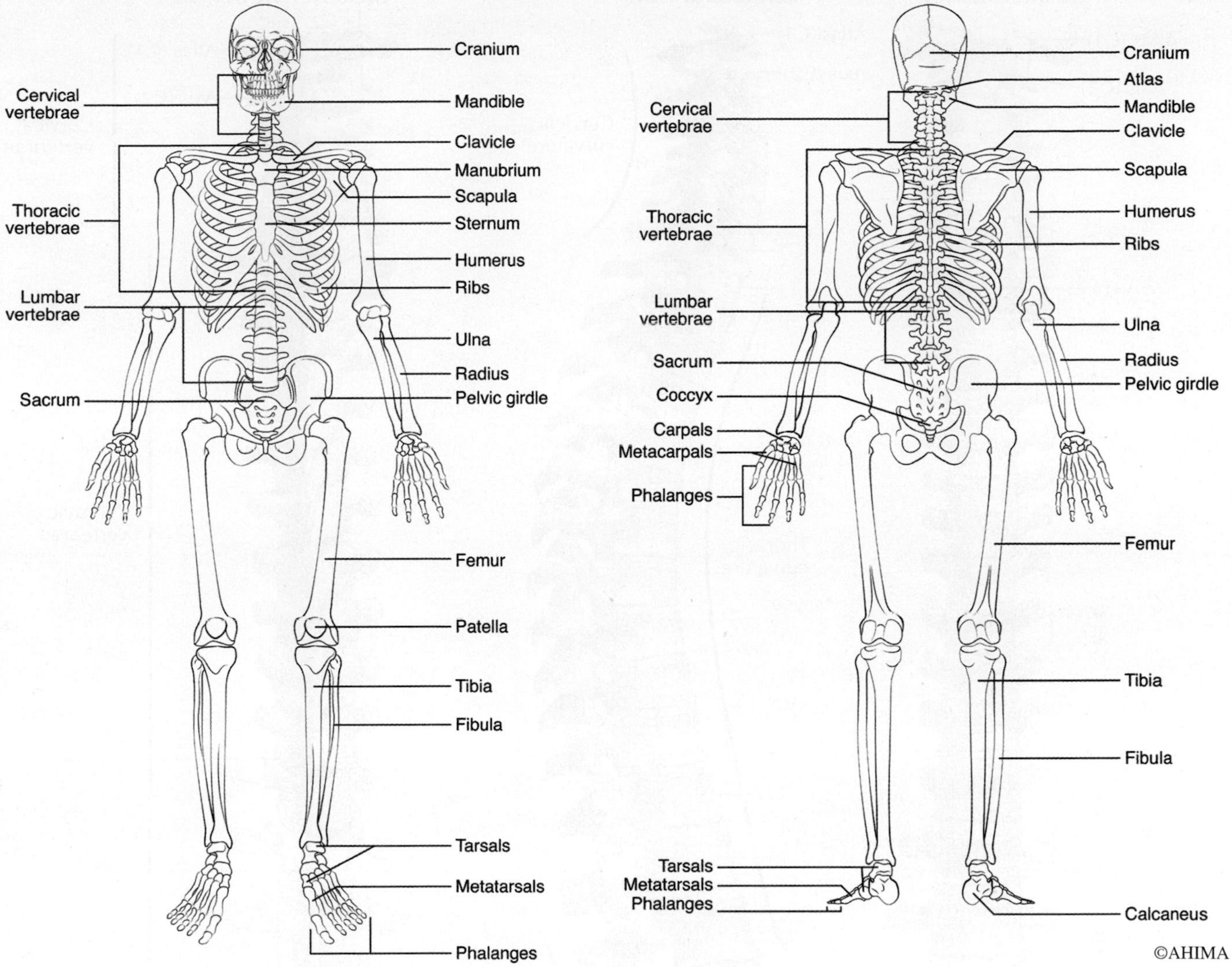
Cranium
Cervical vertebrae
Mandible
Clavicle
Thoracic vertebrae
Manubrium
Scapula
Sternum
Humerus
Lumbar vertebrae
Ribs
Ulna
Radius
Sacrum
Pelvic girdle
Femur
Patella
Tibia
Fibula
Tarsals
Metatarsals
Phalanges
Cranium
Atlas
Cervical vertebrae
Mandible
Clavicle
Scapula
Thoracic vertebrae
Humerus
Ribs
Lumbar vertebrae
Ulna
Sacrum
Radius
Pelvic girdle
Coccyx
Carpals
Metacarpals
Phalanges
Femur
Tibia
Fibula
Tarsals
Metatarsals
Phalanges
Calcaneus

Vertebral Column

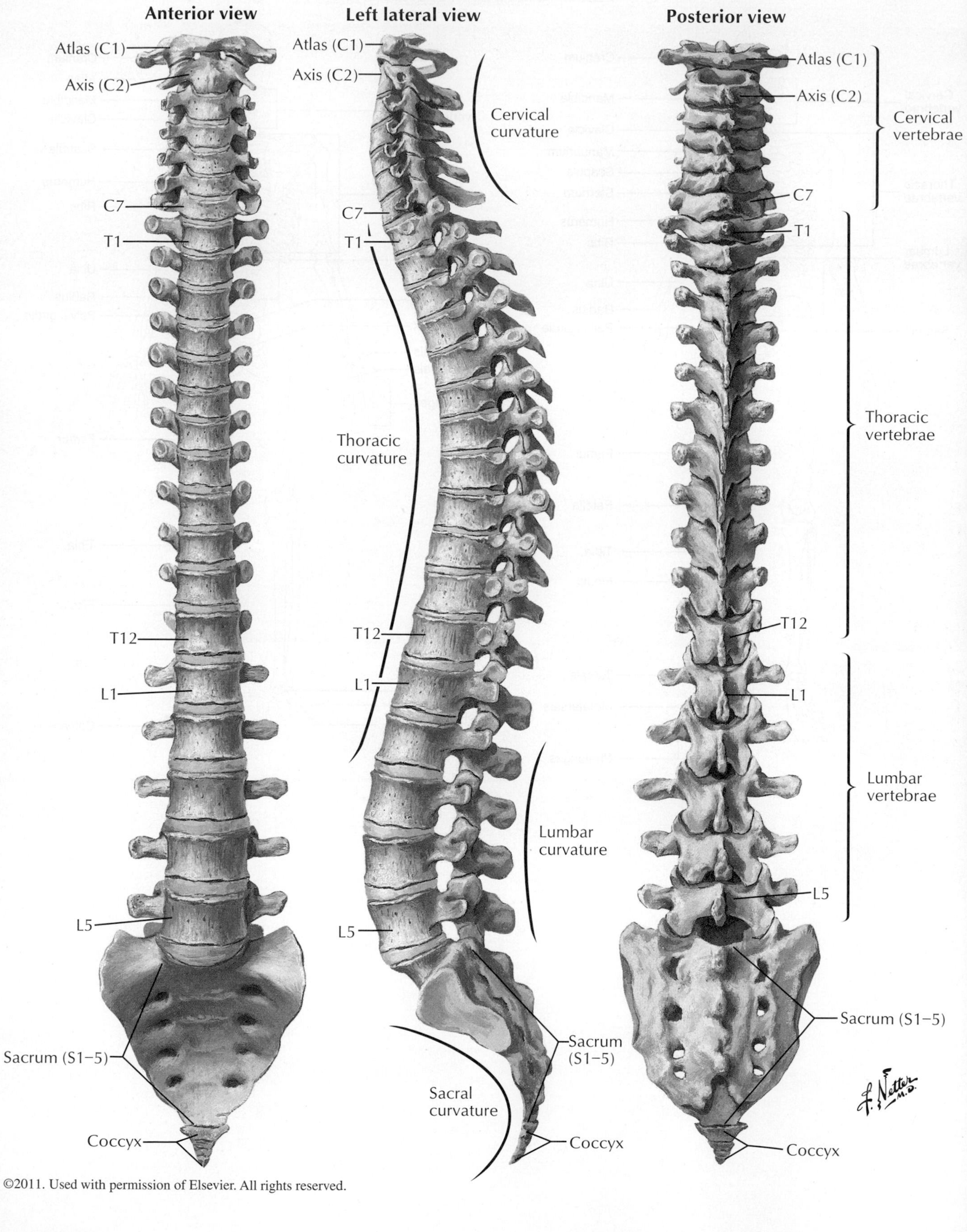

Anterior view
Atlas (C1)
Axis (C2)
C7
T1
T12
L1
L5
Sacrum (S1–5)
Coccyx
Left lateral view
Atlas (C1)
Axis (C2)
Cervical curvature
C7
T1
Thoracic curvature
T12
L1
Lumbar curvature
L5
Sacrum (S1–5)
Sacral curvature
Coccyx
Posterior view
Atlas (C1)
Axis (C2)
Cervical vertebrae
C7
T1
Thoracic vertebrae
T12
L1
Lumbar vertebrae
L5
Sacrum (S1–5)
Coccyx
F. Netter M.D.

Lower Bones Tables 0Q2–0QW

Section 0 **Medical and Surgical**
Body System Q **Lower Bones**
Operation 2 **Change:** Taking out or off a device from a body part and putting back an identical or similar device in or on the same body part without cutting or puncturing the skin or a mucous membrane

Body Part (4th)	Approach (5th)	Device (6th)	Qualifier (7th)
Y Lower Bone	**X** External	**0** Drainage Device **Y** Other Device	**Z** No Qualifier

Section 0 **Medical and Surgical**
Body System Q **Lower Bones**
Operation 5 **Destruction:** Physical eradication of all or a portion of a body part by the direct use of energy, force, or a destructive agent

Body Part (4th)	Approach (5th)	Device (6th)	Qualifier (7th)
0 Lumbar Vertebra **1** Sacrum **2** Pelvic Bone, Right **3** Pelvic Bone, Left **4** Acetabulum, Right **5** Acetabulum, Left **6** Upper Femur, Right **7** Upper Femur, Left **8** Femoral Shaft, Right **9** Femoral Shaft, Left **B** Lower Femur, Right **C** Lower Femur, Left **D** Patella, Right **F** Patella, Left **G** Tibia, Right **H** Tibia, Left **J** Fibula, Right **K** Fibula, Left **L** Tarsal, Right **M** Tarsal, Left **N** Metatarsal, Right **P** Metatarsal, Left **Q** Toe Phalanx, Right **R** Toe Phalanx, Left **S** Coccyx	**0** Open **3** Percutaneous **4** Percutaneous Endoscopic	**Z** No Device	**Z** No Qualifier

Section 0 **Medical and Surgical**
Body System Q **Lower Bones**
Operation 8 **Division:** Cutting into a body part, without draining fluids and/or gases from the body part, in order to separate or transect a body part

Body Part (4th)	Approach (5th)	Device (6th)	Qualifier (7th)
0 Lumbar Vertebra **1** Sacrum **2** Pelvic Bone, Right **3** Pelvic Bone, Left **4** Acetabulum, Right **5** Acetabulum, Left **6** Upper Femur, Right **7** Upper Femur, Left **8** Femoral Shaft, Right **9** Femoral Shaft, Left **B** Lower Femur, Right **C** Lower Femur, Left **D** Patella, Right **F** Patella, Left **G** Tibia, Right **H** Tibia, Left **J** Fibula, Right **K** Fibula, Left **L** Tarsal, Right **M** Tarsal, Left **N** Metatarsal, Right **P** Metatarsal, Left **Q** Toe Phalanx, Right **R** Toe Phalanx, Left **S** Coccyx	**0** Open **3** Percutaneous **4** Percutaneous Endoscopic	**Z** No Device	**Z** No Qualifier

Section 0 **Medical and Surgical**
Body System Q **Lower Bones**
Operation 9 **Drainage:** Taking or letting out fluids and/or gases from a body part

Body Part (4th)	Approach (5th)	Device (6th)	Qualifier (7th)
0 Lumbar Vertebra **1** Sacrum **2** Pelvic Bone, Right **3** Pelvic Bone, Left **4** Acetabulum, Right **5** Acetabulum, Left **6** Upper Femur, Right **7** Upper Femur, Left **8** Femoral Shaft, Right **9** Femoral Shaft, Left **B** Lower Femur, Right **C** Lower Femur, Left **D** Patella, Right **F** Patella, Left **G** Tibia, Right **H** Tibia, Left **J** Fibula, Right **K** Fibula, Left **L** Tarsal, Right **M** Tarsal, Left **N** Metatarsal, Right **P** Metatarsal, Left **Q** Toe Phalanx, Right **R** Toe Phalanx, Left **S** Coccyx	**0** Open **3** Percutaneous **4** Percutaneous Endoscopic	**0** Drainage Device	**Z** No Qualifier

Continued →

Section 0 **Medical and Surgical**
Body System Q **Lower Bones**
Operation 9 **Drainage:** Taking or letting out fluids and/or gases from a body part

Body Part (4th)	Approach (5th)	Device (6th)	Qualifier (7th)
0 Lumbar Vertebra **1** Sacrum **2** Pelvic Bone, Right **3** Pelvic Bone, Left **4** Acetabulum, Right **5** Acetabulum, Left **6** Upper Femur, Right **7** Upper Femur, Left **8** Femoral Shaft, Right **9** Femoral Shaft, Left **B** Lower Femur, Right **C** Lower Femur, Left **D** Patella, Right **F** Patella, Left **G** Tibia, Right **H** Tibia, Left **J** Fibula, Right **K** Fibula, Left **L** Tarsal, Right **M** Tarsal, Left **N** Metatarsal, Right **P** Metatarsal, Left **Q** Toe Phalanx, Right **R** Toe Phalanx, Left **S** Coccyx	**0** Open **3** Percutaneous **4** Percutaneous Endoscopic	**Z** No Device	**X** Diagnostic **Z** No Qualifier

Section 0 **Medical and Surgical**
Body System Q **Lower Bones**
Operation B **Excision:** Cutting out or off, without replacement, a portion of a body part

Body Part (4th)	Approach (5th)	Device (6th)	Qualifier (7th)
0 Lumbar Vertebra **1** Sacrum **2** Pelvic Bone, Right **3** Pelvic Bone, Left **4** Acetabulum, Right **5** Acetabulum, Left **6** Upper Femur, Right **7** Upper Femur, Left **8** Femoral Shaft, Right **9** Femoral Shaft, Left **B** Lower Femur, Right **C** Lower Femur, Left **D** Patella, Right **F** Patella, Left **G** Tibia, Right **H** Tibia, Left **J** Fibula, Right **K** Fibula, Left **L** Tarsal, Right **M** Tarsal, Left **Q** Toe Phalanx, Right **R** Toe Phalanx, Left **S** Coccyx	**0** Open **3** Percutaneous **4** Percutaneous Endoscopic	**Z** No Device	**X** Diagnostic **Z** No Qualifier
N Metatarsal, Right **P** Metatarsal, Left	**0** Open **3** Percutaneous **4** Percutaneous Endoscopic	**Z** No Device	**2** Sesamoid Bone(s) 1st Toe **X** Diagnostic **Z** No Qualifier

Section 0 **Medical and Surgical**
Body System Q **Lower Bones**
Operation C **Extirpation:** Taking or cutting out solid matter from a body part

Body Part (4th)	Approach (5th)	Device (6th)	Qualifier (7th)
0 Lumbar Vertebra **1** Sacrum **2** Pelvic Bone, Right **3** Pelvic Bone, Left **4** Acetabulum, Right **5** Acetabulum, Left **6** Upper Femur, Right **7** Upper Femur, Left **8** Femoral Shaft, Right **9** Femoral Shaft, Left **B** Lower Femur, Right **C** Lower Femur, Left **D** Patella, Right **F** Patella, Left **G** Tibia, Right **H** Tibia, Left **J** Fibula, Right **K** Fibula, Left **L** Tarsal, Right **M** Tarsal, Left **N** Metatarsal, Right **P** Metatarsal, Left **Q** Toe Phalanx, Right **R** Toe Phalanx, Left **S** Coccyx	**0** Open **3** Percutaneous **4** Percutaneous Endoscopic	**Z** No Device	**Z** No Qualifier

Section 0 **Medical and Surgical**
Body System Q **Lower Bones**
Operation D **Extraction:** Pulling or stripping out or off all or a portion of a body part by the use of force

Body Part (4th)	Approach (5th)	Device (6th)	Qualifier (7th)
0 Lumbar Vertebra **1** Sacrum **2** Pelvic Bone, Right **3** Pelvic Bone, Left **4** Acetabulum, Right **5** Acetabulum, Left **6** Upper Femur, Right **7** Upper Femur, Left **8** Femoral Shaft, Right **9** Femoral Shaft, Left **B** Lower Femur, Right **C** Lower Femur, Left **D** Patella, Right **F** Patella, Left **G** Tibia, Right **H** Tibia, Left **J** Fibula, Right **K** Fibula, Left **L** Tarsal, Right **M** Tarsal, Left **N** Metatarsal, Right **P** Metatarsal, Left **Q** Toe Phalanx, Right **R** Toe Phalanx, Left **S** Coccyx	**0** Open	**Z** No Device	**Z** No Qualifier

Section 0 **Medical and Surgical**
Body System Q **Lower Bones**
Operation H **Insertion:** Putting in a nonbiological appliance that monitors, assists, performs, or prevents a physiological function but does not physically take the place of a body part

Body Part (4th)	Approach (5th)	Device (6th)	Qualifier (7th)
0 Lumbar Vertebra **1** Sacrum **2** Pelvic Bone, Right **3** Pelvic Bone, Left **4** Acetabulum, Right **5** Acetabulum, Left **D** Patella, Right **F** Patella, Left **L** Tarsal, Right **M** Tarsal, Left **N** Metatarsal, Right **P** Metatarsal, Left **Q** Toe Phalanx, Right **R** Toe Phalanx, Left **S** Coccyx	**0** Open **3** Percutaneous **4** Percutaneous Endoscopic	**4** Internal Fixation Device **5** External Fixation Device	**Z** No Qualifier
6 Upper Femur, Right **7** Upper Femur, Left **B** Lower Femur, Right **C** Lower Femur, Left **J** Fibula, Right **K** Fibula, Left	**0** Open **3** Percutaneous **4** Percutaneous Endoscopic	**4** Internal Fixation Device **5** External Fixation Device **6** Internal Fixation Device, Intramedullary **8** External Fixation Device, Limb Lengthening **B** External Fixation Device, Monoplanar **C** External Fixation Device, Ring **D** External Fixation Device, Hybrid	**Z** No Qualifier
8 Femoral Shaft, Right **9** Femoral Shaft, Left **G** Tibia, Right **H** Tibia, Left	**0** Open **3** Percutaneous **4** Percutaneous Endoscopic	**4** Internal Fixation Device **5** External Fixation Device **6** Internal Fixation Device, Intramedullary **7** Internal Fixation Device, Intramedullary Limb Lengthening **8** External Fixation Device, Limb Lengthening **B** External Fixation Device, Monoplanar **C** External Fixation Device, Ring **D** External Fixation Device, Hybrid	**Z** No Qualifier
Y Lower Bone	**0** Open **3** Percutaneous **4** Percutaneous Endoscopic	**M** Bone Growth Stimulator	**Z** No Qualifier

Section 0 **Medical and Surgical**
Body System Q **Lower Bones**
Operation J **Inspection:** Visually and/or manually exploring a body part

Body Part (4th)	Approach (5th)	Device (6th)	Qualifier (7th)
Y Lower Bone	**0** Open **3** Percutaneous **4** Percutaneous Endoscopic **X** External	**Z** No Device	**Z** No Qualifier

Section 0 **Medical and Surgical**
Body System Q **Lower Bones**
Operation N **Release:** Freeing a body part from an abnormal physical constraint by cutting or by the use of force

Body Part (4th)	Approach (5th)	Device (6th)	Qualifier (7th)
0 Lumbar Vertebra **1** Sacrum **2** Pelvic Bone, Right **3** Pelvic Bone, Left **4** Acetabulum, Right **5** Acetabulum, Left **6** Upper Femur, Right **7** Upper Femur, Left **8** Femoral Shaft, Right **9** Femoral Shaft, Left **B** Lower Femur, Right **C** Lower Femur, Left **D** Patella, Right **F** Patella, Left **G** Tibia, Right **H** Tibia, Left **J** Fibula, Right **K** Fibula, Left **L** Tarsal, Right **M** Tarsal, Left **N** Metatarsal, Right **P** Metatarsal, Left **Q** Toe Phalanx, Right **R** Toe Phalanx, Left **S** Coccyx	**0** Open **3** Percutaneous **4** Percutaneous Endoscopic	**Z** No Device	**Z** No Qualifier

Section 0 **Medical and Surgical**
Body System Q **Lower Bones**
Operation P **Removal:** Taking out or off a device from a body part

Body Part (4th)	Approach (5th)	Device (6th)	Qualifier (7th)
0 Lumbar Vertebra **1** Sacrum **2** Pelvic Bone, Right **3** Pelvic Bone, Left **4** Acetabulum, Right **5** Acetabulum, Left **6** Upper Femur, Right **7** Upper Femur, Left **8** Femoral Shaft, Right **9** Femoral Shaft, Left **B** Lower Femur, Right **C** Lower Femur, Left **D** Patella, Right **F** Patella, Left **G** Tibia, Right **H** Tibia, Left **J** Fibula, Right **K** Fibula, Left **L** Tarsal, Right **M** Tarsal, Left **N** Metatarsal, Right **P** Metatarsal, Left **Q** Toe Phalanx, Right **R** Toe Phalanx, Left **S** Coccyx	**0** Open **3** Percutaneous **4** Percutaneous Endoscopic	**4** Internal Fixation Device **5** External Fixation Device **7** Autologous Tissue Substitute **J** Synthetic Substitute **K** Nonautologous Tissue Substitute	**Z** No Qualifier

Continued →

Section 0 **Medical and Surgical**
Body System Q **Lower Bones**
Operation P **Removal:** Taking out or off a device from a body part

Body Part (4th)	Approach (5th)	Device (6th)	Qualifier (7th)
0 Lumbar Vertebra **1** Sacrum **2** Pelvic Bone, Right **3** Pelvic Bone, Left **4** Acetabulum, Right **5** Acetabulum, Left **6** Upper Femur, Right **7** Upper Femur, Left **8** Femoral Shaft, Right **9** Femoral Shaft, Left **B** Lower Femur, Right **C** Lower Femur, Left **D** Patella, Right **F** Patella, Left **G** Tibia, Right **H** Tibia, Left **J** Fibula, Right **K** Fibula, Left **L** Tarsal, Right **M** Tarsal, Left **N** Metatarsal, Right **P** Metatarsal, Left **Q** Toe Phalanx, Right **R** Toe Phalanx, Left **S** Coccyx	**X** External	**4** Internal Fixation Device **5** External Fixation Device	**Z** No Qualifier
Y Lower Bone	**0** Open **3** Percutaneous **4** Percutaneous Endoscopic **X** External	**0** Drainage Device **M** Bone Growth Stimulator	**Z** No Qualifier

Section 0 **Medical and Surgical**
Body System Q **Lower Bones**
Operation Q **Repair:** Restoring, to the extent possible, a body part to its normal anatomic structure and function

Body Part (4th)	Approach (5th)	Device (6th)	Qualifier (7th)
0 Lumbar Vertebra **1** Sacrum **2** Pelvic Bone, Right **3** Pelvic Bone, Left **4** Acetabulum, Right **5** Acetabulum, Left **6** Upper Femur, Right **7** Upper Femur, Left **8** Femoral Shaft, Right **9** Femoral Shaft, Left **B** Lower Femur, Right **C** Lower Femur, Left **D** Patella, Right **F** Patella, Left **G** Tibia, Right **H** Tibia, Left **J** Fibula, Right **K** Fibula, Left **L** Tarsal, Right **M** Tarsal, Left **N** Metatarsal, Right **P** Metatarsal, Left **Q** Toe Phalanx, Right **R** Toe Phalanx, Left **S** Coccyx	**0** Open **3** Percutaneous **4** Percutaneous Endoscopic **X** External	**Z** No Device	**Z** No Qualifier

Section 0 **Medical and Surgical**
Body System Q **Lower Bones**
Operation R **Replacement:** Putting in or on biological or synthetic material that physically takes the place and/or function of all or a portion of a body part

Body Part (4th)	Approach (5th)	Device (6th)	Qualifier (7th)
0 Lumbar Vertebra **1** Sacrum **2** Pelvic Bone, Right **3** Pelvic Bone, Left **4** Acetabulum, Right **5** Acetabulum, Left **6** Upper Femur, Right **7** Upper Femur, Left **8** Femoral Shaft, Right **9** Femoral Shaft, Left **B** Lower Femur, Right **C** Lower Femur, Left **D** Patella, Right **F** Patella, Left **G** Tibia, Right **H** Tibia, Left **J** Fibula, Right **K** Fibula, Left **L** Tarsal, Right **M** Tarsal, Left **N** Metatarsal, Right **P** Metatarsal, Left **Q** Toe Phalanx, Right **R** Toe Phalanx, Left **S** Coccyx	**0** Open **3** Percutaneous **4** Percutaneous Endoscopic	**7** Autologous Tissue Substitute **J** Synthetic Substitute **K** Nonautologous Tissue Substitute	**Z** No Qualifier

Section 0 **Medical and Surgical**
Body System Q **Lower Bones**
Operation S **Reposition:** Moving to its normal location, or other suitable location, all or a portion of a body part

Body Part (4th)	Approach (5th)	Device (6th)	Qualifier (7th)
0 Lumbar Vertebra	**0** Open **4** Percutaneous Endoscopic	**3** Spinal Stabilization Device, Vertebral Body Tether **4** Internal Fixation Device **Z** No Device	**Z** No Qualifier
0 Lumbar Vertebra	**3** Percutaneous	**4** Internal Fixation Device **Z** No Device	**Z** No Qualifier
0 Lumbar Vertebra	**X** External	**Z** No Device	**Z** No Qualifier
1 Sacrum **4** Acetabulum, Right **5** Acetabulum, Left **S** Coccyx	**0** Open **3** Percutaneous **4** Percutaneous Endoscopic	**4** Internal Fixation Device **Z** No Device	**Z** No Qualifier
1 Sacrum **4** Acetabulum, Right **5** Acetabulum, Left **S** Coccyx	**X** External	**Z** No Device	**Z** No Qualifier
2 Pelvic Bone, Right **3** Pelvic Bone, Left **D** Patella, Right **F** Patella, Left **L** Tarsal, Right **M** Tarsal, Left **Q** Toe Phalanx, Right **R** Toe Phalanx, Left	**0** Open **3** Percutaneous **4** Percutaneous Endoscopic	**4** Internal Fixation Device **5** External Fixation Device **Z** No Device	**Z** No Qualifier

Continued →

Section 0 **Medical and Surgical**
Body System Q **Lower Bones**
Operation S **Reposition:** Moving to its normal location, or other suitable location, all or a portion of a body part

Body Part (4th)	Approach (5th)	Device (6th)	Qualifier (7th)
2 Pelvic Bone, Right **3** Pelvic Bone, Left **D** Patella, Right **F** Patella, Left **L** Tarsal, Right **M** Tarsal, Left **Q** Toe Phalanx, Right **R** Toe Phalanx, Left	**X** External	**Z** No Device	**Z** No Qualifier
6 Upper Femur, Right **7** Upper Femur, Left **8** Femoral Shaft, Right **9** Femoral Shaft, Left **B** Lower Femur, Right **C** Lower Femur, Left **G** Tibia, Right **H** Tibia, Left **J** Fibula, Right **K** Fibula, Left	**0** Open **3** Percutaneous **4** Percutaneous Endoscopic	**4** Internal Fixation Device **5** External Fixation Device **6** Internal Fixation Device, Intramedullary **B** External Fixation Device, Monoplanar **C** External Fixation Device, Ring **D** External Fixation Device, Hybrid **Z** No Device	**Z** No Qualifier
6 Upper Femur, Right **7** Upper Femur, Left **8** Femoral Shaft, Right **9** Femoral Shaft, Left **B** Lower Femur, Right **C** Lower Femur, Left **G** Tibia, Right **H** Tibia, Left **J** Fibula, Right **K** Fibula, Left	**X** External	**Z** No Device	**Z** No Qualifier
N Metatarsal, Right **P** Metatarsal, Left	**0** Open **3** Percutaneous **4** Percutaneous Endoscopic	**4** Internal Fixation Device **5** External Fixation Device **Z** No Device	**2** Sesamoid Bone(s) 1st Toe **Z** No Qualifier
N Metatarsal, Right **P** Metatarsal, Left	**X** External	**Z** No Device	**2** Sesamoid Bone(s) 1st Toe **Z** No Qualifier

Section 0 **Medical and Surgical**
Body System Q **Lower Bones**
Operation T **Resection:** Cutting out or off, without replacement, all of a body part

Body Part (4th)	Approach (5th)	Device (6th)	Qualifier (7th)
2 Pelvic Bone, Right **3** Pelvic Bone, Left **4** Acetabulum, Right **5** Acetabulum, Left **6** Upper Femur, Right **7** Upper Femur, Left **8** Femoral Shaft, Right **9** Femoral Shaft, Left **B** Lower Femur, Right **C** Lower Femur, Left **D** Patella, Right **F** Patella, Left **G** Tibia, Right **H** Tibia, Left **J** Fibula, Right **K** Fibula, Left **L** Tarsal, Right **M** Tarsal, Left **N** Metatarsal, Right **P** Metatarsal, Left **Q** Toe Phalanx, Right **R** Toe Phalanx, Left **S** Coccyx	**0** Open	**Z** No Device	**Z** No Qualifier

Section 0 **Medical and Surgical**
Body System Q **Lower Bones**
Operation U **Supplement:** Putting in or on biological or synthetic material that physically reinforces and/or augments the function of a portion of a body part

Body Part (4th)	Approach (5th)	Device (6th)	Qualifier (7th)
0 Lumbar Vertebra **1** Sacrum **2** Pelvic Bone, Right **3** Pelvic Bone, Left **4** Acetabulum, Right **5** Acetabulum, Left **6** Upper Femur, Right **7** Upper Femur, Left **8** Femoral Shaft, Right **9** Femoral Shaft, Left **B** Lower Femur, Right **C** Lower Femur, Left **D** Patella, Right **F** Patella, Left **G** Tibia, Right **H** Tibia, Left **J** Fibula, Right **K** Fibula, Left **L** Tarsal, Right **M** Tarsal, Left **N** Metatarsal, Right **P** Metatarsal, Left **Q** Toe Phalanx, Right **R** Toe Phalanx, Left **S** Coccyx	**0** Open **3** Percutaneous **4** Percutaneous Endoscopic	**7** Autologous Tissue Substitute **J** Synthetic Substitute **K** Nonautologous Tissue Substitute	**Z** No Qualifier

Section 0 **Medical and Surgical**
Body System Q **Lower Bones**
Operation W **Revision:** Correcting, to the extent possible, a portion of a malfunctioning device or the position of a displaced device

Body Part (4th)	Approach (5th)	Device (6th)	Qualifier (7th)
0 Lumbar Vertebra **1** Sacrum **4** Acetabulum, Right **5** Acetabulum, Left **S** Coccyx	**0** Open **3** Percutaneous **4** Percutaneous Endoscopic **X** External	**4** Internal Fixation Device **7** Autologous Tissue Substitute **J** Synthetic Substitute **K** Nonautologous Tissue Substitute	**Z** No Qualifier
2 Pelvic Bone, Right **3** Pelvic Bone, Left **6** Upper Femur, Right **7** Upper Femur, Left **8** Femoral Shaft, Right **9** Femoral Shaft, Left **B** Lower Femur, Right **C** Lower Femur, Left **D** Patella, Right **F** Patella, Left **G** Tibia, Right **H** Tibia, Left **J** Fibula, Right **K** Fibula, Left **L** Tarsal, Right **M** Tarsal, Left **N** Metatarsal, Right **P** Metatarsal, Left **Q** Toe Phalanx, Right **R** Toe Phalanx, Left	**0** Open **3** Percutaneous **4** Percutaneous Endoscopic **X** External	**4** Internal Fixation Device **5** External Fixation Device **7** Autologous Tissue Substitute **J** Synthetic Substitute **K** Nonautologous Tissue Substitute	**Z** No Qualifier

Continued →

Section 0 **Medical and Surgical**
Body System Q **Lower Bones**
Operation W **Revision:** Correcting, to the extent possible, a portion of a malfunctioning device or the position of a displaced device

Body Part (4th)	Approach (5th)	Device (6th)	Qualifier (7th)
Y Lower Bone	**0** Open **3** Percutaneous **4** Percutaneous Endoscopic **X** External	**0** Drainage Device **M** Bone Growth Stimulator	**Z** No Qualifier

AHA Coding Clinic

0Q830ZZ Division of Left Pelvic Bone, Open Approach—AHA CC: 2Q, 2016, 32
0QB10ZZ Excision of Sacrum, Open Approach—AHA CC: 2Q, 2020, 26
0QB20ZZ Excision of Right Pelvic Bone, Open Approach—AHA CC: 2Q, 2014, 6-7: 4Q, 2018, 12-13
0QB30ZZ Excision of Left Pelvic Bone, Open Approach—AHA CC: 2Q, 2019, 19-20
0QB74ZZ Excision of Left Upper Femur, Percutaneous Endoscopic Approach—AHA CC: 4Q, 2014, 25-26
0QBJ0ZZ Excision of Right Fibula, Open Approach—AHA CC: 1Q, 2017, 23-24
0QBK0ZZ Excision of Left Fibula, Open Approach—AHA CC: 2Q, 2013, 39-40
0QBL0ZZ Excision of Right Tarsal, Open Approach—AHA CC: 3Q, 2018, 17-18
0QBN0ZZ Excision of Right Metatarsal, Open Approach—AHA CC: 2Q, 2021, 18-19
0QH204Z Insertion of Internal Fixation Device into Right Pelvic Bone, Open Approach—AHA CC: 1Q, 2017, 21-22
0QH304Z Insertion of Internal Fixation Device into Left Pelvic Bone, Open Approach—AHA CC: 1Q, 2017, 21-22
0QHG04Z Insertion of Internal Fixation Device into Right Tibia, Open Approach—AHA CC: 3Q, 2016, 34-35
0QHJ04Z Insertion of Internal Fixation Device into Right Fibula, Open Approach—AHA CC: 3Q, 2016, 34-35
0QP004Z Removal of Internal Fixation Device from Lumbar Vertebra, Open Approach—AHA CC: 4Q, 2017, 75
0QPG04Z Removal of Internal Fixation Device from Right Tibia, Open Approach—AHA CC: 2Q, 2015, 6-7
0QQ10ZZ Repair Sacrum, Open Approach—AHA CC: 3Q, 2014, 24
0QQ20ZZ Repair Right Pelvic Bone, Open Approach—AHA CC: 1Q, 2018, 15
0QQ30ZZ Repair Left Pelvic Bone, Open Approach—AHA CC: 1Q, 2018, 15
0QS004Z Reposition Lumbar Vertebra with Internal Fixation Device, Open Approach—AHA CC: 1Q, 2020, 33-34
0QS504Z Reposition Left Acetabulum with Internal Fixation Device, Open Approach—AHA CC: 2Q, 2016, 32; 1Q, 2018, 25
0QS904Z Reposition Left Femoral Shaft with Internal Fixation Device, Open Approach—AHA CC: 3Q, 2019, 26
0QSC04Z Reposition Left Lower Femur with Internal Fixation Device, Open Approach—AHA CC: 4Q, 2014, 31
0QSF04Z Reposition Left Patella with Internal Fixation Device, Open Approach—AHA CC: 3Q, 2016, 34-35
0QSH04Z Reposition Left Tibia with Internal Fixation Device, Open Approach—AHA CC: 4Q, 2014, 30-31; 3Q, 2016, 34-35
0QSK0ZZ Reposition Left Fibula, Open Approach—AHA CC: 3Q, 2016, 34-35
0QSL04Z Reposition Right Tarsal with Internal Fixation Device, Open Approach—AHA CC: 1Q, 2018, 13
0QSM04Z Reposition Left Tarsal with Internal Fixation Device, Open Approach—AHA CC: 1Q, 2018, 13
0QT60ZZ Resection of Right Upper Femur, Open Approach—AHA CC: 3Q, 2016, 30-31
0QT70ZZ Resection of Left Upper Femur, Open Approach—AHA CC: 3Q, 2015, 26; 3Q, 2016, 30-31
0QTC0ZZ Resection of Left Lower Femur, Open Approach—AHA CC: 4Q, 2014, 30-31
0QU03JZ Supplement Lumbar Vertebra with Synthetic Substitute, Percutaneous Approach—AHA CC: 2Q, 2014, 12-13; 2Q, 2019, 35
0QU20JZ Supplement Right Pelvic Bone with Synthetic Substitute, Open Approach—AHA CC: 2Q, 2013, 35-36
0QU50JZ Supplement Left Acetabulum with Synthetic Substitute, Open Approach—AHA CC: 3Q, 2015, 18-19
0QU90KZ Supplement Left Femoral Shaft with Nonautologous Tissue Substitute, Open Approach—AHA CC: 3Q, 2019, 26
0QUC0KZ Supplement Left Lower Femur with—Nonautologous Tissue Substitute, Open Approach—AHA CC: 4Q, 2014, 31
0QW034Z Revision of Internal Fixation Device in Lumbar Vertebra, Percutaneous Approach—AHA CC: 4Q, 2017, 75

Intervertebral Joint

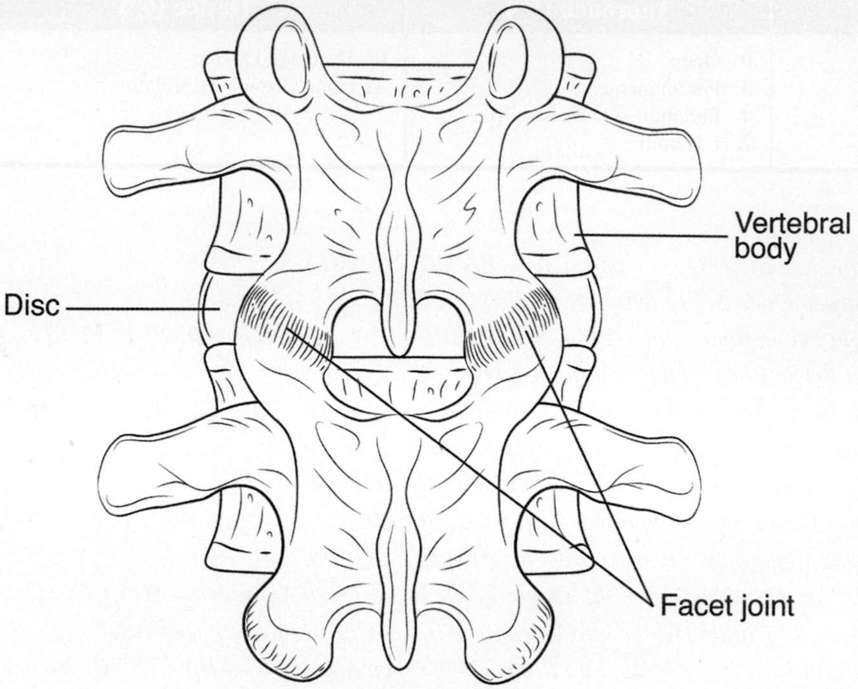
Vertebral body
Disc
Facet joint

©AHIMA

Shoulder

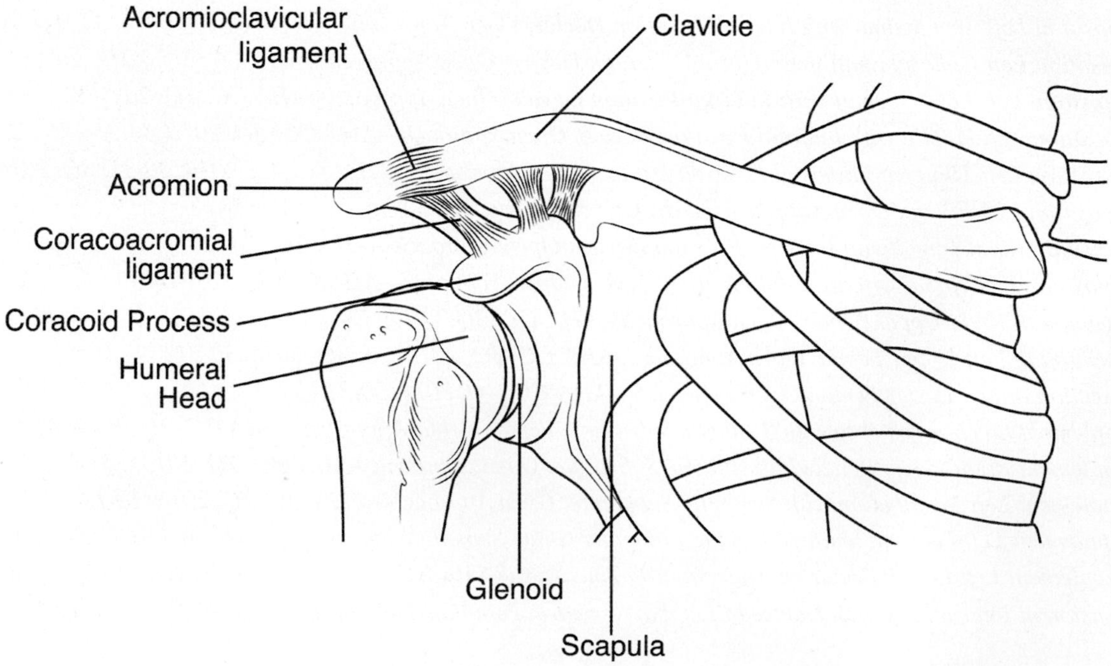
Acromioclavicular ligament
Clavicle
Acromion
Coracoacromial ligament
Coracoid Process
Humeral Head
Glenoid
Scapula

©AHIMA

Cervical Spine Injury: Anterior Interbody Fusion by Dowel Graft (Cloward)

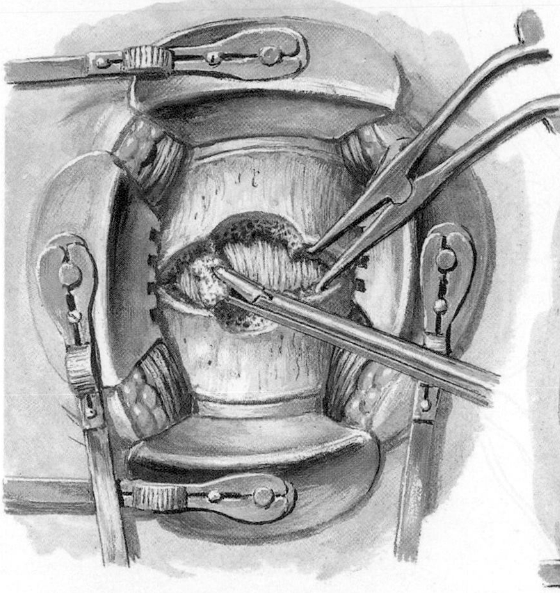

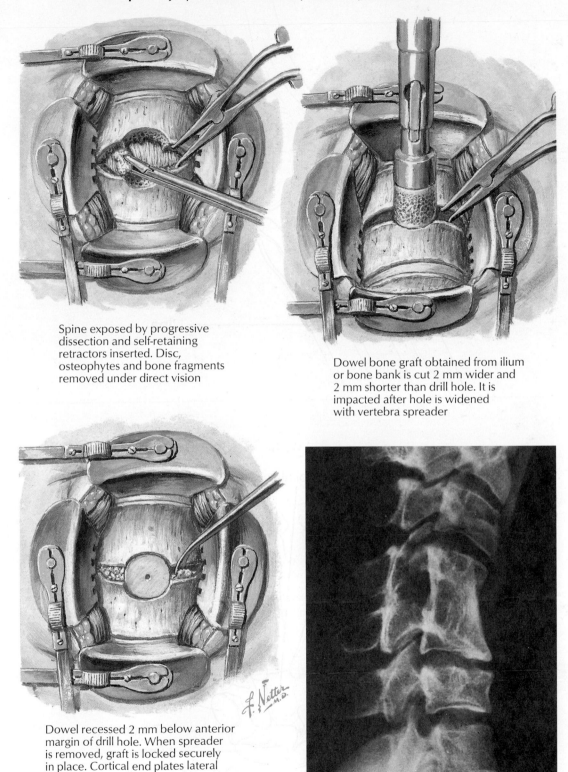

Spine exposed by progressive dissection and self-retaining retractors inserted. Disc, osteophytes and bone fragments removed under direct vision

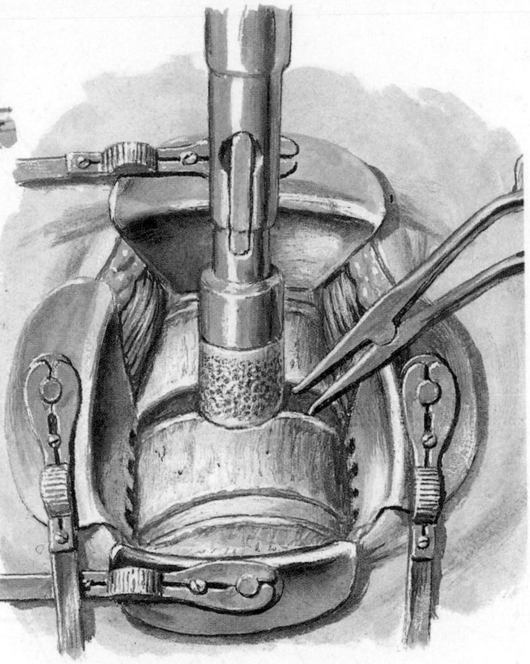

Dowel bone graft obtained from ilium or bone bank is cut 2 mm wider and 2 mm shorter than drill hole. It is impacted after hole is widened with vertebra spreader

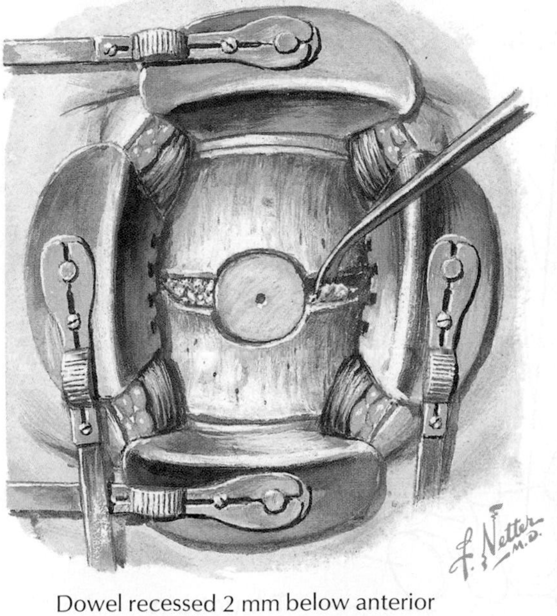

Dowel recessed 2 mm below anterior margin of drill hole. When spreader is removed, graft is locked securely in place. Cortical end plates lateral to dowel are perforated and interspace packed with bone dust removed from drill

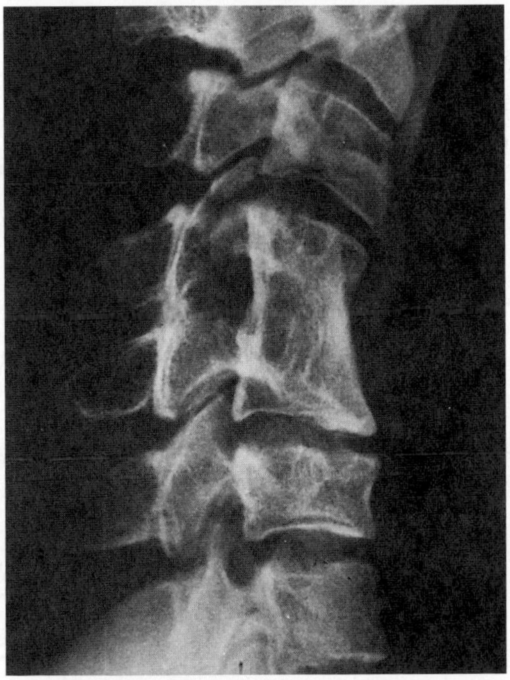

Follow-up x-ray film. Dowel graft fusion of C5-6 with good union

Elbow

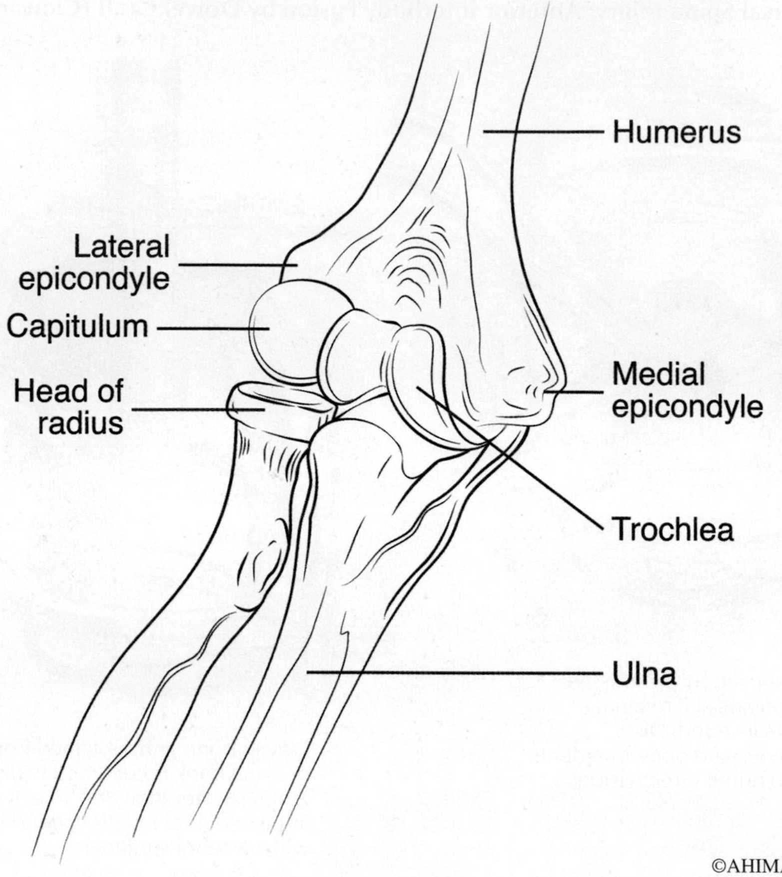

Humerus
Lateral epicondyle
Capitulum
Head of radius
Medial epicondyle
Trochlea
Ulna

Wrist

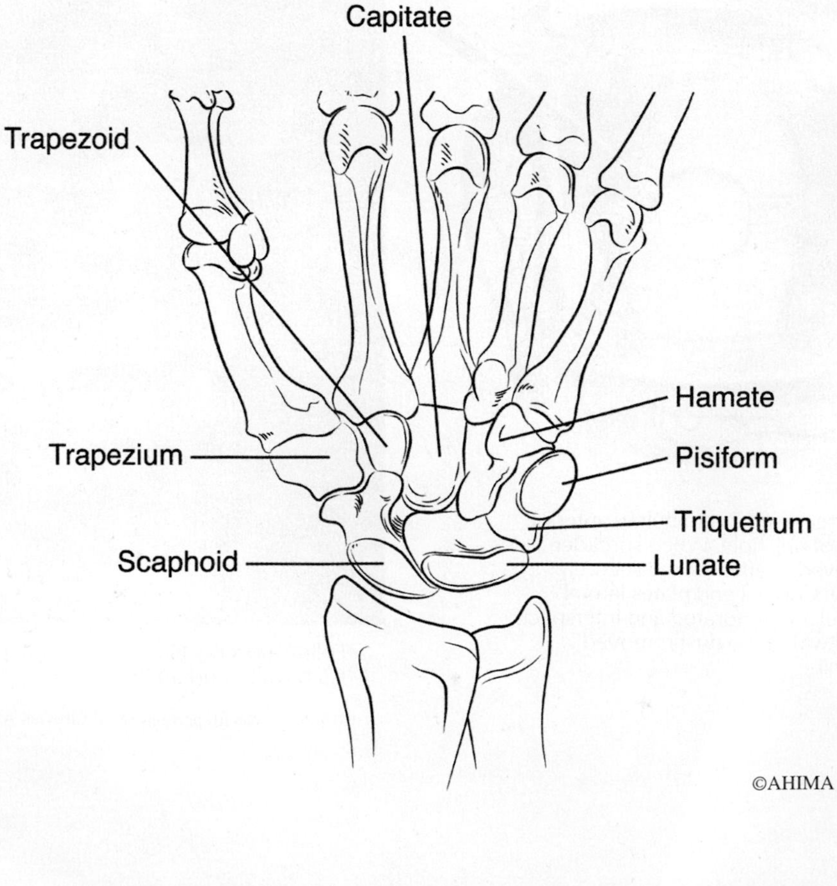

Capitate
Trapezoid
Hamate
Trapezium
Pisiform
Triquetrum
Scaphoid
Lunate

Section 0 **Medical and Surgical**
Body System R **Upper Joints**
Operation 2 **Change:** Taking out or off a device from a body part and putting back an identical or similar device in or on the same body part without cutting or puncturing the skin or a mucous membrane

Body Part (4th)	Approach (5th)	Device (6th)	Qualifier (7th)
Y Upper Joint	**X** External	**0** Drainage Device **Y** Other Device	**Z** No Qualifier

Section 0 **Medical and Surgical**
Body System R **Upper Joints**
Operation 5 **Destruction:** Physical eradication of all or a portion of a body part by the direct use of energy, force, or a destructive agent

Body Part (4th)	Approach (5th)	Device (6th)	Qualifier (7th)
0 Occipital-cervical Joint **1** Cervical Vertebral Joint **3** Cervical Vertebral Disc **4** Cervicothoracic Vertebral Joint **5** Cervicothoracic Vertebral Disc **6** Thoracic Vertebral Joint **9** Thoracic Vertebral Disc **A** Thoracolumbar Vertebral Joint **B** Thoracolumbar Vertebral Disc **C** Temporomandibular Joint, Right **D** Temporomandibular Joint, Left **E** Sternoclavicular Joint, Right **F** Sternoclavicular Joint, Left **G** Acromioclavicular Joint, Right **H** Acromioclavicular Joint, Left **J** Shoulder Joint, Right **K** Shoulder Joint, Left **L** Elbow Joint, Right **M** Elbow Joint, Left **N** Wrist Joint, Right **P** Wrist Joint, Left **Q** Carpal Joint, Right **R** Carpal Joint, Left **S** Carpometacarpal Joint, Right **T** Carpometacarpal Joint, Left **U** Metacarpophalangeal Joint, Right **V** Metacarpophalangeal Joint, Left **W** Finger Phalangeal Joint, Right **X** Finger Phalangeal Joint, Left	**0** Open **3** Percutaneous **4** Percutaneous Endoscopic	**Z** No Device	**Z** No Qualifier

Section 0 **Medical and Surgical**
Body System R **Upper Joints**
Operation 9 **Drainage:** Taking or letting out fluids and/or gases from a body part

Body Part (4th)	Approach (5th)	Device (6th)	Qualifier (7th)
0 Occipital-cervical Joint **1** Cervical Vertebral Joint **3** Cervical Vertebral Disc **4** Cervicothoracic Vertebral Joint **5** Cervicothoracic Vertebral Disc **6** Thoracic Vertebral Joint **9** Thoracic Vertebral Disc **A** Thoracolumbar Vertebral Joint **B** Thoracolumbar Vertebral Disc **C** Temporomandibular Joint, Right **D** Temporomandibular Joint, Left **E** Sternoclavicular Joint, Right **F** Sternoclavicular Joint, Left **G** Acromioclavicular Joint, Right **H** Acromioclavicular Joint, Left **J** Shoulder Joint, Right **K** Shoulder Joint, Left **L** Elbow Joint, Right **M** Elbow Joint, Left **N** Wrist Joint, Right **P** Wrist Joint, Left **Q** Carpal Joint, Right **R** Carpal Joint, Left **S** Carpometacarpal Joint, Right **T** Carpometacarpal Joint, Left **U** Metacarpophalangeal Joint, Right **V** Metacarpophalangeal Joint, Left **W** Finger Phalangeal Joint, Right **X** Finger Phalangeal Joint, Left	**0** Open **3** Percutaneous **4** Percutaneous Endoscopic	**0** Drainage Device	**Z** No Qualifier
0 Occipital-cervical Joint **1** Cervical Vertebral Joint **3** Cervical Vertebral Disc **4** Cervicothoracic Vertebral Joint **5** Cervicothoracic Vertebral Disc **6** Thoracic Vertebral Joint **9** Thoracic Vertebral Disc **A** Thoracolumbar Vertebral Joint **B** Thoracolumbar Vertebral Disc **C** Temporomandibular Joint, Right **D** Temporomandibular Joint, Left **E** Sternoclavicular Joint, Right **F** Sternoclavicular Joint, Left **G** Acromioclavicular Joint, Right **H** Acromioclavicular Joint, Left **J** Shoulder Joint, Right **K** Shoulder Joint, Left **L** Elbow Joint, Right **M** Elbow Joint, Left [illegible] Wrist Joint, Right [illegible]ist Joint, Left [illegible]l Joint, Right [illegible]int, Left [illegible]pal Joint, Right [illegible]l Joint, Left [illegible]al Joint, Right [illegible]Joint, Left [illegible]Right [illegible]	**0** Open **3** Percutaneous **4** Percutaneous Endoscopic	**Z** No Device	**X** Diagnostic **Z** No Qualifier

Section	**0**	**Medical and Surgical**
Body System	**R**	**Upper Joints**
Operation	**B**	**Excision:** Cutting out or off, without replacement, a portion of a body part

Body Part (4th)	Approach (5th)	Device (6th)	Qualifier (7th)
0 Occipital-cervical Joint **1** Cervical Vertebral Joint **3** Cervical Vertebral Disc **4** Cervicothoracic Vertebral Joint **5** Cervicothoracic Vertebral Disc **6** Thoracic Vertebral Joint **9** Thoracic Vertebral Disc **A** Thoracolumbar Vertebral Joint **B** Thoracolumbar Vertebral Disc **C** Temporomandibular Joint, Right **D** Temporomandibular Joint, Left **E** Sternoclavicular Joint, Right **F** Sternoclavicular Joint, Left **G** Acromioclavicular Joint, Right **H** Acromioclavicular Joint, Left **J** Shoulder Joint, Right **K** Shoulder Joint, Left **L** Elbow Joint, Right **M** Elbow Joint, Left **N** Wrist Joint, Right **P** Wrist Joint, Left **Q** Carpal Joint, Right **R** Carpal Joint, Left **S** Carpometacarpal Joint, Right **T** Carpometacarpal Joint, Left **U** Metacarpophalangeal Joint, Right **V** Metacarpophalangeal Joint, Left **W** Finger Phalangeal Joint, Right **X** Finger Phalangeal Joint, Left	**0** Open **3** Percutaneous **4** Percutaneous Endoscopic	**Z** No Device	**X** Diagnostic **Z** No Qualifier

Section 0 **Medical and Surgical**
Body System R **Upper Joints**
Operation C **Extirpation:** Taking or cutting out solid matter from a body part

Body Part (4th)	Approach (5th)	Device (6th)	Qualifier (7th)
0 Occipital-cervical Joint **1** Cervical Vertebral Joint **3** Cervical Vertebral Disc **4** Cervicothoracic Vertebral Joint **5** Cervicothoracic Vertebral Disc **6** Thoracic Vertebral Joint **9** Thoracic Vertebral Disc **A** Thoracolumbar Vertebral Joint **B** Thoracolumbar Vertebral Disc **C** Temporomandibular Joint, Right **D** Temporomandibular Joint, Left **E** Sternoclavicular Joint, Right **F** Sternoclavicular Joint, Left **G** Acromioclavicular Joint, Right **H** Acromioclavicular Joint, Left **J** Shoulder Joint, Right **K** Shoulder Joint, Left **L** Elbow Joint, Right **M** Elbow Joint, Left **N** Wrist Joint, Right **P** Wrist Joint, Left **Q** Carpal Joint, Right **R** Carpal Joint, Left **S** Carpometacarpal Joint, Right **T** Carpometacarpal Joint, Left **U** Metacarpophalangeal Joint, Right **V** Metacarpophalangeal Joint, Left **W** Finger Phalangeal Joint, Right **X** Finger Phalangeal Joint, Left	**0** Open **3** Percutaneous **4** Percutaneous Endoscopic	**Z** No Device	**Z** No Qualifier

Section 0 **Medical and Surgical**
Body System R **Upper Joints**
Operation G **Fusion:** Joining together portions of an articular body part rendering the articular body part immobile

Body Part (4th)	Approach (5th)	Device (6th)	Qualifier (7th)
0 Occipital-cervical Joint **1** Cervical Vertebral Joint **2** Cervical Vertebral Joints, 2 or more **4** Cervicothoracic Vertebral Joint **6** Thoracic Vertebral Joint **7** Thoracic Vertebral Joints, 2 to 7 **8** Thoracic Vertebral Joints, 8 or more **A** Thoracolumbar Vertebral Joint	**0** Open **3** Percutaneous **4** Percutaneous Endoscopic	**7** Autologous Tissue Substitute **J** Synthetic Substitute **K** Nonautologous Tissue Substitute	**0** Anterior Approach, Anterior Column **1** Posterior Approach, Posterior Column **J** Posterior Approach, Anterior Column
0 Occipital-cervical Joint **1** Cervical Vertebral Joint **2** Cervical Vertebral Joints, 2 or more **4** Cervicothoracic Vertebral Joint **6** Thoracic Vertebral Joint **7** Thoracic Vertebral Joints, 2 to 7 **8** Thoracic Vertebral Joints, 8 or more **A** Thoracolumbar Vertebral Joint	**0** Open **3** Percutaneous **4** Percutaneous Endoscopic	**A** Interbody Fusion Device	**0** Anterior Approach, Anterior Column **J** Posterior Approach, Anterior Column
C Temporomandibular Joint, Right **D** Temporomandibular Joint, Left **E** Sternoclavicular Joint, Right **F** Sternoclavicular Joint, Left **G** Acromioclavicular Joint, Right **H** Acromioclavicular Joint, Left **J** Shoulder Joint, Right **K** Shoulder Joint, Left	**0** Open **3** Percutaneous **4** Percutaneous Endoscopic	**4** Internal Fixation Device **7** Autologous Tissue Substitute **J** Synthetic Substitute **K** Nonautologous Tissue Substitute	**Z** No Qualifier

Continued →

Section 0 **Medical and Surgical**
Body System R **Upper Joints**
Operation G **Fusion:** Joining together portions of an articular body part rendering the articular body part immobile

Body Part (4th)	Approach (5th)	Device (6th)	Qualifier (7th)
L Elbow Joint, Right **M** Elbow Joint, Left **N** Wrist Joint, Right **P** Wrist Joint, Left **Q** Carpal Joint, Right **R** Carpal Joint, Left **S** Carpometacarpal Joint, Right **T** Carpometacarpal Joint, Left **U** Metacarpophalangeal Joint, Right **V** Metacarpophalangeal Joint, Left **W** Finger Phalangeal Joint, Right **X** Finger Phalangeal Joint, Left	**0** Open **3** Percutaneous **4** Percutaneous Endoscopic	**3** Internal Fixation Device, Sustained Compression **4** Internal Fixation Device **5** External Fixation Device **7** Autologous Tissue Substitute **J** Synthetic Substitute **K** Nonautologous Tissue Substitute	**Z** No Qualifier

Section 0 **Medical and Surgical**
Body System R **Upper Joints**
Operation H **Insertion:** Putting in a nonbiological appliance that monitors, assists, performs, or prevents a physiological function but does not physically take the place of a body part

Body Part (4th)	Approach (5th)	Device (6th)	Qualifier (7th)
0 Occipital-cervical Joint **1** Cervical Vertebral Joint **4** Cervicothoracic Vertebral Joint **6** Thoracic Vertebral Joint **A** Thoracolumbar Vertebral Joint	**0** Open **3** Percutaneous **4** Percutaneous Endoscopic	**3** Infusion Device **4** Internal Fixation Device **8** Spacer **B** Spinal Stabilization Device, Interspinous Process **C** Spinal Stabilization Device, Pedicle-Based **D** Spinal Stabilization Device, Facet Replacement	**Z** No Qualifier
3 Cervical Vertebral Disc **5** Cervicothoracic Vertebral Disc **9** Thoracic Vertebral Disc **B** Thoracolumbar Vertebral Disc	**0** Open **3** Percutaneous **4** Percutaneous Endoscopic	**3** Infusion Device	**Z** No Qualifier
C Temporomandibular Joint, Right **D** Temporomandibular Joint, Left **E** Sternoclavicular Joint, Right **F** Sternoclavicular Joint, Left **G** Acromioclavicular Joint, Right **H** Acromioclavicular Joint, Left **J** Shoulder Joint, Right **K** Shoulder Joint, Left	**0** Open **3** Percutaneous **4** Percutaneous Endoscopic	**3** Infusion Device **4** Internal Fixation Device **8** Spacer	**Z** No Qualifier
L Elbow Joint, Right **M** Elbow Joint, Left **N** Wrist Joint, Right **P** Wrist Joint, Left **Q** Carpal Joint, Right **R** Carpal Joint, Left **S** Carpometacarpal Joint, Right **T** Carpometacarpal Joint, Left **U** Metacarpophalangeal Joint, Right **V** Metacarpophalangeal Joint, Left **W** Finger Phalangeal Joint, Right **X** Finger Phalangeal Joint, Left	**0** Open **3** Percutaneous **4** Percutaneous Endoscopic	**3** Infusion Device **4** Internal Fixation Device **5** External Fixation Device **8** Spacer	**Z** No Qualifier

Section 0 **Medical and Surgical**
Body System R **Upper Joints**
Operation J **Inspection:** Visually and/or manually exploring a body part

Body Part (4th)	Approach (5th)	Device (6th)	Qualifier (7th)
0 Occipital-cervical Joint 1 Cervical Vertebral Joint 3 Cervical Vertebral Disc 4 Cervicothoracic Vertebral Joint 5 Cervicothoracic Vertebral Disc 6 Thoracic Vertebral Joint 9 Thoracic Vertebral Disc A Thoracolumbar Vertebral Joint B Thoracolumbar Vertebral Disc C Temporomandibular Joint, Right D Temporomandibular Joint, Left E Sternoclavicular Joint, Right F Sternoclavicular Joint, Left G Acromioclavicular Joint, Right H Acromioclavicular Joint, Left J Shoulder Joint, Right K Shoulder Joint, Left L Elbow Joint, Right M Elbow Joint, Left N Wrist Joint, Right P Wrist Joint, Left Q Carpal Joint, Right R Carpal Joint, Left S Carpometacarpal Joint, Right T Carpometacarpal Joint, Left U Metacarpophalangeal Joint, Right V Metacarpophalangeal Joint, Left W Finger Phalangeal Joint, Right X Finger Phalangeal Joint, Left	0 Open 3 Percutaneous 4 Percutaneous Endoscopic X External	Z No Device	Z No Qualifier

Section 0 **Medical and Surgical**
Body System R **Upper Joints**
Operation N **Release:** Freeing a body part from an abnormal physical constraint by cutting or by the use of force

Body Part (4th)	Approach (5th)	Device (6th)	Qualifier (7th)
0 Occipital-cervical Joint 1 Cervical Vertebral Joint 3 Cervical Vertebral Disc 4 Cervicothoracic Vertebral Joint 5 Cervicothoracic Vertebral Disc 6 Thoracic Vertebral Joint 9 Thoracic Vertebral Disc A Thoracolumbar Vertebral Joint B Thoracolumbar Vertebral Disc C Temporomandibular Joint, Right D Temporomandibular Joint, Left E Sternoclavicular Joint, Right F Sternoclavicular Joint, Left G Acromioclavicular Joint, Right H Acromioclavicular Joint, Left J Shoulder Joint, Right K Shoulder Joint, Left L Elbow Joint, Right M Elbow Joint, Left N Wrist Joint, Right P Wrist Joint, Left Q Carpal Joint, Right R Carpal Joint, Left S Carpometacarpal Joint, Right T Carpometacarpal Joint, Left U Metacarpophalangeal Joint, Right V Metacarpophalangeal Joint, Left W Finger Phalangeal Joint, Right X Finger Phalangeal Joint, Left	0 Open 3 Percutaneous 4 Percutaneous Endoscopic X External	Z No Device	Z No Qualifier

Section 0 **Medical and Surgical**
Body System R **Upper Joints**
Operation P **Removal:** Taking out or off a device from a body part

Body Part (4th)	Approach (5th)	Device (6th)	Qualifier (7th)
0 Occipital-cervical Joint **1** Cervical Vertebral Joint **4** Cervicothoracic Vertebral Joint **6** Thoracic Vertebral Joint **A** Thoracolumbar Vertebral Joint	**0** Open **3** Percutaneous **4** Percutaneous Endoscopic	**0** Drainage Device **3** Infusion Device **4** Internal Fixation Device **7** Autologous Tissue Substitute **8** Spacer **A** Interbody Fusion Device **J** Synthetic Substitute **K** Nonautologous Tissue Substitute	**Z** No Qualifier
0 Occipital-cervical Joint **1** Cervical Vertebral Joint **4** Cervicothoracic Vertebral Joint **6** Thoracic Vertebral Joint **A** Thoracolumbar Vertebral Joint	**X** External	**0** Drainage Device **3** Infusion Device **4** Internal Fixation Device	**Z** No Qualifier
3 Cervical Vertebral Disc **5** Cervicothoracic Vertebral Disc **9** Thoracic Vertebral Disc **B** Thoracolumbar Vertebral Disc	**0** Open **3** Percutaneous **4** Percutaneous Endoscopic	**0** Drainage Device **3** Infusion Device **7** Autologous Tissue Substitute **J** Synthetic Substitute **K** Nonautologous Tissue Substitute	**Z** No Qualifier
3 Cervical Vertebral Disc **5** Cervicothoracic Vertebral Disc **9** Thoracic Vertebral Disc **B** Thoracolumbar Vertebral Disc	**X** External	**0** Drainage Device **3** Infusion Device	**Z** No Qualifier
C Temporomandibular Joint, Right **D** Temporomandibular Joint, Left **E** Sternoclavicular Joint, Right **F** Sternoclavicular Joint, Left **G** Acromioclavicular Joint, Right **H** Acromioclavicular Joint, Left	**0** Open **3** Percutaneous **4** Percutaneous Endoscopic	**0** Drainage Device **3** Infusion Device **4** Internal Fixation Device **7** Autologous Tissue Substitute **8** Spacer **J** Synthetic Substitute **K** Nonautologous Tissue Substitute	**Z** No Qualifier
C Temporomandibular Joint, Right **D** Temporomandibular Joint, Left **E** Sternoclavicular Joint, Right **F** Sternoclavicular Joint, Left **G** Acromioclavicular Joint, Right **H** Acromioclavicular Joint, Left	**X** External	**0** Drainage Device **3** Infusion Device **4** Internal Fixation Device	**Z** No Qualifier
J Shoulder Joint, Right **K** Shoulder Joint, Left	**0** Open **3** Percutaneous **4** Percutaneous Endoscopic	**0** Drainage Device **3** Infusion Device **4** Internal Fixation Device **7** Autologous Tissue Substitute **8** Spacer **K** Nonautologous Tissue Substitute	**Z** No Qualifier
J Shoulder Joint, Right **K** Shoulder Joint, Left	**0** Open **3** Percutaneous **4** Percutaneous Endoscopic	**J** Synthetic Substitute	**6** Humeral Surface **7** Glenoid Surface **Z** No Device
J Shoulder Joint, Right **K** Shoulder Joint, Left	**X** External	**0** Drainage Device **3** Infusion Device **4** Internal Fixation Device	**Z** No Qualifier

Continued →

Section **0** **Medical and Surgical**
Body System **R** **Upper Joints**
Operation **P** **Removal:** Taking out or off a device from a body part

Body Part (4th)	Approach (5th)	Device (6th)	Qualifier (7th)
L Elbow Joint, Right **M** Elbow Joint, Left **N** Wrist Joint, Right **P** Wrist Joint, Left **Q** Carpal Joint, Right **R** Carpal Joint, Left **S** Carpometacarpal Joint, Right **T** Carpometacarpal Joint, Left **U** Metacarpophalangeal Joint, Right **V** Metacarpophalangeal Joint, Left **W** Finger Phalangeal Joint, Right **X** Finger Phalangeal Joint, Left	**0** Open **3** Percutaneous **4** Percutaneous Endoscopic	**0** Drainage Device **3** Infusion Device **4** Internal Fixation Device **5** External Fixation Device **7** Autologous Tissue Substitute **8** Spacer **J** Synthetic Substitute **K** Nonautologous Tissue Substitute	**Z** No Qualifier
L Elbow Joint, Right **M** Elbow Joint, Left **N** Wrist Joint, Right **P** Wrist Joint, Left **Q** Carpal Joint, Right **R** Carpal Joint, Left **S** Carpometacarpal Joint, Right **T** Carpometacarpal Joint, Left **U** Metacarpophalangeal Joint, Right **V** Metacarpophalangeal Joint, Left **W** Finger Phalangeal Joint, Right **X** Finger Phalangeal Joint, Left	**X** External	**0** Drainage Device **3** Infusion Device **4** Internal Fixation Device **5** External Fixation Device	**Z** No Qualifier

Section **0** **Medical and Surgical**
Body System **R** **Upper Joints**
Operation **Q** **Repair:** Restoring, to the extent possible, a body part to its normal anatomic structure and function

Body Part (4th)	Approach (5th)	Device (6th)	Qualifier (7th)
0 Occipital-cervical Joint **1** Cervical Vertebral Joint **3** Cervical Vertebral Disc **4** Cervicothoracic Vertebral Joint **5** Cervicothoracic Vertebral Disc **6** Thoracic Vertebral Joint **9** Thoracic Vertebral Disc **A** Thoracolumbar Vertebral Joint **B** Thoracolumbar Vertebral Disc **C** Temporomandibular Joint, Right **D** Temporomandibular Joint, Left **E** Sternoclavicular Joint, Right **F** Sternoclavicular Joint, Left **G** Acromioclavicular Joint, Right **H** Acromioclavicular Joint, Left **J** Shoulder Joint, Right **K** Shoulder Joint, Left **L** Elbow Joint, Right **M** Elbow Joint, Left **N** Wrist Joint, Right **P** Wrist Joint, Left **Q** Carpal Joint, Right **R** Carpal Joint, Left **S** Carpometacarpal Joint, Right **T** Carpometacarpal Joint, Left **U** Metacarpophalangeal Joint, Right **V** Metacarpophalangeal Joint, Left **W** Finger Phalangeal Joint, Right **X** Finger Phalangeal Joint, Left	**0** Open **3** Percutaneous **4** Percutaneous Endoscopic **X** External	**Z** No Device	**Z** No Qualifier

Section 0 **Medical and Surgical**
Body System R **Upper Joints**
Operation R **Replacement:** Putting in or on biological or synthetic material that physically takes the place and/or function of all or a portion of a body part

Body Part (4th)	Approach (5th)	Device (6th)	Qualifier (7th)
0 Occipital-cervical Joint **1** Cervical Vertebral Joint **3** Cervical Vertebral Disc **4** Cervicothoracic Vertebral Joint **5** Cervicothoracic Vertebral Disc **6** Thoracic Vertebral Joint **9** Thoracic Vertebral Disc **A** Thoracolumbar Vertebral Joint **B** Thoracolumbar Vertebral Disc **C** Temporomandibular Joint, Right **D** Temporomandibular Joint, Left **E** Sternoclavicular Joint, Right **F** Sternoclavicular Joint, Left **G** Acromioclavicular Joint, Right **H** Acromioclavicular Joint, Left **L** Elbow Joint, Right **M** Elbow Joint, Left **N** Wrist Joint, Right **P** Wrist Joint, Left **Q** Carpal Joint, Right **R** Carpal Joint, Left **S** Carpometacarpal Joint, Right **T** Carpometacarpal Joint, Left **U** Metacarpophalangeal Joint, Right **V** Metacarpophalangeal Joint, Left **W** Finger Phalangeal Joint, Right **X** Finger Phalangeal Joint, Left	**0** Open	**7** Autologous Tissue Substitute **J** Synthetic Substitute **K** Nonautologous Tissue Substitute	**Z** No Qualifier
J Shoulder Joint, Right **K** Shoulder Joint, Left	**0** Open	**0** Synthetic Substitute, Reverse Ball and Socket **7** Autologous Tissue Substitute **K** Nonautologous Tissue Substitute	**Z** No Qualifier
J Shoulder Joint, Right **K** Shoulder Joint, Left	**0** Open	**J** Synthetic Substitute	**6** Humeral Surface **7** Glenoid Surface **Z** No Qualifier

Section 0 **Medical and Surgical**
Body System R **Upper Joints**
Operation S **Reposition:** Moving to its normal location, or other suitable location, all or a portion of a body part

Body Part (4th)	Approach (5th)	Device (6th)	Qualifier (7th)
0 Occipital-cervical Joint **1** Cervical Vertebral Joint **4** Cervicothoracic Vertebral Joint **6** Thoracic Vertebral Joint **A** Thoracolumbar Vertebral Joint **C** Temporomandibular Joint, Right **D** Temporomandibular Joint, Left **E** Sternoclavicular Joint, Right **F** Sternoclavicular Joint, Left **G** Acromioclavicular Joint, Right **H** Acromioclavicular Joint, Left **J** Shoulder Joint, Right **K** Shoulder Joint, Left	**0** Open **3** Percutaneous **4** Percutaneous Endoscopic **X** External	**4** Internal Fixation Device **Z** No Device	**Z** No Qualifier

Continued →

Section 0 **Medical and Surgical**
Body System R **Upper Joints**
Operation S **Reposition:** Moving to its normal location, or other suitable location, all or a portion of a body part

Body Part (4th)	Approach (5th)	Device (6th)	Qualifier (7th)
L Elbow Joint, Right **M** Elbow Joint, Left **N** Wrist Joint, Right **P** Wrist Joint, Left **Q** Carpal Joint, Right **R** Carpal Joint, Left **S** Carpometacarpal Joint, Right **T** Carpometacarpal Joint, Left **U** Metacarpophalangeal Joint, Right **V** Metacarpophalangeal Joint, Left **W** Finger Phalangeal Joint, Right **X** Finger Phalangeal Joint, Left	**0** Open **3** Percutaneous **4** Percutaneous Endoscopic **X** External	**4** Internal Fixation Device **5** External Fixation Device **Z** No Device	**Z** No Qualifier

Section 0 **Medical and Surgical**
Body System R **Upper Joints**
Operation T **Resection:** Cutting out or off, without replacement, all of a body part

Body Part (4th)	Approach (5th)	Device (6th)	Qualifier (7th)
3 Cervical Vertebral Disc **4** Cervicothoracic Vertebral Joint **5** Cervicothoracic Vertebral Disc **9** Thoracic Vertebral Disc **B** Thoracolumbar Vertebral Disc **C** Temporomandibular Joint, Right **D** Temporomandibular Joint, Left **E** Sternoclavicular Joint, Right **F** Sternoclavicular Joint, Left **G** Acromioclavicular Joint, Right **H** Acromioclavicular Joint, Left **J** Shoulder Joint, Right **K** Shoulder Joint, Left **L** Elbow Joint, Right **M** Elbow Joint, Left **N** Wrist Joint, Right **P** Wrist Joint, Left **Q** Carpal Joint, Right **R** Carpal Joint, Left **S** Carpometacarpal Joint, Right **T** Carpometacarpal Joint, Left **U** Metacarpophalangeal Joint, Right **V** Metacarpophalangeal Joint, Left **W** Finger Phalangeal Joint, Right **X** Finger Phalangeal Joint, Left	**0** Open	**Z** No Device	**Z** No Qualifier

Section 0 **Medical and Surgical**
Body System R **Upper Joints**
Operation U **Supplement:** Putting in or on biological or synthetic material that physically reinforces and/or augments the function of a portion of a body part

Body Part (4th)	Approach (5th)	Device (6th)	Qualifier (7th)
0 Occipital-cervical Joint **1** Cervical Vertebral Joint **3** Cervical Vertebral Disc **4** Cervicothoracic Vertebral Joint **5** Cervicothoracic Vertebral Disc **6** Thoracic Vertebral Joint **9** Thoracic Vertebral Disc **A** Thoracolumbar Vertebral Joint **B** Thoracolumbar Vertebral Disc **C** Temporomandibular Joint, Right **D** Temporomandibular Joint, Left **E** Sternoclavicular Joint, Right **F** Sternoclavicular Joint, Left **G** Acromioclavicular Joint, Right **H** Acromioclavicular Joint, Left **J** Shoulder Joint, Right **K** Shoulder Joint, Left **L** Elbow Joint, Right **M** Elbow Joint, Left **N** Wrist Joint, Right **P** Wrist Joint, Left **Q** Carpal Joint, Right **R** Carpal Joint, Left **S** Carpometacarpal Joint, Right **T** Carpometacarpal Joint, Left **U** Metacarpophalangeal Joint, Right **V** Metacarpophalangeal Joint, Left **W** Finger Phalangeal Joint, Right **X** Finger Phalangeal Joint, Left	**0** Open **3** Percutaneous **4** Percutaneous Endoscopic	**7** Autologous Tissue Substitute **J** Synthetic Substitute **K** Nonautologous Tissue Substitute	**Z** No Qualifier

Section 0 **Medical and Surgical**
Body System R **Upper Joints**
Operation W **Revision:** Correcting, to the extent possible, a portion of a malfunctioning device or the position of a displaced device

Body Part (4th)	Approach (5th)	Device (6th)	Qualifier (7th)
0 Occipital-cervical Joint **1** Cervical Vertebral Joint **4** Cervicothoracic Vertebral Joint **6** Thoracic Vertebral Joint **A** Thoracolumbar Vertebral Joint	**0** Open **3** Percutaneous **4** Percutaneous Endoscopic **X** External	**0** Drainage Device **3** Infusion Device **4** Internal Fixation Device **7** Autologous Tissue Substitute **8** Spacer **A** Interbody Fusion Device **J** Synthetic Substitute **K** Nonautologous Tissue Substitute	**Z** No Qualifier
3 Cervical Vertebral Disc **5** Cervicothoracic Vertebral Disc **9** Thoracic Vertebral Disc **B** Thoracolumbar Vertebral Disc	**0** Open **3** Percutaneous **4** Percutaneous Endoscopic **X** External	**0** Drainage Device **3** Infusion Device **7** Autologous Tissue Substitute **J** Synthetic Substitute **K** Nonautologous Tissue Substitute	**Z** No Qualifier
C Temporomandibular Joint, Right **D** Temporomandibular Joint, Left **E** Sternoclavicular Joint, Right **F** Sternoclavicular Joint, Left **G** Acromioclavicular Joint, Right **H** Acromioclavicular Joint, Left	**0** Open **3** Percutaneous **4** Percutaneous Endoscopic **X** External	**0** Drainage Device **3** Infusion Device **4** Internal Fixation Device **7** Autologous Tissue Substitute **8** Spacer **J** Synthetic Substitute **K** Nonautologous Tissue Substitute	**Z** No Qualifier

Continued →

Section	**0**	**Medical and Surgical**
Body System	**R**	**Upper Joints**
Operation	**W**	**Revision:** Correcting, to the extent possible, a portion of a malfunctioning device or the position of a displaced device

Body Part (4th)	Approach (5th)	Device (6th)	Qualifier (7th)
J Shoulder Joint, Right **K** Shoulder Joint, Left	**0** Open **3** Percutaneous **4** Percutaneous Endoscopic **X** External	**0** Drainage Device **3** Infusion Device **4** Internal Fixation Device **7** Autologous Tissue Substitute **8** Spacer **K** Nonautologous Tissue Substitute	**Z** No Qualifier
J Shoulder Joint, Right **K** Shoulder Joint, Left	**0** Open **3** Percutaneous **4** Percutaneous Endoscopic **X** External	**J** Synthetic Substitute	**6** Humeral Surface **7** Glenoid Surface **Z** No Device
L Elbow Joint, Right **M** Elbow Joint, Left **N** Wrist Joint, Right **P** Wrist Joint, Left **Q** Carpal Joint, Right **R** Carpal Joint, Left **S** Carpometacarpal Joint, Right **T** Carpometacarpal Joint, Left **U** Metacarpophalangeal Joint, Right **V** Metacarpophalangeal Joint, Left **W** Finger Phalangeal Joint, Right **X** Finger Phalangeal Joint, Left	**0** Open **3** Percutaneous **4** Percutaneous Endoscopic **X** External	**0** Drainage Device **3** Infusion Device **4** Internal Fixation Device **5** External Fixation Device **7** Autologous Tissue Substitute **8** Spacer **J** Synthetic Substitute **K** Nonautologous Tissue Substitute	**Z** No Qualifier

AHA Coding Clinic

0RG20A0 Fusion of 2 or more Cervical Vertebral Joints with Interbody Fusion Device, Anterior Approach, Anterior Column, Open Approach—AHA CC: 3Q, 2019, 28

0RG2371 Fusion of 2 or more Cervical Vertebral Joints with Autologous Tissue Substitute, Posterior Approach, Posterior Column, Percutaneous Approach—AHA CC: 2Q, 2019, 19-20

0RG40A0 Fusion of Cervicothoracic Vertebral Joint with Interbody Fusion Device, Anterior Approach, Anterior Column, Open Approach—AHA CC: 1Q, 2013, 29-30; 2Q, 2014, 7-8

0RG7071 Fusion of 2 to 7 Thoracic Vertebral Joints with Autologous Tissue Substitute, Posterior Approach, Posterior Column, Open Approach—AHA CC: 1Q, 2013, 21-23

0RGA071 Fusion of Thoracolumbar Vertebral Joint with Autologous Tissue Substitute, Posterior Approach, Posterior Column, Open Approach—AHA CC: 1Q, 2013, 21-23

0RGW04Z Fusion of Right Finger Phalangeal Joint with Internal Fixation Device, Open Approach—AHA CC: 4Q, 2017, 62

0RHJ04Z Insertion of Internal Fixation Device into Right Shoulder Joint, Open Approach—AHA CC: 3Q, 2016, 32-33

0RNJ4ZZ Release Right Shoulder Joint, Percutaneous Endoscopic Approach—AHA CC: 3Q, 2016, 32-33

0RNK4ZZ Release Left Shoulder Joint, Percutaneous Endoscopic Approach—AHA CC: 2Q, 2015, 22-23

0RQJ4ZZ Repair Right Shoulder Joint, Percutaneous Endoscopic Approach—AHA CC: 1Q, 2016, 30-31

0RRJ00Z Replacement of Right Shoulder Joint with Reverse Ball and Socket Synthetic Substitute, Open Approach—AHA CC: 1Q, 2015, 27

0RRK0J6 Replacement of Left Shoulder Joint with Synthetic Substitute, Humeral Surface, Open Approach—AHA CC: 3Q, 2015, 14-15

0RSH04Z Reposition Left Acromioclavicular Joint with Internal Fixation Device, Open Approach—AHA CC: 3Q, 2019, 26-27

0RSPXZZ Reposition Left Wrist Joint, External Approach—AHA CC: 4Q, 2014, 32-33

0RSR04Z Reposition Left Carpal Joint with Internal Fixation Device, Open Approach—AHA CC: 3Q, 2014, 33-34

0RT50ZZ Resection of Cervicothoracic Vertebral Disc, Open Approach—AHA CC: 2Q, 2014, 7-8

0RUH0KZ Supplement Left Acromioclavicular Joint with Nonautologous Tissue Substitute, Open Approach—AHA CC: 3Q, 2019, 26-27

0RUT07Z Supplement Left Carpometacarpal Joint with Autologous Tissue Substitute, Open Approach—AHA CC: 3Q, 2015, 26-27

Intervertebral Joint

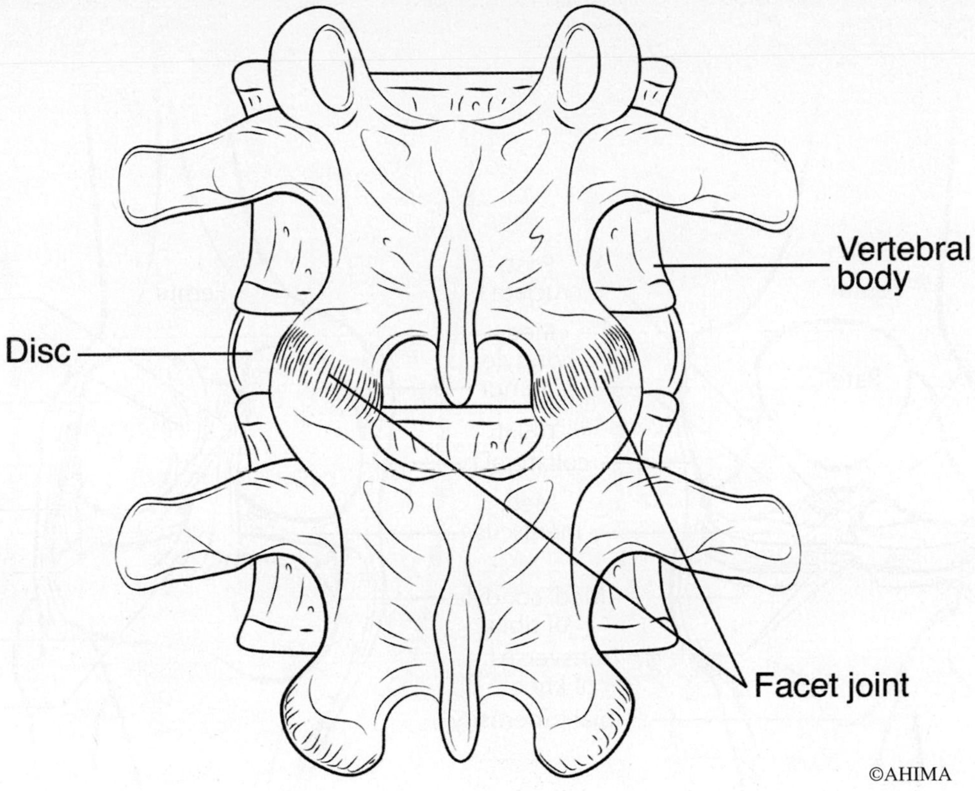
Vertebral body
Disc
Facet joint

Hip

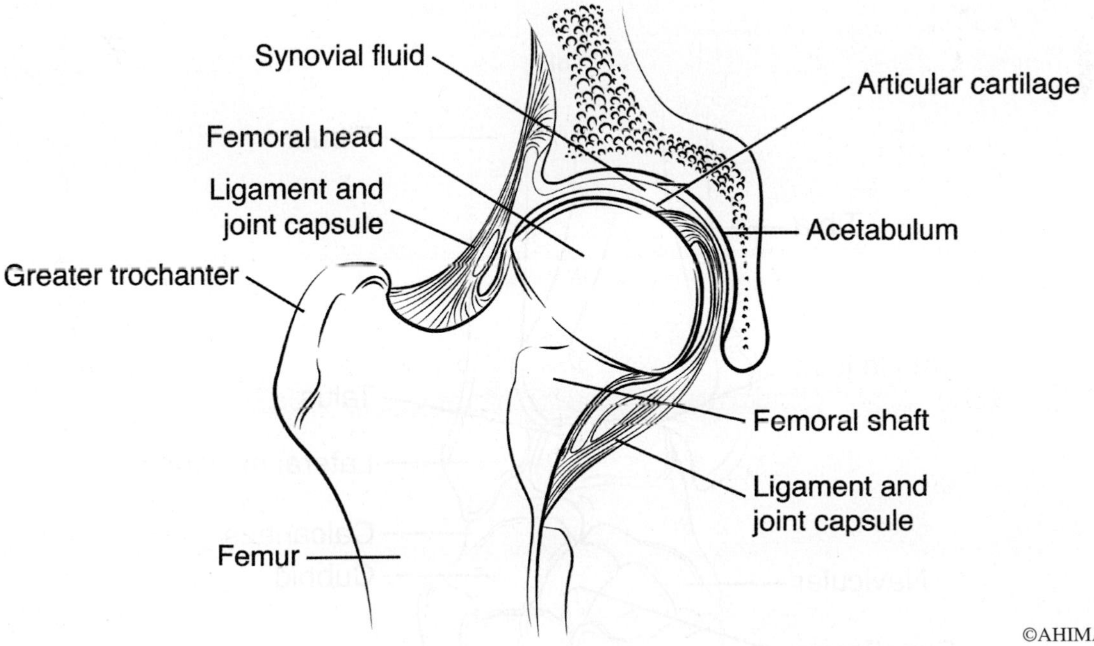
Synovial fluid
Articular cartilage
Femoral head
Ligament and joint capsule
Acetabulum
Greater trochanter
Femoral shaft
Ligament and joint capsule
Femur

Knee Joint

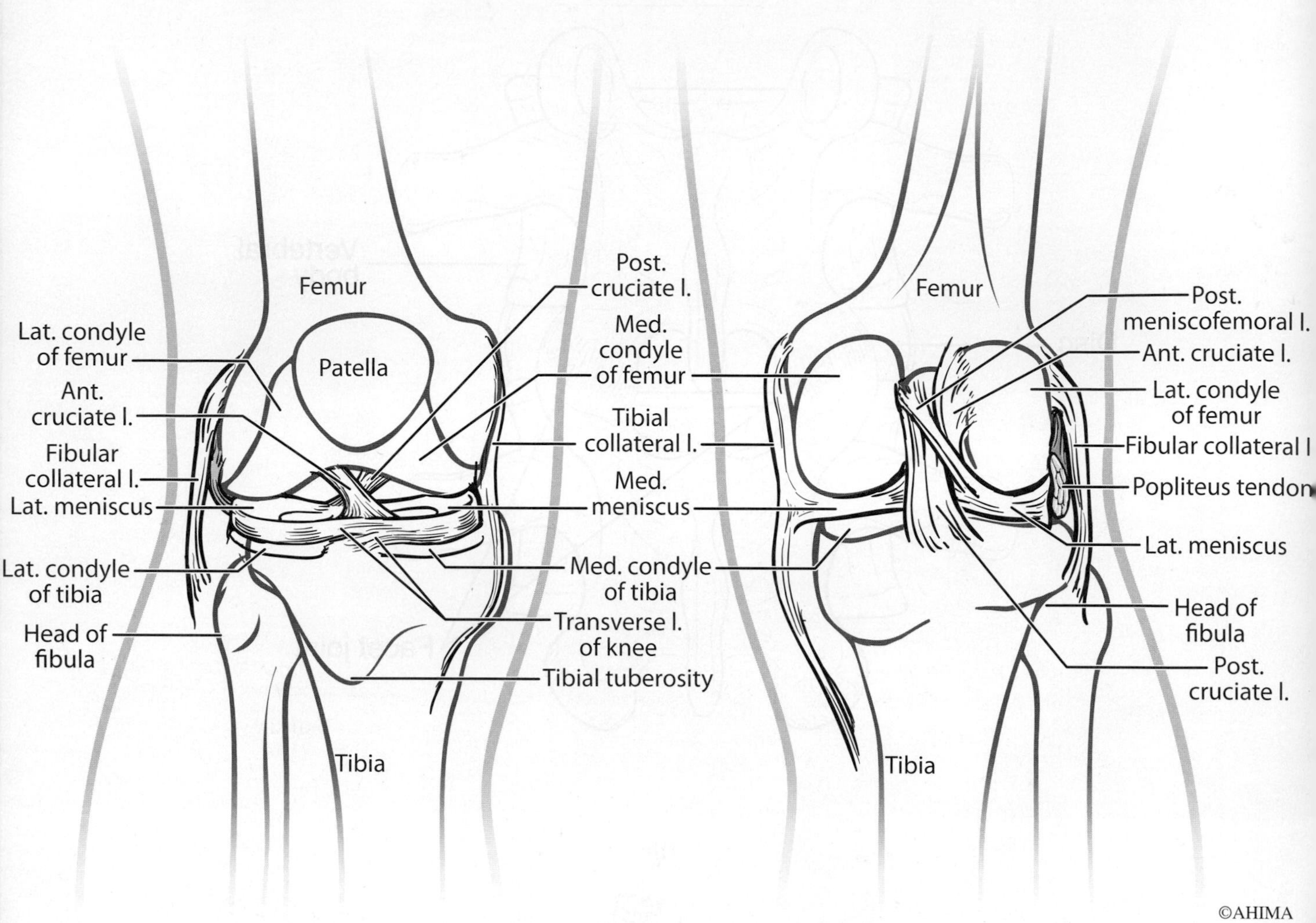
ANTERIOR
POSTERIOR
Femur
Patella
Lat. condyle of femur
Ant. cruciate l.
Fibular collateral l.
Lat. meniscus
Lat. condyle of tibia
Head of fibula
Post. cruciate l.
Med. condyle of femur
Tibial collateral l.
Med. meniscus
Med. condyle of tibia
Transverse l. of knee
Tibial tuberosity
Tibia
Femur
Post. meniscofemoral l.
Ant. cruciate l.
Lat. condyle of femur
Fibular collateral l
Popliteus tendon
Lat. meniscus
Head of fibula
Post. cruciate l.
Tibia

Ankle

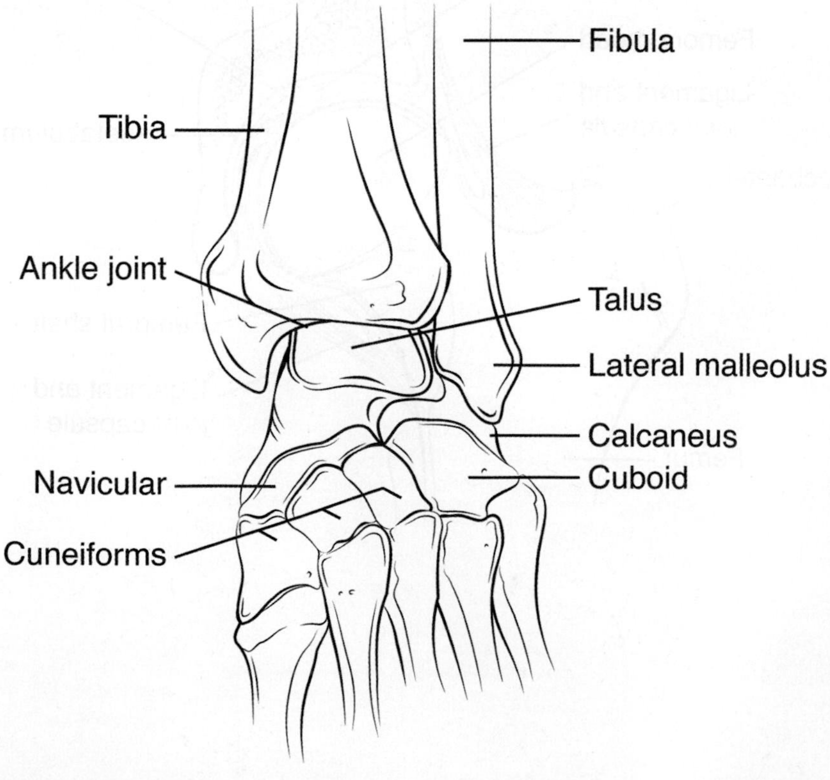
Fibula
Tibia
Ankle joint
Talus
Lateral malleolus
Calcaneus
Navicular
Cuboid
Cuneiforms

Total Knee Replacement Technique: Steps 1-5

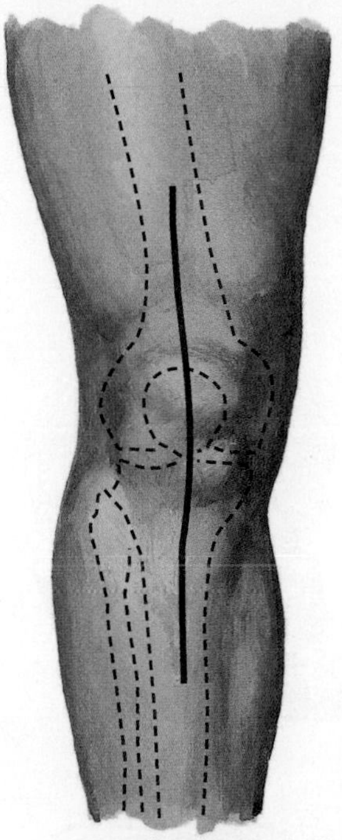

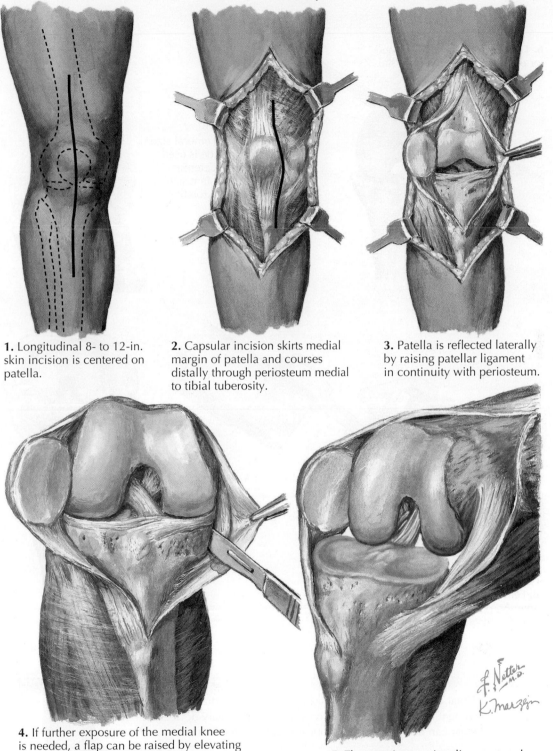

1. Longitudinal 8- to 12-in. skin incision is centered on patella.

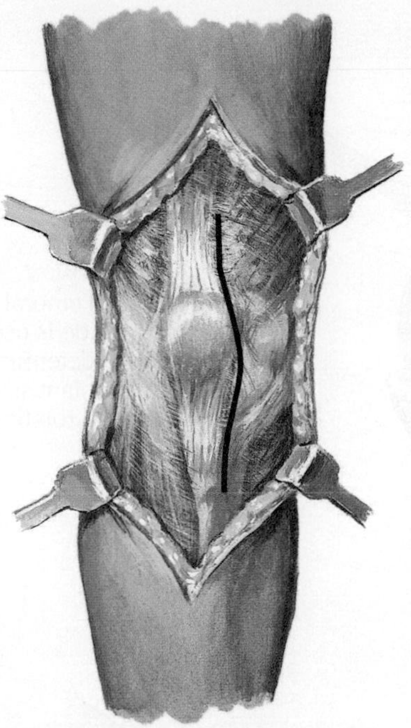

2. Capsular incision skirts medial margin of patella and courses distally through periosteum medial to tibial tuberosity.

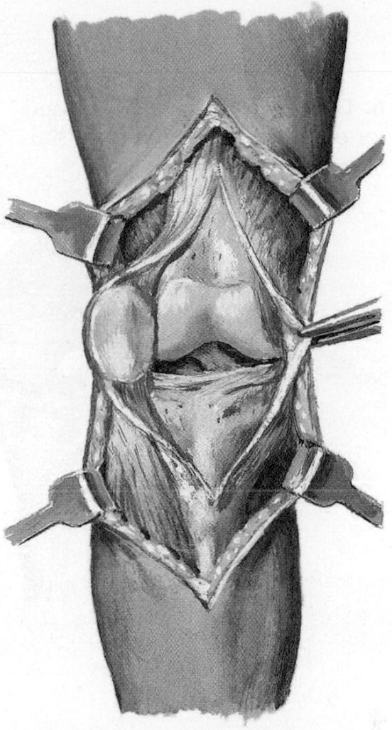

3. Patella is reflected laterally by raising patellar ligament in continuity with periosteum.

4. If further exposure of the medial knee is needed, a flap can be raised by elevating the deep medial collateral ligament and pes anserinus subperiosteally, aided by external rotation of the tibia.

5. The anterior cruciate ligament and both menisci are excised, and the tibia is subluxated anteriorly.

Total Knee Replacement Technique: Steps 6-9

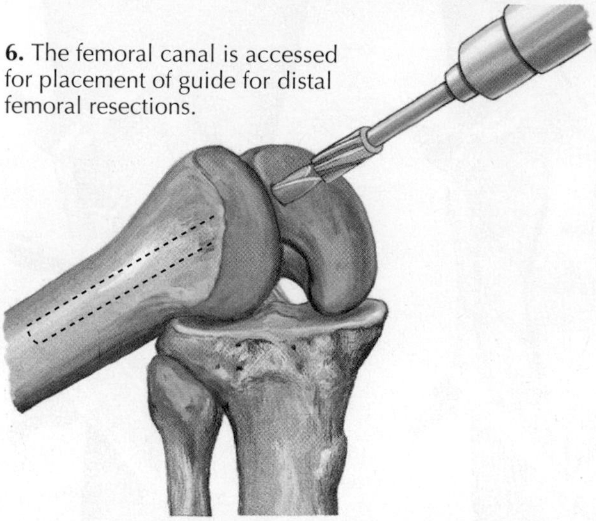

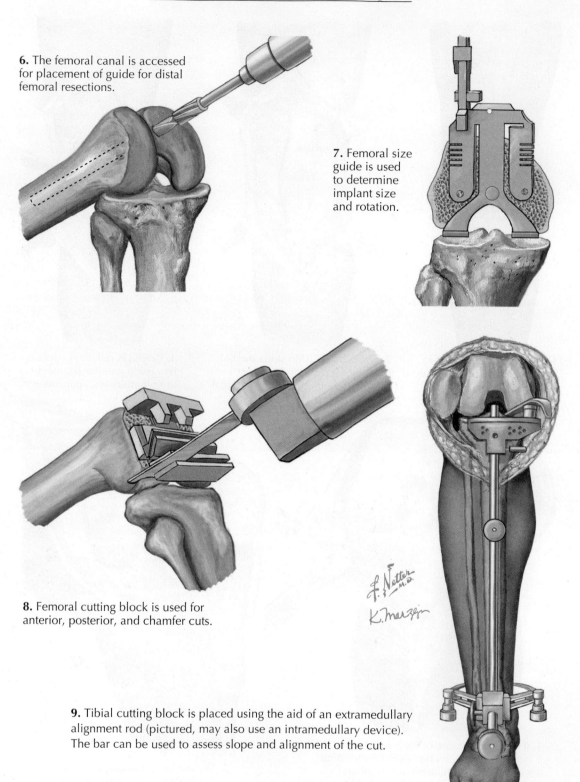

6. The femoral canal is accessed for placement of guide for distal femoral resections.

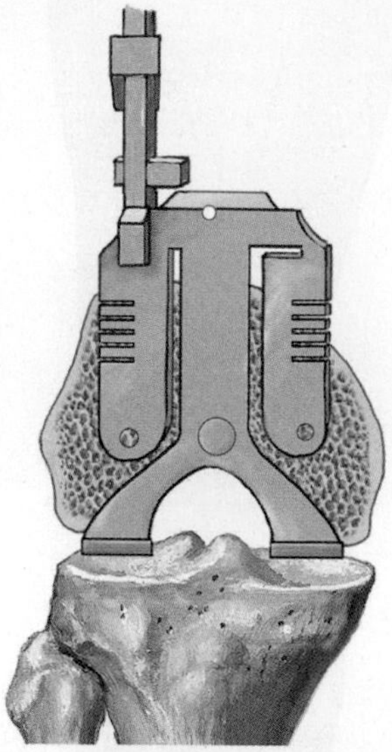

7. Femoral size guide is used to determine implant size and rotation.

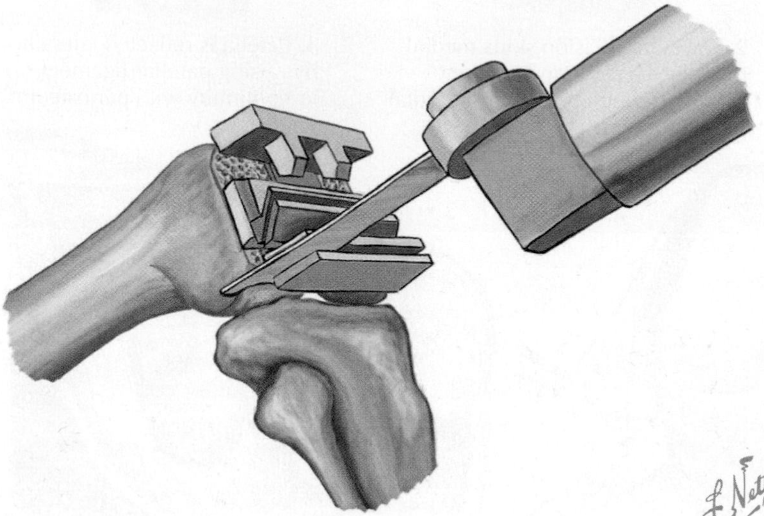

8. Femoral cutting block is used for anterior, posterior, and chamfer cuts.

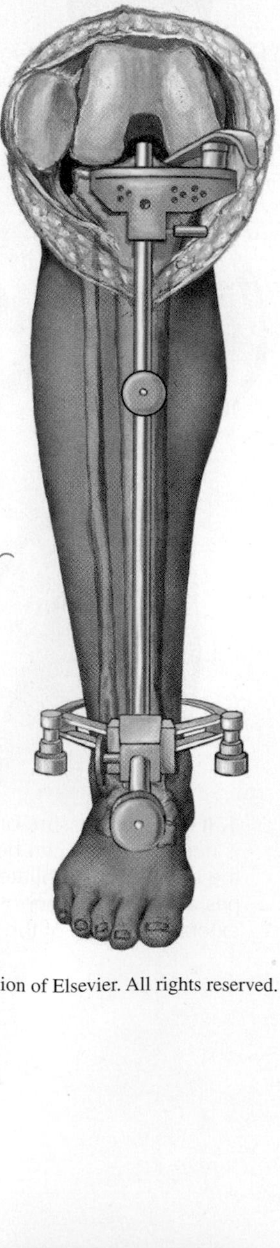

9. Tibial cutting block is placed using the aid of an extramedullary alignment rod (pictured, may also use an intramedullary device). The bar can be used to assess slope and alignment of the cut.

Total Knee Replacement Technique: Steps 10-14

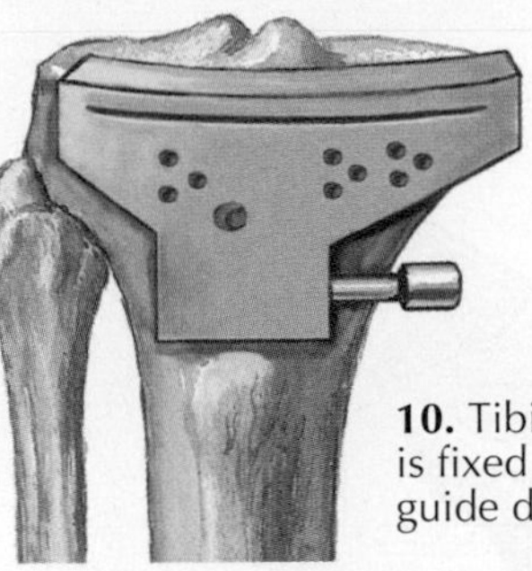

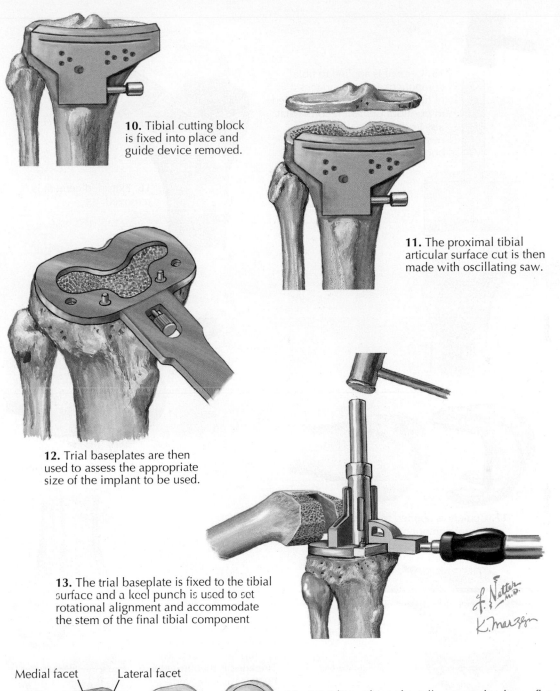

10. Tibial cutting block is fixed into place and guide device removed.

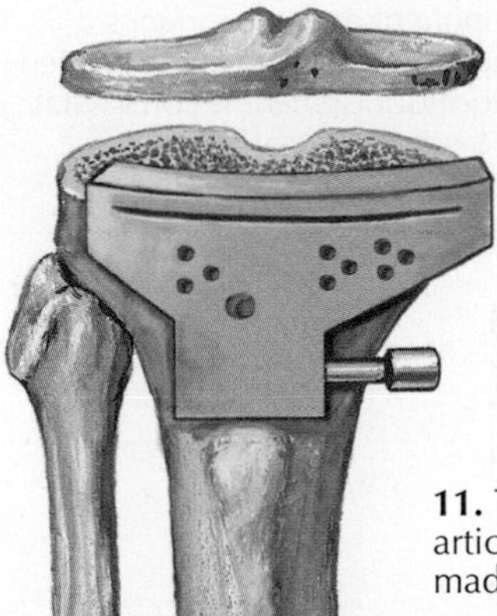

11. The proximal tibial articular surface cut is then made with oscillating saw.

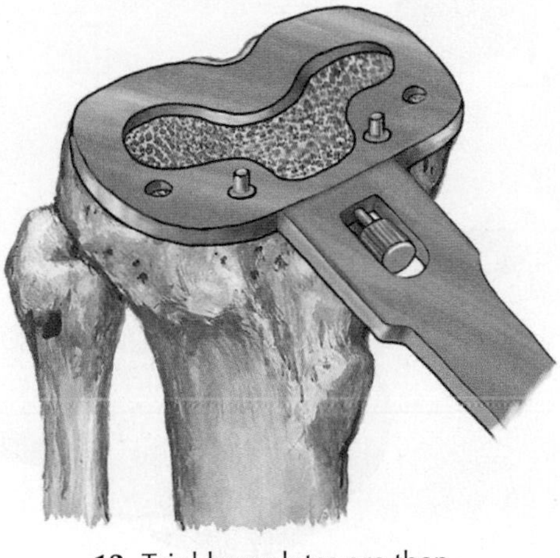

12. Trial baseplates are then used to assess the appropriate size of the implant to be used.

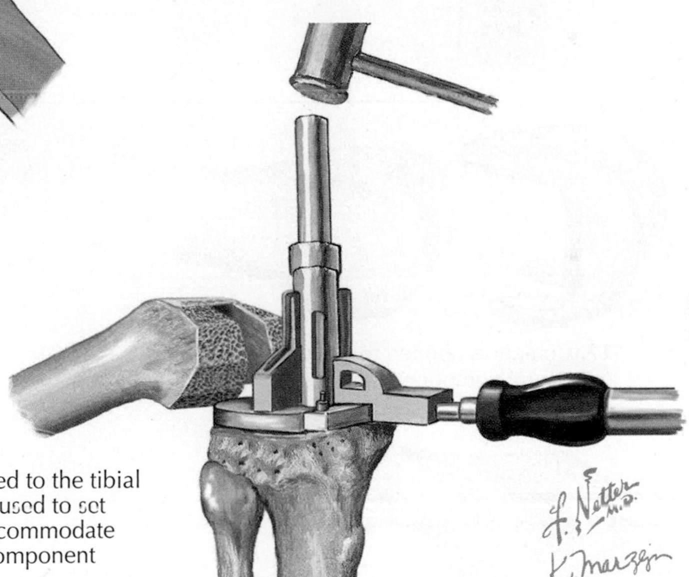

13. The trial baseplate is fixed to the tibial surface and a keel punch is used to set rotational alignment and accommodate the stem of the final tibial component

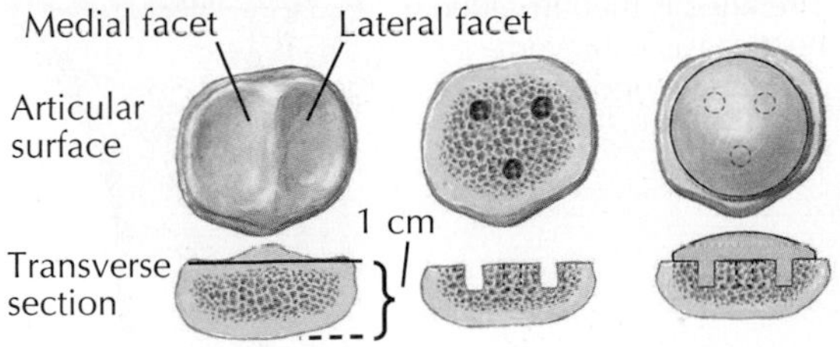
Medial facet
Lateral facet
Articular surface
1 cm
Transverse section

14. Articular surface of patella resected to leave flat surface. Equal amounts to be removed from medial and lateral facets, but at least 1 cm of bone must be left to ensure adequate strength. Using a patella drill template, three holes are drilled into the surface to accommodate the final patellar component, which is cemented in place.

Total Knee Replacement Technique: Steps 15-20

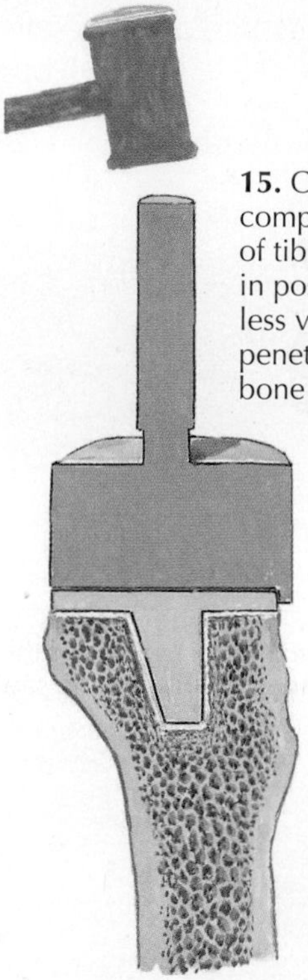

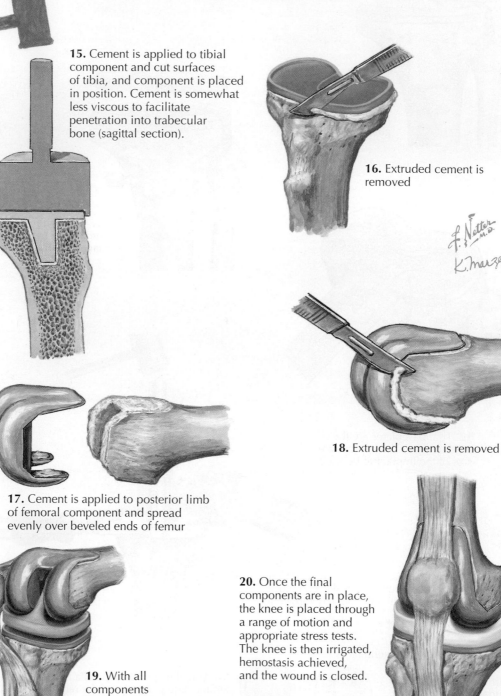

15. Cement is applied to tibial component and cut surfaces of tibia, and component is placed in position. Cement is somewhat less viscous to facilitate penetration into trabecular bone (sagittal section).

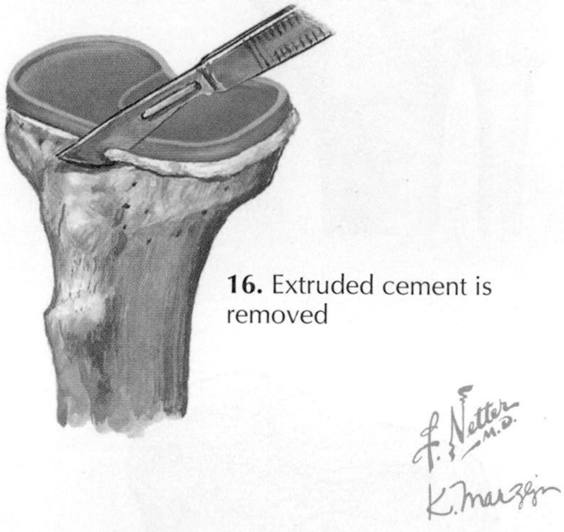

16. Extruded cement is removed

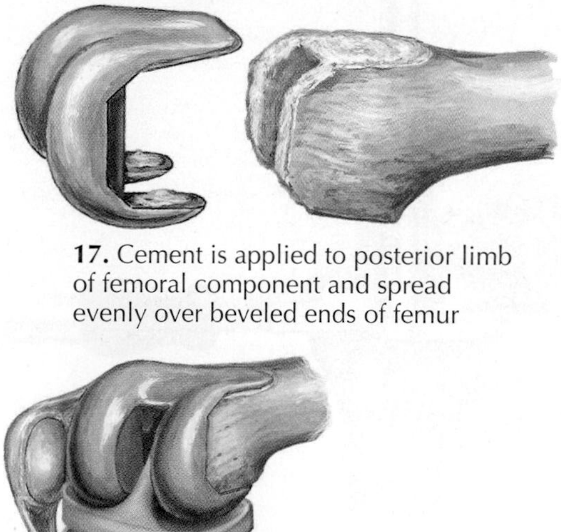

17. Cement is applied to posterior limb of femoral component and spread evenly over beveled ends of femur

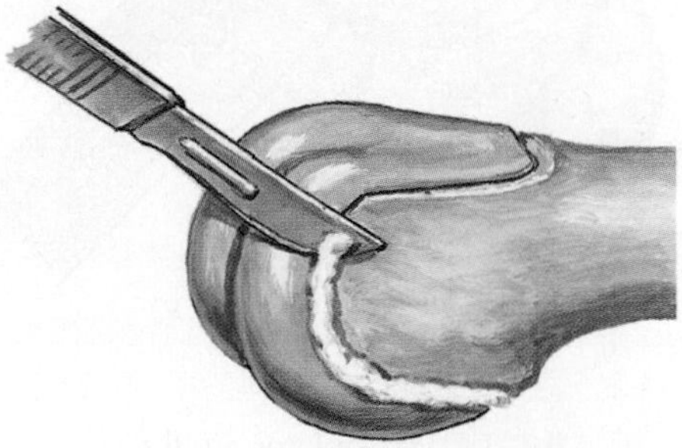

18. Extruded cement is removed

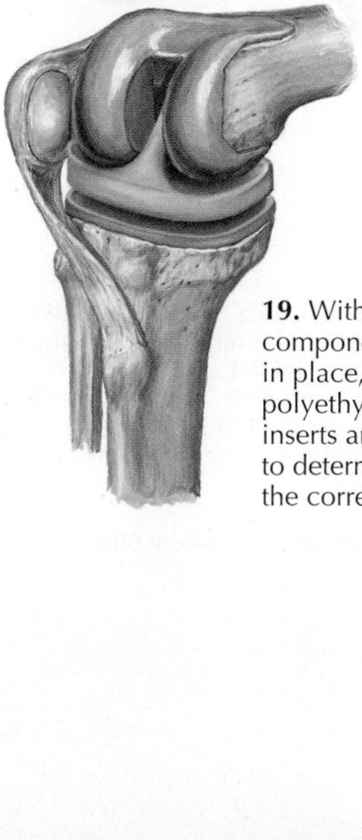

19. With all components in place, trial polyethylene inserts are used to determine the correct size.

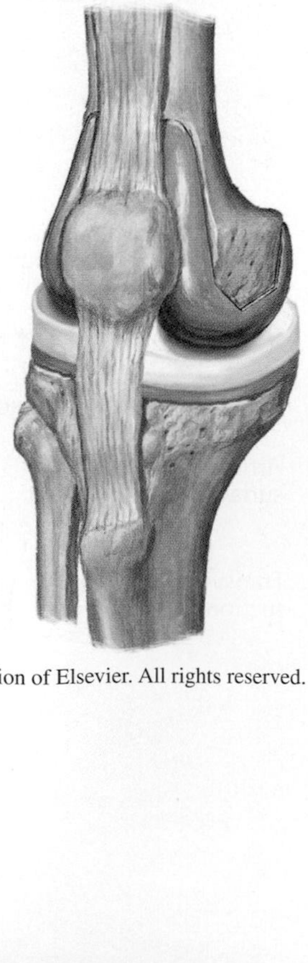

20. Once the final components are in place, the knee is placed through a range of motion and appropriate stress tests. The knee is then irrigated, hemostasis achieved, and the wound is closed.

Section 0 **Medical and Surgical**
Body System S **Lower Joints**
Operation 2 **Change:** Taking out or off a device from a body part and putting back an identical or similar device in or on the same body part without cutting or puncturing the skin or a mucous membrane

Body Part (4th)	Approach (5th)	Device (6th)	Qualifier (7th)
Y Lower Joint	**X** External	**0** Drainage Device **Y** Other Device	**Z** No Qualifier

Section 0 **Medical and Surgical**
Body System S **Lower Joints**
Operation 5 **Destruction:** Physical eradication of all or a portion of a body part by the direct use of energy, force, or a destructive agent

Body Part (4th)	Approach (5th)	Device (6th)	Qualifier (7th)
0 Lumbar Vertebral Joint **2** Lumbar Vertebral Disc **3** Lumbosacral Joint **4** Lumbosacral Disc **5** Sacrococcygeal Joint **6** Coccygeal Joint **7** Sacroiliac Joint, Right **8** Sacroiliac Joint, Left **9** Hip Joint, Right **B** Hip Joint, Left **C** Knee Joint, Right **D** Knee Joint, Left **F** Ankle Joint, Right **G** Ankle Joint, Left **H** Tarsal Joint, Right **J** Tarsal Joint, Left **K** Tarsometatarsal Joint, Right **L** Tarsometatarsal Joint, Left **M** Metatarsal-Phalangeal Joint, Right **N** Metatarsal-Phalangeal Joint, Left **P** Toe Phalangeal Joint, Right **Q** Toe Phalangeal Joint, Left	**0** Open **3** Percutaneous **4** Percutaneous Endoscopic	**Z** No Device	**Z** No Qualifier

Section 0 **Medical and Surgical**
Body System S **Lower Joints**
Operation 9 **Drainage:** Taking or letting out fluids and/or gases from a body part

Body Part (4th)	Approach (5th)	Device (6th)	Qualifier (7th)
0 Lumbar Vertebral Joint **2** Lumbar Vertebral Disc **3** Lumbosacral Joint **4** Lumbosacral Disc **5** Sacrococcygeal Joint **6** Coccygeal Joint **7** Sacroiliac Joint, Right **8** Sacroiliac Joint, Left **9** Hip Joint, Right **B** Hip Joint, Left **C** Knee Joint, Right **D** Knee Joint, Left **F** Ankle Joint, Right **G** Ankle Joint, Left **H** Tarsal Joint, Right **J** Tarsal Joint, Left **K** Tarsometatarsal Joint, Right **L** Tarsometatarsal Joint, Left **M** Metatarsal-Phalangeal Joint, Right **N** Metatarsal-Phalangeal Joint, Left **P** Toe Phalangeal Joint, Right **Q** Toe Phalangeal Joint, Left	**0** Open **3** Percutaneous **4** Percutaneous Endoscopic	**0** Drainage Device	**Z** No Qualifier
0 Lumbar Vertebral Joint **2** Lumbar Vertebral Disc **3** Lumbosacral Joint **4** Lumbosacral Disc **5** Sacrococcygeal Joint **6** Coccygeal Joint **7** Sacroiliac Joint, Right **8** Sacroiliac Joint, Left **9** Hip Joint, Right **B** Hip Joint, Left **C** Knee Joint, Right **D** Knee Joint, Left **F** Ankle Joint, Right **G** Ankle Joint, Left **H** Tarsal Joint, Right **J** Tarsal Joint, Left **K** Tarsometatarsal Joint, Right **L** Tarsometatarsal Joint, Left **M** Metatarsal-Phalangeal Joint, Right **N** Metatarsal-Phalangeal Joint, Left **P** Toe Phalangeal Joint, Right **Q** Toe Phalangeal Joint, Left	**0** Open **3** Percutaneous **4** Percutaneous Endoscopic	**Z** No Device	**X** Diagnostic **Z** No Qualifier

Section 0 **Medical and Surgical**
Body System S **Lower Joints**
Operation B **Excision:** Cutting out or off, without replacement, a portion of a body part

Body Part (4th)	Approach (5th)	Device (6th)	Qualifier (7th)
0 Lumbar Vertebral Joint 2 Lumbar Vertebral Disc 3 Lumbosacral Joint 4 Lumbosacral Disc 5 Sacrococcygeal Joint 6 Coccygeal Joint 7 Sacroiliac Joint, Right 8 Sacroiliac Joint, Left 9 Hip Joint, Right B Hip Joint, Left C Knee Joint, Right D Knee Joint, Left F Ankle Joint, Right G Ankle Joint, Left H Tarsal Joint, Right J Tarsal Joint, Left K Tarsometatarsal Joint, Right L Tarsometatarsal Joint, Left M Metatarsal-Phalangeal Joint, Right N Metatarsal-Phalangeal Joint, Left P Toe Phalangeal Joint, Right Q Toe Phalangeal Joint, Left	0 Open 3 Percutaneous 4 Percutaneous Endoscopic	Z No Device	X Diagnostic Z No Qualifier

Section 0 **Medical and Surgical**
Body System S **Lower Joints**
Operation C **Extirpation:** Taking or cutting out solid matter from a body part

Body Part (4th)	Approach (5th)	Device (6th)	Qualifier (7th)
0 Lumbar Vertebral Joint 2 Lumbar Vertebral Disc 3 Lumbosacral Joint 4 Lumbosacral Disc 5 Sacrococcygeal Joint 6 Coccygeal Joint 7 Sacroiliac Joint, Right 8 Sacroiliac Joint, Left 9 Hip Joint, Right B Hip Joint, Left C Knee Joint, Right D Knee Joint, Left F Ankle Joint, Right G Ankle Joint, Left H Tarsal Joint, Right J Tarsal Joint, Left K Tarsometatarsal Joint, Right L Tarsometatarsal Joint, Left M Metatarsal-Phalangeal Joint, Right N Metatarsal-Phalangeal Joint, Left P Toe Phalangeal Joint, Right Q Toe Phalangeal Joint, Left	0 Open 3 Percutaneous 4 Percutaneous Endoscopic	Z No Device	Z No Qualifier

Section 0 **Medical and Surgical**
Body System S **Lower Joints**
Operation G **Fusion:** Joining together portions of an articular body part rendering the articular body part immobile

Body Part (4th)	Approach (5th)	Device (6th)	Qualifier (7th)
0 Lumbar Vertebral Joint **1** Lumbar Vertebral Joints, 2 or more **3** Lumbosacral Joint	**0** Open **3** Percutaneous **4** Percutaneous Endoscopic	**7** Autologous Tissue Substitute **J** Synthetic Substitute **K** Nonautologous Tissue Substitute	**0** Anterior Approach, Anterior Column **1** Posterior Approach, Posterior Column **J** Posterior Approach, Anterior Column
0 Lumbar Vertebral Joint **1** Lumbar Vertebral Joints, 2 or more **3** Lumbosacral Joint	**0** Open **3** Percutaneous **4** Percutaneous Endoscopic	**A** Interbody Fusion Device	**0** Anterior Approach, Anterior Column **J** Posterior Approach, Anterior Column
5 Sacrococcygeal Joint **6** Coccygeal Joint **7** Sacroiliac Joint, Right **8** Sacroiliac Joint, Left	**0** Open **3** Percutaneous **4** Percutaneous Endoscopic	**4** Internal Fixation Device **7** Autologous Tissue Substitute **J** Synthetic Substitute **K** Nonautologous Tissue Substitute	**Z** No Qualifier
9 Hip Joint, Right **B** Hip Joint, Left **C** Knee Joint, Right **D** Knee Joint, Left **F** Ankle Joint, Right **G** Ankle Joint, Left **H** Tarsal Joint, Right **J** Tarsal Joint, Left **K** Tarsometatarsal Joint, Right **L** Tarsometatarsal Joint, Left **M** Metatarsal-Phalangeal Joint, Right **N** Metatarsal-Phalangeal Joint, Left **P** Toe Phalangeal Joint, Right **Q** Toe Phalangeal Joint, Left	**0** Open **3** Percutaneous **4** Percutaneous Endoscopic	**3** Internal Fixation Device, Sustained Compression **4** Internal Fixation Device **5** External Fixation Device **7** Autologous Tissue Substitute **J** Synthetic Substitute **K** Nonautologous Tissue Substitute	**Z** No Qualifier

Section 0 **Medical and Surgical**
Body System S **Lower Joints**
Operation H **Insertion:** Putting in a nonbiological appliance that monitors, assists, performs, or prevents a physiological function but does not physically take the place of a body part

Body Part (4th)	Approach (5th)	Device (6th)	Qualifier (7th)
0 Lumbar Vertebral Joint **3** Lumbosacral Joint	**0** Open **3** Percutaneous **4** Percutaneous Endoscopic	**3** Infusion Device **4** Internal Fixation Device **8** Spacer **B** Spinal Stabilization Device, Interspinous Process **C** Spinal Stabilization Device, Pedicle-Based **D** Spinal Stabilization Device, Facet Replacement	**Z** No Qualifier
2 Lumbar Vertebral Disc **4** Lumbosacral Disc	**0** Open **3** Percutaneous **4** Percutaneous Endoscopic	**3** Infusion Device **8** Spacer	**Z** No Qualifier
5 Sacrococcygeal Joint **6** Coccygeal Joint **7** Sacroiliac Joint, Right **8** Sacroiliac Joint, Left	**0** Open **3** Percutaneous **4** Percutaneous Endoscopic	**3** Infusion Device **4** Internal Fixation Device **8** Spacer	**Z** No Qualifier

Continued →

Section 0 Medical and Surgical
Body System S Lower Joints
Operation H **Insertion:** Putting in a nonbiological appliance that monitors, assists, performs, or prevents a physiological function but does not physically take the place of a body part

Body Part (4th)	Approach (5th)	Device (6th)	Qualifier (7th)
9 Hip Joint, Right **B** Hip Joint, Left **C** Knee Joint, Right **D** Knee Joint, Left **F** Ankle Joint, Right **G** Ankle Joint, Left **H** Tarsal Joint, Right **J** Tarsal Joint, Left **K** Tarsometatarsal Joint, Right **L** Tarsometatarsal Joint, Left **M** Metatarsal-Phalangeal Joint, Right **N** Metatarsal-Phalangeal Joint, Left **P** Toe Phalangeal Joint, Right **Q** Toe Phalangeal Joint, Left	**0** Open **3** Percutaneous **4** Percutaneous Endoscopic	**3** Infusion Device **4** Internal Fixation Device **5** External Fixation Device **8** Spacer	**Z** No Qualifier

Section 0 Medical and Surgical
Body System S Lower Joints
Operation J **Inspection:** Visually and/or manually exploring a body part

Body Part (4th)	Approach (5th)	Device (6th)	Qualifier (7th)
0 Lumbar Vertebral Joint **2** Lumbar Vertebral Disc **3** Lumbosacral Joint **4** Lumbosacral Disc **5** Sacrococcygeal Joint **6** Coccygeal Joint **7** Sacroiliac Joint, Right **8** Sacroiliac Joint, Left **9** Hip Joint, Right **B** Hip Joint, Left **C** Knee Joint, Right **D** Knee Joint, Left **F** Ankle Joint, Right **G** Ankle Joint, Left **H** Tarsal Joint, Right **J** Tarsal Joint, Left **K** Tarsometatarsal Joint, Right **L** Tarsometatarsal Joint, Left **M** Metatarsal-Phalangeal Joint, Right **N** Metatarsal-Phalangeal Joint, Left **P** Toe Phalangeal Joint, Right **Q** Toe Phalangeal Joint, Left	**0** Open **3** Percutaneous **4** Percutaneous Endoscopic **X** External	**Z** No Device	**Z** No Qualifier

Section 0 **Medical and Surgical**
Body System S **Lower Joints**
Operation N **Release:** Freeing a body part from an abnormal physical constraint by cutting or by the use of force

Body Part (4th)	Approach (5th)	Device (6th)	Qualifier (7th)
0 Lumbar Vertebral Joint 2 Lumbar Vertebral Disc 3 Lumbosacral Joint 4 Lumbosacral Disc 5 Sacrococcygeal Joint 6 Coccygeal Joint 7 Sacroiliac Joint, Right 8 Sacroiliac Joint, Left 9 Hip Joint, Right B Hip Joint, Left C Knee Joint, Right D Knee Joint, Left F Ankle Joint, Right G Ankle Joint, Left H Tarsal Joint, Right J Tarsal Joint, Left K Tarsometatarsal Joint, Right L Tarsometatarsal Joint, Left M Metatarsal-Phalangeal Joint, Right N Metatarsal-Phalangeal Joint, Left P Toe Phalangeal Joint, Right Q Toe Phalangeal Joint, Left	0 Open 3 Percutaneous 4 Percutaneous Endoscopic X External	Z No Device	Z No Qualifier

Section 0 **Medical and Surgical**
Body System S **Lower Joints**
Operation P **Removal:** Taking out or off a device from a body part

Body Part (4th)	Approach (5th)	Device (6th)	Qualifier (7th)
0 Lumbar Vertebral Joint 3 Lumbosacral Joint	0 Open 3 Percutaneous 4 Percutaneous Endoscopic	0 Drainage Device 3 Infusion Device 4 Internal Fixation Device 7 Autologous Tissue Substitute 8 Spacer A Interbody Fusion Device J Synthetic Substitute K Nonautologous Tissue Substitute	Z No Qualifier
0 Lumbar Vertebral Joint 3 Lumbosacral Joint	X External	0 Drainage Device 3 Infusion Device 4 Internal Fixation Device	Z No Qualifier
2 Lumbar Vertebral Disc 4 Lumbosacral Disc	0 Open 3 Percutaneous 4 Percutaneous Endoscopic	0 Drainage Device 3 Infusion Device 7 Autologous Tissue Substitute J Synthetic Substitute K Nonautologous Tissue Substitute	Z No Qualifier
2 Lumbar Vertebral Disc 4 Lumbosacral Disc	X External	0 Drainage Device 3 Infusion Device	Z No Qualifier
5 Sacrococcygeal Joint 6 Coccygeal Joint 7 Sacroiliac Joint, Right 8 Sacroiliac Joint, Left	0 Open 3 Percutaneous 4 Percutaneous Endoscopic	0 Drainage Device 3 Infusion Device 4 Internal Fixation Device 7 Autologous Tissue Substitute 8 Spacer J Synthetic Substitute K Nonautologous Tissue Substitute	Z No Qualifier

Continued →

Section 0 Medical and Surgical
Body System S Lower Joints
Operation P **Removal:** Taking out or off a device from a body part

Body Part (4th)	Approach (5th)	Device (6th)	Qualifier (7th)
5 Sacrococcygeal Joint **6** Coccygeal Joint **7** Sacroiliac Joint, Right **8** Sacroiliac Joint, Left	**X** External	**0** Drainage Device **3** Infusion Device **4** Internal Fixation Device	**Z** No Qualifier
9 Hip Joint, Right **B** Hip Joint, Left	**0** Open	**0** Drainage Device **3** Infusion Device **4** Internal Fixation Device **5** External Fixation Device **7** Autologous Tissue Substitute **8** Spacer **9** Liner **B** Resurfacing Device **E** Articulating Spacer **J** Synthetic Substitute **K** Nonautologous Tissue Substitute	**Z** No Qualifier
9 Hip Joint, Right **B** Hip Joint, Left	**3** Percutaneous **4** Percutaneous Endoscopic	**0** Drainage Device **3** Infusion Device **4** Internal Fixation Device **5** External Fixation Device **7** Autologous Tissue Substitute **8** Spacer **J** Synthetic Substitute **K** Nonautologous Tissue Substitute	**Z** No Qualifier
9 Hip Joint, Right **B** Hip Joint, Left	**X** External	**0** Drainage Device **3** Infusion Device **4** Internal Fixation Device **5** External Fixation Device	**Z** No Qualifier
A Hip Joint, Acetabular Surface, Right **E** Hip Joint, Acetabular Surface, Left **R** Hip Joint, Femoral Surface, Right **S** Hip Joint, Femoral Surface, Left **T** Knee Joint, Femoral Surface, Right **U** Knee Joint, Femoral Surface, Left **V** Knee Joint, Tibial Surface, Right **W** Knee Joint, Tibial Surface, Left	**0** Open **3** Percutaneous **4** Percutaneous Endoscopic	**J** Synthetic Substitute	**Z** No Qualifier
C Knee Joint, Right **D** Knee Joint, Left	**0** Open	**0** Drainage Device **3** Infusion Device **4** Internal Fixation Device **5** External Fixation Device **7** Autologous Tissue Substitute **8** Spacer **9** Liner **E** Articulating Spacer **K** Nonautologous Tissue Substitute **L** Synthetic Substitute, Unicondylar Medial **M** Synthetic Substitute, Unicondylar Lateral **N** Synthetic Substitute, Unicondylar Patellofemoral	**Z** No Qualifier
C Knee Joint, Right **D** Knee Joint, Left	**0** Open	**J** Synthetic Substitute	**C** Patellar Surface **Z** No Qualifier

Continued →

Section **0** **Medical and Surgical** *0SP Continued*
Body System **S** **Lower Joints**
Operation **P** **Removal:** Taking out or off a device from a body part

Body Part (4th)	Approach (5th)	Device (6th)	Qualifier (7th)
C Knee Joint, Right **D** Knee Joint, Left	**3** Percutaneous **4** Percutaneous Endoscopic	**0** Drainage Device **3** Infusion Device **4** Internal Fixation Device **5** External Fixation Device **7** Autologous Tissue Substitute **8** Spacer **K** Nonautologous Tissue Substitute **L** Synthetic Substitute, Unicondylar Medial **M** Synthetic Substitute, Unicondylar Lateral **N** Synthetic Substitute, Unicondylar Patellofemoral	**Z** No Qualifier
C Knee Joint, Right **D** Knee Joint, Left	**3** Percutaneous **4** Percutaneous Endoscopic	**J** Synthetic Substitute	**C** Patellar Surface **Z** No Qualifier
C Knee Joint, Right **D** Knee Joint, Left	**X** External	**0** Drainage Device **3** Infusion Device **4** Internal Fixation Device **5** External Fixation Device	**Z** No Qualifier
F Ankle Joint, Right **G** Ankle Joint, Left **H** Tarsal Joint, Right **J** Tarsal Joint, Left **K** Tarsometatarsal Joint, Right **L** Tarsometatarsal Joint, Left **M** Metatarsal-Phalangeal Joint, Right **N** Metatarsal-Phalangeal Joint, Left **P** Toe Phalangeal Joint, Right **Q** Toe Phalangeal Joint, Left	**0** Open **3** Percutaneous **4** Percutaneous Endoscopic	**0** Drainage Device **3** Infusion Device **4** Internal Fixation Device **5** External Fixation Device **7** Autologous Tissue Substitute **8** Spacer **J** Synthetic Substitute **K** Nonautologous Tissue Substitute	**Z** No Qualifier
F Ankle Joint, Right **G** Ankle Joint, Left **H** Tarsal Joint, Right **J** Tarsal Joint, Left **K** Tarsometatarsal Joint, Right **L** Tarsometatarsal Joint, Left **M** Metatarsal-Phalangeal Joint, Right **N** Metatarsal-Phalangeal Joint, Left **P** Toe Phalangeal Joint, Right **Q** Toe Phalangeal Joint, Left	**X** External	**0** Drainage Device **3** Infusion Device **4** Internal Fixation Device **5** External Fixation Device	**Z** No Qualifier

Section 0 **Medical and Surgical**
Body System S **Lower Joints**
Operation Q **Repair:** Restoring, to the extent possible, a body part to its normal anatomic structure and function

Body Part (4th)	Approach (5th)	Device (6th)	Qualifier (7th)
0 Lumbar Vertebral Joint **2** Lumbar Vertebral Disc **3** Lumbosacral Joint **4** Lumbosacral Disc **5** Sacrococcygeal Joint **6** Coccygeal Joint **7** Sacroiliac Joint, Right **8** Sacroiliac Joint, Left **9** Hip Joint, Right **B** Hip Joint, Left **C** Knee Joint, Right **D** Knee Joint, Left **F** Ankle Joint, Right **G** Ankle Joint, Left **H** Tarsal Joint, Right **J** Tarsal Joint, Left **K** Tarsometatarsal Joint, Right **L** Tarsometatarsal Joint, Left **M** Metatarsal-Phalangeal Joint, Right **N** Metatarsal-Phalangeal Joint, Left **P** Toe Phalangeal Joint, Right **Q** Toe Phalangeal Joint, Left	**0** Open **3** Percutaneous **4** Percutaneous Endoscopic **X** External	**Z** No Device	**Z** No Qualifier

Section 0 **Medical and Surgical**
Body System S **Lower Joints**
Operation R **Replacement:** Putting in or on biological or synthetic material that physically takes the place and/or function of all or a portion of a body part

Body Part (4th)	Approach (5th)	Device (6th)	Qualifier (7th)
0 Lumbar Vertebral Joint **2** Lumbar Vertebral Disc **3** Lumbosacral Joint **4** Lumbosacral Disc **5** Sacrococcygeal Joint **6** Coccygeal Joint **7** Sacroiliac Joint, Right **8** Sacroiliac Joint, Left **H** Tarsal Joint, Right **J** Tarsal Joint, Left **K** Tarsometatarsal Joint, Right **L** Tarsometatarsal Joint, Left **M** Metatarsal-Phalangeal Joint, Right **N** Metatarsal-Phalangeal Joint, Left **P** Toe Phalangeal Joint, Right **Q** Toe Phalangeal Joint, Left	**0** Open	**7** Autologous Tissue Substitute **J** Synthetic Substitute **K** Nonautologous Tissue Substitute	**Z** No Qualifier
9 Hip Joint, Right **B** Hip Joint, Left	**0** Open	**1** Synthetic Substitute, Metal **2** Synthetic Substitute, Metal on Polyethylene **3** Synthetic Substitute, Ceramic **4** Synthetic Substitute, Ceramic on Polyethylene **6** Synthetic Substitute, Oxidized Zirconium on Polyethylene **J** Synthetic Substitute	**9** Cemented **A** Uncemented **Z** No Qualifier
9 Hip Joint, Right **B** Hip Joint, Left	**0** Open	**7** Autologous Tissue Substitute **E** Articulating Spacer **K** Nonautologous Tissue Substitute	**Z** No Qualifier
A Hip Joint, Acetabular Surface, Right **E** Hip Joint, Acetabular Surface, Left	**0** Open	**0** Synthetic Substitute, Polyethylene **1** Synthetic Substitute, Metal **3** Synthetic Substitute, Ceramic **J** Synthetic Substitute	**9** Cemented **A** Uncemented **Z** No Qualifier

Continued →

Section 0 **Medical and Surgical**
Body System S **Lower Joints**
Operation R **Replacement:** Putting in or on biological or synthetic material that physically takes the place and/or function of all or a portion of a body part

Body Part (4th)	Approach (5th)	Device (6th)	Qualifier (7th)
A Hip Joint, Acetabular Surface, Right **E** Hip Joint, Acetabular Surface, Left	**0** Open	**7** Autologous Tissue Substitute **K** Nonautologous Tissue Substitute	**Z** No Qualifier
C Knee Joint, Right **D** Knee Joint, Left	**0** Open	**6** Synthetic Substitute, Oxidized Zirconium on Polyethylene **J** Synthetic Substitute **L** Synthetic Substitute, Unicondylar Medial **M** Synthetic Substitute, Unicondylar Lateral **N** Synthetic Substitute, Unicondylar Patellofemoral	**9** Cemented **A** Uncemented **Z** No Qualifier
C Knee Joint, Right **D** Knee Joint, Left	**0** Open	**7** Autologous Tissue Substitute **E** Articulating Spacer **K** Nonautologous Tissue Substitute	**Z** No Qualifier
F Ankle Joint, Right **G** Ankle Joint, Left **T** Knee Joint, Femoral Surface, Right **U** Knee Joint, Femoral Surface, Left **V** Knee Joint, Tibial Surface, Right **W** Knee Joint, Tibial Surface, Left	**0** Open	**7** Autologous Tissue Substitute **K** Nonautologous Tissue Substitute	**Z** No Qualifier
F Ankle Joint, Right **G** Ankle Joint, Left **T** Knee Joint, Femoral Surface, Right **U** Knee Joint, Femoral Surface, Left **V** Knee Joint, Tibial Surface, Right **W** Knee Joint, Tibial Surface, Left	**0** Open	**J** Synthetic Substitute	**9** Cemented **A** Uncemented **Z** No Qualifier
R Hip Joint, Femoral Surface, Right **S** Hip Joint, Femoral Surface, Left	**0** Open	**1** Synthetic Substitute, Metal **3** Synthetic Substitute, Ceramic **J** Synthetic Substitute	**9** Cemented **A** Uncemented **Z** No Qualifier
R Hip Joint, Femoral Surface, Right **S** Hip Joint, Femoral Surface, Left	**0** Open	**7** Autologous Tissue Substitute **K** Nonautologous Tissue Substitute	**Z** No Qualifier

Section 0 **Medical and Surgical**
Body System S **Lower Joints**
Operation S **Reposition:** Moving to its normal location, or other suitable location, all or a portion of a body part

Body Part (4th)	Approach (5th)	Device (6th)	Qualifier (7th)
0 Lumbar Vertebral Joint **3** Lumbosacral Joint **5** Sacrococcygeal Joint **6** Coccygeal Joint **7** Sacroiliac Joint, Right **8** Sacroiliac Joint, Left	**0** Open **3** Percutaneous **4** Percutaneous Endoscopic **X** External	**4** Internal Fixation Device **Z** No Device	**Z** No Qualifier
9 Hip Joint, Right **B** Hip Joint, Left **C** Knee Joint, Right **D** Knee Joint, Left **F** Ankle Joint, Right **G** Ankle Joint, Left **H** Tarsal Joint, Right **J** Tarsal Joint, Left **K** Tarsometatarsal Joint, Right **L** Tarsometatarsal Joint, Left **M** Metatarsal-Phalangeal Joint, Right **N** Metatarsal-Phalangeal Joint, Left **P** Toe Phalangeal Joint, Right **Q** Toe Phalangeal Joint, Left	**0** Open **3** Percutaneous **4** Percutaneous Endoscopic **X** External	**4** Internal Fixation Device **5** External Fixation Device **Z** No Device	**Z** No Qualifier

Section 0 **Medical and Surgical**
Body System S **Lower Joints**
Operation T **Resection:** Cutting out or off, without replacement, all of a body part

Body Part (4th)	Approach (5th)	Device (6th)	Qualifier (7th)
2 Lumbar Vertebral Disc **4** Lumbosacral Disc **5** Sacrococcygeal Joint **6** Coccygeal Joint **7** Sacroiliac Joint, Right **8** Sacroiliac Joint, Left **9** Hip Joint, Right **B** Hip Joint, Left **C** Knee Joint, Right **D** Knee Joint, Left **F** Ankle Joint, Right **G** Ankle Joint, Left **H** Tarsal Joint, Right **J** Tarsal Joint, Left **K** Tarsometatarsal Joint, Right **L** Tarsometatarsal Joint, Left **M** Metatarsal-Phalangeal Joint, Right **N** Metatarsal-Phalangeal Joint, Left **P** Toe Phalangeal Joint, Right **Q** Toe Phalangeal Joint, Left	**0** Open	**Z** No Device	**Z** No Qualifier

Section 0 **Medical and Surgical**
Body System S **Lower Joints**
Operation U **Supplement:** Putting in or on biological or synthetic material that physically reinforces and/or augments the function of a portion of a body part

Body Part (4th)	Approach (5th)	Device (6th)	Qualifier (7th)
0 Lumbar Vertebral Joint **2** Lumbar Vertebral Disc **3** Lumbosacral Joint **4** Lumbosacral Disc **5** Sacrococcygeal Joint **6** Coccygeal Joint **7** Sacroiliac Joint, Right **8** Sacroiliac Joint, Left **F** Ankle Joint, Right **G** Ankle Joint, Left **H** Tarsal Joint, Right **J** Tarsal Joint, Left **K** Tarsometatarsal Joint, Right **L** Tarsometatarsal Joint, Left **M** Metatarsal-Phalangeal Joint, Right **N** Metatarsal-Phalangeal Joint, Left **P** Toe Phalangeal Joint, Right **Q** Toe Phalangeal Joint, Left	**0** Open **3** Percutaneous **4** Percutaneous Endoscopic	**7** Autologous Tissue Substitute **J** Synthetic Substitute **K** Nonautologous Tissue Substitute	**Z** No Qualifier
9 Hip Joint, Right **B** Hip Joint, Left	**0** Open	**7** Autologous Tissue Substitute **9** Liner **B** Resurfacing Device **J** Synthetic Substitute **K** Nonautologous Tissue Substitute	**Z** No Qualifier
9 Hip Joint, Right **B** Hip Joint, Left	**3** Percutaneous **4** Percutaneous Endoscopic	**7** Autologous Tissue Substitute **J** Synthetic Substitute **K** Nonautologous Tissue Substitute	**Z** No Qualifier
A Hip Joint, Acetabular Surface, Right **E** Hip Joint, Acetabular Surface, Left **R** Hip Joint, Femoral Surface, Right **S** Hip Joint, Femoral Surface, Left	**0** Open	**9** Liner **B** Resurfacing Device	**Z** No Qualifier

Continued →

Section 0 **Medical and Surgical**
Body System S **Lower Joints**
Operation U **Supplement:** Putting in or on biological or synthetic material that physically reinforces and/or augments the function of a portion of a body part

Body Part (4th)	Approach (5th)	Device (6th)	Qualifier (7th)
C Knee Joint, Right **D** Knee Joint, Left	**0** Open	**7** Autologous Tissue Substitute **J** Synthetic Substitute **K** Nonautologous Tissue Substitute	**Z** No Qualifier
C Knee Joint, Right **D** Knee Joint, Left	**0** Open	**9** Liner	**C** Patellar Surface **Z** No Qualifier
C Knee Joint, Right **D** Knee Joint, Left	**3** Percutaneous **4** Percutaneous Endoscopic	**7** Autologous Tissue Substitute **J** Synthetic Substitute **K** Nonautologous Tissue Substitute	**Z** No Qualifier
T Knee Joint, Femoral Surface, Right **U** Knee Joint, Femoral Surface, Left **V** Knee Joint, Tibial Surface, Right **W** Knee Joint, Tibial Surface, Left	**0** Open	**9** Liner	**Z** No Qualifier

Section 0 **Medical and Surgical**
Body System S **Lower Joints**
Operation W **Revision:** Correcting, to the extent possible, a portion of a malfunctioning device or the position of a displaced device

Body Part (4th)	Approach (5th)	Device (6th)	Qualifier (7th)
0 Lumbar Vertebral Joint **3** Lumbosacral Joint	**0** Open **3** Percutaneous **4** Percutaneous Endoscopic **X** External	**0** Drainage Device **3** Infusion Device **4** Internal Fixation Device **7** Autologous Tissue Substitute **8** Spacer **A** Interbody Fusion Device **J** Synthetic Substitute **K** Nonautologous Tissue Substitute	**Z** No Qualifier
2 Lumbar Vertebral Disc **4** Lumbosacral Disc	**0** Open **3** Percutaneous **4** Percutaneous Endoscopic **X** External	**0** Drainage Device **3** Infusion Device **7** Autologous Tissue Substitute **J** Synthetic Substitute **K** Nonautologous Tissue Substitute	**Z** No Qualifier
5 Sacrococcygeal Joint **6** Coccygeal Joint **7** Sacroiliac Joint, Right **8** Sacroiliac Joint, Left	**0** Open **3** Percutaneous **4** Percutaneous Endoscopic **X** External	**0** Drainage Device **3** Infusion Device **4** Internal Fixation Device **7** Autologous Tissue Substitute **8** Spacer **J** Synthetic Substitute **K** Nonautologous Tissue Substitute	**Z** No Qualifier
9 Hip Joint, Right **B** Hip Joint, Left	**0** Open	**0** Drainage Device **3** Infusion Device **4** Internal Fixation Device **5** External Fixation Device **7** Autologous Tissue Substitute **8** Spacer **9** Liner **B** Resurfacing Device **J** Synthetic Substitute **K** Nonautologous Tissue Substitute	**Z** No Qualifier

Continued →

Section 0 **Medical and Surgical**
Body System S **Lower Joints**
Operation W **Revision:** Correcting, to the extent possible, a portion of a malfunctioning device or the position of a displaced device

Body Part (4th)	Approach (5th)	Device (6th)	Qualifier (7th)
9 Hip Joint, Right **B** Hip Joint, Left	**3** Percutaneous **4** Percutaneous Endoscopic **X** External	**0** Drainage Device **3** Infusion Device **4** Internal Fixation Device **5** External Fixation Device **7** Autologous Tissue Substitute **8** Spacer **J** Synthetic Substitute **K** Nonautologous Tissue Substitute	**Z** No Qualifier
A Hip Joint, Acetabular Surface, Right **E** Hip Joint, Acetabular Surface, Left **R** Hip Joint, Femoral Surface, Right **S** Hip Joint, Femoral Surface, Left **T** Knee Joint, Femoral Surface, Right **U** Knee Joint, Femoral Surface, Left **V** Knee Joint, Tibial Surface, Right **W** Knee Joint, Tibial Surface, Left	**0** Open **3** Percutaneous **4** Percutaneous Endoscopic **X** External	**J** Synthetic Substitute	**Z** No Qualifier
C Knee Joint, Right **D** Knee Joint, Left	**0** Open	**0** Drainage Device **3** Infusion Device **4** Internal Fixation Device **5** External Fixation Device **7** Autologous Tissue Substitute **8** Spacer **9** Liner **K** Nonautologous Tissue Substitute	**Z** No Qualifier
C Knee Joint, Right **D** Knee Joint, Left	**0** Open	**J** Synthetic Substitute	**C** Patellar Surface **Z** No Qualifier
C Knee Joint, Right **D** Knee Joint, Left	**3** Percutaneous **4** Percutaneous Endoscopic **X** External	**0** Drainage Device **3** Infusion Device **4** Internal Fixation Device **5** External Fixation Device **7** Autologous Tissue Substitute **8** Spacer **K** Nonautologous Tissue Substitute	**Z** No Qualifier
C Knee Joint, Right **E** Knee Joint, Left	**3** Percutaneous **4** Percutaneous Endoscopic **X** External	**J** Synthetic Substitute	**C** Patellar Surface **Z** No Qualifier
F Ankle Joint, Right **G** Ankle Joint, Left **H** Tarsal Joint, Right **J** Tarsal Joint, Left **K** Tarsometatarsal Joint, Right **L** Tarsometatarsal Joint, Left **M** Metatarsal-Phalangeal Joint, Right **N** Metatarsal-Phalangeal Joint, Left **P** Toe Phalangeal Joint, Right **Q** Toe Phalangeal Joint, Left	**0** Open **3** Percutaneous **4** Percutaneous Endoscopic **X** External	**0** Drainage Device **3** Infusion Device **4** Internal Fixation Device **5** External Fixation Device **7** Autologous Tissue Substitute **8** Spacer **J** Synthetic Substitute **K** Nonautologous Tissue Substitute	**Z** No Qualifier

AHA Coding Clinic

0S9D4ZZ Drainage of Left Knee Joint, Percutaneous Endoscopic Approach— AHA CC: 2Q, 2018, 17

0SB20ZZ Excision of Lumbar Vertebral Disc, Open Approach—AHA CC: 2Q, 2014, 6-7; 2Q, 2016, 16; 4Q, 2017, 76-77

0SB40ZZ Excision of Lumbosacral Disc, Open Approach—AHA CC: 4Q, 2017, 76-77

0SBD4ZZ Excision of Left Knee Joint, Percutaneous Endoscopic Approach—AHA CC: 1Q, 2015, 34

0SG0071 Fusion of Lumbar Vertebral Joint with Autologous Tissue Substitute, Posterior Approach, Posterior Column, Open Approach—AHA CC: 1Q, 2013, 21-23; 3Q, 2013, 25-26

0SG00AJ Fusion of Lumbar Vertebral Joint with Interbody Fusion Device, Posterior Approach, Anterior Column, Open Approach—AHA CC: 3Q, 2013, 25-26

0SG107J Fusion of 2 or more Lumbar Vertebral Joints with Autologous Tissue Substitute, Posterior Approach, Anterior Column, Open Approach—AHA CC: 3Q, 2014, 36

0SGG04Z Fusion of Left Ankle Joint with Internal Fixation Device, Open Approach—AHA CC: 2Q, 2013, 39-40

0SGG07Z Fusion of Left Ankle Joint with Autologous Tissue Substitute, Open Approach—AHA CC: 2Q, 2013, 39-40

0SH408Z Insertion of Spacer into Lumbosacral Disc, Open Approach—AHA CC: 1Q, 2021, 18-19

0SJG3ZZ Inspection of Left Ankle Joint, Percutaneous Approach—AHA CC: 1Q, 2017, 50

0SNC4ZZ Release Right Knee Joint, Percutaneous Endoscopic Approach—AHA CC: 2Q, 2020, 26-27

0SP909Z Removal of Liner from Right Hip Joint, Open Approach—AHA CC: 2Q, 2015, 19-20; 4Q, 2016, 111-112

0SP90JZ Removal of Synthetic Substitute from Right Hip Joint, Open Approach—AHA CC: 2Q, 2015, 19-20

0SPC0JZ Removal of Synthetic Substitute from Right Knee Joint, Open Approach—AHA CC: 2Q, 2015, 18-19

0SPF0JZ Removal of Synthetic Substitute from Right Ankle Joint, Open Approach—AHA CC: 4Q, 2017, 107-108; 1Q, 2021, 17-18

0SPG04Z Removal of Internal Fixation Device from Left Ankle Joint, Open Approach—AHA CC: 2Q, 2013, 39-40

0SPR0JZ Removal of Synthetic Substitute from Right Hip Joint, Femoral Surface, Open Approach—AHA CC: 4Q, 2016, 111-112

0SPW0JZ Removal of Synthetic Substitute from Left Knee Joint, Tibial Surface, Open Approach—AHA CC: 2Q, 2018, 16-17

0SQB4ZZ Repair Left Hip Joint, Percutaneous Endoscopic Approach—AHA CC: 4Q, 2014, 25-26

0SR9029 Replacement of Right Hip Joint with Metal on Polyethylene Synthetic Substitute, Cemented, Open Approach—AHA CC: 3Q, 2020, 33-34

0SRB06Z Replacement of Left Hip Joint with Oxidized Zirconium on Polyethylene Synthetic Substitute, Open Approach—AHA CC: 4Q, 2017, 39

0SRB0J9 Replacement of Left Hip Joint with Synthetic Substitute, Cemented, Open Approach—AHA CC: 3Q, 2015, 18-19

0SRC0J9 Replacement of Right Knee Joint with Synthetic Substitute, Cemented, Open Approach—AHA CC: 2Q, 2015, 18-19

0SRD0JZ Replacement of Left Knee Joint with Synthetic Substitute, Open Approach—AHA CC: 4Q, 2016, 109-110

0SRD0LZ Replacement of Left Knee Joint with Unicondylar Synthetic Substitute, Open Approach—AHA CC: 4Q, 2016, 110

0SRF0JA Replacement of Right Ankle Joint with Synthetic Substitute, Uncemented, Open Approach—AHA CC: 4Q, 2017, 107-108

0SRR03A Replacement of Right Hip Joint, Femoral Surface with Ceramic Synthetic Substitute, Uncemented, Open Approach—AHA CC: 2Q, 2015, 19-20

0SRR0J9 Replacement of Right Hip Joint, Femoral Surface with Synthetic Substitute, Cemented, Open Approach—AHA CC: 4Q, 2016, 111-112

0SRW0JZ Replacement of Left Knee Joint, Tibial Surface with Synthetic Substitute, Open Approach—AHA CC: 2Q, 2018, 16-17

0SSB04Z Reposition Left Hip Joint with Internal Fixation Device, Open Approach—AHA CC: 2Q, 2016, 32

0STD0ZZ Resection of Left Knee Joint, Open Approach—AHA CC: 4Q, 2014, 30-31

0STM0ZZ Resection of Right Metatarsal-Phalangeal Joint, Open Approach—AHA CC: 1Q, 2016, 20-21

0SUA09Z Supplement Right Hip Joint, Acetabular Surface with Liner, Open Approach—AHA CC: 2Q, 2015, 19-20; 4Q, 2016, 111-112

0SUF0JZ Supplement Right Ankle Joint with Synthetic Substitute, Open Approach—AHA CC: 1Q, 2021, 17-18

0SWF0JZ Revision of Synthetic Substitute in Right Ankle Joint, Open Approach—AHA CC: 4Q, 2017, 107-108

0SWW0JZ Revision of Synthetic Substitute in Left Knee Joint, Tibial Surface, Open Approach—AHA CC: 4Q, 2016, 112

Urinary System

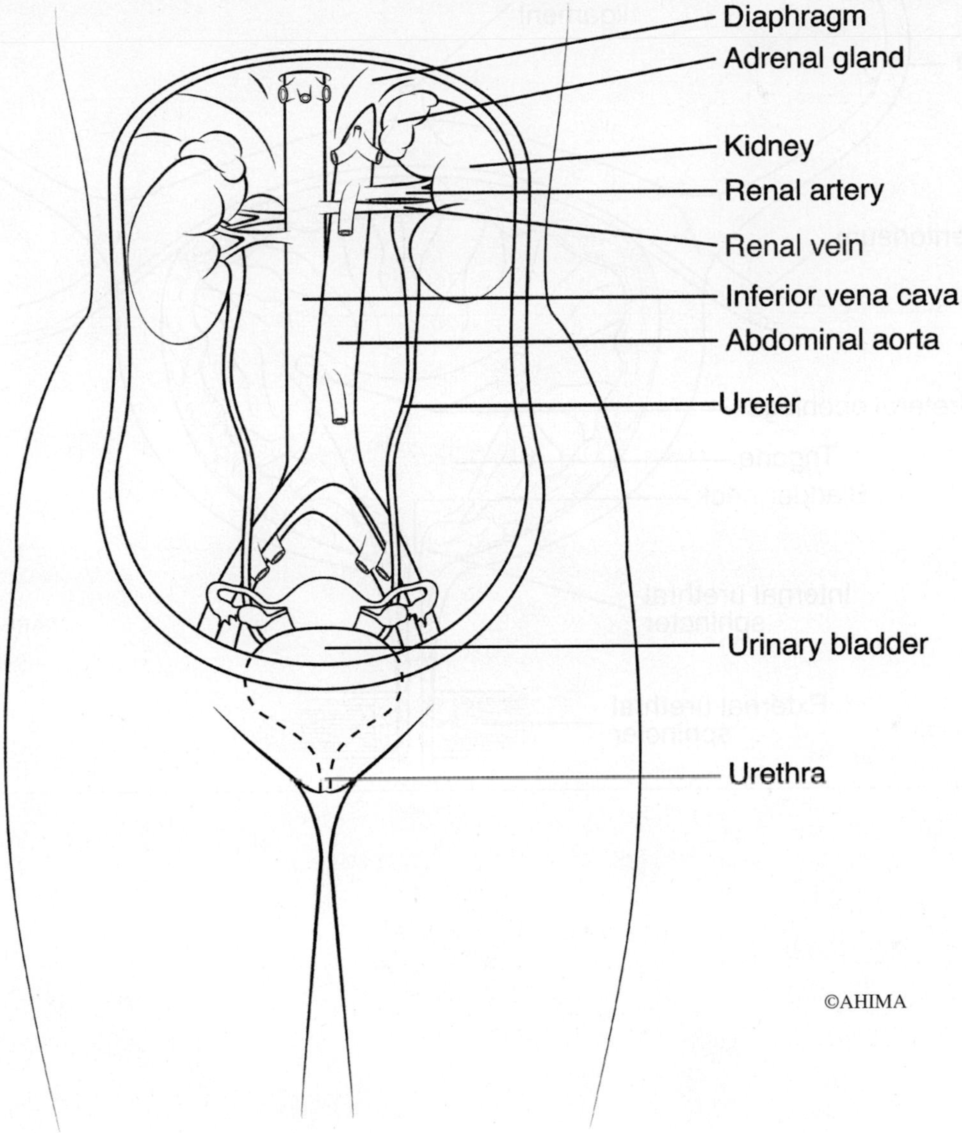
Diaphragm
Adrenal gland
Kidney
Renal artery
Renal vein
Inferior vena cava
Abdominal aorta
Ureter
Urinary bladder
Urethra
©AHIMA

Lower Urinary Tract

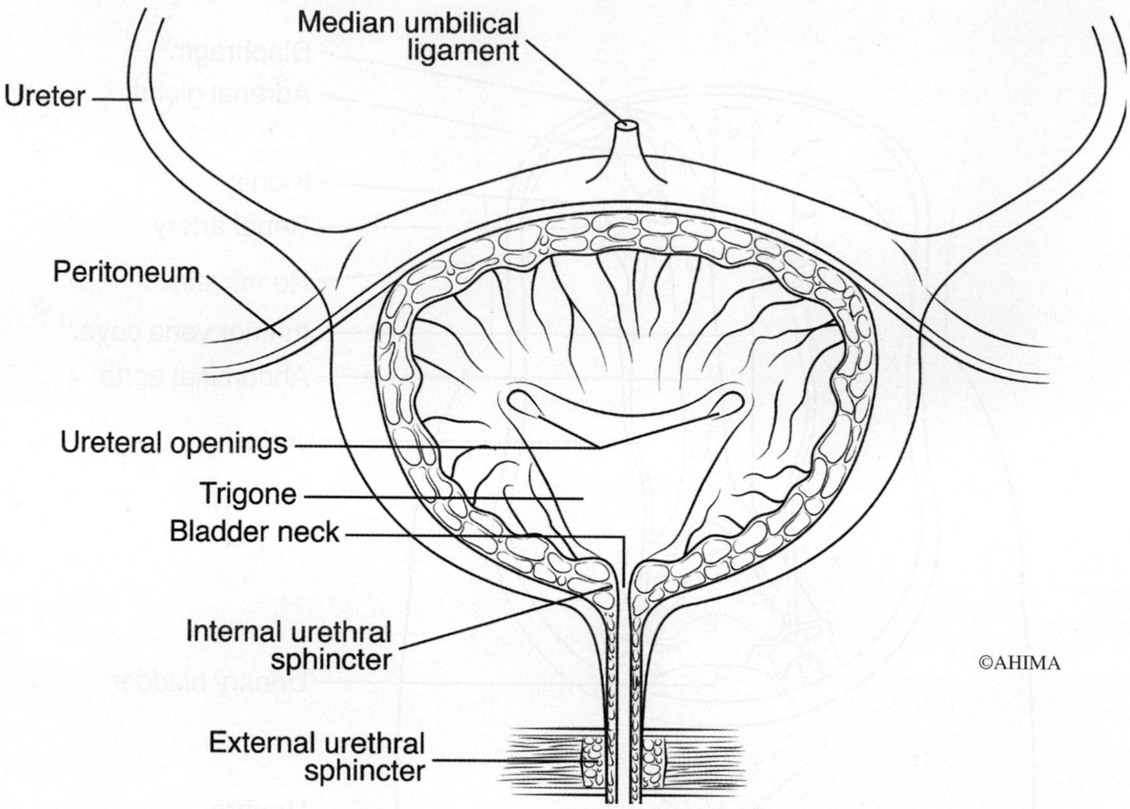

Median umbilical ligament
Ureter
Peritoneum
Ureteral openings
Trigone
Bladder neck
Internal urethral sphincter
External urethral sphincter
©AHIMA

Kidney

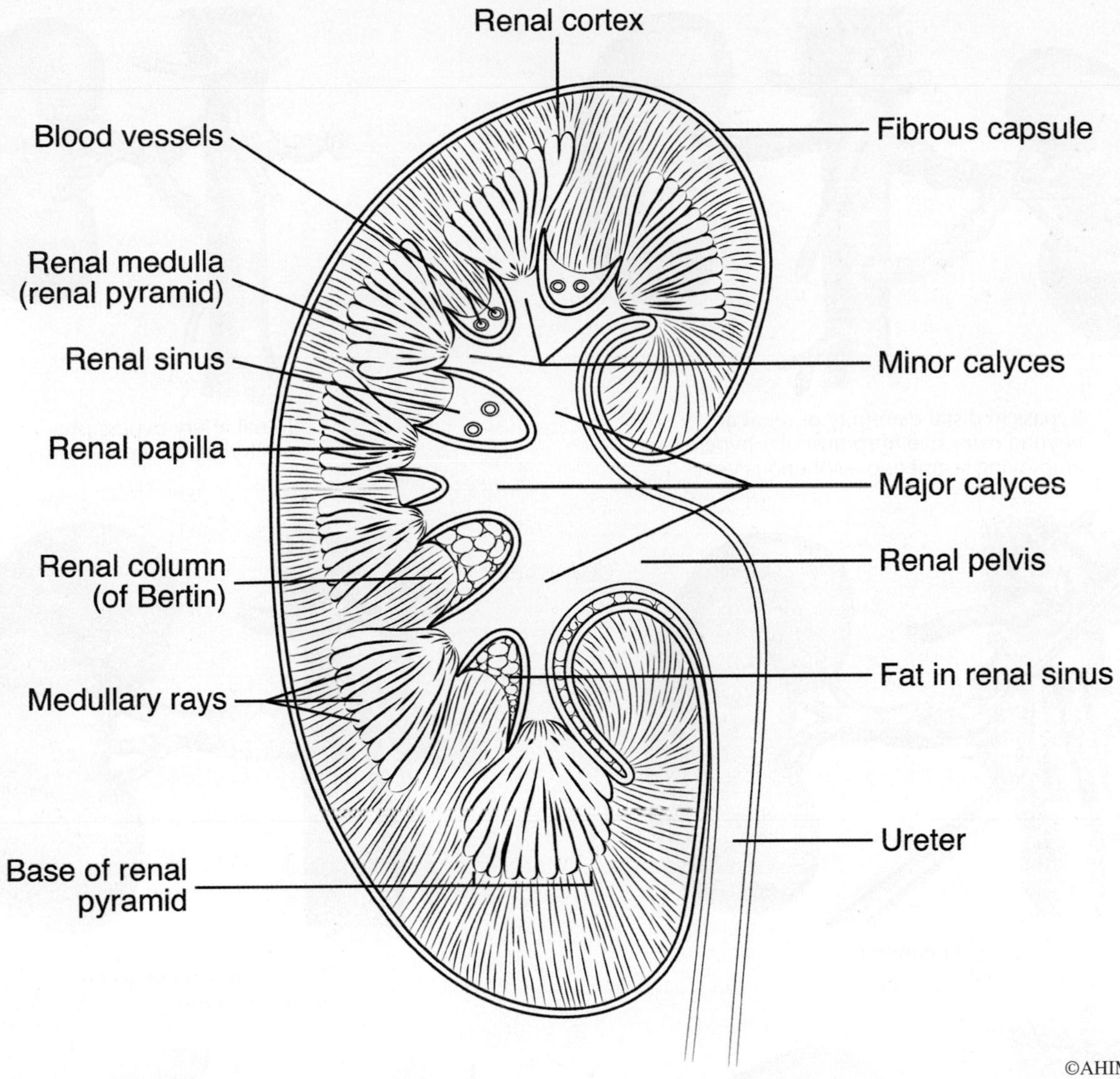

Renal cortex
Blood vessels
Fibrous capsule
Renal medulla (renal pyramid)
Renal sinus
Minor calyces
Renal papilla
Major calyces
Renal column (of Bertin)
Renal pelvis
Fat in renal sinus
Medullary rays
Ureter
Base of renal pyramid

Renal Revascularization

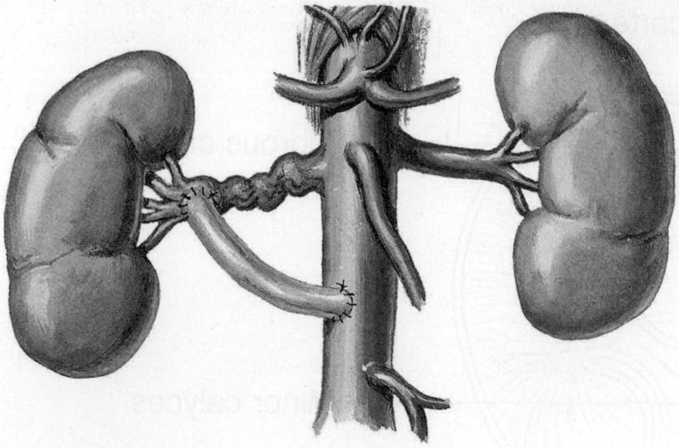

Bypass to distal extremity of renal artery beyond extensive fibromuscular hyperplasia, employing segment of saphenous vein

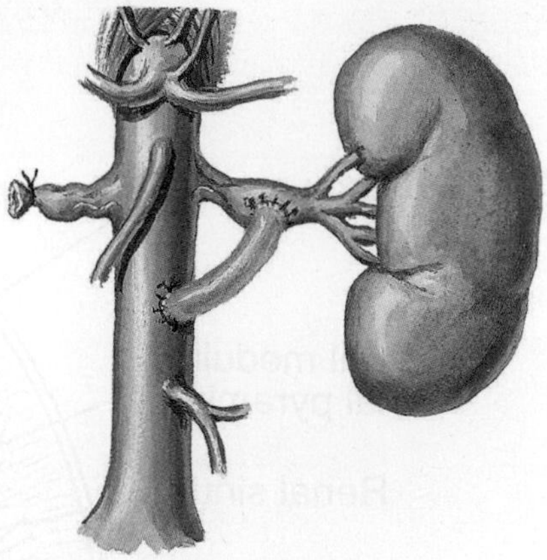

Renal artery bypass plus contralateral nephrectomy

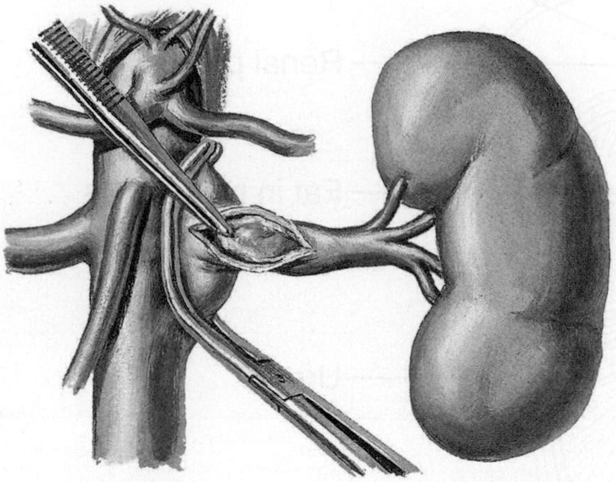

Endarterectomy

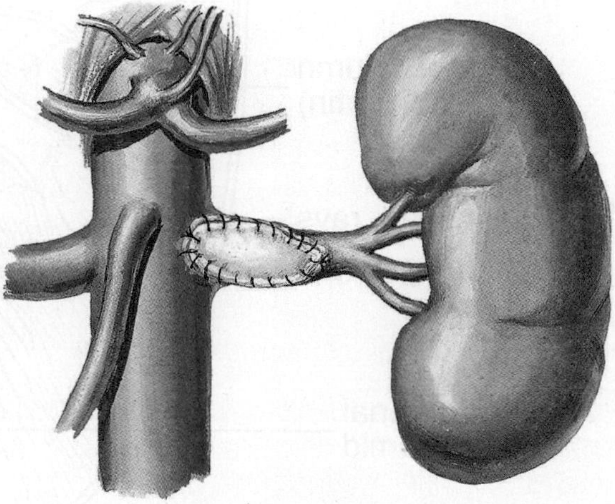

Patch graft with or without endarterectomy

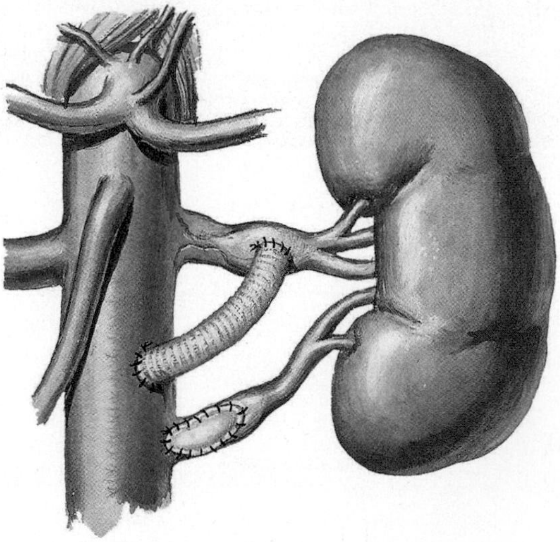

Renal artery bypass plus patch graft to accessory renal artery

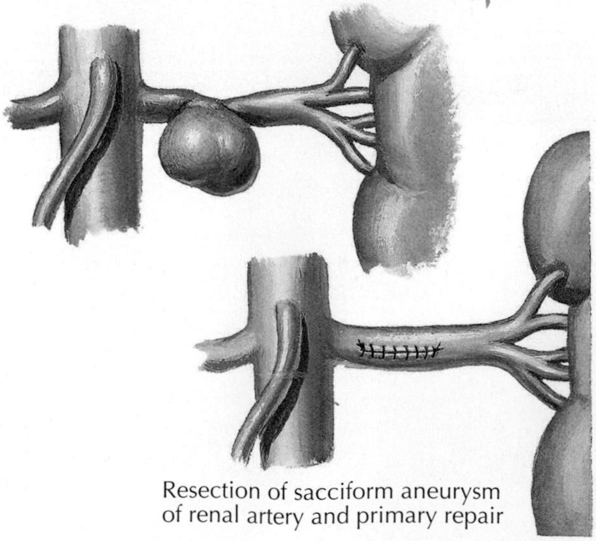

Resection of sacciform aneurysm of renal artery and primary repair

Urinary System Tables 0T1–0TY

Section 0 **Medical and Surgical**
Body System T **Urinary System**
Operation 1 **Bypass:** Altering the route of passage of the contents of a tubular body part

Body Part (4th)	Approach (5th)	Device (6th)	Qualifier (7th)
3 Kidney Pelvis, Right **4** Kidney Pelvis, Left	**0** Open **4** Percutaneous Endoscopic	**7** Autologous Tissue Substitute **J** Synthetic Substitute **K** Nonautologous Tissue Substitute **Z** No Device	**3** Kidney Pelvis, Right **4** Kidney Pelvis, Left **6** Ureter, Right **7** Ureter, Left **8** Colon **9** Colocutaneous **A** Ileum **B** Bladder **C** Ileocutaneous **D** Cutaneous
3 Kidney Pelvis, Right **4** Kidney Pelvis, Left	**3** Percutaneous	**J** Synthetic Substitute	**D** Cutaneous
6 Ureter, Right **7** Ureter, Left **8** Ureters, Bilateral	**0** Open **4** Percutaneous Endoscopic	**7** Autologous Tissue Substitute **J** Synthetic Substitute **K** Nonautologous Tissue Substitute **Z** No Device	**6** Ureter, Right **7** Ureter, Left **8** Colon **9** Colocutaneous **A** Ileum **B** Bladder **C** Ileocutaneous **D** Cutaneous
6 Ureter, Right **7** Ureter, Left **8** Ureters, Bilateral	**3** Percutaneous	**J** Synthetic Substitute	**D** Cutaneous
B Bladder	**0** Open **4** Percutaneous Endoscopic	**7** Autologous Tissue Substitute **J** Synthetic Substitute **K** Nonautologous Tissue Substitute **Z** No Device	**9** Colocutaneous **C** Ileocutaneous **D** Cutaneous
B Bladder	**3** Percutaneous	**J** Synthetic Substitute	**D** Cutaneous

Section 0 **Medical and Surgical**
Body System T **Urinary System**
Operation 2 **Change:** Taking out or off a device from a body part and putting back an identical or similar device in or on the same body part without cutting or puncturing the skin or a mucous membrane

Body Part (4th)	Approach (5th)	Device (6th)	Qualifier (7th)
5 Kidney **9** Ureter **B** Bladder **D** Urethra	**X** External	**0** Drainage Device **Y** Other Device	**Z** No Qualifier

Section 0 **Medical and Surgical**
Body System T **Urinary System**
Operation 5 **Destruction:** Physical eradication of all or a portion of a body part by the direct use of energy, force, or a destructive agent

Body Part (4th)	Approach (5th)	Device (6th)	Qualifier (7th)
0 Kidney, Right **1** Kidney, Left **3** Kidney Pelvis, Right **4** Kidney Pelvis, Left **6** Ureter, Right **7** Ureter, Left **B** Bladder **C** Bladder Neck	**0** Open **3** Percutaneous **4** Percutaneous Endoscopic **7** Via Natural or Artificial Opening **8** Via Natural or Artificial Opening Endoscopic	**Z** No Device	**Z** No Qualifier

Continued →

Section 0 Medical and Surgical
Body System T Urinary System
Operation 5 **Destruction:** Physical eradication of all or a portion of a body part by the direct use of energy, force, or a destructive agent

Body Part (4th)	Approach (5th)	Device (6th)	Qualifier (7th)
D Urethra	0 Open 3 Percutaneous 4 Percutaneous Endoscopic 7 Via Natural or Artificial Opening 8 Via Natural or Artificial Opening Endoscopic X External	Z No Device	Z No Qualifier

Section 0 Medical and Surgical
Body System T Urinary System
Operation 7 **Dilation:** Expanding an orifice or the lumen of a tubular body part

Body Part (4th)	Approach (5th)	Device (6th)	Qualifier (7th)
3 Kidney Pelvis, Right 4 Kidney Pelvis, Left 6 Ureter, Right 7 Ureter, Left 8 Ureters, Bilateral B Bladder C Bladder Neck D Urethra	0 Open 3 Percutaneous 4 Percutaneous Endoscopic 7 Via Natural or Artificial Opening 8 Via Natural or Artificial Opening Endoscopic	D Intraluminal Device Z No Device	Z No Qualifier

Section 0 Medical and Surgical
Body System T Urinary System
Operation 8 **Division:** Cutting into a body part, without draining fluids and/or gases from the body part, in order to separate or transect a body part

Body Part (4th)	Approach (5th)	Device (6th)	Qualifier (7th)
2 Kidneys, Bilateral C Bladder Neck	0 Open 3 Percutaneous 4 Percutaneous Endoscopic	Z No Device	Z No Qualifier

Section 0 Medical and Surgical
Body System T Urinary System
Operation 9 **Drainage:** Taking or letting out fluids and/or gases from a body part

Body Part (4th)	Approach (5th)	Device (6th)	Qualifier (7th)
0 Kidney, Right 1 Kidney, Left 3 Kidney Pelvis, Right 4 Kidney Pelvis, Left 6 Ureter, Right 7 Ureter, Left 8 Ureters, Bilateral B Bladder C Bladder Neck	0 Open 3 Percutaneous 4 Percutaneous Endoscopic 7 Via Natural or Artificial Opening 8 Via Natural or Artificial Opening Endoscopic	0 Drainage Device	Z No Qualifier
0 Kidney, Right 1 Kidney, Left 3 Kidney Pelvis, Right 4 Kidney Pelvis, Left 6 Ureter, Right 7 Ureter, Left 8 Ureters, Bilateral B Bladder C Bladder Neck	0 Open 3 Percutaneous 4 Percutaneous Endoscopic 7 Via Natural or Artificial Opening 8 Via Natural or Artificial Opening Endoscopic	Z No Device	X Diagnostic Z No Qualifier

Continued →

Section 0 Medical and Surgical
Body System T Urinary System
Operation 9 **Drainage:** Taking or letting out fluids and/or gases from a body part

Body Part (4th)	Approach (5th)	Device (6th)	Qualifier (7th)
D Urethra	0 Open 3 Percutaneous 4 Percutaneous Endoscopic 7 Via Natural or Artificial Opening 8 Via Natural or Artificial Opening Endoscopic X External	0 Drainage Device	Z No Qualifier
D Urethra	0 Open 3 Percutaneous 4 Percutaneous Endoscopic 7 Via Natural or Artificial Opening 8 Via Natural or Artificial Opening Endoscopic X External	Z No Device	X Diagnostic Z No Qualifier

Section 0 Medical and Surgical
Body System T Urinary System
Operation B **Excision:** Cutting out or off, without replacement, a portion of a body part

Body Part (4th)	Approach (5th)	Device (6th)	Qualifier (7th)
0 Kidney, Right 1 Kidney, Left 3 Kidney Pelvis, Right 4 Kidney Pelvis, Left 6 Ureter, Right 7 Ureter, Left B Bladder C Bladder Neck	0 Open 3 Percutaneous 4 Percutaneous Endoscopic 7 Via Natural or Artificial Opening 8 Via Natural or Artificial Opening Endoscopic	Z No Device	X Diagnostic Z No Qualifier
D Urethra	0 Open 3 Percutaneous 4 Percutaneous Endoscopic 7 Via Natural or Artificial Opening 8 Via Natural or Artificial Opening Endoscopic X External	Z No Device	X Diagnostic Z No Qualifier

Section 0 Medical and Surgical
Body System T Urinary System
Operation C **Extirpation:** Taking or cutting out solid matter from a body part

Body Part (4th)	Approach (5th)	Device (6th)	Qualifier (7th)
0 Kidney, Right 1 Kidney, Left 3 Kidney Pelvis, Right 4 Kidney Pelvis, Left 6 Ureter, Right 7 Ureter, Left B Bladder C Bladder Neck	0 Open 3 Percutaneous 4 Percutaneous Endoscopic 7 Via Natural or Artificial Opening 8 Via Natural or Artificial Opening Endoscopic	Z No Device	Z No Qualifier
D Urethra	0 Open 3 Percutaneous 4 Percutaneous Endoscopic 7 Via Natural or Artificial Opening 8 Via Natural or Artificial Opening Endoscopic X External	Z No Device	Z No Qualifier

Section 0 **Medical and Surgical**
Body System T **Urinary System**
Operation D **Extraction:** Pulling or stripping out or off all or a portion of a body part by the use of force

Body Part (4th)	Approach (5th)	Device (6th)	Qualifier (7th)
0 Kidney, Right **1** Kidney, Left	**0** Open **3** Percutaneous **4** Percutaneous Endoscopic	**Z** No Device	**Z** No Qualifier

Section 0 **Medical and Surgical**
Body System T **Urinary System**
Operation F **Fragmentation:** Breaking solid matter in a body part into pieces

Body Part (4th)	Approach (5th)	Device (6th)	Qualifier (7th)
3 Kidney Pelvis, Right **4** Kidney Pelvis, Left **6** Ureter, Right **7** Ureter, Left **B** Bladder **C** Bladder Neck **D** Urethra	**0** Open **3** Percutaneous **4** Percutaneous Endoscopic **7** Via Natural or Artificial Opening **8** Via Natural or Artificial Opening Endoscopic **X** External	**Z** No Device	**Z** No Qualifier

Section 0 **Medical and Surgical**
Body System T **Urinary System**
Operation H **Insertion:** Putting in a nonbiological appliance that monitors, assists, performs, or prevents a physiological function but does not physically take the place of a body part

Body Part (4th)	Approach (5th)	Device (6th)	Qualifier (7th)
5 Kidney	**0** Open **3** Percutaneous **4** Percutaneous Endoscopic **7** Via Natural or Artificial Opening **8** Via Natural or Artificial Opening Endoscopic	**1** Radioactive Element **2** Monitoring Device **3** Infusion Device **Y** Other Device	**Z** No Qualifier
9 Ureter	**0** Open **3** Percutaneous **4** Percutaneous Endoscopic **7** Via Natural or Artificial Opening **8** Via Natural or Artificial Opening Endoscopic	**1** Radioactive Element **2** Monitoring Device **3** Infusion Device **M** Stimulator Lead **Y** Other Device	**Z** No Qualifier
B Bladder	**0** Open **3** Percutaneous **4** Percutaneous Endoscopic **7** Via Natural or Artificial Opening **8** Via Natural or Artificial Opening Endoscopic	**1** Radioactive Element **2** Monitoring Device **3** Infusion Device **L** Artificial Sphincter **M** Stimulator Lead **Y** Other Device	**Z** No Qualifier
C Bladder Neck	**0** Open **3** Percutaneous **4** Percutaneous Endoscopic **7** Via Natural or Artificial Opening **8** Via Natural or Artificial Opening Endoscopic	**L** Artificial Sphincter	**Z** No Qualifier
D Urethra	**0** Open **3** Percutaneous **4** Percutaneous Endoscopic **7** Via Natural or Artificial Opening **8** Via Natural or Artificial Opening Endoscopic	**1** Radioactive Element **2** Monitoring Device **3** Infusion Device **L** Artificial Sphincter **Y** Other Device	**Z** No Qualifier
D Urethra	**X** External	**2** Monitoring Device **3** Infusion Device **L** Artificial Sphincter	**Z** No Qualifier

Section 0 **Medical and Surgical**
Body System T **Urinary System**
Operation J **Inspection:** Visually and/or manually exploring a body part

Body Part (4th)	Approach (5th)	Device (6th)	Qualifier (7th)
5 Kidney **9** Ureter **B** Bladder **D** Urethra	**0** Open **3** Percutaneous **4** Percutaneous Endoscopic **7** Via Natural or Artificial Opening **8** Via Natural or Artificial Opening Endoscopic **X** External	**Z** No Device	**Z** No Qualifier

Section 0 **Medical and Surgical**
Body System T **Urinary System**
Operation L **Occlusion:** Completely closing an orifice or the lumen of a tubular body part

Body Part (4th)	Approach (5th)	Device (6th)	Qualifier (7th)
3 Kidney Pelvis, Right **4** Kidney Pelvis, Left **6** Ureter, Right **7** Ureter, Left **B** Bladder **C** Bladder Neck	**0** Open **3** Percutaneous **4** Percutaneous Endoscopic	**C** Extraluminal Device **D** Intraluminal Device **Z** No Device	**Z** No Qualifier
3 Kidney Pelvis, Right **4** Kidney Pelvis, Left **6** Ureter, Right **7** Ureter, Left **B** Bladder **C** Bladder Neck	**7** Via Natural or Artificial Opening **8** Via Natural or Artificial Opening Endoscopic	**D** Intraluminal Device **Z** No Device	**Z** No Qualifier
D Urethra	**0** Open **3** Percutaneous **4** Percutaneous Endoscopic **X** External	**C** Extraluminal Device **D** Intraluminal Device **Z** No Device	**Z** No Qualifier
D Urethra	**7** Via Natural or Artificial Opening **8** Via Natural or Artificial Opening Endoscopic	**D** Intraluminal Device **Z** No Device	**Z** No Qualifier

Section 0 **Medical and Surgical**
Body System T **Urinary System**
Operation M **Reattachment:** Putting back in or on all or a portion of a separated body part to its normal location or other suitable location

Body Part (4th)	Approach (5th)	Device (6th)	Qualifier (7th)
0 Kidney, Right **1** Kidney, Left **2** Kidneys, Bilateral **3** Kidney Pelvis, Right **4** Kidney Pelvis, Left **6** Ureter, Right **7** Ureter, Left **8** Ureters, Bilateral **B** Bladder **C** Bladder Neck **D** Urethra	**0** Open **4** Percutaneous Endoscopic	**Z** No Device	**Z** No Qualifier

Section 0 **Medical and Surgical**
Body System T **Urinary System**
Operation N **Release:** Freeing a body part from an abnormal physical constraint by cutting or by the use of force

Body Part (4th)	Approach (5th)	Device (6th)	Qualifier (7th)
0 Kidney, Right **1** Kidney, Left **3** Kidney Pelvis, Right **4** Kidney Pelvis, Left **6** Ureter, Right **7** Ureter, Left **B** Bladder **C** Bladder Neck	**0** Open **3** Percutaneous **4** Percutaneous Endoscopic **7** Via Natural or Artificial Opening **8** Via Natural or Artificial Opening Endoscopic	**Z** No Device	**Z** No Qualifier
D Urethra	**0** Open **3** Percutaneous **4** Percutaneous Endoscopic **7** Via Natural or Artificial Opening **8** Via Natural or Artificial Opening Endoscopic **X** External	**Z** No Device	**Z** No Qualifier

Section 0 **Medical and Surgical**
Body System T **Urinary System**
Operation P **Removal:** Taking out or off a device from a body part

Body Part (4th)	Approach (5th)	Device (6th)	Qualifier (7th)
5 Kidney	**0** Open **3** Percutaneous **4** Percutaneous Endoscopic **7** Via Natural or Artificial Opening **8** Via Natural or Artificial Opening Endoscopic	**0** Drainage Device **2** Monitoring Device **3** Infusion Device **7** Autologous Tissue Substitute **C** Extraluminal Device **D** Intraluminal Device **J** Synthetic Substitute **K** Nonautologous Tissue Substitute **Y** Other Device	**Z** No Qualifier
5 Kidney	**X** External	**0** Drainage Device **2** Monitoring Device **3** Infusion Device **D** Intraluminal Device	**Z** No Qualifier
9 Ureter	**0** Open **3** Percutaneous **4** Percutaneous Endoscopic **7** Via Natural or Artificial Opening **8** Via Natural or Artificial Opening Endoscopic	**0** Drainage Device **2** Monitoring Device **3** Infusion Device **7** Autologous Tissue Substitute **C** Extraluminal Device **D** Intraluminal Device **J** Synthetic Substitute **K** Nonautologous Tissue Substitute **M** Stimulator Lead **Y** Other Device	**Z** No Qualifier
9 Ureter	**X** External	**0** Drainage Device **2** Monitoring Device **3** Infusion Device **D** Intraluminal Device **M** Stimulator Lead	**Z** No Qualifier

Continued →

Section 0 **Medical and Surgical**
Body System T **Urinary System**
Operation P **Removal:** Taking out or off a device from a body part

Body Part (4th)	Approach (5th)	Device (6th)	Qualifier (7th)
B Bladder	**0** Open **3** Percutaneous **4** Percutaneous Endoscopic **7** Via Natural or Artificial Opening **8** Via Natural or Artificial Opening Endoscopic	**0** Drainage Device **2** Monitoring Device **3** Infusion Device **7** Autologous Tissue Substitute **C** Extraluminal Device **D** Intraluminal Device **J** Synthetic Substitute **K** Nonautologous Tissue Substitute **L** Artificial Sphincter **M** Stimulator Lead **Y** Other Device	**Z** No Qualifier
B Bladder	**X** External	**0** Drainage Device **2** Monitoring Device **3** Infusion Device **D** Intraluminal Device **L** Artificial Sphincter **M** Stimulator Lead	**Z** No Qualifier
D Urethra	**0** Open **3** Percutaneous **4** Percutaneous Endoscopic **7** Via Natural or Artificial Opening **8** Via Natural or Artificial Opening Endoscopic	**0** Drainage Device **2** Monitoring Device **3** Infusion Device **7** Autologous Tissue Substitute **C** Extraluminal Device **D** Intraluminal Device **J** Synthetic Substitute **K** Nonautologous Tissue Substitute **L** Artificial Sphincter **Y** Other Device	**Z** No Qualifier
D Urethra	**X** External	**0** Drainage Device **2** Monitoring Device **3** Infusion Device **D** Intraluminal Device **L** Artificial Sphincter	**Z** No Qualifier

Section 0 **Medical and Surgical**
Body System T **Urinary System**
Operation Q **Repair:** Restoring, to the extent possible, a body part to its normal anatomic structure and function

Body Part (4th)	Approach (5th)	Device (6th)	Qualifier (7th)
0 Kidney, Right **1** Kidney, Left **3** Kidney Pelvis, Right **4** Kidney Pelvis, Left **6** Ureter, Right **7** Ureter, Left **B** Bladder **C** Bladder Neck	**0** Open **3** Percutaneous **4** Percutaneous Endoscopic **7** Via Natural or Artificial Opening **8** Via Natural or Artificial Opening Endoscopic	**Z** No Device	**Z** No Qualifier
D Urethra	**0** Open **3** Percutaneous **4** Percutaneous Endoscopic **7** Via Natural or Artificial Opening **8** Via Natural or Artificial Opening Endoscopic **X** External	**Z** No Device	**Z** No Qualifier

Section 0 **Medical and Surgical**
Body System T **Urinary System**
Operation R **Replacement:** Putting in or on biological or synthetic material that physically takes the place and/or function of all or a portion of a body part

Body Part (4th)	Approach (5th)	Device (6th)	Qualifier (7th)
3 Kidney Pelvis, Right **4** Kidney Pelvis, Left **6** Ureter, Right **7** Ureter, Left **B** Bladder **C** Bladder Neck	**0** Open **4** Percutaneous Endoscopic **7** Via Natural or Artificial Opening **8** Via Natural or Artificial Opening Endoscopic	**7** Autologous Tissue Substitute **J** Synthetic Substitute **K** Nonautologous Tissue Substitute	**Z** No Qualifier
D Urethra	**0** Open **4** Percutaneous Endoscopic **7** Via Natural or Artificial Opening **8** Via Natural or Artificial Opening Endoscopic **X** External	**7** Autologous Tissue Substitute **J** Synthetic Substitute **K** Nonautologous Tissue Substitute	**Z** No Qualifier

Section 0 **Medical and Surgical**
Body System T **Urinary System**
Operation S **Reposition:** Moving to its normal location, or other suitable location, all or a portion of a body part

Body Part (4th)	Approach (5th)	Device (6th)	Qualifier (7th)
0 Kidney, Right **1** Kidney, Left **2** Kidneys, Bilateral **3** Kidney Pelvis, Right **4** Kidney Pelvis, Left **6** Ureter, Right **7** Ureter, Left **8** Ureters, Bilateral **B** Bladder **C** Bladder Neck **D** Urethra	**0** Open **4** Percutaneous Endoscopic	**Z** No Device	**Z** No Qualifier

Section 0 **Medical and Surgical**
Body System T **Urinary System**
Operation T **Resection:** Cutting out or off, without replacement, all of a body part

Body Part (4th)	Approach (5th)	Device (6th)	Qualifier (7th)
0 Kidney, Right **1** Kidney, Left **2** Kidneys, Bilateral	**0** Open **4** Percutaneous Endoscopic	**Z** No Device	**Z** No Qualifier
3 Kidney Pelvis, Right **4** Kidney Pelvis, Left **6** Ureter, Right **7** Ureter, Left **B** Bladder **C** Bladder Neck **D** Urethra	**0** Open **4** Percutaneous Endoscopic **7** Via Natural or Artificial Opening **8** Via Natural or Artificial Opening Endoscopic	**Z** No Device	**Z** No Qualifier

Section 0 **Medical and Surgical**
Body System T **Urinary System**
Operation U **Supplement:** Putting in or on biological or synthetic material that physically reinforces and/or augments the function of a portion of a body part

Body Part (4th)	Approach (5th)	Device (6th)	Qualifier (7th)
3 Kidney Pelvis, Right **4** Kidney Pelvis, Left **6** Ureter, Right **7** Ureter, Left **B** Bladder **C** Bladder Neck	**0** Open **4** Percutaneous Endoscopic **7** Via Natural or Artificial Opening **8** Via Natural or Artificial Opening Endoscopic	**7** Autologous Tissue Substitute **J** Synthetic Substitute **K** Nonautologous Tissue Substitute	**Z** No Qualifier
D Urethra	**0** Open **4** Percutaneous Endoscopic **7** Via Natural or Artificial Opening **8** Via Natural or Artificial Opening Endoscopic **X** External	**7** Autologous Tissue Substitute **J** Synthetic Substitute **K** Nonautologous Tissue Substitute	**Z** No Qualifier

Section 0 **Medical and Surgical**
Body System T **Urinary System**
Operation V **Restriction:** Partially closing an orifice or the lumen of a tubular body part

Body Part (4th)	Approach (5th)	Device (6th)	Qualifier (7th)
3 Kidney Pelvis, Right **4** Kidney Pelvis, Left **6** Ureter, Right **7** Ureter, Left **B** Bladder **C** Bladder Neck	**0** Open **3** Percutaneous **4** Percutaneous Endoscopic	**C** Extraluminal Device **D** Intraluminal Device **Z** No Device	**Z** No Qualifier
3 Kidney Pelvis, Right **4** Kidney Pelvis, Left **6** Ureter, Right **7** Ureter, Left **B** Bladder **C** Bladder Neck	**7** Via Natural or Artificial Opening **8** Via Natural or Artificial Opening Endoscopic	**D** Intraluminal Device **Z** No Device	**Z** No Qualifier
D Urethra	**0** Open **3** Percutaneous **4** Percutaneous Endoscopic	**C** Extraluminal Device **D** Intraluminal Device **Z** No Device	**Z** No Qualifier
D Urethra	**7** Via Natural or Artificial Opening **8** Via Natural or Artificial Opening Endoscopic	**D** Intraluminal Device **Z** No Device	**Z** No Qualifier
D Urethra	**X** External	**Z** No Device	**Z** No Qualifier

Section 0 **Medical and Surgical**
Body System T **Urinary System**
Operation W **Revision:** Correcting, to the extent possible, a portion of a malfunctioning device or the position of a displaced device

Body Part (4th)	Approach (5th)	Device (6th)	Qualifier (7th)
5 Kidney	**0** Open **3** Percutaneous **4** Percutaneous Endoscopic **7** Via Natural or Artificial Opening **8** Via Natural or Artificial Opening Endoscopic	**0** Drainage Device **2** Monitoring Device **3** Infusion Device **7** Autologous Tissue Substitute **C** Extraluminal Device **D** Intraluminal Device **J** Synthetic Substitute **K** Nonautologous Tissue Substitute **Y** Other Device	**Z** No Qualifier

Continued →

Section 0 **Medical and Surgical**
Body System T **Urinary System**
Operation W **Revision:** Correcting, to the extent possible, a portion of a malfunctioning device or the position of a displaced device

Body Part (4th)	Approach (5th)	Device (6th)	Qualifier (7th)
5 Kidney	**X** External	**0** Drainage Device **2** Monitoring Device **3** Infusion Device **7** Autologous Tissue Substitute **C** Extraluminal Device **D** Intraluminal Device **J** Synthetic Substitute **K** Nonautologous Tissue Substitute	**Z** No Qualifier
9 Ureter	**0** Open **3** Percutaneous **4** Percutaneous Endoscopic **7** Via Natural or Artificial Opening **8** Via Natural or Artificial Opening Endoscopic	**0** Drainage Device **2** Monitoring Device **3** Infusion Device **7** Autologous Tissue Substitute **C** Extraluminal Device **D** Intraluminal Device **J** Synthetic Substitute **K** Nonautologous Tissue Substitute **M** Stimulator Lead **Y** Other Device	**Z** No Qualifier
9 Ureter	**X** External	**0** Drainage Device **2** Monitoring Device **3** Infusion Device **7** Autologous Tissue Substitute **C** Extraluminal Device **D** Intraluminal Device **J** Synthetic Substitute **K** Nonautologous Tissue Substitute **M** Stimulator Lead	**Z** No Qualifier
B Bladder	**0** Open **3** Percutaneous **4** Percutaneous Endoscopic **7** Via Natural or Artificial Opening **8** Via Natural or Artificial Opening Endoscopic	**0** Drainage Device **2** Monitoring Device **3** Infusion Device **7** Autologous Tissue Substitute **C** Extraluminal Device **D** Intraluminal Device **J** Synthetic Substitute **K** Nonautologous Tissue Substitute **L** Artificial Sphincter **M** Stimulator Lead **Y** Other Device	**Z** No Qualifier
B Bladder	**X** External	**0** Drainage Device **2** Monitoring Device **3** Infusion Device **7** Autologous Tissue Substitute **C** Extraluminal Device **D** Intraluminal Device **J** Synthetic Substitute **K** Nonautologous Tissue Substitute **L** Artificial Sphincter **M** Stimulator Lead	**Z** No Qualifier
D Urethra	**0** Open **3** Percutaneous **4** Percutaneous Endoscopic **7** Via Natural or Artificial Opening **8** Via Natural or Artificial Opening Endoscopic	**0** Drainage Device **2** Monitoring Device **3** Infusion Device **7** Autologous Tissue Substitute **C** Extraluminal Device **D** Intraluminal Device **J** Synthetic Substitute **K** Nonautologous Tissue Substitute **L** Artificial Sphincter **Y** Other Device	**Z** No Qualifier

Continued →

Section 0 **Medical and Surgical**
Body System T **Urinary System**
Operation W **Revision:** Correcting, to the extent possible, a portion of a malfunctioning device or the position of a displaced device

Body Part (4th)	Approach (5th)	Device (6th)	Qualifier (7th)
D Urethra	**X** External	**0** Drainage Device **2** Monitoring Device **3** Infusion Device **7** Autologous Tissue Substitute **C** Extraluminal Device **D** Intraluminal Device **J** Synthetic Substitute **K** Nonautologous Tissue Substitute **L** Artificial Sphincter	**Z** No Qualifier

Section 0 **Medical and Surgical**
Body System T **Urinary System**
Operation Y **Transplantation:** Putting in or on all or a portion of a living body part taken from another individual or animal to physically take the place and/or function of all or a portion of a similar body part

Body Part (4th)	Approach (5th)	Device (6th)	Qualifier (7th)
0 Kidney, Right **1** Kidney, Left	**0** Open	**Z** No Device	**0** Allogeneic **1** Syngeneic **2** Zooplastic

AHA Coding Clinic

0T170ZB Bypass Left Ureter to Bladder, Open Approach—AHA CC: 3Q, 2015, 34-35

0T180ZC Bypass Bilateral Ureters to Ileocutaneous, Open Approach—AHA CC: 3Q, 2017, 20-21

0T1B0Z9 Bypass Bladder to Colocutaneous, Open Approach—AHA CC: 3Q, 2017, 21-22

0T768DZ Dilation of Right Ureter with Intraluminal Device, Via Natural or Artificial Opening Endoscopic—AHA CC: 2Q, 2016, 27-28; 4Q, 2017, 111

0T778DZ Dilation of Left Ureter with Intraluminal Device, Via Natural or Artificial Opening Endoscopic—AHA CC: 2Q, 2015, 8-9

0T7D8DZ Dilation of Urethra with Intraluminal Device, Via Natural or Artificial Opening Endoscopic—AHA CC: 4Q, 2013, 123

0T9680Z Drainage of Right Ureter with Drainage Device, Via Natural or Artificial Opening Endoscopic—AHA CC: 3Q, 2017, 19-20

0TBB8ZX Excision of Bladder, Via Natural or Artificial Opening Endoscopic, Diagnostic—AHA CC: 1Q, 2016, 19

0TBB8ZZ Excision of Bladder, Via Natural or Artificial Opening Endoscopic—AHA CC: 2Q, 2014, 8

0TBD8ZZ Excision of Urethra, Via Natural or Artificial Opening Endoscopic—AHA CC: 3Q, 2015, 34

0TC18ZZ Extirpation of Matter from Left Kidney, Via Natural or Artificial Opening Endoscopic—AHA CC: 2Q, 2015, 8-9

0TC48ZZ Extirpation of Matter from Left Kidney Pelvis, Via Natural or Artificial Opening Endoscopic—AHA CC: 2Q, 2015, 7-8

0TC68ZZ Extirpation of Matter from Right Ureter, Via Natural or Artificial Opening Endoscopic—AHA CC: 4Q, 2013, 122-123

0TC78ZZ Extirpation of Matter from Left Ureter, Via Natural or Artificial Opening Endoscopic—AHA CC: 2Q, 2015, 8-9

0TCB8ZZ Extirpation of Matter from Bladder, Via Natural or Artificial Opening Endoscopic—AHA CC: 2Q, 2015, 8-9; 3Q, 2016, 23-24; 3Q, 2019, 4

0TF3XZZ Fragmentation in Right Kidney Pelvis, External Approach—AHA CC: 4Q, 2013, 122

0TP98DZ Removal of Intraluminal Device from Ureter, Via Natural or Artificial Opening Endoscopic—AHA CC: 2Q, 2016, 27-28

0TQD0ZZ Repair Urethra, Open Approach—AHA CC: 1Q, 2017, 37-38

0TRB07Z Replacement of Bladder with Autologous Tissue Substitute, Open Approach—AHA CC: 3Q, 2017, 20-21

0TS60ZZ Reposition Right Ureter, Open Approach—AHA CC: 1Q, 2017, 36-37; 1Q, 2019, 29-30

0TSD0ZZ Reposition Urethra, Open Approach—AHA CC: 1Q, 2016, 15-16

0TT10ZZ Resection of Left Kidney, Open Approach—AHA CC: 3Q, 2014, 16

0TT70ZZ Resection of Left Ureter, Open Approach—AHA CC: 3Q, 2014, 16

0TUB07Z Supplement Bladder with Autologous Tissue Substitute, Open Approach—AHA CC: 3Q, 2017, 21-22

0TUD07Z Supplement Urethra with Autologous Tissue Substitute, Open Approach—AHA CC: 1Q, 2019, 29-30

0TV68ZZ Restriction of Right Ureter, Via Natural or Artificial Opening Endoscopic—AHA CC: 2Q, 2015, 11-12

0TV78ZZ Restriction of Left Ureter, Via Natural or Artificial Opening Endoscopic—AHA CC: 2Q, 2015, 11-12

Female Reproductive System

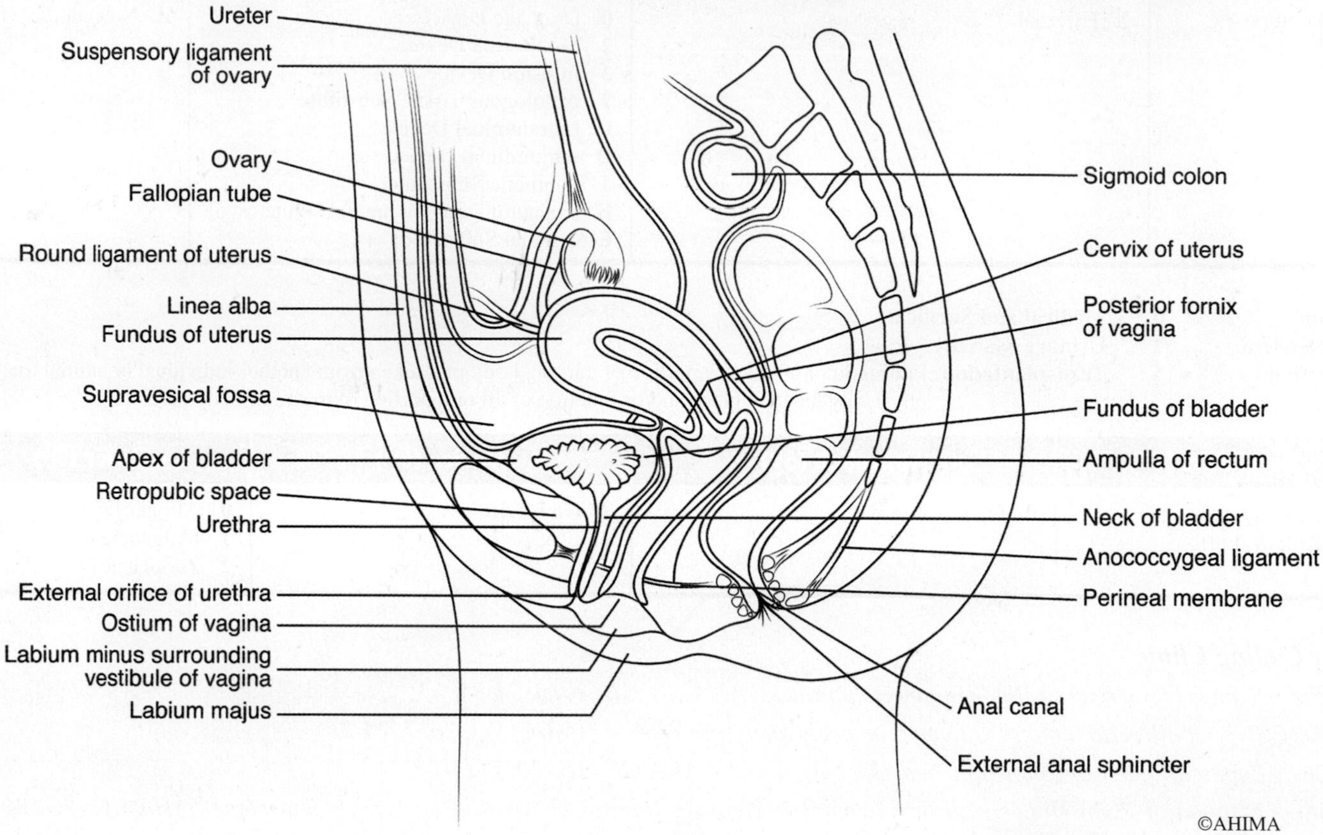
Ureter
Suspensory ligament of ovary
Ovary
Fallopian tube
Round ligament of uterus
Linea alba
Fundus of uterus
Supravesical fossa
Apex of bladder
Retropubic space
Urethra
External orifice of urethra
Ostium of vagina
Labium minus surrounding vestibule of vagina
Labium majus
Sigmoid colon
Cervix of uterus
Posterior fornix of vagina
Fundus of bladder
Ampulla of rectum
Neck of bladder
Anococcygeal ligament
Perineal membrane
Anal canal
External anal sphincter

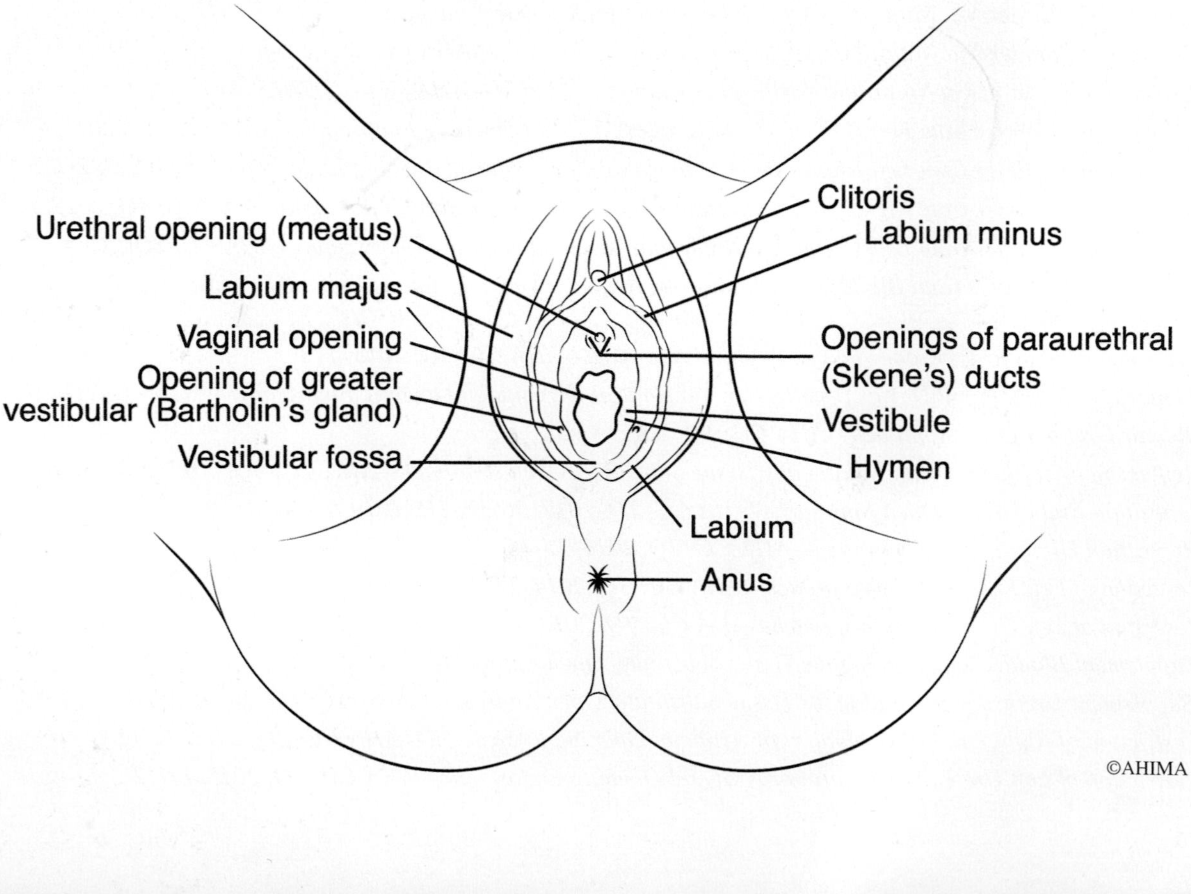
Urethral opening (meatus)
Labium majus
Vaginal opening
Opening of greater vestibular (Bartholin's gland)
Vestibular fossa
Clitoris
Labium minus
Openings of paraurethral (Skene's) ducts
Vestibule
Hymen
Labium
Anus

Uterus, Ovaries and Uterine Tubes

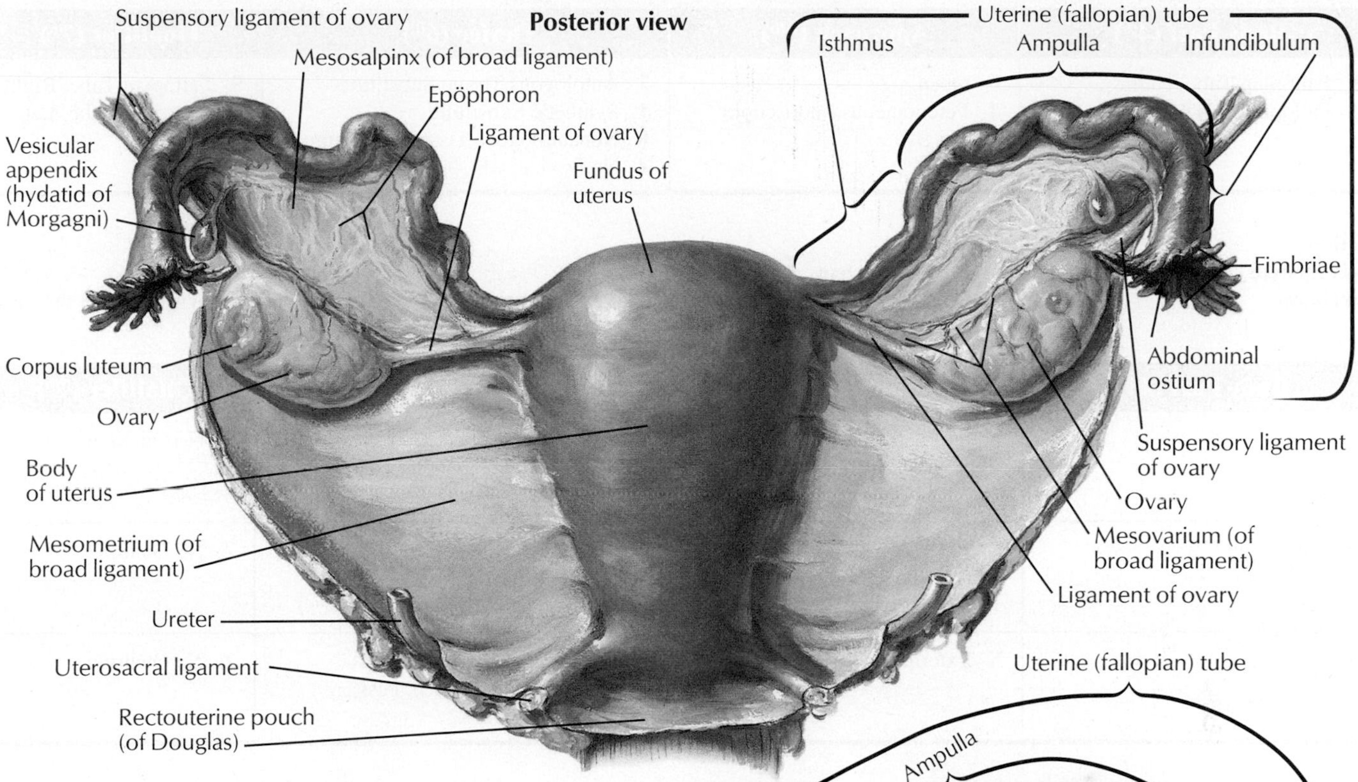

Posterior view
Suspensory ligament of ovary
Mesosalpinx (of broad ligament)
Epöphoron
Ligament of ovary
Fundus of uterus
Vesicular appendix (hydatid of Morgagni)
Corpus luteum
Ovary
Body of uterus
Mesometrium (of broad ligament)
Ureter
Uterosacral ligament
Rectouterine pouch (of Douglas)
Uterine (fallopian) tube
Isthmus
Ampulla
Infundibulum
Fimbriae
Abdominal ostium
Suspensory ligament of ovary
Ovary
Mesovarium (of broad ligament)
Ligament of ovary

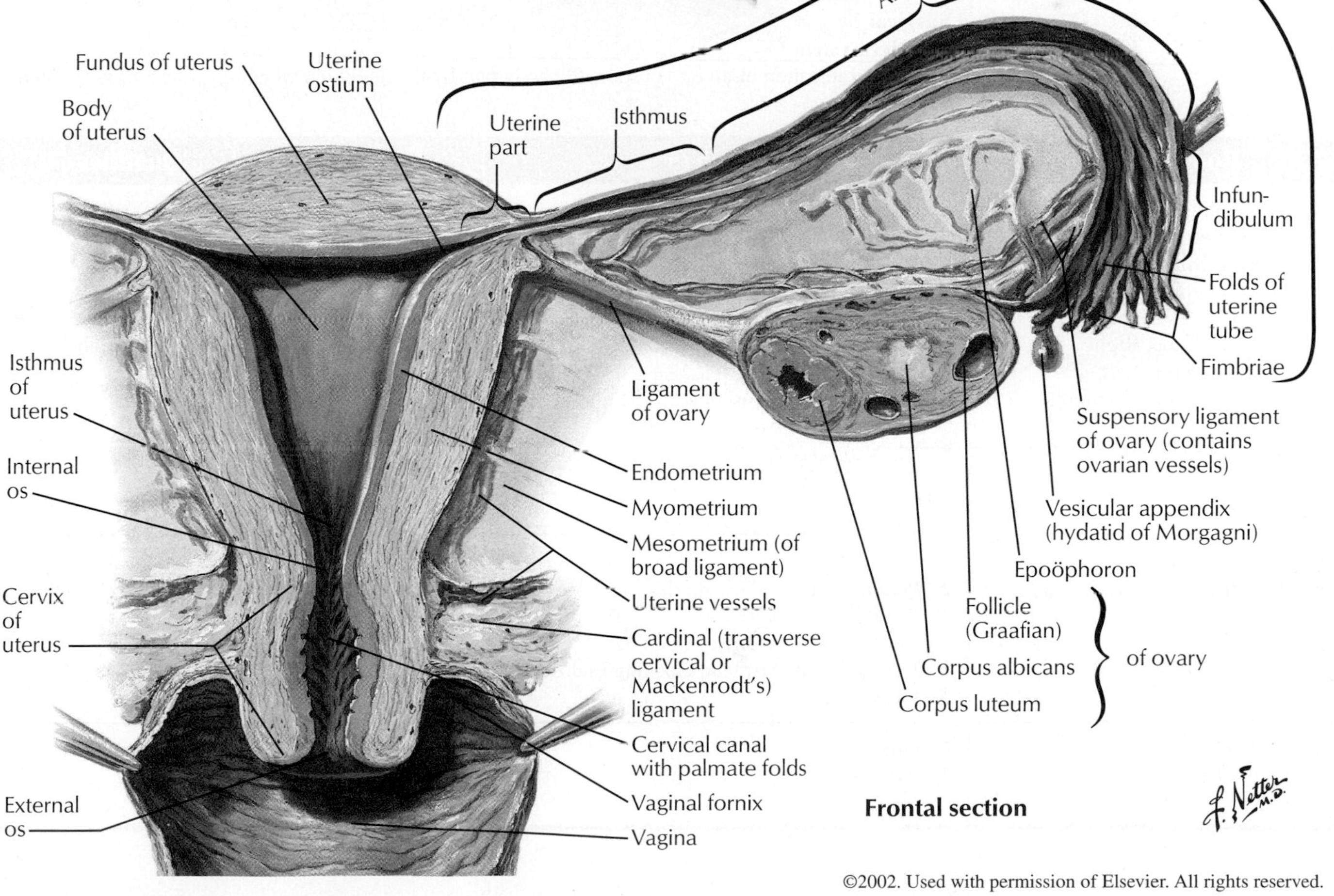

Uterine (fallopian) tube
Ampulla
Fundus of uterus
Uterine ostium
Body of uterus
Uterine part
Isthmus
Infun-dibulum
Folds of uterine tube
Fimbriae
Isthmus of uterus
Internal os
Ligament of ovary
Suspensory ligament of ovary (contains ovarian vessels)
Endometrium
Myometrium
Mesometrium (of broad ligament)
Uterine vessels
Vesicular appendix (hydatid of Morgagni)
Epoöphoron
Cervix of uterus
Cardinal (transverse cervical or Mackenrodt's) ligament
Follicle (Graafian)
Corpus albicans
Corpus luteum
of ovary
Cervical canal with palmate folds
Vaginal fornix
External os
Vagina
Frontal section
F. Netter M.D.

Female Reproductive System Tables 0U1–0UY

Section 0 **Medical and Surgical**
Body System U **Female Reproductive System**
Operation 1 **Bypass:** Altering the route of passage of the contents of a tubular body part

Body Part (4th)	Approach (5th)	Device (6th)	Qualifier (7th)
5 Fallopian Tube, Right **6** Fallopian Tube, Left	**0** Open **4** Percutaneous Endoscopic	**7** Autologous Tissue Substitute **J** Synthetic Substitute **K** Nonautologous Tissue Substitute **Z** No Device	**5** Fallopian Tube, Right **6** Fallopian Tube, Left **9** Uterus

Section 0 **Medical and Surgical**
Body System U **Female Reproductive System**
Operation 2 **Change:** Taking out or off a device from a body part and putting back an identical or similar device in or on the same body part without cutting or puncturing the skin or a mucous membrane

Body Part (4th)	Approach (5th)	Device (6th)	Qualifier (7th)
3 Ovary **8** Fallopian Tube **M** Vulva	**X** External	**0** Drainage Device **Y** Other Device	**Z** No Qualifier
D Uterus and Cervix	**X** External	**0** Drainage Device **H** Contraceptive Device **Y** Other Device	**Z** No Qualifier
H Vagina and Cul-de-sac	**X** External	**0** Drainage Device **G** Intraluminal Device, Pessary **Y** Other Device	**Z** No Qualifier

Section 0 **Medical and Surgical**
Body System U **Female Reproductive System**
Operation 5 **Destruction:** Physical eradication of all or a portion of a body part by the direct use of energy, force, or a destructive agent

Body Part (4th)	Approach (5th)	Device (6th)	Qualifier (7th)
0 Ovary, Right **1** Ovary, Left **2** Ovaries, Bilateral **4** Uterine Supporting Structure	**0** Open **3** Percutaneous **4** Percutaneous Endoscopic **8** Via Natural or Artificial Opening Endoscopic	**Z** No Device	**Z** No Qualifier
5 Fallopian Tube, Right **6** Fallopian Tube, Left **7** Fallopian Tubes, Bilateral **9** Uterus **B** Endometrium **C** Cervix **F** Cul-de-sac	**0** Open **3** Percutaneous **4** Percutaneous Endoscopic **7** Via Natural or Artificial Opening **8** Via Natural or Artificial Opening Endoscopic	**Z** No Device	**Z** No Qualifier
G Vagina **K** Hymen	**0** Open **3** Percutaneous **4** Percutaneous Endoscopic **7** Via Natural or Artificial Opening **8** Via Natural or Artificial Opening Endoscopic **X** External	**Z** No Device	**Z** No Qualifier
J Clitoris **L** Vestibular Gland **M** Vulva	**0** Open **X** External	**Z** No Device	**Z** No Qualifier

Section 0 **Medical and Surgical**
Body System U **Female Reproductive System**
Operation 7 **Dilation:** Expanding an orifice or the lumen of a tubular body part

Body Part (4th)	Approach (5th)	Device (6th)	Qualifier (7th)
5 Fallopian Tube, Right 6 Fallopian Tube, Left 7 Fallopian Tubes, Bilateral 9 Uterus C Cervix G Vagina	0 Open 3 Percutaneous 4 Percutaneous Endoscopic 7 Via Natural or Artificial Opening 8 Via Natural or Artificial Opening Endoscopic	D Intraluminal Device Z No Device	Z No Qualifier
K Hymen	0 Open 3 Percutaneous 4 Percutaneous Endoscopic 7 Via Natural or Artificial Opening 8 Via Natural or Artificial Opening Endoscopic X External	D Intraluminal Device Z No Device	Z No Qualifier

Section 0 **Medical and Surgical**
Body System U **Female Reproductive System**
Operation 8 **Division:** Cutting into a body part, without draining fluids and/or gases from the body part, in order to separate or transect a body part

Body Part (4th)	Approach (5th)	Device (6th)	Qualifier (7th)
0 Ovary, Right 1 Ovary, Left 2 Ovaries, Bilateral 4 Uterine Supporting Structure	0 Open 3 Percutaneous 4 Percutaneous Endoscopic	Z No Device	Z No Qualifier
K Hymen	7 Via Natural or Artificial Opening 8 Via Natural or Artificial Opening Endoscopic X External	Z No Device	Z No Qualifier

Section 0 **Medical and Surgical**
Body System U **Female Reproductive System**
Operation 9 **Drainage:** Taking or letting out fluids and/or gases from a body part

Body Part (4th)	Approach (5th)	Device (6th)	Qualifier (7th)
0 Ovary, Right 1 Ovary, Left 2 Ovaries, Bilateral	0 Open 3 Percutaneous 4 Percutaneous Endoscopic 8 Via Natural or Artificial Opening Endoscopic	0 Drainage Device	Z No Qualifier
0 Ovary, Right 1 Ovary, Left 2 Ovaries, Bilateral	0 Open 3 Percutaneous 4 Percutaneous Endoscopic 8 Via Natural or Artificial Opening Endoscopic	Z No Device	X Diagnostic Z No Qualifier
0 Ovary, Right 1 Ovary, Left 2 Ovaries, Bilateral	X External	Z No Device	Z No Qualifier
4 Uterine Supporting Structure	0 Open 3 Percutaneous 4 Percutaneous Endoscopic 8 Via Natural or Artificial Opening Endoscopic	0 Drainage Device	Z No Qualifier
4 Uterine Supporting Structure	0 Open 3 Percutaneous 4 Percutaneous Endoscopic 8 Via Natural or Artificial Opening Endoscopic	Z No Device	X Diagnostic Z No Qualifier

Continued →

Section 0 **Medical and Surgical**
Body System U **Female Reproductive System**
Operation 9 **Drainage:** Taking or letting out fluids and/or gases from a body part

Body Part (4th)	Approach (5th)	Device (6th)	Qualifier (7th)
5 Fallopian Tube, Right **6** Fallopian Tube, Left **7** Fallopian Tubes, Bilateral **9** Uterus **C** Cervix **F** Cul-de-sac	**0** Open **3** Percutaneous **4** Percutaneous Endoscopic **7** Via Natural or Artificial Opening **8** Via Natural or Artificial Opening Endoscopic	**0** Drainage Device	**Z** No Qualifier
5 Fallopian Tube, Right **6** Fallopian Tube, Left **7** Fallopian Tubes, Bilateral **9** Uterus **C** Cervix **F** Cul-de-sac	**0** Open **3** Percutaneous **4** Percutaneous Endoscopic **7** Via Natural or Artificial Opening **8** Via Natural or Artificial Opening Endoscopic	**Z** No Device	**X** Diagnostic **Z** No Qualifier
G Vagina **K** Hymen	**0** Open **3** Percutaneous **4** Percutaneous Endoscopic **7** Via Natural or Artificial Opening **8** Via Natural or Artificial Opening Endoscopic **X** External	**0** Drainage Device	**Z** No Qualifier
G Vagina **K** Hymen	**0** Open **3** Percutaneous **4** Percutaneous Endoscopic **7** Via Natural or Artificial Opening **8** Via Natural or Artificial Opening Endoscopic **X** External	**Z** No Device	**X** Diagnostic **Z** No Qualifier
J Clitoris **L** Vestibular Gland **M** Vulva	**0** Open **X** External	**0** Drainage Device	**Z** No Qualifier
J Clitoris **L** Vestibular Gland **M** Vulva	**0** Open **X** External	**Z** No Device	**X** Diagnostic **Z** No Qualifier

Section 0 **Medical and Surgical**
Body System U **Female Reproductive System**
Operation B **Excision:** Cutting out or off, without replacement, a portion of a body part

Body Part (4th)	Approach (5th)	Device (6th)	Qualifier (7th)
0 Ovary, Right **1** Ovary, Left **2** Ovaries, Bilateral **4** Uterine Supporting Structure **5** Fallopian Tube, Right **6** Fallopian Tube, Left **7** Fallopian Tubes, Bilateral **9** Uterus **C** Cervix **F** Cul-de-sac	**0** Open **3** Percutaneous **4** Percutaneous Endoscopic **7** Via Natural or Artificial Opening **8** Via Natural or Artificial Opening Endoscopic	**Z** No Device	**X** Diagnostic **Z** No Qualifier

Continued →

Section 0 **Medical and Surgical**
Body System U **Female Reproductive System**
Operation B **Excision:** Cutting out or off, without replacement, a portion of a body part

Body Part (4th)	Approach (5th)	Device (6th)	Qualifier (7th)
G Vagina **K** Hymen	**0** Open **3** Percutaneous **4** Percutaneous Endoscopic **7** Via Natural or Artificial Opening **8** Via Natural or Artificial Opening Endoscopic **X** External	**Z** No Device	**X** Diagnostic **Z** No Qualifier
J Clitoris **L** Vestibular Gland **M** Vulva	**0** Open **X** External	**Z** No Device	**X** Diagnostic **Z** No Qualifier

Section 0 **Medical and Surgical**
Body System U **Female Reproductive System**
Operation C **Extirpation:** Taking or cutting out solid matter from a body part

Body Part (4th)	Approach (5th)	Device (6th)	Qualifier (7th)
0 Ovary, Right **1** Ovary, Left **2** Ovaries, Bilateral **4** Uterine Supporting Structure	**0** Open **3** Percutaneous **4** Percutaneous Endoscopic **8** Via Natural or Artificial Opening Endoscopic	**Z** No Device	**Z** No Qualifier
5 Fallopian Tube, Right **6** Fallopian Tube, Left **7** Fallopian Tubes, Bilateral **9** Uterus **B** Endometrium **C** Cervix **F** Cul-de-sac	**0** Open **3** Percutaneous **4** Percutaneous Endoscopic **7** Via Natural or Artificial Opening **8** Via Natural or Artificial Opening Endoscopic	**Z** No Device	**Z** No Qualifier
G Vagina **K** Hymen	**0** Open **3** Percutaneous **4** Percutaneous Endoscopic **7** Via Natural or Artificial Opening **8** Via Natural or Artificial Opening Endoscopic **X** External	**Z** No Device	**Z** No Qualifier
J Clitoris **L** Vestibular Gland **M** Vulva	**0** Open **X** External	**Z** No Device	**Z** No Qualifier

Section 0 **Medical and Surgical**
Body System U **Female Reproductive System**
Operation D **Extraction:** Pulling or stripping out or off all or a portion of a body part by the use of force

Body Part (4th)	Approach (5th)	Device (6th)	Qualifier (7th)
B Endometrium	**7** Via Natural or Artificial Opening **8** Via Natural or Artificial Opening Endoscopic	**Z** No Device	**X** Diagnostic **Z** No Qualifier
N Ova	**0** Open **3** Percutaneous **4** Percutaneous Endoscopic	**Z** No Device	**Z** No Qualifier

Section 0 **Medical and Surgical**
Body System U **Female Reproductive System**
Operation F **Fragmentation:** Breaking solid matter in a body part into pieces

Body Part (4th)	Approach (5th)	Device (6th)	Qualifier (7th)
5 Fallopian Tube, Right **6** Fallopian Tube, Left **7** Fallopian Tubes, Bilateral **9** Uterus	**0** Open **3** Percutaneous **4** Percutaneous Endoscopic **7** Via Natural or Artificial Opening **8** Via Natural or Artificial Opening Endoscopic **X** External	**Z** No Device	**Z** No Qualifier

Section 0 **Medical and Surgical**
Body System U **Female Reproductive System**
Operation H **Insertion:** Putting in a nonbiological appliance that monitors, assists, performs, or prevents a physiological function but does not physically take the place of a body part

Body Part (4th)	Approach (5th)	Device (6th)	Qualifier (7th)
3 Ovary	**0** Open **3** Percutaneous **4** Percutaneous Endoscopic	**1** Radioactive Element **3** Infusion Device **Y** Other Device	**Z** No Qualifier
3 Ovary	**7** Via Natural or Artificial Opening **8** Via Natural or Artificial Opening Endoscopic	**1** Radioactive Element **Y** Other Device	**Z** No Qualifier
8 Fallopian Tube **D** Uterus and Cervix **H** Vagina and Cul-de-sac	**0** Open **3** Percutaneous **4** Percutaneous Endoscopic **7** Via Natural or Artificial Opening **8** Via Natural or Artificial Opening Endoscopic	**3** Infusion Device **Y** Other Device	**Z** No Qualifier
9 Uterus	**0** Open **7** Via Natural or Artificial Opening **8** Via Natural or Artificial Opening Endoscopic	**1** Radioactive Element **H** Contraceptive Device	**Z** No Qualifier
C Cervix	**0** Open **3** Percutaneous **4** Percutaneous Endoscopic	**1** Radioactive Element	**Z** No Qualifier
C Cervix	**7** Via Natural or Artificial Opening **8** Via Natural or Artificial Opening Endoscopic	**1** Radioactive Element **H** Contraceptive Device	**Z** No Qualifier
F Cul-de-sac	**7** Via Natural or Artificial Opening **8** Via Natural or Artificial Opening Endoscopic	**G** Intraluminal Device, Pessary	**Z** No Qualifier
G Vagina	**0** Open **3** Percutaneous **4** Percutaneous Endoscopic **X** External	**1** Radioactive Element	**Z** No Qualifier
G Vagina	**7** Via Natural or Artificial Opening **8** Via Natural or Artificial Opening Endoscopic	**1** Radioactive Element **G** Intraluminal Device, Pessary	**Z** No Qualifier

Section 0 **Medical and Surgical**
Body System U **Female Reproductive System**
Operation J **Inspection:** Visually and/or manually exploring a body part

Body Part (4th)	Approach (5th)	Device (6th)	Qualifier (7th)
3 Ovary	**0** Open **3** Percutaneous **4** Percutaneous Endoscopic **8** Via Natural or Artificial Opening Endoscopic **X** External	**Z** No Device	**Z** No Qualifier

Continued →

Section 0 **Medical and Surgical**
Body System U **Female Reproductive System**
Operation J **Inspection:** Visually and/or manually exploring a body part

Body Part (4th)	Approach (5th)	Device (6th)	Qualifier (7th)
8 Fallopian Tube **D** Uterus and Cervix **H** Vagina and Cul-de-sac	**0** Open **3** Percutaneous **4** Percutaneous Endoscopic **7** Via Natural or Artificial Opening **8** Via Natural or Artificial Opening Endoscopic **X** External	**Z** No Device	**Z** No Qualifier
M Vulva	**0** Open **X** External	**Z** No Device	**Z** No Qualifier

Section 0 **Medical and Surgical**
Body System U **Female Reproductive System**
Operation L **Occlusion:** Completely closing an orifice or the lumen of a tubular body part

Body Part (4th)	Approach (5th)	Device (6th)	Qualifier (7th)
5 Fallopian Tube, Right **6** Fallopian Tube, Left **7** Fallopian Tubes, Bilateral	**0** Open **3** Percutaneous **4** Percutaneous Endoscopic	**C** Extraluminal Device **D** Intraluminal Device **Z** No Device	**Z** No Qualifier
5 Fallopian Tube, Right **6** Fallopian Tube, Left **7** Fallopian Tubes, Bilateral	**7** Via Natural or Artificial Opening **8** Via Natural or Artificial Opening Endoscopic	**D** Intraluminal Device **Z** No Device	**Z** No Qualifier
F Cul-de-sac **G** Vagina	**7** Via Natural or Artificial Opening **8** Via Natural or Artificial Opening Endoscopic	**D** Intraluminal Device **Z** No Device	**Z** No Qualifier

Section 0 **Medical and Surgical**
Body System U **Female Reproductive System**
Operation M **Reattachment:** Putting back in or on all or a portion of a separated body part to its normal location or other suitable location

Body Part (4th)	Approach (5th)	Device (6th)	Qualifier (7th)
0 Ovary, Right **1** Ovary, Left **2** Ovaries, Bilateral **4** Uterine Supporting Structure **5** Fallopian Tube, Right **6** Fallopian Tube, Left **7** Fallopian Tubes, Bilateral **9** Uterus **C** Cervix **F** Cul-de-sac **G** Vagina	**0** Open **4** Percutaneous Endoscopic	**Z** No Device	**Z** No Qualifier
J Clitoris **M** Vulva	**X** External	**Z** No Device	**Z** No Qualifier
K Hymen	**0** Open **4** Percutaneous Endoscopic **X** External	**Z** No Device	**Z** No Qualifier

Section 0 **Medical and Surgical**
Body System U **Female Reproductive System**
Operation N **Release:** Freeing a body part from an abnormal physical constraint by cutting or by the use of force

Body Part (4th)	Approach (5th)	Device (6th)	Qualifier (7th)
0 Ovary, Right **1** Ovary, Left **2** Ovaries, Bilateral **4** Uterine Supporting Structure	**0** Open **3** Percutaneous **4** Percutaneous Endoscopic **8** Via Natural or Artificial Opening Endoscopic	**Z** No Device	**Z** No Qualifier
5 Fallopian Tube, Right **6** Fallopian Tube, Left **7** Fallopian Tubes, Bilateral **9** Uterus **C** Cervix **F** Cul-de-sac	**0** Open **3** Percutaneous **4** Percutaneous Endoscopic **7** Via Natural or Artificial Opening **8** Via Natural or Artificial Opening Endoscopic	**Z** No Device	**Z** No Qualifier
G Vagina **K** Hymen	**0** Open **3** Percutaneous **4** Percutaneous Endoscopic **7** Via Natural or Artificial Opening **8** Via Natural or Artificial Opening Endoscopic **X** External	**Z** No Device	**Z** No Qualifier
J Clitoris **L** Vestibular Gland **M** Vulva	**0** Open **X** External	**Z** No Device	**Z** No Qualifier

Section 0 **Medical and Surgical**
Body System U **Female Reproductive System**
Operation P **Removal:** Taking out or off a device from a body part

Body Part (4th)	Approach (5th)	Device (6th)	Qualifier (7th)
3 Ovary	**0** Open **3** Percutaneous **4** Percutaneous Endoscopic	**0** Drainage Device **3** Infusion Device **Y** Other Device	**Z** No Qualifier
3 Ovary	**7** Via Natural or Artificial Opening **8** Via Natural or Artificial Opening Endoscopic	**Y** Other Device	**Z** No Qualifier
3 Ovary	**X** External	**0** Drainage Device **3** Infusion Device	**Z** No Qualifier
8 Fallopian Tube	**0** Open **3** Percutaneous **4** Percutaneous Endoscopic **7** Via Natural or Artificial Opening **8** Via Natural or Artificial Opening Endoscopic	**0** Drainage Device **3** Infusion Device **7** Autologous Tissue Substitute **C** Extraluminal Device **D** Intraluminal Device **J** Synthetic Substitute **K** Nonautologous Tissue Substitute **Y** Other Device	**Z** No Qualifier
8 Fallopian Tube	**X** External	**0** Drainage Device **3** Infusion Device **D** Intraluminal Device	**Z** No Qualifier
D Uterus and Cervix	**0** Open **3** Percutaneous **4** Percutaneous Endoscopic **7** Via Natural or Artificial Opening **8** Via Natural or Artificial Opening Endoscopic	**0** Drainage Device **1** Radioactive Element **3** Infusion Device **7** Autologous Tissue Substitute **C** Extraluminal Device **D** Intraluminal Device **H** Contraceptive Device **J** Synthetic Substitute **K** Nonautologous Tissue Substitute **Y** Other Device	**Z** No Qualifier

Continued →

Section 0 **Medical and Surgical**
Body System U **Female Reproductive System**
Operation P **Removal:** Taking out or off a device from a body part

Body Part (4th)	Approach (5th)	Device (6th)	Qualifier (7th)
D Uterus and Cervix	**X** External	**0** Drainage Device **3** Infusion Device **D** Intraluminal Device **H** Contraceptive Device	**Z** No Qualifier
H Vagina and Cul-de-sac	**0** Open **3** Percutaneous **4** Percutaneous Endoscopic **7** Via Natural or Artificial Opening **8** Via Natural or Artificial Opening Endoscopic	**0** Drainage Device **1** Radioactive Element **3** Infusion Device **7** Autologous Tissue Substitute **D** Intraluminal Device **J** Synthetic Substitute **K** Nonautologous Tissue Substitute **Y** Other Device	**Z** No Qualifier
H Vagina and Cul-de-sac	**X** External	**0** Drainage Device **1** Radioactive Element **3** Infusion Device **D** Intraluminal Device	**Z** No Qualifier
M Vulva	**0** Open	**0** Drainage Device **7** Autologous Tissue Substitute **J** Synthetic Substitute **K** Nonautologous Tissue Substitute	**Z** No Qualifier
M Vulva	**X** External	**0** Drainage Device	**Z** No Qualifier

Section 0 **Medical and Surgical**
Body System U **Female Reproductive System**
Operation Q **Repair:** Restoring, to the extent possible, a body part to its normal anatomic structure and function

Body Part (4th)	Approach (5th)	Device (6th)	Qualifier (7th)
0 Ovary, Right **1** Ovary, Left **2** Ovaries, Bilateral **4** Uterine Supporting Structure	**0** Open **3** Percutaneous **4** Percutaneous Endoscopic **8** Via Natural or Artificial Opening Endoscopic	**Z** No Device	**Z** No Qualifier
5 Fallopian Tube, Right **6** Fallopian Tube, Left **7** Fallopian Tubes, Bilateral **9** Uterus **C** Cervix **F** Cul-de-sac	**0** Open **3** Percutaneous **4** Percutaneous Endoscopic **7** Via Natural or Artificial Opening **8** Via Natural or Artificial Opening Endoscopic	**Z** No Device	**Z** No Qualifier
G Vagina **K** Hymen	**0** Open **3** Percutaneous **4** Percutaneous Endoscopic **7** Via Natural or Artificial Opening **8** Via Natural or Artificial Opening Endoscopic **X** External	**Z** No Device	**Z** No Qualifier
J Clitoris **L** Vestibular Gland **M** Vulva	**0** Open **X** External	**Z** No Device	**Z** No Qualifier

Section 0 **Medical and Surgical**
Body System U **Female Reproductive System**
Operation S **Reposition:** Moving to its normal location, or other suitable location, all or a portion of a body part

Body Part (4th)	Approach (5th)	Device (6th)	Qualifier (7th)
0 Ovary, Right **1** Ovary, Left **2** Ovaries, Bilateral **4** Uterine Supporting Structure **5** Fallopian Tube, Right **6** Fallopian Tube, Left **7** Fallopian Tubes, Bilateral **C** Cervix **F** Cul-de-sac	**0** Open **4** Percutaneous Endoscopic **8** Via Natural or Artificial Opening Endoscopic	**Z** No Device	**Z** No Qualifier
9 Uterus **G** Vagina	**0** Open **4** Percutaneous Endoscopic **7** Via Natural or Artificial Opening **8** Via Natural or Artificial Opening Endoscopic **X** External	**Z** No Device	**Z** No Qualifier

Section 0 **Medical and Surgical**
Body System U **Female Reproductive System**
Operation T **Resection:** Cutting out or off, without replacement, all of a body part

Body Part (4th)	Approach (5th)	Device (6th)	Qualifier (7th)
0 Ovary, Right **1** Ovary, Left **2** Ovaries, Bilateral **5** Fallopian Tube, Right **6** Fallopian Tube, Left **7** Fallopian Tubes, Bilateral	**0** Open **4** Percutaneous Endoscopic **7** Via Natural or Artificial Opening **8** Via Natural or Artificial Opening Endoscopic **F** Via Natural or Artificial Opening With Percutaneous Endoscopic Assistance	**Z** No Device	**Z** No Qualifier
4 Uterine Supporting Structure **C** Cervix **F** Cul-de-sac **G** Vagina	**0** Open **4** Percutaneous Endoscopic **7** Via Natural or Artificial Opening **8** Via Natural or Artificial Opening Endoscopic	**Z** No Device	**Z** No Qualifier
9 Uterus	**0** Open **4** Percutaneous Endoscopic **7** Via Natural or Artificial Opening **8** Via Natural or Artificial Opening Endoscopic **F** Via Natural or Artificial Opening with Percutaneous Endoscopic Assistance	**Z** No Device	**L** Supracervical **Z** No Qualifier
J Clitoris **L** Vestibular Gland **M** Vulva	**0** Open **X** External	**Z** No Device	**Z** No Qualifier
K Hymen	**0** Open **4** Percutaneous Endoscopic **7** Via Natural or Artificial Opening **8** Via Natural or Artificial Opening Endoscopic **X** External	**Z** No Device	**Z** No Qualifier

Section 0 **Medical and Surgical**
Body System U **Female Reproductive System**
Operation U **Supplement:** Putting in or on biological or synthetic material that physically reinforces and/or augments the function of a portion of a body part

Body Part (4th)	Approach (5th)	Device (6th)	Qualifier (7th)
4 Uterine Supporting Structure	**0** Open **4** Percutaneous Endoscopic	**7** Autologous Tissue Substitute **J** Synthetic Substitute **K** Nonautologous Tissue Substitute	**Z** No Qualifier
5 Fallopian Tube, Right **6** Fallopian Tube, Left **7** Fallopian Tubes, Bilateral **F** Cul-de-sac	**0** Open **4** Percutaneous Endoscopic **7** Via Natural or Artificial Opening **8** Via Natural or Artificial Opening Endoscopic	**7** Autologous Tissue Substitute **J** Synthetic Substitute **K** Nonautologous Tissue Substitute	**Z** No Qualifier
G Vagina **K** Hymen	**0** Open **4** Percutaneous Endoscopic **7** Via Natural or Artificial Opening **8** Via Natural or Artificial Opening Endoscopic **X** External	**7** Autologous Tissue Substitute **J** Synthetic Substitute **K** Nonautologous Tissue Substitute	**Z** No Qualifier
J Clitoris **M** Vulva	**0** Open **X** External	**7** Autologous Tissue Substitute **J** Synthetic Substitute **K** Nonautologous Tissue Substitute	**Z** No Qualifier

Section 0 **Medical and Surgical**
Body System U **Female Reproductive System**
Operation V **Restriction:** Partially closing an orifice or the lumen of a tubular body part

Body Part (4th)	Approach (5th)	Device (6th)	Qualifier (7th)
C Cervix	**0** Open **3** Percutaneous **4** Percutaneous Endoscopic	**C** Extraluminal Device **D** Intraluminal Device **Z** No Device	**Z** No Qualifier
C Cervix	**7** Via Natural or Artificial Opening **8** Via Natural or Artificial Opening Endoscopic	**D** Intraluminal Device **Z** No Device	**Z** No Qualifier

Section 0 **Medical and Surgical**
Body System U **Female Reproductive System**
Operation W **Revision:** Correcting, to the extent possible, a portion of a malfunctioning device or the position of a displaced device

Body Part (4th)	Approach (5th)	Device (6th)	Qualifier (7th)
3 Ovary	**0** Open **3** Percutaneous **4** Percutaneous Endoscopic	**0** Drainage Device **3** Infusion Device **Y** Other Device	**Z** No Qualifier
3 Ovary	**7** Via Natural or Artificial Opening **8** Via Natural or Artificial Opening Endoscopic	**Y** Other Device	**Z** No Qualifier
3 Ovary	**X** External	**0** Drainage Device **3** Infusion Device	**Z** No Qualifier
8 Fallopian Tube	**0** Open **3** Percutaneous **4** Percutaneous Endoscopic **7** Via Natural or Artificial Opening **8** Via Natural or Artificial Opening Endoscopic **X** External	**0** Drainage Device **3** Infusion Device **7** Autologous Tissue Substitute **C** Extraluminal Device **D** Intraluminal Device **J** Synthetic Substitute **K** Nonautologous Tissue Substitute **Y** Other Device	**Z** No Qualifier

Continued →

Section 0 **Medical and Surgical**
Body System U **Female Reproductive System**
Operation W **Revision:** Correcting, to the extent possible, a portion of a malfunctioning device or the position of a displaced device

Body Part (4th)	Approach (5th)	Device (6th)	Qualifier (7th)
8 Fallopian Tube	**X** External	**0** Drainage Device **3** Infusion Device **7** Autologous Tissue Substitute **C** Extraluminal Device **D** Intraluminal Device **J** Synthetic Substitute **K** Nonautologous Tissue Substitute	**Z** No Qualifier
D Uterus and Cervix	**0** Open **3** Percutaneous **4** Percutaneous Endoscopic **7** Via Natural or Artificial Opening **8** Via Natural or Artificial Opening Endoscopic	**0** Drainage Device **1** Radioactive Element **3** Infusion Device **7** Autologous Tissue Substitute **C** Extraluminal Device **D** Intraluminal Device **H** Contraceptive Device **J** Synthetic Substitute **K** Nonautologous Tissue Substitute **Y** Other Device	**Z** No Qualifier
D Uterus and Cervix	**X** External	**0** Drainage Device **3** Infusion Device **7** Autologous Tissue Substitute **C** Extraluminal Device **D** Intraluminal Device **H** Contraceptive Device **J** Synthetic Substitute **K** Nonautologous Tissue Substitute	**Z** No Qualifier
H Vagina and Cul-de-sac	**0** Open **3** Percutaneous **4** Percutaneous Endoscopic **7** Via Natural or Artificial Opening **8** Via Natural or Artificial Opening Endoscopic	**0** Drainage Device **1** Radioactive Element **3** Infusion Device **7** Autologous Tissue Substitute **D** Intraluminal Device **J** Synthetic Substitute **K** Nonautologous Tissue Substitute **Y** Other Device	**Z** No Qualifier
H Vagina and Cul-de-sac	**X** External	**0** Drainage Device **3** Infusion Device **7** Autologous Tissue Substitute **D** Intraluminal Device **J** Synthetic Substitute **K** Nonautologous Tissue Substitute	**Z** No Qualifier
M Vulva	**0** Open **X** External	**0** Drainage Device **7** Autologous Tissue Substitute **J** Synthetic Substitute **K** Nonautologous Tissue Substitute	**Z** No Qualifier

Section 0 **Medical and Surgical**
Body System U **Female Reproductive System**
Operation Y
Transplantation: Putting in or on all or a portion of a living body part taken from another individual or animal to physically take the place and/or function of all or a portion of a similar body part

Body Part (4th)	Approach (5th)	Device (6th)	Qualifier (7th)
0 Ovary, Right **1** Ovary, Left **9** Uterus	**0** Open	**Z** No Device	**0** Allogeneic **1** Syngeneic **2** Zooplastic

AHA Coding Clinic

0U7C7ZZ Dilation of Cervix, Via Natural or Artificial Opening—AHA CC: 2Q, 2020, 30

0U9G7ZZ Drainage of Vagina, Via Natural or Artificial Opening—AHA CC: 4Q, 2016, 58-59

0UB64ZZ Excision of Left Fallopian Tube, Percutaneous Endoscopic Approach—AHA CC: 3Q, 2015, 31-32

0UB70ZZ Excision of Bilateral Fallopian Tubes, Open Approach—AHA CC: 3Q, 2015, 31

0UB90ZZ Excision of Uterus, Open Approach—AHA CC: 4Q, 2014, 16

0UBMXZZ Excision of Vulva, External Approach—AHA CC: 3Q, 2014, 12

0UC97ZZ Extirpation of Matter from Uterus, Via Natural or Artificial Opening—AHA CC: 2Q, 2013, 38

0UCC7ZZ Extirpation of Matter from Cervix, Via Natural or Artificial Opening—AHA CC: 3Q, 2015, 30

0UCC8ZZ Extirpation of Matter from Cervix, Via Natural or Artificial Opening Endoscopic—AHA CC: 3Q, 2015, 30-31

0UH97HZ Insertion of Contraceptive Device into Uterus, Via Natural or Artificial Opening—AHA CC: 2Q, 2013, 34

0UHD7YZ Insertion of Other Device into Uterus and Cervix, Via Natural or Artificial Opening—AHA CC: 4Q, 2017, 104; 1Q, 2018, 25

0UJD4ZZ Inspection of Uterus and Cervix, Percutaneous Endoscopic Approach—AHA CC: 1Q, 2015, 33-34

0UQ60ZZ Repair Left Fallopian Tube, Open Approach—AHA CC: 4Q, 2020, 60

0UQJXZZ Repair Clitoris, External Approach—AHA CC: 4Q, 2013, 120-121

0UQMXZZ Repair Vulva, External Approach—AHA CC: 4Q, 2014, 18-19

0US9XZZ Reposition Uterus, External Approach—AHA CC: 1Q, 2016, 9

0UT00ZZ Resection of Right Ovary, Open Approach—AHA CC: 1Q, 2013, 24

0UT20ZZ Resection of Bilateral Ovaries, Open Approach—AHA CC: 1Q, 2015, 33-34

0UT70ZZ Resection of Bilateral Fallopian Tubes, Open Approach—AHA CC: 1Q, 2015, 33-34

0UT90ZZ Resection of Uterus, Open Approach—AHA CC: 3Q, 2013, 28; 1Q, 2015, 33-34; 4Q, 2017, 68

0UT97ZL Resection of Uterus, Supracervical, Via Natural or Artificial Opening—AHA CC: 4Q, 2017, 68

0UTC0ZZ Resection of Cervix, Open Approach—AHA CC: 3Q, 2013, 28; 1Q, 2015, 33-34

0UVC7ZZ Restriction of Cervix, Via Natural or Artificial Opening—AHA CC: 3Q, 2015, 30

Male Reproductive System

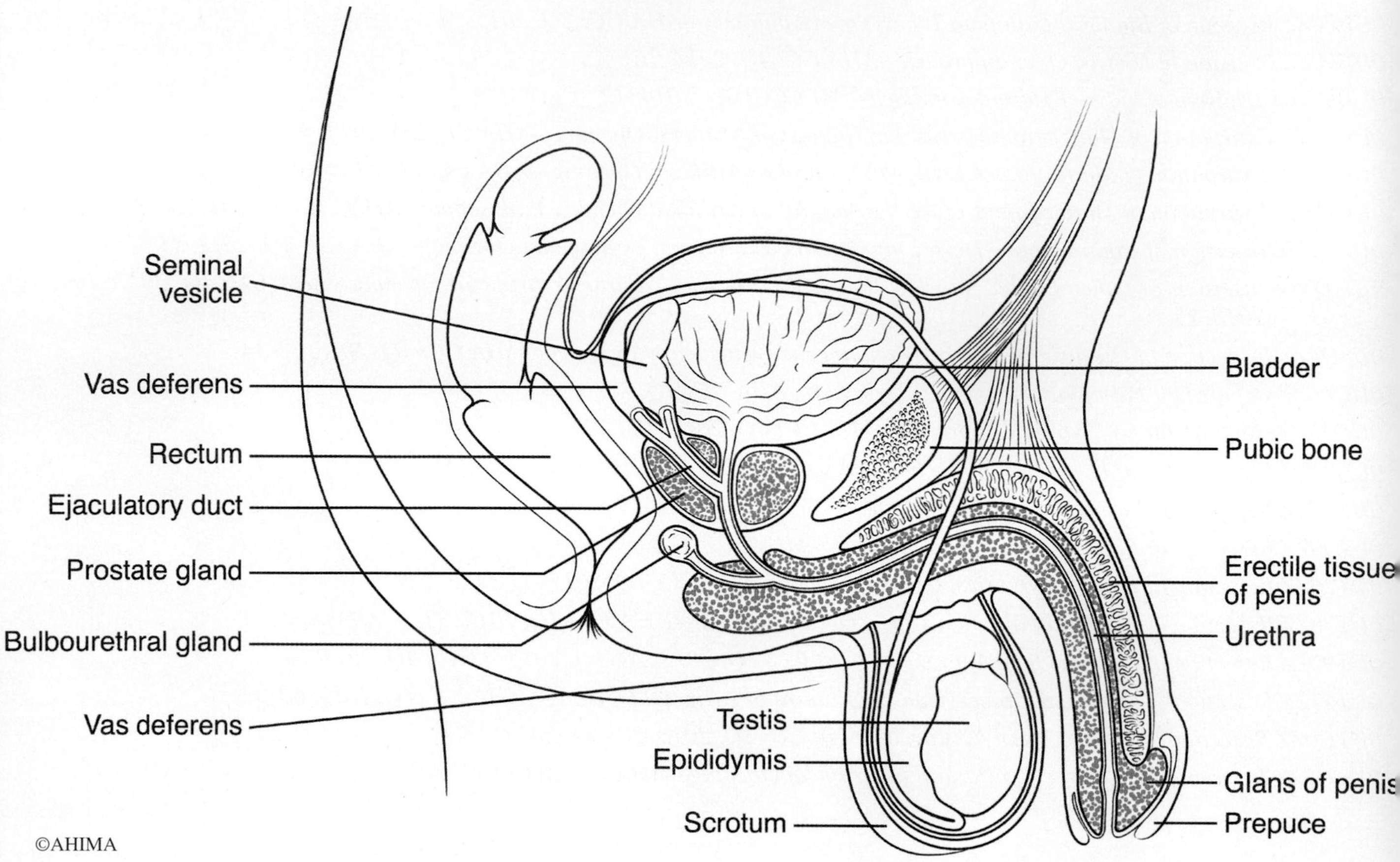
Seminal vesicle
Vas deferens
Rectum
Ejaculatory duct
Prostate gland
Bulbourethral gland
Vas deferens
Testis
Epididymis
Scrotum
Bladder
Pubic bone
Erectile tissue of penis
Urethra
Glans of penis
Prepuce

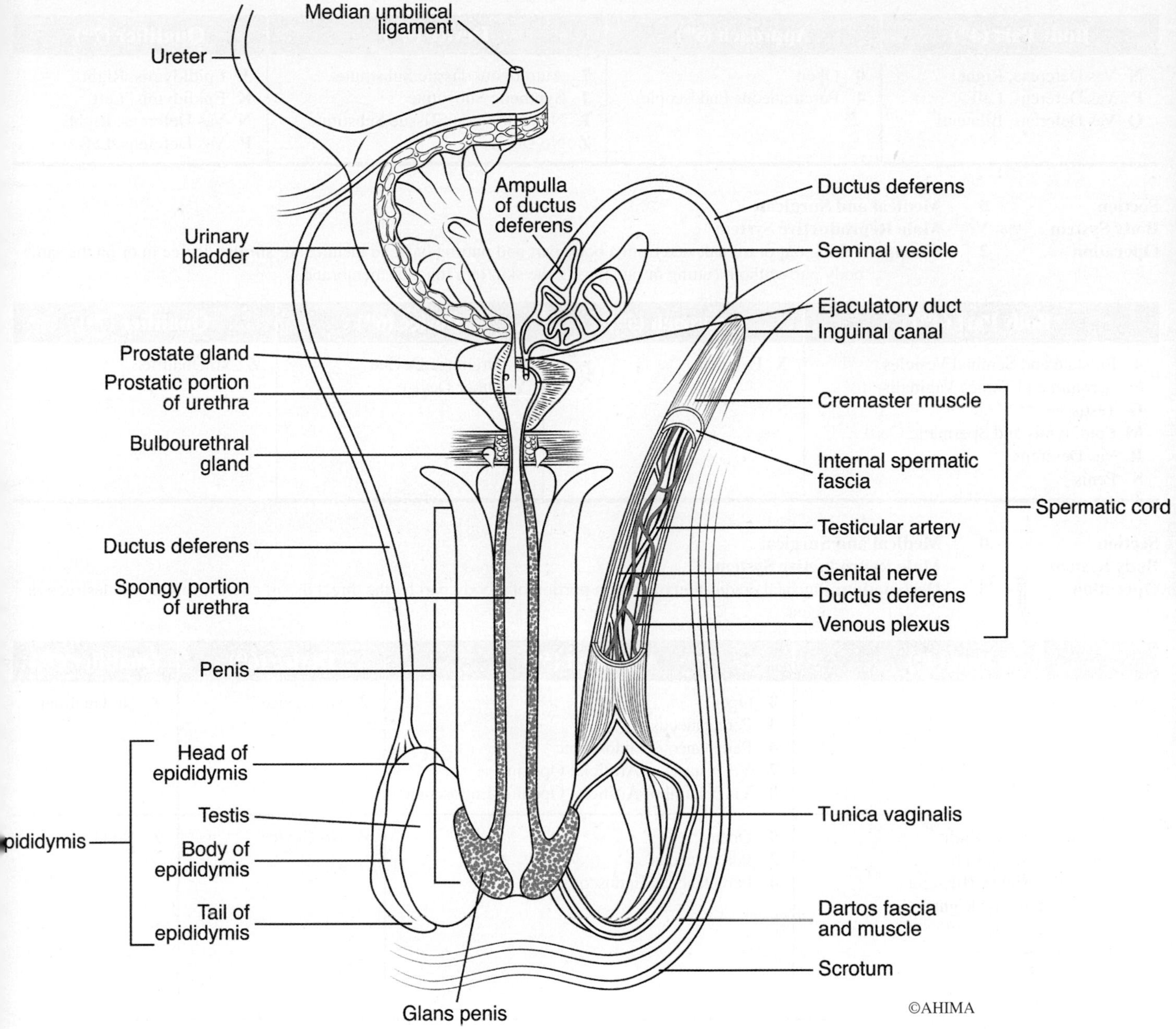
Median umbilical ligament
Ureter
Ampulla of ductus deferens
Ductus deferens
Seminal vesicle
Urinary bladder
Ejaculatory duct
Inguinal canal
Prostate gland
Prostatic portion of urethra
Cremaster muscle
Bulbourethral gland
Internal spermatic fascia
Spermatic cord
Testicular artery
Ductus deferens
Genital nerve
Ductus deferens
Spongy portion of urethra
Venous plexus
Penis
Head of epididymis
Testis
Tunica vaginalis
pididymis
Body of epididymis
Tail of epididymis
Dartos fascia and muscle
Scrotum
Glans penis

Male Reproductive System Tables 0V1–0VY

Section 0 **Medical and Surgical**
Body System V **Male Reproductive System**
Operation 1 **Bypass:** Altering the route of passage of the contents of a tubular body part

Body Part (4th)	Approach (5th)	Device (6th)	Qualifier (7th)
N Vas Deferens, Right **P** Vas Deferens, Left **Q** Vas Deferens, Bilateral	**0** Open **4** Percutaneous Endoscopic	**7** Autologous Tissue Substitute **J** Synthetic Substitute **K** Nonautologous Tissue Substitute **Z** No Device	**J** Epididymis, Right **K** Epididymis, Left **N** Vas Deferens, Right **P** Vas Deferens, Left

Section 0 **Medical and Surgical**
Body System V **Male Reproductive System**
Operation 2 **Change:** Taking out or off a device from a body part and putting back an identical or similar device in or on the same body part without cutting or puncturing the skin or a mucous membrane

Body Part (4th)	Approach (5th)	Device (6th)	Qualifier (7th)
4 Prostate and Seminal Vesicles **8** Scrotum and Tunica Vaginalis **D** Testis **M** Epididymis and Spermatic Cord **R** Vas Deferens **S** Penis	**X** External	**0** Drainage Device **Y** Other Device	**Z** No Qualifier

Section 0 **Medical and Surgical**
Body System V **Male Reproductive System**
Operation 5 **Destruction:** Physical eradication of all or a portion of a body part by the direct use of energy, force, or a destructive agent

Body Part (4th)	Approach (5th)	Device (6th)	Qualifier (7th)
0 Prostate	**0** Open **3** Percutaneous **4** Percutaneous Endoscopic **7** Via Natural or Artificial Opening **8** Via Natural or Artificial Opening Endoscopic	**Z** No Device	**Z** No Qualifier
1 Seminal Vesicle, Right **2** Seminal Vesicle, Left **3** Seminal Vesicles, Bilateral **6** Tunica Vaginalis, Right **7** Tunica Vaginalis, Left **9** Testis, Right **B** Testis, Left **C** Testes, Bilateral	**0** Open **3** Percutaneous **4** Percutaneous Endoscopic	**Z** No Device	**Z** No Qualifier
5 Scrotum **S** Penis **T** Prepuce	**0** Open **3** Percutaneous **4** Percutaneous Endoscopic **X** External	**Z** No Device	**Z** No Qualifier
F Spermatic Cord, Right **G** Spermatic Cord, Left **H** Spermatic Cords, Bilateral **J** Epididymis, Right **K** Epididymis, Left **L** Epididymis, Bilateral **N** Vas Deferens, Right **P** Vas Deferens, Left **Q** Vas Deferens, Bilateral	**0** Open **3** Percutaneous **4** Percutaneous Endoscopic **8** Via Natural or Artificial Opening Endoscopic	**Z** No Device	**Z** No Qualifier

Section 0 **Medical and Surgical**
Body System V **Male Reproductive System**
Operation 7 **Dilation:** Expanding an orifice or the lumen of a tubular body part

Body Part (4th)	Approach (5th)	Device (6th)	Qualifier (7th)
N Vas Deferens, Right **P** Vas Deferens, Left **Q** Vas Deferens, Bilateral	**0** Open **3** Percutaneous **4** Percutaneous Endoscopic	**D** Intraluminal Device **Z** No Device	**Z** No Qualifier

Section 0 **Medical and Surgical**
Body System V **Male Reproductive System**
Operation 9 **Drainage:** Taking or letting out fluids and/or gases from a body part

Body Part (4th)	Approach (5th)	Device (6th)	Qualifier (7th)
0 Prostate	**0** Open **3** Percutaneous **4** Percutaneous Endoscopic **7** Via Natural or Artificial Opening **8** Via Natural or Artificial Opening Endoscopic	**0** Drainage Device	**Z** No Qualifier
0 Prostate	**0** Open **3** Percutaneous **4** Percutaneous Endoscopic **7** Via Natural or Artificial Opening **8** Via Natural or Artificial Opening Endoscopic	**Z** No Device	**X** Diagnostic **Z** No Qualifier
1 Seminal Vesicle, Right **2** Seminal Vesicle, Left **3** Seminal Vesicles, Bilateral **6** Tunica Vaginalis, Right **7** Tunica Vaginalis, Left **9** Testis, Right **B** Testis, Left **C** Testes, Bilateral **F** Spermatic Cord, Right **G** Spermatic Cord, Left **H** Spermatic Cords, Bilateral **J** Epididymis, Right **K** Epididymis, Left **L** Epididymis, Bilateral **N** Vas Deferens, Right **P** Vas Deferens, Left **Q** Vas Deferens, Bilateral	**0** Open **3** Percutaneous **4** Percutaneous Endoscopic	**0** Drainage Device	**Z** No Qualifier
1 Seminal Vesicle, Right **2** Seminal Vesicle, Left **3** Seminal Vesicles, Bilateral **6** Tunica Vaginalis, Right **7** Tunica Vaginalis, Left **9** Testis, Right **B** Testis, Left **C** Testes, Bilateral **F** Spermatic Cord, Right **G** Spermatic Cord, Left **H** Spermatic Cords, Bilateral **J** Epididymis, Right **K** Epididymis, Left **L** Epididymis, Bilateral **N** Vas Deferens, Right **P** Vas Deferens, Left **Q** Vas Deferens, Bilateral	**0** Open **3** Percutaneous **4** Percutaneous Endoscopic	**Z** No Device	**X** Diagnostic **Z** No Qualifier
5 Scrotum **S** Penis **T** Prepuce	**0** Open **3** Percutaneous **4** Percutaneous Endoscopic **X** External	**0** Drainage Device	**Z** No Qualifier

Continued →

Section 0 Medical and Surgical
Body System V Male Reproductive System
Operation 9 **Drainage:** Taking or letting out fluids and/or gases from a body part

0V9 Continued

Body Part (4th)	Approach (5th)	Device (6th)	Qualifier (7th)
5 Scrotum S Penis T Prepuce	0 Open 3 Percutaneous 4 Percutaneous Endoscopic X External	Z No Device	X Diagnostic Z No Qualifier

Section 0 Medical and Surgical
Body System V Male Reproductive System
Operation B **Excision:** Cutting out or off, without replacement, a portion of a body part

Body Part (4th)	Approach (5th)	Device (6th)	Qualifier (7th)
0 Prostate	0 Open 3 Percutaneous 4 Percutaneous Endoscopic 7 Via Natural or Artificial Opening 8 Via Natural or Artificial Opening Endoscopic	Z No Device	X Diagnostic Z No Qualifier
1 Seminal Vesicle, Right 2 Seminal Vesicle, Left 3 Seminal Vesicles, Bilateral 6 Tunica Vaginalis, Right 7 Tunica Vaginalis, Left 9 Testis, Right B Testis, Left C Testes, Bilateral	0 Open 3 Percutaneous 4 Percutaneous Endoscopic	Z No Device	X Diagnostic Z No Qualifier
5 Scrotum S Penis T Prepuce	0 Open 3 Percutaneous 4 Percutaneous Endoscopic X External	Z No Device	X Diagnostic Z No Qualifier
F Spermatic Cord, Right G Spermatic Cord, Left H Spermatic Cords, Bilateral J Epididymis, Right K Epididymis, Left L Epididymis, Bilateral N Vas Deferens, Right P Vas Deferens, Left Q Vas Deferens, Bilateral	0 Open 3 Percutaneous 4 Percutaneous Endoscopic 8 Via Natural or Artificial Opening Endoscopic	Z No Device	X Diagnostic Z No Qualifier

Section 0 Medical and Surgical
Body System V Male Reproductive System
Operation C **Extirpation:** Taking or cutting out solid matter from a body part

Body Part (4th)	Approach (5th)	Device (6th)	Qualifier (7th)
0 Prostate	0 Open 3 Percutaneous 4 Percutaneous Endoscopic 7 Via Natural or Artificial Opening 8 Via Natural or Artificial Opening Endoscopic	Z No Device	Z No Qualifier

Continued →

Section 0 **Medical and Surgical**
Body System V **Male Reproductive System**
Operation C **Extirpation:** Taking or cutting out solid matter from a body part

Body Part (4th)	Approach (5th)	Device (6th)	Qualifier (7th)
1 Seminal Vesicle, Right 2 Seminal Vesicle, Left 3 Seminal Vesicles, Bilateral 6 Tunica Vaginalis, Right 7 Tunica Vaginalis, Left 9 Testis, Right B Testis, Left C Testes, Bilateral F Spermatic Cord, Right G Spermatic Cord, Left H Spermatic Cords, Bilateral J Epididymis, Right K Epididymis, Left L Epididymis, Bilateral N Vas Deferens, Right P Vas Deferens, Left Q Vas Deferens, Bilateral	0 Open 3 Percutaneous 4 Percutaneous Endoscopic	Z No Device	Z No Qualifier
5 Scrotum S Penis T Prepuce	0 Open 3 Percutaneous 4 Percutaneous Endoscopic X External	Z No Device	Z No Qualifier

Section 0 **Medical and Surgical**
Body System V **Male Reproductive System**
Operation H **Insertion:** Putting in a nonbiological appliance that monitors, assists, performs, or prevents a physiological function but does not physically take the place of a body part

Body Part (4th)	Approach (5th)	Device (6th)	Qualifier (7th)
0 Prostate	0 Open 3 Percutaneous 4 Percutaneous Endoscopic 7 Via Natural or Artificial Opening 8 Via Natural or Artificial Opening Endoscopic	1 Radioactive Element	Z No Qualifier
4 Prostate and Seminal Vesicles 8 Scrotum and Tunica Vaginalis M Epididymis and Spermatic Cord R Vas Deferens	0 Open 3 Percutaneous 4 Percutaneous Endoscopic 7 Via Natural or Artificial Opening 8 Via Natural or Artificial Opening Endoscopic	3 Infusion Device Y Other Device	Z No Qualifier
D Testis	0 Open 3 Percutaneous 4 Percutaneous Endoscopic 7 Via Natural or Artificial Opening 8 Via Natural or Artificial Opening Endoscopic	1 Radioactive Element 3 Infusion Device Y Other Device	Z No Qualifier
S Penis	0 Open 3 Percutaneous 4 Percutaneous Endoscopic	3 Infusion Device Y Other Device	Z No Qualifier
S Penis	7 Via Natural or Artificial Opening 8 Via Natural or Artificial Opening Endoscopic	Y Other Device	Z No Qualifier
S Penis	X External	3 Infusion Device	Z No Qualifier

Section 0 **Medical and Surgical**
Body System V **Male Reproductive System**
Operation J **Inspection:** Visually and/or manually exploring a body part

Body Part (4th)	Approach (5th)	Device (6th)	Qualifier (7th)
4 Prostate and Seminal Vesicles **8** Scrotum and Tunica Vaginalis **D** Testis **M** Epididymis and Spermatic Cord **R** Vas Deferens **S** Penis	**0** Open **3** Percutaneous **4** Percutaneous Endoscopic **X** External	**Z** No Device	**Z** No Qualifier

Section 0 **Medical and Surgical**
Body System V **Male Reproductive System**
Operation L **Occlusion:** Completely closing an orifice or the lumen of a tubular body part

Body Part (4th)	Approach (5th)	Device (6th)	Qualifier (7th)
F Spermatic Cord, Right **G** Spermatic Cord, Left **H** Spermatic Cords, Bilateral **N** Vas Deferens, Right **P** Vas Deferens, Left **Q** Vas Deferens, Bilateral	**0** Open **3** Percutaneous **4** Percutaneous Endoscopic **8** Via Natural or Artificial Opening Endoscopic	**C** Extraluminal Device **D** Intraluminal Device **Z** No Device	**Z** No Qualifier

Section 0 **Medical and Surgical**
Body System V **Male Reproductive System**
Operation M **Reattachment:** Putting back in or on all or a portion of a separated body part to its normal location or other suitable location

Body Part (4th)	Approach (5th)	Device (6th)	Qualifier (7th)
5 Scrotum **S** Penis	**X** External	**Z** No Device	**Z** No Qualifier
6 Tunica Vaginalis, Right **7** Tunica Vaginalis, Left **9** Testis, Right **B** Testis, Left **C** Testes, Bilateral **F** Spermatic Cord, Right **G** Spermatic Cord, Left **H** Spermatic Cords, Bilateral	**0** Open **4** Percutaneous Endoscopic	**Z** No Device	**Z** No Qualifier

Section 0 **Medical and Surgical**
Body System V **Male Reproductive System**
Operation N **Release:** Freeing a body part from an abnormal physical constraint by cutting or by the use of force

Body Part (4th)	Approach (5th)	Device (6th)	Qualifier (7th)
0 Prostate	**0** Open **3** Percutaneous **4** Percutaneous Endoscopic **7** Via Natural or Artificial Opening **8** Via Natural or Artificial Opening Endoscopic	**Z** No Device	**Z** No Qualifier
1 Seminal Vesicle, Right **2** Seminal Vesicle, Left **3** Seminal Vesicles, Bilateral **6** Tunica Vaginalis, Right **7** Tunica Vaginalis, Left **9** Testis, Right **B** Testis, Left **C** Testes, Bilateral	**0** Open **3** Percutaneous **4** Percutaneous Endoscopic	**Z** No Device	**Z** No Qualifier

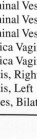

Continued →

Section 0 Medical and Surgical
Body System V Male Reproductive System
Operation N **Release:** Freeing a body part from an abnormal physical constraint by cutting or by the use of force

Body Part (4th)	Approach (5th)	Device (6th)	Qualifier (7th)
5 Scrotum **S** Penis **T** Prepuce	**0** Open **3** Percutaneous **4** Percutaneous Endoscopic **X** External	**Z** No Device	**Z** No Qualifier
F Spermatic Cord, Right **G** Spermatic Cord, Left **H** Spermatic Cords, Bilateral **J** Epididymis, Right **K** Epididymis, Left **L** Epididymis, Bilateral **N** Vas Deferens, Right **P** Vas Deferens, Left **Q** Vas Deferens, Bilateral	**0** Open **3** Percutaneous **4** Percutaneous Endoscopic **8** Via Natural or Artificial Opening Endoscopic	**Z** No Device	**Z** No Qualifier

Section 0 Medical and Surgical
Body System V Male Reproductive System
Operation P **Removal:** Taking out or off a device from a body part

Body Part (4th)	Approach (5th)	Device (6th)	Qualifier (7th)
4 Prostate and Seminal Vesicles	**0** Open **3** Percutaneous **4** Percutaneous Endoscopic **7** Via Natural or Artificial Opening **8** Via Natural or Artificial Opening Endoscopic	**0** Drainage Device **1** Radioactive Element **3** Infusion Device **7** Autologous Tissue Substitute **J** Synthetic Substitute **K** Nonautologous Tissue Substitute **Y** Other Device	**Z** No Qualifier
4 Prostate and Seminal Vesicles	**X** External	**0** Drainage Device **1** Radioactive Element **3** Infusion Device	**Z** No Qualifier
8 Scrotum and Tunica Vaginalis **D** Testis **S** Penis	**0** Open **3** Percutaneous **4** Percutaneous Endoscopic **7** Via Natural or Artificial Opening **8** Via Natural or Artificial Opening Endoscopic	**0** Drainage Device **3** Infusion Device **7** Autologous Tissue Substitute **J** Synthetic Substitute **K** Nonautologous Tissue Substitute **Y** Other Device	**Z** No Qualifier
8 Scrotum and Tunica Vaginalis **D** Testis **S** Penis	**X** External	**0** Drainage Device **3** Infusion Device	**Z** No Qualifier
M Epididymis and Spermatic Cord	**0** Open **3** Percutaneous **4** Percutaneous Endoscopic **7** Via Natural or Artificial Opening **8** Via Natural or Artificial Opening Endoscopic	**0** Drainage Device **3** Infusion Device **7** Autologous Tissue Substitute **C** Extraluminal Device **J** Synthetic Substitute **K** Nonautologous Tissue Substitute **Y** Other Device	**Z** No Qualifier
M Epididymis and Spermatic Cord	**X** External	**0** Drainage Device **3** Infusion Device	**Z** No Qualifier

Continued →

Section 0 **Medical and Surgical**
Body System V **Male Reproductive System**
Operation P **Removal:** Taking out or off a device from a body part

Body Part (4th)	Approach (5th)	Device (6th)	Qualifier (7th)
R Vas Deferens	**0** Open **3** Percutaneous **4** Percutaneous Endoscopic **7** Via Natural or Artificial Opening **8** Via Natural or Artificial Opening Endoscopic	**0** Drainage Device **3** Infusion Device **7** Autologous Tissue Substitute **C** Extraluminal Device **D** Intraluminal Device **J** Synthetic Substitute **K** Nonautologous Tissue Substitute **Y** Other Device	**Z** No Qualifier
R Vas Deferens	**X** External	**0** Drainage Device **3** Infusion Device **D** Intraluminal Device	**Z** No Qualifier

Section 0 **Medical and Surgical**
Body System V **Male Reproductive System**
Operation Q **Repair:** Restoring, to the extent possible, a body part to its normal anatomic structure and function

Body Part (4th)	Approach (5th)	Device (6th)	Qualifier (7th)
0 Prostate	**0** Open **3** Percutaneous **4** Percutaneous Endoscopic **7** Via Natural or Artificial Opening **8** Via Natural or Artificial Opening Endoscopic	**Z** No Device	**Z** No Qualifier
1 Seminal Vesicle, Right **2** Seminal Vesicle, Left **3** Seminal Vesicles, Bilateral **6** Tunica Vaginalis, Right **7** Tunica Vaginalis, Left **9** Testis, Right **B** Testis, Left **C** Testes, Bilateral	**0** Open **3** Percutaneous **4** Percutaneous Endoscopic	**Z** No Device	**Z** No Qualifier
5 Scrotum **S** Penis **T** Prepuce	**0** Open **3** Percutaneous **4** Percutaneous Endoscopic **X** External	**Z** No Device	**Z** No Qualifier
F Spermatic Cord, Right **G** Spermatic Cord, Left **H** Spermatic Cords, Bilateral **J** Epididymis, Right **K** Epididymis, Left **L** Epididymis, Bilateral **N** Vas Deferens, Right **P** Vas Deferens, Left **Q** Vas Deferens, Bilateral	**0** Open **3** Percutaneous **4** Percutaneous Endoscopic **8** Via Natural or Artificial Opening Endoscopic	**Z** No Device	**Z** No Qualifier

Section 0 **Medical and Surgical**
Body System V **Male Reproductive System**
Operation R **Replacement:** Putting in or on biological or synthetic material that physically takes the place and/or function of all or a portion of a body part

Body Part (4th)	Approach (5th)	Device (6th)	Qualifier (7th)
9 Testis, Right **B** Testis, Left **C** Testes, Bilateral	**0** Open	**J** Synthetic Substitute	**Z** No Qualifier

Section 0 **Medical and Surgical**
Body System V **Male Reproductive System**
Operation S **Reposition:** Moving to its normal location, or other suitable location, all or a portion of a body part

Body Part (4th)	Approach (5th)	Device (6th)	Qualifier (7th)
9 Testis, Right **B** Testis, Left **C** Testes, Bilateral **F** Spermatic Cord, Right **G** Spermatic Cord, Left **H** Spermatic Cords, Bilateral	**0** Open **3** Percutaneous **4** Percutaneous Endoscopic **8** Via Natural or Artificial Opening Endoscopic	**Z** No Device	**Z** No Qualifier

Section 0 **Medical and Surgical**
Body System V **Male Reproductive System**
Operation T **Resection:** Cutting out or off, without replacement, all of a body part

Body Part (4th)	Approach (5th)	Device (6th)	Qualifier (7th)
0 Prostate	**0** Open **4** Percutaneous Endoscopic **7** Via Natural or Artificial Opening **8** Via Natural or Artificial Opening Endoscopic	**Z** No Device	**Z** No Qualifier
1 Seminal Vesicle, Right **2** Seminal Vesicle, Left **3** Seminal Vesicles, Bilateral **6** Tunica Vaginalis, Right **7** Tunica Vaginalis, Left **9** Testis, Right **B** Testis, Left **C** Testes, Bilateral **F** Spermatic Cord, Right **G** Spermatic Cord, Left **H** Spermatic Cords, Bilateral **J** Epididymis, Right **K** Epididymis, Left **L** Epididymis, Bilateral **N** Vas Deferens, Right **P** Vas Deferens, Left **Q** Vas Deferens, Bilateral	**0** Open **4** Percutaneous Endoscopic	**Z** No Device	**Z** No Qualifier
5 Scrotum **S** Penis **T** Prepuce	**0** Open **4** Percutaneous Endoscopic **X** External	**Z** No Device	**Z** No Qualifier

Section 0 **Medical and Surgical**
Body System V **Male Reproductive System**
Operation U **Supplement:** Putting in or on biological or synthetic material that physically reinforces and/or augments the function of a portion of a body part

Body Part (4th)	Approach (5th)	Device (6th)	Qualifier (7th)
1 Seminal Vesicle, Right **2** Seminal Vesicle, Left **3** Seminal Vesicles, Bilateral **6** Tunica Vaginalis, Right **7** Tunica Vaginalis, Left **F** Spermatic Cord, Right **G** Spermatic Cord, Left **H** Spermatic Cords, Bilateral **J** Epididymis, Right **K** Epididymis, Left **L** Epididymis, Bilateral **N** Vas Deferens, Right **P** Vas Deferens, Left **Q** Vas Deferens, Bilateral	**0** Open **4** Percutaneous Endoscopic **8** Via Natural or Artificial Opening Endoscopic	**7** Autologous Tissue Substitute **J** Synthetic Substitute **K** Nonautologous Tissue Substitute	**Z** No Qualifier

Continued →

Section 0 **Medical and Surgical**
Body System V **Male Reproductive System**
Operation U **Supplement:** Putting in or on biological or synthetic material that physically reinforces and/or augments the function of a portion of a body part

Body Part (4th)	Approach (5th)	Device (6th)	Qualifier (7th)
5 Scrotum **S** Penis **T** Prepuce	**0** Open **4** Percutaneous Endoscopic **X** External	**7** Autologous Tissue Substitute **J** Synthetic Substitute **K** Nonautologous Tissue Substitute	**Z** No Qualifier
9 Testis, Right **B** Testis, Left **C** Testes, Bilateral	**0** Open	**7** Autologous Tissue Substitute **J** Synthetic Substitute **K** Nonautologous Tissue Substitute	**Z** No Qualifier

Section 0 **Medical and Surgical**
Body System V **Male Reproductive System**
Operation W **Revision:** Correcting, to the extent possible, a portion of a malfunctioning device or the position of a displaced device

Body Part (4th)	Approach (5th)	Device (6th)	Qualifier (7th)
4 Prostate and Seminal Vesicles **8** Scrotum and Tunica Vaginalis **D** Testis **S** Penis	**0** Open **3** Percutaneous **4** Percutaneous Endoscopic **7** Via Natural or Artificial Opening **8** Via Natural or Artificial Opening Endoscopic	**0** Drainage Device **3** Infusion Device **7** Autologous Tissue Substitute **J** Synthetic Substitute **K** Nonautologous Tissue Substitute **Y** Other Device	**Z** No Qualifier
4 Prostate and Seminal Vesicles **8** Scrotum and Tunica Vaginalis **D** Testis **S** Penis	**X** External	**0** Drainage Device **3** Infusion Device **7** Autologous Tissue Substitute **J** Synthetic Substitute **K** Nonautologous Tissue Substitute	**Z** No Qualifier
M Epididymis and Spermatic Cord	**0** Open **3** Percutaneous **4** Percutaneous Endoscopic **7** Via Natural or Artificial Opening **8** Via Natural or Artificial Opening Endoscopic	**0** Drainage Device **3** Infusion Device **7** Autologous Tissue Substitute **C** Extraluminal Device **J** Synthetic Substitute **K** Nonautologous Tissue Substitute **Y** Other Device	**Z** No Qualifier
M Epididymis and Spermatic Cord	**X** External	**0** Drainage Device **3** Infusion Device **7** Autologous Tissue Substitute **C** Extraluminal Device **J** Synthetic Substitute **K** Nonautologous Tissue Substitute	**Z** No Qualifier
R Vas Deferens	**0** Open **3** Percutaneous **4** Percutaneous Endoscopic **7** Via Natural or Artificial Opening **8** Via Natural or Artificial Opening Endoscopic	**0** Drainage Device **3** Infusion Device **7** Autologous Tissue Substitute **C** Extraluminal Device **D** Intraluminal Device **J** Synthetic Substitute **K** Nonautologous Tissue Substitute **Y** Other Device	**Z** No Qualifier
R Vas Deferens	**X** External	**0** Drainage Device **3** Infusion Device **7** Autologous Tissue Substitute **C** Extraluminal Device **C** Intraluminal Device **J** Synthetic Substitute **K** Nonautologous Tissue Substitute	**Z** No Qualifier

Section	0	Medical and Surgical
Body System	V	Male Reproductive System
Operation	X	**Transfer:** Moving, without taking out, all or a portion of a body part to another location to take over the function of all or a portion of a body part

Body Part (4th)	Approach (5th)	Device (6th)	Qualifier (7th)
T Prepuce	**0** Open **X** External	**Z** No Device	**D** Urethra **S** Penis

Section	0	Medical and Surgical
Body System	V	Male Reproductive System
Operation	Y	**Transplantation:** Putting in or on all or a portion of a living body part taken from another individual or animal to physically take the place and/or function of all or a portion of a similar body part

Body Part (4th)	Approach (5th)	Device (6th)	Qualifier (7th)
5 Scrotum **6** Penis	**0** Open	**Z** No Device	**0** Allogeneic **1** Syngeneic **2** Zooplastic

AHA Coding Clinic

0VBQ4ZZ Excision of Bilateral Vas Deferens, Percutaneous Endoscopic Approach—AHA CC: 4Q, 2014, 33-34; 1Q, 2016, 23

0VPS0JZ Removal of Synthetic Substitute from Penis, Open Approach—AHA CC: 2Q, 2016, 28-29

0VQS3ZZ Repair Penis, Percutaneous Approach—AHA CC: 3Q, 2018, 12

0VT04ZZ Resection of Prostate, Percutaneous Endoscopic Approach— AHA CC: 4Q, 2014, 33-34

0VT34ZZ Resection of Bilateral Seminal Vesicles, Percutaneous Endoscopic Approach—AHA CC: 4Q, 2014, 33-34

0VUS07Z Supplement Penis with Autologous Tissue Substitute, Open Approach—AHA CC: 1Q, 2020, 31-32

0VUS0JZ Supplement Penis with Synthetic Substitute, Open Approach—AHA CC: 3Q, 2015, 25; 2Q, 2016, 28-29

0VY50Z0 Transplantation of Scrotum, Allogeneic, Open Approach—AHA CC: 4Q, 2020, 58-59

0VYS0Z0 Transplantation of Penis, Allogeneic, Open Approach—AHA CC: 4Q, 2020, 58-59

Body Cavities

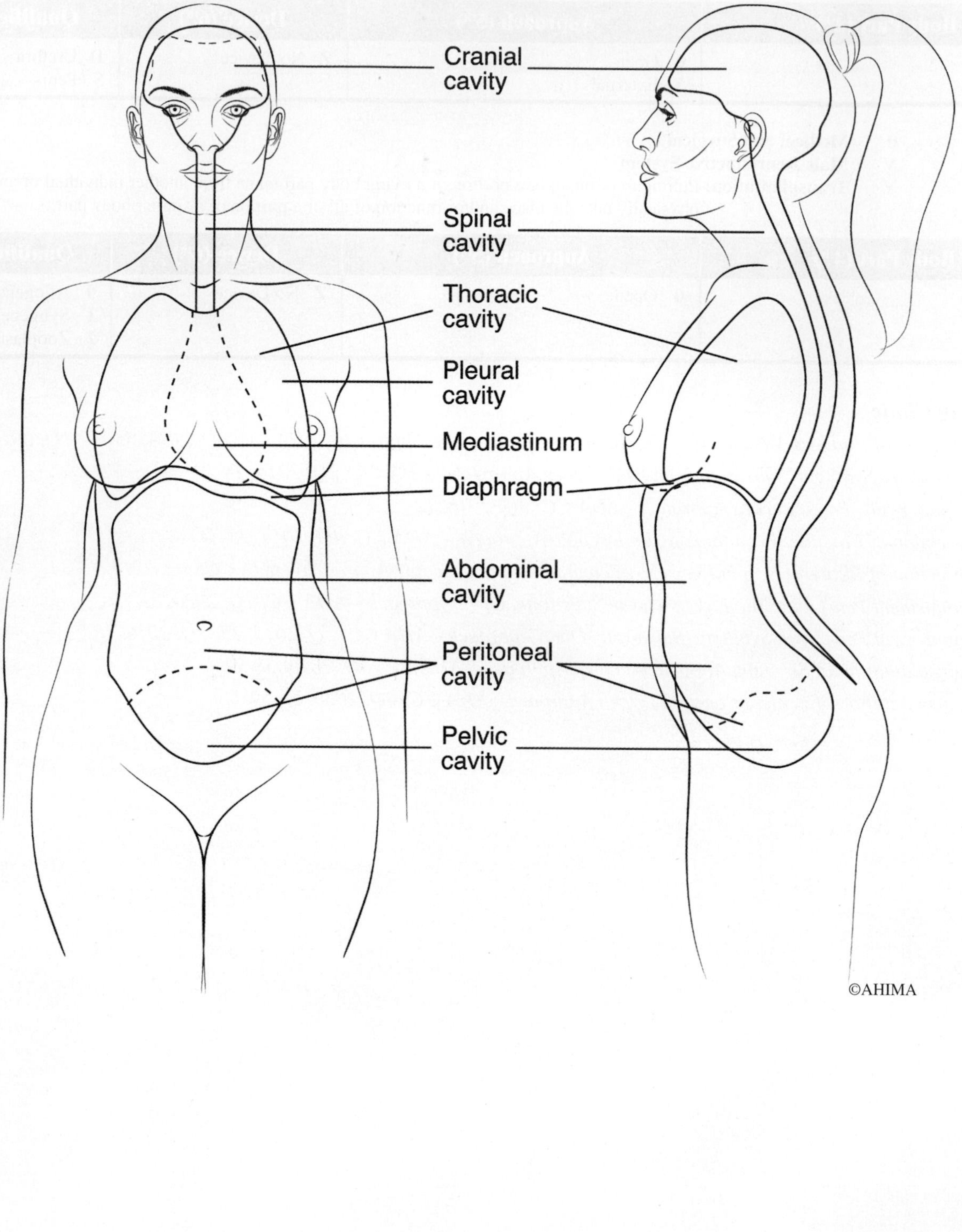
Cranial cavity
Spinal cavity
Thoracic cavity
Pleural cavity
Mediastinum
Diaphragm
Abdominal cavity
Peritoneal cavity
Pelvic cavity
©AHIMA

Body Areas

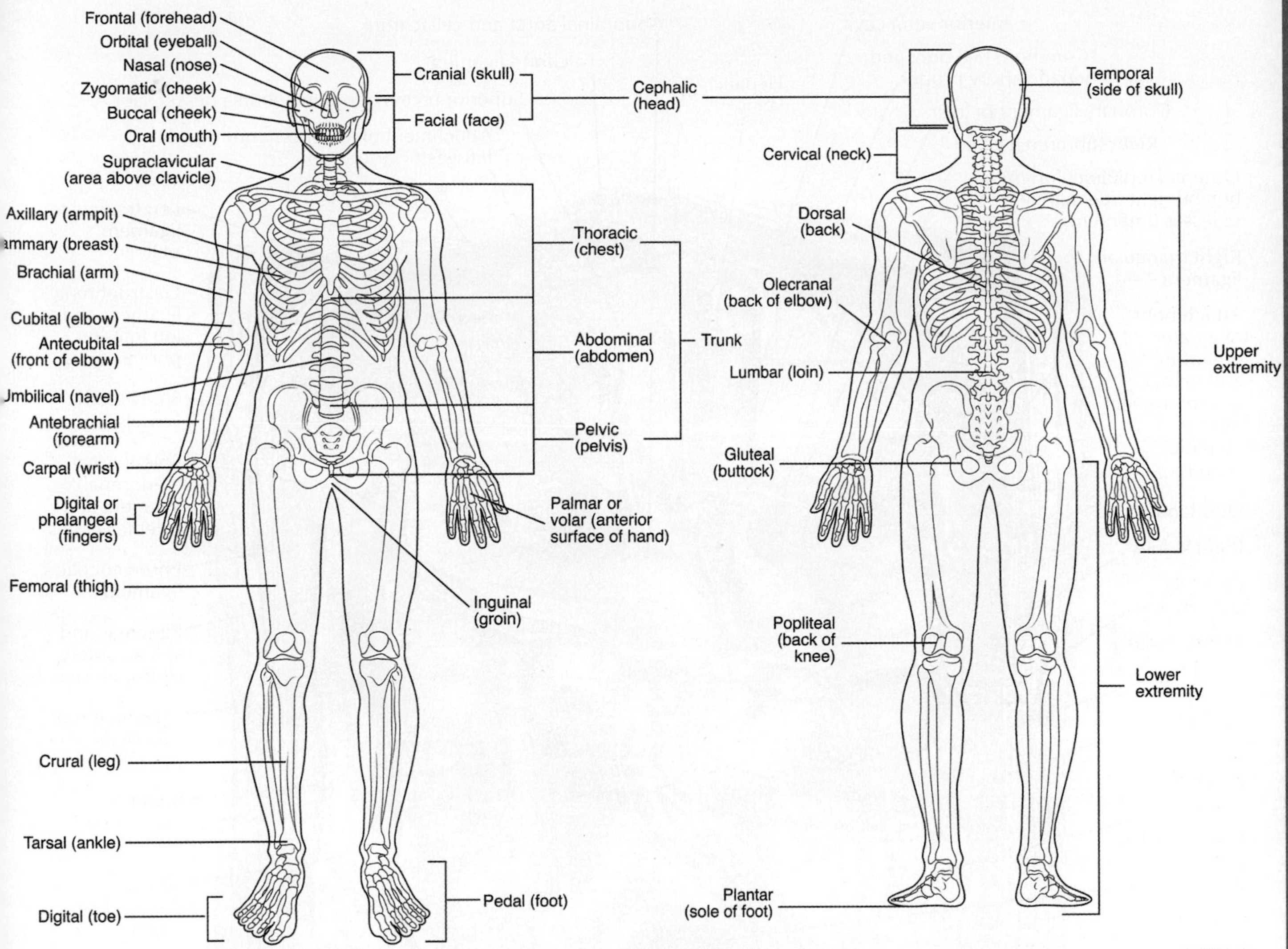
Frontal (forehead)
Orbital (eyeball)
Nasal (nose)
Zygomatic (cheek)
Buccal (cheek)
Oral (mouth)
Supraclavicular (area above clavicle)
Axillary (armpit)
ammary (breast)
Brachial (arm)
Cubital (elbow)
Antecubital (front of elbow)
Jmbilical (navel)
Antebrachial (forearm)
Carpal (wrist)
Digital or phalangeal (fingers)
Femoral (thigh)
Crural (leg)
Tarsal (ankle)
Digital (toe)
Cranial (skull)
Facial (face)
Cephalic (head)
Thoracic (chest)
Abdominal (abdomen)
Trunk
Pelvic (pelvis)
Palmar or volar (anterior surface of hand)
Inguinal (groin)
Pedal (foot)
Temporal (side of skull)
Cervical (neck)
Dorsal (back)
Olecranal (back of elbow)
Lumbar (loin)
Upper extremity
Gluteal (buttock)
Popliteal (back of knee)
Lower extremity
Plantar (sole of foot)

Peritoneum of Posterior Abdominal Wall

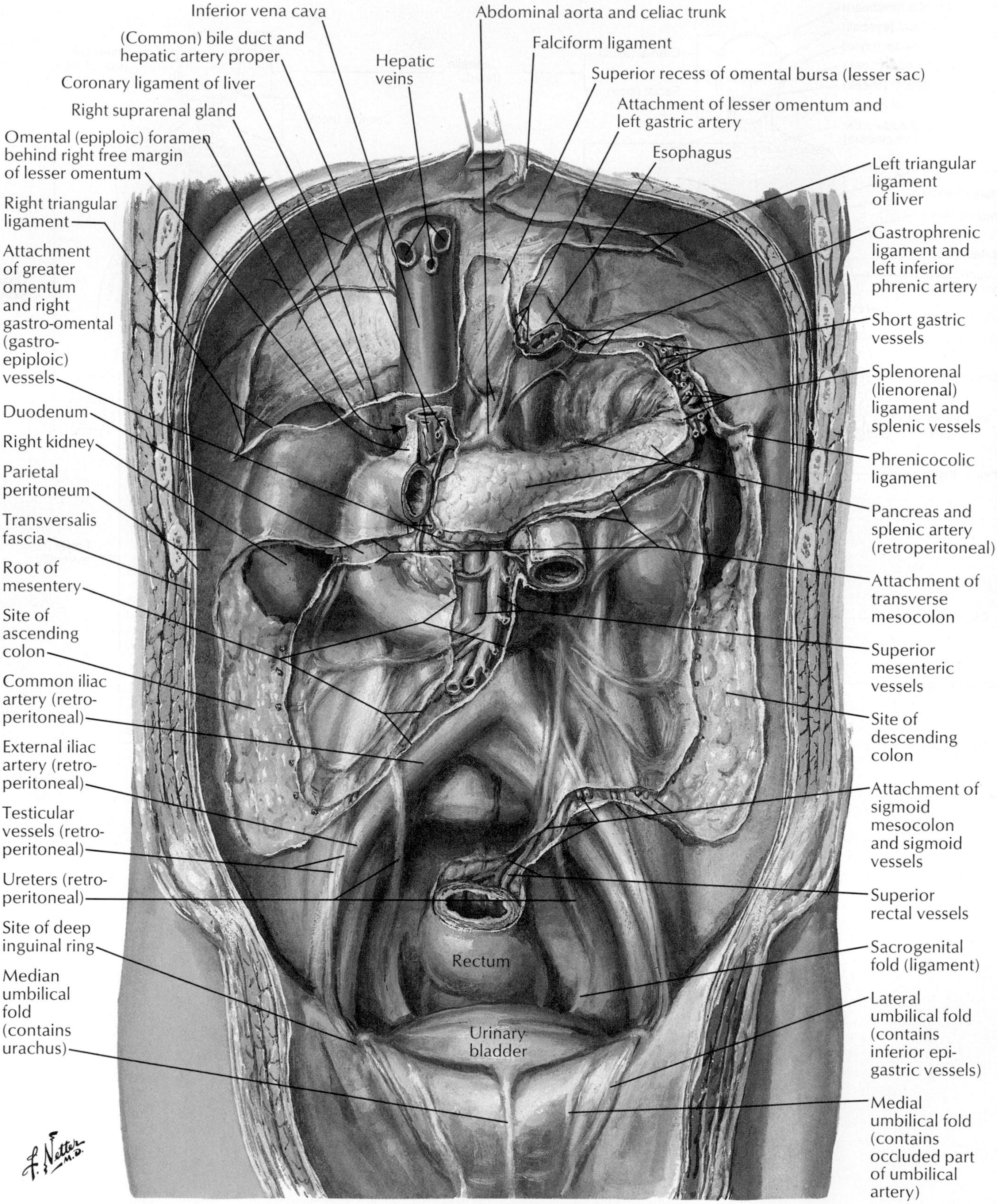
Inferior vena cava
(Common) bile duct and hepatic artery proper
Coronary ligament of liver
Right suprarenal gland
Omental (epiploic) foramen behind right free margin of lesser omentum
Right triangular ligament
Attachment of greater omentum and right gastro-omental (gastro-epiploic) vessels
Duodenum
Right kidney
Parietal peritoneum
Transversalis fascia
Root of mesentery
Site of ascending colon
Common iliac artery (retro-peritoneal)
External iliac artery (retro-peritoneal)
Testicular vessels (retro-peritoneal)
Ureters (retro-peritoneal)
Site of deep inguinal ring
Median umbilical fold (contains urachus)
Hepatic veins
Abdominal aorta and celiac trunk
Falciform ligament
Superior recess of omental bursa (lesser sac)
Attachment of lesser omentum and left gastric artery
Esophagus
Left triangular ligament of liver
Gastrophrenic ligament and left inferior phrenic artery
Short gastric vessels
Splenorenal (lienorenal) ligament and splenic vessels
Phrenicocolic ligament
Pancreas and splenic artery (retroperitoneal)
Attachment of transverse mesocolon
Superior mesenteric vessels
Site of descending colon
Attachment of sigmoid mesocolon and sigmoid vessels
Superior rectal vessels
Sacrogenital fold (ligament)
Lateral umbilical fold (contains inferior epi-gastric vessels)
Medial umbilical fold (contains occluded part of umbilical artery)
Rectum
Urinary bladder
F. Netter M.D.

Hernia I – Indirect and Direct Inguinal Hernias

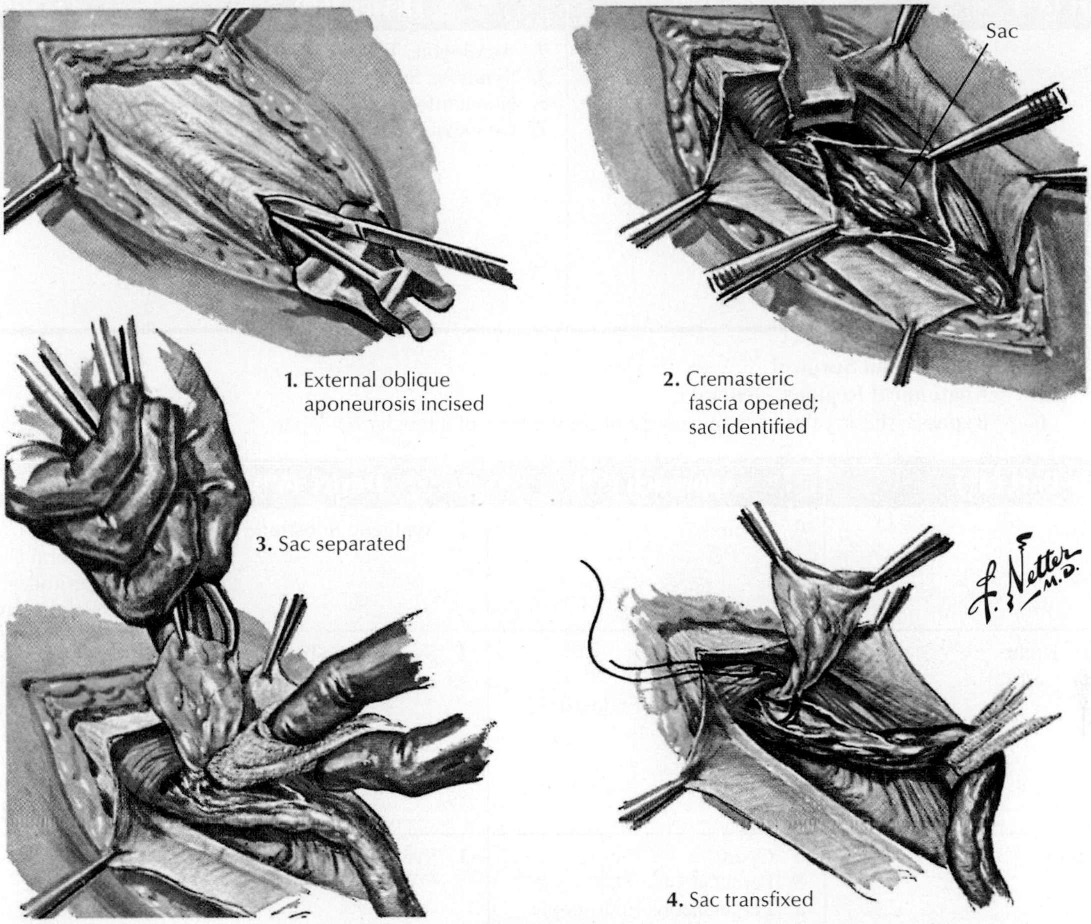
Sac
1. External oblique aponeurosis incised
2. Cremasteric fascia opened; sac identified
3. Sac separated
4. Sac transfixed
F. Netter M.D.

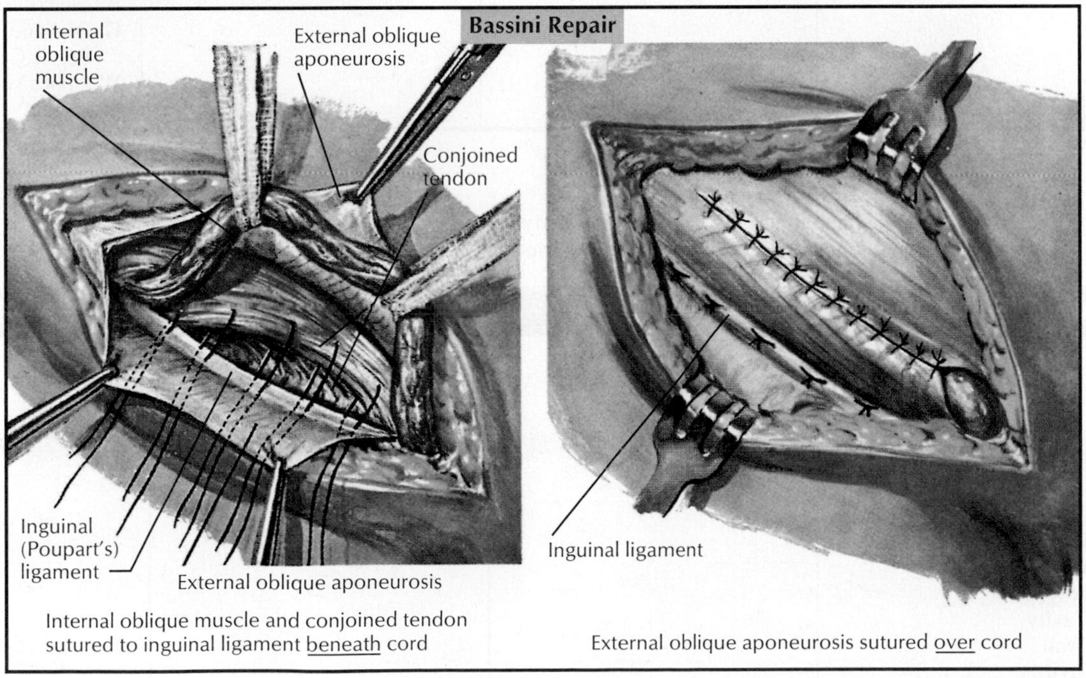
Bassini Repair
Internal oblique muscle
External oblique aponeurosis
Conjoined tendon
Inguinal (Poupart's) ligament
External oblique aponeurosis
Internal oblique muscle and conjoined tendon sutured to inguinal ligament beneath cord
Inguinal ligament
External oblique aponeurosis sutured over cord

Anatomical Regions, General Tables 0W0–0WY

Section 0 **Medical and Surgical**
Body System W **Anatomical Regions, General**
Operation 0 **Alteration:** Modifying the anatomic structure of a body part without affecting the function of the body part

Body Part (4th)	Approach (5th)	Device (6th)	Qualifier (7th)
0 Head 2 Face 4 Upper Jaw 5 Lower Jaw 6 Neck 8 Chest Wall F Abdominal Wall K Upper Back L Lower Back M Perineum, Male N Perineum, Female	0 Open 3 Percutaneous 4 Percutaneous Endoscopic	7 Autologous Tissue Substitute J Synthetic Substitute K Nonautologous Tissue Substitute Z No Device	Z No Qualifier

Section 0 **Medical and Surgical**
Body System W **Anatomical Regions, General**
Operation 1 **Bypass:** Altering the route of passage of the contents of a tubular body part

Body Part (4th)	Approach (5th)	Device (6th)	Qualifier (7th)
1 Cranial Cavity	0 Open	J Synthetic Substitute	9 Pleural Cavity, Right B Pleural Cavity, Left G Peritoneal Cavity J Pelvic Cavity
9 Pleural Cavity, Right B Pleural Cavity, Left J Pelvic Cavity	0 Open 3 Percutaneous 4 Percutaneous Endoscopic	J Synthetic Substitute	4 Cutaneous 9 Pleural Cavity, Right B Pleural Cavity, Left G Peritoneal Cavity J Pelvic Cavity W Upper Vein Y Lower Vein
G Peritoneal Cavity	0 Open 3 Percutaneous 4 Percutaneous Endoscopic	J Synthetic Substitute	4 Cutaneous 6 Bladder 9 Pleural Cavity, Right B Pleural Cavity, Left G Peritoneal Cavity J Pelvic Cavity W Upper Vein Y Lower Vein

Section 0 **Medical and Surgical**
Body System W **Anatomical Regions, General**
Operation 2 **Change:** Taking out or off a device from a body part and putting back an identical or similar device in or on the same body part without cutting or puncturing the skin or a mucous membrane

Body Part (4th)	Approach (5th)	Device (6th)	Qualifier (7th)
0 Head 1 Cranial Cavity 2 Face 4 Upper Jaw 5 Lower Jaw 6 Neck 8 Chest Wall 9 Pleural Cavity, Right B Pleural Cavity, Left C Mediastinum D Pericardial Cavity F Abdominal Wall G Peritoneal Cavity H Retroperitoneum J Pelvic Cavity K Upper Back L Lower Back M Perineum, Male N Perineum, Female	X External	0 Drainage Device Y Other Device	Z No Qualifier

Section 0 **Medical and Surgical**
Body System W **Anatomical Regions, General**
Operation 3 **Control:** Stopping, or attempting to stop, postprocedural or other acute bleeding

Body Part (4th)	Approach (5th)	Device (6th)	Qualifier (7th)
0 Head **1** Cranial Cavity **2** Face **4** Upper Jaw **5** Lower Jaw **6** Neck **8** Chest Wall **9** Pleural Cavity, Right **B** Pleural Cavity, Left **C** Mediastinum **D** Pericardial Cavity **F** Abdominal Wall **G** Peritoneal Cavity **H** Retroperitoneum **J** Pelvic Cavity **K** Upper Back **L** Lower Back **M** Perineum, Male **N** Perineum, Female	**0** Open **3** Percutaneous **4** Percutaneous Endoscopic	**Z** No Device	**Z** No Qualifier
3 Oral Cavity and Throat	**0** Open **3** Percutaneous **4** Percutaneous Endoscopic **7** Via Natural or Artificial Opening **8** Via Natural or Artificial Opening Endoscopic **X** External	**Z** No Device	**Z** No Qualifier
P Gastrointestinal Tract **Q** Respiratory Tract **R** Genitourinary Tract	**0** Open **3** Percutaneous **4** Percutaneous Endoscopic **7** Via Natural or Artificial Opening **8** Via Natural or Artificial Opening Endoscopic	**Z** No Device	**Z** No Qualifier

Section 0 **Medical and Surgical**
Body System W **Anatomical Regions, General**
Operation 4 **Creation:** Putting in or on biological or synthetic material to form a new body part that to the extent possible replicates the anatomic structure or function of an absent body part

Body Part (4th)	Approach (5th)	Device (6th)	Qualifier (7th)
M Perineum, Male	**0** Open	**7** Autologous Tissue Substitute **J** Synthetic Substitute **K** Nonautologous Tissue Substitute	**0** Vagina
N Perineum, Female	**0** Open	**7** Autologous Tissue Substitute **J** Synthetic Substitute **K** Nonautologous Tissue Substitute	**1** Penis

Section 0 **Medical and Surgical**
Body System W **Anatomical Regions, General**
Operation 8 **Division:** Cutting into a body part, without draining fluids and/or gases from the body part, in order to separate or transect a body part

Body Part (4th)	Approach (5th)	Device (6th)	Qualifier (7th)
N Perineum, Female	**X** External	**Z** No Device	**Z** No Qualifier

Section 0 **Medical and Surgical**
Body System W **Anatomical Regions, General**
Operation 9 **Drainage:** Taking or letting out fluids and/or gases from a body part

Body Part (4th)	Approach (5th)	Device (6th)	Qualifier (7th)
0 Head **1** Cranial Cavity **2** Face **3** Oral Cavity and Throat **4** Upper Jaw **5** Lower Jaw **6** Neck **8** Chest Wall **9** Pleural Cavity, Right **B** Pleural Cavity, Left **C** Mediastinum **D** Pericardial Cavity **F** Abdominal Wall **G** Peritoneal Cavity **H** Retroperitoneum **K** Upper Back **L** Lower Back **M** Perineum, Male **N** Perineum, Female	**0** Open **3** Percutaneous **4** Percutaneous Endoscopic	**0** Drainage Device	**Z** No Qualifier
0 Head **1** Cranial Cavity **2** Face **3** Oral Cavity and Throat **4** Upper Jaw **5** Lower Jaw **6** Neck **8** Chest Wall **9** Pleural Cavity, Right **B** Pleural Cavity, Left **C** Mediastinum **D** Pericardial Cavity **F** Abdominal Wall **G** Peritoneal Cavity **H** Retroperitoneum **K** Upper Back **L** Lower Back **M** Perineum, Male **N** Perineum, Female	**0** Open **3** Percutaneous **4** Percutaneous Endoscopic	**Z** No Device	**X** Diagnostic **Z** No Qualifier
J Pelvic Cavity	**0** Open **3** Percutaneous **4** Percutaneous Endoscopic **7** Via Natural or Artificial Opening **8** Via Natural or Artificial Opening Endoscopic	**0** Drainage Device	**Z** No Qualifier
J Pelvic Cavity	**0** Open **3** Percutaneous **4** Percutaneous Endoscopic **7** Via Natural or Artificial Opening **8** Via Natural or Artificial Opening Endoscopic	**Z** No Device	**X** Diagnostic **Z** No Qualifier

Section 0 **Medical and Surgical**
Body System W **Anatomical Regions, General**
Operation B **Excision:** Cutting out or off, without replacement, a portion of a body part

Body Part (4th)	Approach (5th)	Device (6th)	Qualifier (7th)
0 Head **2** Face **3** Oral Cavity and Throat **4** Upper Jaw **5** Lower Jaw **8** Chest Wall **K** Upper Back **L** Lower Back **M** Perineum, Male **N** Perineum, Female	**0** Open **3** Percutaneous **4** Percutaneous Endoscopic **X** External	**Z** No Device	**X** Diagnostic **Z** No Qualifier

Continued →

Section 0 **Medical and Surgical**
Body System W **Anatomical Regions, General**
Operation B **Excision:** Cutting out or off, without replacement, a portion of a body part

Body Part (4th)	Approach (5th)	Device (6th)	Qualifier (7th)
6 Neck **F** Abdominal Wall	**0** Open **3** Percutaneous **4** Percutaneous Endoscopic	**Z** No Device	**X** Diagnostic **Z** No Qualifier
6 Neck **F** Abdominal Wall	**X** External	**Z** No Device	**2** Stoma **X** Diagnostic **Z** No Qualifier
C Mediastinum **H** Retroperitoneum	**0** Open **3** Percutaneous **4** Percutaneous Endoscopic	**Z** No Device	**X** Diagnostic **Z** No Qualifier

Section 0 **Medical and Surgical**
Body System W **Anatomical Regions, General**
Operation C **Extirpation:** Taking or cutting out solid matter from a body part

Body Part (4th)	Approach (5th)	Device (6th)	Qualifier (7th)
1 Cranial Cavity **3** Oral Cavity and Throat **9** Pleural Cavity, Right **B** Pleural Cavity, Left **C** Mediastinum **D** Pericardial Cavity **G** Peritoneal Cavity **H** Retroperitoneum **J** Pelvic Cavity	**0** Open **3** Percutaneous **4** Percutaneous Endoscopic **X** External	**Z** No Device	**Z** No Qualifier
4 Upper Jaw **5** Lower Jaw	**0** Open **3** Percutaneous **4** Percutaneous Endoscopic	**Z** No Device	**Z** No Qualifier
P Gastrointestinal Tract **Q** Respiratory Tract **R** Genitourinary Tract	**0** Open **3** Percutaneous **4** Percutaneous Endoscopic **7** Via Natural or Artificial Opening **8** Via Natural or Artificial Opening Endoscopic **X** External	**Z** No Device	**Z** No Qualifier

Section 0 **Medical and Surgical**
Body System W **Anatomical Regions, General**
Operation F **Fragmentation:** Breaking solid matter in a body part into pieces

Body Part (4th)	Approach (5th)	Device (6th)	Qualifier (7th)
1 Cranial Cavity **3** Oral Cavity and Throat **9** Pleural Cavity, Right **B** Pleural Cavity, Left **C** Mediastinum **D** Pericardial Cavity **G** Peritoneal Cavity **J** Pelvic Cavity	**0** Open **3** Percutaneous **4** Percutaneous Endoscopic **X** External	**Z** No Device	**Z** No Qualifier
P Gastrointestinal Tract **Q** Respiratory Tract **R** Genitourinary Tract	**0** Open **3** Percutaneous **4** Percutaneous Endoscopic **7** Via Natural or Artificial Opening **8** Via Natural or Artificial Opening Endoscopic **X** External	**Z** No Device	**Z** No Qualifier

Section 0 **Medical and Surgical**
Body System W **Anatomical Regions, General**
Operation H **Insertion:** Putting in a nonbiological appliance that monitors, assists, performs, or prevents a physiological function but does not physically take the place of a body part

Body Part (4th)	Approach (5th)	Device (6th)	Qualifier (7th)
0 Head **1** Cranial Cavity **2** Face **3** Oral Cavity and Throat **4** Upper Jaw **5** Lower Jaw **6** Neck **8** Chest Wall **9** Pleural Cavity, Right **B** Pleural Cavity, Left **C** Mediastinum **D** Pericardial Cavity **F** Abdominal Wall **G** Peritoneal Cavity **H** Retroperitoneum **J** Pelvic Cavity **K** Upper Back **L** Lower Back **M** Perineum, Male **N** Perineum, Female	**0** Open **3** Percutaneous **4** Percutaneous Endoscopic	**1** Radioactive Element **3** Infusion Device **Y** Other Device	**Z** No Qualifier
P Gastrointestinal Tract **Q** Respiratory Tract **R** Genitourinary Tract	**0** Open **3** Percutaneous **4** Percutaneous Endoscopic **7** Via Natural or Artificial Opening **8** Via Natural or Artificial Opening Endoscopic	**1** Radioactive Element **3** Infusion Device **Y** Other Device	**Z** No Qualifier

Section 0 **Medical and Surgical**
Body System W **Anatomical Regions, General**
Operation J **Inspection:** Visually and/or manually exploring a body part

Body Part (4th)	Approach (5th)	Device (6th)	Qualifier (7th)
0 Head **2** Face **3** Oral Cavity and Throat **4** Upper Jaw **5** Lower Jaw **6** Neck **8** Chest Wall **F** Abdominal Wall **K** Upper Back **L** Lower Back **M** Perineum, Male **N** Perineum, Female	**0** Open **3** Percutaneous **4** Percutaneous Endoscopic **X** External	**Z** No Device	**Z** No Qualifier
1 Cranial Cavity **9** Pleural Cavity, Right **B** Pleural Cavity, Left **C** Mediastinum **D** Pericardial Cavity **G** Peritoneal Cavity **H** Retroperitoneum **J** Pelvic Cavity	**0** Open **3** Percutaneous **4** Percutaneous Endoscopic	**Z** No Device	**Z** No Qualifier
P Gastrointestinal Tract **Q** Respiratory Tract **R** Genitourinary Tract	**0** Open **3** Percutaneous **4** Percutaneous Endoscopic **7** Via Natural or Artificial Opening **8** Via Natural or Artificial Opening Endoscopic	**Z** No Device	**Z** No Qualifier

Section 0 **Medical and Surgical**
Body System W **Anatomical Regions, General**
Operation M **Reattachment:** Putting back in or on all or a portion of a separated body part to its normal location or other suitable location

Body Part (4th)	Approach (5th)	Device (6th)	Qualifier (7th)
2 Face 4 Upper Jaw 5 Lower Jaw 6 Neck 8 Chest Wall F Abdominal Wall K Upper Back L Lower Back M Perineum, Male N Perineum, Female	0 Open	Z No Device	Z No Qualifier

Section 0 **Medical and Surgical**
Body System W **Anatomical Regions, General**
Operation P **Removal:** Taking out or off a device from a body part

Body Part (4th)	Approach (5th)	Device (6th)	Qualifier (7th)
0 Head 2 Face 4 Upper Jaw 5 Lower Jaw 6 Neck 8 Chest Wall C Mediastinum F Abdominal Wall K Upper Back L Lower Back M Perineum, Male N Perineum, Female	0 Open 3 Percutaneous 4 Percutaneous Endoscopic X External	0 Drainage Device 1 Radioactive Element 3 Infusion Device 7 Autologous Tissue Substitute J Synthetic Substitute K Nonautologous Tissue Substitute Y Other Device	Z No Qualifier
1 Cranial Cavity 9 Pleural Cavity, Right B Pleural Cavity, Left G Peritoneal Cavity J Pelvic Cavity	0 Open 3 Percutaneous 4 Percutaneous Endoscopic	0 Drainage Device 1 Radioactive Element 3 Infusion Device J Synthetic Substitute Y Other Device	Z No Qualifier
1 Cranial Cavity 9 Pleural Cavity, Right B Pleural Cavity, Left G Peritoneal Cavity J Pelvic Cavity	X External	0 Drainage Device 1 Radioactive Element 3 Infusion Device	Z No Qualifier
D Pericardial Cavity H Retroperitoneum	0 Open 3 Percutaneous 4 Percutaneous Endoscopic	0 Drainage Device 1 Radioactive Element 3 Infusion Device Y Other Device	Z No Qualifier
D Pericardial Cavity H Retroperitoneum	X External	0 Drainage Device 1 Radioactive Element 3 Infusion Device	Z No Qualifier
P Gastrointestinal Tract Q Respiratory Tract R Genitourinary Tract	0 Open 3 Percutaneous 4 Percutaneous Endoscopic 7 Via Natural or Artificial Opening 8 Via Natural or Artificial Opening Endoscopic X External	1 Radioactive Element 3 Infusion Device Y Other Device	Z No Qualifier

Section 0 **Medical and Surgical**
Body System W **Anatomical Regions, General**
Operation Q **Repair:** Restoring, to the extent possible, a body part to its normal anatomic structure and function

Body Part (4th)	Approach (5th)	Device (6th)	Qualifier (7th)
0 Head 2 Face 3 Oral Cavity and Throat 4 Upper Jaw 5 Lower Jaw 8 Chest Wall K Upper Back L Lower Back M Perineum, Male N Perineum, Female	0 Open 3 Percutaneous 4 Percutaneous Endoscopic X External	Z No Device	Z No Qualifier
6 Neck F Abdominal Wall	0 Open 3 Percutaneous 4 Percutaneous Endoscopic	Z No Device	Z No Qualifier
6 Neck F Abdominal Wall	X External	Z No Device	2 Stoma Z No Qualifier
C Mediastinum	0 Open 3 Percutaneous 4 Percutaneous Endoscopic	Z No Device	Z No Qualifier

Section 0 **Medical and Surgical**
Body System W **Anatomical Regions, General**
Operation U **Supplement:** Putting in or on biological or synthetic material that physically reinforces and/or augments the function of a portion of a body part

Body Part (4th)	Approach (5th)	Device (6th)	Qualifier (7th)
0 Head 2 Face 4 Upper Jaw 5 Lower Jaw 6 Neck 8 Chest Wall C Mediastinum F Abdominal Wall K Upper Back L Lower Back M Perineum, Male N Perineum, Female	0 Open 4 Percutaneous Endoscopic	7 Autologous Tissue Substitute J Synthetic Substitute K Nonautologous Tissue Substitute	Z No Qualifier

Section 0 **Medical and Surgical**
Body System W **Anatomical Regions, General**
Operation W **Revision:** Correcting, to the extent possible, a portion of a malfunctioning device or the position of a displaced device

Body Part (4th)	Approach (5th)	Device (6th)	Qualifier (7th)
0 Head 2 Face 4 Upper Jaw 5 Lower Jaw 6 Neck 8 Chest Wall C Mediastinum F Abdominal Wall K Upper Back L Lower Back M Perineum, Male N Perineum, Female	0 Open 3 Percutaneous 4 Percutaneous Endoscopic X External	0 Drainage Device 1 Radioactive Element 3 Infusion Device 7 Autologous Tissue Substitute J Synthetic Substitute K Nonautologous Tissue Substitute Y Other Device	Z No Qualifier
1 Cranial Cavity 9 Pleural Cavity, Right B Pleural Cavity, Left G Peritoneal Cavity J Pelvic Cavity	0 Open 3 Percutaneous 4 Percutaneous Endoscopic X External	0 Drainage Device 1 Radioactive Element 3 Infusion Device J Synthetic Substitute Y Other Device	Z No Qualifier

Continued →

Section 0 **Medical and Surgical**
Body System W **Anatomical Regions, General**
Operation W **Revision:** Correcting, to the extent possible, a portion of a malfunctioning device or the position of a displaced device

Body Part (4th)	Approach (5th)	Device (6th)	Qualifier (7th)
D Pericardial Cavity H Retroperitoneum	0 Open 3 Percutaneous 4 Percutaneous Endoscopic X External	0 Drainage Device 1 Radioactive Element 3 Infusion Device Y Other Device	Z No Qualifier
P Gastrointestinal Tract Q Respiratory Tract R Genitourinary Tract	0 Open 3 Percutaneous 4 Percutaneous Endoscopic 7 Via Natural or Artificial Opening 8 Via Natural or Artificial Opening Endoscopic X External	1 Radioactive Element 3 Infusion Device Y Other Device	Z No Qualifier

Section 0 **Medical and Surgical**
Body System W **Anatomical Regions, General**
Operation Y **Transplantation:** Putting in or on all or a portion of a living body part taken from another individual or animal to physically take the place and/or function of all or a portion of a similar body part

Body Part (4th)	Approach (5th)	Device (6th)	Qualifier (7th)
2 Face	0 Open	Z No Device	0 Allogeneic 1 Syngeneic

AHA Coding Clinic

0W020ZZ Alteration of Face, Open Approach—AHA CC: 1Q, 2015, 31
0W1G3J4 Bypass Peritoneal Cavity to Cutaneous with Synthetic Substitute, Percutaneous Approach—AHA CC: 4Q, 2013, 126-127
0W1G3J6 Bypass Peritoneal Cavity to Bladder with Synthetic Substitute, Percutaneous Approach—AHA CC: 4Q, 2020, 55
0W1G3JW Bypass Peritoneal Cavity to Upper Vein with Synthetic Substitute, Percutaneous Approach—AHA CC: 4Q, 2018, 42-43
0W310ZZ Control Bleeding in Cranial Cavity, Open Approach—AHA CC: 3Q, 2019, 4-5
0W3F0ZZ Control Bleeding in Abdominal Wall, Open Approach—AHA CC: 4Q, 2016, 100-101
0W3P8ZZ Control Bleeding in Gastrointestinal Tract, Via Natural or Artificial Opening Endoscopic—AHA CC: 4Q, 2016, 99-100; 4Q, 2017, 105; 1Q, 2018, 19
0W3Q7ZZ Control Bleeding in Respiratory Tract, Via Natural or Artificial Opening—AHA CC: 4Q, 2017, 106
0W3Q8ZZ Control Bleeding in Respiratory Tract, Via Natural or Artificial Opening Endoscopic—AHA CC: 1Q, 2018, 19-20
0W3R7ZZ Control Bleeding in Genitourinary Tract, Via Natural or Artificial Opening—AHA CC: 4Q, 2014, 44
0W930ZZ Drainage of Oral Cavity and Throat, Open Approach—AHA CC: 2Q, 2017, 16-17
0W9G3ZZ Drainage of Peritoneal Cavity, Percutaneous Approach—AHA CC: 3Q, 2017, 12-13
0WBF4ZZ Excision of Abdominal Wall, Percutaneous Endoscopic Approach—AHA CC: 1Q, 2016, 21-22
0WBH0ZZ Excision of Retroperitoneum, Open Approach—AHA CC: 1Q, 2019, 27
0WBNXZZ Excision of Female Perineum, External Approach—AHA CC: 4Q, 2013, 119-120
0WC30ZZ Extirpation of Matter from Oral Cavity and Throat, Open Approach—AHA CC: 2Q, 2017, 16
0WHG03Z Insertion of Infusion Device into Peritoneal Cavity, Open Approach—AHA CC: 2Q, 2021, 14
0WHG33Z Insertion of Infusion Device into Peritoneal Cavity, Percutaneous Approach—AHA CC: 2Q, 2015, 36; 2Q, 2016, 14
0WHJ01Z Insertion of Radioactive Element into Pelvic Cavity, Open Approach—AHA CC: 4Q, 2019, 43-44
0WJC0ZZ Inspection of Mediastinum, Open Approach—AHA CC: 3Q, 2018, 29
0WJG4ZZ Inspection of Peritoneal Cavity, Percutaneous Endoscopic Approach—AHA CC: 2Q, 2013, 36-37; 1Q, 2019, 4-5, 25; 2Q, 2021, 19-20
0WJJ4ZZ Inspection of Pelvic Cavity, Percutaneous Endoscopic Approach—AHA CC: 4Q, 2016, 58-59
0WQF0ZZ Repair Abdominal Wall, Open Approach—AHA CC: 4Q, 2014, 38-39; 3Q, 2014, 28-29; 3Q, 2016, 6; 3Q, 2017, 8-9
0WU80JZ Supplement Chest Wall with Synthetic Substitute, Open Approach—AHA CC: 4Q, 2012, 101-102
0WUF07Z Supplement Abdominal Wall with Autologous Tissue Substitute, Open Approach—AHA CC: 3Q, 2016, 40-41
0WUF0JZ Supplement Abdominal Wall with Synthetic Substitute, Open Approach—AHA CC: 4Q, 2014, 39-40; 3Q, 2017, 8
0WWG4JZ Revision of Synthetic Substitute in Peritoneal Cavity, Percutaneous Endoscopic Approach—AHA CC: 2Q, 2015, 9-10

Anatomical Regions, Upper Extremities Tables 0X0–0XY

Section 0 **Medical and Surgical**
Body System X **Anatomical Regions, Upper Extremities**
Operation 0 **Alteration:** Modifying the anatomic structure of a body part without affecting the function of the body part

Body Part (4th)	Approach (5th)	Device (6th)	Qualifier (7th)
2 Shoulder Region, Right **3** Shoulder Region, Left **4** Axilla, Right **5** Axilla, Left **6** Upper Extremity, Right **7** Upper Extremity, Left **8** Upper Arm, Right **9** Upper Arm, Left **B** Elbow Region, Right **C** Elbow Region, Left **D** Lower Arm, Right **F** Lower Arm, Left **G** Wrist Region, Right **H** Wrist Region, Left	**0** Open **3** Percutaneous **4** Percutaneous Endoscopic	**7** Autologous Tissue Substitute **J** Synthetic Substitute **K** Nonautologous Tissue Substitute **Z** No Device	**Z** No Qualifier

Section 0 **Medical and Surgical**
Body System X **Anatomical Regions, Upper Extremities**
Operation 2 **Change:** Taking out or off a device from a body part and putting back an identical or similar device in or on the same body part without cutting or puncturing the skin or a mucous membrane

Body Part (4th)	Approach (5th)	Device (6th)	Qualifier (7th)
6 Upper Extremity, Right **7** Upper Extremity, Left	**X** External	**0** Drainage Device **Y** Other Device	**Z** No Qualifier

Section 0 **Medical and Surgical**
Body System X **Anatomical Regions, Upper Extremities**
Operation 3 **Control:** Stopping, or attempting to stop, postprocedural or other acute bleeding

Body Part (4th)	Approach (5th)	Device (6th)	Qualifier (7th)
2 Shoulder Region, Right **3** Shoulder Region, Left **4** Axilla, Right **5** Axilla, Left **6** Upper Extremity, Right **7** Upper Extremity, Left **8** Upper Arm, Right **9** Upper Arm, Left **B** Elbow Region, Right **C** Elbow Region, Left **D** Lower Arm, Right **F** Lower Arm, Left **G** Wrist Region, Right **H** Wrist Region, Left **J** Hand, Right **K** Hand, Left	**0** Open **3** Percutaneous **4** Percutaneous Endoscopic	**Z** No Device	**Z** No Qualifier

Section 0 **Medical and Surgical**
Body System X **Anatomical Regions, Upper Extremities**
Operation 6 **Detachment:** Cutting off all or a portion of the upper or lower extremities

Body Part (4th)	Approach (5th)	Device (6th)	Qualifier (7th)
0 Forequarter, Right **1** Forequarter, Left **2** Shoulder Region, Right **3** Shoulder Region, Left **B** Elbow Region, Right **C** Elbow Region, Left	**0** Open	**Z** No Device	**Z** No Qualifier
8 Upper Arm, Right **9** Upper Arm, Left **D** Lower Arm, Right **F** Lower Arm, Left	**0** Open	**Z** No Device	**1** High **2** Mid **3** Low
J Hand, Right **K** Hand, Left	**0** Open	**Z** No Device	**0** Complete **4** Complete 1st Ray **5** Complete 2nd Ray **6** Complete 3rd Ray **7** Complete 4th Ray **8** Complete 5th Ray **9** Partial 1st Ray **B** Partial 2nd Ray **C** Partial 3rd Ray **D** Partial 4th Ray **F** Partial 5th Ray
L Thumb, Right **M** Thumb, Left **N** Index Finger, Right **P** Index Finger, Left **Q** Middle Finger, Right **R** Middle Finger, Left **S** Ring Finger, Right **T** Ring Finger, Left **V** Little Finger, Right **W** Little Finger, Left	**0** Open	**Z** No Device	**0** Complete **1** High **2** Mid **3** Low

Section 0 **Medical and Surgical**
Body System X **Anatomical Regions, Upper Extremities**
Operation 9 **Drainage:** Taking or letting out fluids and/or gases from a body part

Body Part (4th)	Approach (5th)	Device (6th)	Qualifier (7th)
2 Shoulder Region, Right **3** Shoulder Region, Left **4** Axilla, Right **5** Axilla, Left **6** Upper Extremity, Right **7** Upper Extremity, Left **8** Upper Arm, Right **9** Upper Arm, Left **B** Elbow Region, Right **C** Elbow Region, Left **D** Lower Arm, Right **F** Lower Arm, Left **G** Wrist Region, Right **H** Wrist Region, Left **J** Hand, Right **K** Hand, Left	**0** Open **3** Percutaneous **4** Percutaneous Endoscopic	**0** Drainage Device	**Z** No Qualifier

Continued →

Section 0 **Medical and Surgical**
Body System X **Anatomical Regions, Upper Extremities**
Operation 9 **Drainage:** Taking or letting out fluids and/or gases from a body part

Body Part (4th)	Approach (5th)	Device (6th)	Qualifier (7th)
2 Shoulder Region, Right **3** Shoulder Region, Left **4** Axilla, Right **5** Axilla, Left **6** Upper Extremity, Right **7** Upper Extremity, Left **8** Upper Arm, Right **9** Upper Arm, Left **B** Elbow Region, Right **C** Elbow Region, Left **D** Lower Arm, Right **F** Lower Arm, Left **G** Wrist Region, Right **H** Wrist Region, Left **J** Hand, Right **K** Hand, Left	**0** Open **3** Percutaneous **4** Percutaneous Endoscopic	**Z** No Device	**X** Diagnostic **Z** No Qualifier

Section 0 **Medical and Surgical**
Body System X **Anatomical Regions, Upper Extremities**
Operation B **Excision:** Cutting out or off, without replacement, a portion of a body part

Body Part (4th)	Approach (5th)	Device (6th)	Qualifier (7th)
2 Shoulder Region, Right **3** Shoulder Region, Left **4** Axilla, Right **5** Axilla, Left **6** Upper Extremity, Right **7** Upper Extremity, Left **8** Upper Arm, Right **9** Upper Arm, Left **B** Elbow Region, Right **C** Elbow Region, Left **D** Lower Arm, Right **F** Lower Arm, Left **G** Wrist Region, Right **H** Wrist Region, Left **J** Hand, Right **K** Hand, Left	**0** Open **3** Percutaneous **4** Percutaneous Endoscopic	**Z** No Device	**X** Diagnostic **Z** No Qualifier

Section 0 **Medical and Surgical**
Body System X **Anatomical Regions, Upper Extremities**
Operation H **Insertion:** Putting in a nonbiological appliance that monitors, assists, performs, or prevents a physiological function but does not physically take the place of a body part

Body Part (4th)	Approach (5th)	Device (6th)	Qualifier (7th)
2 Shoulder Region, Right **3** Shoulder Region, Left **4** Axilla, Right **5** Axilla, Left **6** Upper Extremity, Right **7** Upper Extremity, Left **8** Upper Arm, Right **9** Upper Arm, Left **B** Elbow Region, Right **C** Elbow Region, Left **D** Lower Arm, Right **F** Lower Arm, Left **G** Wrist Region, Right **H** Wrist Region, Left **J** Hand, Right **K** Hand, Left	**0** Open **3** Percutaneous **4** Percutaneous Endoscopic	**1** Radioactive Element **3** Infusion Device **Y** Other Device	**Z** No Qualifier

Section 0 **Medical and Surgical**
Body System X **Anatomical Regions, Upper Extremities**
Operation J **Inspection:** Visually and/or manually exploring a body part

Body Part (4th)	Approach (5th)	Device (6th)	Qualifier (7th)
2 Shoulder Region, Right **3** Shoulder Region, Left **4** Axilla, Right **5** Axilla, Left **6** Upper Extremity, Right **7** Upper Extremity, Left **8** Upper Arm, Right **9** Upper Arm, Left **B** Elbow Region, Right **C** Elbow Region, Left **D** Lower Arm, Right **F** Lower Arm, Left **G** Wrist Region, Right **H** Wrist Region, Left **J** Hand, Right **K** Hand, Left	**0** Open **3** Percutaneous **4** Percutaneous Endoscopic **X** External	**Z** No Device	**Z** No Qualifier

Section 0 **Medical and Surgical**
Body System X **Anatomical Regions, Upper Extremities**
Operation M **Reattachment:** Putting back in or on all or a portion of a separated body part to its normal location or other suitable location

Body Part (4th)	Approach (5th)	Device (6th)	Qualifier (7th)
0 Forequarter, Right **1** Forequarter, Left **2** Shoulder Region, Right **3** Shoulder Region, Left **4** Axilla, Right **5** Axilla, Left **6** Upper Extremity, Right **7** Upper Extremity, Left **8** Upper Arm, Right **9** Upper Arm, Left **B** Elbow Region, Right **C** Elbow Region, Left **D** Lower Arm, Right **F** Lower Arm, Left **G** Wrist Region, Right **H** Wrist Region, Left **J** Hand, Right **K** Hand, Left **L** Thumb, Right **M** Thumb, Left **N** Index Finger, Right **P** Index Finger, Left **Q** Middle Finger, Right **R** Middle Finger, Left **S** Ring Finger, Right **T** Ring Finger, Left **V** Little Finger, Right **W** Little Finger, Left	**0** Open	**Z** No Device	**Z** No Qualifier

Section 0 Medical and Surgical
Body System X Anatomical Regions, Upper Extremities
Operation P **Removal:** Taking out or off a device from a body part

Body Part (4th)	Approach (5th)	Device (6th)	Qualifier (7th)
6 Upper Extremity, Right 7 Upper Extremity, Left	0 Open 3 Percutaneous 4 Percutaneous Endoscopic X External	0 Drainage Device 1 Radioactive Element 3 Infusion Device 7 Autologous Tissue Substitute J Synthetic Substitute K Nonautologous Tissue Substitute Y Other Device	Z No Qualifier

Section 0 Medical and Surgical
Body System X Anatomical Regions, Upper Extremities
Operation Q **Repair:** Restoring, to the extent possible, a body part to its normal anatomic structure and function

Body Part (4th)	Approach (5th)	Device (6th)	Qualifier (7th)
2 Shoulder Region, Right 3 Shoulder Region, Left 4 Axilla, Right 5 Axilla, Left 6 Upper Extremity, Right 7 Upper Extremity, Left 8 Upper Arm, Right 9 Upper Arm, Left B Elbow Region, Right C Elbow Region, Left D Lower Arm, Right F Lower Arm, Left G Wrist Region, Right H Wrist Region, Left J Hand, Right K Hand, Left L Thumb, Right M Thumb, Left N Index Finger, Right P Index Finger, Left Q Middle Finger, Right R Middle Finger, Left S Ring Finger, Right T Ring Finger, Left V Little Finger, Right W Little Finger, Left	0 Open 3 Percutaneous 4 Percutaneous Endoscopic X External	Z No Device	Z No Qualifier

Section 0 Medical and Surgical
Body System X Anatomical Regions, Upper Extremities
Operation R **Replacement:** Putting in or on biological or synthetic material that physically takes the place and/or function of all or a portion of a body part

Body Part (4th)	Approach (5th)	Device (6th)	Qualifier (7th)
L Thumb, Right M Thumb, Left	0 Open 4 Percutaneous Endoscopic	7 Autologous Tissue Substitute	N Toe, Right P Toe, Left

Section 0 Medical and Surgical
Body System X Anatomical Regions, Upper Extremities
Operation U **Supplement:** Putting in or on biological or synthetic material that physically reinforces and/or augments the function of a portion of a body part

Body Part (4th)	Approach (5th)	Device (6th)	Qualifier (7th)
2 Shoulder Region, Right **3** Shoulder Region, Left **4** Axilla, Right **5** Axilla, Left **6** Upper Extremity, Right **7** Upper Extremity, Left **8** Upper Arm, Right **9** Upper Arm, Left **B** Elbow Region, Right **C** Elbow Region, Left **D** Lower Arm, Right **F** Lower Arm, Left **G** Wrist Region, Right **H** Wrist Region, Left **J** Hand, Right **K** Hand, Left **L** Thumb, Right **M** Thumb, Left **N** Index Finger, Right **P** Index Finger, Left **Q** Middle Finger, Right **R** Middle Finger, Left **S** Ring Finger, Right **T** Ring Finger, Left **V** Little Finger, Right **W** Little Finger, Left	**0** Open **4** Percutaneous Endoscopic	**7** Autologous Tissue Substitute **J** Synthetic Substitute **K** Nonautologous Tissue Substitute	**Z** No Qualifier

Section 0 Medical and Surgical
Body System X Anatomical Regions, Upper Extremities
Operation W **Revision:** Correcting, to the extent possible, a portion of a malfunctioning device or the position of a displaced device

Body Part (4th)	Approach (5th)	Device (6th)	Qualifier (7th)
6 Upper Extremity, Right **7** Upper Extremity, Left	**0** Open **3** Percutaneous **4** Percutaneous Endoscopic **X** External	**0** Drainage Device **3** Infusion Device **7** Autologous Tissue Substitute **J** Synthetic Substitute **K** Nonautologous Tissue Substitute **Y** Other Device	**Z** No Qualifier

Section 0 Medical and Surgical
Body System X Anatomical Regions, Upper Extremities
Operation X **Transfer:** Moving, without taking out, all or a portion of a body part to another location to take over the function of all or a portion of a body part

Body Part (4th)	Approach (5th)	Device (6th)	Qualifier (7th)
N Index Finger, Right	**0** Open	**Z** No Device	**L** Thumb, Right
P Index Finger, Left	**0** Open	**Z** No Device	**M** Thumb, Left

Section 0 Medical and Surgical
Body System X Anatomical Regions, Upper Extremities
Operation Y **Transplantation:** Putting in or on all or a portion of a living body part taken from another individual or animal to physically take the place and/or function of all or a portion of a similar body part

Body Part (4th)	Approach (5th)	Device (6th)	Qualifier (7th)
J Hand, Right **K** Hand, Left	**0** Open	**Z** No Device	**0** Allogeneic **1** Syngeneic

AHA Coding Clinic

0X370ZZ Control Bleeding in Left Upper Extremity, Open Approach—AHA CC: 1Q, 2015, 35

0X6M0Z3 Detachment at Left Thumb, Low, Open Approach—AHA CC: 3Q, 2016, 33-34; 1Q, 2017, 52

0X6T0Z3 Detachment at Left Ring Finger, Low, Open Approach—AHA CC: 3Q, 2016, 33-34; 1Q, 2017, 52

0X6V0Z0 Detachment at Right Little Finger, Complete, Open Approach—AHA CC: 2Q, 2017, 18-19

0X6W0Z3 Detachment at Left Little Finger, Low, Open Approach—AHA CC: 3Q, 2016, 33-34; 1Q, 2017, 52

0XH90YZ Insertion of Other Device into Left Upper Arm, Open Approach—AHA CC: 2Q, 2017, 20-21

0XP70YZ Removal of Other Device from Left Upper Extremity, Open Approach—AHA CC: 2Q, 2017, 20-21

Anatomical Regions, Lower Extremities 0Y0–0YW

Section 0 **Medical and Surgical**
Body System Y **Anatomical Regions, Lower Extremities**
Operation 0 **Alteration:** Modifying the anatomic structure of a body part without affecting the function of the body part

Body Part (4th)	Approach (5th)	Device (6th)	Qualifier (7th)
0 Buttock, Right **1** Buttock, Left **9** Lower Extremity, Right **B** Lower Extremity, Left **C** Upper Leg, Right **D** Upper Leg, Left **F** Knee Region, Right **G** Knee Region, Left **H** Lower Leg, Right **J** Lower Leg, Left **K** Ankle Region, Right **L** Ankle Region, Left	**0** Open **3** Percutaneous **4** Percutaneous Endoscopic	**7** Autologous Tissue Substitute **J** Synthetic Substitute **K** Nonautologous Tissue Substitute **Z** No Device	**Z** No Qualifier

Section 0 **Medical and Surgical**
Body System Y **Anatomical Regions, Lower Extremities**
Operation 2 **Change:** Taking out or off a device from a body part and putting back an identical or similar device in or on the same body part without cutting or puncturing the skin or a mucous membrane

Body Part (4th)	Approach (5th)	Device (6th)	Qualifier (7th)
9 Lower Extremity, Right **B** Lower Extremity, Left	**X** External	**0** Drainage Device **Y** Other Device	**Z** No Qualifier

Section 0 **Medical and Surgical**
Body System Y **Anatomical Regions, Lower Extremities**
Operation 3 **Control:** Stopping, or attempting to stop, postprocedural or other acute bleeding

Body Part (4th)	Approach (5th)	Device (6th)	Qualifier (7th)
0 Buttock, Right **1** Buttock, Left **5** Inguinal Region, Right **6** Inguinal Region, Left **7** Femoral Region, Right **8** Femoral Region, Left **9** Lower Extremity, Right **B** Lower Extremity, Left **C** Upper Leg, Right **D** Upper Leg, Left **F** Knee Region, Right **G** Knee Region, Left **H** Lower Leg, Right **J** Lower Leg, Left **K** Ankle Region, Right **L** Ankle Region, Left **M** Foot, Right **N** Foot, Left	**0** Open **3** Percutaneous **4** Percutaneous Endoscopic	**Z** No Device	**Z** No Qualifier

Section 0 **Medical and Surgical**
Body System Y **Anatomical Regions, Lower Extremities**
Operation 6 **Detachment:** Cutting off all or a portion of the upper or lower extremities

Body Part (4th)	Approach (5th)	Device (6th)	Qualifier (7th)
2 Hindquarter, Right **3** Hindquarter, Left **4** Hindquarter, Bilateral **7** Femoral Region, Right **8** Femoral Region, Left **F** Knee Region, Right **G** Knee Region, Left	**0** Open	**Z** No Device	**Z** No Qualifier
C Upper Leg, Right **D** Upper Leg, Left **H** Lower Leg, Right **J** Lower Leg, Left	**0** Open	**Z** No Device	**1** High **2** Mid **3** Low
M Foot, Right **N** Foot, Left	**0** Open	**Z** No Device	**0** Complete **4** Complete 1st Ray **5** Complete 2nd Ray **6** Complete 3rd Ray **7** Complete 4th Ray **8** Complete 5th Ray **9** Partial 1st Ray **B** Partial 2nd Ray **C** Partial 3rd Ray **D** Partial 4th Ray **F** Partial 5th Ray
P 1st Toe, Right **Q** 1st Toe, Left **R** 2nd Toe, Right **S** 2nd Toe, Left **T** 3rd Toe, Right **U** 3rd Toe, Left **V** 4th Toe, Right **W** 4th Toe, Left **X** 5th Toe, Right **Y** 5th Toe, Left	**0** Open	**Z** No Device	**0** Complete **1** High **2** Mid **3** Low

Section 0 **Medical and Surgical**
Body System Y **Anatomical Regions, Lower Extremities**
Operation 9 **Drainage:** Taking or letting out fluids and/or gases from a body part

Body Part (4th)	Approach (5th)	Device (6th)	Qualifier (7th)
0 Buttock, Right **1** Buttock, Left **5** Inguinal Region, Right **6** Inguinal Region, Left **7** Femoral Region, Right **8** Femoral Region, Left **9** Lower Extremity, Right **B** Lower Extremity, Left **C** Upper Leg, Right **D** Upper Leg, Left **F** Knee Region, Right **G** Knee Region, Left **H** Lower Leg, Right **J** Lower Leg, Left **K** Ankle Region, Right **L** Ankle Region, Left **M** Foot, Right **N** Foot, Left	**0** Open **3** Percutaneous **4** Percutaneous Endoscopic	**0** Drainage Device	**Z** No Qualifier

Continued →

Section 0 **Medical and Surgical**
Body System Y **Anatomical Regions, Lower Extremities**
Operation 9 **Drainage:** Taking or letting out fluids and/or gases from a body part

Body Part (4th)	Approach (5th)	Device (6th)	Qualifier (7th)
0 Buttock, Right **1** Buttock, Left **5** Inguinal Region, Right **6** Inguinal Region, Left **7** Femoral Region, Right **8** Femoral Region, Left **9** Lower Extremity, Right **B** Lower Extremity, Left **C** Upper Leg, Right **D** Upper Leg, Left **F** Knee Region, Right **G** Knee Region, Left **H** Lower Leg, Right **J** Lower Leg, Left **K** Ankle Region, Right **L** Ankle Region, Left **M** Foot, Right **N** Foot, Left	**0** Open **3** Percutaneous **4** Percutaneous Endoscopic	**Z** No Device	**X** Diagnostic **Z** No Qualifier

Section 0 **Medical and Surgical**
Body System Y **Anatomical Regions, Lower Extremities**
Operation B **Excision:** Cutting out or off, without replacement, a portion of a body part

Body Part (4th)	Approach (5th)	Device (6th)	Qualifier (7th)
0 Buttock, Right **1** Buttock, Left **5** Inguinal Region, Right **6** Inguinal Region, Left **7** Femoral Region, Right **8** Femoral Region, Left **9** Lower Extremity, Right **B** Lower Extremity, Left **C** Upper Leg, Right **D** Upper Leg, Left **F** Knee Region, Right **G** Knee Region, Left **H** Lower Leg, Right **J** Lower Leg, Left **K** Ankle Region, Right **L** Ankle Region, Left **M** Foot, Right **N** Foot, Left	**0** Open **3** Percutaneous **4** Percutaneous Endoscopic	**Z** No Device	**X** Diagnostic **Z** No Qualifier

Section 0 **Medical and Surgical**
Body System Y **Anatomical Regions, Lower Extremities**
Operation H **Insertion:** Putting in a nonbiological appliance that monitors, assists, performs, or prevents a physiological function but does not physically take the place of a body part

Body Part (4th)	Approach (5th)	Device (6th)	Qualifier (7th)
0 Buttock, Right **1** Buttock, Left **5** Inguinal Region, Right **6** Inguinal Region, Left **7** Femoral Region, Right **8** Femoral Region, Left **9** Lower Extremity, Right **B** Lower Extremity, Left **C** Upper Leg, Right **D** Upper Leg, Left **F** Knee Region, Right **G** Knee Region, Left **H** Lower Leg, Right **J** Lower Leg, Left **K** Ankle Region, Right **L** Ankle Region, Left **M** Foot, Right **N** Foot, Left	**0** Open **3** Percutaneous **4** Percutaneous Endoscopic	**1** Radioactive Element **3** Infusion Device **Y** Other Device	**Z** No Qualifier

Section 0 **Medical and Surgical**
Body System Y **Anatomical Regions, Lower Extremities**
Operation J **Inspection:** Visually and/or manually exploring a body part

Body Part (4th)	Approach (5th)	Device (6th)	Qualifier (7th)
0 Buttock, Right **1** Buttock, Left **5** Inguinal Region, Right **6** Inguinal Region, Left **7** Femoral Region, Right **8** Femoral Region, Left **9** Lower Extremity, Right **A** Inguinal Region, Bilateral **B** Lower Extremity, Left **C** Upper Leg, Right **D** Upper Leg, Left **E** Femoral Region, Bilateral **F** Knee Region, Right **G** Knee Region, Left **H** Lower Leg, Right **J** Lower Leg, Left **K** Ankle Region, Right **L** Ankle Region, Left **M** Foot, Right **N** Foot, Left	**0** Open **3** Percutaneous **4** Percutaneous Endoscopic **X** External	**Z** No Device	**Z** No Qualifier

Section 0 **Medical and Surgical**
Body System Y **Anatomical Regions, Lower Extremities**
Operation M **Reattachment:** Putting back in or on all or a portion of a separated body part to its normal location or other suitable location

Body Part (4th)	Approach (5th)	Device (6th)	Qualifier (7th)
0 Buttock, Right **1** Buttock, Left **2** Hindquarter, Right **3** Hindquarter, Left **4** Hindquarter, Bilateral **5** Inguinal Region, Right **6** Inguinal Region, Left **7** Femoral Region, Right **8** Femoral Region, Left **9** Lower Extremity, Right **B** Lower Extremity, Left **C** Upper Leg, Right **D** Upper Leg, Left **F** Knee Region, Right **G** Knee Region, Left **H** Lower Leg, Right **J** Lower Leg, Left **K** Ankle Region, Right **L** Ankle Region, Left **M** Foot, Right **N** Foot, Left **P** 1st Toe, Right **Q** 1st Toe, Left **R** 2nd Toe, Right **S** 2nd Toe, Left **T** 3rd Toe, Right **U** 3rd Toe, Left **V** 4th Toe, Right **W** 4th Toe, Left **X** 5th Toe, Right **Y** 5th Toe, Left	**0** Open	**Z** No Device	**Z** No Qualifier

Section 0 **Medical and Surgical**
Body System Y **Anatomical Regions, Lower Extremities**
Operation P **Removal:** Taking out or off a device from a body part

Body Part (4th)	Approach (5th)	Device (6th)	Qualifier (7th)
9 Lower Extremity, Right **B** Lower Extremity, Left	**0** Open **3** Percutaneous **4** Percutaneous Endoscopic **X** External	**0** Drainage Device **1** Radioactive Element **3** Infusion Device **7** Autologous Tissue Substitute **J** Synthetic Substitute **K** Nonautologous Tissue Substitute **Y** Other Device	**Z** No Qualifier

Section 0 **Medical and Surgical**
Body System Y **Anatomical Regions, Lower Extremities**
Operation Q **Repair:** Restoring, to the extent possible, a body part to its normal anatomic structure and function

Body Part (4th)	Approach (5th)	Device (6th)	Qualifier (7th)
0 Buttock, Right **1** Buttock, Left **5** Inguinal Region, Right **6** Inguinal Region, Left **7** Femoral Region, Right **8** Femoral Region, Left **9** Lower Extremity, Right **A** Inguinal Region, Bilateral **B** Lower Extremity, Left **C** Upper Leg, Right **D** Upper Leg, Left **E** Femoral Region, Bilateral **F** Knee Region, Right **G** Knee Region, Left **H** Lower Leg, Right **J** Lower Leg, Left **K** Ankle Region, Right **L** Ankle Region, Left **M** Foot, Right **N** Foot, Left **P** 1st Toe, Right **Q** 1st Toe, Left **R** 2nd Toe, Right **S** 2nd Toe, Left **T** 3rd Toe, Right **U** 3rd Toe, Left **V** 4th Toe, Right **W** 4th Toe, Left **X** 5th Toe, Right **Y** 5th Toe, Left	**0** Open **3** Percutaneous **4** Percutaneous Endoscopic **X** External	**Z** No Device	**Z** No Qualifier

Section 0 Medical and Surgical
Body System Y Anatomical Regions, Lower Extremities
Operation U **Supplement:** Putting in or on biological or synthetic material that physically reinforces and/or augments the function of a portion of a body part

Body Part (4th)	Approach (5th)	Device (6th)	Qualifier (7th)
0 Buttock, Right **1** Buttock, Left **5** Inguinal Region, Right **6** Inguinal Region, Left **7** Femoral Region, Right **8** Femoral Region, Left **9** Lower Extremity, Right **A** Inguinal Region, Bilateral **B** Lower Extremity, Left **C** Upper Leg, Right **D** Upper Leg, Left **E** Femoral Region, Bilateral **F** Knee Region, Right **G** Knee Region, Left **H** Lower Leg, Right **J** Lower Leg, Left **K** Ankle Region, Right **L** Ankle Region, Left **M** Foot, Right **N** Foot, Left **P** 1st Toe, Right **Q** 1st Toe, Left **R** 2nd Toe, Right **S** 2nd Toe, Left **T** 3rd Toe, Right **U** 3rd Toe, Left **V** 4th Toe, Right **W** 4th Toe, Left **X** 5th Toe, Right **Y** 5th Toe, Left	**0** Open **4** Percutaneous Endoscopic	**7** Autologous Tissue Substitute **J** Synthetic Substitute **K** Nonautologous Tissue Substitute	**Z** No Qualifier

Section 0 Medical and Surgical
Body System Y Anatomical Regions, Lower Extremities
Operation W **Revision:** Correcting, to the extent possible, a portion of a malfunctioning device or the position of a displaced device

Body Part (4th)	Approach (5th)	Device (6th)	Qualifier (7th)
9 Lower Extremity, Right **B** Lower Extremity, Left	**0** Open **3** Percutaneous **4** Percutaneous Endoscopic **X** External	**0** Drainage Device **3** Infusion Device **7** Autologous Tissue Substitute **J** Synthetic Substitute **K** Nonautologous Tissue Substitute **Y** Other Device	**Z** No Qualifier

AHA Coding Clinic

0Y6N0Z0 Detachment at Left Foot, Complete, Open Approach—AHA CC: 1Q, 2015, 28; 1Q, 2017, 22-23

0Y6P0Z3 Detachment at Right 1st Toe, Low, Open Approach—AHA CC: 2Q, 2015, 28-29

0Y6Q0Z3 Detachment at Left 1st Toe, Low, Open Approach—AHA CC: 2Q, 2015, 28-29

0Y950ZZ Drainage of Right Inguinal Region, Open Approach—AHA CC: 1Q, 2015, 23

0Y980ZZ Drainage of Left Femoral Region, Open Approach—AHA CC: 1Q, 2015, 22

Obstetrics Section (102–10Y)

Within each section of ICD-10-PCS the characters have different meanings. The seven character meanings for the Obstetrics section are illustrated here through the procedure example of *Manually-assisted delivery*.

Section	Body System	Root Operation	Body Part	Approach	Device	Qualifier
Obstetrics	Pregnancy	Delivery	Products of Conception	External	None	None
1	0	E	0	X	Z	Z

Section (Character 1)

All Obstetric procedure codes have a first character value of 1.

Body System (Character 2)

The alphanumeric character for the body system is placed in the second position. The body system applicable to the Obstetrics section is Pregnancy and has a character value of 0.

Root Operations (Character 3)

The alphanumeric character value for root operations is placed in the third position. Listed below are the root operations applicable to the Obstetrics section with their associated meaning.

Character Value	Root Operation	Root Operation Definition
2	Change	Taking out or off a device from a body part and putting back an identical or similar device in or on the same body part without cutting or puncturing the skin or a mucous membrane
9	Drainage	Taking or letting out fluids and/or gases from a body part
A	Abortion	Artificially terminating a pregnancy
D	Extraction	Pulling or stripping out or off all or a portion of a body part by the use of force
E	Delivery	Assisting the passage of the products of conception from the genital canal
H	Insertion	Putting in a nonbiological appliance that monitors, assists, performs, or prevents a physiological function but does not physically take the place of a body part
J	Inspection	Visually and/or manually exploring a body part
P	Removal	Taking out or off a device from a body part, region or orifice
Q	Repair	Restoring, to the extent possible, a body part to its normal anatomic structure and function
S	Reposition	Moving to its normal location, or other suitable location, all or a portion of a body part
T	Resection	Cutting out or off, without replacement, all of a body part
Y	Transplantation	Putting in or on all or a portion of a living body part taken from another individual or animal to physically take the place and/or function of all or a portion of a similar body part

Body Part (Character 4)

For each body system the applicable body part character values will be available for procedure code construction. An example of a body part is Products of Conception.

Approach (Character 5)

The approach is the technique used to reach the procedure site. The following are the approach character values for the Obstetrics section with the associated definitions.

Character Value	Approach	Approach Definition
0	Open	Cutting through the skin or mucous membrane and any other body layers necessary to expose the site of the procedure
3	Percutaneous	Entry, by puncture or minor incision, of instrumentation through the skin or mucous membrane and any other body layers necessary to reach the site of the procedure

Continued →

Character Value	Approach	Approach Definition
4	Percutaneous Endoscopic	Entry, by puncture or minor incision, of instrumentation through the skin or mucous membrane and any other body layers necessary to reach and visualize the site of the procedure
7	Via Natural or Artificial Opening	Entry of instrumentation through a natural or artificial external opening to reach the site of the procedure
8	Via Natural or Artificial Opening Endoscopic	Entry of instrumentation through a natural or artificial external opening to reach and visualize the site of the procedure
X	External	Procedures performed directly on the skin or mucous membrane and procedures performed indirectly by the application of external force through the skin or mucous membrane

Device (Character 6)

Depending on the procedure performed there may or may not be a device used. There are two types of devices included in the Obstetrics section: monitoring electrode and other device. When a device is not utilized during the procedure, the placeholder Z is the character value that should be reported.

Qualifier (Character 7)

The qualifier represents an additional attribute for the procedure when applicable. For example, drainage procedures in this section include several qualifiers including fetal cerebrospinal fluid that is reported with the character value of A. If there is no qualifier for a procedure, the placeholder Z is the character valve that should be reported.

Obstetric Section Guidelines (section 1)

C. Obstetrics Section

Products of Conception

C1. Procedures performed on the products of conception are coded to the Obstetrics section. Procedures performed on the pregnant female other than the products of conception are coded to the appropriate root operation in the Medical and Surgical section.

Example: Amniocentesis is coded to the products of conception body part in the Obstetrics section. Repair of obstetric urethral laceration is coded to the urethra body part in the Medical and Surgical section.

Procedures following delivery or abortion

C2. Procedures performed following a delivery or abortion for curettage of the endometrium or evacuation of retained products of conception are all coded in the Obstetrics section, to the root operation Extraction and the body part Products of Conception, Retained. Diagnostic or therapeutic dilation and curettage performed during times other than the postpartum or post-abortion period are all coded in the Medical and Surgical section, to the root operation Extraction and the body part Endometrium.

Coding Guidelines References

The table below links ICD-10-PCS coding guidelines to Obstetrics section body system tables. The guidelines identified in the table are provided in order to remind users to reference the coding guidelines prior to code reporting. It is imperative to review the ICD-10-PCS coding guidelines to ensure the procedure code being reported is accurate and complete.

Table References

Table	Root Operation	Coding Guideline(s)
102	Change	C1
10D	Extraction	C2

Obstetrics Section Tables

Obstetrics Tables 102–10Y

Section 1 **Obstetrics**
Body System 0 **Pregnancy**
Operation 2 **Change:** Taking out or off a device from a body part and putting back an identical or similar device in or on the same body part without cutting or puncturing the skin or a mucous membrane

Body Part (4th)	Approach (5th)	Device (6th)	Qualifier (7th)
0 Products of Conception	**7** Via Natural or Artificial Opening	**3** Monitoring Electrode **Y** Other Device	**Z** No Qualifier

Section 1 **Obstetrics**
Body System 0 **Pregnancy**
Operation 9 **Drainage:** Taking or letting out fluids and/or gases from a body part

Body Part (4th)	Approach (5th)	Device (6th)	Qualifier (7th)
0 Products of Conception	**0** Open **3** Percutaneous **4** Percutaneous Endoscopic **7** Via Natural or Artificial Opening **8** Via Natural or Artificial Opening Endoscopic	**Z** No Device	**9** Fetal Blood **A** Fetal Cerebrospinal Fluid **B** Fetal Fluid, Other **C** Amniotic Fluid, Therapeutic **D** Fluid, Other **U** Amniotic Fluid, Diagnostic

Section 1 **Obstetrics**
Body System 0 **Pregnancy**
Operation A **Abortion:** Artificially terminating a pregnancy

Body Part (4th)	Approach (5th)	Device (6th)	Qualifier (7th)
0 Products of Conception	**0** Open **3** Percutaneous **4** Percutaneous Endoscopic **8** Via Natural or Artificial Opening Endoscopic	**Z** No Device	**Z** No Qualifier
0 Products of Conception	**7** Via Natural or Artificial Opening	**Z** No Device	**6** Vacuum **W** Laminaria **X** Abortifacient **Z** No Qualifier

Section 1 **Obstetrics**
Body System 0 **Pregnancy**
Operation D **Extraction:** Pulling or stripping out or off all or a portion of a body part by the use of force

Body Part (4th)	Approach (5th)	Device (6th)	Qualifier (7th)
0 Products of Conception	**0** Open	**Z** No Device	**0** High **1** Low **2** Extraperitoneal
0 Products of Conception	**7** Via Natural or Artificial Opening	**Z** No Device	**3** Low Forceps **4** Mid Forceps **5** High Forceps **6** Vacuum **7** Internal Version **8** Other

Continued →

Section	1	Obstetrics
Body System	0	Pregnancy
Operation	D	**Extraction:** Pulling or stripping out or off all or a portion of a body part by the use of force

Body Part (4th)	Approach (5th)	Device (6th)	Qualifier (7th)
1 Products of Conception, Retained	7 Via Natural or Artificial Opening 8 Via Natural or Artificial Opening Endoscopic	Z No Device	9 Manual Z No Qualifier
2 Products of Conception, Ectopic	0 Open 4 Percutaneous Endoscopic 7 Via Natural or Artificial Opening 8 Via Natural or Artificial Opening Endoscopic	Z No Device	Z No Qualifier

Section	1	Obstetrics
Body System	0	Pregnancy
Operation	E	**Delivery:** Assisting the passage of the products of conception from the genital canal

Body Part (4th)	Approach (5th)	Device (6th)	Qualifier (7th)
0 Products of Conception	X External	Z No Device	Z No Qualifier

Section	1	Obstetrics
Body System	0	Pregnancy
Operation	H	**Insertion:** Putting in a nonbiological appliance that monitors, assists, performs, or prevents a physiological function but does not physically take the place of a body part

Body Part (4th)	Approach (5th)	Device (6th)	Qualifier (7th)
0 Products of Conception	0 Open 7 Via Natural or Artificial Opening	3 Monitoring Electrode Y Other Device	Z No Qualifier

Section	1	Obstetrics
Body System	0	Pregnancy
Operation	J	**Inspection:** Visually and/or manually exploring a body part

Body Part (4th)	Approach (5th)	Device (6th)	Qualifier (7th)
0 Products of Conception 1 Products of Conception, Retained 2 Products of Conception, Ectopic	0 Open 3 Percutaneous 4 Percutaneous Endoscopic 7 Via Natural or Artificial Opening 8 Via Natural or Artificial Opening Endoscopic X External	Z No Device	Z No Qualifier

Section	1	Obstetrics
Body System	0	Pregnancy
Operation	P	**Removal:** Taking out or off a device from a body part, region or orifice

Body Part (4th)	Approach (5th)	Device (6th)	Qualifier (7th)
0 Products of Conception	0 Open 7 Via Natural or Artificial Opening	3 Monitoring Electrode Y Other Device	Z No Qualifier

Section 1 **Obstetrics**
Body System 0 **Pregnancy**
Operation Q **Repair:** Restoring, to the extent possible, a body part to its normal anatomic structure and function

Body Part (4th)	Approach (5th)	Device (6th)	Qualifier (7th)
0 Products of Conception	**0** Open **3** Percutaneous **4** Percutaneous Endoscopic **7** Via Natural or Artificial Opening **8** Via Natural or Artificial Opening Endoscopic	**Y** Other Device **Z** No Device	**E** Nervous System **F** Cardiovascular System **G** Lymphatics and Hemic **H** Eye **J** Ear, Nose and Sinus **K** Respiratory System **L** Mouth and Throat **M** Gastrointestinal System **N** Hepatobiliary and Pancreas **P** Endocrine System **Q** Skin **R** Musculoskeletal System **S** Urinary System **T** Female Reproductive System **V** Male Reproductive System **Y** Other Body System

Section 1 **Obstetrics**
Body System 0 **Pregnancy**
Operation S **Reposition:** Moving to its normal location, or other suitable location, all or a portion of a body part

Body Part (4th)	Approach (5th)	Device (6th)	Qualifier (7th)
0 Products of Conception	**7** Via Natural or Artificial Opening **X** External	**Z** No Device	**Z** No Qualifier
2 Products of Conception, Ectopic	**0** Open **3** Percutaneous **4** Percutaneous Endoscopic **7** Via Natural or Artificial Opening **8** Via Natural or Artificial Opening Endoscopic	**Z** No Device	**Z** No Qualifier

Section 1 **Obstetrics**
Body System 0 **Pregnancy**
Operation T **Resection:** Cutting out or off, without replacement, all of a body part

Body Part (4th)	Approach (5th)	Device (6th)	Qualifier (7th)
2 Products of Conception, Ectopic	**0** Open **3** Percutaneous **4** Percutaneous Endoscopic **7** Via Natural or Artificial Opening **8** Via Natural or Artificial Opening Endoscopic	**Z** No Device	**Z** No Qualifier

Section 1 **Obstetrics**
Body System 0 **Pregnancy**
Operation Y **Transplantation:** Putting in or on all or a portion of a living body part taken from another individual or animal to physically take the place and/or function of all or a portion of a similar body part

Body Part (4th)	Approach (5th)	Device (6th)	Qualifier (7th)
0 Products of Conception	**3** Percutaneous **4** Percutaneous Endoscopic **7** Via Natural or Artificial Opening	**Z** No Device	**E** Nervous System **F** Cardiovascular System **G** Lymphatics and Hemic **H** Eye **J** Ear, Nose and Sinus **K** Respiratory System **L** Mouth and Throat **M** Gastrointestinal System **N** Hepatobiliary and Pancreas **P** Endocrine System **Q** Skin **R** Musculoskeletal System **S** Urinary System **T** Female Reproductive System **V** Male Reproductive System **Y** Other Body System

AHA Coding Clinic

10904ZC Drainage of Amniotic Fluid, Therapeutic from Products of Conception, Percutaneous Endoscopic Approach—AHA CC: 3Q, 2014, 12-13

10907ZC Drainage of Amniotic Fluid, Therapeutic from Products of Conception, Via Natural or Artificial Opening—AHA CC: 2Q, 2014, 9-10

10D00Z0 Extraction of Products of Conception, High, Open Approach— AHA CC: 2Q, 2018, 17-18; 4Q, 2018, 51

10D00Z1 Extraction of Products of Conception, Low, Open Approach—AHA CC: 4Q, 2018, 50-51

10D07Z3 Extraction of Products of Conception, Low Forceps, Via Natural or Artificial Opening—AHA CC: 1Q, 2016, 9-10

10D07Z6 Extraction of Products of Conception, Vacuum, Via Natural or Artificial Opening—AHA CC: 4Q, 2014, 43

10D20ZZ Extraction of Products of Conception, Ectopic, Open Approach—AHA CC: 1Q, 2021, 52

10D27ZZ Extraction of Products of Conception, Ectopic, Via Natural or Artificial Opening—AHA CC: 4Q, 2020, 60; 1Q, 2021, 52

10E0XZZ Delivery of Products of Conception, External Approach—AHA CC: 2Q, 2014, 9-10; 4Q, 2014, 17-18; 2Q, 2016, 34-35; 3Q, 2017, 5

10H07YZ Insertion of Other Device into Products of Conception, Via Natural or Artificial Opening—AHA CC: 2Q, 2013, 36

10Q00ZK Repair Respiratory System in Products of Conception, Open Approach—AHA CC: 2Q, 2021, 21-22

10Q04ZY Repair Other Body System in Products of Conception, Percutaneous Endoscopic Approach—AHA CC: 3Q, 2014, 12-13

10T24ZZ Resection of Products of Conception, Ectopic, Percutaneous Endoscopic Approach—AHA CC: 3Q, 2015, 32; 3Q, 2020, 47

Placement Section (2W0–2Y5)

Within each section of ICD-10-PCS the characters have different meanings. The seven character meanings for the Placement section are illustrated below through the procedure example of *Placement of pressure dressing on abdominal wall.*

Section	Body System	Root Operation	Body Region	Approach	Device	Qualifier
Placement	Anatomical Regions	Compression	Abdominal Wall	External	Pressure Dressing	None
2	W	1	3	X	6	Z

Section (Character 1)

All Placement procedure codes have a first character value of 2.

Body System (Character 2)

The alphanumeric character for the body system is placed in the second position. There are two character values applicable for the Placement section. The character value of W is reported for anatomical regions. The character value Y is reported for anatomical orifices.

Root Operations (Character 3)

The alphanumeric character value for root operations is placed in the third position. The following are the root operations applicable to the Placement section with their associated meaning.

Character Value	Root Operation	Root Operation Definition
0	Change	Taking out or off a device from a body part and putting back an identical or similar device in or on the same body part without cutting or puncturing the skin or a mucous membrane
1	Compression	Putting pressure on a body region
2	Dressing	Putting material on a body region for protection
3	Immobilization	Limiting or preventing motion of a body region
4	Packing	Putting material in a body region or orifice
5	Removal	Taking out or off a device from a body part
6	Traction	Exerting a pulling force on a body region in a distal direction

Body Region (Character 4)

For each body system the applicable body part character values will be available for procedure code construction. An example of a body region is Chest Wall.

Approach (Character 5)

The only approach technique utilized for the Placement section is External approach and is reported with the character value of X.

Character Value	Approach	Approach Definition
X	External	Procedures performed directly on the skin or mucous membrane and procedures performed indirectly by the application of external force through the skin or mucous membrane

Device (Character 6)

Depending on the procedure performed there may or may not be a device used. There are several types of devices included in the Placement section. Here is a sample list of the devices included in this section:

- Cast
- Packing material
- Pressure dressing
- Traction apparatus

When a device is not utilized during the procedure, the placeholder Z is the character value that should be reported.

Qualifier (Character 7)

The qualifier represents an additional attribute for the procedure when applicable. Currently, there are no qualifiers in the Placement section; therefore, the placeholder character value of Z should be reported.

Coding Guideline References

Before reporting Change and Removal procedures in this section users should review coding guideline B6.1c.

Placement Section Tables

Placement Tables 2W0–2Y5

Section	2	**Placement**
Body System	W	**Anatomical Regions**
Operation	0	**Change:** Taking out or off a device from a body part and putting back an identical or similar device in or on the same body part without cutting or puncturing the skin or a mucous membrane

Body Region (4th)	Approach (5th)	Device (6th)	Qualifier (7th)
0 Head **2** Neck **3** Abdominal Wall **4** Chest Wall **5** Back **6** Inguinal Region, Right **7** Inguinal Region, Left **8** Upper Extremity, Right **9** Upper Extremity, Left **A** Upper Arm, Right **B** Upper Arm, Left **C** Lower Arm, Right **D** Lower Arm, Left **E** Hand, Right **F** Hand, Left **G** Thumb, Right **H** Thumb, Left **J** Finger, Right **K** Finger, Left **L** Lower Extremity, Right **M** Lower Extremity, Left **N** Upper Leg, Right **P** Upper Leg, Left **Q** Lower Leg, Right **R** Lower Leg, Left **S** Foot, Right **T** Foot, Left **U** Toe, Right **V** Toe, Left	**X** External	**0** Traction Apparatus **1** Splint **2** Cast **3** Brace **4** Bandage **5** Packing Material **6** Pressure Dressing **7** Intermittent Pressure Device **Y** Other Device	**Z** No Qualifier
1 Face	**X** External	**0** Traction Apparatus **1** Splint **2** Cast **3** Brace **4** Bandage **5** Packing Material **6** Pressure Dressing **7** Intermittent Pressure Device **9** Wire **Y** Other Device	**Z** No Qualifier

Section 2 **Placement**
Body System W **Anatomical Regions**
Operation 1 **Compression:** Putting pressure on a body region

Body Region (4th)	Approach (5th)	Device (6th)	Qualifier (7th)
0 Head **1** Face **2** Neck **3** Abdominal Wall **4** Chest Wall **5** Back **6** Inguinal Region, Right **7** Inguinal Region, Left **8** Upper Extremity, Right **9** Upper Extremity, Left **A** Upper Arm, Right **B** Upper Arm, Left **C** Lower Arm, Right **D** Lower Arm, Left **E** Hand, Right **F** Hand, Left **G** Thumb, Right **H** Thumb, Left **J** Finger, Right **K** Finger, Left **L** Lower Extremity, Right **M** Lower Extremity, Left **N** Upper Leg, Right **P** Upper Leg, Left **Q** Lower Leg, Right **R** Lower Leg, Left **S** Foot, Right **T** Foot, Left **U** Toe, Right **V** Toe, Left	**X** External	**6** Pressure Dressing **7** Intermittent Pressure Device	**Z** No Qualifier

Section 2 **Placement**
Body System W **Anatomical Regions**
Operation 2 **Dressing:** Putting material on a body region for protection

Body Region (4th)	Approach (5th)	Device (6th)	Qualifier (7th)
0 Head **1** Face **2** Neck **3** Abdominal Wall **4** Chest Wall **5** Back **6** Inguinal Region, Right **7** Inguinal Region, Left **8** Upper Extremity, Right **9** Upper Extremity, Left **A** Upper Arm, Right **B** Upper Arm, Left **C** Lower Arm, Right **D** Lower Arm, Left **E** Hand, Right **F** Hand, Left **G** Thumb, Right **H** Thumb, Left **J** Finger, Right **K** Finger, Left **L** Lower Extremity, Right **M** Lower Extremity, Left **N** Upper Leg, Right **P** Upper Leg, Left **Q** Lower Leg, Right **R** Lower Leg, Left **S** Foot, Right **T** Foot, Left **U** Toe, Right **V** Toe, Left	**X** External	**4** Bandage	**Z** No Qualifier

Section 2 **Placement**
Body System W **Anatomical Regions**
Operation 3 **Immobilization:** Limiting or preventing motion of a body region

Body Region (4th)	Approach (5th)	Device (6th)	Qualifier (7th)
0 Head **2** Neck **3** Abdominal Wall **4** Chest Wall **5** Back **6** Inguinal Region, Right **7** Inguinal Region, Left **8** Upper Extremity, Right **9** Upper Extremity, Left **A** Upper Arm, Right **B** Upper Arm, Left **C** Lower Arm, Right **D** Lower Arm, Left **E** Hand, Right **F** Hand, Left **G** Thumb, Right **H** Thumb, Left **J** Finger, Right **K** Finger, Left **L** Lower Extremity, Right **M** Lower Extremity, Left **N** Upper Leg, Right **P** Upper Leg, Left **Q** Lower Leg, Right **R** Lower Leg, Left **S** Foot, Right **T** Foot, Left **U** Toe, Right **V** Toe, Left	**X** External	**1** Splint **2** Cast **3** Brace **Y** Other Device	**Z** No Qualifier
1 Face	**X** External	**1** Splint **2** Cast **3** Brace **9** Wire **Y** Other Device	**Z** No Qualifier

Section 2 **Placement**
Body System W **Anatomical Regions**
Operation 4 **Packing:** Putting material in a body region or orifice

Body Region (4th)	Approach (5th)	Device (6th)	Qualifier (7th)
0 Head **1** Face **2** Neck **3** Abdominal Wall **4** Chest Wall **5** Back **6** Inguinal Region, Right **7** Inguinal Region, Left **8** Upper Extremity, Right **9** Upper Extremity, Left **A** Upper Arm, Right **B** Upper Arm, Left **C** Lower Arm, Right **D** Lower Arm, Left **E** Hand, Right **F** Hand, Left **G** Thumb, Right **H** Thumb, Left **J** Finger, Right **K** Finger, Left **L** Lower Extremity, Right **M** Lower Extremity, Left **N** Upper Leg, Right **P** Upper Leg, Left **Q** Lower Leg, Right **R** Lower Leg, Left **S** Foot, Right **T** Foot, Left **U** Toe, Right **V** Toe, Left	**X** External	**5** Packing Material	**Z** No Qualifier

Section 2 **Placement**
Body System W **Anatomical Regions**
Operation 5 **Removal:** Taking out or off a device from a body part

Body Region (4th)	Approach (5th)	Device (6th)	Qualifier (7th)
0 Head **2** Neck **3** Abdominal Wall **4** Chest Wall **5** Back **6** Inguinal Region, Right **7** Inguinal Region, Left **8** Upper Extremity, Right **9** Upper Extremity, Left **A** Upper Arm, Right **B** Upper Arm, Left **C** Lower Arm, Right **D** Lower Arm, Left **E** Hand, Right **F** Hand, Left **G** Thumb, Right **H** Thumb, Left **J** Finger, Right **K** Finger, Left **L** Lower Extremity, Right **M** Lower Extremity, Left **N** Upper Leg, Right **P** Upper Leg, Left **Q** Lower Leg, Right **R** Lower Leg, Left **S** Foot, Right **T** Foot, Left **U** Toe, Right **V** Toe, Left	**X** External	**0** Traction Apparatus **1** Splint **2** Cast **3** Brace **4** Bandage **5** Packing Material **6** Pressure Dressing **7** Intermittent Pressure Device **Y** Other Device	**Z** No Qualifier
1 Face	**X** External	**0** Traction Apparatus **1** Splint **2** Cast **3** Brace **4** Bandage **5** Packing Material **6** Pressure Dressing **7** Intermittent Pressure Device **9** Wire **Y** Other Device	**Z** No Qualifier

Section 2 **Placement**
Body System W **Anatomical Regions**
Operation 6 **Traction:** Exerting a pulling force on a body region in a distal direction

Body Region (4th)	Approach (5th)	Device (6th)	Qualifier (7th)
0 Head **1** Face **2** Neck **3** Abdominal Wall **4** Chest Wall **5** Back **6** Inguinal Region, Right **7** Inguinal Region, Left **8** Upper Extremity, Right **9** Upper Extremity, Left **A** Upper Arm, Right **B** Upper Arm, Left **C** Lower Arm, Right **D** Lower Arm, Left **E** Hand, Right **F** Hand, Left **G** Thumb, Right **H** Thumb, Left **J** Finger, Right **K** Finger, Left **L** Lower Extremity, Right **M** Lower Extremity, Left **N** Upper Leg, Right **P** Upper Leg, Left **Q** Lower Leg, Right **R** Lower Leg, Left **S** Foot, Right **T** Foot, Left **U** Toe, Right **V** Toe, Left	**X** External	**0** Traction Apparatus **Z** No Device	**Z** No Qualifier

Section 2 **Placement**
Body System Y **Anatomical Orifices**
Operation 0 **Change:** Taking out or off a device from a body part and putting back an identical or similar device in or on the same body part without cutting or puncturing the skin or a mucous membrane

Body Region (4th)	Approach (5th)	Device (6th)	Qualifier (7th)
0 Mouth and Pharynx **1** Nasal **2** Ear **3** Anorectal **4** Female Genital Tract **5** Urethra	**X** External	**5** Packing Material	**Z** No Qualifier

Section 2 **Placement**
Body System Y **Anatomical Orifices**
Operation 4 **Packing:** Putting material in a body region or orifice

Body Region (4th)	Approach (5th)	Device (6th)	Qualifier (7th)
0 Mouth and Pharynx **1** Nasal **2** Ear **3** Anorectal **4** Female Genital Tract **5** Urethra	**X** External	**5** Packing Material	**Z** No Qualifier

Section 2 **Placement**
Body System Y **Anatomical Orifices**
Operation 5 **Removal:** Taking out or off a device from a body part

Body Region (4th)	Approach (5th)	Device (6th)	Qualifier (7th)
0 Mouth and Pharynx **1** Nasal **2** Ear **3** Anorectal **4** Female Genital Tract **5** Urethra	**X** External	**5** Packing Material	**Z** No Qualifier

AHA Coding Clinic

2W60X0Z Traction of Head using Traction Apparatus—AHA CC: 2Q, 2013, 39

2W62X0Z Traction of Neck using Traction Apparatus—AHA CC: 2Q, 2015, 35

2Y41X5Z Packing of Nasal Region using Packing Material—AHA CC: 4Q, 2017, 106; 4Q, 2018, 38

Within each section of ICD-10-PCS, the characters have different meanings. The seven character meanings for the Administration section are illustrated here through the procedure example of *Nerve block injection to median nerve*.

Section	Body System	Root Operation	Body System/ Region	Approach	Substance	Qualifier
Administration	Physiological System and Anatomical Region	Introduction	Peripheral Nerves and Plexi	Percutaneous	Regional Anesthetic	None
3	E	0	T	3	C	Z

Section (Character 1)

All Administration procedure codes have a first character value of 3.

Body System (Character 2)

The alphanumeric character for the body system is placed in the second position. There are three character values applicable for the Administration section.

Character Value	Character Value Description
0	Circulatory
C	Indwelling Device
E	Physiological System and Anatomical Region

Root Operations (Character 3)

The alphanumeric character value for root operations is placed in the third position. Listed here are the root operations applicable to the Administration section with their associated meaning.

Character Value	Root Operation	Root Operation Definition
0	Introduction	Putting in or on a therapeutic, diagnostic, nutritional, physiological, or prophylactic substance except blood or blood products
1	Irrigation	Putting in or on a cleansing substance
2	Transfusion	Putting in blood or blood products

Body System/Region (Character 4)

For each body system the applicable body part character values will be available for procedure code construction. An example of a body region is upper GI.

Approach (Character 5)

The approach is the technique used to reach the procedure site. Listed here are the approach character values for the Administration with the associated definitions.

Character Value	Approach	Approach Definition
0	Open	Cutting through the skin or mucous membrane and any other body layers necessary to expose the site of the procedure
3	Percutaneous	Entry, by puncture or minor incision, of instrumentation through the skin or mucous membrane and any other body layers necessary to reach the site of the procedure
4	Percutaneous Endoscopic	Entry, by puncture or minor incision, of instrumentation through the skin or mucous membrane and any other body layers necessary to reach and visualize the site of the procedure
7	Via Natural or Artificial Opening	Entry of instrumentation through a natural or artificial external opening to reach the site of the procedure
8	Via Natural or Artificial Opening Endoscopic	Entry of instrumentation through a natural or artificial external opening to reach and visualize the site of the procedure
X	External	Procedures performed directly on the skin or mucous membrane and procedures performed indirectly by the application of external force through the skin or mucous membrane

Substance (Character 6)

In the Administration section a substance is always utilized. The substance is reported in the sixth character position by the type of substance utilized. The following is a sample list of the substances included in this section:

- Anti-inflammatory
- Antineoplastic
- Bone marrow
- Platelet inhibitor
- Whole blood

Qualifier (Character 7)

The qualifier represents an additional attribute for the procedure when applicable. There are several qualifiers included in the Administration section. For example, transfusion procedures in this section include qualifiers including Autologous and Nonautologous that are reported with the character values of 0 and 1, respectively. If there is no qualifier for a procedure, the placeholder Z is the character value that should be reported.

If a coder is unsure of which option to select for the substance qualifier utilized during the procedure, Appendix F can be used to guide the selection. It is important to note that not all substance qualifier categories are provided by CMS in Appendix F. However, for example, the coding scenario indicates that Clolar was introduced percutaneously via the peripheral vein. The coder references Table 3E0 (Introduction in Physiological Systems and Anatomical Regions) under the peripheral vein, percutaneous approach, anti-neoplastic. Clolar is not a substance qualifier choice. However, the coder can then locate the substance qualifier categories in Appendix F. The category Clofarabine includes Clolar. Therefore, the coder should select P - Clofarabine for the 7th character.

Important Definitions for the Administration Section

Administration Root Operation	Qualifier	Definition
Transfusion (302)	0 - Autologous	Derived or transferred from the same individual's body*
	1 - Nonautologous	Derived or transferred from another individual's body

*Taken from The Free Dictionary by Farlex at www.thefreedictionary.com

Coding Guideline References

Before reporting Transfusion procedures for embryonic stem cells (6th character A), bone marrow (6th character G), cord blood stem cells (6th character X) or hematopoietic stem cells (6th character Y) users should review coding guideline B3.16.

Before reporting Administration codes for all Biliary and Pancreatic Tract (4th character value of J) procedures with a 6th character value of U (Pancreatic Islet Cells), users should review coding guideline B3.16.

Before reporting Irrigation procedures in this section, users should review coding guideline B6.1c.

Administration Tables 302–3E1

Section	**3**	**Administration**
Body System	**0**	**Circulatory**
Operation	**2**	**Transfusion:** Putting in blood or blood products

Body System / Region (4th)	Approach (5th)	Substance (6th)	Qualifier (7th)
3 Peripheral Vein **4** Central Vein	**3** Percutaneous	**A** Stem Cells, Embryonic	**Z** No Qualifier
3 Peripheral Vein **4** Central Vein	**3** Percutaneous	**C** Hematopoietic Stem/Progenitor Cells, Genetically Modified	**0** Autologous
3 Peripheral Vein **4** Central Vein	**3** Percutaneous	**D** Pathogen Reduced Cryoprecipitated Fibrinogen Complex	**1** Nonautologous
3 Peripheral Vein **4** Central Vein	**3** Percutaneous	**G** Bone Marrow **X** Stem Cells, Cord Blood **Y** Stem Cells, Hematopoietic	**0** Autologous **2** Allogeneic, Related **3** Allogeneic, Unrelated **4** Allogeneic, Unspecified
3 Peripheral Vein **4** Central Vein	**3** Percutaneous	**H** Whole Blood **J** Serum Albumin **K** Frozen Plasma **L** Fresh Plasma **M** Plasma Cryoprecipitate **N** Red Blood Cells **P** Frozen Red Cells **Q** White Cells **R** Platelets **S** Globulin **T** Fibrinogen **V** Antihemophilic Factors **W** Factor IX	**0** Autologous **1** Nonautologous
3 Peripheral Vein **4** Central Vein	**3** Percutaneous	**U** Stem Cells, T-cell Depleted Hematopoietic	**2** Allogeneic, Related **3** Allogeneic, Unrelated **4** Allogeneic, Unspecified
7 Products of Conception, Circulatory	**3** Percutaneous **7** Via Natural or Artificial Opening	**H** Whole Blood **J** Serum Albumin **K** Frozen Plasma **L** Fresh Plasma **M** Plasma Cryoprecipitate **N** Red Blood Cells **P** Frozen Red Cells **Q** White Cells **R** Platelets **S** Globulin **T** Fibrinogen **V** Antihemophilic Factors **W** Factor IX	**1** Nonautologous
8 Vein	**3** Percutaneous	**B** 4-Factor Prothrombin Complex Concentrate	**1** Nonautologous

Section	**3**	**Administration**
Body System	**C**	**Indwelling Device**
Operation	**1**	**Irrigation:** Putting in or on a cleansing substance

Body System / Region (4th)	Approach (5th)	Substance (6th)	Qualifier (7th)
Z None	**X** External	**8** Irrigating Substance	**Z** No Qualifier

Section	**3**	**Administration**
Body System	**E**	**Physiological Systems and Anatomical Regions**
Operation	**0**	**Introduction:** Putting in or on a therapeutic, diagnostic, nutritional, physiological, or prophylactic substance except blood or blood products

Body System / Region (4th)	Approach (5th)	Substance (6th)	Qualifier (7th)
0 Skin and Mucous Membranes	**X** External	**0** Antineoplastic	**5** Other Antineoplastic **M** Monoclonal Antibody
0 Skin and Mucous Membranes	**X** External	**2** Anti-infective	**8** Oxazolidinones **9** Other Anti-infective
0 Skin and Mucous Membranes	**X** External	**3** Anti-inflammatory **B** Anesthetic Agent **K** Other Diagnostic Substance **M** Pigment **N** Analgesics, Hypnotics, Sedatives **T** Destructive Agent	**Z** No Qualifier
0 Skin and Mucous Membranes	**X** External	**G** Other Therapeutic Substance	**C** Other Substance
1 Subcutaneous Tissue	**0** Open	**2** Anti-infective	**A** Anti-Infective Envelope
1 Subcutaneous Tissue	**3** Percutaneous	**0** Antineoplastic	**5** Other Antineoplastic **M** Monoclonal Antibody
1 Subcutaneous Tissue	**3** Percutaneous	**2** Anti-infective	**8** Oxazolidinones **9** Other Anti-infective **A** Anti-Infective Envelope
1 Subcutaneous Tissue	**3** Percutaneous	**3** Anti-inflammatory **6** Nutritional Substance **7** Electrolytic and Water Balance Substance **B** Anesthetic Agent **H** Radioactive Substance **K** Other Diagnostic Substance **N** Analgesics, Hypnotics, Sedatives **T** Destructive Agent	**Z** No Qualifier
1 Subcutaneous Tissue	**3** Percutaneous	**4** Serum, Toxoid and Vaccine	**0** Influenza Vaccine **Z** No Qualifier
1 Subcutaneous Tissue	**3** Percutaneous	**G** Other Therapeutic Substance	**C** Other Substance
1 Subcutaneous Tissue	**3** Percutaneous	**V** Hormone	**G** Insulin **J** Other Hormone
2 Muscle	**3** Percutaneous	**0** Antineoplastic	**5** Other Antineoplastic **M** Monoclonal Antibody
2 Muscle	**3** Percutaneous	**2** Anti-infective	**8** Oxazolidinones **9** Other Anti-infective
2 Muscle	**3** Percutaneous	**3** Anti-inflammatory **6** Nutritional Substance **7** Electrolytic and Water Balance Substance **B** Anesthetic Agent **H** Radioactive Substance **K** Other Diagnostic Substance **N** Analgesics, Hypnotics, Sedatives **T** Destructive Agent	**Z** No Qualifier
2 Muscle	**3** Percutaneous	**4** Serum, Toxoid and Vaccine	**0** Influenza Vaccine **Z** No Qualifier
2 Muscle	**3** Percutaneous	**G** Other Therapeutic Substance	**C** Other Substance

Continued →

Body System / Region (4th)	Approach (5th)	Substance (6th)	Qualifier (7th)
3 Peripheral Vein	**0** Open	**0** Antineoplastic	**2** High-dose Interleukin-2 **3** Low-dose Interleukin-2 **5** Other Antineoplastic **M** Monoclonal Antibody **P** Clofarabine
3 Peripheral Vein	**0** Open	**1** Thrombolytic	**6** Recombinant Human-activated Protein C **7** Other Thrombolytic
3 Peripheral Vein	**0** Open	**2** Anti-infective	**8** Oxazolidinones **9** Other Anti-infective
3 Peripheral Vein	**0** Open	**3** Anti-inflammatory **4** Serum, Toxoid and Vaccine **6** Nutritional Substance **7** Electrolytic and Water Balance Substance **F** Intracirculatory Anesthetic **H** Radioactive Substance **K** Other Diagnostic Substance **N** Analgesics, Hypnotics, Sedatives **P** Platelet Inhibitor **R** Antiarrhythmic **T** Destructive Agent **X** Vasopressor	**Z** No Qualifier
3 Peripheral Vein	**0** Open	**G** Other Therapeutic Substance	**C** Other Substance **N** Blood Brain Barrier Disruption
3 Peripheral Vein	**0** Open	**U** Pancreatic Islet Cells	**0** Autologous **1** Nonautologous
3 Peripheral Vein	**0** Open	**V** Hormone	**G** Insulin **H** Human B-type Natriuretic Peptide **J** Other Hormone
3 Peripheral Vein	**0** Open	**W** Immunotherapeutic	**K** Immunostimulator **L** Immunosuppressive
3 Peripheral Vein	**3** Percutaneous	**0** Antineoplastic	**2** High-dose Interleukin-2 **3** Low-dose Interleukin-2 **5** Other Antineoplastic **M** Monoclonal Antibody **P** Clofarabine
3 Peripheral Vein	**3** Percutaneous	**1** Thrombolytic	**6** Recombinant Human-activated Protein C **7** Other Thrombolytic
3 Peripheral Vein	**3** Percutaneous	**2** Anti-infective	**8** Oxazolidinones **9** Other Anti-infective
3 Peripheral Vein	**3** Percutaneous	**3** Anti-inflammatory **4** Serum, Toxoid and Vaccine **6** Nutritional Substance **7** Electrolytic and Water Balance Substance **F** Intracirculatory Anesthetic **H** Radioactive Substance **K** Other Diagnostic Substance **N** Analgesics, Hypnotics, Sedatives **P** Platelet Inhibitor **R** Antiarrhythmic **T** Destructive Agent **X** Vasopressor	**Z** No Qualifier

Continued →

Section 3 **Administration**
Body System E **Physiological Systems and Anatomical Regions**
Operation 0 **Introduction:** Putting in or on a therapeutic, diagnostic, nutritional, physiological, or prophylactic substance except blood or blood products

Body System / Region (4th)	Approach (5th)	Substance (6th)	Qualifier (7th)
3 Peripheral Vein	**3** Percutaneous	**G** Other Therapeutic Substance	**C** Other Substance **N** Blood Brain Barrier Disruption **Q** Glucarpidase
3 Peripheral Vein	**3** Percutaneous	**U** Pancreatic Islet Cells	**0** Autologous **1** Nonautologous
3 Peripheral Vein	**3** Percutaneous	**V** Hormone	**G** Insulin **H** Human B-type Natriuretic Peptide **J** Other Hormone
3 Peripheral Vein	**3** Percutaneous	**W** Immunotherapeutic	**K** Immunostimulator **L** Immunosuppressive
4 Central Vein	**0** Opcn	**0** Antineoplastic	**2** High-dose Interleukin-2 **3** Low-dose Interleukin-2 **5** Other Antineoplastic **M** Monoclonal Antibody **P** Clofarabine
4 Central Vein	**0** Open	**1** Thrombolytic	**6** Recombinant Human-activated Protein C **7** Other Thrombolytic
4 Central Vein	**0** Open	**2** Anti-infective	**8** Oxazolidinones **9** Other Anti-infective
4 Central Vein	**0** Open	**3** Anti-inflammatory **4** Serum, Toxoid and Vaccine **6** Nutritional Substance **7** Electrolytic and Water Balance Substance **F** Intracirculatory Anesthetic **H** Radioactive Substance **K** Other Diagnostic Substance **N** Analgesics, Hypnotics, Sedatives **P** Platelet Inhibitor **R** Antiarrhythmic **T** Destructive Agent **X** Vasopressor	**Z** No Qualifier
4 Central Vein	**0** Open	**G** Other Therapeutic Substance	**C** Other Substance **N** Blood Brain Barrier Disruption
4 Central Vein	**0** Open	**V** Hormone	**G** Insulin **H** Human B-type Natriuretic Peptide **J** Other Hormone
4 Central Vein	**0** Open	**W** Immunotherapeutic	**K** Immunostimulator **L** Immunosuppressive
4 Central Vein	**3** Percutaneous	**0** Antineoplastic	**2** High-dose Interleukin-2 **3** Low-dose Interleukin-2 **5** Other Antineoplastic **M** Monoclonal Antibody **P** Clofarabine
4 Central Vein	**3** Percutaneous	**1** Thrombolytic	**6** Recombinant Human-activated Protein C **7** Other Thrombolytic

Continued →

Body System / Region (4th)	Approach (5th)	Substance (6th)	Qualifier (7th)
4 Central Vein	3 Percutaneous	2 Anti-infective	8 Oxazolidinones 9 Other Anti-infective
4 Central Vein	3 Percutaneous	3 Anti-inflammatory 4 Serum, Toxoid and Vaccine 6 Nutritional Substance 7 Electrolytic and Water Balance Substance F Intracirculatory Anesthetic H Radioactive Substance K Other Diagnostic Substance N Analgesics, Hypnotics, Sedatives P Platelet Inhibitor R Antiarrhythmic T Destructive Agent X Vasopressor	Z No Qualifier
4 Central Vein	3 Percutaneous	G Other Therapeutic Substance	C Other Substance N Blood Brain Barrier Disruption Q Glucarpidase
4 Central Vein	3 Percutaneous	V Hormone	G Insulin H Human B-type Natriuretic Peptide J Other Hormone
4 Central Vein	3 Percutaneous	W Immunotherapeutic	K Immunostimulator L Immunosuppressive
5 Peripheral Artery 6 Central Artery	0 Open 3 Percutaneous	0 Antineoplastic	2 High-dose Interleukin-2 3 Low-dose Interleukin-2 5 Other Antineoplastic M Monoclonal Antibody P Clofarabine
5 Peripheral Artery 6 Central Artery	0 Open 3 Percutaneous	1 Thrombolytic	6 Recombinant Human-activated Protein C 7 Other Thrombolytic
5 Peripheral Artery 6 Central Artery	0 Open 3 Percutaneous	2 Anti-infective	8 Oxazolidinones 9 Other Anti-infective
5 Peripheral Artery 6 Central Artery	0 Open 3 Percutaneous	3 Anti-inflammatory 4 Serum, Toxoid and Vaccine 6 Nutritional Substance 7 Electrolytic and Water Balance Substance F Intracirculatory Anesthetic H Radioactive Substance K Other Diagnostic Substance N Analgesics, Hypnotics, Sedatives P Platelet Inhibitor R Antiarrhythmic T Destructive Agent X Vasopressor	Z No Qualifier
5 Peripheral Artery 6 Central Artery	0 Open 3 Percutaneous	G Other Therapeutic Substance	C Other Substance N Blood Brain Barrier Disruption
5 Peripheral Artery 6 Central Artery	0 Open 3 Percutaneous	V Hormone	G Insulin H Human B-type Natriuretic Peptide J Other Hormone

Continued →

Section 3 **Administration**
Body System E **Physiological Systems and Anatomical Regions**
Operation 0 **Introduction:** Putting in or on a therapeutic, diagnostic, nutritional, physiological, or prophylactic substance except blood or blood products

Body System / Region (4th)	Approach (5th)	Substance (6th)	Qualifier (7th)
5 Peripheral Artery **6** Central Artery	**0** Open **3** Percutaneous	**W** Immunotherapeutic	**K** Immunostimulator **L** Immunosuppressive
7 Coronary Artery **8** Heart	**0** Open **3** Percutaneous	**1** Thrombolytic	**6** Recombinant Human-activated Protein C **7** Other Thrombolytic
7 Coronary Artery **8** Heart	**0** Open **3** Percutaneous	**G** Other Therapeutic Substance	**C** Other Substance
7 Coronary Artery **8** Heart	**0** Open **3** Percutaneous	**K** Other Diagnostic Substance **P** Platelet Inhibitor	**Z** No Qualifier
7 Coronary Artery **8** Heart	**4** Percutaneous Endoscopic	**G** Other Therapeutic Substance	**C** Other Substance
9 Nose	**3** Percutaneous **7** Via Natural or Artificial Opening **X** External	**0** Antineoplastic	**5** Other Antineoplastic **M** Monoclonal Antibody
9 Nose	**3** Percutaneous **7** Via Natural or Artificial Opening **X** External	**2** Anti-infective	**8** Oxazolidinones **9** Other Anti-infective
9 Nose	**3** Percutaneous **7** Via Natural or Artificial Opening **X** External	**3** Anti-inflammatory **4** Serum, Toxoid and Vaccine **B** Anesthetic Agent **H** Radioactive Substance **K** Other Diagnostic Substance **N** Analgesics, Hypnotics, Sedatives **T** Destructive Agent	**Z** No Qualifier
9 Nose	**3** Percutaneous **7** Via Natural or Artificial Opening **X** External	**G** Other Therapeutic Substance	**C** Other Substance
A Bone Marrow	**3** Percutaneous	**0** Antineoplastic	**5** Other Antineoplastic **M** Monoclonal Antibody
A Bone Marrow	**3** Percutaneous	**G** Other Therapeutic Substance	**C** Other Substance
B Ear	**3** Percutaneous **7** Via Natural or Artificial Opening **X** External	**0** Antineoplastic	**4** Liquid Brachytherapy Radioisotope **5** Other Antineoplastic **M** Monoclonal Antibody
B Ear	**3** Percutaneous **7** Via Natural or Artificial Opening **X** External	**2** Anti-infective	**8** Oxazolidinones **9** Other Anti-infective
B Ear	**3** Percutaneous **7** Via Natural or Artificial Opening **X** External	**3** Anti-inflammatory **B** Anesthetic Agent **H** Radioactive Substance **K** Other Diagnostic Substance **N** Analgesics, Hypnotics, Sedatives **T** Destructive Agent	**Z** No Qualifier

Continued →

Section 3 Administration
Body System E Physiological Systems and Anatomical Regions
Operation 0 Introduction: Putting in or on a therapeutic, diagnostic, nutritional, physiological, or prophylactic substance except blood or blood products

Body System / Region (4th)	Approach (5th)	Substance (6th)	Qualifier (7th)
B Ear	**3** Percutaneous **7** Via Natural or Artificial Opening **X** External	**G** Other Therapeutic Substance	**C** Other Substance
C Eye	**3** Percutaneous **7** Via Natural or Artificial Opening **X** External	**0** Antineoplastic	**4** Liquid Brachytherapy Radioisotope **5** Other Antineoplastic **M** Monoclonal Antibody
C Eye	**3** Percutaneous **7** Via Natural or Artificial Opening **X** External	**2** Anti-infective	**8** Oxazolidinones **9** Other Anti-infective
C Eye	**3** Percutaneous **7** Via Natural or Artificial Opening **X** External	**3** Anti-inflammatory **B** Anesthetic Agent **H** Radioactive Substance **K** Other Diagnostic Substance **M** Pigment **N** Analgesics, Hypnotics, Sedatives **T** Destructive Agent	**Z** No Qualifier
C Eye	**3** Percutaneous **7** Via Natural or Artificial Opening **X** External	**G** Other Therapeutic Substance	**C** Other Substance
C Eye	**3** Percutaneous **7** Via Natural or Artificial Opening **X** External	**S** Gas	**F** Other Gas
D Mouth and Pharynx	**3** Percutaneous **7** Via Natural or Artificial Opening **X** External	**0** Antineoplastic	**4** Liquid Brachytherapy Radioisotope **5** Other Antineoplastic **M** Monoclonal Antibody
D Mouth and Pharynx	**3** Percutaneous **7** Via Natural or Artificial Opening **X** External	**2** Anti-infective	**8** Oxazolidinones **9** Other Anti-infective
D Mouth and Pharynx	**3** Percutaneous **7** Via Natural or Artificial Opening **X** External	**3** Anti-inflammatory **4** Serum, Toxoid and Vaccine **6** Nutritional Substance **7** Electrolytic and Water Balance Substance **B** Anesthetic Agent **H** Radioactive Substance **K** Other Diagnostic Substance **N** Analgesics, Hypnotics, Sedatives **R** Antiarrhythmic **T** Destructive Agent	**Z** No Qualifier
D Mouth and Pharynx	**3** Percutaneous **7** Via Natural or Artificial Opening **X** External	**G** Other Therapeutic Substance	**C** Other Substance

Continued →

Section 3 **Administration**
Body System E **Physiological Systems and Anatomical Regions**
Operation 0 **Introduction:** Putting in or on a therapeutic, diagnostic, nutritional, physiological, or prophylactic substance except blood or blood products

Body System / Region (4th)	Approach (5th)	Substance (6th)	Qualifier (7th)
E Products of Conception **G** Upper GI **H** Lower GI **K** Genitourinary Tract **N** Male Reproductive	**3** Percutaneous **7** Via Natural or Artificial Opening **8** Via Natural or Artificial Opening Endoscopic	**0** Antineoplastic	**4** Liquid Brachytherapy Radioisotope **5** Other Antineoplastic **M** Monoclonal Antibody
E Products of Conception **G** Upper GI **H** Lower GI **K** Genitourinary Tract **N** Male Reproductive	**3** Percutaneous **7** Via Natural or Artificial Opening **8** Via Natural or Artificial Opening Endoscopic	**2** Anti-infective	**8** Oxazolidinones **9** Other Anti-infective
E Products of Conception **G** Upper GI **H** Lower GI **K** Genitourinary Tract **N** Male Reproductive	**3** Percutaneous **7** Via Natural or Artificial Opening **8** Via Natural or Artificial Opening Endoscopic	**3** Anti-inflammatory **6** Nutritional Substance **7** Electrolytic and Water Balance Substance **B** Anesthetic Agent **H** Radioactive Substance **K** Other Diagnostic Substance **N** Analgesics, Hypnotics, Sedatives **T** Destructive Agent	**Z** No Qualifier
E Products of Conception **G** Upper GI **H** Lower GI **K** Genitourinary Tract **N** Male Reproductive	**3** Percutaneous **7** Via Natural or Artificial Opening **8** Via Natural or Artificial Opening Endoscopic	**G** Other Therapeutic Substance	**C** Other Substance
E Products of Conception **G** Upper GI **H** Lower GI **K** Genitourinary Tract **N** Male Reproductive	**3** Percutaneous **7** Via Natural or Artificial Opening **8** Via Natural or Artificial Opening Endoscopic	**S** Gas	**F** Other Gas
E Products of Conception **G** Upper GI **H** Lower GI **K** Genitourinary Tract **N** Male Reproductive	**4** Percutaneous Endoscopic	**G** Other Therapeutic Substance	**C** Other Substance
F Respiratory Tract	**3** Percutaneous **7** Via Natural or Artificial Opening **8** Via Natural or Artificial Opening Endoscopic	**0** Antineoplastic	**4** Liquid Brachytherapy Radioisotope **5** Other Antineoplastic **M** Monoclonal Antibody
F Respiratory Tract	**3** Percutaneous **7** Via Natural or Artificial Opening **8** Via Natural or Artificial Opening Endoscopic	**2** Anti-infective	**8** Oxazolidinones **9** Other Anti-infective
F Respiratory Tract	**3** Percutaneous **7** Via Natural or Artificial Opening **8** Via Natural or Artificial Opening Endoscopic	**3** Anti-inflammatory **6** Nutritional Substance **7** Electrolytic and Water Balance Substance **B** Anesthetic Agent **H** Radioactive Substance **K** Other Diagnostic Substance **N** Analgesics, Hypnotics, Sedatives **T** Destructive Agent	**Z** No Qualifier

Continued →

Section 3 Administration
Body System E Physiological Systems and Anatomical Regions
Operation 0 Introduction: Putting in or on a therapeutic, diagnostic, nutritional, physiological, or prophylactic substance except blood or blood products

Body System / Region (4th)	Approach (5th)	Substance (6th)	Qualifier (7th)
F Respiratory Tract	**3** Percutaneous **7** Via Natural or Artificial Opening **8** Via Natural or Artificial Opening Endoscopic	**G** Other Therapeutic Substance	**C** Other Substance
F Respiratory Tract	**3** Percutaneous **7** Via Natural or Artificial Opening **8** Via Natural or Artificial Opening Endoscopic	**S** Gas	**D** Nitric Oxide **F** Other Gas
F Respiratory Tract	**4** Percutaneous Endoscopic	**G** Other Therapeutic Substance	**C** Other Substance
J Biliary and Pancreatic Tract	**3** Percutaneous **7** Via Natural or Artificial Opening **8** Via Natural or Artificial Opening Endoscopic	**0** Antineoplastic	**4** Liquid Brachytherapy Radioisotope **5** Other Antineoplastic **M** Monoclonal Antibody
J Biliary and Pancreatic Tract	**3** Percutaneous **7** Via Natural or Artificial Opening **8** Via Natural or Artificial Opening Endoscopic	**2** Anti-infective	**8** Oxazolidinones **9** Other Anti-infective
J Biliary and Pancreatic Tract	**3** Percutaneous **7** Via Natural or Artificial Opening **8** Via Natural or Artificial Opening Endoscopic	**3** Anti-inflammatory **6** Nutritional Substance **7** Electrolytic and Water Balance Substance **B** Anesthetic Agent **H** Radioactive Substance **K** Other Diagnostic Substance **N** Analgesics, Hypnotics, Sedatives **T** Destructive Agent	**Z** No Qualifier
J Biliary and Pancreatic Tract	**3** Percutaneous **7** Via Natural or Artificial Opening **8** Via Natural or Artificial Opening Endoscopic	**G** Other Therapeutic Substance	**C** Other Substance
J Biliary and Pancreatic Tract	**3** Percutaneous **7** Via Natural or Artificial Opening **8** Via Natural or Artificial Opening Endoscopic	**S** Gas	**F** Other Gas
J Biliary and Pancreatic Tract	**3** Percutaneous **7** Via Natural or Artificial Opening **8** Via Natural or Artificial Opening Endoscopic	**U** Pancreatic Islet Cells	**0** Autologous **1** Nonautologous
J Biliary and Pancreatic Tract	**4** Percutaneous Endoscopic	**G** Other Therapeutic Substance	**C** Other Substance

Continued →

Section	**3**	**Administration**	
Body System	**E**	**Physiological Systems and Anatomical Regions**	
Operation	**0**	**Introduction:** Putting in or on a therapeutic, diagnostic, nutritional, physiological, or prophylactic substance except blood or blood products	

Body System / Region (4th)	Approach (5th)	Substance (6th)	Qualifier (7th)
L Pleural Cavity	**0** Open	**5** Adhesion Barrier	**Z** No Qualifier
L Pleural Cavity	**3** Percutaneous	**0** Antineoplastic	**4** Liquid Brachytherapy Radioisotope **5** Other Antineoplastic **M** Monoclonal Antibody
L Pleural Cavity	**3** Percutaneous	**2** Anti-infective	**8** Oxazolidinones **9** Other Anti-infective
L Pleural Cavity	**3** Percutaneous	**3** Anti-inflammatory **5** Adhesion Barrier **6** Nutritional Substance **7** Electrolytic and Water Balance Substance **B** Anesthetic Agent **H** Radioactive Substance **K** Other Diagnostic Substance **N** Analgesics, Hypnotics, Sedatives **T** Destructive Agent	**Z** No Qualifier
L Pleural Cavity	**3** Percutaneous	**G** Other Therapeutic Substance	**C** Other Substance
L Pleural Cavity	**3** Percutaneous	**S** Gas	**F** Other Gas
L Pleural Cavity	**4** Percutaneous Endoscopic	**5** Adhesion Barrier	**Z** No Qualifier
L Pleural Cavity	**4** Percutaneous Endoscopic	**G** Other Therapeutic Substance	**C** Other Substance
L Pleural Cavity	**7** Via Natural or Artificial Opening	**0** Antineoplastic	**4** Liquid Brachytherapy Radioisotope **5** Other Antineoplastic **M** Monoclonal Antibody
L Pleural Cavity	**7** Via Natural or Artificial Opening	**S** Gas	**F** Other Gas
M Peritoneal Cavity	**0** Open	**5** Adhesion Barrier	**Z** No Qualifier
M Peritoneal Cavity	**3** Percutaneous	**0** Antineoplastic	**4** Liquid Brachytherapy Radioisotope **5** Other Antineoplastic **M** Monoclonal Antibody **Y** Hyperthermic
M Peritoneal Cavity	**3** Percutaneous	**2** Anti-infective	**8** Oxazolidinones **9** Other Anti-infective
M Peritoneal Cavity	**3** Percutaneous	**3** Anti-inflammatory **5** Adhesion Barrier **6** Nutritional Substance **7** Electrolytic and Water Balance Substance **B** Anesthetic Agent **H** Radioactive Substance **K** Other Diagnostic Substance **N** Analygesics, Hypnotics, Sedatives **T** Destructive Agent	**Z** No Qualifier
M Peritoneal Cavity	**3** Percutaneous	**G** Other Therapeutic Substance	**C** Other Substance
M Peritoneal Cavity	**3** Percutaneous	**S** Gas	**F** Other Gas
M Peritoneal Cavity	**4** Percutaneous Endoscopic	**5** Adhesion Barrier	**Z** No Qualifier

Continued →

Body System / Region (4th)	Approach (5th)	Substance (6th)	Qualifier (7th)
M Peritoneal Cavity	**4** Percutaneous Endoscopic	**G** Other Therapeutic Substance	**C** Other Substance
M Peritoneal Cavity	**7** Via Natural or Artificial Opening	**0** Antineoplastic	**4** Liquid Brachytherapy Radioisotope **5** Other Antineoplastic **M** Monoclonal Antibody
M Peritoneal Cavity	**7** Via Natural or Artificial Opening	**S** Gas	**F** Other Gas
P Female Reproductive	**0** Open	**5** Adhesion Barrier	**Z** No Qualifier
P Female Reproductive	**3** Percutaneous	**0** Antineoplastic	**4** Liquid Brachytherapy Radioisotope **5** Other Antineoplastic **M** Monoclonal Antibody
P Female Reproductive	**3** Percutaneous	**2** Anti-infective	**8** Oxazolidinones **9** Other Anti-infective
P Female Reproductive	**3** Percutaneous	**3** Anti-inflammatory **5** Adhesion Barrier **6** Nutritional Substance **7** Electrolytic and Water Balance Substance **B** Anesthetic Agent **H** Radioactive Substance **K** Other Diagnostic Substance **L** Sperm **N** Analgesics, Hypnotics, Sedatives **T** Destructive Agent **V** Hormone	**Z** No Qualifier
P Female Reproductive	**3** Percutaneous	**G** Other Therapeutic Substance	**C** Other Substance
P Female Reproductive	**3** Percutaneous	**Q** Fertilized Ovum	**0** Autologous **1** Nonautologous
P Female Reproductive	**3** Percutaneous	**S** Gas	**F** Other Gas
P Female Reproductive	**4** Percutaneous Endoscopic	**5** Adhesion Barrier	**Z** No Qualifier
P Female Reproductive	**4** Percutaneous Endoscopic	**G** Other Therapeutic Substance	**C** Other Substance
P Female Reproductive	**7** Via Natural or Artificial Opening	**0** Antineoplastic	**4** Liquid Brachytherapy Radioisotope **5** Other Antineoplastic **M** Monoclonal Antibody
P Female Reproductive	**7** Via Natural or Artificial Opening	**2** Anti-infective	**8** Oxazolidinones **9** Other Anti-infective
P Female Reproductive	**7** Via Natural or Artificial Opening	**5** Adhesion Barrier **6** Nutritional Substance **7** Electrolytic and Water Balance Substance **B** Anesthetic Agent **H** Radioactive Substance **K** Other Diagnostic Substance **L** Sperm **N** Analgestics, Hypnotics, Sedatives **T** Destructive Agent **V** Hormone	**Z** No Qualifier
P Female Reproductive	**7** Via Natural or Artificial Opening	**G** Other Therapeutic Substance	**C** Other Substance

Continued →

Section 3 **Administration**
Body System E **Physiological Systems and Anatomical Regions**
Operation 0 **Introduction:** Putting in or on a therapeutic, diagnostic, nutritional, physiological, or prophylactic substance except blood or blood products

3E0 Continued

Body System / Region (4th)	Approach (5th)	Substance (6th)	Qualifier (7th)
P Female Reproductive	**7** Via Natural or Artificial Opening	**Q** Fertilized Ovum	**0** Autologous **1** Nonautologous
P Female Reproductive	**7** Via Natural or Artificial Opening	**S** Gas	**F** Other Gas
P Female Reproductive	**8** Via Natural or Artificial Opening Endoscopic	**0** Antineoplastic	**4** Liquid Brachytherapy Radioisotope **5** Other Antineoplastic **M** Monoclonal Antibody
P Female Reproductive	**8** Via Natural or Artificial Opening Endoscopic	**2** Anti-infective	**8** Oxazolidinones **9** Other Anti-infective
P Female Reproductive	**8** Via Natural or Artificial Opening Endoscopic	**3** Anti-inflammatory **6** Nutritional Substance **7** Electrolytic and Water Balance Substance **B** Anesthetic Agent **H** Radioactive Substance **K** Other Diagnostic Substance **N** Analgesics, Hypnotics, Sedatives **T** Destructive Agent	**Z** No Qualifier
P Female Reproductive	**8** Via Natural or Artificial Opening Endoscopic	**G** Other Therapeutic Substance	**C** Other Substance
P Female Reproductive	**8** Via Natural or Artificial Opening Endoscopic	**S** Gas	**F** Other Gas
Q Cranial Cavity and Brain	**0** Open **3** Percutaneous	**0** Antineoplastic	**4** Liquid Brachytherapy Radioisotope **5** Other Antineoplastic **M** Monoclonal Antibody
Q Cranial Cavity and Brain	**0** Open **3** Percutaneous	**2** Anti-infective	**8** Oxazolidinones **9** Other Anti-infective
Q Cranial Cavity and Brain	**0** Open **3** Percutaneous	**3** Anti-inflammatory **6** Nutritional Substitute **7** Electrolytic and Water Balance Substitute **A** Stem Cells, Embryonic **B** Anesthetic Agent **H** Radioactive Substance **K** Other Diagnostic Substance **N** Analgesics, Hypnotics, Sedatives **T** Destructive Agent	**Z** No Qualifier
Q Cranial Cavity and Brain	**0** Open **3** Percutaneous	**E** Stem Cells, Somatic	**0** Autologous **1** Nonautologous
Q Cranial Cavity and Brain	**0** Open **3** Percutaneous	**G** Other Therapeutic Substance	**C** Other Substance
Q Cranial Cavity and Brain	**0** Open **3** Percutaneous	**S** Gas	**F** Other Gas
Q Cranial Cavity and Brain	**7** Via Natural or Artificial Opening	**0** Antineoplastic	**4** Liquid Brachytherapy Radioisotope **5** Other Antineoplastic **M** Monoclonal Antibody
Q Cranial Cavity and Brain	**7** Via Natural or Artificial Opening	**S** Gas	**F** Other Gas

Continued →

Body System / Region (4th)	Approach (5th)	Substance (6th)	Qualifier (7th)
R Spinal Canal	**0** Open	**A** Stem Cells, Embryonic	**Z** No Qualifier
R Spinal Canal	**0** Open	**E** Stem Cells, Somatic	**0** Autologous **1** Nonautologous
R Spinal Canal	**3** Percutaneous	**0** Antineoplastic	**2** High-dose Interleukin-2 **3** Low-dose Interleukin-2 **4** Liquid Brachytherapy Radioisotope **5** Other Antineoplastic **M** Monoclonal Antibody
R Spinal Canal	**3** Percutaneous	**2** Anti-infective	**8** Oxazolidinones **9** Other Anti-infective
R Spinal Canal	**3** Percutaneous	**3** Anti-inflammatory **6** Nutritional Substance **7** Electrolytic and Water Balance Substance **A** Stem Cells, Embryonic **B** Anesthetic Agent **H** Radioactive Substance **K** Other Diagnostic Substance **N** Analgesics, Hypnotics, Sedatives **T** Destructive Agent	**Z** No Qualifier
R Spinal Canal	**3** Percutaneous	**E** Stem Cells, Somatic	**0** Autologous **1** Nonautologous
R Spinal Canal	**3** Percutaneous	**G** Other Therapeutic Substance	**C** Other Substance
R Spinal Canal	**3** Percutaneous	**S** Gas	**F** Other Gas
R Spinal Canal	**7** Via Natural or Artificial Opening	**S** Gas	**F** Other Gas
S Epidural Space	**3** Percutaneous	**0** Antineoplastic	**2** High-dose Interleukin-2 **3** Low-dose Interleukin-2 **4** Liquid Brachytherapy Radioisotope **5** Other Antineoplastic **M** Monoclonal Antibody
S Epidural Space	**3** Percutaneous	**2** Anti-infective	**8** Oxazolidinones **9** Other Anti-infective
S Epidural Space	**3** Percutaneous	**3** Anti-inflammatory **6** Nutritional Substance **7** Electrolytic and Water Balance Substance **B** Anesthetic Agent **H** Radioactive Substance **K** Other Diagnostic Substance **N** Analgesics, Hypnotics, Sedatives **T** Destructive Agent	**Z** No Qualifier
S Epidural Space	**3** Percutaneous	**G** Other Therapeutic Substance	**C** Other Substance
S Epidural Space	**3** Percutaneous	**S** Gas	**F** Other Gas
S Epidural Space	**7** Via Natural or Artificial Opening	**S** Gas	**F** Other Gas
T Peripheral Nerves and Plexi **X** Cranial Nerves	**3** Percutaneous	**3** Anti-inflammatory **B** Anesthetic Agent **T** Destructive Agent	**Z** No Qualifier

Continued →

Section 3 **Administration**
Body System E **Physiological Systems and Anatomical Regions**
Operation 0 **Introduction:** Putting in or on a therapeutic, diagnostic, nutritional, physiological, or prophylactic substance except blood or blood products

Body System / Region (4th)	Approach (5th)	Substance (6th)	Qualifier (7th)
T Peripheral Nerves and Plexi **X** Cranial Nerves	**3** Percutaneous	**G** Other Therapeutic Substance	**C** Other Substance
U Joints	**0** Open	**2** Anti-infective	**8** Oxazolidinones **9** Other Anti-infective
U Joints	**0** Open	**G** Other Therapeutic Substance	**B** Recombinant Bone Morphogenetic Protein
U Joints	**3** Percutaneous	**0** Antineoplastic	**4** Liquid Brachytherapy Radioisotope **5** Other Antineoplastic **M** Monoclonal Antibody
U Joints	**3** Percutaneous	**2** Anti-infective	**8** Oxazolidinones **9** Other Anti-infective
U Joints	**3** Percutaneous	**3** Anti-inflammatory **6** Nutritional Substance **7** Electrolytic and Water Balance Substance **B** Anesthetic Agent **H** Radioactive Substance **K** Other Diagnostic Substance **N** Analgesics, Hypnotics, Sedatives **T** Destructive Agent	**Z** No Qualifier
U Joints	**3** Percutaneous	**G** Other Therapeutic Substance	**B** Recombinant Bone Morphogenetic Protein **C** Other Substance
U Joints	**3** Percutaneous	**S** Gas	**F** Other Gas
U Joints	**4** Percutaneous Endoscopic	**G** Other Therapeutic Substance	**C** Other Substance
V Bones	**0** Open	**G** Other Therapeutic Substance	**B** Recombinant Bone Morphogenetic Protein
V Bones	**3** Percutaneous	**0** Antineoplastic	**5** Other Antineoplastic **M** Monoclonal Antibody
V Bones	**3** Percutaneous	**2** Anti-infective	**8** Oxazolidinones **9** Other Anti-infective
V Bones	**3** Percutaneous	**3** Anti-inflammatory **6** Nutritional Substance **7** Electrolytic and Water Balance Substance **B** Anesthetic Agent **H** Radioactive Substance **K** Other Diagnostic Substance **N** Analgesics, Hypnotics, Sedatives **T** Destructive Agent	**Z** No Qualifier
V Bones	**3** Percutaneous	**G** Other Therapeutic Substance	**B** Recombinant Bone Morphogenetic Protein **C** Other Substance
W Lymphatics	**3** Percutaneous	**0** Antineoplastic	**5** Other Antineoplastic **M** Monoclonal Antibody
W Lymphatics	**3** Percutaneous	**2** Anti-infective	**8** Oxazolidinones **9** Other Anti-infective

Continued →

Section 3 **Administration**
Body System E **Physiological Systems and Anatomical Regions**
Operation 0 **Introduction:** Putting in or on a therapeutic, diagnostic, nutritional, physiological, or prophylactic substance except blood or blood products

Body System / Region (4th)	Approach (5th)	Substance (6th)	Qualifier (7th)
W Lymphatics	**3** Percutaneous	**3** Anti-inflammatory **6** Nutritional Substance **7** Electrolytic and Water Balance Substance **B** Anesthetic Agent **H** Radioactive Substance **K** Other Diagnostic Substance **N** Analgesics, Hypnotics, Sedatives **T** Destructive Agent	**Z** No Qualifier
W Lymphatics	**3** Percutaneous	**G** Other Therapeutic Substance	**C** Other Substance
Y Pericardial Cavity	**3** Percutaneous	**0** Antineoplastic	**4** Liquid Brachytherapy Radioisotope **5** Other Antineoplastic **M** Monoclonal Antibody
Y Pericardial Cavity	**3** Percutaneous	**2** Anti-infective	**8** Oxazolidinones **9** Other Anti-infective
Y Pericardial Cavity	**3** Percutaneous	**3** Anti-inflammatory **6** Nutritional Substance **7** Electrolytic and Water Balance Substance **B** Anesthetic Agent **H** Radioactive Substance **K** Other Diagnostic Substance **N** Analgesics, Hypnotics, Sedatives **T** Destructive Agent	**Z** No Qualifier
Y Pericardial Cavity	**3** Percutaneous	**G** Other Therapeutic Substance	**C** Other Substance
Y Pericardial Cavity	**3** Percutaneous	**S** Gas	**F** Other Gas
Y Pericardial Cavity	**4** Percutaneous Endoscopic	**G** Other Therapeutic Substance	**C** Other Substance
Y Pericardial Cavity	**7** Via Natural or Artificial Opening	**0** Antineoplastic	**4** Liquid Brachytherapy Radioisotope **5** Other Antineoplastic **M** Monoclonal Antibody
Y Pericardial Cavity	**7** Via Natural or Artificial Opening	**S** Gas	**F** Other Gas

Section 3 **Administration**
Body System E **Physiological Systems and Anatomical Regions**
Operation 1 **Irrigation:** Putting in or on a cleansing substance

Body System / Region (4th)	Approach (5th)	Substance (6th)	Qualifier (7th)
0 Skin and Mucous Membranes **C** Eye	**3** Percutaneous **X** External	**8** Irrigating Substance	**X** Diagnostic **Z** No Qualifier
9 Nose **B** Ear **F** Respiratory Tract **G** Upper GI **H** Lower GI **J** Biliary and Pancreatic Tract **K** Genitourinary Tract **N** Male Reproductive **P** Female Reproductive	**3** Percutaneous **7** Via Natural or Artificial Opening **8** Via Natural or Artificial Opening Endoscopic	**8** Irrigating Substance	**X** Diagnostic **Z** No Qualifier

Continued →

Section 3 Administration **3E1 Continued**
Body System E Physiological Systems and Anatomical Regions
Operation 1 Irrigation: Putting in or on a cleansing substance

Body System / Region (4th)	Approach (5th)	Substance (6th)	Qualifier (7th)
L Pleural Cavity Q Cranial Cavity and Brain R Spinal Canal S Epidural Space Y Pericardial Cavity	3 Percutaneous	8 Irrigating Substance	X Diagnostic Z No Qualifier
M Peritoneal Cavity	3 Percutaneous	8 Irrigating Substance	X Diagnostic Z No Qualifier
M Peritoneal Cavity	3 Percutaneous	9 Dialysate	Z No Qualifier
M Peritoneal Cavity	4 Percutaneous Endoscopic	8 Irrigating Substance	X Diagnostic Z No Qualifier
U Joints	3 Percutaneous 4 Percutaneous Endoscopic	8 Irrigating Substance	X Diagnostic Z No Qualifier

AHA Coding Clinic

3E013GC Introduction of Other Therapeutic Substance into Subcutaneous Tissue, Percutaneous Approach—AHA CC: 2Q, 2014, 10
3E0234Z Introduction of Serum, Toxoid and Vaccine into Muscle, Percutaneous Approach—AHA CC: 4Q, 2014, 16
3E03317 Introduction of Other Thrombolytic into Peripheral Vein, Percutaneous Approach—AHA CC: 4Q, 2013, 124; 4Q, 2020, 49-50
3E033VJ Introduction of Other Hormone into Peripheral Vein, Percutaneous Approach—AHA CC: 4Q, 2014, 17-18
3E04317 Introduction of Other Thrombolytic into Central Vein, Percutaneous Approach—AHA CC: 4Q, 2020, 49-50
3E05305 Introduction of Other Antineoplastic into Peripheral Artery, Percutaneous Approach—AHA CC: 1Q, 2015, 38
3E05317 Introduction of Other Thrombolytic into Peripheral Artery, Percutaneous Approach—AHA CC: 4Q, 2020, 49-50
3E06305 Introduction of Other Antineoplastic into Central Artery, Percutaneous Approach—AHA CC: 3Q, 2014 26-27
3E06317 Introduction of Other Thrombolytic into Central Artery, Percutaneous Approach—AHA CC: 4Q, 2014, 19-20; 4Q, 2020, 49-50
3E073GC Introduction of Other Therapeutic Substance into Coronary Artery, Percutaneous Approach—AHA CC: 3Q, 2018. 7-8
3E0G76Z Introduction of Nutritional Substance into Upper GI, Via Natural or Artificial Opening—AHA CC: 2Q, 2015, 29
3E0G8GC Introduction of Other Therapeutic Substance into Upper GI, via Natural or Artificial Opening Endoscopic—AHA CC: 3Q, 2015, 24-25
3E0G8TZ Introduction of Destructive Agent into Upper GI, Via Natural or Artificial Opening Endoscopic—AHA CC: 1Q, 2013, 27
3E0H3GC Introduction of Other Therapeutic Substance into Lower GI, Percutaneous Approach—AHA CC: 1Q, 2017, 37
3E0L3GC Introduction of Other Therapeutic Substance into Pleural Cavity, Percutaneous Approach—AHA CC: 2Q, 2015, 31; 2Q, 2017, 14-15
3E0M30Y Introduction of Hyperthermic Antineoplastic into Peritoneal Cavity, Percutaneous Approach—AHA CC: 4Q, 2019, 37
3E0M3GC Introduction of Other Therapeutic Substance into Peritoneal Cavity, Percutaneous Approach—AHA CC: 4Q, 2014, 38
3E0P7GC Introduction of Other Therapeutic Substance into Female Reproductive, Via Natural or Artificial Opening—AHA CC: 2Q, 2014, 8-9
3E0Q005 Introduction of Other Antineoplastic into Cranial Cavity and Brain, Open Approach—AHA CC: 4Q, 2016, 114
3E0Q305 Introduction of Other Antineoplastic into Cranial Cavity and Brain, Percutaneous Approach—AHA CC: 4Q, 2014, 34-35
3E0R305 Introduction of Other Antineoplastic into Spinal Canal, Percutaneous Approach—AHA CC: 1Q, 2015, 31
3E0U0GB Introduction of Recombinant Bone Morphogenetic Protein into Joints, Open Approach—AHA CC: 1Q, 2018, 8
3E0V0GB Introduction of Recombinant Bone Morphogenetic Protein into Bones, Open Approach—AHA CC: 3Q, 2016, 29-30

Measurement and Monitoring Section (4A0–4B0)

Within each section of ICD-10-PCS the characters have different meanings. The seven character meanings for the Measurement and Monitoring section are illustrated here through the procedure example of *External electrocardiogram (EKG), single reading*.

Section	Body System	Root Operation	Body System	Approach	Function / Device	Qualifier
Measurement and Monitoring	Physiological Systems	Measurement	Cardiac	External	Electrical Activity	None
4	A	0	2	X	4	Z

Section (Character 1)

All Measurement and Monitoring procedure codes have a first character value of 4.

Body System (Character 2)

The alphanumeric character for the body system is placed in the second position. There are two character values applicable for the Measurement and Monitoring section. The character value of A is reported for physiological systems. The character value B is reported for physiological devices.

Root Operations (Character 3)

The alphanumeric character value for root operations is placed in the third position. Listed here are the root operations applicable to the Measurement and Monitoring section with their associated meaning.

Character Value	Root Operation	Root Operation Definition
0	Measurement	Determining the level of a physiological or physical function at a point in time
1	Monitoring	Determining the level of a physiological or physical function repetitively over a period of time

Body System/Region (Character 4)

For each body system the applicable body part character values will be available for procedure code construction. An example of a body region for this section is Respiratory.

Approach (Character 5)

The approach is the technique used to reach the procedure site. The following are the approach character values for the Measurement and Monitoring section with the associated definitions.

Character Value	Approach	Approach Definition
0	Open	Cutting through the skin or mucous membrane and any other body layers necessary to expose the site of the procedure
3	Percutaneous	Entry, by puncture or minor incision, of instrumentation through the skin or mucous membrane and any other body layers necessary to reach the site of the procedure
4	Percutaneous Endoscopic	Entry, by puncture or minor incision, of instrumentation through the skin or mucous membrane and any other body layers necessary to reach and visualize the site of the procedure
7	Via Natural or Artificial Opening	Entry of instrumentation through a natural or artificial external opening to reach the site of the procedure
8	Via Natural or Artificial Opening Endoscopic	Entry of instrumentation through a natural or artificial external opening to reach and visualize the site of the procedure
X	External	Procedures performed directly on the skin or mucous membrane and procedures performed indirectly by the application of external force through the skin or mucous membrane

Function/Device (Character 6)

In the Measurement and Monitoring section a function or device is always utilized. The function or device is reported in the sixth character position by the type of function monitored or measured or by the device utilized. The following is a sample list of the functions and devices included in this section:

- Conductivity
- Flow
- Metabolism
- Pressure
- Sound

Qualifier (Character 7)

The qualifier represents an additional attribute for the procedure when applicable. There are several qualifiers included in the Measurement and Monitoring section. For example, measurement procedures in this section include several qualifiers including stress that is reported with the character value of 4. If there is no qualifier for a procedure, the placeholder Z is the character valve that should be reported.

Measurement and Monitoring Section Tables

Measurement and Monitoring Tables 4A0–4B0

Section 4 **Measurement and Monitoring**
Body System A **Physiological Systems**
Operation 0 **Measurement:** Determining the level of a physiological or physical function at a point in time

Body System (4th)	Approach (5th)	Function / Device (6th)	Qualifier (7th)
0 Central Nervous	**0** Open	**2** Conductivity **4** Electrical Activity **B** Pressure	**Z** No Qualifier
0 Central Nervous	**3** Percutaneous **7** Via Natural or Artificial Opening **8** Via Natural or Artificial Opening Endoscopic	**4** Electrical Activity	**Z** No Qualifier
0 Central Nervous	**3** Percutaneous **7** Via Natural or Artificial Opening **8** Via Natural or Artificial Opening Endoscopic	**B** Pressure **K** Temperature **R** Saturation	**D** Intracranial
0 Central Nervous	**X** External	**2** Conductivity **4** Electrical Activity	**Z** No Qualifier
1 Peripheral Nervous	**0** Open **3** Percutaneous **7** Via Natural or Artificial Opening **8** Via Natural or Artificial Opening Endoscopic **X** External	**2** Conductivity	**9** Sensory **B** Motor
1 Peripheral Nervous	**0** Open **3** Percutaneous **7** Via Natural or Artificial Opening **8** Via Natural or Artificial Opening Endoscopic **X** External	**4** Electrical Activity	**Z** No Qualifier
2 Cardiac	**0** Open **3** Percutaneous **7** Via Natural or Artificial Opening **8** Via Natural or Artificial Opening Endoscopic	**4** Electrical Activity **9** Output **C** Rate **F** Rhythm **H** Sound **P** Action Currents	**Z** No Qualifier
2 Cardiac	**0** Open **3** Percutaneous **7** Via Natural or Artificial Opening **8** Via Natural or Artificial Opening Endoscopic	**N** Sampling and Pressure	**6** Right Heart **7** Left Heart **8** Bilateral
2 Cardiac	**X** External	**4** Electrical Activity	**A** Guidance **Z** No Qualifier

Continued →

Section 4 **Measurement and Monitoring**
Body System A **Physiological Systems**
Operation 0 **Measurement:** Determining the level of a physiological or physical function at a point in time

Body System (4th)	Approach (5th)	Function / Device (6th)	Qualifier (7th)
2 Cardiac	**X** External	**9** Output **C** Rate **F** Rhythm **H** Sound **P** Action Currents	**Z** No Qualifier
2 Cardiac	**X** External	**M** Total Activity	**4** Stress
3 Arterial	**0** Open **3** Percutaneous	**5** Flow **J** Pulse	**1** Peripheral **3** Pulmonary **C** Coronary
3 Arterial	**0** Open **3** Percutaneous	**B** Pressure	**1** Peripheral **3** Pulmonary **C** Coronary **F** Other Thoracic
3 Arterial	**0** Open **3** Percutaneous	**H** Sound **R** Saturation	**1** Peripheral
3 Arterial	**X** External	**5** Flow	**1** Peripheral **D** Intracranial
3 Arterial	**X** External	**B** Pressure **H** Sound **J** Pulse **R** Saturation	**1** Peripheral
4 Venous	**0** Open **3** Percutaneous	**5** Flow **B** Pressure **J** Pulse	**0** Central **1** Peripheral **2** Portal **3** Pulmonary
4 Venous	**0** Open **3** Percutaneous	**R** Saturation	**1** Peripheral
4 Venous	**4** Percutaneous Endoscopic	**B** Pressure	**2** Portal
4 Venous	**X** External	**5** Flow **B** Pressure **J** Pulse **R** Saturation	**1** Peripheral
5 Circulatory	**X** External	**L** Volume	**Z** No Qualifier
6 Lymphatic	**0** Open **3** Percutaneous **7** Via Natural or Artificial Opening **8** Via Natural or Artificial Opening Endoscopic	**5** Flow **B** Pressure	**Z** No Qualifier
7 Visual	**X** External	**0** Acuity **7** Mobility **B** Pressure	**Z** No Qualifier
8 Olfactory	**X** External	**0** Acuity	**Z** No Qualifier
9 Respiratory	**7** Via Natural or Artificial Opening **8** Via Natural or Artificial Opening Endoscopic **X** External	**1** Capacity **5** Flow **C** Rate **D** Resistance **L** Volume **M** Total Activity	**Z** No Qualifier
B Gastrointestinal	**7** Via Natural or Artificial Opening **8** Via Natural or Artificial Opening Endoscopic	**8** Motility **B** Pressure **G** Secretion	**Z** No Qualifier

Continued →

Section 4 **Measurement and Monitoring**
Body System A **Physiological Systems**
Operation 0 **Measurement:** Determining the level of a physiological or physical function at a point in time

Body System (4th)	Approach (5th)	Function / Device (6th)	Qualifier (7th)
C Biliary	**3** Percutaneous **4** Percutaneous Endoscopic **7** Via Natural or Artificial Opening **8** Via Natural or Artificial Opening Endoscopic	**5** Flow **B** Pressure	**Z** No Qualifier
D Urinary	**7** Via Natural or Artificial Opening **8** Via Natural or Artificial Opening Endoscopic	**3** Contractility **5** Flow **B** Pressure **D** Resistance **L** Volume	**Z** No Qualifier
F Musculoskeletal	**3** Percutaneous	**3** Contractility	**Z** No Qualifier
F Musculoskeletal	**3** Percutaneous	**B** Pressure	**E** Compartment
F Musculoskeletal	**X** External	**3** Contractility	**Z** No Qualifier
H Products of Conception, Cardiac	**7** Via Natural or Artificial Opening **8** Via Natural or Artificial Opening Endoscopic **X** External	**4** Electrical Activity **C** Rate **F** Rhythm **H** Sound	**Z** No Qualifier
J Products of Conception, Nervous	**7** Via Natural or Artificial Opening **8** Via Natural or Artificial Opening Endoscopic **X** External	**2** Conductivity **4** Electrical Activity **B** Pressure	**Z** No Qualifier
Z None	**7** Via Natural or Artificial Opening	**6** Metabolism **K** Temperature	**Z** No Qualifier
Z None	**X** External	**6** Metabolism **K** Temperature **Q** Sleep	**Z** No Qualifier

Section 4 **Measurement and Monitoring**
Body System A **Physiological Systems**
Operation 1 **Monitoring:** Determining the level of a physiological or physical function repetitively over a period of time

Body System (4th)	Approach (5th)	Function / Device (6th)	Qualifier (7th)
0 Central Nervous	**0** Open	**2** Conductivity **B** Pressure	**Z** No Qualifier
0 Central Nervous	**0** Open	**4** Electrical Activity	**G** Intraoperative **Z** No Qualifier
0 Central Nervous	**3** Percutaneous **7** Via Natural or Artificial Opening **8** Via Natural or Artificial Opening Endoscopic	**4** Electrical Activity	**G** Intraoperative **Z** No Qualifier
0 Central Nervous	**3** Percutaneous **7** Via Natural or Artificial Opening **8** Via Natural or Artificial Opening Endoscopic	**B** Pressure **K** Temperature **R** Saturation	**D** Intracranial
0 Central Nervous	**X** External	**2** Conductivity	**Z** No Qualifier
0 Central Nervous	**X** External	**4** Electrical Activity	**G** Intraoperative **Z** No Qualifier
1 Peripheral Nervous	**0** Open **3** Percutaneous **7** Via Natural or Artificial Opening **8** Via Natural or Artificial Opening Endoscopic **X** External	**2** Conductivity	**9** Sensory **B** Motor

Continued →

Body System (4th)	Approach (5th)	Function / Device (6th)	Qualifier (7th)
1 Peripheral Nervous	0 Open 3 Percutaneous 7 Via Natural or Artificial Opening 8 Via Natural or Artificial Opening Endoscopic X External	4 Electrical Activity	G Intraoperative Z No Qualifier
2 Cardiac	0 Open 3 Percutaneous 7 Via Natural or Artificial Opening 8 Via Natural or Artificial Opening Endoscopic	4 Electrical Activity 9 Output C Rate F Rhythm H Sound	Z No Qualifier
2 Cardiac	X External	4 Electrical Activity	5 Ambulatory Z No Qualifier
2 Cardiac	X External	9 Output C Rate F Rhythm H Sound	Z No Qualifier
2 Cardiac	X External	M Total Activity	4 Stress
2 Cardiac	X External	S Vascular Perfusion	H Indocyanine Green Dye
3 Arterial	0 Open 3 Percutaneous	5 Flow B Pressure J Pulse	1 Peripheral 3 Pulmonary C Coronary
3 Arterial	0 Open 3 Percutaneous	H Sound R Saturation	1 Peripheral
3 Arterial	X External	5 Flow B Pressure H Sound J Pulse R Saturation	1 Peripheral
4 Venous	0 Open 3 Percutaneous	5 Flow B Pressure J Pulse	0 Central 1 Peripheral 2 Portal 3 Pulmonary
4 Venous	0 Open 3 Percutaneous	R Saturation	0 Central 2 Portal 3 Pulmonary
4 Venous	X External	5 Flow B Pressure J Pulse	1 Peripheral
6 Lymphatic	0 Open 3 Percutaneous 7 Via Natural or Artificial Opening 8 Via Natural or Artificial Opening Endoscopic	5 Flow	H Indocyanine Green Dye Z No Qualifier
6 Lymphatic	0 Open 3 Percutaneous 7 Via Natural or Artificial Opening 8 Via Natural or Artificial Opening Endoscopic	B Pressure	Z No Qualifier
9 Respiratory	7 Via Natural or Artificial Opening X External	1 Capacity 5 Flow C Rate D Resistance L Volume	Z No Qualifier
B Gastrointestinal	7 Via Natural or Artificial Opening 8 Via Natural or Artificial Opening Endoscopic	8 Motility B Pressure G Secretion	Z No Qualifier

Continued →

Section	4	Measurement and Monitoring
Body System	A	Physiological Systems
Operation	1	**Monitoring:** Determining the level of a physiological or physical function repetitively over a period of time

Body System (4th)	Approach (5th)	Function / Device (6th)	Qualifier (7th)
B Gastrointestinal	**X** External	**S** Vascular Perfusion	**H** Indocyanine Green Dye
D Urinary	**7** Via Natural or Artificial Opening **8** Via Natural or Artificial Opening Endoscopic	**3** Contractility **5** Flow **B** Pressure **D** Resistance **L** Volume	**Z** No Qualifier
G Skin and Breast	**X** External	**S** Vascular Perfusion	**H** Indocyanine Green Dye
H Products of Conception, Cardiac	**7** Via Natural or Artificial Opening **8** Via Natural or Artificial Opening Endoscopic **X** External	**4** Electrical Activity **C** Rate **F** Rhythm **H** Sound	**Z** No Qualifier
J Products of Conception, Nervous	**7** Via Natural or Artificial Opening **8** Via Natural or Artificial Opening Endoscopic **X** External	**2** Conductivity **4** Electrical Activity **B** Pressure	**Z** No Qualifier
Z None	**7** Via Natural or Artificial Opening	**K** Temperature	**Z** No Qualifier
Z None	**X** External	**K** Temperature **Q** Sleep	**Z** No Qualifier

Section	4	Measurement and Monitoring
Body System	B	Physiological Devices
Operation	0	**Measurement:** Determining the level of a physiological or physical function at a point in time

Body System (4th)	Approach (5th)	Function / Device (6th)	Qualifier (7th)
0 Central Nervous	**X** External	**V** Stimulator	**Z** No Qualifier
0 Central Nervous	**X** External	**W** Cerebrospinal Fluid Shunt	**0** Wireless Sensor
1 Peripheral Nervous **F** Musculoskeletal	**X** External	**V** Stimulator	**Z** No Qualifier
2 Cardiac	**X** External	**S** Pacemaker **T** Defibrillator	**Z** No Qualifier
9 Respiratory	**X** External	**S** Pacemaker	**Z** No Qualifier

AHA Coding Clinic

4A023N6 Measurement of Cardiac Sampling and Pressure, Right Heart, Percutaneous Approach—AHA CC: 3Q, 2019, 32

4A023N8 Measurement of Cardiac Sampling and Pressure, Bilateral, Percutaneous Approach—AHA CC: 1Q, 2018, 12-13

4A02X4Z Measurement of Cardiac Electrical Activity, External Approach—AHA CC: 3Q, 2015, 29

4A033BC Measurement of Arterial Pressure, Coronary, Percutaneous Approach—AHA CC: 3Q, 2016, 37

4A0F3BE Measurement of Musculoskeletal Pressure, Compartment, Percutaneous Approach—AHA CC: 4Q, 2020, 63-64

4A103BD Monitoring of Intracranial Pressure, Percutaneous Approach—AHA CC: 2Q, 2016, 29

4A1134G Monitoring of Peripheral Nervous Electrical Activity, Intraoperative, Percutaneous Approach—AHA CC: 4Q, 2014, 28-29

4A11X4G Monitoring of Peripheral Nervous Electrical Activity, Intraoperative, External Approach—AHA CC: 1Q, 2015, 26; 2Q, 2015, 14

4A1239Z Monitoring of Cardiac Output, Percutaneous Approach—AHA CC: 3Q, 2015, 35

4A133B1 Monitoring of Arterial Pressure, Peripheral, Percutaneous Approach, for Continuous Monitoring of Pressure—AHA CC: 2Q, 2016, 33

4A133B3 Monitoring of Arterial Pressure, Pulmonary, Percutaneous Approach—AHA CC: 3Q, 2015, 35

4A133J1 Monitoring of Arterial Pulse, Peripheral, Percutaneous Approach, for Continuous Monitoring of Pulse—AHA CC: 2Q, 2016, 33

Extracorporeal or Systemic Assistance and Performance Section (5A0–5A2)

Within each section of ICD-10-PCS the characters have different meanings. The seven character meanings for the Extracorporeal or Systemic Assistance and Performance section are illustrated here through the procedure example of *Hyperbaric oxygenation of wound.*

Section	Body System	Root Operation	Body System	Duration	Function	Qualifier
Extracorporeal or Systemic Assistance and Performance	Physiological Systems	Assistance	Circulatory	Intermittent	Oxygenation	Hyperbaric
5	A	0	5	1	2	1

Section (Character 1)

All Extracorporeal or Systemic Assistance and Performance procedure codes have a first character value of 5.

Body System (Character 2)

The alphanumeric character for the body system is placed in the second position. There is one character value applicable for the Extracorporeal or Systemic Assistance and Performance section. The character value of A is reported for physiological systems.

Root Operations (Character 3)

The alphanumeric character value for root operations is placed in the third position. Listed here are the root operations applicable to the Extracorporeal or Systemic Assistance and Performance section with their associated meaning.

Character Value	Root Operation	Root Operation Definition
0	Assistance	Taking over a portion of a physiological function by extracorporeal means
1	Performance	Completely taking over a physiological function by extracorporeal means
2	Restoration	Returning, or attempting to return, a physiological function to its original state by extracorporeal means

Body System (Character 4)

For each body system, the applicable body part character values will be available for procedure code construction. An example of a body region for this section is respiratory.

Duration (Character 5)

The duration represents the length of time or frequency for which the assistance or performance is utilized. Some examples of duration are Intermittent, Continuous, or Less than 24 consecutive hours.

Function (Character 6)

In the Extracorporeal or Systemic Assistance and Performance section a function is always reported. The function is reported in the sixth character position. The following is a sample list of the functions utilized in this section:

- Output
- Oxygenation
- Pacing
- Ventilation

Qualifier (Character 7)

The qualifier represents an additional attribute for the procedure when applicable. There are several qualifiers included in the Extracorporeal or Systemic Assistance and Performance section. For example, assistance procedures in this section include several qualifiers including Balloon Pump, which is reported with the character value of 0. If there is no qualifier for a procedure, the placeholder Z is the character valve that should be reported.

Extracorporeal or Systemic Assistance and Performance Section Tables

Extracorporeal or Systemic Assistance and Performance Tables 5A0–5A2

Section 5 **Extracorporeal or Systemic Assistance and Performance**
Body System A **Physiological Systems**
Operation 0 **Assistance:** Taking over a portion of a physiological function by extracorporeal means

Body System (4th)	Duration (5th)	Function (6th)	Qualifier (7th)
2 Cardiac	1 Intermittent 2 Continuous	1 Output	0 Balloon Pump 5 Pulsatile Compression 6 Other Pump D Impeller Pump
5 Circulatory	1 Intermittent 2 Continuous	2 Oxygenation	1 Hyperbaric C Supersaturated
9 Respiratory	2 Continuous	0 Filtration	Z No Qualifier
9 Respiratory	3 Less than 24 Consecutive Hours 4 24-96 Consecutive Hours 5 Greater than 96 Consecutive Hours	5 Ventilation	7 Continuous Positive Airway Pressure 8 Intermittent Positive Airway Pressure 9 Continuous Negative Airway Pressure A High Nasal Flow/Velocity B Intermittent Negative Airway Pressure Z No Qualifier

Section 5 **Extracorporeal or Systemic Assistance and Performance**
Body System A **Physiological Systems**
Operation 1 **Performance:** Completely taking over a physiological function by extracorporeal means

Body System (4th)	Duration (5th)	Function (6th)	Qualifier (7th)
2 Cardiac	0 Single	1 Output	2 Manual
2 Cardiac	1 Intermittent	3 Pacing	Z No Qualifier
2 Cardiac	2 Continuous	1 Output	J Automated Z No Qualifier
2 Cardiac	2 Continuous	3 Pacing	Z No Qualifier
5 Circulatory	2 Continuous A Intraoperative	2 Oxygenation	F Membrane, Central G Membrane, Peripheral Veno-arterial H Membrane, Peripheral Veno-venous
9 Respiratory	0 Single	5 Ventilation	4 Nonmechanical
9 Respiratory	3 Less than 24 Consecutive Hours 4 24-96 Consecutive Hours 5 Greater than 96 Consecutive Hours	5 Ventilation	Z No Qualifier
C Biliary	0 Single 6 Multiple	0 Filtration	Z No Qualifier
D Urinary	7 Intermittent, Less than 6 Hours Per Day 8 Prolonged Intermittent, 6-18 Hours Per Day 9 Continuous, Greater than 18 Hours Per Day	0 Filtration	Z No Qualifier

Section 5 **Extracorporeal or Systemic Assistance and Performance**
Body System A **Physiological Systems**
Operation 2 **Restoration:** Returning, or attempting to return, a physiological function to its original state by extracorporeal means.

Body System (4th)	Duration (5th)	Function (6th)	Qualifier (7th)
2 Cardiac	0 Single	4 Rhythm	Z No Qualifier

AHA Coding Clinic

5A02210 Assistance with Cardiac Output using Balloon Pump, Continuous—AHA CC: 3Q, 2013, 18-19; 2Q, 2018, 4-5; 2Q, 2021, 12

5A0221D Assistance with Cardiac Output using Impeller Pump, Continuous—AHA CC: 3Q, 2014, 19; 4Q, 2016, 138-139; 1Q, 2017, 11-12; 4Q, 2017, 43-45

5A09357 Assistance with Respiratory Ventilation, <24 Hrs, CPAP—AHA CC: 4Q, 2014, 9-10; 1Q, 2020, 10-11

5A09457 Assistance with Respiratory Ventilation, 24-96 Hrs, CPAP—AHA CC: 4Q, 2014, 9-10

5A09557 Assistance with Respiratory Ventilation, >96 Hrs, CPAP—AHA CC: 4Q, 2014, 9-10

5A1221Z Performance of Cardiac Output, Continuous—AHA CC: 3Q, 2013, 18-19; 1Q, 2014, 10-11; 3Q, 2014, 16-17, 20-21; 4Q, 2015, 22-25; 1Q, 2016, 27-28; 1Q, 2017, 19-20; 3Q, 2017, 7-8

ECMO, Extracorporeal Oxygenation, Membrane—AHA CC: 3Q, 2019, 19-23; 4Q, 2019, 39-41

5A1223Z Performance of Cardiac Pacing, Continuous—AHA CC: 3Q, 2013, 18-19

5A1522F Extracorporeal Oxygenation, Membrane, Central—AHA CC: 2Q, 2019, 36

5A1522G Extracorporeal Oxygenation, Membrane, Peripheral Veno-arterial—AHA CC: 4Q, 2018, 53-54

5A1522H Extracorporeal Oxygenation, Membrane, Peripheral Veno-venous—AHA CC: 4Q, 2018. 53-54

5A15A2G Extracorporeal Oxygenation, Membrane, Peripheral Veno-arterial, Intraoperative—AHA CC: 4Q, 2019, 39-40

5A1935Z Respiratory Ventilation, Less than 24 Consecutive Hours—AHA CC: 4Q, 2014, 3-15; 1Q, 2018, 13-14

5A1945Z Respiratory Ventilation, 24-96 Consecutive Hours—AHA CC: 4Q, 2014, 3-15

5A1955Z Respiratory Ventilation, Greater than 96 Consecutive Hours—AHA CC: 4Q, 2014, 3-15

5A1C00Z Performance of Biliary Filtration, Single—AHA CC: 1Q, 2016, 28-29

5A1D60Z Performance of Urinary Filtration, Multiple—AHA CC: 1Q, 2016, 29

5A1D70Z Performance of Urinary Filtration, Intermittent, Less than 6 Hours Per Day—AHA CC: 4Q, 2017, 72-73

5A1D80Z Performance of Urinary Filtration, Prolonged Intermittent, 6-18 hours Per Day—AHA CC: 4Q, 2017, 72

5A1D90Z Performance of Urinary Filtration, Continuous, Greater than 18 hours Per Day—AHA CC: 4Q, 2017, 72-73

Extracorporeal or Systemic Therapies Section (6A0–6AB)

Within each section of ICD-10-PCS the characters have different meanings. The seven character meanings for the Extracorporeal or Systemic Therapies section are illustrated here through the procedure example of *Ultraviolet light phototherapy, series treatment.*

Section	Body System	Root Operation	Body System	Duration	Qualifier	Qualifier
Extracorporeal or Systemic Therapies	Physiological Systems	UV Light Therapy	Skin	Multiple	None	None
6	A	8	0	1	Z	Z

Section (Character 1)

All Extracorporeal or Systemic Therapies procedure codes have a first character value of 6.

Body System (Character 2)

The alphanumeric character for the body system is placed in the second position. There is one character value applicable for the Extracorporeal or Systemic Therapies section. The character value of A is reported for physiological systems.

Root Operations (Character 3)

The alphanumeric character value for root operations is placed in the third position. Listed below are the root operations applicable to the Extracorporeal or Systemic Therapies section with their associated meaning.

Character Value	Root Operation	Root Operation Definition
0	Atmospheric Control	Extracorporeal control of atmospheric pressure and composition
1	Decompression	Extracorporeal elimination of undissolved gas from body fluids
2	Electromagnetic Therapy	Extracorporeal treatment by electromagnetic rays
3	Hyperthermia	Extracorporeal raising of body temperature
4	Hypothermia	Extracorporeal lowering of body temperature
5	Pheresis	Extracorporeal separation of blood products
6	Phototherapy	Extracorporeal treatment by light rays
7	Ultrasound Therapy	Extracorporeal treatment by ultrasound
8	Ultraviolet Light Therapy	Extracorporeal treatment by ultraviolet light
9	Shock Wave Therapy	Extracorporeal treatment by shock waves
B	Perfusion	Extracorporeal treatment by diffusion of therapeutic fluid

Body System (Character 4)

For each body system the applicable body part character values will be available for procedure code construction. An example of a body region for this section is Skin.

Duration (Character 5)

The duration represents the number of therapy sessions performed. Single is reported with character value 0; Multiple is reported with character value 1.

Qualifier (Character 6)

Character 6 is the first of two qualifier characters for the Extracorporeal or Systemic Therapies section. The qualifier represents an additional attribute for the procedure when applicable. There are currently no qualifier values for the sixth character position, so the character value of Z is always reported.

Qualifier (Character 7)

Character 7 is the second of two qualifier characters for the Extracorporeal or Systemic Therapies section. The qualifier represents an additional attribute for the procedure when applicable. There are some qualifiers included in the Extracorporeal or Systemic Therapies section. For example, pheresis procedures in this section include several qualifiers including Plasma that is reported with the character value of 3. If there is no qualifier for a procedure, the placeholder Z is the character valve that should be reported.

Extracorporeal or Systemic Therapies Section Tables

Extracorporeal or Systemic Therapies Tables 6A0–6AB

Section 6 **Extracorporeal or Systemic Therapies**
Body System A **Physiological Systems**
Operation 0 **Atmospheric Control:** Extracorporeal control of atmospheric pressure and composition

Body System (4th)	Duration (5th)	Qualifier (6th)	Qualifier (7th)
Z None	**0** Single **1** Multiple	**Z** No Qualifier	**Z** No Qualifier

Section 6 **Extracorporeal or Systemic Therapies**
Body System A **Physiological Systems**
Operation 1 **Decompression:** Extracorporeal elimination of undissolved gas from body fluids

Body System (4th)	Duration (5th)	Qualifier (6th)	Qualifier (7th)
5 Circulatory	**0** Single **1** Multiple	**Z** No Qualifier	**Z** No Qualifier

Section 6 **Extracorporeal or Systemic Therapies**
Body System A **Physiological Systems**
Operation 2 **Electromagnetic Therapy:** Extracorporeal treatment by electromagnetic rays

Body System (4th)	Duration (5th)	Qualifier (6th)	Qualifier (7th)
1 Urinary **2** Central Nervous	**0** Single **1** Multiple	**Z** No Qualifier	**Z** No Qualifier

Section 6 **Extracorporeal or Systemic Therapies**
Body System A **Physiological Systems**
Operation 3 **Hyperthermia:** Extracorporeal raising of body temperature

Body System (4th)	Duration (5th)	Qualifier (6th)	Qualifier (7th)
Z None	**0** Single **1** Multiple	**Z** No Qualifier	**Z** No Qualifier

Section 6 **Extracorporeal or Systemic Therapies**
Body System A **Physiological Systems**
Operation 4 **Hypothermia:** Extracorporeal lowering of body temperature

Body System (4th)	Duration (5th)	Qualifier (6th)	Qualifier (7th)
Z None	**0** Single **1** Multiple	**Z** No Qualifier	**Z** No Qualifier

Section 6 **Extracorporeal or Systemic Therapies**
Body System A **Physiological Systems**
Operation 5 **Pheresis:** Extracorporeal separation of blood products

Body System (4th)	Duration (5th)	Qualifier (6th)	Qualifier (7th)
5 Circulatory	**0** Single **1** Multiple	**Z** No Qualifier	**0** Erythrocytes **1** Leukocytes **2** Platelets **3** Plasma **T** Stem Cells, Cord Blood **V** Stem Cells, Hematopoietic

Section	6	Extracorporeal or Systemic Therapies
Body System	A	Physiological Systems
Operation	6	**Phototherapy:** Extracorporeal treatment by light rays

Body System (4th)	Duration (5th)	Qualifier (6th)	Qualifier (7th)
0 Skin **5** Circulatory	**0** Single **1** Multiple	**Z** No Qualifier	**Z** No Qualifier

Section	6	Extracorporeal or Systemic Therapies
Body System	A	Physiological Systems
Operation	7	**Ultrasound Therapy:** Extracorporeal treatment by ultrasound

Body System (4th)	Duration (5th)	Qualifier (6th)	Qualifier (7th)
5 Circulatory	**0** Single **1** Multiple	**Z** No Qualifier	**4** Head and Neck Vessels **5** Heart **6** Peripheral Vessels **7** Other Vessels **Z** No Qualifier

Section	6	Extracorporeal or Systemic Therapies
Body System	A	Physiological Systems
Operation	8	**Ultraviolet Light Therapy:** Extracorporeal treatment by ultraviolet light

Body System (4th)	Duration (5th)	Qualifier (6th)	Qualifier (7th)
0 Skin	**0** Single **1** Multiple	**Z** No Qualifier	**Z** No Qualifier

Section	6	Extracorporeal or Systemic Therapies
Body System	A	Physiological Systems
Operation	9	**Shock Wave Therapy:** Extracorporeal treatment by shock waves

Body System (4th)	Duration (5th)	Qualifier (6th)	Qualifier (7th)
3 Musculoskeletal	**0** Single **1** Multiple	**Z** No Qualifier	**Z** No Qualifier

Section	6	Extracorporeal or Systemic Therapies
Body System	A	Physiological Systems
Operation	B	**Perfusion:** Extracorporeal treatment by diffusion of therapeutic fluid

Body System (4th)	Duration (5th)	Qualifier (6th)	Qualifier (7th)
5 Circulatory **B** Respiratory System **F** Hepatobiliary System and Pancreas **T** Urinary System	**0** Single	**B** Donor Organ	**Z** No Qualifier

AHA Coding Clinic

6A4Z0ZZ Hypothermia, Single—AHA CC: 2Q, 2019, 17-18

6A750Z7 Ultrasound Therapy of Other Vessels, Single—AHA CC: 4Q, 2014, 19-20

Osteopathic Section (7W0)

Within each section of ICD-10-PCS, the characters have different meanings. The seven character meanings for the Osteopathic section are illustrated below through the procedure example of Indirect osteopathic treatment of sacrum.

Section	Body System	Root Operation	Body Region	Approach	Method	Qualifier
Osteopathic	Anatomical Regions	Treatment	Sacrum	External	Indirect	None
7	W	0	4	X	4	Z

Section (Character 1)

All Osteopathic procedure codes have a first character value of 7.

Body System (Character 2)

The alphanumeric character for the body system is placed in the second position. There is one character value applicable for the Osteopathic section. The character value of W is reported for anatomical regions.

Root Operations (Character 3)

The alphanumeric character value for root operations is placed in the third position. Listed here is the root operation applicable to the Osteopathic section with its associated meaning.

Character Value	Root Operation	Root Operation Definition
0	Treatment	Manual treatment to eliminate or alleviate somatic dysfunction and related disorders

Body Region (Character 4)

For each body region the applicable body part character values will be available for procedure code construction. An example of a body region for this section is Head.

Approach (Character 5)

The approach is the technique used to reach the procedure site. The following are the approach character values for the Osteopathic section with the associated definitions.

Character Value	Approach	Approach Definition
X	External	Procedures performed directly on the skin or mucous membrane and procedures performed indirectly by the application of external force through the skin or mucous membrane

Method (Character 6)

The method identifies the treatment method used to complete the osteopathic procedure. The available methods are:

- Articulatory-Raising
- Fascial Release
- General Mobilization
- High Velocity-Low Amplitude
- Indirect
- Low Velocity-High Amplitude
- Lymphatic Pump
- Muscle Energy-Isometric
- Muscle Energy-Isotonic
- Other

Qualifier (Character 7)

The qualifier represents an additional attribute for the procedure when applicable. Currently, there are no qualifiers in the Osteopathic section; therefore, the placeholder character value of Z should be reported.

Osteopathic Section Table

Osteopathic Table 7W0

Section	7	**Osteopathic**
Body System	W	**Anatomical Regions**
Operation	0	**Treatment:** Manual treatment to eliminate or alleviate somatic dysfunction and related disorders

Body Region (4th)	Approach (5th)	Method (6th)	Qualifier (7th)
0 Head **1** Cervical **2** Thoracic **3** Lumbar **4** Sacrum **5** Pelvis **6** Lower Extremities **7** Upper Extremities **8** Rib Cage **9** Abdomen	**X** External	**0** Articulatory-Raising **1** Fascial Release **2** General Mobilization **3** High Velocity-Low Amplitude **4** Indirect **5** Low Velocity-High Amplitude **6** Lymphatic Pump **7** Muscle Energy-Isometric **8** Muscle Energy-Isotonic **9** Other Method	**Z** None

AHA Coding Clinic

No references have been issued for the Osteopathic Section.

Other Procedures Section (8C0–8E0)

Within each section of ICD-10-PCS the characters have different meanings. The seven character meanings for the Other Procedures section are illustrated here through the procedure example of Yoga therapy.

Section	Body System	Root Operation	Body Region	Approach	Method	Qualifier
Other Procedures	Physiological Systems and Anatomical Regions	Other Procedures	None	External	Other Method	Yoga Therapy
8	E	0	Z	X	Y	4

Section (Character 1)

All Other Procedures codes have a first character value of 8.

Body System (Character 2)

The alphanumeric character for the body system is placed in the second position. There are two character values applicable for the Other Procedures section. The character value of C is reported for indwelling device. The character value of E is reported for physiological system and anatomical regions.

Root Operations (Character 3)

The alphanumeric character value for root operations is placed in the third position. Listed here is the root operation applicable to the Other Procedures section with its associated meaning.

Character Value	Root Operation	Root Operation Definition
0	Other Procedures	Methodologies which attempt to remediate or cure a disorder or disease

Body Region (Character 4)

For each body region the applicable body part character values will be available for procedure code construction. An example of a body region for this section is Lower Extremity.

Approach (Character 5)

The approach is the technique used to reach the procedure site. The following are the approach character values for the Other Procedures section with the associated definitions.

Character Value	Approach	Approach Definition
0	Open	Cutting through the skin or mucous membrane and any other body layers necessary to expose the site of the procedure
3	Percutaneous	Entry, by puncture or minor incision, of instrumentation through the skin or mucous membrane and any other body layers necessary to reach the site of the procedure
4	Percutaneous Endoscopic	Entry, by puncture or minor incision, of instrumentation through the skin or mucous membrane and any other body layers necessary to reach and visualize the site of the procedure
7	Via Natural or Artificial Opening	Entry of instrumentation through a natural or artificial external opening to reach the site of the procedure
8	Via Natural or Artificial Opening Endoscopic	Entry of instrumentation through a natural or artificial external opening to reach and visualize the site of the procedure
X	External	Procedures performed directly on the skin or mucous membrane and procedures performed indirectly by the application of external force through the skin or mucous membrane

Method (Character 6)

The method identifies the treatment method used to complete the other procedure. The available methods are:

- Acupuncture
- Collection
- Computer Assisted Procedure
- Near Infrared Spectroscopy
- Robotic Assisted procedure
- Therapeutic Massage
- Other

Qualifier (Character 7)

The qualifier represents an additional attribute for the procedure when applicable. In the preceding example of Yoga therapy, the qualifier of 4 was used to report that the other procedure was Yoga therapy. If there is no qualifier for a procedure, the placeholder Z is the character valve that should be reported.

Other Procedures Section Tables

Other Procedures Tables 8C0–8E0

Section 8 **Other Procedures**
Body System C **Indwelling Device**
Operation 0 **Other Procedures:** Methodologies which attempt to remediate or cure a disorder or disease

Body Region (4th)	Approach (5th)	Method (6th)	Qualifier (7th)
1 Nervous System	**X** External	**6** Collection	**J** Cerebrospinal Fluid **L** Other Fluid
2 Circulatory System	**X** External	**6** Collection	**K** Blood **L** Other Fluid

Section 8 **Other Procedures**
Body System E **Physiological Systems and Anatomical Regions**
Operation 0 **Other Procedures:** Methodologies which attempt to remediate or cure a disorder or disease

Body Region (4th)	Approach (5th)	Method (6th)	Qualifier (7th)
1 Nervous System **U** Female Reproductive System	**X** External	**Y** Other Method	**7** Examination
2 Circulatory System	**3** Percutaneous **X** External	**D** Near Infrared Spectroscopy	**Z** No Qualifier
9 Head and Neck Region	**0** Open	**C** Robotic Assisted Procedure	**Z** No Qualifier
9 Head and Neck Region	**0** Open	**E** Fluorescence Guided Procedure	**M** Aminolevulinic Acid **Z** No Qualifier
9 Head and Neck Region	**3** Percutaneous **4** Percutaneous Endoscopic **7** Via Natural or Artificial Opening **8** Via Natural or Artificial Opening Endoscopic	**C** Robotic Assisted Procedure **E** Fluorescence Guided Procedure	**Z** No Qualifier
9 Head and Neck Region	**X** External	**B** Computer Assisted Procedure	**F** With Fluoroscopy **G** With Computerized Tomography **H** With Magnetic Resonance Imaging **Z** No Qualifier
9 Head and Neck Region	**X** External	**C** Robotic Assisted Procedure	**Z** No Qualifier
9 Head and Neck Region	**X** External	**Y** Other Method	**8** Suture Removal

Continued →

Section 8 **Other Procedures**
Body System E **Physiological Systems and Anatomical Regions**
Operation 0 **Other Procedures:** Methodologies which attempt to remediate or cure a disorder or disease

Body Region (4th)	Approach (5th)	Method (6th)	Qualifier (7th)
H Integumentary System and Breast	**3** Percutaneous	**0** Acupuncture	**0** Anesthesia **Z** No Qualifier
H Integumentary System and Breast	**X** External	**6** Collection	**2** Breast Milk
H Integumentary System and Breast	**X** External	**Y** Other Method	**9** Piercing
K Musculoskeletal System	**X** External	**1** Therapeutic Massage	**Z** No Qualifier
K Musculoskeletal System	**X** External	**Y** Other Method	**7** Examination
V Male Reproductive System	**X** External	**1** Therapeutic Massage	**C** Prostate **D** Rectum
V Male Reproductive System	**X** External	**6** Collection	**3** Sperm
W Trunk Region	**0** Open **3** Percutaneous **4** Percutaneous Endoscopic **7** Via Natural or Artificial Opening **8** Via Natural or Artificial Opening Endoscopic	**C** Robotic Assisted Procedure **E** Fluorescence Guided Procedure	**Z** No Qualifier
W Trunk Region	**X** External	**B** Computer Assisted Procedure	**F** With Fluoroscopy **G** With Computerized Tomography **H** With Magnetic Resonance Imaging **Z** No Qualifier
W Trunk Region	**X** External	**C** Robotic Assisted Procedure	**Z** No Qualifier
W Trunk Region	**X** External	**Y** Other Method	**8** Suture Removal
X Upper Extremity **Y** Lower Extremity	**0** Open **3** Percutaneous **4** Percutaneous Endoscopic	**C** Robotic Assisted Procedure **E** Fluorescence Guided Procedure	**Z** No Qualifier
X Upper Extremity **Y** Lower Extremity	**X** External	**B** Computer Assisted Procedure	**F** With Fluoroscopy **G** With Computerized Tomography **H** With Magnetic Resonance Imaging **Z** No Qualifier
X Upper Extremity **Y** Lower Extremity	**X** External	**C** Robotic Assisted Procedure	**Z** No Qualifier
X Upper Extremity **Y** Lower Extremity	**X** External	**Y** Other Method	**8** Suture Removal
Z None	**X** External	**Y** Other Method	**1** In Vitro Fertilization **4** Yoga Therapy **5** Meditation **6** Isolation

AHA Coding Clinic

8E09XBZ Computer Assisted Procedure of Head and Neck Region—AHA CC: 2Q, 2021, 19-20

8E0W4CZ Robotic Assisted Procedure of Trunk Region, Percutaneous Endoscopic Approach—AHA CC: 4Q, 2014, 33-34; 1Q, 2015, 33-34; 1Q, 2019, 30-31; 4Q, 2020, 53-54

Chiropractic Section (9WB)

Within each section of ICD-10-PCS the characters have different meanings. The seven character meanings for the Chiropractic section are illustrated here through the procedure example of Chiropractic treatment of cervical spine, short lever specific contact.

Section	Body System	Root Operation	Body Region	Approach	Method	Qualifier
Chiropractic	Anatomical Regions	Manipulation	Cervical	External	Short Lever Specific Contact	None
9	W	B	1	X	H	Z

Section (Character 1)

All Chiropractic procedure codes have a first character value of 9.

Body System (Character 2)

The alphanumeric character for the body system is placed in the second position. There is one character value applicable for the Chiropractic section. The character value of W is reported for anatomical regions.

Root Operations (Character 3)

The alphanumeric character value for root operations is placed in the third position. The following is the root operation applicable to the Chiropractic section with its associated meaning.

Character Value	Root Operation	Root Operation Definition
B	Manipulation	Manual procedure that involves a directed thrust to move a joint past the physiological range of motion, without exceeding the anatomical limit

Body Region (Character 4)

For each body region the applicable body part character values will be available for procedure code construction. An example of a body region for this section is Rib Cage.

Approach (Character 5)

The approach is the technique used to reach the procedure site. The following are the approach character values for the Chiropractic section with the associated definitions.

Character Value	Approach	Approach Definition
X	External	Procedures performed directly on the skin or mucous membrane and procedures performed indirectly by the application of external force through the skin or mucous membrane

Method (Character 6)

The method identifies the treatment method used to complete the chiropractic procedure. The available methods are:

- Non-Manual
- Indirect Visceral
- Extra-Articular
- Direct-Visual
- Long Lever Specific Contact
- Short Lever Specific Contact
- Long and Short Lever Specific Contact
- Mechanically Assisted
- Other

Qualifier (Character 7)

The qualifier represents an additional attribute for the procedure when applicable. Currently, there are no qualifiers in the Chiropractic section; therefore, the placeholder character value of Z should be reported.

Chiropractic Section Table

Chiropractic Table 9WB

Section	**9**	**Chiropractic**
Body System	**W**	**Anatomical Regions**
Operation	**B**	**Manipulation:** Manual procedure that involves a directed thrust to move a joint past the physiological range of motion, without exceeding the anatomical limit

Body Region (4th)	Approach (5th)	Method (6th)	Qualifier (7th)
0 Head **1** Cervical **2** Thoracic **3** Lumbar **4** Sacrum **5** Pelvis **6** Lower Extremities **7** Upper Extremities **8** Rib Cage **9** Abdomen	**X** External	**B** Non-Manual **C** Indirect Visceral **D** Extra-Articular **F** Direct Visceral **G** Long Lever Specific Contact **H** Short Lever Specific Contact **J** Long and Short Lever Specific Contact **K** Mechanically Assisted **L** Other Method	**Z** None

AHA Coding Clinic

No references have been issued for the Chiropractic Section.

Imaging Section (B00–BY4)

Within each section of ICD-10-PCS the characters have different meanings. The seven character meanings for the Imaging section are illustrated here through the procedure example of X-ray right clavicle, limited study.

Section	Body System	Root Type	Body Part	Contrast	Qualifier	Qualifier
Imaging	Non-Axial Upper Bones	Plain Radiography	Clavicle, right	None	None	None
B	P	0	4	Z	Z	Z

Section (Character 1)

All Imaging procedure codes have a first character value of B.

Body System (Character 2)

The alphanumeric character for the body system is placed in the second position. The following are the body systems applicable to the Imaging section.

Character Value	Character Value Description
0	Central Nervous System
2	Heart
3	Upper Arteries
4	Lower Arteries
5	Veins
7	Lymphatic System
8	Eye
9	Ear, Nose, Mouth and Throat
B	Respiratory System
D	Gastrointestinal System
F	Hepatobiliary System and Pancreas
G	Endocrine System
H	Skin, Subcutaneous Tissue and Breast
L	Connective Tissue
N	Skull and Facial Bones
P	Non-Axial Upper Bones
Q	Non-Axial Lower Bones
R	Axial Skeleton, Except Skull and Facial Bones
T	Urinary System
U	Female Reproductive System
V	Male Reproductive System
W	Anatomical Regions
Y	Fetus and Obstetrical

Root Types (Character 3)

The alphanumeric character value for root types is placed in the third position. Listed here are the root types applicable to the Imaging section with their associated meaning.

Character Value	Root Type	Root Type Definition
0	Plain Radiography	Planar display of an image developed from the capture of external ionizing radiation on photographic or photoconductive plate
1	Fluoroscopy	Single plane or bi-plane real time display of an image developed from the capture of external ionizing radiation on a fluorescent screen. The image may also be stored by either digital or analog means

Continued →

Character Value	Root Type	Root Type Definition
2	Computerized Tomography (CT Scan)	Computer reformatted digital display of multiplanar images developed from the capture of multiple exposures of external ionizing radiation
3	Magnetic Resonance Imaging (MRI)	Computer reformatted digital display of multiplanar images developed from the capture of radiofrequency signals emitted by nuclei in a body site excited within a magnetic field
4	Ultrasonography	Real time display of images of anatomy or flow information developed from the capture of reflected and attenuated high frequency sound waves
5	Other Imaging	Other specified modality for visualizing a body part

Body Part (Character 4)

For each body part the applicable body part character values will be available for procedure code construction. An example of a body part for this section is Spinal Cord.

Contrast (Character 5)

When contrast is utilized during an imaging procedure, the corresponding contrast character value should be reported in the fifth character position. The following are the contrast character values for the Imaging section:

- High Osmolar
- Low Osmolar
- Other Contrast

If contrast is not utilized, the placeholder character value of Z should be reported.

Qualifier (Character 6)

This qualifier character specifies when an image taken without contrast is followed by one with contrast. The character value of 0 is reported for Unenhanced and Enhanced.

Qualifier (Character 7)

The qualifier represents an additional attribute for the procedure when applicable. For example, ultrasonography procedures in this section include the qualifier Densitometry that is reported with the character value of 1 for some body parts. If there is no qualifier for a procedure, the placeholder Z is the character valve that should be reported.

Imaging Section Tables

Imaging Tables B00–BY4

Section B **Imaging**
Body System 0 **Central Nervous System**
Type 0 **Plain Radiography:** Planar display of an image developed from the capture of external ionizing radiation on photographic or photoconductive plate

Body Part (4th)	Contrast (5th)	Qualifier (6th)	Qualifier (7th)
B Spinal Cord	**0** High Osmolar **1** Low Osmolar **Y** Other Contrast **Z** None	**Z** None	**Z** None

Section B **Imaging**
Body System 0 **Central Nervous System**
Type 1 **Fluoroscopy:** Single plane or bi-plane real time display of an image developed from the capture of external ionizing radiation on a fluorescent screen. The image may also be stored by either digital or analog means

Body Part (4th)	Contrast (5th)	Qualifier (6th)	Qualifier (7th)
B Spinal Cord	**0** High Osmolar **1** Low Osmolar **Y** Other Contrast **Z** None	**Z** None	**Z** None

Section B **Imaging**
Body System 0 **Central Nervous System**
Type 2 **Computerized Tomography (CT Scan):** Computer reformatted digital display of multiplanar images developed from the capture of multiple exposures of external ionizing radiation

Body Part (4th)	Contrast (5th)	Qualifier (6th)	Qualifier (7th)
0 Brain 7 Cisterna 8 Cerebral Ventricle(s) 9 Sella Turcica/Pituitary Gland B Spinal Cord	0 High Osmolar 1 Low Osmolar Y Other Contrast	0 Unenhanced and Enhanced Z None	Z None
0 Brain 7 Cisterna 8 Cerebral Ventricle(s) 9 Sella Turcica/Pituitary Gland B Spinal Cord	Z None	Z None	Z None

Section B **Imaging**
Body System 0 **Central Nervous System**
Type 3 **Magnetic Resonance Imaging (MRI):** Computer reformatted digital display of multiplanar images developed from the capture of radiofrequency signals emitted by nuclei in a body site excited within a magnetic field

Body Part (4th)	Contrast (5th)	Qualifier (6th)	Qualifier (7th)
0 Brain 9 Sella Turcica/Pituitary Gland B Spinal Cord C Acoustic Nerves	Y Other Contrast	0 Unenhanced and Enhanced Z None	Z None
0 Brain 9 Sella Turcica/Pituitary Gland B Spinal Cord C Acoustic Nerves	Z None	Z None	Z None

Section B **Imaging**
Body System 0 **Central Nervous System**
Type 4 **Ultrasonography:** Real time display of images of anatomy or flow information developed from the capture of reflected and attenuated high frequency sound waves

Body Part (4th)	Contrast (5th)	Qualifier (6th)	Qualifier (7th)
0 Brain B Spinal Cord	Z None	Z None	Z None

Section B **Imaging**
Body System 2 **Heart**
Type 0 **Plain Radiography:** Planar display of an image developed from the capture of external ionizing radiation on photographic or photoconductive plate

Body Part (4th)	Contrast (5th)	Qualifier (6th)	Qualifier (7th)
0 Coronary Artery, Single 1 Coronary Arteries, Multiple 2 Coronary Artery Bypass Graft, Single 3 Coronary Artery Bypass Grafts, Multiple 4 Heart, Right 5 Heart, Left 6 Heart, Right and Left 7 Internal Mammary Bypass Graft, Right 8 Internal Mammary Bypass Graft, Left F Bypass Graft, Other	0 High Osmolar 1 Low Osmolar Y Other Contrast	Z None	Z None

Section B **Imaging**
Body System 2 **Heart**
Type 1 **Fluoroscopy:** Single plane or bi-plane real time display of an image developed from the capture of external ionizing radiation on a fluorescent screen. The image may also be stored by either digital or analog means

Body Part (4th)	Contrast (5th)	Qualifier (6th)	Qualifier (7th)
0 Coronary Artery, Single **1** Coronary Arteries, Multiple **2** Coronary Artery Bypass Graft, Single **3** Coronary Artery Bypass Grafts, Multiple	**0** High Osmolar **1** Low Osmolar **Y** Other Contrast	**1** Laser	**0** Intraoperative
0 Coronary Artery, Single **1** Coronary Arteries, Multiple **2** Coronary Artery Bypass Graft, Single **3** Coronary Artery Bypass Grafts, Multiple	**0** High Osmolar **1** Low Osmolar **Y** Other Contrast	**Z** None	**Z** None
4 Heart, Right **5** Heart, Left **6** Heart, Right and Left **7** Internal Mammary Bypass Graft, Right **8** Internal Mammary Bypass Graft, Left **F** Bypass Graft, Other	**0** High Osmolar **1** Low Osmolar **Y** Other Contrast	**Z** None	**Z** None

Section B **Imaging**
Body System 2 **Heart**
Type 2 **Computerized Tomography (CT Scan):** Computer reformatted digital display of multiplanar images developed from the capture of multiple exposures of external ionizing radiation

Body Part (4th)	Contrast (5th)	Qualifier (6th)	Qualifier (7th)
1 Coronary Arteries, Multiple **3** Coronary Artery Bypass Grafts, Multiple **6** Heart, Right and Left	**0** High Osmolar **1** Low Osmolar **Y** Other Contrast	**0** Unenhanced and Enhanced **Z** None	**Z** None
1 Coronary Arteries, Multiple **3** Coronary Artery Bypass Grafts, Multiple **6** Heart, Right and Left	**Z** None	**2** Intravascular Optical Coherence **Z** None	**Z** None

Section B **Imaging**
Body System 2 **Heart**
Type 3 **Magnetic Resonance Imaging (MRI):** Computer reformatted digital display of multiplanar images developed from the capture of radiofrequency signals emitted by nuclei in a body site excited within a magnetic field

Body Part (4th)	Contrast (5th)	Qualifier (6th)	Qualifier (7th)
1 Coronary Arteries, Multiple **3** Coronary Artery Bypass Grafts, Multiple **6** Heart, Right and Left	**Y** Other Contrast	**0** Unenhanced and Enhanced **Z** None	**Z** None
1 Coronary Arteries, Multiple **3** Coronary Artery Bypass Grafts, Multiple **6** Heart, Right and Left	**Z** None	**Z** None	**Z** None

Section B **Imaging**
Body System 2 **Heart**
Type 4 **Ultrasonography:** Real time display of images of anatomy or flow information developed from the capture of reflected and attenuated high frequency sound waves

Body Part (4th)	Contrast (5th)	Qualifier (6th)	Qualifier (7th)
0 Coronary Artery, Single **1** Coronary Arteries, Multiple **4** Heart, Right **5** Heart, Left **6** Heart, Right and Left **B** Heart with Aorta **C** Pericardium **D** Pediatric Heart	**Y** Other Contrast	**Z** None	**Z** None
0 Coronary Artery, Single **1** Coronary Arteries, Multiple **4** Heart, Right **5** Heart, Left **6** Heart, Right and Left **B** Heart with Aorta **C** Pericardium **D** Pediatric Heart	**Z** None	**Z** None	**3** Intravascular **4** Transesophageal **Z** None

Section B **Imaging**
Body System 3 **Upper Arteries**
Type 0 **Plain Radiography:** Planar display of an image developed from the capture of external ionizing radiation on photographic or photoconductive plate

Body Part (4th)	Contrast (5th)	Qualifier (6th)	Qualifier (7th)
0 Thoracic Aorta **1** Brachiocephalic-Subclavian Artery, Right **2** Subclavian Artery, Left **3** Common Carotid Artery, Right **4** Common Carotid Artery, Left **5** Common Carotid Arteries, Bilateral **6** Internal Carotid Artery, Right **7** Internal Carotid Artery, Left **8** Internal Carotid Arteries, Bilateral **9** External Carotid Artery, Right **B** External Carotid Artery, Left **C** External Carotid Arteries, Bilateral **D** Vertebral Artery, Right **F** Vertebral Artery, Left **G** Vertebral Arteries, Bilateral **H** Upper Extremity Arteries, Right **J** Upper Extremity Arteries, Left **K** Upper Extremity Arteries, Bilateral **L** Intercostal and Bronchial Arteries **M** Spinal Arteries **N** Upper Arteries, Other **P** Thoraco-Abdominal Aorta **Q** Cervico-Cerebral Arch **R** Intracranial Arteries **S** Pulmonary Artery, Right **T** Pulmonary Artery, Left	**0** High Osmolar **1** Low Osmolar **Y** Other Contrast **Z** None	**Z** None	**Z** None

Section B **Imaging**
Body System 3 **Upper Arteries**
Type 1 **Fluoroscopy:** Single plane or bi-plane real time display of an image developed from the capture of external ionizing radiation on a fluorescent screen. The image may also be stored by either digital or analog means

Body Part (4th)	Contrast (5th)	Qualifier (6th)	Qualifier (7th)
0 Thoracic Aorta **1** Brachiocephalic-Subclavian Artery, Right **2** Subclavian Artery, Left **3** Common Carotid Artery, Right **4** Common Carotid Artery, Left **5** Common Carotid Arteries, Bilateral **6** Internal Carotid Artery, Right **7** Internal Carotid Artery, Left **8** Internal Carotid Arteries, Bilateral **9** External Carotid Artery, Right **B** External Carotid Artery, Left **C** External Carotid Arteries, Bilateral **D** Vertebral Artery, Right **F** Vertebral Artery, Left **G** Vertebral Arteries, Bilateral **H** Upper Extremity Arteries, Right **J** Upper Extremity Arteries, Left **K** Upper Extremity Arteries, Bilateral **L** Intercostal and Bronchial Arteries **M** Spinal Arteries **N** Upper Arteries, Other **P** Thoraco-Abdominal Aorta **Q** Cervico-Cerebral Arch **R** Intracranial Arteries **S** Pulmonary Artery, Right **T** Pulmonary Artery, Left **U** Pulmonary Trunk	**0** High Osmolar **1** Low Osmolar **Y** Other Contrast	**1** Laser	**0** Intraoperative
0 Thoracic Aorta **1** Brachiocephalic-Subclavian Artery, Right **2** Subclavian Artery, Left **3** Common Carotid Artery, Right **4** Common Carotid Artery, Left **5** Common Carotid Arteries, Bilateral **6** Internal Carotid Artery, Right **7** Internal Carotid Artery, Left **8** Internal Carotid Arteries, Bilateral **9** External Carotid Artery, Right **B** External Carotid Artery, Left **C** External Carotid Arteries, Bilateral **D** Vertebral Artery, Right **F** Vertebral Artery, Left **G** Vertebral Arteries, Bilateral **H** Upper Extremity Arteries, Right **J** Upper Extremity Arteries, Left **K** Upper Extremity Arteries, Bilateral **L** Intercostal and Bronchial Arteries **M** Spinal Arteries **N** Upper Arteries, Other **P** Thoraco-Abdominal Aorta **Q** Cervico-Cerebral Arch **R** Intracranial Arteries **S** Pulmonary Artery, Right **T** Pulmonary Artery, Left **U** Pulmonary Trunk	**0** High Osmolar **1** Low Osmolar **Y** Other Contrast	**Z** None	**Z** None

Continued →

Section B **Imaging**
Body System 3 **Upper Arteries**
Type 1 **Fluoroscopy:** Single plane or bi-plane real time display of an image developed from the capture of external ionizing radiation on a fluorescent screen. The image may also be stored by either digital or analog means

Body Part (4th)	Contrast (5th)	Qualifier (6th)	Qualifier (7th)
0 Thoracic Aorta **1** Brachiocephalic-Subclavian Artery, Right **2** Subclavian Artery, Left **3** Common Carotid Artery, Right **4** Common Carotid Artery, Left **5** Common Carotid Arteries, Bilateral **6** Internal Carotid Artery, Right **7** Internal Carotid Artery, Left **8** Internal Carotid Arteries, Bilateral **9** External Carotid Artery, Right **B** External Carotid Artery, Left **C** External Carotid Arteries, Bilateral **D** Vertebral Artery, Right **F** Vertebral Artery, Left **G** Vertebral Arteries, Bilateral **H** Upper Extremity Arteries, Right **J** Upper Extremity Arteries, Left **K** Upper Extremity Arteries, Bilateral **L** Intercostal and Bronchial Arteries **M** Spinal Arteries **N** Upper Arteries, Other **P** Thoraco-Abdominal Aorta **Q** Cervico-Cerebral Arch **R** Intracranial Arteries **S** Pulmonary Artery, Right **T** Pulmonary Artery, Left **U** Pulmonary Trunk	**Z** None	**Z** None	**Z** None

Section B **Imaging**
Body System 3 **Upper Arteries**
Type 2 **Computerized Tomography (CT Scan):** Computer reformatted digital display of multiplanar images developed from the capture of multiple exposures of external ionizing radiation

Body Part (4th)	Contrast (5th)	Qualifier (6th)	Qualifier (7th)
0 Thoracic Aorta **5** Common Carotid Arteries, Bilateral **8** Internal Carotid Arteries, Bilateral **G** Vertebral Arteries, Bilateral **R** Intracranial Arteries **S** Pulmonary Artery, Right **T** Pulmonary Artery, Left	**0** High Osmolar **1** Low Osmolar **Y** Other Contrast	**Z** None	**Z** None
0 Thoracic Aorta **5** Common Carotid Arteries, Bilateral **8** Internal Carotid Arteries, Bilateral **G** Vertebral Arteries, Bilateral **R** Intracranial Arteries **S** Pulmonary Artery, Right **T** Pulmonary Artery, Left	**Z** None	**2** Intravascular Optical Coherence **Z** None	**Z** None

Section B Imaging
Body System 3 Upper Arteries
Type 3 **Magnetic Resonance Imaging (MRI):** Computer reformatted digital display of multiplanar images developed from the capture of radiofrequency signals emitted by nuclei in a body site excited within a magnetic field

Body Part (4th)	Contrast (5th)	Qualifier (6th)	Qualifier (7th)
0 Thoracic Aorta **5** Common Carotid Arteries, Bilateral **8** Internal Carotid Arteries, Bilateral **G** Vertebral Arteries, Bilateral **H** Upper Extremity Arteries, Right **J** Upper Extremity Arteries, Left **K** Upper Extremity Arteries, Bilateral **M** Spinal Arteries **Q** Cervico-Cerebral Arch **R** Intracranial Arteries	**Y** Other Contrast	**0** Unenhanced and Enhanced **Z** None	**Z** None
0 Thoracic Aorta **5** Common Carotid Arteries, Bilateral **8** Internal Carotid Arteries, Bilateral **G** Vertebral Arteries, Bilateral **H** Upper Extremity Arteries, Right **J** Upper Extremity Arteries, Left **K** Upper Extremity Arteries, Bilateral **M** Spinal Arteries **Q** Cervico-Cerebral Arch **R** Intracranial Arteries	**Z** None	**Z** None	**Z** None

Section B Imaging
Body System 3 Upper Arteries
Type 4 **Ultrasonography:** Real time display of images of anatomy or flow information developed from the capture of reflected and attenuated high frequency sound waves

Body Part (4th)	Contrast (5th)	Qualifier (6th)	Qualifier (7th)
0 Thoracic Aorta **1** Brachiocephalic-Subclavian Artery, Right **2** Subclavian Artery, Left **3** Common Carotid Artery, Right **4** Common Carotid Artery, Left **5** Common Carotid Arteries, Bilateral **6** Internal Carotid Artery, Right **7** Internal Carotid Artery, Left **8** Internal Carotid Arteries, Bilateral **H** Upper Extremity Arteries, Right **J** Upper Extremity Arteries, Left **K** Upper Extremity Arteries, Bilateral **R** Intracranial Arteries **S** Pulmonary Artery, Right **T** Pulmonary Artery, Left **V** Ophthalmic Arteries	**Z** None	**Z** None	**3** Intravascular **Z** None

Section B **Imaging**
Body System 4 **Lower Arteries**
Type 0 **Plain Radiography:** Planar display of an image developed from the capture of external ionizing radiation on photographic or photoconductive plate

Body Part (4th)	Contrast (5th)	Qualifier (6th)	Qualifier (7th)
0 Abdominal Aorta **2** Hepatic Artery **3** Splenic Arteries **4** Superior Mesenteric Artery **5** Inferior Mesenteric Artery **6** Renal Artery, Right **7** Renal Artery, Left **8** Renal Arteries, Bilateral **9** Lumbar Arteries **B** Intra-Abdominal Arteries, Other **C** Pelvic Arteries **D** Aorta and Bilateral Lower Extremity Arteries **F** Lower Extremity Arteries, Right **G** Lower Extremity Arteries, Left **J** Lower Arteries, Other **M** Renal Artery Transplant	**0** High Osmolar **1** Low Osmolar **Y** Other Contrast	**Z** None	**Z** None

Section B **Imaging**
Body System 4 **Lower Arteries**
Type 1 **Fluoroscopy:** Single plane or bi-plane real time display of an image developed from the capture of external ionizing radiation on a fluorescent screen. The image may also be stored by either digital or analog means

Body Part (4th)	Contrast (5th)	Qualifier (6th)	Qualifier (7th)
0 Abdominal Aorta **2** Hepatic Artery **3** Splenic Arteries **4** Superior Mesenteric Artery **5** Inferior Mesenteric Artery **6** Renal Artery, Right **7** Renal Artery, Left **8** Renal Arteries, Bilateral **9** Lumbar Arteries **B** Intra-Abdominal Arteries, Other **C** Pelvic Arteries **D** Aorta and Bilateral Lower Extremity Arteries **F** Lower Extremity Arteries, Right **G** Lower Extremity Arteries, Left **J** Lower Arteries, Other	**0** High Osmolar **1** Low Osmolar **Y** Other Contrast	**1** Laser	**0** Intraoperative
0 Abdominal Aorta **2** Hepatic Artery **3** Splenic Arteries **4** Superior Mesenteric Artery **5** Inferior Mesenteric Artery **6** Renal Artery, Right **7** Renal Artery, Left **8** Renal Arteries, Bilateral **9** Lumbar Arteries **B** Intra-Abdominal Arteries, Other **C** Pelvic Arteries **D** Aorta and Bilateral Lower Extremity Arteries **F** Lower Extremity Arteries, Right **G** Lower Extremity Arteries, Left **J** Lower Arteries, Other	**0** High Osmolar **1** Low Osmolar **Y** Other Contrast	**Z** None	**Z** None

Continued →

Section B **Imaging**
Body System 4 **Lower Arteries**
Type 1 **Fluoroscopy:** Single plane or bi-plane real time display of an image developed from the capture of external ionizing radiation on a fluorescent screen. The image may also be stored by either digital or analog means

Body Part (4th)	Contrast (5th)	Qualifier (6th)	Qualifier (7th)
0 Abdominal Aorta **2** Hepatic Artery **3** Splenic Arteries **4** Superior Mesenteric Artery **5** Inferior Mesenteric Artery **6** Renal Artery, Right **7** Renal Artery, Left **8** Renal Arteries, Bilateral **9** Lumbar Arteries **B** Intra-Abdominal Arteries, Other **C** Pelvic Arteries **D** Aorta and Bilateral Lower Extremity Arteries **F** Lower Extremity Arteries, Right **G** Lower Extremity Arteries, Left **J** Lower Arteries, Other	**Z** None	**Z** None	**Z** None

Section B **Imaging**
Body System 4 **Lower Arteries**
Type 2 **Computerized Tomography (CT Scan):** Computer reformatted digital display of multiplanar images developed from the capture of multiple exposures of external ionizing radiation

Body Part (4th)	Contrast (5th)	Qualifier (6th)	Qualifier (7th)
0 Abdominal Aorta **1** Celiac Artery **4** Superior Mesenteric Artery **8** Renal Arteries, Bilateral **C** Pelvic Arteries **F** Lower Extremity Arteries, Right **G** Lower Extremity Arteries, Left **H** Lower Extremity Arteries, Bilateral **M** Renal Artery Transplant	**0** High Osmolar **1** Low Osmolar **Y** Other Contrast	**Z** None	**Z** None
0 Abdominal Aorta **1** Celiac Artery **4** Superior Mesenteric Artery **8** Renal Arteries, Bilateral **C** Pelvic Arteries **F** Lower Extremity Arteries, Right **G** Lower Extremity Arteries, Left **H** Lower Extremity Arteries, Bilateral **M** Renal Artery Transplant	**Z** None	**2** Intravascular Optical Coherence **Z** None	**Z** None

Section B **Imaging**
Body System 4 **Lower Arteries**
Type 3 **Magnetic Resonance Imaging (MRI):** Computer reformatted digital display of multiplanar images developed from the capture of radiofrequency signals emitted by nuclei in a body site excited within a magnetic field

Body Part (4th)	Contrast (5th)	Qualifier (6th)	Qualifier (7th)
0 Abdominal Aorta **1** Celiac Artery **4** Superior Mesenteric Artery **8** Renal Arteries, Bilateral **C** Pelvic Arteries **F** Lower Extremity Arteries, Right **G** Lower Extremity Arteries, Left **H** Lower Extremity Arteries, Bilateral	**Y** Other Contrast	**0** Unenhanced and Enhanced **Z** None	**Z** None

Continued →

Section B **Imaging**
Body System 4 **Lower Arteries**
Type 3 **Magnetic Resonance Imaging (MRI):** Computer reformatted digital display of multiplanar images developed from the capture of radiofrequency signals emitted by nuclei in a body site excited within a magnetic field

Body Part (4th)	Contrast (5th)	Qualifier (6th)	Qualifier (7th)
0 Abdominal Aorta **1** Celiac Artery **4** Superior Mesenteric Artery **8** Renal Arteries, Bilateral **C** Pelvic Arteries **F** Lower Extremity Arteries, Right **G** Lower Extremity Arteries, Left **H** Lower Extremity Arteries, Bilateral	**Z** None	**Z** None	**Z** None

Section B **Imaging**
Body System 4 **Lower Arteries**
Type 4 **Ultrasonography:** Real time display of images of anatomy or flow information developed from the capture of reflected and attenuated high frequency sound waves

Body Part (4th)	Contrast (5th)	Qualifier (6th)	Qualifier (7th)
0 Abdominal Aorta **4** Superior Mesenteric Artery **5** Inferior Mesenteric Artery **6** Renal Artery, Right **7** Renal Artery, Left **8** Renal Arteries, Bilateral **B** Intra-Abdominal Arteries, Other **F** Lower Extremity Arteries, Right **G** Lower Extremity Arteries, Left **H** Lower Extremity Arteries, Bilateral **K** Celiac and Mesenteric Arteries **L** Femoral Artery **N** Penile Arteries	**Z** None	**Z** None	**3** Intravascular **Z** None

Section B Imaging
Body System 5 Veins
Type 0 **Plain Radiography:** Planar display of an image developed from the capture of external ionizing radiation on photographic or photoconductive plate

Body Part (4th)	Contrast (5th)	Qualifier (6th)	Qualifier (7th)
0 Epidural Veins **1** Cerebral and Cerebellar Veins **2** Intracranial Sinuses **3** Jugular Veins, Right **4** Jugular Veins, Left **5** Jugular Veins, Bilateral **6** Subclavian Vein, Right **7** Subclavian Vein, Left **8** Superior Vena Cava **9** Inferior Vena Cava **B** Lower Extremity Veins, Right **C** Lower Extremity Veins, Left **D** Lower Extremity Veins, Bilateral **F** Pelvic (Iliac) Veins, Right **G** Pelvic (Iliac) Veins, Left **H** Pelvic (Iliac) Veins, Bilateral **J** Renal Vein, Right **K** Renal Vein, Left **L** Renal Veins, Bilateral **M** Upper Extremity Veins, Right **N** Upper Extremity Veins, Left **P** Upper Extremity Veins, Bilateral **Q** Pulmonary Vein, Right **R** Pulmonary Vein, Left **S** Pulmonary Veins, Bilateral **T** Portal and Splanchnic Veins **V** Veins, Other **W** Dialysis Shunt/Fistula	**0** High Osmolar **1** Low Osmolar **Y** Other Contrast	**Z** None	**Z** None

Section B Imaging
Body System 5 Veins
Type 1 **Fluoroscopy:** Single plane or bi-plane real time display of an image developed from the capture of external ionizing radiation on a fluorescent screen. The image may also be stored by either digital or analog means

Body Part (4th)	Contrast (5th)	Qualifier (6th)	Qualifier (7th)
0 Epidural Veins **1** Cerebral and Cerebellar Veins **2** Intracranial Sinuses **3** Jugular Veins, Right **4** Jugular Veins, Left **5** Jugular Veins, Bilateral **6** Subclavian Vein, Right **7** Subclavian Vein, Left **8** Superior Vena Cava **9** Inferior Vena Cava **B** Lower Extremity Veins, Right **C** Lower Extremity Veins, Left **D** Lower Extremity Veins, Bilateral **F** Pelvic (Iliac) Veins, Right **G** Pelvic (Iliac) Veins, Left **H** Pelvic (Iliac) Veins, Bilateral **J** Renal Vein, Right **K** Renal Vein, Left **L** Renal Veins, Bilateral **M** Upper Extremity Veins, Right **N** Upper Extremity Veins, Left **P** Upper Extremity Veins, Bilateral **Q** Pulmonary Vein, Right **R** Pulmonary Vein, Left **S** Pulmonary Veins, Bilateral **T** Portal and Splanchnic Veins **V** Veins, Other **W** Dialysis Shunt/Fistula	**0** High Osmolar **1** Low Osmolar **Y** Other Contrast **Z** None	**Z** None	**A** Guidance **Z** None

Section B Imaging
Body System 5 Veins
Type 2 **Computerized Tomography (CT Scan):** Computer reformatted digital display of multiplanar images developed from the capture of multiple exposures of external ionizing radiation

Body Part (4th)	Contrast (5th)	Qualifier (6th)	Qualifier (7th)
2 Intracranial Sinuses **8** Superior Vena Cava **9** Inferior Vena Cava **F** Pelvic (Iliac) Veins, Right **G** Pelvic (Iliac) Veins, Left **H** Pelvic (Iliac) Veins, Bilateral **J** Renal Vein, Right **K** Renal Vein, Left **L** Renal Veins, Bilateral **Q** Pulmonary Vein, Right **R** Pulmonary Vein, Left **S** Pulmonary Veins, Bilateral **T** Portal and Splanchnic Veins	**0** High Osmolar **1** Low Osmolar **Y** Other Contrast	**0** Unenhanced and Enhanced **Z** None	**Z** None
2 Intracranial Sinuses **8** Superior Vena Cava **9** Inferior Vena Cava **F** Pelvic (Iliac) Veins, Right **G** Pelvic (Iliac) Veins, Left **H** Pelvic (Iliac) Veins, Bilateral **J** Renal Vein, Right	**Z** None	**2** Intravascular Optical Coherence **Z** None	**Z** None
K Renal Vein, Left **L** Renal Veins, Bilateral **Q** Pulmonary Vein, Right **R** Pulmonary Vein, Left **S** Pulmonary Veins, Bilateral **T** Portal and Splanchnic Veins			

Section B Imaging
Body System 5 Veins
Type 3 **Magnetic Resonance Imaging (MRI):** Computer reformatted digital display of multiplanar images developed from the capture of radiofrequency signals emitted by nuclei in a body site excited within a magnetic field

Body Part (4th)	Contrast (5th)	Qualifier (6th)	Qualifier (7th)
1 Cerebral and Cerebellar Veins **2** Intracranial Sinuses **5** Jugular Veins, Bilateral **8** Superior Vena Cava **9** Inferior Vena Cava **B** Lower Extremity Veins, Right **C** Lower Extremity Veins, Left **D** Lower Extremity Veins, Bilateral **H** Pelvic (Iliac) Veins, Bilateral **L** Renal Veins, Bilateral **M** Upper Extremity Veins, Right **N** Upper Extremity Veins, Left **P** Upper Extremity Veins, Bilateral **S** Pulmonary Veins, Bilateral **T** Portal and Splanchnic Veins **V** Veins, Other	**Y** Other Contrast	**0** Unenhanced and Enhanced **Z** None	**Z** None

Continued →

Section B **Imaging**
Body System 5 **Veins**
Type 3 **Magnetic Resonance Imaging (MRI):** Computer reformatted digital display of multiplanar images developed from the capture of radiofrequency signals emitted by nuclei in a body site excited within a magnetic field

Body Part (4th)	Contrast (5th)	Qualifier (6th)	Qualifier (7th)
1 Cerebral and Cerebellar Veins **2** Intracranial Sinuses **5** Jugular Veins, Bilateral **8** Superior Vena Cava **9** Inferior Vena Cava **B** Lower Extremity Veins, Right **C** Lower Extremity Veins, Left **D** Lower Extremity Veins, Bilateral **H** Pelvic (Iliac) Veins, Bilateral **L** Renal Veins, Bilateral **M** Upper Extremity Veins, Right **N** Upper Extremity Veins, Left **P** Upper Extremity Veins, Bilateral **S** Pulmonary Veins, Bilateral **T** Portal and Splanchnic Veins **V** Veins, Other	**Z** None	**Z** None	**Z** None

Section B **Imaging**
Body System 5 **Veins**
Type 4 **Ultrasonography:** Real time display of images of anatomy or flow information developed from the capture of reflected and attenuated high frequency sound waves

Body Part (4th)	Contrast (5th)	Qualifier (6th)	Qualifier (7th)
3 Jugular Veins, Right **4** Jugular Veins, Left **6** Subclavian Vein, Right **7** Subclavian Vein, Left **8** Superior Vena Cava **9** Inferior Vena Cava **B** Lower Extremity Veins, Right **C** Lower Extremity Veins, Left **D** Lower Extremity Veins, Bilateral **J** Renal Vein, Right **K** Renal Vein, Left **L** Renal Veins, Bilateral **M** Upper Extremity Veins, Right **N** Upper Extremity Veins, Left **P** Upper Extremity Veins, Bilateral **T** Portal and Splanchnic Veins	**Z** None	**Z** None	**3** Intravascular **A** Guidance **Z** None

Section B **Imaging**
Body System 7 **Lymphatic System**
Type 0 **Plain Radiography:** Planar display of an image developed from the capture of external ionizing radiation on photographic or photoconductive plate

Body Part (4th)	Contrast (5th)	Qualifier (6th)	Qualifier (7th)
0 Abdominal/Retroperitoneal Lymphatics, Unilateral **1** Abdominal/Retroperitoneal Lymphatics, Bilateral **4** Lymphatics, Head and Neck **5** Upper Extremity Lymphatics, Right **6** Upper Extremity Lymphatics, Left **7** Upper Extremity Lymphatics, Bilateral **8** Lower Extremity Lymphatics, Right **9** Lower Extremity Lymphatics, Left **B** Lower Extremity Lymphatics, Bilateral **C** Lymphatics, Pelvic	**0** High Osmolar **1** Low Osmolar **Y** Other Contrast	**Z** None	**Z** None

Section B **Imaging**
Body System 8 **Eye**
Type 0 **Plain Radiography:** Planar display of an image developed from the capture of external ionizing radiation on photographic or photoconductive plate

Body Part (4th)	Contrast (5th)	Qualifier (6th)	Qualifier (7th)
0 Lacrimal Duct, Right 1 Lacrimal Duct, Left 2 Lacrimal Ducts, Bilateral	0 High Osmolar 1 Low Osmolar Y Other Contrast	Z None	Z None
3 Optic Foramina, Right 4 Optic Foramina, Left 5 Eye, Right 6 Eye, Left 7 Eyes, Bilateral	Z None	Z None	Z None

Section B **Imaging**
Body System 8 **Eye**
Type 2 **Computerized Tomography (CT Scan):** Computer reformatted digital display of multiplanar images developed from the capture of multiple exposures of external ionizing radiation

Body Part (4th)	Contrast (5th)	Qualifier (6th)	Qualifier (7th)
5 Eye, Right 6 Eye, Left 7 Eyes, Bilateral	0 High Osmolar 1 Low Osmolar Y Other Contrast	0 Unenhanced and Enhanced Z None	Z None
5 Eye, Right 6 Eye, Left 7 Eyes, Bilateral	Z None	Z None	Z None

Section B **Imaging**
Body System 8 **Eye**
Type 3 **Magnetic Resonance Imaging (MRI):** Computer reformatted digital display of multiplanar images developed from the capture of radiofrequency signals emitted by nuclei in a body site excited within a magnetic field

Body Part (4th)	Contrast (5th)	Qualifier (6th)	Qualifier (7th)
5 Eye, Right 6 Eye, Left 7 Eyes, Bilateral	Y Other Contrast	0 Unenhanced and Enhanced Z None	Z None
5 Eye, Right 6 Eye, Left 7 Eyes, Bilateral	Z None	Z None	Z None

Section B **Imaging**
Body System 8 **Eye**
Type 4 **Ultrasonography:** Real time display of images of anatomy or flow information developed from the capture of reflected and attenuated high frequency sound waves

Body Part (4th)	Contrast (5th)	Qualifier (6th)	Qualifier (7th)
5 Eye, Right 6 Eye, Left 7 Eyes, Bilateral	Z None	Z None	Z None

Section B **Imaging**
Body System 9 **Ear, Nose, Mouth and Throat**
Type 0 **Plain Radiography:** Planar display of an image developed from the capture of external ionizing radiation on photographic or photoconductive plate

Body Part (4th)	Contrast (5th)	Qualifier (6th)	Qualifier (7th)
2 Paranasal Sinuses F Nasopharynx/Oropharynx H Mastoids	Z None	Z None	Z None
4 Parotid Gland, Right 5 Parotid Gland, Left 6 Parotid Glands, Bilateral 7 Submandibular Gland, Right 8 Submandibular Gland, Left 9 Submandibular Glands, Bilateral B Salivary Gland, Right C Salivary Gland, Left D Salivary Glands, Bilateral	0 High Osmolar 1 Low Osmolar Y Other Contrast	Z None	Z None

Section B **Imaging**
Body System 9 **Ear, Nose, Mouth and Throat**
Type 1 **Fluoroscopy:** Single plane or bi-plane real time display of an image developed from the capture of external ionizing radiation on a fluorescent screen. The image may also be stored by either digital or analog means

Body Part (4th)	Contrast (5th)	Qualifier (6th)	Qualifier (7th)
G Pharynx and Epiglottis J Larynx	Y Other Contrast Z None	Z None	Z None

Section B **Imaging**
Body System 9 **Ear, Nose, Mouth and Throat**
Type 2 **Computerized Tomography (CT Scan):** Computer reformatted digital display of multiplanar images developed from the capture of multiple exposures of external ionizing radiation

Body Part (4th)	Contrast (5th)	Qualifier (6th)	Qualifier (7th)
0 Ear 2 Paranasal Sinuses 6 Parotid Glands, Bilateral 9 Submandibular Glands, Bilateral D Salivary Glands, Bilateral F Nasopharynx/Oropharynx J Larynx	0 High Osmolar 1 Low Osmolar Y Other Contrast	0 Unenhanced and Enhanced Z None	Z None
0 Ear 2 Paranasal Sinuses 6 Parotid Glands, Bilateral 9 Submandibular Glands, Bilateral D Salivary Glands, Bilateral F Nasopharynx/Oropharynx J Larynx	Z None	Z None	Z None

Section B **Imaging**
Body System 9 **Ear, Nose, Mouth and Throat**
Type 3 **Magnetic Resonance Imaging (MRI):** Computer reformatted digital display of multiplanar images developed from the capture of radiofrequency signals emitted by nuclei in a body site excited within a magnetic field

Body Part (4th)	Contrast (5th)	Qualifier (6th)	Qualifier (7th)
0 Ear 2 Paranasal Sinuses 6 Parotid Glands, Bilateral 9 Submandibular Glands, Bilateral D Salivary Glands, Bilateral F Nasopharynx/Oropharynx J Larynx	Y Other Contrast	0 Unenhanced and Enhanced Z None	Z None

Continued →

Section **B** **Imaging**
Body System **9** **Ear, Nose, Mouth and Throat**
Type **3** **Magnetic Resonance Imaging (MRI):** Computer reformatted digital display of multiplanar images developed from the capture of radiofrequency signals emitted by nuclei in a body site excited within a magnetic field

Body Part (4th)	Contrast (5th)	Qualifier (6th)	Qualifier (7th)
0 Ear **2** Paranasal Sinuses **6** Parotid Glands, Bilateral **9** Submandibular Glands, Bilateral **D** Salivary Glands, Bilateral **F** Nasopharynx/Oropharynx **J** Larynx	**Z** None	**Z** None	**Z** None

Section **B** **Imaging**
Body System **B** **Respiratory System**
Type **0** **Plain Radiography:** Planar display of an image developed from the capture of external ionizing radiation on photographic or photoconductive plate

Body Part (4th)	Contrast (5th)	Qualifier (6th)	Qualifier (7th)
7 Tracheobronchial Tree, Right **8** Tracheobronchial Tree, Left **9** Tracheobronchial Trees, Bilateral	**Y** Other Contrast	**Z** None	**Z** None
D Upper Airways	**Z** None	**Z** None	**Z** None

Section **B** **Imaging**
Body System **B** **Respiratory System**
Type **1** **Fluoroscopy:** Single plane or bi-plane real time display of an image developed from the capture of external ionizing radiation on a fluorescent screen. The image may also be stored by either digital or analog means

Body Part (4th)	Contrast (5th)	Qualifier (6th)	Qualifier (7th)
2 Lung, Right **3** Lung, Left **4** Lungs, Bilateral **6** Diaphragm **C** Mediastinum **D** Upper Airways	**Z** None	**Z** None	**Z** None
7 Tracheobronchial Tree, Right **8** Tracheobronchial Tree, Left **9** Tracheobronchial Trees, Bilateral	**Y** Other Contrast	**Z** None	**Z** None

Section **B** **Imaging**
Body System **B** **Respiratory System**
Type **2** **Computerized Tomography (CT Scan):** Computer reformatted digital display of multiplanar images developed from the capture of multiple exposures of external ionizing radiation

Body Part (4th)	Contrast (5th)	Qualifier (6th)	Qualifier (7th)
4 Lungs, Bilateral **7** Tracheobronchial Tree, Right **8** Tracheobronchial Tree, Left **9** Tracheobronchial Trees, Bilateral **F** Trachea/Airways	**0** High Osmolar **1** Low Osmolar **Y** Other Contrast	**0** Unenhanced and Enhanced **Z** None	**Z** None
4 Lungs, Bilateral **7** Tracheobronchial Tree, Right **8** Tracheobronchial Tree, Left **9** Tracheobronchial Trees, Bilateral **F** Trachea/Airways	**Z** None	**Z** None	**Z** None

Section B **Imaging**
Body System B **Respiratory System**
Type 3 **Magnetic Resonance Imaging (MRI):** Computer reformatted digital display of multiplanar images developed from the capture of radiofrequency signals emitted by nuclei in a body site excited within a magnetic field

Body Part (4th)	Contrast (5th)	Qualifier (6th)	Qualifier (7th)
G Lung Apices	**Y** Other Contrast	**0** Unenhanced and Enhanced **Z** None	**Z** None
G Lung Apices	**Z** None	**Z** None	**Z** None

Section B **Imaging**
Body System B **Respiratory System**
Type 4 **Ultrasonography:** Real time display of images of anatomy or flow information developed from the capture of reflected and attenuated high frequency sound waves

Body Part (4th)	Contrast (5th)	Qualifier (6th)	Qualifier (7th)
B Pleura **C** Mediastinum	**Z** None	**Z** None	**Z** None

Section B **Imaging**
Body System D **Gastrointestinal System**
Type 1 **Fluoroscopy:** Single plane or bi-plane real time display of an image developed from the capture of external ionizing radiation on a fluorescent screen. The image may also be stored by either digital or analog means

Body Part (4th)	Contrast (5th)	Qualifier (6th)	Qualifier (7th)
1 Esophagus **2** Stomach **3** Small Bowel **4** Colon **5** Upper GI **6** Upper GI and Small Bowel **9** Duodenum **B** Mouth/Oropharynx	**Y** Other Contrast **Z** None	**Z** None	**Z** None

Section B **Imaging**
Body System D **Gastrointestinal System**
Type 2 **Computerized Tomography (CT Scan):** Computer reformatted digital display of multiplanar images developed from the capture of multiple exposures of external ionizing radiation

Body Part (4th)	Contrast (5th)	Qualifier (6th)	Qualifier (7th)
4 Colon	**0** High Osmolar **1** Low Osmolar **Y** Other Contrast	**0** Unenhanced and Enhanced **Z** None	**Z** None
4 Colon	**Z** None	**Z** None	**Z** None

Section B **Imaging**
Body System D **Gastrointestinal System**
Type 4 **Ultrasonography:** Real time display of images of anatomy or flow information developed from the capture of reflected and attenuated high frequency sound waves

Body Part (4th)	Contrast (5th)	Qualifier (6th)	Qualifier (7th)
1 Esophagus **2** Stomach **7** Gastrointestinal Tract **8** Appendix **9** Duodenum **C** Rectum	**Z** None	**Z** None	**Z** None

Section B **Imaging**
Body System F **Hepatobiliary System and Pancreas**
Type 0 **Plain Radiography:** Planar display of an image developed from the capture of external ionizing radiation on photographic or photoconductive plate

Body Part (4th)	Contrast (5th)	Qualifier (6th)	Qualifier (7th)
0 Bile Ducts **3** Gallbladder and Bile Ducts **C** Hepatobiliary System, All	**0** High Osmolar **1** Low Osmolar **Y** Other Contrast	**Z** None	**Z** None

Section B **Imaging**
Body System F **Hepatobiliary System and Pancreas**
Type 1 **Fluoroscopy:** Single plane or bi-plane real time display of an image developed from the capture of external ionizing radiation on a fluorescent screen. The image may also be stored by either digital or analog means

Body Part (4th)	Contrast (5th)	Qualifier (6th)	Qualifier (7th)
0 Bile Ducts **1** Biliary and Pancreatic Ducts **2** Gallbladder **3** Gallbladder and Bile Ducts **4** Gallbladder, Bile Ducts and Pancreatic Ducts **8** Pancreatic Ducts	**0** High Osmolar **1** Low Osmolar **Y** Other Contrast	**Z** None	**Z** None
5 Liver	**0** High Osmolar **1** Low Osmolar **Y** Other Contrast	**Z** None	**Z** None
5 Liver	**Z** None	**Z** None	**A** Guidance

Section B **Imaging**
Body System F **Hepatobiliary System and Pancreas**
Type 2 **Computerized Tomography (CT Scan):** Computer reformatted digital display of multiplanar images developed from the capture of multiple exposures of external ionizing radiation

Body Part (4th)	Contrast (5th)	Qualifier (6th)	Qualifier (7th)
5 Liver **6** Liver and Spleen **7** Pancreas **C** Hepatobiliary System, All	**0** High Osmolar **1** Low Osmolar **Y** Other Contrast	**0** Unenhanced and Enhanced **Z** None	**Z** None
5 Liver **6** Liver and Spleen **7** Pancreas **C** Hepatobiliary System, All	**Z** None	**Z** None	**Z** None

Section B **Imaging**
Body System F **Hepatobiliary System and Pancreas**
Type 3 **Magnetic Resonance Imaging (MRI):** Computer reformatted digital display of multiplanar images developed from the capture of radiofrequency signals emitted by nuclei in a body site excited within a magnetic field

Body Part (4th)	Contrast (5th)	Qualifier (6th)	Qualifier (7th)
5 Liver **6** Liver and Spleen **7** Pancreas	**Y** Other Contrast	**0** Unenhanced and Enhanced **Z** None	**Z** None
5 Liver **6** Liver and Spleen **7** Pancreas	**Z** None	**Z** None	**Z** None

Section B **Imaging**
Body System F **Hepatobiliary System and Pancreas**
Type 4 **Ultrasonography:** Real time display of images of anatomy or flow information developed from the capture of reflected and attenuated high frequency sound waves

Body Part (4th)	Contrast (5th)	Qualifier (6th)	Qualifier (7th)
0 Bile Ducts **2** Gallbladder **3** Gallbladder and Bile Ducts **5** Liver **6** Liver and Spleen **7** Pancreas **C** Hepatobiliary System, All	**Z** None	**Z** None	**Z** None

Section B **Imaging**
Body System F **Hepatobiliary System and Pancreas**
Type 5 **Other Imaging:** Other specified modality for visualizing a body part

Body Part (4th)	Contrast (5th)	Qualifier (6th)	Qualifier (7th)
0 Bile Ducts **2** Gallbladder **3** Gallbladder and Bile Ducts **5** Liver **6** Liver and Spleen **7** Pancreas **C** Hepatobiliary System, All	**2** Fluorescing Agent	**0** Indocyanine Green Dye **Z** None	**0** Intraoperative **Z** None

Section B **Imaging**
Body System G **Endocrine System**
Type 2 **Computerized Tomography (CT Scan):** Computer reformatted digital display of multiplanar images developed from the capture of multiple exposures of external ionizing radiation

Body Part (4th)	Contrast (5th)	Qualifier (6th)	Qualifier (7th)
2 Adrenal Glands, Bilateral **3** Parathyroid Glands **4** Thyroid Gland	**0** High Osmolar **1** Low Osmolar **Y** Other Contrast	**0** Unenhanced and Enhanced **Z** None	**Z** None
2 Adrenal Glands, Bilateral **3** Parathyroid Glands **4** Thyroid Gland	**Z** None	**Z** None	**Z** None

Section B **Imaging**
Body System G **Endocrine System**
Type 3 **Magnetic Resonance Imaging (MRI):** Computer reformatted digital display of multiplanar images developed from the capture of radiofrequency signals emitted by nuclei in a body site excited within a magnetic field

Body Part (4th)	Contrast (5th)	Qualifier (6th)	Qualifier (7th)
2 Adrenal Glands, Bilateral **3** Parathyroid Glands **4** Thyroid Gland	**Y** Other Contrast	**0** Unenhanced and Enhanced **Z** None	**Z** None
2 Adrenal Glands, Bilateral **3** Parathyroid Glands **4** Thyroid Gland	**Z** None	**Z** None	**Z** None

Section B **Imaging**
Body System G **Endocrine System**
Type 4 **Ultrasonography:** Real time display of images of anatomy or flow information developed from the capture of reflected and attenuated high frequency sound waves

Body Part (4th)	Contrast (5th)	Qualifier (6th)	Qualifier (7th)
0 Adrenal Gland, Right **1** Adrenal Gland, Left **2** Adrenal Glands, Bilateral **3** Parathyroid Glands **4** Thyroid Gland	**Z** None	**Z** None	**Z** None

Section B **Imaging**
Body System H **Skin, Subcutaneous Tissue and Breast**
Type 0 **Plain Radiography:** Planar display of an image developed from the capture of external ionizing radiation on photographic or photoconductive plate

Body Part (4th)	Contrast (5th)	Qualifier (6th)	Qualifier (7th)
0 Breast, Right **1** Breast, Left **2** Breasts, Bilateral	**Z** None	**Z** None	**Z** None
3 Single Mammary Duct, Right **4** Single Mammary Duct, Left **5** Multiple Mammary Ducts, Right **6** Multiple Mammary Ducts, Left	**0** High Osmolar **1** Low Osmolar **Y** Other Contrast **Z** None	**Z** None	**Z** None

Section B **Imaging**
Body System H **Skin, Subcutaneous Tissue and Breast**
Type 3 **Magnetic Resonance Imaging (MRI):** Computer reformatted digital display of multiplanar images developed from the capture of radiofrequency signals emitted by nuclei in a body site excited within a magnetic field

Body Part (4th)	Contrast (5th)	Qualifier (6th)	Qualifier (7th)
0 Breast, Right **1** Breast, Left **2** Breasts, Bilateral **D** Subcutaneous Tissue, Head/Neck **F** Subcutaneous Tissue, Upper Extremity **G** Subcutaneous Tissue, Thorax **H** Subcutaneous Tissue, Abdomen and Pelvis **J** Subcutaneous Tissue, Lower Extremity	**Y** Other Contrast	**0** Unenhanced and Enhanced **Z** None	**Z** None
0 Breast, Right **1** Breast, Left **2** Breasts, Bilateral **D** Subcutaneous Tissue, Head/Neck **F** Subcutaneous Tissue, Upper Extremity **G** Subcutaneous Tissue, Thorax **H** Subcutaneous Tissue, Abdomen and Pelvis **J** Subcutaneous Tissue, Lower Extremity	**Z** None	**Z** None	**Z** None

Section B **Imaging**
Body System H **Skin, Subcutaneous Tissue and Breast**
Type 4 **Ultrasonography:** Real time display of images of anatomy or flow information developed from the capture of reflected and attenuated high frequency sound waves

Body Part (4th)	Contrast (5th)	Qualifier (6th)	Qualifier (7th)
0 Breast, Right **1** Breast, Left **2** Breasts, Bilateral **7** Extremity, Upper **8** Extremity, Lower **9** Abdominal Wall **B** Chest Wall **C** Head and Neck	**Z** None	**Z** None	**Z** None

Section B **Imaging**
Body System L **Connective Tissue**
Type 3 **Magnetic Resonance Imaging (MRI):** Computer reformatted digital display of multiplanar images developed from the capture of radiofrequency signals emitted by nuclei in a body site excited within a magnetic field

Body Part (4th)	Contrast (5th)	Qualifier (6th)	Qualifier (7th)
0 Connective Tissue, Upper Extremity **1** Connective Tissue, Lower Extremity **2** Tendons, Upper Extremity **3** Tendons, Lower Extremity	**Y** Other Contrast	**0** Unenhanced and Enhanced **Z** None	**Z** None
0 Connective Tissue, Upper Extremity **1** Connective Tissue, Lower Extremity **2** Tendons, Upper Extremity **3** Tendons, Lower Extremity	**Z** None	**Z** None	**Z** None

Section B **Imaging**
Body System L **Connective Tissue**
Type 4 **Ultrasonography:** Real time display of images of anatomy or flow information developed from the capture of reflected and attenuated high frequency sound waves

Body Part (4th)	Contrast (5th)	Qualifier (6th)	Qualifier (7th)
0 Connective Tissue, Upper Extremity **1** Connective Tissue, Lower Extremity **2** Tendons, Upper Extremity **3** Tendons, Lower Extremity	**Z** None	**Z** None	**Z** None

Section B **Imaging**
Body System N **Skull and Facial Bones**
Type 0 **Plain Radiography:** Planar display of an image developed from the capture of external ionizing radiation on photographic or photoconductive plate

Body Part (4th)	Contrast (5th)	Qualifier (6th)	Qualifier (7th)
0 Skull **1** Orbit, Right **2** Orbit, Left **3** Orbits, Bilateral **4** Nasal Bones **5** Facial Bones **6** Mandible **B** Zygomatic Arch, Right **C** Zygomatic Arch, Left **D** Zygomatic Arches, Bilateral **G** Tooth, Single **H** Teeth, Multiple **J** Teeth, All	**Z** None	**Z** None	**Z** None
7 Temporomandibular Joint, Right **8** Temporomandibular Joint, Left **9** Temporomandibular Joints, Bilateral	**0** High Osmolar **1** Low Osmolar **Y** Other Contrast **Z** None	**Z** None	**Z** None

Section B **Imaging**
Body System N **Skull and Facial Bones**
Type 1 **Fluoroscopy:** Single plane or bi-plane real time display of an image developed from the capture of external ionizing radiation on a fluorescent screen. The image may also be stored by either digital or analog means

Body Part (4th)	Contrast (5th)	Qualifier (6th)	Qualifier (7th)
7 Temporomandibular Joint, Right **8** Temporomandibular Joint, Left **9** Temporomandibular Joints, Bilateral	**0** High Osmolar **1** Low Osmolar **Y** Other Contrast **Z** None	**Z** None	**Z** None

Section B **Imaging**
Body System N **Skull and Facial Bones**
Type 2 **Computerized Tomography (CT Scan):** Computer reformatted digital display of multiplanar images developed from the capture of multiple exposures of external ionizing radiation

Body Part (4th)	Contrast (5th)	Qualifier (6th)	Qualifier (7th)
0 Skull **3** Orbits, Bilateral **5** Facial Bones **6** Mandible **9** Temporomandibular Joints, Bilateral **F** Temporal Bones	**0** High Osmolar **1** Low Osmolar **Y** Other Contrast **Z** None	**Z** None	**Z** None

Section B **Imaging**
Body System N **Skull and Facial Bones**
Type 3 **Magnetic Resonance Imaging (MRI):** Computer reformatted digital display of multiplanar images developed from the capture of radiofrequency signals emitted by nuclei in a body site excited within a magnetic field

Body Part (4th)	Contrast (5th)	Qualifier (6th)	Qualifier (7th)
9 Temporomandibular Joints, Bilateral	**Y** Other Contrast **Z** None	**Z** None	**Z** None

Section B **Imaging**
Body System P **Non-Axial Upper Bones**
Type 0 **Plain Radiography:** Planar display of an image developed from the capture of external ionizing radiation on photographic or photoconductive plate

Body Part (4th)	Contrast (5th)	Qualifier (6th)	Qualifier (7th)
0 Sternoclavicular Joint, Right **1** Sternoclavicular Joint, Left **2** Sternoclavicular Joints, Bilateral **3** Acromioclavicular Joints, Bilateral **4** Clavicle, Right **5** Clavicle, Left **6** Scapula, Right **7** Scapula, Left **A** Humerus, Right **B** Humerus, Left **E** Upper Arm, Right **F** Upper Arm, Left **J** Forearm, Right **K** Forearm, Left **N** Hand, Right **P** Hand, Left **R** Finger(s), Right **S** Finger(s), Left **X** Ribs, Right **Y** Ribs, Left	**Z** None	**Z** None	**Z** None
8 Shoulder, Right **9** Shoulder, Left **C** Hand/Finger Joint, Right **D** Hand/Finger Joint, Left **G** Elbow, Right **H** Elbow, Left **L** Wrist, Right **M** Wrist, Left	**0** High Osmolar **1** Low Osmolar **Y** Other Contrast **Z** None	**Z** None	**Z** None

Section	**B**	**Imaging**
Body System	**P**	**Non-Axial Upper Bones**
Type	**1**	**Fluoroscopy:** Single plane or bi-plane real time display of an image developed from the capture of external ionizing radiation on a fluorescent screen. The image may also be stored by either digital or analog means

Body Part (4th)	Contrast (5th)	Qualifier (6th)	Qualifier (7th)
0 Sternoclavicular Joint, Right **1** Sternoclavicular Joint, Left **2** Sternoclavicular Joints, Bilateral **3** Acromioclavicular Joints, Bilateral **4** Clavicle, Right **5** Clavicle, Left **6** Scapula, Right **7** Scapula, Left **A** Humerus, Right **B** Humerus, Left **E** Upper Arm, Right **F** Upper Arm, Left **J** Forearm, Right **K** Forearm, Left **N** Hand, Right **P** Hand, Left **R** Finger(s), Right **S** Finger(s), Left **X** Ribs, Right **Y** Ribs, Left	**Z** None	**Z** None	**Z** None
8 Shoulder, Right **9** Shoulder, Left **L** Wrist, Right **M** Wrist, Left	**0** High Osmolar **1** Low Osmolar **Y** Other Contrast **Z** None	**Z** None	**Z** None
C Hand/Finger Joint, Right **D** Hand/Finger Joint, Left **G** Elbow, Right **H** Elbow, Left	**0** High Osmolar **1** Low Osmolar **Y** Other Contrast	**Z** None	**Z** None

Section	**B**	**Imaging**
Body System	**P**	**Non-Axial Upper Bones**
Type	**2**	**Computerized Tomography (CT Scan):** Computer reformatted digital display of multiplanar images developed from the capture of multiple exposures of external ionizing radiation

Body Part (4th)	Contrast (5th)	Qualifier (6th)	Qualifier (7th)
0 Sternoclavicular Joint, Right **1** Sternoclavicular Joint, Left **W** Thorax	**0** High Osmolar **1** Low Osmolar **Y** Other Contrast	**Z** None	**Z** None

Continued →

BP2 Continued

Section B **Imaging**
Body System P **Non-Axial Upper Bones**
Type 2 **Computerized Tomography (CT Scan):** Computer reformatted digital display of multiplanar images developed from the capture of multiple exposures of external ionizing radiation

Body Part (4th)	Contrast (5th)	Qualifier (6th)	Qualifier (7th)
2 Sternoclavicular Joints, Bilateral **3** Acromioclavicular Joints, Bilateral **4** Clavicle, Right **5** Clavicle, Left **6** Scapula, Right **7** Scapula, Left **8** Shoulder, Right **9** Shoulder, Left **A** Humerus, Right **B** Humerus, Left **E** Upper Arm, Right **F** Upper Arm, Left **G** Elbow, Right **H** Elbow, Left **J** Forearm, Right **K** Forearm, Left **L** Wrist, Right **M** Wrist, Left **N** Hand, Right **P** Hand, Left **Q** Hands and Wrists, Bilateral **R** Finger(s), Right **S** Finger(s), Left **T** Upper Extremity, Right **U** Upper Extremity, Left **V** Upper Extremities, Bilateral **X** Ribs, Right **Y** Ribs, Left	**0** High Osmolar **1** Low Osmolar **Y** Other Contrast **Z** None	**Z** None	**Z** None
C Hand/Finger Joint, Right **D** Hand/Finger Joint, Left	**Z** None	**Z** None	**Z** None

Section B **Imaging**
Body System P **Non-Axial Upper Bones**
Type 3 **Magnetic Resonance Imaging (MRI):** Computer reformatted digital display of multiplanar images developed from the capture of radiofrequency signals emitted by nuclei in a body site excited within a magnetic field

Body Part (4th)	Contrast (5th)	Qualifier (6th)	Qualifier (7th)
8 Shoulder, Right **9** Shoulder, Left **C** Hand/Finger Joint, Right **D** Hand/Finger Joint, Left **E** Upper Arm, Right **F** Upper Arm, Left **G** Elbow, Right **H** Elbow, Left **J** Forearm, Right **K** Forearm, Left **L** Wrist, Right **M** Wrist, Left	**Y** Other Contrast	**0** Unenhanced and Enhanced **Z** None	**Z** None

Continued →

Section B **Imaging**
Body System P **Non-Axial Upper Bones**
Type 3 **Magnetic Resonance Imaging (MRI):** Computer reformatted digital display of multiplanar images developed from the capture of radiofrequency signals emitted by nuclei in a body site excited within a magnetic field

Body Part (4th)	Contrast (5th)	Qualifier (6th)	Qualifier (7th)
8 Shoulder, Right **9** Shoulder, Left **C** Hand/Finger Joint, Right **D** Hand/Finger Joint, Left **E** Upper Arm, Right **F** Upper Arm, Left **G** Elbow, Right **H** Elbow, Left **J** Forearm, Right **K** Forearm, Left **L** Wrist, Right **M** Wrist, Left	**Z** None	**Z** None	**Z** None

Section B **Imaging**
Body System P **Non-Axial Upper Bones**
Type 4 **Ultrasonography:** Real time display of images of anatomy or flow information developed from the capture of reflected and attenuated high frequency sound waves

Body Part (4th)	Contrast (5th)	Qualifier (6th)	Qualifier (7th)
8 Shoulder, Right **9** Shoulder, Left **G** Elbow, Right **H** Elbow, Left **L** Wrist, Right **M** Wrist, Left **N** Hand, Right **P** Hand, Left	**Z** None	**Z** None	**1** Densitometry **Z** None

Section B **Imaging**
Body System Q **Non-Axial Lower Bones**
Type 0 **Plain Radiography:** Planar display of an image developed from the capture of external ionizing radiation on photographic or photoconductive plate

Body Part (4th)	Contrast (5th)	Qualifier (6th)	Qualifier (7th)
0 Hip, Right **1** Hip, Left	**0** High Osmolar **1** Low Osmolar **Y** Other Contrast	**Z** None	**Z** None
0 Hip, Right **1** Hip, Left	**Z** None	**Z** None	**1** Densitometry **Z** None
3 Femur, Right **4** Femur, Left	**Z** None	**Z** None	**1** Densitometry **Z** None
7 Knee, Right **8** Knee, Left **G** Ankle, Right **H** Ankle, Left	**0** High Osmolar **1** Low Osmolar **Y** Other Contrast **Z** None	**Z** None	**Z** None
D Lower Leg, Right **F** Lower Leg, Left **J** Calcaneus, Right **K** Calcaneus, Left **L** Foot, Right **M** Foot, Left **P** Toe(s), Right **Q** Toe(s), Left **V** Patella, Right **W** Patella, Left	**Z** None	**Z** None	**Z** None

Continued →

Section B **Imaging**
Body System Q **Non-Axial Lower Bones**
Type 0 **Plain Radiography:** Planar display of an image developed from the capture of external ionizing radiation on photographic or photoconductive plate

Body Part (4th)	Contrast (5th)	Qualifier (6th)	Qualifier (7th)
X Foot/Toe Joint, Right **Y** Foot/Toe Joint, Left	**0** High Osmolar **1** Low Osmolar **Y** Other Contrast	**Z** None	**Z** None

Section B **Imaging**
Body System Q **Non-Axial Lower Bones**
Type 1 **Fluoroscopy:** Single plane or bi-plane real time display of an image developed from the capture of external ionizing radiation on a fluorescent screen. The image may also be stored by either digital or analog means

Body Part (4th)	Contrast (5th)	Qualifier (6th)	Qualifier (7th)
0 Hip, Right **1** Hip, Left **7** Knee, Right **8** Knee, Left **G** Ankle, Right **H** Ankle, Left **X** Foot/Toe Joint, Right **Y** Foot/Toe Joint, Left	**0** High Osmolar **1** Low Osmolar **Y** Other Contrast **Z** None	**Z** None	**Z** None
3 Femur, Right **4** Femur, Left **D** Lower Leg, Right **F** Lower Leg, Left **J** Calcaneus, Right **K** Calcaneus, Left **L** Foot, Right **M** Foot, Left **P** Toe(s), Right **Q** Toe(s), Left **V** Patella, Right **W** Patella, Left	**Z** None	**Z** None	**Z** None

Section B **Imaging**
Body System Q **Non-Axial Lower Bones**
Type 2 **Computerized Tomography (CT Scan):** Computer reformatted digital display of multiplanar images developed from the capture of multiple exposures of external ionizing radiation

Body Part (4th)	Contrast (5th)	Qualifier (6th)	Qualifier (7th)
0 Hip, Right **1** Hip, Left **3** Femur, Right **4** Femur, Left **7** Knee, Right **8** Knee, Left **D** Lower Leg, Right **F** Lower Leg, Left **G** Ankle, Right **H** Ankle, Left **J** Calcaneus, Right **K** Calcaneus, Left **L** Foot, Right **M** Foot, Left **P** Toe(s), Right **Q** Toe(s), Left **R** Lower Extremity, Right **S** Lower Extremity, Left **V** Patella, Right **W** Patella, Left **X** Foot/Toe Joint, Right **Y** Foot/Toe Joint, Left	**0** High Osmolar **1** Low Osmolar **Y** Other Contrast **Z** None	**Z** None	**Z** None

Continued →

Section B Imaging
Body System Q Non-Axial Lower Bones
Type 2 Computerized Tomography (CT Scan): Computer reformatted digital display of multiplanar images developed from the capture of multiple exposures of external ionizing radiation

Body Part (4th)	Contrast (5th)	Qualifier (6th)	Qualifier (7th)
B Tibia/Fibula, Right **C** Tibia/Fibula, Left	**0** High Osmolar **1** Low Osmolar **Y** Other Contrast	**Z** None	**Z** None

Section B Imaging
Body System Q Non-Axial Lower Bones
Type 3 Magnetic Resonance Imaging (MRI): Computer reformatted digital display of multiplanar images developed from the capture of radiofrequency signals emitted by nuclei in a body site excited within a magnetic field

Body Part (4th)	Contrast (5th)	Qualifier (6th)	Qualifier (7th)
0 Hip, Right **1** Hip, Left **3** Femur, Right **4** Femur, Left **7** Knee, Right **8** Knee, Left **D** Lower Leg, Right **F** Lower Leg, Left **G** Ankle, Right **H** Ankle, Left **J** Calcaneus, Right **K** Calcaneus, Left **L** Foot, Right **M** Foot, Left **P** Toe(s), Right **Q** Toe(s), Left **V** Patella, Right **W** Patella, Left	**Y** Other Contrast	**0** Unenhanced and Enhanced **Z** None	**Z** None
0 Hip, Right **1** Hip, Left **3** Femur, Right **4** Femur, Left **7** Knee, Right **8** Knee, Left **D** Lower Leg, Right **F** Lower Leg, Left **G** Ankle, Right **H** Ankle, Left **J** Calcaneus, Right **K** Calcaneus, Left **L** Foot, Right **M** Foot, Left **P** Toe(s), Right **Q** Toe(s), Left **V** Patella, Right **W** Patella, Left	**Z** None	**Z** None	**Z** None

Section B **Imaging**
Body System Q **Non-Axial Lower Bones**
Type 4 **Ultrasonography:** Real time display of images of anatomy or flow information developed from the capture of reflected and attenuated high frequency sound waves

Body Part (4th)	Contrast (5th)	Qualifier (6th)	Qualifier (7th)
0 Hip, Right 1 Hip, Left 2 Hips, Bilateral 7 Knee, Right 8 Knee, Left 9 Knees, Bilateral	Z None	Z None	Z None

Section B **Imaging**
Body System R **Axial Skeleton, Except Skull and Facial Bones**
Type 0 **Plain Radiography:** Planar display of an image developed from the capture of external ionizing radiation on photographic or photoconductive plate

Body Part (4th)	Contrast (5th)	Qualifier (6th)	Qualifier (7th)
0 Cervical Spine 7 Thoracic Spine 9 Lumbar Spine G Whole Spine	Z None	Z None	1 Densitometry Z None
1 Cervical Disc(s) 2 Thoracic Disc(s) 3 Lumbar Disc(s) 4 Cervical Facet Joint(s) 5 Thoracic Facet Joint(s) 6 Lumbar Facet Joint(s) D Sacroiliac Joints	0 High Osmolar 1 Low Osmolar Y Other Contrast Z None	Z None	Z None
8 Thoracolumbar Joint B Lumbosacral Joint C Pelvis F Sacrum and Coccyx H Sternum	Z None	Z None	Z None

Section B **Imaging**
Body System R **Axial Skeleton, Except Skull and Facial Bones**
Type 1 **Fluoroscopy:** Single plane or bi-plane real time display of an image developed from the capture of external ionizing radiation on a fluorescent screen. The image may also be stored by either digital or analog means

Body Part (4th)	Contrast (5th)	Qualifier (6th)	Qualifier (7th)
0 Cervical Spine 1 Cervical Disc(s) 2 Thoracic Disc(s) 3 Lumbar Disc(s) 4 Cervical Facet Joint(s) 5 Thoracic Facet Joint(s) 6 Lumbar Facet Joint(s) 7 Thoracic Spine 8 Thoracolumbar Joint 9 Lumbar Spine B Lumbosacral Joint C Pelvis D Sacroiliac Joints F Sacrum and Coccyx G Whole Spine H Sternum	0 High Osmolar 1 Low Osmolar Y Other Contrast Z None	Z None	Z None

Section B **Imaging**
Body System R **Axial Skeleton, Except Skull and Facial Bones**
Type 2 **Computerized Tomography (CT Scan):** Computer reformatted digital display of multiplanar images developed from the capture of multiple exposures of external ionizing radiation

Body Part (4th)	Contrast (5th)	Qualifier (6th)	Qualifier (7th)
0 Cervical Spine **7** Thoracic Spine **9** Lumbar Spine **C** Pelvis **D** Sacroiliac Joints **F** Sacrum and Coccyx	**0** High Osmolar **1** Low Osmolar **Y** Other Contrast **Z** None	**Z** None	**Z** None

Section B **Imaging**
Body System R **Axial Skeleton, Except Skull and Facial Bones**
Type 3 **Magnetic Resonance Imaging (MRI):** Computer reformatted digital display of multiplanar images developed from the capture of radiofrequency signals emitted by nuclei in a body site excited within a magnetic field

Body Part (4th)	Contrast (5th)	Qualifier (6th)	Qualifier (7th)
0 Cervical Spine **1** Cervical Disc(s) **2** Thoracic Disc(s) **3** Lumbar Disc(s) **7** Thoracic Spine **9** Lumbar Spine **C** Pelvis **F** Sacrum and Coccyx	**Y** Other Contrast	**0** Unenhanced and Enhanced **Z** None	**Z** None
0 Cervical Spine **1** Cervical Disc(s) **2** Thoracic Disc(s) **3** Lumbar Disc(s) **7** Thoracic Spine **9** Lumbar Spine **C** Pelvis **F** Sacrum and Coccyx	**Z** None	**Z** None	**Z** None

Section B **Imaging**
Body System R **Axial Skeleton, Except Skull and Facial Bones**
Type 4 **Ultrasonography:** Real time display of images of anatomy or flow information developed from the capture of reflected and attenuated high frequency sound waves

Body Part (4th)	Contrast (5th)	Qualifier (6th)	Qualifier (7th)
0 Cervical Spine **7** Thoracic Spine **9** Lumbar Spine **F** Sacrum and Coccyx	**Z** None	**Z** None	**Z** None

Section B **Imaging**
Body System T **Urinary System**
Type 0 **Plain Radiography:** Planar display of an image developed from the capture of external ionizing radiation on photographic or photoconductive plate

Body Part (4th)	Contrast (5th)	Qualifier (6th)	Qualifier (7th)
0 Bladder **1** Kidney, Right **2** Kidney, Left **3** Kidneys, Bilateral **4** Kidneys, Ureters and Bladder **5** Urethra **6** Ureter, Right **7** Ureter, Left **8** Ureters, Bilateral **B** Bladder and Urethra **C** Ileal Diversion Loop	**0** High Osmolar **1** Low Osmolar **Y** Other Contrast **Z** None	**Z** None	**Z** None

Section B **Imaging**
Body System T **Urinary System**
Type 1 **Fluoroscopy:** Single plane or bi-plane real time display of an image developed from the capture of external ionizing radiation on a fluorescent screen. The image may also be stored by either digital or analog means

Body Part (4th)	Contrast (5th)	Qualifier (6th)	Qualifier (7th)
0 Bladder 1 Kidney, Right 2 Kidney, Left 3 Kidneys, Bilateral 4 Kidneys, Ureters and Bladder 5 Urethra 6 Ureter, Right 7 Ureter, Left B Bladder and Urethra C Ileal Diversion Loop D Kidney, Ureter and Bladder, Right F Kidney, Ureter and Bladder, Left G Ileal Loop, Ureters and Kidneys	0 High Osmolar 1 Low Osmolar Y Other Contrast Z None	Z None	Z None

Section B **Imaging**
Body System T **Urinary System**
Type 2 **Computerized Tomography (CT Scan):** Computer reformatted digital display of multiplanar images developed from the capture of multiple exposures of external ionizing radiation

Body Part (4th)	Contrast (5th)	Qualifier (6th)	Qualifier (7th)
0 Bladder 1 Kidney, Right 2 Kidney, Left 3 Kidneys, Bilateral 9 Kidney Transplant	0 High Osmolar 1 Low Osmolar Y Other Contrast	0 Unenhanced and Enhanced Z None	Z None
0 Bladder 1 Kidney, Right 2 Kidney, Left 3 Kidneys, Bilateral 9 Kidney Transplant	Z None	Z None	Z None

Section B **Imaging**
Body System T **Urinary System**
Type 3 **Magnetic Resonance Imaging (MRI):** Computer reformatted digital display of multiplanar images developed from the capture of radiofrequency signals emitted by nuclei in a body site excited within a magnetic field

Body Part (4th)	Contrast (5th)	Qualifier (6th)	Qualifier (7th)
0 Bladder 1 Kidney, Right 2 Kidney, Left 3 Kidneys, Bilateral 9 Kidney Transplant	Y Other Contrast	0 Unenhanced and Enhanced Z None	Z None
0 Bladder 1 Kidney, Right 2 Kidney, Left 3 Kidneys, Bilateral 9 Kidney Transplant	Z None	Z None	Z None

Section B **Imaging**
Body System T **Urinary System**
Type 4 **Ultrasonography:** Real time display of images of anatomy or flow information developed from the capture of reflected and attenuated high frequency sound waves

Body Part (4th)	Contrast (5th)	Qualifier (6th)	Qualifier (7th)
0 Bladder 1 Kidney, Right 2 Kidney, Left 3 Kidneys, Bilateral 5 Urethra 6 Ureter, Right 7 Ureter, Left 8 Ureters, Bilateral 9 Kidney Transplant J Kidneys and Bladder	Z None	Z None	Z None

Section B **Imaging**
Body System U **Female Reproductive System**
Type 0 **Plain Radiography:** Planar display of an image developed from the capture of external ionizing radiation on photographic or photoconductive plate

Body Part (4th)	Contrast (5th)	Qualifier (6th)	Qualifier (7th)
0 Fallopian Tube, Right 1 Fallopian Tube, Left 2 Fallopian Tubes, Bilateral 6 Uterus 8 Uterus and Fallopian Tubes 9 Vagina	0 High Osmolar 1 Low Osmolar Y Other Contrast	Z None	Z None

Section B **Imaging**
Body System U **Female Reproductive System**
Type 1 **Fluoroscopy:** Single plane or bi-plane real time display of an image developed from the capture of external ionizing radiation on a fluorescent screen. The image may also be stored by either digital or analog means

Body Part (4th)	Contrast (5th)	Qualifier (6th)	Qualifier (7th)
0 Fallopian Tube, Right 1 Fallopian Tube, Left 2 Fallopian Tubes, Bilateral 6 Uterus 8 Uterus and Fallopian Tubes 9 Vagina	0 High Osmolar 1 Low Osmolar Y Other Contrast Z None	Z None	Z None

Section B **Imaging**
Body System U **Female Reproductive System**
Type 3 **Magnetic Resonance Imaging (MRI):** Computer reformatted digital display of multiplanar images developed from the capture of radiofrequency signals emitted by nuclei in a body site excited within a magnetic field

Body Part (4th)	Contrast (5th)	Qualifier (6th)	Qualifier (7th)
3 Ovary, Right 4 Ovary, Left 5 Ovaries, Bilateral 6 Uterus 9 Vagina B Pregnant Uterus C Uterus and Ovaries	Y Other Contrast	0 Unenhanced and Enhanced Z None	Z None
3 Ovary, Right 4 Ovary, Left 5 Ovaries, Bilateral 6 Uterus 9 Vagina B Pregnant Uterus C Uterus and Ovaries	Z None	Z None	Z None

Section B **Imaging**
Body System U **Female Reproductive System**
Type 4 **Ultrasonography:** Real time display of images of anatomy or flow information developed from the capture of reflected and attenuated high frequency sound waves

Body Part (4th)	Contrast (5th)	Qualifier (6th)	Qualifier (7th)
0 Fallopian Tube, Right **1** Fallopian Tube, Left **2** Fallopian Tubes, Bilateral **3** Ovary, Right **4** Ovary, Left **5** Ovaries, Bilateral **6** Uterus **C** Uterus and Ovaries	**Y** Other Contrast **Z** None	**Z** None	**Z** None

Section B **Imaging**
Body System V **Male Reproductive System**
Type 0 **Plain Radiography:** Planar display of an image developed from the capture of external ionizing radiation on photographic or photoconductive plate

Body Part (4th)	Contrast (5th)	Qualifier (6th)	Qualifier (7th)
0 Corpora Cavernosa **1** Epididymis, Right **2** Epididymis, Left **3** Prostate **5** Testicle, Right **6** Testicle, Left **8** Vasa Vasorum	**0** High Osmolar **1** Low Osmolar **Y** Other Contrast	**Z** None	**Z** None

Section B **Imaging**
Body System V **Male Reproductive System**
Type 1 **Fluoroscopy:** Single plane or bi-plane real time display of an image developed from the capture of external ionizing radiation on a fluorescent screen. The image may also be stored by either digital or analog means

Body Part (4th)	Contrast (5th)	Qualifier (6th)	Qualifier (7th)
0 Corpora Cavernosa **8** Vasa Vasorum	**0** High Osmolar **1** Low Osmolar **Y** Other Contrast **Z** None	**Z** None	**Z** None

Section B **Imaging**
Body System V **Male Reproductive System**
Type 2 **Computerized Tomography (CT Scan):** Computer reformatted digital display of multiplanar images developed from the capture of multiple exposures of external ionizing radiation

Body Part (4th)	Contrast (5th)	Qualifier (6th)	Qualifier (7th)
3 Prostate	**0** High Osmolar **1** Low Osmolar **Y** Other Contrast	**0** Unenhanced and Enhanced **Z** None	**Z** None
3 Prostate	**Z** None	**Z** None	**Z** None

Section B Imaging
Body System V Male Reproductive System
Type 3 Magnetic Resonance Imaging (MRI): Computer reformatted digital display of multiplanar images developed from the capture of radiofrequency signals emitted by nuclei in a body site excited within a magnetic field

Body Part (4th)	Contrast (5th)	Qualifier (6th)	Qualifier (7th)
0 Corpora Cavernosa 3 Prostate 4 Scrotum 5 Testicle, Right 6 Testicle, Left 7 Testicles, Bilateral	Y Other Contrast	0 Unenhanced and Enhanced Z None	Z None
0 Corpora Cavernosa 3 Prostate 4 Scrotum 5 Testicle, Right 6 Testicle, Left 7 Testicles, Bilateral	Z None	Z None	Z None

Section B Imaging
Body System V Male Reproductive System
Type 4 Ultrasonography: Real time display of images of anatomy or flow information developed from the capture of reflected and attenuated high frequency sound waves

Body Part (4th)	Contrast (5th)	Qualifier (6th)	Qualifier (7th)
4 Scrotum 9 Prostate and Seminal Vesicles B Penis	Z None	Z None	Z None

Section B Imaging
Body System W Anatomical Regions
Type 0 Plain Radiography: Planar display of an image developed from the capture of external ionizing radiation on photographic or photoconductive plate

Body Part (4th)	Contrast (5th)	Qualifier (6th)	Qualifier (7th)
0 Abdomen 1 Abdomen and Pelvis 3 Chest B Long Bones, All C Lower Extremity J Upper Extremity K Whole Body L Whole Skeleton M Whole Body, Infant	Z None	Z None	Z None

Section B Imaging
Body System W Anatomical Regions
Type 1 Fluoroscopy: Single plane or bi-plane real time display of an image developed from the capture of external ionizing radiation on a fluorescent screen. The image may also be stored by either digital or analog means

Body Part (4th)	Contrast (5th)	Qualifier (6th)	Qualifier (7th)
1 Abdomen and Pelvis 9 Head and Neck C Lower Extremity J Upper Extremity	0 High Osmolar 1 Low Osmolar Y Other Contrast Z None	Z None	Z None

Section B **Imaging**
Body System W **Anatomical Regions**
Type 2 **Computerized Tomography (CT Scan):** Computer reformatted digital display of multiplanar images developed from the capture of multiple exposures of external ionizing radiation

Body Part (4th)	Contrast (5th)	Qualifier (6th)	Qualifier (7th)
0 Abdomen **1** Abdomen and Pelvis **4** Chest and Abdomen **5** Chest, Abdomen and Pelvis **8** Head **9** Head and Neck **F** Neck **G** Pelvic Region	**0** High Osmolar **1** Low Osmolar **Y** Other Contrast	**0** Unenhanced and Enhanced **Z** None	**Z** None
0 Abdomen **1** Abdomen and Pelvis **4** Chest and Abdomen **5** Chest, Abdomen and Pelvis **8** Head **9** Head and Neck **F** Neck **G** Pelvic Region	**Z** None	**Z** None	**Z** None

Section B **Imaging**
Body System W **Anatomical Regions**
Type 3 **Magnetic Resonance Imaging (MRI):** Computer reformatted digital display of multiplanar images developed from the capture of radiofrequency signals emitted by nuclei in a body site excited within a magnetic field

Body Part (4th)	Contrast (5th)	Qualifier (6th)	Qualifier (7th)
0 Abdomen **8** Head **F** Neck **G** Pelvic Region **H** Retroperitoneum **P** Brachial Plexus	**Y** Other Contrast	**0** Unenhanced and Enhanced **Z** None	**Z** None
0 Abdomen **8** Head **F** Neck **G** Pelvic Region **H** Retroperitoneum **P** Brachial Plexus	**Z** None	**Z** None	**Z** None
3 Chest	**Y** Other Contrast	**0** Unenhanced and Enhanced **Z** None	**Z** None

Section B **Imaging**
Body System W **Anatomical Regions**
Type 4 **Ultrasonography:** Real time display of images of anatomy or flow information developed from the capture of reflected and attenuated high frequency sound waves

Body Part (4th)	Contrast (5th)	Qualifier (6th)	Qualifier (7th)
0 Abdomen **1** Abdomen and Pelvis **F** Neck **G** Pelvic Region	**Z** None	**Z** None	**Z** None

Section B **Imaging**
Body System W **Anatomical Regions**
Type 5 **Other Imaging:** Other specified modality for visualizing a body part

Body Part (4th)	Contrast (5th)	Qualifier (6th)	Qualifier (7th)
2 Trunk **9** Head and Neck **C** Lower Extremity **J** Upper Extremi	**Z** None	**1** Bacterial Autofluorescence	**Z** None

Section B **Imaging**
Body System Y **Fetus and Obstetrical**
Type 3 **Magnetic Resonance Imaging (MRI):** Computer reformatted digital display of multiplanar images developed from the capture of radiofrequency signals emitted by nuclei in a body site excited within a magnetic field

Body Part (4th)	Contrast (5th)	Qualifier (6th)	Qualifier (7th)
0 Fetal Head **1** Fetal Heart **2** Fetal Thorax **3** Fetal Abdomen **4** Fetal Spine **5** Fetal Extremities **6** Whole Fetus	**Y** Other Contrast	**0** Unenhanced and Enhanced **Z** None	**Z** None
0 Fetal Head **1** Fetal Heart **2** Fetal Thorax **3** Fetal Abdomen **4** Fetal Spine **5** Fetal Extremities **6** Whole Fetus	**Z** None	**Z** None	**Z** None

Section B **Imaging**
Body System Y **Fetus and Obstetrical**
Type 4 **Ultrasonography:** Real time display of images of anatomy or flow information developed from the capture of reflected and attenuated high frequency sound waves

Body Part (4th)	Contrast (5th)	Qualifier (6th)	Qualifier (7th)
7 Fetal Umbilical Cord **8** Placenta **9** First Trimester, Single Fetus **B** First Trimester, Multiple Gestation **C** Second Trimester, Single Fetus **D** Second Trimester, Multiple Gestation **F** Third Trimester, Single Fetus **G** Third Trimester, Multiple Gestation	**Z** None	**Z** None	**Z** None

AHA Coding Clinic

B2151ZZ Fluoroscopy of Left Heart using Low Osmolar Contrast—AHA CC: 1Q, 2018, 12-13

B518ZZA Fluoroscopy of Superior Vena Cava, Guidance, for Fluoroscopic Guidance used to Place the Renal Dialysis Catheter—AHA CC: 4Q, 2015, 30

BF50200 Other Imaging of Bile Ducts using Fluorescing Agent, Indocyanine Green Dye, Intraoperative—AHA CC: 4Q, 2020, 67-68

Nuclear Medicine Section (C01–CW7)

Within each section of ICD-10-PCS the characters have different meanings. The seven character meanings for the Nuclear Medicine section are illustrated here through the procedure example of *Technetium tomo scan of liver*.

Section	Body System	Root Type	Body Part	Radionuclide	Qualifier	Qualifier
Nuclear Medicine	Hepatobiliary and Pancreas	Tomographic (Tomo)	Liver	Technetium 99m	None	None
C	F	2	5	1	Z	Z

Section (Character 1)

All Nuclear Medicine procedure codes have a first character value of C.

Body System (Character 2)

The alphanumeric character for the body system is placed in the second position. The following are the body systems applicable to the Nuclear Medicine section.

Character Value	Character Value Description
0	Central Nervous System
2	Heart
5	Veins
7	Lymphatic System
8	Eye
9	Ear, Nose, Mouth and Throat
B	Respiratory System
D	Gastrointestinal System
F	Hepatobiliary System and Pancreas
G	Endocrine System
H	Skin, Subcutaneous Tissue and Breast
P	Musculoskeletal
T	Urinary System
V	Male Reproductive System
W	Anatomical Regions

Root Types (Character 3)

The alphanumeric character value for root types is placed in the third position. The following are the root types applicable to the Nuclear Medicine section with their associated meaning.

Character Value	Root Type	Root Type Definition
1	Planar Nuclear Medicine Imaging	Introduction of radioactive materials into the body for single plane display of images developed from the capture of radioactive emissions
2	Tomographic (Tomo) Nuclear Medicine Imaging	Introduction of radioactive materials into the body for three dimensional display of images developed from the capture of radioactive emissions
3	Positron Emission Tomographic (PET) Imaging	Introduction of radioactive materials into the body for three dimensional display of images developed from the simultaneous capture, 180 degrees apart, of radioactive emissions
4	Nonimaging Nuclear Medicine Uptake	Introduction of radioactive materials into the body for measurements of organ function, from the detection of radioactive emissions
5	Nonimaging Nuclear Medicine Probe	Introduction of radioactive materials into the body for the study of distribution and fate of certain substances by the detection of radioactive emissions; or, alternatively, measurement of absorption of radioactive emissions from an external source

Continued →

Character Value	Root Type	Root Type Definition
6	Nonimaging Nuclear Medicine Assay	Introduction of radioactive materials into the body for the study of body fluids and blood elements, by the detection of radioactive emissions
7	Systemic Nuclear Medicine Therapy	Introduction of unsealed radioactive materials into the body for treatment

Body Part (Character 4)

For each body part the applicable body part character values will be available for procedure code construction. An example of a body part is Cerebrospinal Fluid.

Radionuclide (Character 5)

When radionuclide is utilized during a nuclear medicine procedure, the corresponding radionuclide character value should be reported in the fifth character position. The following are examples of the radionuclide character values available for the Nuclear Medicine section.

- Krypton (Kr-81m)
- Technetium 99m (Tc-99m)
- Xenon 127 (Xe-127)
- Xenon 133 (Xe-133)
- Other Radionuclide

If radionuclide is not utilized, the placeholder character value of Z should be reported.

Qualifier (Character 6)

The qualifier represents an additional attribute for the procedure when applicable. Currently, there are no qualifiers in the Nuclear Medicine section; therefore, the placeholder character value of Z should be reported.

Qualifier (Character 7)

The qualifier represents an additional attribute for the procedure when applicable. Currently, there are no qualifiers in the Nuclear Medicine section; therefore, the placeholder character value of Z should be reported.

Nuclear Medicine Section Tables

Nuclear Medicine Tables C01–CW7

Section C **Nuclear Medicine**
Body System 0 **Central Nervous System**
Type 1 **Planar Nuclear Medicine Imaging:** Introduction of radioactive materials into the body for single plane display of images developed from the capture of radioactive emissions

Body Part (4th)	Radionuclide (5th)	Qualifier (6th)	Qualifier (7th)
0 Brain	**1** Technetium 99m (Tc-99m) **Y** Other Radionuclide	**Z** None	**Z** None
5 Cerebrospinal Fluid	**D** Indium 111 (In-111) **Y** Other Radionuclide	**Z** None	**Z** None
Y Central Nervous System	**Y** Other Radionuclide	**Z** None	**Z** None

Section C **Nuclear Medicine**
Body System 0 **Central Nervous System**
Type 2 **Tomographic (Tomo) Nuclear Medicine Imaging:** Introduction of radioactive materials into the body for three dimensional display of images developed from the capture of radioactive emissions

Body Part (4th)	Radionuclide (5th)	Qualifier (6th)	Qualifier (7th)
0 Brain	**1** Technetium 99m (Tc-99m) **F** Iodine 123 (I-123) **S** Thallium 201 (Tl-201) **Y** Other Radionuclide	**Z** None	**Z** None
5 Cerebrospinal Fluid	**D** Indium 111 (In-111) **Y** Other Radionuclide	**Z** None	**Z** None
Y Central Nervous System	**Y** Other Radionuclide	**Z** None	**Z** None

Section C **Nuclear Medicine**
Body System 0 **Central Nervous System**
Type 3 **Positron Emission Tomographic (PET) Imaging:** Introduction of radioactive materials into the body for three dimensional display of images developed from the simultaneous capture, 180 degrees apart, of radioactive emissions

Body Part (4th)	Radionuclide (5th)	Qualifier (6th)	Qualifier (7th)
0 Brain	**B** Carbon 11 (C-11) **K** Fluorine 18 (F-18) **M** Oxygen 15 (O-15) **Y** Other Radionuclide	**Z** None	**Z** None
Y Central Nervous System	**Y** Other Radionuclide	**Z** None	**Z** None

Section C **Nuclear Medicine**
Body System 0 **Central Nervous System**
Type 5 **Nonimaging Nuclear Medicine Probe:** Introduction of radioactive materials into the body for the study of distribution and fate of certain substances by the detection of radioactive emissions; or, alternatively, measurement of absorption of radioactive emissions from an external source

Body Part (4th)	Radionuclide (5th)	Qualifier (6th)	Qualifier (7th)
0 Brain	**V** Xenon 133 (Xe-133) **Y** Other Radionuclide	**Z** None	**Z** None
Y Central Nervous System	**Y** Other Radionuclide	**Z** None	**Z** None

Section C **Nuclear Medicine**
Body System 2 **Heart**
Type 1 **Planar Nuclear Medicine Imaging:** Introduction of radioactive materials into the body for single plane display of images developed from the capture of radioactive emissions

Body Part (4th)	Radionuclide (5th)	Qualifier (6th)	Qualifier (7th)
6 Heart, Right and Left	**1** Technetium 99m (Tc-99m) **Y** Other Radionuclide	**Z** None	**Z** None
G Myocardium	**1** Technetium 99m (Tc-99m) **D** Indium 111 (In-111) **S** Thallium 201 (Tl-201) **Y** Other Radionuclide **Z** None	**Z** None	**Z** None
Y Heart	**Y** Other Radionuclide	**Z** None	**Z** None

Section C Nuclear Medicine
Body System 2 Heart
Type 2 Tomographic (Tomo) Nuclear Medicine Imaging: Introduction of radioactive materials into the body for three dimensional display of images developed from the capture of radioactive emissions

Body Part (4th)	Radionuclide (5th)	Qualifier (6th)	Qualifier (7th)
6 Heart, Right and Left	1 Technetium 99m (Tc-99m) Y Other Radionuclide	Z None	Z None
G Myocardium	1 Technetium 99m (Tc-99m) D Indium 111 (In-111) K Fluorine 18 (F-18) S Thallium 201 (Tl-201) Y Other Radionuclide Z None	Z None	Z None
Y Heart	Y Other Radionuclide	Z None	Z None

Section C Nuclear Medicine
Body System 2 Heart
Type 3 Positron Emission Tomographic (PET) Imaging: Introduction of radioactive materials into the body for three dimensional display of images developed from the simultaneous capture, 180 degrees apart, of radioactive emissions

Body Part (4th)	Radionuclide (5th)	Qualifier (6th)	Qualifier (7th)
G Myocardium	K Fluorine 18 (F-18) M Oxygen 15 (O-15) Q Rubidium 82 (Rb-82) R Nitrogen 13 (N-13) Y Other Radionuclide	Z None	Z None
Y Heart	Y Other Radionuclide	Z None	Z None

Section C Nuclear Medicine
Body System 2 Heart
Type 5 Nonimaging Nuclear Medicine Probe: Introduction of radioactive materials into the body for the study of distribution and fate of certain substances by the detection of radioactive emissions; or, alternatively, measurement of absorption of radioactive emissions from an external source

Body Part (4th)	Radionuclide (5th)	Qualifier (6th)	Qualifier (7th)
6 Heart, Right and Left	1 Technetium 99m (Tc-99m) Y Other Radionuclide	Z None	Z None
Y Heart	Y Other Radionuclide	Z None	Z None

Section C Nuclear Medicine
Body System 5 Veins
Type 1 Planar Nuclear Medicine Imaging: Introduction of radioactive materials into the body for single plane display of images developed from the capture of radioactive emissions

Body Part (4th)	Radionuclide (5th)	Qualifier (6th)	Qualifier (7th)
B Lower Extremity Veins, Right C Lower Extremity Veins, Left D Lower Extremity Veins, Bilateral N Upper Extremity Veins, Right P Upper Extremity Veins, Left Q Upper Extremity Veins, Bilateral R Central Veins	1 Technetium 99m (Tc-99m) Y Other Radionuclide	Z None	Z None
Y Veins	Y Other Radionuclide	Z None	Z None

Section C **Nuclear Medicine**
Body System 7 **Lymphatic and Hematologic System**
Type 1 **Planar Nuclear Medicine Imaging:** Introduction of radioactive materials into the body for single plane display of images developed from the capture of radioactive emissions

Body Part (4th)	Radionuclide (5th)	Qualifier (6th)	Qualifier (7th)
0 Bone Marrow	**1** Technetium 99m (Tc-99m) **D** Indium 111 (In-111) **Y** Other Radionuclide	**Z** None	**Z** None
2 Spleen **5** Lymphatics, Head and Neck **D** Lymphatics, Pelvic **J** Lymphatics, Head **K** Lymphatics, Neck **L** Lymphatics, Upper Chest **M** Lymphatics, Trunk **N** Lymphatics, Upper Extremity **P** Lymphatics, Lower Extremity	**1** Technetium 99m (Tc-99m) **Y** Other Radionuclide	**Z** None	**Z** None
3 Blood	**D** Indium 111 (In-111) **Y** Other Radionuclide	**Z** None	**Z** None
Y Lymphatic and Hematologic System	**Y** Other Radionuclide	**Z** None	**Z** None

Section C **Nuclear Medicine**
Body System 7 **Lymphatic and Hematologic System**
Type 2 **Tomographic (Tomo) Nuclear Medicine Imaging:** Introduction of radioactive materials into the body for three dimensional display of images developed from the capture of radioactive emissions

Body Part (4th)	Radionuclide (5th)	Qualifier (6th)	Qualifier (7th)
2 Spleen	**1** Technetium 99m (Tc-99m) **Y** Other Radionuclide	**Z** None	**Z** None
Y Lymphatic and Hematologic System	**Y** Other Radionuclide	**Z** None	**Z** None

Section C **Nuclear Medicine**
Body System 7 **Lymphatic and Hematologic System**
Type 5 **Nonimaging Nuclear Medicine Probe:** Introduction of radioactive materials into the body for the study of distribution and fate of certain substances by the detection of radioactive emissions; or, alternatively, measurement of absorption of radioactive emissions from an external source

Body Part (4th)	Radionuclide (5th)	Qualifier (6th)	Qualifier (7th)
5 Lymphatics, Head and Neck **D** Lymphatics, Pelvic **J** Lymphatics, Head **K** Lymphatics, Neck **L** Lymphatics, Upper Chest **M** Lymphatics, Trunk **N** Lymphatics, Upper Extremity **P** Lymphatics, Lower Extremity	**1** Technetium 99m (Tc-99m) **Y** Other Radionuclide	**Z** None	**Z** None
Y Lymphatic and Hematologic System	**Y** Other Radionuclide	**Z** None	**Z** None

Section C Nuclear Medicine
Body System 7 Lymphatic and Hematologic System
Type 6 Nonimaging Nuclear Medicine Assay: Introduction of radioactive materials into the body for the study of body fluids and blood elements, by the detection of radioactive emissions

Body Part (4th)	Radionuclide (5th)	Qualifier (6th)	Qualifier (7th)
3 Blood	1 Technetium 99m (Tc-99m) 7 Cobalt 58 (Co-58) C Cobalt 57 (Co-57) D Indium 111 (In-111) H Iodine 125 (I-125) W Chromium (Cr-51) Y Other Radionuclide	Z None	Z None
Y Lymphatic and Hematologic System	Y Other Radionuclide	Z None	Z None

Section C Nuclear Medicine
Body System 8 Eye
Type 1 Planar Nuclear Medicine Imaging: Introduction of radioactive materials into the body for single plane display of images developed from the capture of radioactive emissions

Body Part (4th)	Radionuclide (5th)	Qualifier (6th)	Qualifier (7th)
9 Lacrimal Ducts, Bilateral	1 Technetium 99m (Tc-99m) Y Other Radionuclide	Z None	Z None
Y Eye	Y Other Radionuclide	Z None	Z None

Section C Nuclear Medicine
Body System 9 Ear, Nose, Mouth and Throat
Type 1 Planar Nuclear Medicine Imaging: Introduction of radioactive materials into the body for single plane display of images developed from the capture of radioactive emissions

Body Part (4th)	Radionuclide (5th)	Qualifier (6th)	Qualifier (7th)
B Salivary Glands, Bilateral	1 Technetium 99m (Tc-99m) Y Other Radionuclide	Z None	Z None
Y Ear, Nose, Mouth and Throat	Y Other Radionuclide	Z None	Z None

Section C Nuclear Medicine
Body System B Respiratory System
Type 1 Planar Nuclear Medicine Imaging: Introduction of radioactive materials into the body for single plane display of images developed from the capture of radioactive emissions

Body Part (4th)	Radionuclide (5th)	Qualifier (6th)	Qualifier (7th)
2 Lungs and Bronchi	1 Technetium 99m (Tc-99m) 9 Krypton (Kr-81m) T Xenon 127 (Xe-127) V Xenon 133 (Xe-133) Y Other Radionuclide	Z None	Z None
Y Respiratory System	Y Other Radionuclide	Z None	Z None

Section C Nuclear Medicine
Body System B Respiratory System
Type 2 Tomographic (Tomo) Nuclear Medicine Imaging: Introduction of radioactive materials into the body for three dimensional display of images developed from the capture of radioactive emissions

Body Part (4th)	Radionuclide (5th)	Qualifier (6th)	Qualifier (7th)
2 Lungs and Bronchi	1 Technetium 99m (Tc-99m) 9 Krypton (Kr-81m) Y Other Radionuclide	Z None	Z None
Y Respiratory System	Y Other Radionuclide	Z Nonc	Z None

Section C **Nuclear Medicine**
Body System B **Respiratory System**
Type 3 **Positron Emission Tomographic (PET) Imaging:** Introduction of radioactive materials into the body for three dimensional display of images developed from the simultaneous capture, 180 degrees apart, of radioactive emissions

Body Part (4th)	Radionuclide (5th)	Qualifier (6th)	Qualifier (7th)
2 Lungs and Bronchi	K Fluorine 18 (F-18) Y Other Radionuclide	Z None	Z None
Y Respiratory System	Y Other Radionuclide	Z None	Z None

Section C **Nuclear Medicine**
Body System D **Gastrointestinal System**
Type 1 **Planar Nuclear Medicine Imaging:** Introduction of radioactive materials into the body for single plane display of images developed from the capture of radioactive emissions

Body Part (4th)	Radionuclide (5th)	Qualifier (6th)	Qualifier (7th)
5 Upper Gastrointestinal Tract 7 Gastrointestinal Tract	1 Technetium 99m (Tc-99m) D Indium 111 (In-111) Y Other Radionuclide	Z None	Z None
Y Digestive System	Y Other Radionuclide	Z None	Z None

Section C **Nuclear Medicine**
Body System D **Gastrointestinal System**
Type 2 **Tomographic (Tomo) Nuclear Medicine Imaging:** Introduction of radioactive materials into the body for three dimensional display of images developed from the capture of radioactive emissions

Body Part (4th)	Radionuclide (5th)	Qualifier (6th)	Qualifier (7th)
7 Gastrointestinal Tract	1 Technetium 99m (Tc-99m) D Indium 111 (In-111) Y Other Radionuclide	Z None	Z None
Y Digestive System	Y Other Radionuclide	Z None	Z None

Section C **Nuclear Medicine**
Body System F **Hepatobiliary System and Pancreas**
Type 1 **Planar Nuclear Medicine Imaging:** Introduction of radioactive materials into the body for single plane display of images developed from the capture of radioactive emissions

Body Part (4th)	Radionuclide (5th)	Qualifier (6th)	Qualifier (7th)
4 Gallbladder 5 Liver 6 Liver and Spleen C Hepatobiliary System, All	1 Technetium 99m (Tc-99m) Y Other Radionuclide	Z None	Z None
Y Hepatobiliary System and Pancreas	Y Other Radionuclide	Z None	Z None

Section C **Nuclear Medicine**
Body System F **Hepatobiliary System and Pancreas**
Type 2 **Tomographic (Tomo) Nuclear Medicine Imaging:** Introduction of radioactive materials into the body for three dimensional display of images developed from the capture of radioactive emissions

Body Part (4th)	Radionuclide (5th)	Qualifier (6th)	Qualifier (7th)
4 Gallbladder 5 Liver 6 Liver and Spleen	1 Technetium 99m (Tc-99m) Y Other Radionuclide	Z None	Z None
Y Hepatobiliary System and Pancreas	Y Other Radionuclide	Z None	Z None

Section C Nuclear Medicine
Body System G Endocrine System
Type 1 Planar Nuclear Medicine Imaging: Introduction of radioactive materials into the body for single plane display of images developed from the capture of radioactive emissions

Body Part (4th)	Radionuclide (5th)	Qualifier (6th)	Qualifier (7th)
1 Parathyroid Glands	1 Technetium 99m (Tc-99m) S Thallium 201 (Tl-201) Y Other Radionuclide	Z None	Z None
2 Thyroid Gland	1 Technetium 99m (Tc-99m) F Iodine 123 (I-123) G Iodine 131 (I-131) Y Other Radionuclide	Z None	Z None
4 Adrenal Glands, Bilateral	G Iodine 131 (I-131) Y Other Radionuclide	Z None	Z None
Y Endocrine System	Y Other Radionuclide	Z None	Z None

Section C Nuclear Medicine
Body System G Endocrine System
Type 2 Tomographic (Tomo) Nuclear Medicine Imaging: Introduction of radioactive materials into the body for three dimensional display of images developed from the capture of radioactive emissions

Body Part (4th)	Radionuclide (5th)	Qualifier (6th)	Qualifier (7th)
1 Parathyroid Glands	1 Technetium 99m (Tc-99m) S Thallium 201 (Tl-201) Y Other Radionuclide	Z None	Z None
Y Endocrine System	Y Other Radionuclide	Z None	Z None

Section C Nuclear Medicine
Body System G Endocrine System
Type 4 Nonimaging Nuclear Medicine Uptake: Introduction of radioactive materials into the body for measurements of organ function, from the detection of radioactive emissions

Body Part (4th)	Radionuclide (5th)	Qualifier (6th)	Qualifier (7th)
2 Thyroid Gland	1 Technetium 99m (Tc-99m) F Iodine 123 (I-123) G Iodine 131 (I-131) Y Other Radionuclide	Z None	Z None
Y Endocrine System	Y Other Radionuclide	Z None	Z None

Section C Nuclear Medicine
Body System H Skin, Subcutaneous Tissue and Breast
Type 1 Planar Nuclear Medicine Imaging: Introduction of radioactive materials into the body for single plane display of images developed from the capture of radioactive emissions

Body Part (4th)	Radionuclide (5th)	Qualifier (6th)	Qualifier (7th)
0 Breast, Right 1 Breast, Left 2 Breasts, Bilateral	1 Technetium 99m (Tc-99m) S Thallium 201 (Tl-201) Y Other Radionuclide	Z None	Z None
Y Skin, Subcutaneous Tissue and Breast	Y Other Radionuclide	Z None	Z None

Section C **Nuclear Medicine**
Body System H **Skin, Subcutaneous Tissue and Breast**
Type 2 **Tomographic (Tomo) Nuclear Medicine Imaging:** Introduction of radioactive materials into the body for three dimensional display of images developed from the capture of radioactive emissions

Body Part (4th)	Radionuclide (5th)	Qualifier (6th)	Qualifier (7th)
0 Breast, Right 1 Breast, Left 2 Breasts, Bilateral	1 Technetium 99m (Tc-99m) S Thallium 201 (Tl-201) Y Other Radionuclide	Z None	Z None
Y Skin, Subcutaneous Tissue and Breast	Y Other Radionuclide	Z None	Z None

Section C **Nuclear Medicine**
Body System P **Musculoskeletal System**
Type 1 **Planar Nuclear Medicine Imaging:** Introduction of radioactive materials into the body for single plane display of images developed from the capture of radioactive emissions

Body Part (4th)	Radionuclide (5th)	Qualifier (6th)	Qualifier (7th)
1 Skull 4 Thorax 5 Spine 6 Pelvis 7 Spine and Pelvis 8 Upper Extremity, Right 9 Upper Extremity, Left B Upper Extremities, Bilateral C Lower Extremity, Right D Lower Extremity, Left F Lower Extremities, Bilateral Z Musculoskeletal System, All	1 Technetium 99m (Tc-99m) Y Other Radionuclide	Z None	Z None
Y Musculoskeletal System, Other	Y Other Radionuclide	Z None	Z None

Section C **Nuclear Medicine**
Body System P **Musculoskeletal System**
Type 2 **Tomographic (Tomo) Nuclear Medicine Imaging:** Introduction of radioactive materials into the body for three dimensional display of images developed from the capture of radioactive emissions

Body Part (4th)	Radionuclide (5th)	Qualifier (6th)	Qualifier (7th)
1 Skull 2 Cervical Spine 3 Skull and Cervical Spine 4 Thorax 6 Pelvis 7 Spine and Pelvis 8 Upper Extremity, Right 9 Upper Extremity, Left B Upper Extremities, Bilateral C Lower Extremity, Right D Lower Extremity, Left F Lower Extremities, Bilateral G Thoracic Spine H Lumbar Spine J Thoracolumbar Spine	1 Technetium 99m (Tc-99m) Y Other Radionuclide	Z None	Z None
Y Musculoskeletal System, Other	Y Other Radionuclide	Z None	Z None

Section C **Nuclear Medicine**
Body System P **Musculoskeletal System**
Type 5 **Nonimaging Nuclear Medicine Probe:** Introduction of radioactive materials into the body for the study of distribution and fate of certain substances by the detection of radioactive emissions; or, alternatively, measurement of absorption of radioactive emissions from an external source

Body Part (4th)	Radionuclide (5th)	Qualifier (6th)	Qualifier (7th)
5 Spine **N** Upper Extremities **P** Lower Extremities	**Z** None	**Z** None	**Z** None
Y Musculoskeletal System, Other	**Y** Other Radionuclide	**Z** None	**Z** None

Section C **Nuclear Medicine**
Body System T **Urinary System**
Type 1 **Planar Nuclear Medicine Imaging:** Introduction of radioactive materials into the body for single plane display of images developed from the capture of radioactive emissions

Body Part (4th)	Radionuclide (5th)	Qualifier (6th)	Qualifier (7th)
3 Kidneys, Ureters and Bladder	**1** Technetium 99m (Tc-99m) **F** Iodine 123 (I-123) **G** Iodine 131 (I-131) **Y** Other Radionuclide	**Z** None	**Z** None
H Bladder and Ureters	**1** Technetium 99m (Tc-99m) **Y** Other Radionuclide	**Z** None	**Z** None
Y Urinary System	**Y** Other Radionuclide	**Z** None	**Z** None

Section C **Nuclear Medicine**
Body System T **Urinary System**
Type 2 **Tomographic (Tomo) Nuclear Medicine Imaging:** Introduction of radioactive materials into the body for three dimensional display of images developed from the capture of radioactive emissions

Body Part (4th)	Radionuclide (5th)	Qualifier (6th)	Qualifier (7th)
3 Kidneys, Ureters and Bladder	**1** Technetium 99m (Tc-99m) **Y** Other Radionuclide	**Z** None	**Z** None
Y Urinary System	**Y** Other Radionuclide	**Z** None	**Z** None

Section C **Nuclear Medicine**
Body System T **Urinary System**
Type 6 **Nonimaging Nuclear Medicine Assay:** Introduction of radioactive materials into the body for the study of body fluids and blood elements, by the detection of radioactive emissions

Body Part (4th)	Radionuclide (5th)	Qualifier (6th)	Qualifier (7th)
3 Kidneys, Ureters and Bladder	**1** Technetium 99m (Tc-99m) **F** Iodine 123 (I-123) **G** Iodine 131 (I-131) **H** Iodine 125 (I-125) **Y** Other Radionuclide	**Z** None	**Z** None
Y Urinary System	**Y** Other Radionuclide	**Z** None	**Z** None

Section C **Nuclear Medicine**
Body System V **Male Reproductive System**
Type 1 **Planar Nuclear Medicine Imaging:** Introduction of radioactive materials into the body for single plane display of images developed from the capture of radioactive emissions

Body Part (4th)	Radionuclide (5th)	Qualifier (6th)	Qualifier (7th)
9 Testicles, Bilateral	1 Technetium 99m (Tc-99m) Y Other Radionuclide	Z None	Z None
Y Male Reproductive System	Y Other Radionuclide	Z None	Z None

Section C **Nuclear Medicine**
Body System W **Anatomical Regions**
Type 1 **Planar Nuclear Medicine Imaging:** Introduction of radioactive materials into the body for single plane display of images developed from the capture of radioactive emissions

Body Part (4th)	Radionuclide (5th)	Qualifier (6th)	Qualifier (7th)
0 Abdomen 1 Abdomen and Pelvis 4 Chest and Abdomen 6 Chest and Neck B Head and Neck D Lower Extremity J Pelvic Region M Upper Extremity N Whole Body	1 Technetium 99m (Tc-99m) D Indium 111 (In-111) F Iodine 123 (I-123) G Iodine 131 (I-131) L Gallium 67 (Ga-67) S Thallium 201 (Tl-201) Y Other Radionuclide	Z None	Z None
3 Chest	1 Technetium 99m (Tc-99m) D Indium 111 (In-111) F Iodine 123 (I-123) G Iodine 131 (I-131) K Fluorine 18 (F-18) L Gallium 67 (Ga-67) S Thallium 201 (Tl-201) Y Other Radionuclide	Z None	Z None
Y Anatomical Regions, Multiple	Y Other Radionuclide	Z None	Z None
Z Anatomical Region, Other	Z None	Z None	Z None

Section C **Nuclear Medicine**
Body System W **Anatomical Regions**
Type 2 **Tomographic (Tomo) Nuclear Medicine Imaging:** Introduction of radioactive materials into the body for three dimensional display of images developed from the capture of radioactive emissions

Body Part (4th)	Radionuclide (5th)	Qualifier (6th)	Qualifier (7th)
0 Abdomen 1 Abdomen and Pelvis 3 Chest 4 Chest and Abdomen 6 Chest and Neck B Head and Neck D Lower Extremity J Pelvic Region M Upper Extremity	1 Technetium 99m (Tc-99m) D Indium 111 (In-111) F Iodine 123 (I-123) G Iodine 131 (I-131) K Fluorine 18 (F-18) L Gallium 67 (Ga-67) S Thallium 201 (Tl-201) Y Other Radionuclide	Z None	Z None
Y Anatomical Regions, Multiple	Y Other Radionuclide	Z None	Z None

Section C **Nuclear Medicine**
Body System W **Anatomical Regions**
Type 3 **Positron Emission Tomographic (PET) Imaging:** Introduction of radioactive materials into the body for three dimensional display of images developed from the simultaneous capture, 180 degrees apart, of radioactive emissions

Body Part (4th)	Radionuclide (5th)	Qualifier (6th)	Qualifier (7th)
N Whole Body	Y Other Radionuclide	Z None	Z None

Section C **Nuclear Medicine**
Body System W **Anatomical Regions**
Type 5 **Nonimaging Nuclear Medicine Probe:** Introduction of radioactive materials into the body for the study of distribution and fate of certain substances by the detection of radioactive emissions; or, alternatively, measurement of absorption of radioactive emissions from an external source

Body Part (4th)	Radionuclide (5th)	Qualifier (6th)	Qualifier (7th)
0 Abdomen 1 Abdomen and Pelvis 3 Chest 4 Chest and Abdomen 6 Chest and Neck B Head and Neck D Lower Extremity J Pelvic Region M Upper Extremity	1 Technetium 99m (Tc-99m) D Indium 111 (In-111) Y Other Radionuclide	Z None	Z None

Section C **Nuclear Medicine**
Body System W **Anatomical Regions**
Type 7 **Systemic Nuclear Medicine Therapy:** Introduction of unsealed radioactive materials into the body for treatment

Body Part (4th)	Radionuclide (5th)	Qualifier (6th)	Qualifier (7th)
0 Abdomen 3 Chest	N Phosphorus 32 (P-32) Y Other Radionuclide	Z None	Z None
G Thyroid	G Iodine 131 (I-131) Y Other Radionuclide	Z None	Z None
N Whole Body	8 Samarium 153 (Sm-153) G Iodine 131 (I-131) N Phosphorus 32 (P-32) P Strontium 89 (Sr-89) Y Other Radionuclide	Z None	Z None
Y Anatomical Regions, Multiple	Y Other Radionuclide	Z None	Z None

AHA Coding Clinic

No references have been issued for the Nuclear Medicine section.

Radiation Therapy Section (D00–DWY)

Within each section of ICD-10-PCS the characters have different meanings. The seven character meanings for the Radiation Therapy section are illustrated here through the procedure example of *HDR brachytherapy of prostate using Palladium 103*.

Section	Body System	Modality	Treatment Site	Modality Qualifier	Isotope	Qualifier
Radiation Therapy	Male Reproductive System	Brachytherapy	Prostate	High Dose Rate (HDR)	Palladium 103	None
D	V	1	0	9	B	Z

Section (Character 1)

All Radiation Therapy procedure codes have a first character value of D.

Body System (Character 2)

The alphanumeric character for the body system is placed in the second position. The following are the body systems applicable to the Radiation Therapy section.

Character Value	Character Value Description
0	Central and Peripheral Nervous System
7	Lymphatic and Hematologic System
8	Eye
9	Ear, Nose, Mouth and Throat
B	Respiratory System
D	Gastrointestinal System
F	Hepatobiliary System and Pancreas
G	Endocrine System
H	Skin
M	Breast
P	Musculoskeletal
T	Urinary System
U	Female Reproductive System
V	Male Reproductive System
W	Anatomical Regions

Modality (Character 3)

The alphanumeric character value for root types is placed in the third position. The following are the root types applicable to the Radiation Therapy section with their associated meaning.

Character Value	Modality	Modality Definition
0	Beam Radiation	The external use of high-energy radiation such as x-rays, photons, electrons, or protons
1	Brachytherapy	The use of radioactive sources placed directly into a tumor bearing area to generate local regions of high intensity radiation
2	Stereotactic Radiosurgery	The use of external radiation sources either from a linear accelerator or a special Cobalt-60 irradiator to deliver many beams of radiation directly to an internal structure in a single fraction
Y	Other Radiation	Other types of radiation therapy such as hyperthermia, contact radiation and plaque radiation. *See Modality qualifier, character 5, for specified types of other radiation.*

Source: CSI Navigator for Radiation Oncology, 2010

Treatment Site (Character 4)

For each treatment site the applicable body part character values will be available for procedure code construction. An example of a treatment site for this section is Brain Stem.

Modality Qualifier (Character 5)

The modality qualifier further specifies the treatment modality. The following are examples of the modality qualifier values available for the Radiation Therapy section:

- Photons >10 MeV
- Neutrons
- Electrons
- High Dose Rate
- Hyperthermia

Isotope (Character 6)

When an isotope is utilized during a radiation oncology procedure, the corresponding isotope character value should be reported in the sixth character position. The following are examples of the isotope character values available for the Radiation Therapy section:

- Iridium 192 (Ir-192)
- Iodine 125 (I-125)
- Californium 252 (Cf-252)

Qualifier (Character 7)

The qualifier represents an additional attribute for the procedure when applicable. For example, beam radiation procedures in this section include the qualifier Intraoperative that is reported with the character value of 0 for some body parts. If there is no qualifier for a procedure, the placeholder Z is the character value that should be reported.

Radiation Therapy Section Guidelines (section D)

D. Radiation Therapy Section

Brachytherapy

D1.a

Brachytherapy is coded to the modality Brachytherapy in the Radiation Therapy section. When a radioactive brachytherapy source is left in the body at the end of the procedure, it is coded separately to the root operation Insertion with the device value Radioactive Element.

Example: Brachytherapy with implantation of a low dose rate brachytherapy source left in the body at the end of the procedure is coded to the applicable treatment site in section D, Radiation Therapy, with the modality Brachytherapy, the modality qualifier value, Low Dose Rate, and the applicable isotope value and qualifier value. The implantation of the brachytherapy source is coded separately to the device value Radioactive Element in the appropriate Insertion table of the Medical and Surgical section. The Radiation Therapy section code identifies the specific modality and isotope of the brachytherapy, and the root operation Insertion code identifies the implantation of the brachytherapy source that remain in the body at the end of the procedure.

Exception: Implantation of Cesium-131 brachytherapy seeds embedded in a collagen matrix to the treatment site after resection of brain tumor is coded to the root operation Insertion with the device value Radioactive Element, Cesium-131 Collagen Implant. The procedure is coded to the root operation Insertion only, because the device value identifies both the implantation of the radioactive element and a specific brachytherapy isotope that is not included in the Radiation Therapy section tables.

D1.b

A separate procedure to place a temporary applicator for delivering the brachytherapy is coded to the root operation Insertion and the device value Other Device.

Examples: Intrauterine brachytherapy applicator placed as a separate procedure from the brachytherapy procedure is coded to Insertion of Other Device, and the brachytherapy is coded separately using the modality Brachytherapy in the Radiation Therapy section. Intrauterine brachytherapy applicator placed concomitantly with delivery of the brachytherapy dose is coded with a single code using the modality Brachytherapy in the Radiation Therapy section.

Radiation Therapy Section Tables

Radiation Therapy Tables D00–DWY

Section D **Radiation Therapy**
Body System 0 **Central and Peripheral Nervous System**
Modality 0 **Beam Radiation**

Treatment Site (4th)	Modality Qualifier (5th)	Isotope (6th)	Qualifier (7th)
0 Brain **1** Brain Stem **6** Spinal Cord **7** Peripheral Nerve	**0** Photons <1 MeV **1** Photons 1 - 10 MeV **2** Photons >10 MeV **4** Heavy Particles (Protons,Ions) **5** Neutrons **6** Neutron Capture	**Z** None	**Z** None
0 Brain **1** Brain Stem **6** Spinal Cord **7** Peripheral Nerve	**3** Electrons	**Z** None	**0** Intraoperative **Z** None

Section D **Radiation Therapy**
Body System 0 **Central and Peripheral Nervous System**
Modality 1 **Brachytherapy**

Treatment Site (4th)	Modality Qualifier (5th)	Isotope (6th)	Qualifier (7th)
0 Brain **1** Brain Stem **6** Spinal Cord **7** Peripheral Nerve	**9** High Dose Rate (HDR)	**7** Cesium 137 (Cs-137) **8** Iridium 192 (Ir-192) **9** Iodine 125 (I-125) **B** Palladium 103 (Pd-103) **C** Californium 252 (Cf-252) **Y** Other Isotope	**Z** None
0 Brain **1** Brain Stem **6** Spinal Cord **7** Peripheral Nerve	**B** Low Dose Rate (LDR)	**6** Cesium 131 (Cs-131) **7** Cesium 137 (Cs-137) **8** Iridium 192 (Ir-192) **9** Iodine 125 (I-125) **C** Californium 252 (Cf-252) **Y** Other Isotope	**Z** None
0 Brain **1** Brain Stem **6** Spinal Cord **7** Peripheral Nerve	**B** Low Dose Rate (LDR)	**B** Palladium 103 (Pd-103)	**1** Unidirectional Source **Z** None

Section D **Radiation Therapy**
Body System 0 **Central and Peripheral Nervous System**
Modality 2 **Stereotactic Radiosurgery**

Treatment Site (4th)	Modality Qualifier (5th)	Isotope (6th)	Qualifier (7th)
0 Brain **1** Brain Stem **6** Spinal Cord **7** Peripheral Nerve	**D** Stereotactic Other Photon Radiosurgery **H** Stereotactic Particulate Radiosurgery **J** Stereotactic Gamma Beam Radiosurgery	**Z** None	**Z** None

Section D **Radiation Therapy**
Body System 0 **Central and Peripheral Nervous System**
Modality Y **Other Radiation**

Treatment Site (4th)	Modality Qualifier (5th)	Isotope (6th)	Qualifier (7th)
0 Brain **1** Brain Stem **6** Spinal Cord **7** Peripheral Nerve	**7** Contact Radiation **8** Hyperthermia **C** Intraoperative Radiation Therapy (IORT) **F** Plaque Radiation **K** Laser Interstitial Thermal Therapy	**Z** None	**Z** None

Section D **Radiation Therapy**
Body System 7 **Lymphatic and Hematologic System**
Modality 0 **Beam Radiation**

Treatment Site (4th)	Modality Qualifier (5th)	Isotope (6th)	Qualifier (7th)
0 Bone Marrow **1** Thymus **2** Spleen **3** Lymphatics, Neck **4** Lymphatics, Axillary **5** Lymphatics, Thorax **6** Lymphatics, Abdomen **7** Lymphatics, Pelvis **8** Lymphatics, Inguinal	**0** Photons <1 MeV **1** Photons 1 - 10 MeV **2** Photons >10 MeV **4** Heavy Particles (Protons,Ions) **5** Neutrons **6** Neutron Capture	**Z** None	**Z** None
0 Bone Marrow **1** Thymus **2** Spleen **3** Lymphatics, Neck **4** Lymphatics, Axillary **5** Lymphatics, Thorax **6** Lymphatics, Abdomen **7** Lymphatics, Pelvis **8** Lymphatics, Inguinal	**3** Electrons	**Z** None	**0** Intraoperative **Z** None

Section D **Radiation Therapy**
Body System 7 **Lymphatic and Hematologic System**
Modality 1 **Brachytherapy**

Treatment Site (4th)	Modality Qualifier (5th)	Isotope (6th)	Qualifier (7th)
0 Bone Marrow **1** Thymus **2** Spleen **3** Lymphatics, Neck **4** Lymphatics, Axillary **5** Lymphatics, Thorax **6** Lymphatics, Abdomen **7** Lymphatics, Pelvis **8** Lymphatics, Inguinal	**9** High Dose Rate (HDR)	**7** Cesium 137 (Cs-137) **8** Iridium 192 (Ir-192) **9** Iodine 125 (I 125) **B** Palladium 103 (Pd-103) **C** Californium 252 (Cf-252) **Y** Other Isotope	**Z** None
0 Bone Marrow **1** Thymus **2** Spleen **3** Lymphatics, Neck **4** Lymphatics, Axillary **5** Lymphatics, Thorax **6** Lymphatics, Abdomen **7** Lymphatics, Pelvis **8** Lymphatics, Inguinal	**B** Low Dose Rate (LDR)	**6** Cesium 131 (Cs-131) **7** Cesium 137 (Cs-137) **8** Iridium 192 (Ir-192) **9** Iodine 125 (I-125) **C** Californium 252 (Cf-252) **Y** Other Isotope	**Z** None
0 Bone Marrow **1** Thymus **2** Spleen **3** Lymphatics, Neck **4** Lymphatics, Axillary **5** Lymphatics, Thorax **6** Lymphatics, Abdomen **7** Lymphatics, Pelvis **8** Lymphatics, Inguinal	**B** Low Dose Rate (LDR)	**B** Palladium 103 (Pd-103)	**1** Unidirectional Source **Z** None

Section D **Radiation Therapy**
Body System 7 **Lymphatic and Hematologic System**
Modality 2 **Stereotactic Radiosurgery**

Treatment Site (4th)	Modality Qualifier (5th)	Isotope (6th)	Qualifier (7th)
0 Bone Marrow 1 Thymus 2 Spleen 3 Lymphatics, Neck 4 Lymphatics, Axillary 5 Lymphatics, Thorax 6 Lymphatics, Abdomen 7 Lymphatics, Pelvis 8 Lymphatics, Inguinal	D Stereotactic Other Photon Radiosurgery H Stereotactic Particulate Radiosurgery J Stereotactic Gamma Beam Radiosurgery	Z None	Z None

Section D **Radiation Therapy**
Body System 7 **Lymphatic and Hematologic System**
Modality Y **Other Radiation**

Treatment Site (4th)	Modality Qualifier (5th)	Isotope (6th)	Qualifier (7th)
0 Bone Marrow 1 Thymus 2 Spleen 3 Lymphatics, Neck 4 Lymphatics, Axillary 5 Lymphatics, Thorax 6 Lymphatics, Abdomen 7 Lymphatics, Pelvis 8 Lymphatics, Inguinal	8 Hyperthermia F Plaque Radiation	Z None	Z None

Section D **Radiation Therapy**
Body System 8 **Eye**
Modality 0 **Beam Radiation**

Treatment Site (4th)	Modality Qualifier (5th)	Isotope (6th)	Qualifier (7th)
0 Eye	0 Photons <1 MeV 1 Photons 1 - 10 MeV 2 Photons >10 MeV 4 Heavy Particles (Protons,Ions) 5 Neutrons 6 Neutron Capture	Z None	Z None
0 Eye	3 Electrons	Z None	0 Intraoperative Z None

Section D **Radiation Therapy**
Body System 8 **Eye**
Modality 1 **Brachytherapy**

Treatment Site (4th)	Modality Qualifier (5th)	Isotope (6th)	Qualifier (7th)
0 Eye	9 High Dose Rate (HDR)	7 Cesium 137 (Cs-137) 8 Iridium 192 (Ir-192) 9 Iodine 125 (I-125) B Palladium 103 (Pd-103) C Californium 252 (Cf-252) Y Other Isotope	Z None
0 Eye	B Low Dose Rate (LDR)	6 Cesium 131 (Cs-131) 7 Cesium 137 (Cs-137) 8 Iridium 192 (Ir-192) 9 Iodine 125 (I-125) C Californium 252 (Cf-252) Y Other Isotope	Z None

Continued →

Section	**D**	**Radiation Therapy**
Body System	**8**	**Eye**
Modality	**1**	**Brachytherapy**

Treatment Site (4th)	Modality Qualifier (5th)	Isotope (6th)	Qualifier (7th)
0 Eye	**B** Low Dose Rate (LDR)	**B** Palladium 103 (Pd-103)	**1** Unidirectional Source **Z** None

Section	**D**	**Radiation Therapy**
Body System	**8**	**Eye**
Modality	**2**	**Stereotactic Radiosurgery**

Treatment Site (4th)	Modality Qualifier (5th)	Isotope (6th)	Qualifier (7th)
0 Eye	**D** Stereotactic Other Photon Radiosurgery **H** Stereotactic Particulate Radiosurgery **J** Stereotactic Gamma Beam Radiosurgery	**Z** None	**Z** None

Section	**D**	**Radiation Therapy**
Body System	**8**	**Eye**
Modality	**Y**	**Other Radiation**

Treatment Site (4th)	Modality Qualifier (5th)	Isotope (6th)	Qualifier (7th)
0 Eye	**7** Contact Radiation **8** Hyperthermia **F** Plaque Radiation	**Z** None	**Z** None

Section	**D**	**Radiation Therapy**
Body System	**9**	**Ear, Nose, Mouth and Throat**
Modality	**0**	**Beam Radiation**

Treatment Site (4th)	Modality Qualifier (5th)	Isotope (6th)	Qualifier (7th)
0 Ear **1** Nose **3** Hypopharynx **4** Mouth **5** Tongue **6** Salivary Glands **7** Sinuses **8** Hard Palate **9** Soft Palate **B** Larynx **D** Nasopharynx **F** Oropharynx	**0** Photons <1 MeV **1** Photons 1 - 10 MeV **2** Photons >10 MeV **4** Heavy Particles (Protons,Ions) **5** Neutrons **6** Neutron Capture	**Z** None	**Z** None
0 Ear **1** Nose **3** Hypopharynx **4** Mouth **5** Tongue **6** Salivary Glands **7** Sinuses **8** Hard Palate **9** Soft Palate **B** Larynx **D** Nasopharynx **F** Oropharynx	**3** Electrons	**Z** None	**0** Intraoperative **Z** None

Section D **Radiation Therapy**
Body System 9 **Ear, Nose, Mouth and Throat**
Modality 1 **Brachytherapy**

Treatment Site (4th)	Modality Qualifier (5th)	Isotope (6th)	Qualifier (7th)
0 Ear **1** Nose **3** Hypopharynx **4** Mouth **5** Tongue **6** Salivary Glands **7** Sinuses **8** Hard Palate **9** Soft Palate **B** Larynx **D** Nasopharynx **F** Oropharynx	**9** High Dose Rate (HDR)	**7** Cesium 137 (Cs-137) **8** Iridium 192 (Ir-192) **9** Iodine 125 (I-125) **B** Palladium 103 (Pd-103) **C** Californium 252 (Cf-252) **Y** Other Isotope	**Z** None
0 Ear **1** Nose **3** Hypopharynx **4** Mouth **5** Tongue **6** Salivary Glands **7** Sinuses **8** Hard Palate **9** Soft Palate **B** Larynx **D** Nasopharynx **F** Oropharynx	**B** Low Dose Rate (LDR)	**6** Cesium 131 (Cs-131) **7** Cesium 137 (Cs-137) **8** Iridium 192 (Ir-192) **9** Iodine 125 (I-125) **C** Californium 252 (Cf-252) **Y** Other Isotope	**Z** None
0 Ear **1** Nose **3** Hypopharynx **4** Mouth **5** Tongue **6** Salivary Glands **7** Sinuses **8** Hard Palate **9** Soft Palate **B** Larynx **D** Nasopharynx **F** Oropharynx	**B** Low Dose Rate (LDR)	**B** Palladium 103 (Pd-103)	**1** Unidirectional Source **Z** None

Section D **Radiation Therapy**
Body System 9 **Ear, Nose, Mouth and Throat**
Modality 2 **Stereotactic Radiosurgery**

Treatment Site (4th)	Modality Qualifier (5th)	Isotope (6th)	Qualifier (7th)
0 Ear **1** Nose **4** Mouth **5** Tongue **6** Salivary Glands **7** Sinuses **8** Hard Palate **9** Soft Palate **B** Larynx **C** Pharynx **D** Nasopharynx	**D** Stereotactic Other Photon Radiosurgery **H** Stereotactic Particulate Radiosurgery **J** Stereotactic Gamma Beam Radiosurgery	**Z** None	**Z** None

Section D **Radiation Therapy**
Body System 9 **Ear, Nose, Mouth and Throat**
Modality Y **Other Radiation**

Treatment Site (4th)	Modality Qualifier (5th)	Isotope (6th)	Qualifier (7th)
0 Ear 1 Nose 5 Tongue 6 Salivary Glands 7 Sinuses 8 Hard Palate 9 Soft Palate	7 Contact Radiation 8 Hyperthermia F Plaque Radiation	Z None	Z None
3 Hypopharynx F Oropharynx	7 Contact Radiation 8 Hyperthermia	Z None	Z None
4 Mouth B Larynx D Nasopharynx	7 Contact Radiation 8 Hyperthermia C Intraoperative Radiation Therapy (IORT) F Plaque Radiation	Z None	Z None
C Pharynx	C Intraoperative Radiation Therapy (IORT) F Plaque Radiation	Z None	Z None

Section D **Radiation Therapy**
Body System B **Respiratory System**
Modality 0 **Beam Radiation**

Treatment Site (4th)	Modality Qualifier (5th)	Isotope (6th)	Qualifier (7th)
0 Trachea 1 Bronchus 2 Lung 5 Pleura 6 Mediastinum 7 Chest Wall 8 Diaphragm	0 Photons <1 MeV 1 Photons 1 - 10 MeV 2 Photons >10 MeV 4 Heavy Particles (Protons,Ions) 5 Neutrons 6 Neutron Capture	Z None	Z None
0 Trachea 1 Bronchus 2 Lung 5 Pleura 6 Mediastinum 7 Chest Wall 8 Diaphragm	3 Electrons	Z None	0 Intraoperative Z None

Section D **Radiation Therapy**
Body System B **Respiratory System**
Modality 1 **Brachytherapy**

Treatment Site (4th)	Modality Qualifier (5th)	Isotope (6th)	Qualifier (7th)
0 Trachea 1 Bronchus 2 Lung 5 Pleura 6 Mediastinum 7 Chest Wall 8 Diaphragm	9 High Dose Rate (HDR)	7 Cesium 137 (Cs-137) 8 Iridium 192 (Ir-192) 9 Iodine 125 (I-125) B Palladium 103 (Pd-103) C Californium 252 (Cf-252) Y Other Isotope	Z None

Continued →

Section D **Radiation Therapy**
Body System B **Respiratory System**
Modality 1 **Brachytherapy**

Treatment Site (4th)	Modality Qualifier (5th)	Isotope (6th)	Qualifier (7th)
0 Trachea **1** Bronchus **2** Lung **5** Pleura **6** Mediastinum **7** Chest Wall **8** Diaphragm	**B** Low Dose Rate (LDR)	**6** Cesium 131 (Cs-131) **7** Cesium 137 (Cs-137) **8** Iridium 192 (Ir-192) **9** Iodine 125 (I-125) **C** Californium 252 (Cf-252) **Y** Other Isotope	**Z** None
0 Trachea **1** Bronchus **2** Lung **5** Pleura **6** Mediastinum **7** Chest Wall **8** Diaphragm	**B** Low Dose Rate (LDR)	**B** Palladium 103 (Pd-103)	**1** Unidirectional Source **Z** None

Section D **Radiation Therapy**
Body System B **Respiratory System**
Modality 2 **Stereotactic Radiosurgery**

Treatment Site (4th)	Modality Qualifier (5th)	Isotope (6th)	Qualifier (7th)
0 Trachea **1** Bronchus **2** Lung **5** Pleura **6** Mediastinum **7** Chest Wall **8** Diaphragm	**D** Stereotactic Other Photon Radiosurgery **H** Stereotactic Particulate Radiosurgery **J** Stereotactic Gamma Beam Radiosurgery	**Z** None	**Z** None

Section D **Radiation Therapy**
Body System B **Respiratory System**
Modality Y **Other Radiation**

Treatment Site (4th)	Modality Qualifier (5th)	Isotope (6th)	Qualifier (7th)
0 Trachea **1** Bronchus **2** Lung **5** Pleura **6** Mediastinum **7** Chest Wall **8** Diaphragm	**7** Contact Radiation **8** Hyperthermia **F** Plaque Radiation **K** Laser Interstitial Thermal Therapy	**Z** None	**Z** None

Section D **Radiation Therapy**
Body System D **Gastrointestinal System**
Modality 0 **Beam Radiation**

Treatment Site (4th)	Modality Qualifier (5th)	Isotope (6th)	Qualifier (7th)
0 Esophagus **1** Stomach **2** Duodenum **3** Jejunum **4** Ileum **5** Colon **7** Rectum	**0** Photons <1 MeV **1** Photons 1 - 10 MeV **2** Photons >10 MeV **4** Heavy Particles (Protons,Ions) **5** Neutrons **6** Neutron Capture	**Z** None	**Z** None

Continued →

Section D **Radiation Therapy**
Body System D **Gastrointestinal System**
Modality 0 **Beam Radiation**

Treatment Site (4th)	Modality Qualifier (5th)	Isotope (6th)	Qualifier (7th)
0 Esophagus 1 Stomach 2 Duodenum 3 Jejunum 4 Ileum 5 Colon 7 Rectum	3 Electrons	Z None	0 Intraoperative Z None

Section D **Radiation Therapy**
Body System D **Gastrointestinal System**
Modality 1 **Brachytherapy**

Treatment Site (4th)	Modality Qualifier (5th)	Isotope (6th)	Qualifier (7th)
0 Esophagus 1 Stomach 2 Duodenum 3 Jejunum 4 Ileum 5 Colon 7 Rectum	9 High Dose Rate (HDR)	7 Cesium 137 (Cs-137) 8 Iridium 192 (Ir-192) 9 Iodine 125 (I-125) B Palladium 103 (Pd-103) C Californium 252 (Cf-252) Y Other Isotope	Z None
0 Esophagus 1 Stomach 2 Duodenum 3 Jejunum 4 Ileum 5 Colon 7 Rectum	B Low Dose Rate (LDR)	6 Cesium 131 (Cs-131) 7 Cesium 137 (Cs-137) 8 Iridium 192 (Ir-192) 9 Iodine 125 (I-125) C Californium 252 (Cf-252) Y Other Isotope	Z None
0 Esophagus 1 Stomach 2 Duodenum 3 Jejunum 4 Ileum 5 Colon 7 Rectum	B Low Dose Rate (LDR)	B Palladium 103 (Pd-103)	1 Unidirectional Source Z None

Section D **Radiation Therapy**
Body System D **Gastrointestinal System**
Modality 2 **Stereotactic Radiosurgery**

Treatment Site (4th)	Modality Qualifier (5th)	Isotope (6th)	Qualifier (7th)
0 Esophagus 1 Stomach 2 Duodenum 3 Jejunum 4 Ileum 5 Colon 7 Rectum	D Stereotactic Other Photon Radiosurgery H Stereotactic Particulate Radiosurgery J Stereotactic Gamma Beam Radiosurgery	Z None	Z None

Section D **Radiation Therapy**
Body System D **Gastrointestinal System**
Modality Y **Other Radiation**

Treatment Site (4th)	Modality Qualifier (5th)	Isotope (6th)	Qualifier (7th)
0 Esophagus	7 Contact Radiation 8 Hyperthermia F Plaque Radiation K Laser Interstitial Thermal Therapy	Z None	Z None

Continued →

Section D **Radiation Therapy**
Body System D **Gastrointestinal System**
Modality Y **Other Radiation**

Treatment Site (4th)	Modality Qualifier (5th)	Isotope (6th)	Qualifier (7th)
1 Stomach 2 Duodenum 3 Jejunum 4 Ileum 5 Colon 7 Rectum	7 Contact Radiation 8 Hyperthermia C Intraoperative Radiation Therapy (IORT) F Plaque Radiation K Laser Interstitial Thermal Therapy	Z None	Z None
8 Anus	C Intraoperative Radiation Therapy (IORT) F Plaque Radiation K Laser Interstitial Thermal Therapy	Z None	Z None

Section D **Radiation Therapy**
Body System F **Hepatobiliary System and Pancreas**
Modality 0 **Beam Radiation**

Treatment Site (4th)	Modality Qualifier (5th)	Isotope (6th)	Qualifier (7th)
0 Liver 1 Gallbladder 2 Bile Ducts 3 Pancreas	0 Photons <1 MeV 1 Photons 1 - 10 MeV 2 Photons >10 MeV 4 Heavy Particles (Protons,Ions) 5 Neutrons 6 Neutron Capture	Z None	Z None
0 Liver 1 Gallbladder 2 Bile Ducts 3 Pancreas	3 Electrons	Z None	0 Intraoperative Z None

Section D **Radiation Therapy**
Body System F **Hepatobiliary System and Pancreas**
Modality 1 **Brachytherapy**

Treatment Site (4th)	Modality Qualifier (5th)	Isotope (6th)	Qualifier (7th)
0 Liver 1 Gallbladder 2 Bile Ducts 3 Pancreas	9 High Dose Rate (HDR)	7 Cesium 137 (Cs-137) 8 Iridium 192 (Ir-192) 9 Iodine 125 (I-125) B Palladium 103 (Pd-103) C Californium 252 (Cf-252) Y Other Isotope	Z None
0 Liver 1 Gallbladder 2 Bile Ducts 3 Pancreas	B Low Dose Rate (LDR)	6 Cesium 131 (Cs-131) 7 Cesium 137 (Cs-137) 8 Iridium 192 (Ir-192) 9 Iodine 125 (I-125) C Californium 252 (Cf-252) Y Other Isotope	Z None
0 Liver 1 Gallbladder 2 Bile Ducts 3 Pancreas	B Low Dose Rate (LDR)	B Palladium 103 (Pd-103)	1 Unidirectional Source Z None

Section D **Radiation Therapy**
Body System F **Hepatobiliary System and Pancreas**
Modality 2 **Stereotactic Radiosurgery**

Treatment Site (4th)	Modality Qualifier (5th)	Isotope (6th)	Qualifier (7th)
0 Liver **1** Gallbladder **2** Bile Ducts **3** Pancreas	**D** Stereotactic Other Photon Radiosurgery **H** Stereotactic Particulate Radiosurgery **J** Stereotactic Gamma Beam Radiosurgery	**Z** None	**Z** None

Section D **Radiation Therapy**
Body System F **Hepatobiliary System and Pancreas**
Modality Y **Other Radiation**

Treatment Site (4th)	Modality Qualifier (5th)	Isotope (6th)	Qualifier (7th)
0 Liver **1** Gallbladder **2** Bile Ducts **3** Pancreas	**7** Contact Radiation **8** Hyperthermia **C** Intraoperative Radiation Therapy (IORT) **F** Plaque Radiation **K** Laser Interstitial Thermal Therapy	**Z** None	**Z** None

Section D **Radiation Therapy**
Body System G **Endocrine System**
Modality 0 **Beam Radiation**

Treatment Site (4th)	Modality Qualifier (5th)	Isotope (6th)	Qualifier (7th)
0 Pituitary Gland **1** Pineal Body **2** Adrenal Glands **4** Parathyroid Glands **5** Thyroid	**0** Photons <1 MeV **1** Photons 1 - 10 MeV **2** Photons >10 MeV **5** Neutrons **6** Neutron Capture	**Z** None	**Z** None
0 Pituitary Gland **1** Pineal Body **2** Adrenal Glands **4** Parathyroid Glands **5** Thyroid	**3** Electrons	**Z** None	**0** Intraoperative **Z** None

Section D **Radiation Therapy**
Body System G **Endocrine System**
Modality 1 **Brachytherapy**

Treatment Site (4th)	Modality Qualifier (5th)	Isotope (6th)	Qualifier (7th)
0 Pituitary Gland **1** Pineal Body **2** Adrenal Glands **4** Parathyroid Glands **5** Thyroid	**9** High Dose Rate (HDR)	**7** Cesium 137 (Cs-137) **8** Iridium 192 (Ir-192) **9** Iodine 125 (I-125) **B** Palladium 103 (Pd-103) **C** Californium 252 (Cf-252) **Y** Other Isotope	**Z** None
0 Pituitary Gland **1** Pineal Body **2** Adrenal Glands **4** Parathyroid Glands **5** Thyroid	**B** Low Dose Rate (LDR)	**6** Cesium 131 (Cs-131) **7** Cesium 137 (Cs-137) **8** Iridium 192 (Ir-192) **9** Iodine 125 (I-125) **C** Californium 252 (Cf-252) **Y** Other Isotope	**Z** None
0 Pituitary Gland **1** Pineal Body **2** Adrenal Glands **4** Parathyroid Glands **5** Thyroid	**B** Low Dose Rate (LDR)	**B** Palladium 103 (Pd-103)	**1** Unidirectional Source **Z** None

Section D **Radiation Therapy**
Body System G **Endocrine System**
Modality 2 **Stereotactic Radiosurgery**

Treatment Site (4th)	Modality Qualifier (5th)	Isotope (6th)	Qualifier (7th)
0 Pituitary Gland 1 Pineal Body 2 Adrenal Glands 4 Parathyroid Glands 5 Thyroid	D Stereotactic Other Photon Radiosurgery H Stereotactic Particulate Radiosurgery J Stereotactic Gamma Beam Radiosurgery	Z None	Z None

Section D **Radiation Therapy**
Body System G **Endocrine System**
Modality Y **Other Radiation**

Treatment Site (4th)	Modality Qualifier (5th)	Isotope (6th)	Qualifier (7th)
0 Pituitary Gland 1 Pineal Body 2 Adrenal Glands 4 Parathyroid Glands 5 Thyroid	7 Contact Radiation 8 Hyperthermia F Plaque Radiation K Laser Interstitial Thermal Therapy	Z None	Z None

Section D **Radiation Therapy**
Body System H **Skin**
Modality 0 **Beam Radiation**

Treatment Site (4th)	Modality Qualifier (5th)	Isotope (6th)	Qualifier (7th)
2 Skin, Face 3 Skin, Neck 4 Skin, Arm 6 Skin, Chest 7 Skin, Back 8 Skin, Abdomen 9 Skin, Buttock B Skin, Leg	0 Photons <1 MeV 1 Photons 1 - 10 MeV 2 Photons >10 MeV 4 Heavy Particles (Protons,Ions) 5 Neutrons 6 Neutron Capture	Z None	Z None
2 Skin, Face 3 Skin, Neck 4 Skin, Arm 6 Skin, Chest 7 Skin, Back 8 Skin, Abdomen 9 Skin, Buttock B Skin, Leg	3 Electrons	Z None	0 Intraoperative Z None

Section D **Radiation Therapy**
Body System H **Skin**
Modality Y **Other Radiation**

Treatment Site (4th)	Modality Qualifier (5th)	Isotope (6th)	Qualifier (7th)
2 Skin, Face 3 Skin, Neck 4 Skin, Arm 6 Skin, Chest 7 Skin, Back 8 Skin, Abdomen 9 Skin, Buttock B Skin, Leg	7 Contact Radiation 8 Hyperthermia F Plaque Radiation	Z None	Z None
5 Skin, Hand C Skin, Foot	F Plaque Radiation	Z None	Z None

Section D Radiation Therapy
Body System M Breast
Modality 0 Beam Radiation

Treatment Site (4th)	Modality Qualifier (5th)	Isotope (6th)	Qualifier (7th)
0 Breast, Left **1** Breast, Right	**0** Photons <1 MeV **1** Photons 1 - 10 MeV **2** Photons >10 MeV **4** Heavy Particles (Protons,Ions) **5** Neutrons **6** Neutron Capture	**Z** None	**Z** None
0 Breast, Left **1** Breast, Right	**3** Electrons	**Z** None	**0** Intraoperative **Z** None

Section D Radiation Therapy
Body System M Breast
Modality 1 Brachytherapy

Treatment Site (4th)	Modality Qualifier (5th)	Isotope (6th)	Qualifier (7th)
0 Breast, Left **1** Breast, Right	**9** High Dose Rate (HDR)	**7** Cesium 137 (Cs-137) **8** Iridium 192 (Ir-192) **9** Iodine 125 (I-125) **B** Palladium 103 (Pd-103) **C** Californium 252 (Cf-252) **Y** Other Isotope	**Z** None
0 Breast, Left **1** Breast, Right	**B** Low Dose Rate (LDR)	**6** Cesium 131 (Cs-131) **7** Cesium 137 (Cs-137) **8** Iridium 192 (Ir-192) **9** Iodine 125 (I-125) **C** Californium 252 (Cf-252) **Y** Other Isotope	**Z** None
0 Breast, Left **1** Breast, Right	**B** Low Dose Rate (LDR)	**B** Palladium 103 (Pd-103)	**1** Unidirectional Source **Z** None

Section D Radiation Therapy
Body System M Breast
Modality 2 Stereotactic Radiosurgery

Treatment Site (4th)	Modality Qualifier (5th)	Isotope (6th)	Qualifier (7th)
0 Breast, Left **1** Breast, Right	**D** Stereotactic Other Photon Radiosurgery **H** Stereotactic Particulate Radiosurgery **J** Stereotactic Gamma Beam Radiosurgery	**Z** None	**Z** None

Section D Radiation Therapy
Body System M Breast
Modality Y Other Radiation

Treatment Site (4th)	Modality Qualifier (5th)	Isotope (6th)	Qualifier (7th)
0 Breast, Left **1** Breast, Right	**7** Contact Radiation **8** Hyperthermia **F** Plaque Radiation **K** Laser Interstitial Thermal Therapy	**Z** None	**Z** None

Section D **Radiation Therapy**
Body System P **Musculoskeletal System**
Modality 0 **Beam Radiation**

Treatment Site (4th)	Modality Qualifier (5th)	Isotope (6th)	Qualifier (7th)
0 Skull **2** Maxilla **3** Mandible **4** Sternum **5** Rib(s) **6** Humerus **7** Radius/Ulna **8** Pelvic Bones **9** Femur **B** Tibia/Fibula **C** Other Bone	**0** Photons <1 MeV **1** Photons 1 - 10 MeV **2** Photons >10 MeV **4** Heavy Particles (Protons,Ions) **5** Neutrons **6** Neutron Capture	**Z** None	**Z** None
0 Skull **2** Maxilla **3** Mandible **4** Sternum **5** Rib(s) **6** Humerus **7** Radius/Ulna **8** Pelvic Bones **9** Femur **B** Tibia/Fibula **C** Other Bone	**3** Electrons	**Z** None	**0** Intraoperative **Z** None

Section D **Radiation Therapy**
Body System P **Musculoskeletal System**
Modality Y **Other Radiation**

Treatment Site (4th)	Modality Qualifier (5th)	Isotope (6th)	Qualifier (7th)
0 Skull **2** Maxilla **3** Mandible **4** Sternum **5** Rib(s) **6** Humerus **7** Radius/Ulna **8** Pelvic Bones **9** Femur **B** Tibia/Fibula **C** Other Bone	**7** Contact Radiation **8** Hyperthermia **F** Plaque Radiation	**Z** None	**Z** None

Section D **Radiation Therapy**
Body System T **Urinary System**
Modality 0 **Beam Radiation**

Treatment Site (4th)	Modality Qualifier (5th)	Isotope (6th)	Qualifier (7th)
0 Kidney **1** Ureter **2** Bladder **3** Urethra	**0** Photons <1 MeV **1** Photons 1 - 10 MeV **2** Photons >10 MeV **4** Heavy Particles (Protons,Ions) **5** Neutrons **6** Neutron Capture	**Z** None	**Z** None
0 Kidney **1** Ureter **2** Bladder **3** Urethra	**3** Electrons	**Z** None	**0** Intraoperative **Z** None

Section D Radiation Therapy
Body System T Urinary System
Modality 1 Brachytherapy

Treatment Site (4th)	Modality Qualifier (5th)	Isotope (6th)	Qualifier (7th)
0 Kidney **1** Ureter **2** Bladder **3** Urethra	**9** High Dose Rate (HDR)	**7** Cesium 137 (Cs-137) **8** Iridium 192 (Ir-192) **9** Iodine 125 (I-125) **B** Palladium 103 (Pd-103) **C** Californium 252 (Cf-252) **Y** Other Isotope	**Z** None
0 Kidney **1** Ureter **2** Bladder **3** Urethra	**B** Low Dose Rate (LDR)	**6** Cesium 131 (Cs-131) **7** Cesium 137 (Cs-137) **8** Iridium 192 (Ir-192) **9** Iodine 125 (I-125) **C** Californium 252 (Cf-252) **Y** Other Isotope	**Z** None
0 Kidney **1** Ureter **2** Bladder **3** Urethra	**B** Low Dose Rate (LDR)	**B** Palladium 103 (Pd-103)	**1** Unidirectional Source **Z** None

Section D Radiation Therapy
Body System T Urinary System
Modality 2 Stereotactic Radiosurgery

Treatment Site (4th)	Modality Qualifier (5th)	Isotope (6th)	Qualifier (7th)
0 Kidney **1** Ureter **2** Bladder **3** Urethra	**D** Stereotactic Other Photon Radiosurgery **H** Stereotactic Particulate Radiosurgery **J** Stereotactic Gamma Beam Radiosurgery	**Z** None	**Z** None

Section D Radiation Therapy
Body System T Urinary System
Modality Y Other Radiation

Treatment Site (4th)	Modality Qualifier (5th)	Isotope (6th)	Qualifier (7th)
0 Kidney **1** Ureter **2** Bladder **3** Urethra	**7** Contact Radiation **8** Hyperthermia **C** Intraoperative Radiation Therapy (IORT) **F** Plaque Radiation	**Z** None	**Z** None

Section D Radiation Therapy
Body System U Female Reproductive System
Modality 0 Beam Radiation

Treatment Site (4th)	Modality Qualifier (5th)	Isotope (6th)	Qualifier (7th)
0 Ovary **1** Cervix **2** Uterus	**0** Photons <1 MeV **1** Photons 1 - 10 MeV **2** Photons >10 MeV **4** Heavy Particles (Protons,Ions) **5** Neutrons **6** Neutron Capture	**Z** None	**Z** None
0 Ovary **1** Cervix **2** Uterus	**3** Electrons	**Z** None	**0** Intraoperative **Z** None

Section D **Radiation Therapy**
Body System U **Female Reproductive System**
Modality 1 **Brachytherapy**

Treatment Site (4th)	Modality Qualifier (5th)	Isotope (6th)	Qualifier (7th)
0 Ovary **1** Cervix **2** Uterus	**9** High Dose Rate (HDR)	**7** Cesium 137 (Cs-137) **8** Iridium 192 (Ir-192) **9** Iodine 125 (I-125) **B** Palladium 103 (Pd-103) **C** Californium 252 (Cf-252) **Y** Other Isotope	**Z** None
0 Ovary **1** Cervix **2** Uterus	**B** Low Dose Rate (LDR)	**6** Cesium 131 (Cs-131) **7** Cesium 137 (Cs-137) **8** Iridium 192 (Ir-192) **9** Iodine 125 (I-125) **C** Californium 252 (Cf-252) **Y** Other Isotope	**Z** None
0 Ovary **1** Cervix **2** Uterus	**B** Low Dose Rate (LDR)	**B** Palladium 103 (Pd-103)	**1** Unidirectional Source **Z** None

Section D **Radiation Therapy**
Body System U **Female Reproductive System**
Modality 2 **Stereotactic Radiosurgery**

Treatment Site (4th)	Modality Qualifier (5th)	Isotope (6th)	Qualifier (7th)
0 Ovary **1** Cervix **2** Uterus	**D** Stereotactic Other Photon Radiosurgery **H** Stereotactic Particulate Radiosurgery **J** Stereotactic Gamma Beam Radiosurgery	**Z** None	**Z** None

Section D **Radiation Therapy**
Body System U **Female Reproductive System**
Modality Y **Other Radiation**

Treatment Site (4th)	Modality Qualifier (5th)	Isotope (6th)	Qualifier (7th)
0 Ovary **1** Cervix **2** Uterus	**7** Contact Radiation **8** Hyperthermia **C** Intraoperative Radiation Therapy (IORT) **F** Plaque Radiation	**Z** None	**Z** None

Section D **Radiation Therapy**
Body System V **Male Reproductive System**
Modality 0 **Beam Radiation**

Treatment Site (4th)	Modality Qualifier (5th)	Isotope (6th)	Qualifier (7th)
0 Prostate **1** Testis	**0** Photons <1 MeV **1** Photons 1 - 10 MeV **2** Photons >10 MeV **4** Heavy Particles (Protons,Ions) **5** Neutrons **6** Neutron Capture	**Z** None	**Z** None
0 Prostate **1** Testis	**3** Electrons	**Z** None	**0** Intraoperative **Z** None

Section D **Radiation Therapy**
Body System V **Male Reproductive System**
Modality 1 **Brachytherapy**

Treatment Site (4th)	Modality Qualifier (5th)	Isotope (6th)	Qualifier (7th)
0 Prostate **1** Testis	**9** High Dose Rate (HDR)	**7** Cesium 137 (Cs-137) **8** Iridium 192 (Ir-192) **9** Iodine 125 (I-125) **B** Palladium 103 (Pd-103) **C** Californium 252 (Cf-252) **Y** Other Isotope	**Z** None
0 Prostate **1** Testis	**B** Low Dose Rate (LDR)	**6** Cesium 131 (Cs-131) **7** Cesium 137 (Cs-137) **8** Iridium 192 (Ir-192) **9** Iodine 125 (I-125) **C** Californium 252 (Cf-252) **Y** Other Isotope	**Z** None
0 Prostate **1** Testis	**B** Low Dose Rate (LDR)	**B** Palladium 103 (Pd-103)	**1** Unidirectional Source **Z** None

Section D **Radiation Therapy**
Body System V **Male Reproductive System**
Modality 2 **Stereotactic Radiosurgery**

Treatment Site (4th)	Modality Qualifier (5th)	Isotope (6th)	Qualifier (7th)
0 Prostate **1** Testis	**D** Stereotactic Other Photon Radiosurgery **H** Stereotactic Particulate Radiosurgery **J** Stereotactic Gamma Beam Radiosurgery	**Z** None	**Z** None

Section D **Radiation Therapy**
Body System V **Male Reproductive System**
Modality Y **Other Radiation**

Treatment Site (4th)	Modality Qualifier (5th)	Isotope (6th)	Qualifier (7th)
0 Prostate	**7** Contact Radiation **8** Hyperthermia **C** Intraoperative Radiation Therapy (IORT) **F** Plaque Radiation **K** Laser Interstitial Thermal Therapy	**Z** None	**Z** None
1 Testis	**7** Contact Radiation **8** Hyperthermia **F** Plaque Radiation	**Z** None	**Z** None

Section D **Radiation Therapy**
Body System W **Anatomical Regions**
Modality 0 **Beam Radiation**

Treatment Site (4th)	Modality Qualifier (5th)	Isotope (6th)	Qualifier (7th)
1 Head and Neck **2** Chest **3** Abdomen **4** Hemibody **5** Whole Body **6** Pelvic Region	**0** Photons <1 MeV **1** Photons 1 - 10 MeV **2** Photons >10 MeV **4** Heavy Particles (Protons,Ions) **5** Neutrons **6** Neutron Capture	**Z** None	**Z** None
1 Head and Neck **2** Chest **3** Abdomen **4** Hemibody **5** Whole Body **6** Pelvic Region	**3** Electrons	**Z** None	**0** Intraoperative **Z** None

Section D **Radiation Therapy**
Body System W **Anatomical Regions**
Modality 1 **Brachytherapy**

Treatment Site (4th)	Modality Qualifier (5th)	Isotope (6th)	Qualifier (7th)
0 Cranial Cavity **K** Upper Back **L** Lower Back **P** Gastrointestinal Track **Q** Respiratory Track **R** Genitourinary Track **X** Upper Extremity **Y** Lower Extremity	**B** Low Dose Rate (LDR)	**B** Palladium 103 (Pd-103)	**1** Unidirectional Source **Z** None
1 Head and Neck **2** Chest **3** Abdomen **6** Pelvic Region	**9** High Dose Rate (HDR)	**7** Cesium 137 (Cs-137) **8** Iridium 192 (Ir-192) **9** Iodine 125 (I-125) **B** Palladium 103 (Pd-103) **C** Californium 252 (Cf-252) **Y** Other Isotope	**Z** None
1 Head and Neck **2** Chest **3** Abdomen **6** Pelvic Region	**B** Low Dose Rate (LDR)	**6** Cesium 131 (Cs-131) **7** Cesium 137 (Cs-137) **8** Iridium 192 (Ir-192) **9** Iodine 125 (I-125) **C** Californium 252 (Cf-252) **Y** Other Isotope	**Z** None
1 Head and Neck **2** Chest **3** Abdomen **6** Pelvic Region	**B** Low Dose Rate (LDR)	**B** Palladium 103 (Pd-103)	**1** Unidirectional Source **Z** None

Section D **Radiation Therapy**
Body System W **Anatomical Regions**
Modality 2 **Stereotactic Radiosurgery**

Treatment Site (4th)	Modality Qualifier (5th)	Isotope (6th)	Qualifier (7th)
1 Head and Neck **2** Chest **3** Abdomen **6** Pelvic Region	**D** Stereotactic Other Photon Radiosurgery **H** Stereotactic Particulate Radiosurgery **J** Stereotactic Gamma Beam Radiosurgery	**Z** None	**Z** None

Section D **Radiation Therapy**
Body System W **Anatomical Regions**
Modality Y **Other Radiation**

Treatment Site (4th)	Modality Qualifier (5th)	Isotope (6th)	Qualifier (7th)
1 Head and Neck **2** Chest **3** Abdomen **4** Hemibody **6** Pelvic Region	**7** Contact Radiation **8** Hyperthermia **F** Plaque Radiation	**Z** None	**Z** None
5 Whole Body	**7** Contact Radiation **8** Hyperthermia **F** Plaque Radiation	**Z** None	**Z** None
5 Whole Body	**G** Isotope Administration	**D** Iodine 131 (I-131) **F** Phosphorus 32 (P-32) **G** Strontium 89 (Sr-89) **H** Strontium 90 (Sr-90) **Y** Other Isotope	**Z** None

AHA Coding Clinic

DU11B7Z Low Dose Rate (LDR) Brachytherapy of Cervix using Cesium 137 (Cs-137)—AHA CC: 4Q, 2017, 104

DW16BB1 Low Dose Rate (LDR) Brachytherapy of Pelvic Region using Palladium 103 (Pd-103), Unidirectional Source—AHA CC: 4Q, 2019, 43-44

DWY38ZZ Hyperthermia of Abdomen—AHA CC: 4Q, 2019, 37

Physical Rehabilitation and Diagnostic Audiology Section (F00–F15)

Within each section of ICD-10-PCS the characters have different meanings. The seven character meanings for the Physical Rehabilitation and Diagnostic Audiology section are illustrated below through the procedure example of *Individual fitting of moveable brace, right knee*.

Section	Section Qualifier	Root Type	Body System/ Region	Type Qualifier	Equipment	Qualifier
Physical Rehabilitation and Diagnostic Audiology	Rehabilitation	Device Fitting	None	Dynamic Orthosis	Orthosis	None
F	0	D	Z	6	E	Z

Section (Character 1)

All Physical Rehabilitation and Diagnostic Audiology procedure codes have a first character value of F.

Section Qualifier (Character 2)

The alphanumeric character in the second character position identifies if the procedure is a physical rehabilitation procedure or a diagnostic audiology procedure. Physical rehabilitation is reported with character value 0, and diagnostic audiology is reported with character value 1.

Root Type (Character 3)

The alphanumeric character value for root types is placed in the third position. The following are the root types applicable to the Physical Rehabilitation and Diagnostic Audiology section with their associated meaning.

Character Value	Root Type	Root Type Definition
0	Speech Assessment	Measurement of speech and related functions
1	Motor and/or Nerve Function Assessment	Measurement of motor, nerve, and related functions
2	Activities of Daily Living Assessment	Measurement of functional level for activities of daily living
3	Hearing Assessment	Measurement of hearing and related functions
4	Hearing Aid Assessment	Measurement of the appropriateness and/or effectiveness of a hearing device
5	Vestibular Assessment	Measurement of the vestibular system and related functions
6	Speech Treatment	Application of techniques to improve, augment, or compensate for speech and related functional impairment
7	Motor Treatment	Exercise or activities to increase or facilitate motor function
8	Activities of Daily Living Treatment	Exercise or activities to facilitate functional competence for activities of daily living
9	Hearing Treatment	Application of techniques to improve, augment, or compensate for hearing and related functional impairment
B	Cochlear Implant Treatment	Application of techniques to improve the communication abilities of individuals with cochlear implant
C	Vestibular Treatment	Application of techniques to improve, augment, or compensate for vestibular and related functional impairment
D	Device Fitting	Fitting of a device designed to facilitate or support achievement of a higher level of function
F	Caregiver Training	Training in activities to support patient's optimal level of function

Body System/Region (Character 4)

For each body system/region the applicable body part character values will be available for procedure code construction. An example of a body region for this section is Musculoskeletal System—Lower Back/Lower Extremity.

Type Qualifier (Character 5)

Type qualifier further specifies the root type procedure. For example, the type qualifier of Gait Training/Functional Ambulation is used with Motor Treatment (character value 7) when applicable.

Equipment (Character 6)

If equipment is utilized during the procedure character six is used to report the type. Some examples of equipment are

- Aerobic Endurance and Conditioning
- Electrotherapeutic
- Mechanical
- Orthosis
- Prosthesis

If equipment is not utilized, the placeholder character value of Z should be reported.

Qualifier (Character 7)

The qualifier represents an additional attribute for the procedure when applicable. Currently, there are no qualifiers in the Physical Rehabilitation and Diagnostic Audiology section; therefore, the placeholder character value of Z should be reported.

Physical Rehabilitation and Diagnostic Audiology Section Tables

Physical Rehabilitation and Diagnostic Audiology Tables F00–F15

Section	**F**	**Physical Rehabilitation and Diagnostic Audiology**
Section Qualifier	**0**	**Rehabilitation**
Type	**0**	**Speech Assessment:** Measurement of speech and related functions

Body System / Region (4th)	Type Qualifier (5th)	Equipment (6th)	Qualifier (7th)
3 Neurological System - Whole Body	**G** Communicative/Cognitive Integration Skills	**K** Audiovisual **M** Augmentative / Alternative Communication **P** Computer **Y** Other Equipment **Z** None	**Z** None
Z None	**0** Filtered Speech **3** Staggered Spondaic Word **Q** Performance Intensity Phonetically Balanced Speech Discrimination **R** Brief Tone Stimuli **S** Distorted Speech **T** Dichotic Stimuli **V** Temporal Ordering of Stimuli **W** Masking Patterns	**1** Audiometer **2** Sound Field / Booth **K** Audiovisual **Z** None	**Z** None
Z None	**1** Speech Threshold **2** Speech/Word Recognition	**1** Audiometer **2** Sound Field / Booth **9** Cochlear Implant **K** Audiovisual **Z** None	**Z** None
Z None	**4** Sensorineural Acuity Level	**1** Audiometer **2** Sound Field / Booth **Z** None	**Z** None
Z None	**5** Synthetic Sentence Identification	**1** Audiometer **2** Sound Field / Booth **9** Cochlear Implant **K** Audiovisual	**Z** None
Z None	**6** Speech and/or Language Screening **7** Nonspoken Language **8** Receptive/Expressive Language **C** Aphasia **G** Communicative/Cognitive Integration Skills **L** Augmentative/Alternative Communication System	**K** Audiovisual **M** Augmentative / Alternative Communication **P** Computer **Y** Other Equipment **Z** None	**Z** None

Continued →

Section **F** **Physical Rehabilitation and Diagnostic Audiology**
Section Qualifier **0** **Rehabilitation**
Type **0** **Speech Assessment:** Measurement of speech and related functions

Body System / Region (4th)	Type Qualifier (5th)	Equipment (6th)	Qualifier (7th)
Z None	**9** Articulation/Phonology	**K** Audiovisual **P** Computer **Q** Speech Analysis **Y** Other Equipment **Z** None	**Z** None
Z None	**B** Motor Speech	**K** Audiovisual **N** Biosensory Feedback **P** Computer **Q** Speech Analysis **T** Aerodynamic Function **Y** Other Equipment **Z** None	**Z** None
Z None	**D** Fluency	**K** Audiovisual **N** Biosensory Feedback **P** Computer **Q** Speech Analysis **S** Voice Analysis **T** Aerodynamic Function **Y** Other Equipment **Z** None	**Z** None
Z None	**F** Voice	**K** Audiovisual **N** Biosensory Feedback **P** Computer **S** Voice Analysis **T** Aerodynamic Function **Y** Other Equipment **Z** None	**Z** None
Z None	**H** Bedside Swallowing and Oral Function **P** Oral Peripheral Mechanism	**Y** Other Equipment **Z** None	**Z** None
Z None	**J** Instrumental Swallowing and Oral Function	**T** Aerodynamic Function **W** Swallowing **Y** Other Equipment	**Z** None
Z None	**K** Orofacial Myofunctional	**K** Audiovisual **P** Computer **Y** Other Equipment **Z** None	**Z** None
Z None	**M** Voice Prosthetic	**K** Audiovisual **P** Computer **S** Voice Analysis **V** Speech Prosthesis **Y** Other Equipment **Z** None	**Z** None
Z None	**N** Non-invasive Instrumental Status	**N** Biosensory Feedback **P** Computer **Q** Speech Analysis **S** Voice Analysis **T** Aerodynamic Function **Y** Other Equipment	**Z** None
Z None	**X** Other Specified Central Auditory Processing	**Z** None	**Z** None

Section F Physical Rehabilitation and Diagnostic Audiology
Section Qualifier 0 Rehabilitation
Type 1 **Motor and/or Nerve Function Assessment:** Measurement of motor, nerve, and related functions

Body System / Region (4th)	Type Qualifier (5th)	Equipment (6th)	Qualifier (7th)
0 Neurological System - Head and Neck **1** Neurological System - Upper Back / Upper Extremity **2** Neurological System - Lower Back / Lower Extremity **3** Neurological System - Whole Body	**0** Muscle Performance	**E** Orthosis **F** Assistive, Adaptive, Supportive or Protective **U** Prosthesis **Y** Other Equipment **Z** None	**Z** None
0 Neurological System - Head and Neck **1** Neurological System - Upper Back / Upper Extremity **2** Neurological System - Lower Back / Lower Extremity **3** Neurological System - Whole Body	**1** Integumentary Integrity **3** Coordination/Dexterity **4** Motor Function **G** Reflex Integrity	**Z** None	**Z** None
0 Neurological System - Head and Neck **1** Neurological System - Upper Back / Upper Extremity **2** Neurological System - Lower Back / Lower Extremity **3** Neurological System - Whole Body	**5** Range of Motion and Joint Integrity **6** Sensory Awareness/ Processing/Integrity	**Y** Other Equipment **Z** None	**Z** None
D Integumentary System - Head and Neck **F** Integumentary System - Upper Back / Upper Extremity **G** Integumentary System - Lower Back / Lower Extremity **H** Integumentary System - Whole Body **J** Musculoskeletal System - Head and Neck **K** Musculoskeletal System - Upper Back / Upper Extremity **L** Musculoskeletal System - Lower Back / Lower Extremity **M** Musculoskeletal System - Whole Body	**0** Muscle Performance	**E** Orthosis **F** Assistive, Adaptive, Supportive or Protective **U** Prosthesis **Y** Other Equipment **Z** None	**Z** None
D Integumentary System - Head and Neck **F** Integumentary System - Upper Back / Upper Extremity **G** Integumentary System - Lower Back / Lower Extremity **H** Integumentary System - Whole Body **J** Musculoskeletal System - Head and Neck **K** Musculoskeletal System - Upper Back / Upper Extremity **L** Musculoskeletal System - Lower Back / Lower Extremity **M** Musculoskeletal System - Whole Body	**1** Integumentary Integrity	**Z** None	**Z** None
D Integumentary System - Head and Neck **F** Integumentary System - Upper Back / Upper Extremity **G** Integumentary System - Lower Back / Lower Extremity **H** Integumentary System - Whole Body **J** Musculoskeletal System - Head and Neck **K** Musculoskeletal System - Upper Back / Upper Extremity **L** Musculoskeletal System - Lower Back / Lower Extremity **M** Musculoskeletal System - Whole Body	**5** Range of Motion and Joint Integrity **6** Sensory Awareness/ Processing/Integrity	**Y** Other Equipment **Z** None	**Z** None

Continued →

Section F **Physical Rehabilitation and Diagnostic Audiology**
Section Qualifier 0 **Rehabilitation**
Type 1 **Motor and/or Nerve Function Assessment:** Measurement of motor, nerve, and related functions

Body System / Region (4th)	Type Qualifier (5th)	Equipment (6th)	Qualifier (7th)
N Genitourinary System	**0** Muscle Performance	**E** Orthosis **F** Assistive, Adaptive, Supportive or Protective **U** Prosthesis **Y** Other Equipment **Z** None	**Z** None
Z None	**2** Visual Motor Integration	**K** Audiovisual **M** Augmentative / Alternative Communication **N** Biosensory Feedback **P** Computer **Q** Speech Analysis **S** Voice Analysis **Y** Other Equipment **Z** None	**Z** None
Z None	**7** Facial Nerve Function	**7** Electrophysiologic	**Z** None
Z None	**9** Somatosensory Evoked Potentials	**J** Somatosensory	**Z** None
Z None	**B** Bed Mobility **C** Transfer **F** Wheelchair Mobility	**E** Orthosis **F** Assistive, Adaptive, Supportive or Protective **U** Prosthesis **Z** None	**Z** None
Z None	**D** Gait and/or Balance	**E** Orthosis **F** Assistive, Adaptive, Supportive or Protective **U** Prosthesis **Y** Other Equipment **Z** None	**Z** None

Section F **Physical Rehabilitation and Diagnostic Audiology**
Section Qualifier 0 **Rehabilitation**
Type 2 **Activities of Daily Living Assessment:** Measurement of functional level for activities of daily living

Body System / Region (4th)	Type Qualifier (5th)	Equipment (6th)	Qualifier (7th)
0 Neurological System - Head and Neck	**9** Cranial Nerve Integrity **D** Neuromotor Development	**Y** Other Equipment **Z** None	**Z** None
1 Neurological System - Upper Back / Upper Extremity **2** Neurological System - Lower Back / Lower Extremity **3** Neurological System - Whole Body	**D** Neuromotor Development	**Y** Other Equipment **Z** None	**Z** None
4 Circulatory System - Head and Neck **5** Circulatory System - Upper Back / Upper Extremity **6** Circulatory System - Lower Back / Lower Extremity **8** Respiratory System - Head and Neck **9** Respiratory System - Upper Back / Upper Extremity **B** Respiratory System - Lower Back / Lower Extremity	**G** Ventilation, Respiration and Circulation	**C** Mechanical **G** Aerobic Endurance and Conditioning **Y** Other Equipment **Z** None	**Z** None

Continued →

Section F Physical Rehabilitation and Diagnostic Audiology
Section Qualifier 0 Rehabilitation
Type 2 **Activities of Daily Living Assessment:** Measurement of functional level for activities of daily living

F02 Continued

Body System / Region (4th)	Type Qualifier (5th)	Equipment (6th)	Qualifier (7th)
7 Circulatory System - Whole Body **C** Respiratory System - Whole Body	**7** Aerobic Capacity and Endurance	**E** Orthosis **G** Aerobic Endurance and Conditioning **U** Prosthesis **Y** Other Equipment **Z** None	**Z** None
7 Circulatory System - Whole Body **C** Respiratory System - Whole Body	**G** Ventilation, Respiration and Circulation	**C** Mechanical **G** Aerobic Endurance and Conditioning **Y** Other Equipment **Z** None	**Z** None
Z None	**0** Bathing/Showering **1** Dressing **3** Grooming/Personal Hygiene **4** Home Management	**E** Orthosis **F** Assistive, Adaptive, Supportive or Protective **U** Prosthesis **Z** None	**Z** None
Z None	**2** Feeding/Eating **8** Anthropometric Characteristics **F** Pain	**Y** Other Equipment **Z** None	**Z** None
Z None	**5** Perceptual Processing	**K** Audiovisual **M** Augmentative / Alternative Communication **N** Biosensory Feedback **P** Computer **Q** Speech Analysis **S** Voice Analysis **Y** Other Equipment **Z** None	**Z** None
Z None	**6** Psychosocial Skills	**Z** None	**Z** None
Z None	**B** Environmental, Home and Work Barriers **C** Ergonomics and Body Mechanics	**E** Orthosis **F** Assistive, Adaptive, Supportive or Protective **U** Prosthesis **Y** Other Equipment **Z** None	**Z** None
Z None	**H** Vocational Activities and Functional Community or Work Reintegration Skills	**E** Orthosis **F** Assistive, Adaptive, Supportive or Protective **G** Aerobic Endurance and Conditioning **U** Prosthesis **Y** Other Equipment **Z** None	**Z** None

Section F Physical Rehabilitation and Diagnostic Audiology
Section Qualifier 0 Rehabilitation
Type 6 **Speech Treatment:** Application of techniques to improve, augment, or compensate for speech and related functional impairment

Body System / Region (4th)	Type Qualifier (5th)	Equipment (6th)	Qualifier (7th)
3 Neurological System - Whole Body	**6** Communicative/Cognitive Integration Skills	**K** Audiovisual **M** Augmentative / Alternative Communication **P** Computer **Y** Other Equipment **Z** None	**Z** None

Continued →

Section F Physical Rehabilitation and Diagnostic Audiology
Section Qualifier 0 Rehabilitation
Type 6 **Speech Treatment:** Application of techniques to improve, augment, or compensate for speech and related functional impairment

Body System / Region (4th)	Type Qualifier (5th)	Equipment (6th)	Qualifier (7th)
Z None	**0** Nonspoken Language **3** Aphasia **6** Communicative/Cognitive Integration Skills	**K** Audiovisual **M** Augmentative / Alternative Communication **P** Computer **Y** Other Equipment **Z** None	**Z** None
Z None	**1** Speech-Language Pathology and Related Disorders Counseling **2** Speech-Language Pathology and Related Disorders Prevention	**K** Audiovisual **Z** None	**Z** None
Z None	**4** Articulation/Phonology	**K** Audiovisual **P** Computer **Q** Speech Analysis **T** Aerodynamic Function **Y** Other Equipment **Z** None	**Z** None
Z None	**5** Aural Rehabilitation	**K** Audiovisual **L** Assistive Listening **M** Augmentative / Alternative Communication **N** Biosensory Feedback **P** Computer **Q** Speech Analysis **S** Voice Analysis **Y** Other Equipment **Z** None	**Z** None
Z None	**7** Fluency	**4** Electroacoustic Immitance / Acoustic Reflex **K** Audiovisual **N** Biosensory Feedback **Q** Speech Analysis **S** Voice Analysis **T** Aerodynamic Function **Y** Other Equipment **Z** None	**Z** None
Z None	**8** Motor Speech	**K** Audiovisual **N** Biosensory Feedback **P** Computer **Q** Speech Analysis **S** Voice Analysis **T** Aerodynamic Function **Y** Other Equipment **Z** None	**Z** None
Z None	**9** Orofacial Myofunctional	**K** Audiovisual **P** Computer **Y** Other Equipment **Z** None	**Z** None
Z None	**B** Receptive/Expressive Language	**K** Audiovisual **L** Assistive Listening **M** Augmentative / Alternative Communication **P** Computer **Y** Other Equipment **Z** None	**Z** None

Continued →

Section F Physical Rehabilitation and Diagnostic Audiology
Section Qualifier 0 Rehabilitation
Type 6 **Speech Treatment:** Application of techniques to improve, augment, or compensate for speech and related functional impairment

Body System / Region (4th)	Type Qualifier (5th)	Equipment (6th)	Qualifier (7th)
Z None	**C** Voice	**K** Audiovisual **N** Biosensory Feedback **P** Computer **S** Voice Analysis **T** Aerodynamic Function **V** Speech Prosthesis **Y** Other Equipment **Z** None	**Z** None
Z None	**D** Swallowing Dysfunction	**M** Augmentative / Alternative Communication **T** Aerodynamic Function **V** Speech Prosthesis **Y** Other Equipment **Z** None	**Z** None

Section F Physical Rehabilitation and Diagnostic Audiology
Section Qualifier 0 Rehabilitation
Type 7 **Motor Treatment:** Exercise or activities to increase or facilitate motor function

Body System / Region (4th)	Type Qualifier (5th)	Equipment (6th)	Qualifier (7th)
0 Neurological System - Head and Neck **1** Neurological System - Upper Back / Upper Extremity **2** Neurological System - Lower Back / Lower Extremity **3** Neurological System - Whole Body **D** Integumentary System - Head and Neck **F** Integumentary System - Upper Back / Upper Extremity **G** Integumentary System - Lower Back / Lower Extremity **H** Integumentary System - Whole Body **J** Musculoskeletal System - Head and Neck **K** Musculoskeletal System - Upper Back / Upper Extremity **L** Musculoskeletal System - Lower Back / Lower Extremity **M** Musculoskeletal System - Whole Body	**0** Range of Motion and Joint Mobility **1** Muscle Performance **2** Coordination/Dexterity **3** Motor Function	**E** Orthosis **F** Assistive, Adaptive, Supportive or Protective **U** Prosthesis **Y** Other Equipment **Z** None	**Z** None
0 Neurological System - Head and Neck **1** Neurological System - Upper Back / Upper Extremity **2** Neurological System - Lower Back / Lower Extremity **3** Neurological System - Whole Body **D** Integumentary System - Head and Neck **F** Integumentary System - Upper Back / Upper Extremity **G** Integumentary System - Lower Back / Lower Extremity **H** Integumentary System - Whole Body **J** Musculoskeletal System - Head and Neck **K** Musculoskeletal System - Upper Back / Upper Extremity **L** Musculoskeletal System - Lower Back / Lower Extremity **M** Musculoskeletal System - Whole Body	**6** Therapeutic Exercise	**B** Physical Agents **C** Mechanical **D** Electrotherapeutic **E** Orthosis **F** Assistive, Adaptive, Supportive or Protective **G** Aerobic Endurance and Conditioning **H** Mechanical or Electromechanical **U** Prosthesis **Y** Other Equipment **Z** None	**Z** None

Continued →

Body System / Region (4th)	Type Qualifier (5th)	Equipment (6th)	Qualifier (7th)
0 Neurological System - Head and Neck **1** Neurological System - Upper Back / Upper Extremity **2** Neurological System - Lower Back / Lower Extremity **3** Neurological System - Whole Body **D** Integumentary System - Head and Neck **F** Integumentary System - Upper Back / Upper Extremity **G** Integumentary System - Lower Back / Lower Extremity **H** Integumentary System - Whole Body **J** Musculoskeletal System - Head and Neck **K** Musculoskeletal System - Upper Back / Upper Extremity **L** Musculoskeletal System - Lower Back / Lower Extremity **M** Musculoskeletal System - Whole Body	**7** Manual Therapy Techniques	**Z** None	**Z** None
4 Circulatory System - Head and Neck **5** Circulatory System - Upper Back / Upper Extremity **6** Circulatory System - Lower Back / Lower Extremity **7** Circulatory System - Whole Body **8** Respiratory System - Head and Neck **9** Respiratory System - Upper Back / Upper Extremity **B** Respiratory System - Lower Back / Lower Extremity **C** Respiratory System - Whole Body	**6** Therapeutic Exercise	**B** Physical Agents **C** Mechanical **D** Electrotherapeutic **E** Orthosis **F** Assistive, Adaptive, Supportive or Protective **G** Aerobic Endurance and Conditioning **H** Mechanical or Electromechanical **U** Prosthesis **Y** Other Equipment **Z** None	**Z** None
N Genitourinary System	**1** Muscle Performance	**E** Orthosis **F** Assistive, Adaptive, Supportive or Protective **U** Prosthesis **Y** Other Equipment **Z** None	**Z** None
N Genitourinary System	**6** Therapeutic Exercise	**B** Physical Agents **C** Mechanical **D** Electrotherapeutic **E** Orthosis **F** Assistive, Adaptive, Supportive or Protective **G** Aerobic Endurance and Conditioning **H** Mechanical or Electromechanical **U** Prosthesis **Y** Other Equipment **Z** None	**Z** None
Z None	**4** Wheelchair Mobility	**D** Electrotherapeutic **E** Orthosis **F** Assistive, Adaptive, Supportive or Protective **U** Prosthesis **Y** Other Equipment **Z** None	**Z** None
Z None	**5** Bed Mobility	**C** Mechanical **E** Orthosis **F** Assistive, Adaptive, Supportive or Protective **U** Prosthesis **Y** Other Equipment **Z** None	**Z** None

Continued →

Section F **Physical Rehabilitation and Diagnostic Audiology**
Section Qualifier 0 **Rehabilitation**
Type 7 **Motor Treatment:** Exercise or activities to increase or facilitate motor function

Body System / Region (4th)	Type Qualifier (5th)	Equipment (6th)	Qualifier (7th)
Z None	**8** Transfer Training	**C** Mechanical **D** Electrotherapeutic **E** Orthosis **F** Assistive, Adaptive, Supportive or Protective **U** Prosthesis **Y** Other Equipment **Z** None	**Z** None
Z None	**9** Gait Training/ Functional Ambulation	**C** Mechanical **D** Electrotherapeutic **E** Orthosis **F** Assistive, Adaptive, Supportive or Protective **G** Aerobic Endurance and Conditioning **U** Prosthesis **Y** Other Equipment **Z** None	**Z** None

Section F **Physical Rehabilitation and Diagnostic Audiology**
Section Qualifier 0 **Rehabilitation**
Type 8 **Activities of Daily Living Treatment:** Exercise or activities to facilitate functional competence for activities of daily living

Body System / Region (4th)	Type Qualifier (5th)	Equipment (6th)	Qualifier (7th)
D Integumentary System - Head and Neck **F** Integumentary System - Upper Back / Upper Extremity **G** Integumentary System - Lower Back / Lower Extremity **H** Integumentary System - Whole Body **J** Musculoskeletal System - Head and Neck **K** Musculoskeletal System - Upper Back / Upper Extremity **L** Musculoskeletal System - Lower Back / Lower Extremity **M** Musculoskeletal System - Whole Body	**5** Wound Management	**B** Physical Agents **C** Mechanical **D** Electrotherapeutic **E** Orthosis **F** Assistive, Adaptive, Supportive or Protective **U** Prosthesis **Y** Other Equipment **Z** None	**Z** None
Z None	**0** Bathing/Showering Techniques **1** Dressing Techniques **2** Grooming/Personal Hygiene	**E** Orthosis **F** Assistive, Adaptive, Supportive or Protective **U** Prosthesis **Y** Other Equipment **Z** None	**Z** None
Z None	**3** Feeding/Eating	**C** Mechanical **D** Electrotherapeutic **E** Orthosis **F** Assistive, Adaptive, Supportive or Protective **U** Prosthesis **Y** Other Equipment **Z** None	**Z** None
Z None	**4** Home Management	**D** Electrotherapeutic **E** Orthosis **F** Assistive, Adaptive, Supportive or Protective **U** Prosthesis **Y** Other Equipment **Z** None	**Z** None

Continued →

Section F **Physical Rehabilitation and Diagnostic Audiology**
Section Qualifier 0 **Rehabilitation**
Type 8 **Activities of Daily Living Treatment:** Exercise or activities to facilitate functional competence for activities of daily living

Body System / Region (4th)	Type Qualifier (5th)	Equipment (6th)	Qualifier (7th)
Z None	**6** Psychosocial Skills	**Z** None	**Z** None
Z None	**7** Vocational Activities and Functional Community or Work Reintegration Skills	**B** Physical Agents **C** Mechanical **D** Electrotherapeutic **E** Orthosis **F** Assistive, Adaptive, Supportive or Protective **G** Aerobic Endurance and Conditioning **U** Prosthesis **Y** Other Equipment **Z** None	**Z** None

Section F **Physical Rehabilitation and Diagnostic Audiology**
Section Qualifier 0 **Rehabilitation**
Type 9 **Hearing Treatment:** Application of techniques to improve, augment, or compensate for hearing and related functional impairment

Body System / Region (4th)	Type Qualifier (5th)	Equipment (6th)	Qualifier (7th)
Z None	**0** Hearing and Related Disorders Counseling **1** Hearing and Related Disorders Prevention	**K** Audiovisual **Z** None	**Z** None
Z None	**2** Auditory Processing	**K** Audiovisual **L** Assistive Listening **P** Computer **Y** Other Equipment **Z** None	**Z** None
Z None	**3** Cerumen Management	**X** Cerumen Management **Z** None	**Z** None

Section F **Physical Rehabilitation and Diagnostic Audiology**
Section Qualifier 0 **Rehabilitation**
Type B **Cochlear Implant Treatment:** Application of techniques to improve the communication abilities of individuals with cochlear implant

Body System / Region (4th)	Type Qualifier (5th)	Equipment (6th)	Qualifier (7th)
Z None	**0** Cochlear Implant Rehabilitation	**1** Audiometer **2** Sound Field / Booth **9** Cochlear Implant **K** Audiovisual **P** Computer **Y** Other Equipment	**Z** None

Section F **Physical Rehabilitation and Diagnostic Audiology**
Section Qualifier 0 **Rehabilitation**
Type C **Vestibular Treatment:** Application of techniques to improve, augment, or compensate for vestibular and related functional impairment

Body System / Region (4th)	Type Qualifier (5th)	Equipment (6th)	Qualifier (7th)
3 Neurological System - Whole Body H Integumentary System - Whole Body M Musculoskeletal System - Whole Body	3 Postural Control	E Orthosis F Assistive, Adaptive, Supportive or Protective U Prosthesis Y Other Equipment Z None	Z None
Z None	0 Vestibular	8 Vestibular / Balance Z None	Z None
Z None	1 Perceptual Processing 2 Visual Motor Integration	K Audiovisual L Assistive Listening N Biosensory Feedback P Computer Q Speech Analysis S Voice Analysis T Aerodynamic Function Y Other Equipment Z None	Z None

Section F **Physical Rehabilitation and Diagnostic Audiology**
Section Qualifier 0 **Rehabilitation**
Type D **Device Fitting:** Fitting of a device designed to facilitate or support achievement of a higher level of function

Body System / Region (4th)	Type Qualifier (5th)	Equipment (6th)	Qualifier (7th)
Z None	0 Tinnitus Masker	5 Hearing Aid Selection / Fitting / Test Z None	Z None
Z None	1 Monaural Hearing Aid 2 Binaural Hearing Aid 5 Assistive Listening Device	1 Audiometer 2 Sound Field / Booth 5 Hearing Aid Selection / Fitting / Test K Audiovisual L Assistive Listening Z None	Z None
Z None	3 Augmentative/Alternative Communication System	M Augmentative / Alternative Communication	Z None
Z None	4 Voice Prosthetic	S Voice Analysis V Speech Prosthesis	Z None
Z None	6 Dynamic Orthosis 7 Static Orthosis 8 Prosthesis 9 Assistive, Adaptive, Supportive or Protective Devices	E Orthosis F Assistive, Adaptive, Supportive or Protective U Prosthesis Z None	Z None

Section F **Physical Rehabilitation and Diagnostic Audiology**
Section Qualifier 0 **Rehabilitation**
Type F **Caregiver Training:** Training in activities to support patient's optimal level of function

Body System / Region (4th)	Type Qualifier (5th)	Equipment (6th)	Qualifier (7th)
Z None	**0** Bathing/Showering Technique **1** Dressing **2** Feeding and Eating **3** Grooming/Personal Hygiene **4** Bed Mobility **5** Transfer **6** Wheelchair Mobility **7** Therapeutic Exercise **8** Airway Clearance Techniques **9** Wound Management **B** Vocational Activities and Functional Community or Work Reintegration Skills **C** Gait Training/Functional Ambulation **D** Application, Proper Use and Care of Devices **F** Application, Proper Use and Care of Orthoses **G** Application, Proper Use and Care of Prosthesis **H** Home Management	**E** Orthosis **F** Assistive, Adaptive, Supportive or Protective **U** Prosthesis **Z** None	**Z** None
Z None	**J** Communication Skills	**K** Audiovisual **L** Assistive Listening **M** Augmentative / Alternative Communication **P** Computer **Z** None	**Z** None

Section F **Physical Rehabilitation and Diagnostic Audiology**
Section Qualifier 1 **Diagnostic Audiology**
Type 3 **Hearing Assessment:** Measurement of hearing and related functions

Body System / Region (4th)	Type Qualifier (5th)	Equipment (6th)	Qualifier (7th)
Z None	**0** Hearing Screening	**0** Occupational Hearing **1** Audiometer **2** Sound Field / Booth **3** Tympanometer **8** Vestibular / Balance **9** Cochlear Implant **Z** None	**Z** None
Z None	**1** Pure Tone Audiometry, Air **2** Pure Tone Audiometry, Air and Bone	**0** Occupational Hearing **1** Audiometer **2** Sound Field / Booth **Z** None	**Z** None
Z None	**3** Bekesy Audiometry **6** Visual Reinforcement Audiometry **9** Short Increment Sensitivity Index **B** Stenger **C** Pure Tone Stenger	**1** Audiometer **2** Sound Field / Booth **Z** None	**Z** None
Z None	**4** Conditioned Play Audiometry **5** Select Picture Audiometry	**1** Audiometer **2** Sound Field / Booth **K** Audiovisual **Z** None	**Z** None
Z None	**7** Alternate Binaural or Monaural Loudness Balance	**1** Audiometer **K** Audiovisual **Z** None	**Z** None

Continued →

Section F **Physical Rehabilitation and Diagnostic Audiology**
Section Qualifier 1 **Diagnostic Audiology**
Type 3 **Hearing Assessment:** Measurement of hearing and related functions

Body System / Region (4th)	Type Qualifier (5th)	Equipment (6th)	Qualifier (7th)
Z None	**8** Tone Decay **D** Tympanometry **F** Eustachian Tube Function **G** Acoustic Reflex Patterns **H** Acoustic Reflex Threshold **J** Acoustic Reflex Decay	**3** Tympanometer **4** Electroacoustic Immitance / Acoustic Reflex **Z** None	**Z** None
Z None	**K** Electrocochleography **L** Auditory Evoked Potentials	**7** Electrophysiologic **Z** None	**Z** None
Z None	**M** Evoked Otoacoustic Emissions, Screening **N** Evoked Otoacoustic Emissions, Diagnostic	**6** Otoacoustic Emission (OAE) **Z** None	**Z** None
Z None	**P** Aural Rehabilitation Status	**1** Audiometer **2** Sound Field / Booth **4** Electroacoustic Immitance / Acoustic Reflex **9** Cochlear Implant **K** Audiovisual **L** Assistive Listening **P** Computer **Z** None	**Z** None
Z None	**Q** Auditory Processing	**K** Audiovisual **P** Computer **Y** Other Equipment **Z** None	**Z** None

Section F **Physical Rehabilitation and Diagnostic Audiology**
Section Qualifier 1 **Diagnostic Audiology**
Type 4 **Hearing Aid Assessment:** Measurement of the appropriateness and/or effectiveness of a hearing device

Body System / Region (4th)	Type Qualifier (5th)	Equipment (6th)	Qualifier (7th)
Z None	**0** Cochlear Implant	**1** Audiometer **2** Sound Field / Booth **3** Tympanometer **4** Electroacoustic Immitance / Acoustic Reflex **5** Hearing Aid Selection / Fitting / Test **7** Electrophysiologic **9** Cochlear Implant **K** Audiovisual **L** Assistive Listening **P** Computer **Y** Other Equipment **Z** None	**Z** None
Z None	**1** Ear Canal Probe Microphone **6** Binaural Electroacoustic Hearing Aid Check **8** Monaural Electroacoustic Hearing Aid Check	**5** Hearing Aid Selection / Fitting / Test **Z** None	**Z** None

Continued →

Section F **Physical Rehabilitation and Diagnostic Audiology**
Section Qualifier 1 **Diagnostic Audiology**
Type 4 **Hearing Aid Assessment:** Measurement of the appropriateness and/or effectiveness of a hearing device

Body System / Region (4th)	Type Qualifier (5th)	Equipment (6th)	Qualifier (7th)
Z None	**2** Monaural Hearing Aid **3** Binaural Hearing Aid	**1** Audiometer **2** Sound Field / Booth **3** Tympanometer **4** Electroacoustic Immitance / Acoustic Reflex **5** Hearing Aid Selection / Fitting / Test **K** Audiovisual **L** Assistive Listening **P** Computer **Z** None	**Z** None
Z None	**4** Assistive Listening System/ Device Selection	**1** Audiometer **2** Sound Field / Booth **3** Tympanometer **4** Electroacoustic Immitance / Acoustic Reflex **K** Audiovisual **L** Assistive Listening **Z** None	**Z** None
Z None	**5** Sensory Aids	**1** Audiometer **2** Sound Field / Booth **3** Tympanometer **4** Electroacoustic Immitance / Acoustic Reflex **5** Hearing Aid Selection / Fitting / Test **K** Audiovisual **L** Assistive Listening **Z** None	**Z** None
Z None	**7** Ear Protector Attentuation	**0** Occupational Hearing **Z** None	**Z** None

Section F **Physical Rehabilitation and Diagnostic Audiology**
Section Qualifier 1 **Diagnostic Audiology**
Type 5 **Vestibular Assessment:** Measurement of the vestibular system and related functions

Body System / Region (4th)	Type Qualifier (5th)	Equipment (6th)	Qualifier (7th)
Z None	**0** Bithermal, Binaural Caloric Irrigation **1** Bithermal, Monaural Caloric Irrigation **2** Unithermal Binaural Screen **3** Oscillating Tracking **4** Sinusoidal Vertical Axis Rotational **5** Dix-Hallpike Dynamic **6** Computerized Dynamic Posturography	**8** Vestibular / Balance **Z** None	**Z** None
Z None	**7** Tinnitus Masker	**5** Hearing Aid Selection / Fitting / Test **Z** None	**Z** None

AHA Coding Clinic

No references have been issued for the Physical Rehabilitation and Diagnostic Audiology section.

Mental Health Section (GZ1–GZJ)

Within each section of ICD-10-PCS the characters have different meanings. The seven character meanings for the Mental Health section are illustrated here through the procedure example of *Crisis intervention*.

Section	Body System	Root Type	Qualifier	Qualifier	Qualifier	Qualifier
Mental Health	None	Crisis Intervention	None	None	None	None
G	Z	2	Z	Z	Z	Z

Section (Character 1)

All Mental Health procedure codes have a first character value of G.

Body System (Character 2)

The body system is not specified for mental health; therefore, the placeholder character value of Z is reported in the second character position.

Root Type (Character 3)

The alphanumeric character value for root types is placed in the third position. Listed below are the root types applicable to the Mental Health section with their associated meaning.

Character Value	Root Type	Root Type Definition
1	Psychological Tests	The administration and interpretation of standardized psychological tests and measurement instruments for the assessment of psychological function
2	Crisis Intervention	Treatment of a traumatized, acutely disturbed or distressed individual for the purpose of short-term stabilization
3	Medication Management	Monitoring and adjusting the use of medications for the treatment of a mental health disorder
5	Individual Psychotherapy	Treatment of an individual with a mental health disorder by behavioral, cognitive, psychoanalytic, psychodynamic or psychophysiological means to improve functioning or well-being
6	Counseling	The application of psychological methods to treat an individual with normal developmental issues and psychological problems in order to increase function, improve well-being, alleviate distress, maladjustment or resolve crises
7	Family Psychotherapy	Treatment that includes one or more family members of an individual with a mental health disorder by behavioral, cognitive, psychoanalytic, psychodynamic or psychophysiological means to improve functioning or well-being
B	Electroconvulsive Therapy	The application of controlled electrical voltages to treat a mental health disorder
C	Biofeedback	Provision of information from the monitoring and regulating of physiological processes in conjunction with cognitive-behavioral techniques to improve patient functioning or well-being
F	Hypnosis	Induction of a state of heightened suggestibility by auditory, visual and tactile techniques to elicit an emotional or behavioral response
G	Narcosynthesis	Administration of intravenous barbiturates in order to release suppressed or repressed thoughts
H	Group Psychotherapy	Treatment of two or more individuals with a mental health disorder by behavioral, cognitive, psychoanalytic, psychodynamic or psychophysiological means to improve functioning or well-being
J	Light Therapy	Application of specialized light treatments to improve functioning or well-being

Qualifier (Character 4)

This qualifier further specifies the root type procedure. For example, the qualifier of Development further specifies the type of Psychological Tests.

Qualifier (Character 5)

The qualifier represents an additional attribute for the procedure when applicable. Currently, there are no qualifiers in the Mental Health section; therefore, the placeholder character value of Z should be reported.

Qualifier (Character 6)

The qualifier represents an additional attribute for the procedure when applicable. Currently, there are no qualifiers in the Mental Health section; therefore, the placeholder character value of Z should be reported.

Qualifier (Character 7)

The qualifier represents an additional attribute for the procedure when applicable. Currently, there are no qualifiers in the Mental Health section; therefore, the placeholder character value of Z should be reported.

Mental Health Section Tables

Mental Health Tables GZ1–GZJ

Section G **Mental Health**
Body System Z **None**
Type 1 **Psychological Tests:** The administration and interpretation of standardized psychological tests and measurement instruments for the assessment of psychological function

Qualifier (4th)	Qualifier (5th)	Qualifier (6th)	Qualifier (7th)
0 Developmental **1** Personality and Behavioral **2** Intellectual and Psychoeducational **3** Neuropsychological **4** Neurobehavioral and Cognitive Status	**Z** None	**Z** None	**Z** None

Section G **Mental Health**
Body System Z **None**
Type 2 **Crisis Intervention:** Treatment of a traumatized, acutely disturbed or distressed individual for the purpose of short-term stabilization

Qualifier (4th)	Qualifier (5th)	Qualifier (6th)	Qualifier (7th)
Z None	**Z** None	**Z** None	**Z** None

Section G **Mental Health**
Body System Z **None**
Type 3 **Medication Management:** Monitoring and adjusting the use of medications for the treatment of a mental health disorder

Qualifier (4th)	Qualifier (5th)	Qualifier (6th)	Qualifier (7th)
Z None	**Z** None	**Z** None	**Z** None

Section G **Mental Health**
Body System Z **None**
Type 5 **Individual Psychotherapy:** Treatment of an individual with a mental health disorder by behavioral, cognitive, psychoanalytic, psychodynamic or psychophysiological means to improve functioning or well-being

Qualifier (4th)	Qualifier (5th)	Qualifier (6th)	Qualifier (7th)
0 Interactive **1** Behavioral **2** Cognitive **3** Interpersonal **4** Psychoanalysis **5** Psychodynamic **6** Supportive **8** Cognitive-Behavioral **9** Psychophysiological	**Z** None	**Z** None	**Z** None

Section G **Mental Health**
Body System Z **None**
Type 6 **Counseling:** The application of psychological methods to treat an individual with normal developmental issues and psychological problems in order to increase function, improve well-being, alleviate distress, maladjustment or resolve crises

Qualifier (4th)	Qualifier (5th)	Qualifier (6th)	Qualifier (7th)
0 Educational **1** Vocational **3** Other Counseling	**Z** None	**Z** None	**Z** None

Section G **Mental Health**
Body System Z **None**
Type 7 **Family Psychotherapy:** Treatment that includes one or more family members of an individual with a mental health disorder by behavioral, cognitive, psychoanalytic, psychodynamic or psychophysiological means to improve functioning or well-being

Qualifier (4th)	Qualifier (5th)	Qualifier (6th)	Qualifier (7th)
2 Other Family Psychotherapy	**Z** None	**Z** None	**Z** None

Section G **Mental Health**
Body System Z **None**
Type B **Electroconvulsive Therapy:** The application of controlled electrical voltages to treat a mental health disorder

Qualifier (4th)	Qualifier (5th)	Qualifier (6th)	Qualifier (7th)
0 Unilateral-Single Seizure **1** Unilateral-Multiple Seizure **2** Bilateral-Single Seizure **3** Bilateral-Multiple Seizure **4** Other Electroconvulsive Therapy	**Z** None	**Z** None	**Z** None

Section G **Mental Health**
Body System Z **None**
Type C **Biofeedback:** Provision of information from the monitoring and regulating of physiological processes in conjunction with cognitive-behavioral techniques to improve patient functioning or well-being

Qualifier (4th)	Qualifier (5th)	Qualifier (6th)	Qualifier (7th)
9 Other Biofeedback	**Z** None	**Z** None	**Z** None

Section G **Mental Health**
Body System Z **None**
Type F **Hypnosis:** Induction of a state of heightened suggestibility by auditory, visual and tactile techniques to elicit an emotional or behavioral response

Qualifier (4th)	Qualifier (5th)	Qualifier (6th)	Qualifier (7th)
Z None	**Z** None	**Z** None	**Z** None

Section G **Mental Health**
Body System Z **None**
Type G **Narcosynthesis:** Administration of intravenous barbiturates in order to release suppressed or repressed thoughts

Qualifier (4th)	Qualifier (5th)	Qualifier (6th)	Qualifier (7th)
Z None	**Z** None	**Z** None	**Z** None

Section G **Mental Health**
Body System Z **None**
Type H **Group Psychotherapy:** Treatment of two or more individuals with a mental health disorder by behavioral, cognitive, psychoanalytic, psychodynamic or psychophysiological means to improve functioning or well-being

Qualifier (4th)	Qualifier (5th)	Qualifier (6th)	Qualifier (7th)
Z None	**Z** None	**Z** None	**Z** None

Section G **Mental Health**
Body System Z **None**
Type J **Light Therapy:** Application of specialized light treatments to improve functioning or well-being

Qualifier (4th)	Qualifier (5th)	Qualifier (6th)	Qualifier (7th)
Z None	**Z** None	**Z** None	**Z** None

AHA Coding Clinic

No references have been issued for the Mental Health section.

Substance Abuse Treatment Section (HZ2–HZ9)

Within each section of ICD-10-PCS the characters have different meanings. The seven character meanings for the Substance Abuse Treatment section are illustrated below through the procedure example of *Substance abuse family counseling*.

Section	Body System	Root Type	Qualifier	Qualifier	Qualifier	Qualifier
Substance Abuse	None	Family Counseling	Other Family Counseling	None	None	None
H	Z	6	3	Z	Z	Z

Section (Character 1)

All Substance Abuse Treatment procedure codes have a first character value of H.

Body System (Character 2)

The body system is not specified for substance abuse treatment; therefore, the placeholder character value of Z is reported in the second character position.

Root Type (Character 3)

The alphanumeric character value for root types is placed in the third position. The following are the root types applicable to the Substance Abuse Treatment section with their associated meaning.

Character Value	Root Type	Root Type Definition
2	Detoxification Services	Detoxification from alcohol and/or drugs
3	Individual Counseling	The application of psychological methods to treat an individual with addictive behavior
4	Group Counseling	The application of psychological methods to treat two or more individuals with addictive behavior
5	Individual Psychotherapy	Treatment of an individual with addictive behavior by behavioral, cognitive, psychoanalytic, psychodynamic or psychophysiological means
6	Family Counseling	The application of psychological methods that includes one or more family members to treat an individual with addictive behavior
8	Medication Management	Monitoring and adjusting the use of replacement medications for the treatment of addiction
9	Pharmacotherapy	The use of replacement medications for the treatment of addiction

Qualifier (Character 4)

This qualifier further specifies the root type procedure. For example, the qualifier of Cognitive further specifies the type of Individual counseling.

Qualifier (Character 5)

The qualifier represents an additional attribute for the procedure when applicable. Currently, there are no qualifiers in the Substance Abuse Treatment section; therefore, the placeholder character value of Z should be reported.

Qualifier (Character 6)

The qualifier represents an additional attribute for the procedure when applicable. Currently, there are no qualifiers in the Substance Abuse Treatment section; therefore, the placeholder character value of Z should be reported.

Qualifier (Character 7)

The qualifier represents an additional attribute for the procedure when applicable. Currently, there are no qualifiers in the Substance Abuse Treatment section; therefore, the placeholder character value of Z should be reported.

Substance Abuse Treatment Section Tables

Substance Abuse Treatment Tables HZ2–HZ9

Section H **Substance Abuse Treatment**
Body System Z **None**
Type 2 **Detoxification Services:** Detoxification from alcohol and/or drugs

Qualifier (4th)	Qualifier (5th)	Qualifier (6th)	Qualifier (7th)
Z None	**Z** None	**Z** None	**Z** None

Section H **Substance Abuse Treatment**
Body System Z **None**
Type 3 **Individual Counseling:** The application of psychological methods to treat an individual with addictive behavior

Qualifier (4th)	Qualifier (5th)	Qualifier (6th)	Qualifier (7th)
0 Cognitive **1** Behavioral **2** Cognitive-Behavioral **3** 12-Step **4** Interpersonal **5** Vocational **6** Psychoeducation **7** Motivational Enhancement **8** Confrontational **9** Continuing Care **B** Spiritual **C** Pre/Post-Test Infectious Disease	**Z** None	**Z** None	**Z** None

Section H **Substance Abuse Treatment**
Body System Z **None**
Type 4 **Group Counseling:** The application of psychological methods to treat two or more individuals with addictive behavior

Qualifier (4th)	Qualifier (5th)	Qualifier (6th)	Qualifier (7th)
0 Cognitive **1** Behavioral **2** Cognitive-Behavioral **3** 12-Step **4** Interpersonal **5** Vocational **6** Psychoeducation **7** Motivational Enhancement **8** Confrontational **9** Continuing Care **B** Spiritual **C** Pre/Post-Test Infectious Disease	**Z** None	**Z** None	**Z** None

Section H **Substance Abuse Treatment**
Body System Z **None**
Type 5 **Individual Psychotherapy:** Treatment of an individual with addictive behavior by behavioral, cognitive, psychoanalytic, psychodynamic or psychophysiological means

Qualifier (4th)	Qualifier (5th)	Qualifier (6th)	Qualifier (7th)
0 Cognitive 1 Behavioral 2 Cognitive-Behavioral 3 12-Step 4 Interpersonal 5 Interactive 6 Psychoeducation 7 Motivational Enhancement 8 Confrontational 9 Supportive B Psychoanalysis C Psychodynamic D Psychophysiological	Z None	Z None	Z None

Section H **Substance Abuse Treatment**
Body System Z **None**
Type 6 **Family Counseling:** The application of psychological methods that includes one or more family members to treat an individual with addictive behavior

Qualifier (4th)	Qualifier (5th)	Qualifier (6th)	Qualifier (7th)
3 Other Family Counseling	Z None	Z None	Z None

Section H **Substance Abuse Treatment**
Body System Z **None**
Type 8 **Medication Management:** Monitoring and adjusting the use of replacement medications for the treatment of addiction

Qualifier (4th)	Qualifier (5th)	Qualifier (6th)	Qualifier (7th)
0 Nicotine Replacement 1 Methadone Maintenance 2 Levo-alpha-acetyl-methadol (LAAM) 3 Antabuse 4 Naltrexone 5 Naloxone 6 Clonidine 7 Bupropion 8 Psychiatric Medication 9 Other Replacement Medication	Z None	Z None	Z None

Section H **Substance Abuse Treatment**
Body System Z **None**
Type 9 **Pharmacotherapy:** The use of replacement medications for the treatment of addiction

Qualifier (4th)	Qualifier (5th)	Qualifier (6th)	Qualifier (7th)
0 Nicotine Replacement 1 Methadone Maintenance 2 Levo-alpha-acetyl-methadol (LAAM) 3 Antabuse 4 Naltrexone 5 Naloxone 6 Clonidine 7 Bupropion 8 Psychiatric Medication 9 Other Replacement Medication	Z None	Z None	Z None

AHA Coding Clinic

HZ2ZZZZ Detoxification Services for Substance Abuse Treatment—AHA CC: 1Q, 2020, 21-22

HZ98ZZZ Pharmacotherapy for Substance Abuse Treatment, Psychiatric Medication—AHA CC: 1Q, 2020, 21-22

Within each section of ICD-10-PCS the characters have different meanings. The seven character meanings for the New Technology section are illustrated below through the procedure example of *Introduction of ceftazidime-avibactam anti-infective into peripheral vein, percutaneous approach.*

Section	Body System	Root Operation	Body Part	Approach	Device / Substance / Technology	Qualifier
New Technology	Anatomical Regions	Introduction	Peripheral Vein	Percutaneous	Ceftazidime-Avibactam Anti-infective	New Technology Group 1
X	W	0	3	3	2	1

Section (Character 1)

All New Technology procedure codes have a first character value of X.

Body System (Character 2)

For each body system the applicable body part character values will be available for procedure code construction.

Root Operations (Character 3)

The alphanumeric character value for root operations is placed in the third position. Listed below are the root operations applicable to the New Technology section with their associated meaning.

Character Value	Root Operation	Root Operation Definition
A	Assistance	Taking over a portion of a physiological function by extracorporeal means
C	Extirpation	Taking or cutting out solid matter from a body part
E	Measurement	Determining a level of a physiological or physical function at a point in time
G	Fusion	Joining together portions of an articular body part rendering the articular body part immobile
H	Insertion	Putting in a nonbiological appliance that monitors, assists, performs, or prevents a physiological function bust does not physically take the place of a body part.
J	Inspection	Visually and/or manually exploring a body part
K	Bypass	Altering the route of passage of the contents of a tubular body part
P	Irrigation	Putting in or on a cleansing substance
R	Replacement	Putting in or on biological or synthetic material that physically takes the place and/or function of all or a portion of a body part
S	Reposition	Moving to its normal location, or other suitable location, all or a portion of a body part
U	Supplement	Putting in or on biological or synthetic material that physically reinforces and/or augments the function of a portion of a body part
V	Restriction	Partially closing an orifice or the lumen of a tubular body part
0	Introduction	Putting in or on a therapeutic, diagnostic, nutritional, physiological, or prophylactic substance except blood or blood products
1	Transfusion In Anatomical Regions	Putting in blood or blood products
2	Monitoring In Joints & Urinary System	Determining the level of a physiological or physical function repetitively
2	Transfusion In Anatomical Regions	Putting in blood or blood products
5	Destruction	Physical eradication of all or a portion of a body part by the direct use of energy, force, or a destructive agent
7	Dilation	Expanding an orifice or the lumen of a tubular body part

Body Part (Character 4)

For each body system the applicable body part character values will be available for procedure code construction.

Approach (Character 5)

The approach is the technique used to reach the procedure site. Listed below are the approach character values for the New Technology section with the associated definitions.

Character Value	Approach	Approach Definition
0	Open	Cutting through the skin or mucous membrane and any other body layers necessary to expo the site of the procedure
3	Percutaneous	Entry, by puncture or minor incision, of instrumentation through the skin or mucous memb and any other body layers necessary to reach the site of the procedure
4	Percutaneous Endoscopic	Entry, by puncture or minor incision, of instrumentation through the skin or mucous memb and any other body layers necessary to reach and visualize the site of the procedure
7	Via Natural or Artificial Opening	Entry of instrumentation through a natural or artificial external opening to reach the site of procedure
8	Via Natural or Artificial Opening Endoscopic	Entry of instrumentation through a natural or artificial external opening to reach and visuali the site of the procedure
X	External	Procedures performed directly on the skin or mucous membrane and procedures performed indirectly by the application of external force through the skin or mucous membrane

Device/Substance/Technology (Character 6)

The New Technology section created a place within ICD-10-PCS to include procedure codes for new services that utilize a specific new device, substance, or technology. Procedures in this section may be part of the Inpatient Prospective Payment System (IPPS) new technology add-on payment mechanism. Depending on the procedure performed there is either a device, substance, or new technology utilized.

Qualifier (Character 7)

The qualifier represents the category year in which the new device, substance, or technology was added to the coding system. In federal fiscal year 2016 (October 1, 2015) the first group of device, substance, and technology was added and therefore are labeled as New Technology Group 1.

New Technology Section Guidelines (section X)

E. New Technology Section

General Guidelines

E1.a Section X codes fully represent the specific procedure described in the code title, and do not require any additional codes from other sections of ICD-10-PCS. When section X contains a code title which describes a specific new technology procedure, and it is the only procedure performed, only the X code is reported for the procedure. There is no need to report an additional code in another section of ICD-10-PCS.

Example: XW043A6 Introduction of Cefiderocol Anti-infective into Central Vein, Percutaneous Approach, New Technology Group 6 can be coded to indicate that Cefiderocol Anti-infective was administered via a central vein. A separate code from table 3E0 in the Administration section of ICD-10-PCS is not coded in addition to this code.

E1.b When multiple procedures are performed, New Technology section X codes are coded following the multiple procedures guideline.

Examples: Dual filter cerebral embolic filtration used during transcatheter aortic valve replacement (TAVR), X2A5312 Cerebral Embolic Filtration, Dual Filter in Innominate Artery and Left Common Carotid Artery, Percutaneous Approach, New Technology Group 2, is coded for the cerebral embolic filtration, along with an ICD-10-PCS code for the TAVR procedure. An extracorporeal flow reversal circuit for embolic neuroprotection placed during a transcarotid arterial revascularization procedure, a code from table X2A, Assistance of the Cardiovascular System is coded for the use of the extracoporeal flow reversal circuit, along with an ICD-10-PCS code for the transcarotid arterial revascularization procedure.

New Technology Section Tables

New Technology Tables X27–XY0

Section X **New Technology**
Body System 2 **Cardiovascular**
Operation 7 **Dilation:** Expanding an orifice or the lumen of a tubular body part

Body Part (4th)	Approach (5th)	Device/Substance/Technology (6th)	Qualifier (7th)
H Femoral Artery, Right **J** Femoral Artery, Left **K** Popliteal Artery, Proximal Right **L** Popliteal Artery, Proximal Left **M** Popliteal Artery, Distal Right **N** Popliteal Artery, Distal Left **P** Anterior Tibial Artery, Right **Q** Anterior Tibial Artery, Left **R** Posterior Tibial Artery, Right **S** Posterior Tibial Artery, Left **T** Peroneal Tibial Artery, Right **U** Peroneal Tibial Artery, Left	**3** Percutaneous	**8** Intraluminal Device, Sustained Release Drug-eluting **9** Intraluminal Device, Sustained Release Drug-eluting, Two **B** Intraluminal Device, Sustained Release Drug-eluting, Three **C** Intraluminal Device, Sustained Release Drug-eluting, Four or More	**5** New Technology Group 5

Section X **New Technology**
Body System 2 **Cardiovascular System**
Operation A **Assistance:** Taking over a portion of a physiological function by extracorporeal means

Body Part (4th)	Approach (5th)	Device/Substance/Technology (6th)	Qualifier (7th)
5 Innominate Artery and Left Common Carotid Artery	**3** Percutaneous	**1** Cerebral Embolic Filtration, Dual Filter	**2** New Technology Group 2
6 Aortic Arch	**3** Percutaneous	**2** Cerebral Embolic Filtration, Single Deflection Filter	**5** New Technology Group 5
H Common Carotid Artery, Right **J** Common Carotid Artery, Left	**3** Percutaneous	**3** Cerebral Embolic Filtration, Extracorporeal Flow Reversal Circuit	**6** New Technology Group 6

Section X **New Technology**
Body System 2 **Cardiovascular System**
Operation C **Extirpation:** Taking or cutting out solid matter from a body part

Body Part (4th)	Approach (5th)	Device/Substance/Technology (6th)	Qualifier (7th)
P Abdominal Aorta **Q** Upper Extremity Vein, Right **R** Upper Extremity Vein, Left **S** Lower Extremity Artery, Right **T** Lower Extremity Artery, Left **U** Lower Extremity Vein, Right **V** Lower Extremity Vein, Left **Y** Great Vessel	**3** Percutaneous	**T** Computer-aided Mechanical Aspiration	**7** New Technology Group 7

Section X **New Technology**
Body System 2 **Cardiovascular System**
Operation J **Inspection:** Visually and/or manually exploring a body part

Body Part (4th)	Approach (5th)	Device/Substance/Technology (6th)	Qualifier (7th)
A Heart	**X** External	**4** Transthoracic Echocardiography Computer-aided Guidance	**7** New Technology Group 7

Section X **New Technology**
Body System 2 **Cardiovascular System**
Operation K **Bypass:** Altering the route of passage of the contents of a tubular body part

Body Part (4th)	Approach (5th)	Device/Substance/Technology (6th)	Qualifier (7th)
B Radial Artery, Right **C** Radial Artery, Left	**3** Percutaneous	**1** Thermal Resistance Energy	**7** New Technology Group 7

Section X **New Technology**
Body System 2 **Cardiovascular System**
Operation R **Replacement:** Putting in or on biological or synthetic material that physically takes the place and/or function of all or a portion of a body part

Body Part (4th)	Approach (5th)	Device/Substance/Technology (6th)	Qualifier (7th)
F Aortic Valve	**0** Open **3** Percutaneous **4** Percutaneous Endoscopic	**3** Zooplastic Tissue, Rapid Deployment Technique	**2** New Technology Group 2
X Thoracic Aorta, Arch	**0** Open	**N** Branched Synthetic Substitute with Intraluminal Device	**7** New Technology Group 7

Section X **New Technology**
Body System 2 **Cardiovascular System**
Operation V **Restriction:** Partially closing an orifice or the lumen of a tubular body part

Body Part (4th)	Approach (5th)	Device/Substance/Technology (6th)	Qualifier (7th)
7 Coronary Sinus	**3** Percutaneous	**Q** Reduction Device	**7** New Technology Group 7
W Thoracic Aorta, Descending	**0** Open	**N** Branched Synthetic Substitute with Intraluminal Device	**7** New Technology Group 7

Section X **New Technology**
Body System D **Gastrointestinal System**
Operation 2 **Monitoring:** Determining the level of a physiological or physical function repetitively over a period of time

Body Part (4th)	Approach (5th)	Device/Substance/Technology (6th)	Qualifier (7th)
G Upper GI **H** Lower GI	**4** Percutaneous Endoscopic **8** Via Natural or Artificial Opening Endoscopic	**V** Oxygen Saturation	**7** New Technology Group 7

Section X **New Technology**
Body System D **Gastrointestinal System**
Operation P **Irrigation:** Putting in or on a cleansing substance

Body Part (4th)	Approach (5th)	Device/Substance/Technology (6th)	Qualifier (7th)
H Lower GI	**8** Via Natural or Artificial Opening Endoscopic	**K** Intraoperative Single-use Oversleeve	**7** New Technology Group 7

Section X **New Technology**
Body System F **Hepatobiliary System and Pancreas**
Operation J **Inspection:** Visually and/or manually exploring a body part

Body Part (4th)	Approach (5th)	Device/Substance/Technology (6th)	Qualifier (7th)
B Hepatobiliary Duct **D** Pancreatic Duct	**8** Via Natural or Artificial Opening Endoscopic	**A** Single-use Duodenoscope	**7** New Technology Group 7

Section X **New Technology**
Body System H **Skin, Subcutaneous Tissue, Fascia and Breast**
Operation R **Replacement:** Putting in or on biological or synthetic material that physically takes the place and/or function of all or a portion of a body part

Body Part (4th)	Approach (5th)	Device/Substance/Technology (6th)	Qualifier (7th)
P Skin	**X** External	**F** Bioengineered Allogeneic Construct	**7** New Technology Group 7
P Skin	**X** External	**L** Skin Substitute, Porcine Liver Derived	**2** New Technology Group 2

Section X **New Technology**
Body System K **Muscles, Tendons, Bursae and Ligaments**
Operation 0 **Introduction:** Putting in or on a therapeutic, diagnostic, nutritional, physiological, or prophylactic substance except blood or blood products

Body Part (4th)	Approach (5th)	Device/Substance/Technology (6th)	Qualifier (7th)
2 Muscle	**3** Percutaneous	**0** Concentrated Bone Marrow Aspirate	**3** New Technology Group 3

Section X **New Technology**
Body System N **Bones**
Operation S **Reposition:** Moving to its normal location, or other suitable location, all or a portion of a body part

Body Part (4th)	Approach (5th)	Device/Substance/Technology (6th)	Qualifier (7th)
0 Lumbar Vertebra	**0** Open	**3** Magnetically Controlled Growth Rod(s)	**2** New Technology Group 2
0 Lumbar Vertebra	**0** Open	**C** Posterior (Dynamic) Distraction Device	**7** New Technology Group 7
0 Lumbar Vertebra	**3** Percutaneous	**3** Magnetically Controlled Growth Rod(s)	**2** New Technology Group 2
0 Lumbar Vertebra	**3** Percutaneous	**C** Posterior (Dynamic) Distraction Device	**7** New Technology Group
3 Cervical Vertebra	**0** Open **3** Percutaneous	**3** Magnetically Controlled Growth Rod(s)	**2** New Technology Group 2
4 Thoracic Vertebra	**0** Open	**3** Magnetically Controlled Growth Rod(s)	**2** New Technology Group 2
4 Thoracic Vertebra	**0** Open	**C** Posterior (Dynamic) Distraction Device	**7** New Technology Group 7
4 Thoracic Vertebra	**3** Percutaneous	**3** Magnetically Controlled Growth Rod(s)	**2** New Technology Group 2
4 Thoracic Vertebra	**3** Percutaneous	**C** Posterior (Dynamic) Distraction Device	**7** New Technology Group 7

Section X **New Technology**
Body System N **Bones**
Operation U **Supplement:** Putting in or on biological or synthetic material that physically reinforces and/or augments the function of a portion of a body part

Body Part (4th)	Approach (5th)	Device/Substance/Technology (6th)	Qualifier (7th)
0 Lumbar Vertebra **4** Thoracic Vertebra	**3** Percutaneous	**5** Synthetic Substitute, Mechanically Expandable (Paired)	**6** New Technology Group 6

Section X **New Technology**
Body System R **Joints**
Operation G **Fusion:** Joining together portions of an articular body part rendering the articular body part immobile

Body Part (4th)	Approach (5th)	Device/Substance/Technology (6th)	Qualifier (7th)
0 Occipital-cervical Joint	**0** Open	**9** Interbody Fusion Device, Nanotextured Surface	**2** New Technology Group 2
0 Occipital-cervical Joint	**0** Open	**F** Interbody Fusion Device, Radiolucent Porous	**3** New Technology Group 3
1 Cervical Vertebral Joint	**0** Open	**9** Interbody Fusion Device, Nanotextured Surface	**2** New Technology Group 2
1 Cervical Vertebral Joint	**0** Open	**F** Interbody Fusion Device, Radiolucent Porous	**3** New Technology Group 3
2 Cervical Vertebral Joints, 2 or More	**0** Open	**9** Interbody Fusion Device, Nanotextured Surface	**2** New Technology Group 2
2 Cervical Vertebral Joints, 2 or More	**0** Open	**F** Interbody Fusion Device, Radiolucent Porous	**3** New Technology Group 3
4 Cervicothoracic Vertebral Joint	**0** Open	**9** Interbody Fusion Device, Nanotextured Surface	**2** New Technology Group 2
4 Cervicothoracic Vertebral Joint	**0** Open	**F** Interbody Fusion Device, Radiolucent Porous	**3** New Technology Group 3
6 Thoracic Vertebral Joint	**0** Open	**9** Interbody Fusion Device, Nanotextured Surface	**2** New Technology Group 2
6 Thoracic Vertebral Joint	**0** Open	**F** Interbody Fusion Device, Radiolucent Porous	**3** New Technology Group 3
7 Thoracic Vertebral Joints, 2 to 7	**0** Open	**9** Interbody Fusion Device, Nanotextured Surface	**2** New Technology Group 2
7 Thoracic Vertebral Joints. 2 to 7	**0** Open	**F** Interbody Fusion Device, Radiolucent Porous	**3** New Technology Group 3
8 Thoracic Vertebral Joints, 8 or More	**0** Open	**9** Interbody Fusion Device, Nanotextured Surface	**2** New Technology Group 2
8 Thoracic Vertebral Joints, 8 or More	**0** Open	**F** Interbody Fusion Device, Radiolucent Porous	**3** New Technology Group 3
A Thoracolumbar Vertebral Joint	**0** Open	**9** Interbody Fusion Device, Nanotextured Surface	**2** New Technology Group 2
A Thoracolumbar Vertebral Joint	**0** Open	**F** Interbody Fusion Device, Radiolucent Porous	**3** New Technology Group 3
A Thoracolumbar Vertebral Joint	**0** Open **3** Percutaneous **4** Percutaneous Endoscopic	**R** Interbody Fusion Device, Customizable	**7** New Technology Group 7
B Lumbar Vertebral Joint	**0** Open	**9** Interbody Fusion Device, Nanotextured Surface	**2** New Technology Group 2
B Lumbar Vertebral Joint	**0** Open	**F** Interbody Fusion Device, Radiolucent Porous	**3** New Technology Group 3
B Lumbar Vertebral Joint	**0** Open **3** Percutaneous **4** Percutaneous Endoscopic	**R** Interbody Fusion Device, Customizable	**7** New Technology Group 7
C Lumbar Vertebral Joints, 2 or More	**0** Open	**9** Interbody Fusion Device, Nanotextured Surface	**2** New Technology Group 2
C Lumbar Vertebral Joints, 2 or More	**0** Open	**F** Interbody Fusion Device, Radiolucent Porous	**3** New Technology Group 3

Continued →

Section X New Technology
Body System R Joints
Operation G **Fusion:** Joining together portions of an articular body part rendering the articular body part immobile

Body Part (4th)	Approach (5th)	Device/Substance/Technology (6th)	Qualifier (7th)
C Lumbar Vertebral Joints, 2 or More	0 Open 3 Percutaneous 4 Percutaneous Endoscopic	R Interbody Fusion Device, Customizable	7 New Technology Group 7
D Lumbosacral Vertebral Joint	0 Open	9 Interbody Fusion Device, Nanotextured Surface	2 New Technology Group 2
D Lumbosacral Vertebral Joint	0 Open	F Interbody Fusion Device, Radiolucent Porous	3 New Technology Group 3
D Lumbarosacral Joint	0 Open 3 Percutaneous 4 Percutaneous Endoscopic	R Interbody Fusion Device, Customizable	7 New Technology Group 7

Section X New Technology
Body System T Urinary System
Operation 2 **Monitoring:** Determining the level of a physiological or physical function repetitively over a period of time

Body Part (4th)	Approach (5th)	Device/Substance/Technology (6th)	Qualifier (7th)
5 Kidney	X External	E Fluorescent Pyrazine	5 New Technology Group 5

Section X New Technology
Body System V Male Reproductive System
Operation 5 **Destruction:** Physical eradication of all or a portion of a body part by the direct use of energy, force, or a destructive agent

Body Part (4th)	Approach (5th)	Device/Substance/Technology (6th)	Qualifier (7th)
0 Prostate	8 Via Natural or Artificial Opening Endoscopic	A Robotic Waterjet Ablation	4 New Technology Group 4

Section X New Technology
Body System W Anatomical Regions
Operation 0 **Introduction:** Putting in or on a therapeutic, diagnostic, nutritional, physiological, or prophylactic substance except blood or blood products

Body Part (4th)	Approach (5th)	Device/Substance/Technology (6th)	Qualifier (7th)
0 Skin	X External	2 Bromelain-enriched Proteolytic Enzyme	7 New Technology Group 7
1 Subcutaneous Tissue	3 Percutaneous	9 Satrailzumab-mwge	7 New Technology Group 7
1 Subcutaneous Tissue	3 Percutaneous	F Other New Technology Therapeutic Substance	5 New Technology Group 5
1 Subcutaneous Tissue	3 Percutaneous	H Other New Technology Monoclonal Antibody K Leronlimab Monoclonal Antibody S COVID-19 Vaccine Dose 1 T COVID-19 Vaccine Dose 2 U COVID-19 Vaccine	6 New Technology Group 6
1 Subcutaneous Tissue	3 Percutaneous	W Caplacizumab	5 New Technology Group 5
1 Subcutaneous Tissue	X External	2 Bromelain-enriched Proteolytic Enzyme	7 New Technology Group 7

Continued →

Section **X** **New Technology**
Body System **W** **Anatomical Regions**
Operation **0** **Introduction:** Putting in or on a therapeutic, diagnostic, nutritional, physiological, or prophylactic substance except blood or blood products

Body Part (4th)	Approach (5th)	Device/Substance/Technology (6th)	Qualifier (7th)
2 Muscle	**3** Percutaneous	**S** COVID-19 Vaccine Dose 1 **T** COVID-19 Vaccine Dose 2 **U** COVID-19 Vaccine	**6** New Technology Group 6
3 Peripheral Vein	**3** Percutaneous	**0** Brexanolone **2** Nerinitide **3** Durvalumab Antineoplastic	**6** New Technology Group 6
3 Peripheral Vein	**3** Percutaneous	**5** Narsoplimab Monoclonal Antibody	**7** New Technology Group 7
3 Peripheral Vein	**3** Percutaneous	**6** Lefamulin Anti-infective	**6** New Technology Group 6
3 Peripheral Vein	**3** Percutaneous	**6** Terlipressin	**7** New Technology Group 7
3 Peripheral Vein	**3** Percutaneous	**7** Coagulation Factor Xa, Inactivated	**2** New Technology Group 2
3 Peripheral Vein	**3** Percutaneous	**7** Trilaciclib **8** Lurbinectedin	**7** New Technology Group 7
3 Peripheral Vein	**3** Percutaneous	**9** Defibrotide Sodium Anticoagulant	**2** New Technology Group 2
3 Peripheral Vein	**3** Percutaneous	**9** Ceftolozane/Tazobactam Anti-infective	**6** New Technology Group 6
3 Peripheral Vein	**3** Percutaneous	**A** Bezlotoxumab Monoclonal Antibody	**3** New Technology Group 3
3 Peripheral Vein	**3** Percutaneous	**A** Cefiderocol Anti-infective	**6** New Technology Group 6
3 Peripheral Vein	**3** Percutaneous	**A** Ciltacabtagene Autoleucel	**7** New Technology Group 7
3 Peripheral Vein	**3** Percutaneous	**B** Cytarabine and Daunorubicin Liposome Antineoplastic	**3** New Technology Group 3
3 Peripheral Vein	**3** Percutaneous	**B** Omadacycline Anti-infective	**6** New Technology Group 6
3 Peripheral Vein	**3** Percutaneous	**B** Amivantamab Monoclonal Antibody	**7** New Technology Group 7
3 Peripheral Vein	**3** Percutaneous	**C** Eculizumab	**6** New Technology Group 6
3 Peripheral Vein	**3** Percutaneous	**C** Engineered Chimeric Antigen Receptor T-cell Immunotherapy, Autologous	**7** New Technology Group 7
3 Peripheral Vein	**3** Percutaneous	**D** Atezolizumab Antineoplastic	**6** New Technology Group 6
3 Peripheral Vein	**3** Percutaneous	**E** Remdesivir Anti-infective	**5** New Technology Group 5
3 Peripheral Vein	**3** Percutaneous	**E** Etesevimab Monoclonal Antibody	**6** New Technology Group 6
3 Peripheral Vein	**3** Percutaneous	**F** Other New Technology Therapeutic Substance	**3** New Technology Group 3
3 Peripheral Vein	**3** Percutaneous	**F** Other New Technology Therapeutic Substance	**5** New Technology Group 5
3 Peripheral Vein	**3** Percutaneous	**F** Bamlanivimab Monoclonal Antibody	**6** New Technology Group 6
3 Peripheral Vein	**3** Percutaneous	**G** Plazomicin Anti-infective	**4** New Technology Group 4
3 Peripheral Vein	**3** Percutaneous	**G** Sarilumab	**5** New Technology Group 5
3 Peripheral Vein	**3** Percutaneous	**G** REGN-COV2 Monoclonal Antibody	**6** New Technology Group 6

Continued →

Section X **New Technology**
Body System W **Anatomical Regions**
Operation 0 **Introduction:** Putting in or on a therapeutic, diagnostic, nutritional, physiological, or prophylactic substance except blood or blood products

Body Part (4th)	Approach (5th)	Device/Substance/Technology (6th)	Qualifier (7th)
3 Peripheral Vein	3 Percutaneous	G Engineered Chimeric Antigen Receptor T-cell Immunotherapy, Allogeneic	7 New Technology Group 7
3 Peripheral Vein	3 Percutaneous	H Synthetic Human Angiotensin II	4 New Technology Group 4
3 Peripheral Vein	3 Percutaneous	H Tocilizumab	5 New Technology Group 5
3 Peripheral Vein	3 Percutaneous	H Other New Technology Monoclonal Antibody	6 New Technology Group 6
3 Peripheral Vein	3 Percutaneous	H Axicabtagene Ciloleucel Immunotherapy J Tisagenlecleucel Immunotherapy	7 New Technology Group 7
3 Peripheral Vein	3 Percutaneous	K Fosfomycin Anti-Infective	5 New Technology Group 5
3 Peripheral Vein	3 Percutaneous	K Idecabtagene Vicleucel Immunotherapy	7 New Technology Group 7
3 Peripheral Vein	3 Percutaneous	L CD24Fc Immunomodulator	6 New Technology Group 6
3 Peripheral Vein	3 Percutaneous	L Lifileucel Immunotherapy M Brexucabtagene Autoleucel Immunotherapy	7 New Technology Group 7
3 Peripheral Vein	3 Percutaneous	N Meropenem-vaborbactam	5 New Technology Group 5
3 Peripheral Vein	3 Percutaneous	N Lisocabtagene Maraleucel Immunotherapy	7 New Technology Group 7
3 Peripheral Vein	3 Percutaneous	Q Tagraxofusp-erzs Antineoplastic S Iobenguane I-131 Antineoplastic U Imipenem-cilastatin-relebactam Anti-infective W Caplacizumab	5 New Technology Group 5
4 Central Vein	3 Percutaneous	0 Brexanolone 2 Nerinitide 3 Durvalumab Antineoplastic	6 New Technology Group 6
4 Central Vein	3 Percutaneous	5 Narsoplimab Monoclonal Antibody	7 New Technology Group 7
4 Central Vein	3 Percutaneous	6 Lefamulin Anti-infective	6 New Technology Group 6
4 Central Vein	3 Percutaneous	6 Terlipressin	7 New Technology Group 7
4 Central Vein	3 Percutaneous	7 Coagulation Factor Xa, Inactivated	2 New Technology Group 2
4 Central Vein	3 Percutaneous	7 Trilaciclib 8 Lurbinectedin	7 New Technology Group 7
4 Central Vein	3 Percutaneous	9 Defibrotide Sodium Anticoagulant	2 New Technology Group 2
4 Central Vein	3 Percutaneous	9 Ceftolozane/Tazobactam Anti-infective	6 New Technology Group 6
4 Central Vein	3 Percutaneous	A Bezlotoxumab Monoclonal Antibody	3 New Technology Group 3
4 Central Vein	3 Percutaneous	A Cefiderocol Anti-infective	6 New Technology Group 6
4 Central Vein	3 Percutaneous	A Ciltacabtagene Autoleucel	7 New Technology Group 7
4 Central Vein	3 Percutaneous	B Cytarabine and Daunorubicin Liposome Antineoplastic	3 New Technology Group 3
4 Central Vein	3 Percutaneous	B Omadacycline Anti-infective	6 New Technology Group 6

Continued →

Section X New Technology
Body System W Anatomical Regions
Operation 0 Introduction: Putting in or on a therapeutic, diagnostic, nutritional, physiological, or prophylactic substance except blood or blood products

Body Part (4th)	Approach (5th)	Device/Substance/Technology (6th)	Qualifier (7th)
4 Central Vein	3 Percutaneous	B Amivantamab Monoclonal Antibody	7 New Technology Group 7
4 Central Vein	3 Percutaneous	C Eculizumab	6 New Technology Group 6
4 Central Vein	3 Percutaneous	C Engineered Chimeric Antigen Receptor T-cell Immunotherapy, Autologous	7 New Technology Group 7
4 Central Vein	3 Percutaneous	D Atezolizumab Antineoplastic	6 New Technology Group 6
4 Central Vein	3 Percutaneous	E Remdesivir Anti-infective	5 New Technology Group 5
4 Central Vein	3 Percutaneous	E Etesevimab Monoclonal Antibody	6 New Technology Group 6
4 Central Vein	3 Percutaneous	F Other New Technology Therapeutic Substance	3 New Technology Group 3
4 Central Vein	3 Percutaneous	F Other New Technology Therapeutic Substance	5 New Technology Group 5
4 Central Vein	3 Percutaneous	F Bamlanivimab Monoclonal Antibody	6 New Technology Group 6
4 Central Vein	3 Percutaneous	G Plazomicin Anti-infective	4 New Technology Group 4
4 Central Vein	3 Percutaneous	G Sarilumab	5 New Technology Group 5
4 Central Vein	3 Percutaneous	G REGN-COV2 Monoclonal Antibody	6 New Technology Group 6
4 Central Vein	3 Percutaneous	G Engineered Chimeric Antigen Receptor T-cell Immunotherapy, Allogeneic	7 New Technology Group 7
4 Central Vein	3 Percutaneous	H Synthetic Human Angiotensin II	4 New Technology Group 4
4 Central Vein	3 Percutaneous	H Tocilizumab	5 New Technology Group 5
4 Central Vein	3 Percutaneous	H Other New Technology Monoclonal Antibody	6 New Technology Group 6
4 Central Vein	3 Percutaneous	H Axicabtagene Ciloleucel Immunotherapy J Tisagenlecleucel Immunotherapy	7 New Technology Group 7
4 Central Vein	3 Percutaneous	K Fosfomycin Anti-Infective	5 New Technology Group 5
4 Central Vein	3 Percutaneous	K Idecabtagene Vicleucel Immunotherapy	7 New Technology Group 7
4 Central Vein	3 Percutaneous	L CD24Fc Immunomodulator	6 New Technology Group 6
4 Central Vein	3 Percutaneous	L Lifileucel Immunotherapy M Brexucabtagene Autoleucel Immunotherapy	7 New Technology Group 7
4 Central Vein	3 Percutaneous	N Meropenem-vaborbactam Anti-infective	5 New Technology Group 5
4 Central Vein	3 Percutaneous	N Lisocabtagene Maraleucel Immunotherapy	7 New Technology Group 7
4 Central Vein	3 Percutaneous	Q Tagraxofusp-erzs Antineoplastic S Iobenguane I-131 Antineoplastic U Imipenem-cilastatin-relebactam Anti-infective W Caplacizumab	5 New Technology Group 5
9 Nose	7 Via Natural or Artificial Opening	M Esketamine Hydrochloride	5 New Technology Group 5
D Mouth and Pharynx	X External	6 Lefamulin Anti-infective	6 New Technology Group 6

Continued →

Section X **New Technology**
Body System W **Anatomical Regions**
Operation 0 **Introduction:** Putting in or on a therapeutic, diagnostic, nutritional, physiological, or prophylactic substance except blood or blood products

Body Part (4th)	Approach (5th)	Device/Substance/Technology (6th)	Qualifier (7th)
D Mouth and Pharynx	**X** External	**8** Uridine Triacetate	**2** New Technology Group 2
D Mouth and Pharynx	**X** External	**F** Other New Technology Therapeutic Substance **J** Apalutamide Antienoplastic **L** Erdafitinib Antineoplastic	**5** New Technology Group 5
D Mouth and Pharynx	**X** External	**M** Baricitinib	**6** New Technology Group 6
D Mouth and Pharynx	**X** External	**R** Venetoclax Antineoplastic **T** Ruxolitinib **V** Gilteritinib Antineoplastic	**5** New Technology Group 5
G Upper GI **H** Lower GI	**7** Via Natural or Artificial Opening	**M** Baricitinib	**6** New Technology Group 6
G Upper GI **H** Lower GI	**8** Via Natural or Artificial Opening Endoscopic	**8** Mineral-based Topical Hemostatic Agent	**6** New Technology Group 6
Q Cranial Cavity and Brain	**3** Percutaneous	**1** Eladocagene exuparvovec	**6** New Technology Group 6
V Bones	**0** Open	**P** Antibiotic-eluting Bone Void Filler	**7** New Technology Group 7

Section X **New Technology**
Body System W **Anatomical Regions**
Operation 1 **Transfusion:** Putting in blood or blood products

Body Part (4th)	Approach (5th)	Device/Substance/Technology (6th)	Qualifier (7th)
3 Peripheral Vein	**3** Percutaneous	**2** Plasma, Convalescent (Nonautologous)	**5** New Technology Group 5
3 Peripheral Vein	**3** Percutaneous	**D** High-Dose Intravenous Immune Globulin **E** Hyperimmune Globulin	**7** New Technology Group 7
4 Central Vein	**3** Percutaneous	**2** Plasma, Convalescent (Nonautologous)	**5** New Technology Group 5
4 Central Vein	**3** Percutaneous	**D** High-Dose Intravenous Immune Globulin **E** Hyperimmune Globulin	**7** New Technology Group 7

Section X **New Technology**
Body System W **Anatomical Regions**
Operation H **Insertion:** Putting in a nonbiological appliance that monitors, assists, performs, or prevents a physiological function but does not physically take the place of a body part

Body Part (4th)	Approach (5th)	Device/Substance/Technology (6th)	Qualifier (7th)
D Mouth and Pharynx	**7** Via Natural or Artificial Opening	**Q** Neurostimulator Lead	**7** New Technology Group 7

Section X **New Technology**
Body System X **Physiological Systems**
Operation E **Measurement:** Determining the level of a physiological or physical function at a point in time

Body Part (4th)	Approach (5th)	Device/Substance/Technology (6th)	Qualifier (7th)
0 Central Nervous	**X** External	**0** Intracranial Vascular Activity, Computer-aided Assessment	**7** New Technology Group 7
3 Arterial	**X** External	**2** Pulmonary Artery Flow, Computer-aided Triage and Notification	**7** New Technology Group 7
5 Circulatory	**X** External	**M** Infection, Whole Blood Nucleic Acid-base Microbial Detection	**5** New Technology Group 5
5 Circulatory	**X** External	**N** Infection, Positive Blood Culture Fluorescence Hybridization for Organism Identification, Concentration and Susceptibility	**6** New Technology Group 6
5 Circulatory	**X** External	**R** Infection, Mechanical Initial Specimen Diversion Technique Using Active Negative Pressure **T** Intracranial Arterial Flow, Whole Blood mRNA **V** Infection, Serum/Plasma Nanoparticle Fluorescence SARS-CoV-2 Antibody Detection	**7** New Technology Group 7
9 Nose	**7** Via Natural or Artificial Opening	**U** Infection, Nasopharyngeal Fluid SARS-CoV-2 Polymerase Chain Reaction	**7** New Technology Group 7
B Respiratory	**X** External	**Q** Infection, Lower Respiratory Fluid Nucleic Acid-base Microbial Detection	**6** New Technology Group 6

Section X **New Technology**
Body System Y **Extracorporeal**
Operation 0 **Introduction:** Putting in or on a therapeutic, diagnostic, nutritional, physiological, or prophylactic substance except blood or blood products

Body Part (4th)	Approach (5th)	Device/Substance/Technology (6th)	Qualifier (7th)
V Vein Graft	**X** External	**8** Endothelial Damage Inhibitor	**3** New Technology Group 3
Y Extracorporeal	**X** External	**3** Nafamostat Anticoagulant	**7** New Technology Group 7

AHA Coding Clinic

X2A5312 Cerebral Embolic Filtration, Dual Filter in Innominate Artery and Left Common Carotid Artery, Percutaneous Approach, New Technology Group 2—AHA CC: 1Q, 2021, 16-17

X2C0361 Extirpation of Matter from Coronary Artery, One Site Using Orbital Atherectomy Technology, Percutaneous Approach, New Technology Group 1—AHA CC: 4Q, 2015, 13-14

XNS0032 Reposition of Lumbar Vertebra using Magnetically Controlled Growth Rod(s), Open Approach, New Technology Group 2—AHA CC: 4Q, 2017, 75

XRGB0F3 Fusion of Lumbar Vertebral Joint using Radiolucent Porous Interbody Fusion Device, Open Approach, New Technology Group 3—AHA CC: 4Q, 2017, 76-77

XRGD0F3 Fusion of Lumbosacral Joint using Radiolucent Porous Interbody Fusion Device, Open Approach, New Technology Group 3—AHA CC: 4Q, 2017, 76-77

XV508A4 Destruction of Prostate using Robotic Waterjet Ablation, Via Natural or Artificial Opening Endoscopic, New Technology Group 4—AHA CC: 4Q, 2018, 55

XW013F5 Introduction of Other New Technology Therapeutic Substance into Subcutaneous Tissue, Percutaneous Approach, New Technology Group 5—AHA CC: 3Q, 2020, 19-20; 1Q, 2021, 49-51

XW033E5 Introduction of Remdesivir Anti-infective into Peripheral Vein, Percutaneous Approach, New Technology Group 5—AHA CC: 3Q, 2020, 18-19

XW033F5 Introduction of Other New Technology Therapeutic Substance into Peripheral Vein, Percutaneous Approach, New Technology Group 5—AHA CC: 3Q, 2020, 19-20; 1Q, 2021, 49-51

XW033G5 Introduction of Sarilumab into Peripheral Vein, Percutaneous Approach, New Technology Group 5—AHA CC: 3Q, 2020, 18-19

XW033H5 Introduction of Tocilizumab into Peripheral Vein, Percutaneous Approach, New Technology Group 5—AHA CC: 3Q, 2020, 18-19

XW04331 Introduction of Idarucizumab, Dabigatran Reversal Agent into Central Vein, Percutaneous Approach, New Technology Group 1—AHA CC: 4Q, 2015, 13

XW04351 Introduction of Blinatumomab Antineoplastic into Central Vein, Percutaneous Approach, New Technology Group 1—AHA CC: 4Q, 2015, 14-15

XW043E5 Introduction of Remdesivir Anti-infective into Central Vein, Percutaneous Approach, New Technology Group 5—AHA CC: 3Q, 2020, 18-19

XW043F5 Introduction of Other New Technology Therapeutic Substance into Central Vein, Percutaneous Approach, New Technology Group 5—AHA CC: 3Q, 2020, 19-20; 1Q, 2021, 49-51

XW043G5 Introduction of Sarilumab into Central Vein, Percutaneous Approach, New Technology Group 5—AHA CC: 3Q, 2020, 18-19

XW043H5 Introduction of Tocilizumab into Central Vein, Percutaneous Approach, New Technology Group 5—AHA CC: 3Q, 2020, 18-19

XW0DXF5 Introduction of Other New Technology Therapeutic Substance into Mouth and Pharynx, External Approach, New Technology Group 5—AHA CC: 3Q, 2020, 19-20; 1Q, 2021, 49-51

XW0Q316 Introduction of Eladocagene exuparvovec into Cranial Cavity and Brain, Percutaneous Approach, New Technology Group 6—AHA CC: 4Q, 2020, 73

XW13325 Transfusion of Convalescent Plasma (Nonautologous) into Peripheral Vein, Percutaneous Approach, New Technology Group 5—AHA CC: 3Q, 2020, 19

XW14325 Transfusion of Convalescent Plasma (Nonautologous) into Central Vein, Percutaneous Approach, New Technology Group 5—AHA CC: 3Q, 2020, 19

Appendix A: Root Operations Definitions

Section 0 - Medical and Surgical — Character 3 - Root Operation	
Alteration (0)	**Definition:** Modifying the anatomic structure of a body part without affecting the function of the body part **Explanation:** Principal purpose is to improve appearance **Includes/Examples:** Face lift, breast augmentation
Bypass (1)	**Definition:** Altering the route of passage of the contents of a tubular body part **Explanation:** Rerouting contents of a body part to a downstream area of the normal route, to a similar route and body part, or to an abnormal route and dissimilar body part. Includes one or more anastomoses, with or without the use of a device **Includes/Examples:** Coronary artery bypass, colostomy formation
Change (2)	**Definition:** Taking out or off a device from a body part and putting back an identical or similar device in or on the same body part without cutting or puncturing the skin or a mucous membrane **Explanation:** All CHANGE procedures are coded using the approach EXTERNAL **Includes/Examples:** Urinary catheter change, gastrostomy tube change
Control (3)	**Definition:** Stopping, or attempting to stop, postprocedural or other acute bleeding **Includes/Examples:** Control of post-prostatectomy hemorrhage, control of intracranial subdural hemorrhage, control of bleeding duodenal ulcer, control of retroperitoneal hemorrhage
Creation (4)	**Definition:** Putting in or on biological or synthetic material to form a new body part that to the extent possible replicates the anatomic structure or function of an absent body part **Explanation:** Used for gender reassignment surgery and corrective procedures in individuals with congenital anomalies **Includes/Examples:** Creation of vagina in a male, creation of right and left atrioventricular valve from common atrioventricular valve
Destruction (5)	**Definition:** Physical eradication of all or a portion of a body part by the direct use of energy, force, or a destructive agent **Explanation:** None of the body part is physically taken out **Includes/Examples:** Fulguration of rectal polyp, cautery of skin lesion
Detachment (6)	**Definition:** Cutting off all or a portion of the upper or lower extremities **Explanation:** The body part value is the site of the detachment, with a qualifier if applicable to further specify the level where the extremity was detached **Includes/Examples:** Below knee amputation, disarticulation of shoulder
Dilation (7)	**Definition:** Expanding an orifice or the lumen of a tubular body part **Explanation:** The orifice can be a natural orifice or an artificially created orifice. Accomplished by stretching a tubular body part using intraluminal pressure or by cutting part of the orifice or wall of the tubular body part **Includes/Examples:** Percutaneous transluminal angioplasty, internal urethrotomy
Division (8)	**Definition:** Cutting into a body part, without draining fluids and/or gases from the body part, in order to separate or transect a body part **Explanation:** All or a portion of the body part is separated into two or more portions **Includes/Examples:** Spinal cordotomy, osteotomy
Drainage (9)	**Definition:** Taking or letting out fluids and/or gases from a body part **Explanation:** The qualifier DIAGNOSTIC is used to identify drainage procedures that are biopsies **Includes/Examples:** Thoracentesis, incision and drainage
Excision (B)	**Definition:** Cutting out or off, without replacement, a portion of a body part **Explanation:** The qualifier DIAGNOSTIC is used to identify excision procedures that are biopsies **Includes/Examples:** Partial nephrectomy, liver biopsy
Extirpation (C)	**Definition:** Taking or cutting out solid matter from a body part **Explanation:** The solid matter may be an abnormal byproduct of a biological function or a foreign body; it may be imbedded in a body part or in the lumen of a tubular body part. The solid matter may or may not have been previously broken into pieces **Includes/Examples:** Thrombectomy, choledocholithotomy
Extraction (D)	**Definition:** Pulling or stripping out or off all or a portion of a body part by the use of force **Explanation:** The qualifier DIAGNOSTIC is used to identify extraction procedures that are biopsies **Includes/Examples:** Dilation and curettage, vein stripping
Fragmentation (F)	**Definition:** Breaking solid matter in a body part into pieces **Explanation:** Physical force (e.g., manual, ultrasonic) applied directly or indirectly is used to break the solid matter into pieces. The solid matter may be an abnormal byproduct of a biological function or a foreign body. The pieces of solid matter are not taken out **Includes/Examples:** Extracorporeal shockwave lithotripsy, transurethral lithotripsy
Fusion (G)	**Definition:** Joining together portions of an articular body part rendering the articular body part immobile **Explanation:** The body part is joined together by fixation device, bone graft, or other means **Includes/Examples:** Spinal fusion, ankle arthrodesis
Insertion (H)	**Definition:** Putting in a nonbiological appliance that monitors, assists, performs, or prevents a physiological function but does not physically take the place of a body part **Includes/Examples:** Insertion of radioactive implant, insertion of central venous catheter

Continued →

Section 0 - Medical and Surgical — Character 3 - Root Operation

Inspection (J)	**Definition:** Visually and/or manually exploring a body part **Explanation:** Visual exploration may be performed with or without optical instrumentation. Manual exploration may be performed directly or through intervening body layers **Includes/Examples:** Diagnostic arthroscopy, exploratory laparotomy
Map (K)	**Definition:** Locating the route of passage of electrical impulses and/or locating functional areas in a body part **Explanation:** Applicable only to the cardiac conduction mechanism and the central nervous system **Includes/Examples:** Cardiac mapping, cortical mapping
Occlusion (L)	**Definition:** Completely closing an orifice or the lumen of a tubular body part **Explanation:** The orifice can be a natural orifice or an artificially created orifice **Includes/Examples:** Fallopian tube ligation, ligation of inferior vena cava
Reattachment (M)	**Definition:** Putting back in or on all or a portion of a separated body part to its normal location or other suitable location **Explanation:** Vascular circulation and nervous pathways may or may not be reestablished **Includes/Examples:** Reattachment of hand, reattachment of avulsed kidney
Release (N)	**Definition:** Freeing a body part from an abnormal physical constraint by cutting or by the use of force **Explanation:** Some of the restraining tissue may be taken out but none of the body part is taken out **Includes/Examples:** Adhesiolysis, carpal tunnel release
Removal (P)	**Definition:** Taking out or off a device from a body part **Explanation:** If a device is taken out and a similar device put in without cutting or puncturing the skin or mucous membrane, the procedure is coded to the root operation CHANGE. Otherwise, the procedure for taking out a device is coded to the root operation REMOVAL **Includes/Examples:** Drainage tube removal, cardiac pacemaker removal
Repair (Q)	**Definition:** Restoring, to the extent possible, a body part to its normal anatomic structure and function **Explanation:** Used only when the method to accomplish the repair is not one of the other root operations **Includes/Examples:** Colostomy takedown, suture of laceration
Replacement (R)	**Definition:** Putting in or on biological or synthetic material that physically takes the place and/or function of all or a portion of a body part **Explanation:** The body part may have been taken out or replaced, or may be taken out, physically eradicated, or rendered nonfunctional during the Replacement procedure. A Removal procedure is coded for taking out the device used in a previous replacement procedure **Includes/Examples:** Total hip replacement, bone graft, free skin graft
Reposition (S)	**Definition:** Moving to its normal location, or other suitable location, all or a portion of a body part **Explanation:** The body part is moved to a new location from an abnormal location, or from a normal location where it is not functioning correctly. The body part may or may not be cut out or off to be moved to the new location **Includes/Examples:** Reposition of undescended testicle, fracture reduction
Resection (T)	**Definition:** Cutting out or off, without replacement, all of a body part **Includes/Examples:** Total nephrectomy, total lobectomy of lung
Restriction (V)	**Definition:** Partially closing an orifice or the lumen of a tubular body part **Explanation:** The orifice can be a natural orifice or an artificially created orifice **Includes/Examples:** Esophagogastric fundoplication, cervical cerclage
Revision (W)	**Definition:** Correcting, to the extent possible, a portion of a malfunctioning device or the position of a displaced device **Explanation:** Revision can include correcting a malfunctioning or displaced device by taking out or putting in components of the device such as a screw or pin **Includes/Examples:** Adjustment of position of pacemaker lead, recementing of hip prosthesis
Supplement (U)	**Definition:** Putting in or on biological or synthetic material that physically reinforces and/or augments the function of a portion of a body part **Explanation:** The biological material is non-living, or is living and from the same individual. The body part may have been previously replaced, and the Supplement procedure is performed to physically reinforce and/or augment the function of the replaced body part **Includes/Examples:** Herniorrhaphy using mesh, mitral valve ring annuloplasty, put a new acetabular liner in a previous hip replacement
Transfer (X)	**Definition:** Moving, without taking out, all or a portion of a body part to another location to take over the function of all or a portion of a body part **Explanation:** The body part transferred remains connected to its vascular and nervous supply **Includes/Examples:** Tendon transfer, skin pedicle flap transfer
Transplantation (Y)	**Definition:** Putting in or on all or a portion of a living body part taken from another individual or animal to physically take the place and/or function of all or a portion of a similar body part **Explanation:** The native body part may or may not be taken out, and the transplanted body part may take over all or a portion of its function **Includes/Examples:** Kidney transplant, heart transplant

Section 1 - Obstetrics — Character 3 - Root Operations Unique to Obstetrics

Abortion (A)	**Definition:** Artificially terminating a pregnancy **Explanation:** Subdivided according to whether an additional device such as a laminaria or abortifacient is used, or whether the abortion was performed by mechanical means **Includes/Example:** Transvaginal abortion using vacuum aspiration technique
Delivery (E)	**Definition:** Assisting the passage of the products of conception from the genital canal **Explanation:** Applies only to manually-assisted, vaginal delivery **Includes/Example:** Manually-assisted delivery

Section 2 - Placement — Character 3 - Root Operation	
Change (0)	**Definition:** Taking out or off a device from a body part and putting back an identical or similar device in or on the same body part without cutting or puncturing the skin or a mucous membrane **Includes/Example:** Change of vaginal packing
Compression (1)	**Definition:** Putting pressure on a body region **Includes/Example:** Placement of pressure dressing on abdominal wall
Dressing (2)	**Definition:** Putting material on a body region for protection **Includes/Example:** Application of sterile dressing to head wound
Immobilization (3)	**Definition:** Limiting or preventing motion of a body region **Includes/Example:** Placement of splint on left finger
Packing (4)	**Definition:** Putting material in a body region or orifice **Includes/Example:** Placement of nasal packing
Removal (5)	**Definition:** Taking out or off a device from a body part **Includes/Example:** Removal of cast from right lower leg
Traction (6)	**Definition:** Exerting a pulling force on a body region in a distal direction **Includes/Example:** Lumbar traction using motorized split-traction table

Section 3 - Administration — Character 3 - Root Operation	
Introduction (0)	**Definition:** Putting in or on a therapeutic, diagnostic, nutritional, physiological, or prophylactic substance except blood or blood products **Includes/Example:** Nerve block injection to median nerve
Irrigation (1)	**Definition:** Putting in or on a cleansing substance **Includes/Example:** Flushing of eye
Transfusion (2)	**Definition:** Putting in blood or blood products **Includes/Example:** Transfusion of cell saver red cells into central venous line

Section 4 - Measurement and Monitoring — Character 3 - Root Operation	
Measurement (0)	**Definition:** Determining the level of a physiological or physical function at a point in time **Includes/Example:** External electrocardiogram (EKG), single reading
Monitoring (1)	**Definition:** Determining the level of a physiological or physical function repetitively over a period of time **Includes/Example:** Urinary pressure monitoring

Section 5 - Extracorporeal Assistance and Performance — Character 3 - Root Operation	
Assistance (0)	**Definition:** Taking over a portion of a physiological function by extracorporeal means **Includes/Example:** Hyperbaric oxygenation of wound
Performance (1)	**Definition:** Completely taking over a physiological function by extracorporeal means **Includes/Example:** Cardiopulmonary bypass in conjunction with CABG
Restoration (2)	**Definition:** Returning, or attempting to return, a physiological function to its original state by extracorporeal means. **Includes/Example:** Attempted cardiac defibrillation, unsuccessful

Section 6 - Extracorporeal Therapies — Character 3 - Root Operation	
Atmospheric Control (0)	**Definition:** Extracorporeal control of atmospheric pressure and composition **Includes/Example:** Atmospheric control, single treatment
Decompression (1)	**Definition:** Extracorporeal elimination of undissolved gas from body fluids **Includes/Example:** Hyperbaric decompression treatment, single
Electromagnetic Therapy (2)	**Definition:** Extracorporeal treatment by electromagnetic rays **Includes/Example:** Electromagnetic therapy, central nervous, multiple treatments
Hyperthermia (3)	**Definition:** Extracorporeal raising of body temperature **Includes/Example:** Hyperthermia, single treatment
Hypothermia (4)	**Definition:** Extracorporeal lowering of body temperature **Includes/Example:** Whole body hypothermia treatment for temperature imbalances, series treatment
Perfusion (B)	**Definition:** Extracorporeal treatment by diffusion of therapeutic fluid
Pheresis (5)	**Definition:** Extracorporeal separation of blood products **Includes/Example:** Therapeutic leukopheresis, single treatment
Phototherapy (6)	**Definition:** Extracorporeal treatment by light rays **Includes/Example:** Phototherapy of circulatory system, series treatment

Continued →

Section 6 - Extracorporeal Therapies — Character 3 - Root Operation

Shock Wave Therapy (7)	**Definition:** Extracorporeal treatment by shock waves **Includes/Example:** Shock wave therapy, musculoskeletal, single treatment
Ultrasound Therapy (8)	**Definition:** Extracorporeal treatment by ultrasound **Includes/Example:** Ultrasound therapy of the heart, single treatment
Ultraviolet Light Therapy (9)	**Definition:** Extracorporeal treatment by ultraviolet light **Includes/Example:** Ultraviolet light phototherapy, series treatment

Section 7 - Osteopathic — Character 3 - Root Operation

Treatment (0)	**Definition:** Manual treatment to eliminate or alleviate somatic dysfunction and related disorders **Includes/Example:** Fascial release of abdomen, osteopathic treatment

Section 8 - Other Procedures — Character 3 - Root Operation

Other Procedures (0)	**Definition:** Methodologies which attempt to remediate or cure a disorder or disease **Includes/Example:** Acupuncture

Section 9 - Chiropractic — Character 3 - Root Operation

Manipulation (B)	**Definition:** Manual procedure that involves a directed thrust to move a joint past the physiological range of motion, without exceeding the anatomical limit **Includes/Example:** Chiropractic treatment of cervical spine, short lever specific contact

Section X - New Technology — Character 3 - Root Operation

Assistance (A)	**Definition:** Taking over a portion of a physiological function by extracorporeal means
Bypass (K)	**Definition:** Altering the route of passage of the contents of a tubular body part
Destruction (5)	**Definition:** Physical eradication of all or a portion of a body part by the direct use of energy, force, or a destructive agent **Explanation:** None of the body part is physically taken out **Includes/Examples:** Fulguration of rectal polyp, cautery of skin lesion
Dilation (7)	**Definition:** Expanding an orifice or the lumen of a tubular body part **Explanation:** The orifice can be a natural orifice or an artificially created orifice. Accomplished by stretching a tubular body part using intraluminal pressure or by cutting part of the orifice or wall of the tubular body part
Extirpation (C)	**Definition:** Taking or cutting out solid matter from a body part **Explanation:** The solid matter may be an abnormal by product of a biological function or a foreign body; it may be imbedded in a body part or in the lumen of a tubular body part. The solid matter may or may not have been previously broken into pieces **Includes/Example:** Thrombectomy, choledocholithotomy
Fusion (G)	**Definition:** Joining together portions of an articular body part rendering the articular body part immobile **Explanation:** The body part is joined together by fixation device, bone graft, or other means **Includes/Examples:** Spinal fusion, ankle arthrodesis
Insertion (H)	**Definition:** Putting in a nonbiological appliance that monitors, assists, performs, or prevents a physiological function bust does not physically take the place of a body part.
Inspection (J)	**Definition:** Visually and/or manually exploring a body part
Introduction (0)	**Definition:** Putting in or on a therapeutic, diagnostic, nutritional, physiological, or prophylactic substance except blood or blood products
Irrigation (P)	**Definition:** Putting in or on a cleansing substance
Measurement (E)	**Definition:** Determining the level of a physiological or physical function at a point in time
Monitoring (2)	**Definition:** Determining the level of a physiological or physical function repetitively over a period of time
Replacement (R)	**Definition:** Putting in or on biological or synthetic material that physically takes the place and/or function of all or a portion of a body part **Explanation:** The body part may have been taken out or replaced, or may be taken out, physically eradicated, or rendered nonfunctional during the Replacement procedure. A Removal procedure is coded for taking out the device used in a previous replacement procedure. **Includes/Examples:** Total hip replacement, bone graft, free skin graft
Reposition (S)	**Definition:** Moving to its normal location, or other suitable location, all or a portion of a body part **Explanation:** The body part is moved to a new location from an abnormal location, or from a normal location where it is not functioning correctly. The body part may or may not be cut out or off to be moved to the new location. **Includes/Examples:** Reposition of undescended testicle, fracture reduction
Restriction (V)	**Definition:** Partially closing an orifice or the lumen of a tubular body part
Supplement (U)	**Definition:** Putting in or on biological or synthetic material that physically reinforces and/or augments the function of a portion of a body part
Transfusion (1&2)	**Definition:** Putting in blood or blood products

Appendix B: Type and Qualifier Definitions

Section B - Imaging — Character 3 - Root Type	
Computerized Tomography (CT Scan) (2)	**Definition:** Computer reformatted digital display of multiplanar images developed from the capture of multiple exposures of external ionizing radiation
Fluoroscopy (1)	**Definition:** Single plane or bi-plane real time display of an image developed from the capture of external ionizing radiation on a fluorescent screen. The image may also be stored by either digital or analog means
Magnetic Resonance Imaging (MRI) (3)	**Definition:** Computer reformatted digital display of multiplanar images developed from the capture of radiofrequency signals emitted by nuclei in a body site excited within a magnetic field
Other Imaging (5)	**Definition:** Other specified modality for visualizing a body part
Plain Radiography (0)	**Definition:** Planar display of an image developed from the capture of external ionizing radiation on photographic or photoconductive plate
Ultrasonography (4)	**Definition:** Real time display of images of anatomy or flow information developed from the capture of reflected and attenuated high frequency sound waves

Section C - Nuclear Medicine — Character 3 - Root Type	
Nonimaging Nuclear Medicine Assay (6)	**Definition:** Introduction of radioactive materials into the body for the study of body fluids and blood elements, by the detection of radioactive emissions
Nonimaging Nuclear Medicine Probe (5)	**Definition:** Introduction of radioactive materials into the body for the study of distribution and fate of certain substances by the detection of radioactive emissions; or, alternatively, measurement of absorption of radioactive emissions from an external source
Nonimaging Nuclear Medicine Uptake (4)	**Definition:** Introduction of radioactive materials into the body for measurements of organ function, from the detection of radioactive emissions
Planar Nuclear Medicine Imaging (1)	**Definition:** Introduction of radioactive materials into the body for single plane display of images developed from the capture of radioactive emissions
Positron Emission Tomographic (PET) Imaging (3)	**Definition:** Introduction of radioactive materials into the body for three dimensional display of images developed from the simultaneous capture, 180 degrees apart, of radioactive emissions
Systemic Nuclear Medicine Therapy (7)	**Definition:** Introduction of unsealed radioactive materials into the body for treatment
Tomographic (Tomo) Nuclear Medicine Imaging (2)	**Definition:** Introduction of radioactive materials into the body for three dimensional display of images developed from the capture of radioactive emissions

Section F - Physical Rehabilitation and Diagnostic Audiology — Character 3 - Root Type	
Activities of Daily Living Assessment	**Definition:** Measurement of functional level for activities of daily living
Activities of Daily Living Treatment	**Definition:** Exercise or activities to facilitate functional competence for activities of daily living
Caregiver Training	**Definition:** Training in activities to support patient's optimal level of function
Cochlear Implant Treatment	**Definition:** Application of techniques to improve the communication abilities of individuals with cochlear implant
Device Fitting	**Definition:** Fitting of a device designed to facilitate or support achievement of a higher level of function
Hearing Aid Assessment	**Definition:** Measurement of the appropriateness and/or effectiveness of a hearing device
Hearing Assessment	**Definition:** Measurement of hearing and related functions
Hearing Treatment	**Definition:** Application of techniques to improve, augment, or compensate for hearing and related functional impairment
Motor and/or Nerve Function Assessment	**Definition:** Measurement of motor, nerve, and related functions
Motor Treatment	**Definition:** Exercise or activities to increase or facilitate motor function
Speech Assessment	**Definition:** Measurement of speech and related functions
Speech Treatment	**Definition:** Application of techniques to improve, augment, or compensate for speech and related functional impairment
Vestibular Assessment	**Definition:** Measurement of the vestibular system and related functions
Vestibular Treatment	**Definition:** Application of techniques to improve, augment, or compensate for vestibular and related functional impairment

Acoustic Reflex Decay	**Definition:** Measures reduction in size/strength of acoustic reflex over time **Includes/Examples:** Includes site of lesion test
Acoustic Reflex Patterns	**Definition:** Defines site of lesion based upon presence/absence of acoustic reflexes with ipsilateral vs. contralateral stimulation
Acoustic Reflex Threshold	**Definition:** Determines minimal intensity that acoustic reflex occurs with ipsilateral and/or contralateral stimulation
Aerobic Capacity and Endurance	**Definition:** Measures autonomic responses to positional changes; perceived exertion, dyspnea or angina during activity; performance during exercise protocols; standard vital signs; and blood gas analysis or oxygen consumption
Alternate Binaural or Monaural Loudness Balance	**Definition:** Determines auditory stimulus parameter that yields the same objective sensation **Includes/Examples:** Sound intensities that yield same loudness perception
Anthropometric Characteristics	**Definition:** Measures edema, body fat composition, height, weight, length and girth
Aphasia (Assessment)	**Definition:** Measures expressive and receptive speech and language function including reading and writing
Aphasia (Treatment)	**Definition:** Applying techniques to improve, augment, or compensate for receptive/expressive language impairments
Articulation/Phonology (Assessment)	**Definition:** Measures speech production
Articulation/Phonology (Treatment)	**Definition:** Applying techniques to correct, improve, or compensate for speech productive impairment
Assistive Listening Device	**Definition:** Assists in use of effective and appropriate assistive listening device/system
Assistive Listening System/Device Selection	**Definition:** Measures the effectiveness and appropriateness of assistive listening systems/devices
Assistive, Adaptive, Supportive or Protective Devices	**Explanation:** Devices to facilitate or support achievement of a higher level of function in wheelchair mobility; bed mobility; transfer or ambulation ability; bath and showering ability; dressing; grooming; personal hygiene; play or leisure
Auditory Evoked Potentials	**Definition:** Measures electric responses produced by the VIIIth cranial nerve and brainstem following auditory stimulation
Auditory Processing (Assessment)	**Definition:** Evaluates ability to receive and process auditory information and comprehension of spoken language
Auditory Processing (Treatment)	**Definition:** Applying techniques to improve the receiving and processing of auditory information and comprehension of spoken language
Augmentative/Alternative Communication System (Assessment)	**Definition:** Determines the appropriateness of aids, techniques, symbols, and/or strategies to augment or replace speech and enhance communication **Includes/Examples:** Includes the use of telephones, writing equipment, emergency equipment, and TDD
Augmentative/Alternative Communication System (Treatment)	**Includes/Examples:** Includes augmentative communication devices and aids
Aural Rehabilitation	**Definition:** Applying techniques to improve the communication abilities associated with hearing loss
Aural Rehabilitation Status	**Definition:** Measures impact of a hearing loss including evaluation of receptive and expressive communication skills
Bathing/Showering	**Includes/Examples:** Includes obtaining and using supplies; soaping, rinsing, and drying body parts; maintaining bathing position; and transferring to and from bathing positions
Bathing/Showering Techniques	**Definition:** Activities to facilitate obtaining and using supplies, soaping, rinsing and drying body parts, maintaining bathing position, and transferring to and from bathing positions
Bed Mobility (Assessment)	**Definition:** Transitional movement within bed
Bed Mobility (Treatment)	**Definition:** Exercise or activities to facilitate transitional movements within bed
Bedside Swallowing and Oral Function	**Includes/Examples:** Bedside swallowing includes assessment of sucking, masticating, coughing, and swallowing. Oral function includes assessment of musculature for controlled movements, structures and functions to determine coordination and phonation
Bekesy Audiometry	**Definition:** Uses an instrument that provides a choice of discrete or continuously varying pure tones; choice of pulsed or continuous signal
Binaural Electroacoustic Hearing Aid Check	**Definition:** Determines mechanical and electroacoustic function of bilateral hearing aids using hearing aid test box
Binaural Hearing Aid (Assessment)	**Definition:** Measures the candidacy, effectiveness, and appropriateness of a hearing aids **Explanation:** Measures bilateral fit

Continued →

Section F - Physical Rehabilitation and Diagnostic Audiology — Character 5 - Type Qualifier

Binaural Hearing Aid (Treatment)	**Explanation:** Assists in achieving maximum understanding and performance
Bithermal, Binaural Caloric Irrigation	**Definition:** Measures the rhythmic eye movements stimulated by changing the temperature of the vestibular system
Bithermal, Monaural Caloric Irrigation	**Definition:** Measures the rhythmic eye movements stimulated by changing the temperature of the vestibular system in one ear
Brief Tone Stimuli	**Definition:** Measures specific central auditory process
Cerumen Management	**Definition:** Includes examination of external auditory canal and tympanic membrane and removal of cerumen from external ear canal
Cochlear Implant	**Definition:** Measures candidacy for cochlear implant
Cochlear Implant Rehabilitation	**Definition:** Applying techniques to improve the communication abilities of individuals with cochlear implant; includes programming the device, providing patients/families with information
Communicative/Cognitive Integration Skills (Assessment)	**Definition:** Measures ability to use higher cortical functions **Includes/Examples:** Includes orientation, recognition, attention span, initiation and termination of activity, memory, sequencing, categorizing, concept formation, spatial operations, judgment, problem solving, generalization and pragmatic communication
Communicative/Cognitive Integration Skills (Treatment)	**Definition:** Activities to facilitate the use of higher cortical functions **Includes/Examples:** Includes level of arousal, orientation, recognition, attention span, initiation and termination of activity, memory sequencing, judgment and problem solving, learning and generalization, and pragmatic communication
Computerized Dynamic Posturography	**Definition:** Measures the status of the peripheral and central vestibular system and the sensory/motor component of balance; evaluates the efficacy of vestibular rehabilitation
Conditioned Play Audiometry	**Definition:** Behavioral measures using nonspeech and speech stimuli to obtain frequency-specific and ear-specific information on auditory status from the patient **Explanation:** Obtains speech reception threshold by having patient point to pictures of spondaic words
Coordination/Dexterity (Assessment)	**Definition:** Measures large and small muscle groups for controlled goal-directed movements **Explanation:** Dexterity includes object manipulation
Coordination/Dexterity (Treatment)	**Definition:** Exercise or activities to facilitate gross coordination and fine coordination
Cranial Nerve Integrity	**Definition:** Measures cranial nerve sensory and motor functions, including tastes, smell and facial expression
Dichotic Stimuli	**Definition:** Measures specific central auditory process
Distorted Speech	**Definition:** Measures specific central auditory process
Dix-Hallpike Dynamic	**Definition:** Measures nystagmus following Dix-Hallpike maneuver
Dressing	**Includes/Examples:** Includes selecting clothing and accessories, obtaining clothing from storage, dressing, fastening and adjusting clothing and shoes, and applying and removing personal devices, prosthesis or orthosis
Dressing Techniques	**Definition:** Activities to facilitate selecting clothing and accessories, dressing and undressing, adjusting clothing and shoes, applying and removing devices, prostheses or orthoses
Dynamic Orthosis	**Includes/Examples:** Includes customized and prefabricated splints, inhibitory casts, spinal and other braces, and protective devices; allows motion through transfer of movement from other body parts or by use of outside forces
Ear Canal Probe Microphone	**Definition:** Real ear measures
Ear Protector Attentuation	**Definition:** Measures ear protector fit and effectiveness
Electrocochleography	**Definition:** Measures the VIIIth cranial nerve action potential
Environmental, Home and Work Barriers	**Definition:** Measures current and potential barriers to optimal function, including safety hazards, access problems and home or office design
Ergonomics and Body Mechanics	**Definition:** Ergonomic measurement of job tasks, work hardening or work conditioning needs; functional capacity; and body mechanics
Eustachian Tube Function	**Definition:** Measures eustachian tube function and patency of eustachian tube
Evoked Otoacoustic Emissions, Diagnostic	**Definition:** Measures auditory evoked potentials in a diagnostic format
Evoked Otoacoustic Emissions, Screening	**Definition:** Measures auditory evoked potentials in a screening format
Facial Nerve Function	**Definition:** Measures electrical activity of the VIIth cranial nerve (facial nerve)
Feeding/Eating (Assessment)	**Includes/Examples:** Includes setting up food, selecting and using utensils and tableware, bringing food or drink to mouth, cleaning face, hands, and clothing, and management of alternative methods of nourishment

Continued →

Feeding/Eating (Treatment)	**Definition:** Exercise or activities to facilitate setting up food, selecting and using utensils and tableware, bringing food or drink to mouth, cleaning face, hands, and clothing, and management of alternative methods of nourishment
Filtered Speech	**Definition:** Uses high or low pass filtered speech stimuli to assess central auditory processing disorders, site of lesion testing
Fluency (Assessment)	**Definition:** Measures speech fluency or stuttering
Fluency (Treatment)	**Definition:** Applying techniques to improve and augment fluent speech
Gait and/or Balance	**Definition:** Measures biomechanical, arthrokinematic and other spatial and temporal characteristics of gait and balance
Gait Training/Functional Ambulation	**Definition:** Exercise or activities to facilitate ambulation on a variety of surfaces and in a variety of environments
Grooming/Personal Hygiene (Assessment)	**Includes/Examples:** Includes ability to obtain and use supplies in a sequential fashion, general grooming, oral hygiene, toilet hygiene, personal care devices, including care for artificial airways
Grooming/Personal Hygiene (Treatment)	**Definition:** Activities to facilitate obtaining and using supplies in a sequential fashion: general grooming, oral hygiene, toilet hygiene, cleaning body, and personal care devices, including artificial airways
Hearing and Related Disorders Counseling	**Definition:** Provides patients/families/caregivers with information, support, referrals to facilitate recovery from a communication disorder **Includes/Examples:** Includes strategies for psychosocial adjustment to hearing loss for clients and families/caregivers
Hearing and Related Disorders Prevention	**Definition:** Provides patients/families/caregivers with information and support to prevent communication disorders
Hearing Screening	**Definition:** Pass/refer measures designed to identify need for further audiologic assessment
Home Management (Assessment)	**Definition:** Obtaining and maintaining personal and household possessions and environment **Includes/Examples:** Includes clothing care, cleaning, meal preparation and cleanup, shopping, money management, household maintenance, safety procedures, and childcare/parenting
Home Management (Treatment)	**Definition:** Activities to facilitate obtaining and maintaining personal household possessions and environment **Includes/Examples:** Includes clothing care, cleaning, meal preparation and clean-up, shopping, money management, household maintenance, safety procedures, childcare/parenting
Instrumental Swallowing and Oral Function	**Definition:** Measures swallowing function using instrumental diagnostic procedures **Explanation:** Methods include videofluoroscopy, ultrasound, manometry, endoscopy
Integumentary Integrity	**Includes/Examples:** Includes burns, skin conditions, ecchymosis, bleeding, blisters, scar tissue, wounds and other traumas, tissue mobility, turgor and texture
Manual Therapy Techniques	**Definition:** Techniques in which the therapist uses his/her hands to administer skilled movements **Includes/Examples:** Includes connective tissue massage, joint mobilization and manipulation, manual lymph drainage, manual traction, soft tissue mobilization and manipulation
Masking Patterns	**Definition:** Measures central auditory processing status
Monaural Electroacoustic Hearing Aid Check	**Definition:** Determines mechanical and electroacoustic function of one hearing aid using hearing aid test box
Monaural Hearing Aid (Assessment)	**Definition:** Measures the candidacy, effectiveness, and appropriateness of a hearing aid **Explanation:** Measures unilateral fit
Monaural Hearing Aid (Treatment)	**Explanation:** Assists in achieving maximum understanding and performance
Motor Function (Assessment)	**Definition:** Measures the body's functional and versatile movement patterns **Includes/Examples:** Includes motor assessment scales, analysis of head, trunk and limb movement, and assessment of motor learning
Motor Function (Treatment)	**Definition:** Exercise or activities to facilitate crossing midline, laterality, bilateral integration, praxis, neuromuscular relaxation, inhibition, facilitation, motor function and motor learning
Motor Speech (Assessment)	**Definition:** Measures neurological motor aspects of speech production
Motor Speech (Treatment)	**Definition:** Applying techniques to improve and augment the impaired neurological motor aspects of speech production
Muscle Performance (Assessment)	**Definition:** Measures muscle strength, power and endurance using manual testing, dynamometry or computer-assisted electromechanical muscle test; functional muscle strength, power and endurance; muscle pain, tone, or soreness; or pelvic-floor musculature **Explanation:** Muscle endurance refers to the ability to contract a muscle repeatedly over time

Continued →

Section F - Physical Rehabilitation and Diagnostic Audiology — Character 5 - Type Qualifier	
Muscle Performance (Treatment)	**Definition:** Exercise or activities to increase the capacity of a muscle to do work in terms of strength, power, and/or endurance **Explanation:** Muscle strength is the force exerted to overcome resistance in one maximal effort. Muscle power is work produced per unit of time, or the product of strength and speed. Muscle endurance is the ability to contract a muscle repeatedly over time
Neuromotor Development	**Definition:** Measures motor development, righting and equilibrium reactions, and reflex and equilibrium reactions
Non-invasive Instrumental Status	**Definition:** Instrumental measures of oral, nasal, vocal, and velopharyngeal functions as they pertain to speech production
Nonspoken Language (Assessment)	**Definition:** Measures nonspoken language (print, sign, symbols) for communication
Nonspoken Language (Treatment)	**Definition:** Applying techniques that improve, augment, or compensate spoken communication
Oral Peripheral Mechanism	**Definition:** Structural measures of face, jaw, lips, tongue, teeth, hard and soft palate, pharynx as related to speech production
Orofacial Myofunctional (Assessment)	**Definition:** Measures orofacial myofunctional patterns for speech and related functions
Orofacial Myofunctional (Treatment)	**Definition:** Applying techniques to improve, alter, or augment impaired orofacial myofunctional patterns and related speech production errors
Oscillating Tracking	**Definition:** Measures ability to visually track
Pain	**Definition:** Measures muscle soreness, pain and soreness with joint movement, and pain perception **Includes/Examples:** Includes questionnaires, graphs, symptom magnification scales or visual analog scales
Perceptual Processing (Assessment)	**Definition:** Measures stereognosis, kinesthesia, body schema, right-left discrimination, form constancy, position in space, visual closure, figure-ground, depth perception, spatial relations and topographical orientation
Perceptual Processing (Treatment)	**Definition:** Exercise and activities to facilitate perceptual processing **Explanation:** Includes stereognosis, kinesthesia, body schema, right-left discrimination, form constancy, position in space, visual closure, figure-ground, depth perception, spatial relations, and topographical orientation **Includes/Examples:** Includes stereognosis, kinesthesia, body schema, right-left discrimination, form constancy, position in space, visual closure, figure-ground, depth perception, spatial relations, and topographical orientation
Performance Intensity Phonetically Balanced Speech Discrimination	**Definition:** Measures word recognition over varying intensity levels
Postural Control	**Definition:** Exercise or activities to increase postural alignment and control
Prosthesis	**Definition:** Artificial substitutes for missing body parts that augment performance or function **Includes/Examples:** Limb prosthesis, ocular prosthesis
Psychosocial Skills (Assessment)	**Definition:** The ability to interact in society and to process emotions **Includes/Examples:** Includes psychological (values, interests, self-concept); social (role performance, social conduct, interpersonal skills, self expression); self-management (coping skills, time management, self-control)
Psychosocial Skills (Treatment)	**Definition:** The ability to interact in society and to process emotions **Includes/Examples:** Includes psychological (values, interests, self-concept); social (role performance, social conduct, interpersonal skills, self expression); self-management (coping skills, time management, self-control)
Pure Tone Audiometry, Air	**Definition:** Air-conduction pure tone threshold measures with appropriate masking
Pure Tone Audiometry, Air and Bone	**Definition:** Air-conduction and bone-conduction pure tone threshold measures with appropriate masking
Pure Tone Stenger	**Definition:** Measures unilateral nonorganic hearing loss based on simultaneous presentation of pure tones of differing volume
Range of Motion and Joint Integrity	**Definition:** Measures quantity, quality, grade, and classification of joint movement and/or mobility **Explanation:** Range of Motion is the space, distance or angle through which movement occurs at a joint or series of joints. Joint integrity is the conformance of joints to expected anatomic, biomechanical and kinematic norms
Range of Motion and Joint Mobility	**Definition:** Exercise or activities to increase muscle length and joint mobility
Receptive/Expressive Language (Assessment)	**Definition:** Measures receptive and expressive language
Receptive/Expressive Language (Treatment)	**Definition:** Applying techniques to improve and augment receptive/expressive language

Continued →

Reflex Integrity	**Definition:** Measures the presence, absence, or exaggeration of developmentally appropriate, pathologic or normal reflexes
Select Picture Audiometry	**Definition:** Establishes hearing threshold levels for speech using pictures
Sensorineural Acuity Level	**Definition:** Measures sensorineural acuity masking presented via bone conduction
Sensory Aids	**Definition:** Determines the appropriateness of a sensory prosthetic device, other than a hearing aid or assistive listening system/device
Sensory Awareness/Processing/Integrity	**Includes/Examples:** Includes light touch, pressure, temperature, pain, sharp/dull, proprioception, vestibular, visual, auditory, gustatory, and olfactory
Short Increment Sensitivity Index	**Definition:** Measures the ear's ability to detect small intensity changes; site of lesion test requiring a behavioral response
Sinusoidal Vertical Axis Rotational	**Definition:** Measures nystagmus following rotation
Somatosensory Evoked Potentials	**Definition:** Measures neural activity from sites throughout the body
Speech and/or Language Screening	**Definition:** Identifies need for further speech and/or language evaluation
Speech Threshold	**Definition:** Measures minimal intensity needed to repeat spondaic words
Speech-Language Pathology and Related Disorders Counseling	**Definition:** Provides patients/families with information, support, referrals to facilitate recovery from a communication disorder
Speech-Language Pathology and Related Disorders Prevention	**Definition:** Applying techniques to avoid or minimize onset and/or development of a communication disorder
Speech/Word Recognition	**Definition:** Measures ability to repeat/identify single syllable words; scores given as a percentage; includes word recognition/speech discrimination
Staggered Spondaic Word	**Definition:** Measures central auditory processing site of lesion based upon dichotic presentation of spondaic words
Static Orthosis	**Includes/Examples:** Includes customized and prefabricated splints, inhibitory casts, spinal and other braces, and protective devices; has no moving parts, maintains joint(s) in desired position
Stenger	**Definition:** Measures unilateral nonorganic hearing loss based on simultaneous presentation of signals of differing volume
Swallowing Dysfunction	**Definition:** Activities to improve swallowing function in coordination with respiratory function **Includes/Examples:** Includes function and coordination of sucking, mastication, coughing, swallowing
Synthetic Sentence Identification	**Definition:** Measures central auditory dysfunction using identification of third order approximations of sentences and competing messages
Temporal Ordering of Stimuli	**Definition:** Measures specific central auditory process
Therapeutic Exercise	**Definition:** Exercise or activities to facilitate sensory awareness, sensory processing, sensory integration, balance training, conditioning, reconditioning **Includes/Examples:** Includes developmental activities, breathing exercises, aerobic endurance activities, aquatic exercises, stretching and ventilatory muscle training
Tinnitus Masker (Assessment)	**Definition:** Determines candidacy for tinnitus masker
Tinnitus Masker (Treatment)	**Explanation:** Used to verify physical fit, acoustic appropriateness, and benefit; assists in achieving maximum benefit
Tone Decay	**Definition:** Measures decrease in hearing sensitivity to a tone; site of lesion test requiring a behavioral response
Transfer	**Definition:** Transitional movement from one surface to another
Transfer Training	**Definition:** Exercise or activities to facilitate movement from one surface to another
Tympanometry	**Definition:** Measures the integrity of the middle ear; measures ease at which sound flows through the tympanic membrane while air pressure against the membrane is varied
Unithermal Binaural Screen	**Definition:** Measures the rhythmic eye movements stimulated by changing the temperature of the vestibular system in both ears using warm water, screening format
Ventilation, Respiration and Circulation	**Definition:** Measures ventilatory muscle strength, power and endurance, pulmonary function and ventilatory mechanics **Includes/Examples:** Includes ability to clear airway, activities that aggravate or relieve edema, pain, dyspnea or other symptoms, chest wall mobility, cardiopulmonary response to performance of ADL and IAD, cough and sputum, standard vital signs
Vestibular	**Definition:** Applying techniques to compensate for balance disorders; includes habituation, exercise therapy, and balance retraining

Continued →

Section F - Physical Rehabilitation and Diagnostic Audiology — Character 5 - Type Qualifier	
Visual Motor Integration (Assessment)	**Definition:** Coordinating the interaction of information from the eyes with body movement during activity
Visual Motor Integration (Treatment)	**Definition:** Exercise or activities to facilitate coordinating the interaction of information from eyes with body movement during activity
Visual Reinforcement Audiometry	**Definition:** Behavioral measures using nonspeech and speech stimuli to obtain frequency/ear-specific information on auditory status **Includes/Examples:** Includes a conditioned response of looking toward a visual reinforcer (e.g., lights, animated toy) every time auditory stimuli are heard
Vocational Activities and Functional Community or Work Reintegration Skills (Assessment)	**Definition:** Measures environmental, home, work (job/school/play) barriers that keep patients from functioning optimally in their environment **Includes/Examples:** Includes assessment of vocational skill and interests, environment of work (job/school/play), injury potential and injury prevention or reduction, ergonomic stressors, transportation skills, and ability to access and use community resources
Vocational Activities and Functional Community or Work Reintegration Skills (Treatment)	**Definition:** Activities to facilitate vocational exploration, body mechanics training, job acquisition, and environmental or work (job/school/play) task adaptation **Includes/Examples:** Includes injury prevention and reduction, ergonomic stressor reduction, job coaching and simulation, work hardening and conditioning, driving training, transportation skills, and use of community resources
Voice (Assessment)	**Definition:** Measures vocal structure, function and production
Voice (Treatment)	**Definition:** Applying techniques to improve voice and vocal function
Voice Prosthetic (Assessment)	**Definition:** Determines the appropriateness of voice prosthetic/adaptive device to enhance or facilitate communication
Voice Prosthetic (Treatment)	**Includes/Examples:** Includes electrolarynx, and other assistive, adaptive, supportive devices
Wheelchair Mobility (Assessment)	**Definition:** Measures fit and functional abilities within wheelchair in a variety of environments
Wheelchair Mobility (Treatment)	**Definition:** Management, maintenance and controlled operation of a wheelchair, scooter or other device, in and on a variety of surfaces and environments
Wound Management	**Includes/Examples:** Includes non-selective and selective debridement (enzymes, autolysis, sharp debridement), dressings (wound coverings, hydrogel, vacuum-assisted closure), topical agents, etc.

Section G - Mental Health — Character 3 - Root Type	
Biofeedback	**Definition:** Provision of information from the monitoring and regulating of physiological processes in conjunction with cognitive-behavioral techniques to improve patient functioning or well-being **Includes/Examples:** Includes EEG, blood pressure, skin temperature or peripheral blood flow, ECG, electrooculogram, EMG, respirometry or capnometry, GSR/EDR, perineometry to monitor/regulate bowel/bladder activity, electrogastrogram to monitor/regulate gastric motility
Counseling	**Definition:** The application of psychological methods to treat an individual with normal developmental issues and psychological problems in order to increase function, improve well-being, alleviate distress, maladjustment or resolve crises
Crisis Intervention	**Definition:** Treatment of a traumatized, acutely disturbed or distressed individual for the purpose of short-term stabilization **Includes/Examples:** Includes defusing, debriefing, counseling, psychotherapy and/or coordination of care with other providers or agencies
Electroconvulsive Therapy	**Definition:** The application of controlled electrical voltages to treat a mental health disorder **Includes/Examples:** Includes appropriate sedation and other preparation of the individual
Family Psychotherapy	**Definition:** Treatment that includes one or more family members of an individual with a mental health disorder by behavioral, cognitive, psychoanalytic, psychodynamic or psychophysiological means to improve functioning or well-being **Explanation:** Remediation of emotional or behavioral problems presented by one or more family members in cases where psychotherapy with more than one family member is indicated
Group Psychotherapy	**Definition:** Treatment of two or more individuals with a mental health disorder by behavioral, cognitive, psychoanalytic, psychodynamic or psychophysiological means to improve functioning or well-being
Hypnosis	**Definition:** Induction of a state of heightened suggestibility by auditory, visual and tactile techniques to elicit an emotional or behavioral response
Individual Psychotherapy	**Definition:** Treatment of an individual with a mental health disorder by behavioral, cognitive, psychoanalytic, psychodynamic or psychophysiological means to improve functioning or well-being
Light Therapy	**Definition:** Application of specialized light treatments to improve functioning or well-being

Continued →

Section G - Mental Health — Character 3 - Root Type

Medication Management	**Definition:** Monitoring and adjusting the use of medications for the treatment of a mental health disorder
Narcosynthesis	**Definition:** Administration of intravenous barbiturates in order to release suppressed or repressed thoughts
Psychological Tests	**Definition:** The administration and interpretation of standardized psychological tests and measurement instruments for the assessment of psychological function

Section G - Mental Health — Character 4 - Type Qualifier

Behavioral	**Definition:** Primarily to modify behavior **Includes/Examples:** Includes modeling and role playing, positive reinforcement of target behaviors, response cost, and training of self-management skills
Cognitive	**Definition:** Primarily to correct cognitive distortions and errors
Cognitive-Behavioral	**Definition:** Combining cognitive and behavioral treatment strategies to improve functioning **Explanation:** Maladaptive responses are examined to determine how cognitions relate to behavior patterns in response to an event. Uses learning principles and information-processing models
Developmental	**Definition:** Age-normed developmental status of cognitive, social and adaptive behavior skills
Intellectual and Psychoeducational	**Definition:** Intellectual abilities, academic achievement and learning capabilities (including behaviors and emotional factors affecting learning)
Interactive	**Definition:** Uses primarily physical aids and other forms of non-oral interaction with a patient who is physically, psychologically or developmentally unable to use ordinary language for communication **Includes/Examples:** Includes the use of toys in symbolic play
Interpersonal	**Definition:** Helps an individual make changes in interpersonal behaviors to reduce psychological dysfunction **Includes/Examples:** Includes exploratory techniques, encouragement of affective expression, clarification of patient statements, analysis of communication patterns, use of therapy relationship and behavior change techniques
Neurobehavioral and Cognitive Status	**Definition:** Includes neurobehavioral status exam, interview(s), and observation for the clinical assessment of thinking, reasoning and judgment, acquired knowledge, attention, memory, visual spatial abilities, language functions, and planning
Neuropsychological	**Definition:** Thinking, reasoning and judgment, acquired knowledge, attention, memory, visual spatial abilities, language functions, planning
Personality and Behavioral	**Definition:** Mood, emotion, behavior, social functioning, psychopathological conditions, personality traits and characteristics
Psychoanalysis	**Definition:** Methods of obtaining a detailed account of past and present mental and emotional experiences to determine the source and eliminate or diminish the undesirable effects of unconscious conflicts **Explanation:** Accomplished by making the individual aware of their existence, origin, and inappropriate expression in emotions and behavior
Psychodynamic	**Definition:** Exploration of past and present emotional experiences to understand motives and drives using insight-oriented techniques to reduce the undesirable effects of internal conflicts on emotions and behavior **Explanation:** Techniques include empathetic listening, clarifying self-defeating behavior patterns, and exploring adaptive alternatives
Psychophysiological	**Definition:** Monitoring and alteration of physiological processes to help the individual associate physiological reactions combined with cognitive and behavioral strategies to gain improved control of these processes to help the individual cope more effectively
Supportive	**Definition:** Formation of therapeutic relationship primarily for providing emotional support to prevent further deterioration in functioning during periods of particular stress **Explanation:** Often used in conjunction with other therapeutic approaches
Vocational	**Definition:** Exploration of vocational interests, aptitudes and required adaptive behavior skills to develop and carry out a plan for achieving a successful vocational placement **Includes/Examples:** Includes enhancing work related adjustment and/or pursuing viable options in training education or preparation

Section H - Substance Abuse Treatment — Character 3 - Root Type

Detoxification Services	**Definition:** Detoxification from alcohol and/or drugs **Explanation:** Not a treatment modality, but helps the patient stabilize physically and psychologically until the body becomes free of drugs and the effects of alcohol
Family Counseling	**Definition:** The application of psychological methods that includes one or more family members to treat an individual with addictive behavior **Explanation:** Provides support and education for family members of addicted individuals. Family member participation is seen as a critical area of substance abuse treatment

Continued →

Section H - Substance Abuse Treatment — Character 3 - Root Type	
Group Counseling	**Definition:** The application of psychological methods to treat two or more individuals with addictive behavior **Explanation:** Provides structured group counseling sessions and healing power through the connection with others
Individual Counseling	**Definition:** The application of psychological methods to treat an individual with addictive behavior **Explanation:** Comprised of several different techniques, which apply various strategies to address drug addiction
Individual Psychotherapy	**Definition:** Treatment of an individual with addictive behavior by behavioral, cognitive, psychoanalytic, psychodynamic or psychophysiological means
Medication Management	**Definition:** Monitoring and adjusting the use of replacement medications for the treatment of addiction
Pharmacotherapy	**Definition:** The use of replacement medications for the treatment of addiction

Appendix C: Approach Definitions

Section 0 - Medical and Surgical — Character 5 - Approach	
External (X)	**Definition:** Procedures performed directly on the skin or mucous membrane and procedures performed indirectly by the application of external force through the skin or mucous membrane
Open (0)	**Definition:** Cutting through the skin or mucous membrane and any other body layers necessary to expose the site of the procedure
Percutaneous (3)	**Definition:** Entry, by puncture or minor incision, of instrumentation through the skin or mucous membrane and any other body layers necessary to reach the site of the procedure
Percutaneous Endoscopic (4)	**Definition:** Entry, by puncture or minor incision, of instrumentation through the skin or mucous membrane and any other body layers necessary to reach and visualize the site of the procedure
Via Natural or Artificial Opening (7)	**Definition:** Entry of instrumentation through a natural or artificial external opening to reach the site of the procedure
Via Natural or Artificial Opening Endoscopic (8)	**Definition:** Entry of instrumentation through a natural or artificial external opening to reach and visualize the site of the procedure
Via Natural or Artificial Opening With Percutaneous Endoscopic Assistance (F)	**Definition:** Entry of instrumentation through a natural or artificial external opening and entry, by puncture or minor incision, of instrumentation through the skin or mucous membrane and any other body layers necessary to aid in the performance of the procedure

Section 1 - Obstetrics — Character 5 - Approach	
External (X)	**Definition:** Procedures performed directly on the skin or mucous membrane and procedures performed indirectly by the application of external force through the skin or mucous membrane
Open (0)	**Definition:** Cutting through the skin or mucous membrane and any other body layers necessary to expose the site of the procedure
Percutaneous (3)	**Definition:** Entry, by puncture or minor incision, of instrumentation through the skin or mucous membrane and any other body layers necessary to reach the site of the procedure
Percutaneous Endoscopic (4)	**Definition:** Entry, by puncture or minor incision, of instrumentation through the skin or mucous membrane and any other body layers necessary to reach and visualize the site of the procedure
Via Natural or Artificial Opening (7)	**Definition:** Entry of instrumentation through a natural or artificial external opening to reach the site of the procedure
Via Natural or Artificial Opening Endoscopic (8)	**Definition:** Entry of instrumentation through a natural or artificial external opening to reach and visualize the site of the procedure

Section 2 - Placement — Character 5 - Approach	
External (X)	**Definition:** Procedures performed directly on the skin or mucous membrane and procedures performed indirectly by the application of external force through the skin or mucous membrane

Section 3 - Administration — Character 5 - Approach	
External (X)	**Definition:** Procedures performed directly on the skin or mucous membrane and procedures performed indirectly by the application of external force through the skin or mucous membrane
Open (0)	**Definition:** Cutting through the skin or mucous membrane and any other body layers necessary to expose the site of the procedure

Continued →

Section 3 - Administration — Character 5 - Approach

Percutaneous (3)	**Definition:** Entry, by puncture or minor incision, of instrumentation through the skin or mucous membrane and any other body layers necessary to reach the site of the procedure
Percutaneous Endoscopic (4)	**Definition:** Entry, by puncture or minor incision, of instrumentation through the skin or mucous membrane and any other body layers necessary to reach and visualize the site of the procedure
Via Natural or Artificial Opening (7)	**Definition:** Entry of instrumentation through a natural or artificial external opening to reach the site of the procedure
Via Natural or Artificial Opening Endoscopic (8)	**Definition:** Entry of instrumentation through a natural or artificial external opening to reach and visualize the site of the procedure

Section 4 - Measurement and Monitoring — Character 5 - Approach

External (X)	**Definition:** Procedures performed directly on the skin or mucous membrane and procedures performed indirectly by the application of external force through the skin or mucous membrane
Open (0)	**Definition:** Cutting through the skin or mucous membrane and any other body layers necessary to expose the site of the procedure
Percutaneous (3)	**Definition:** Entry, by puncture or minor incision, of instrumentation through the skin or mucous membrane and any other body layers necessary to reach the site of the procedure
Percutaneous Endoscopic (4)	**Definition:** Entry, by puncture or minor incision, of instrumentation through the skin or mucous membrane and any other body layers necessary to reach and visualize the site of the procedure
Via Natural or Artificial Opening (7)	**Definition:** Entry of instrumentation through a natural or artificial external opening to reach the site of the procedure
Via Natural or Artificial Opening Endoscopic (8)	**Definition:** Entry of instrumentation through a natural or artificial external opening to reach and visualize the site of the procedure

Section 7 - Osteopathic — Character 5 - Approach

External (X)	**Definition:** Procedures performed directly on the skin or mucous membrane and procedures performed indirectly by the application of external force through the skin or mucous membrane

Section 8 - Other Procedures — Character 5 - Approach

External (X)	**Definition:** Procedures performed directly on the skin or mucous membrane and procedures performed indirectly by the application of external force through the skin or mucous membrane
Open (0)	**Definition:** Cutting through the skin or mucous membrane and any other body layers necessary to expose the site of the procedure
Percutaneous (3)	**Definition:** Entry, by puncture or minor incision, of instrumentation through the skin or mucous membrane and any other body layers necessary to reach the site of the procedure
Percutaneous Endoscopic (4)	**Definition:** Entry, by puncture or minor incision, of instrumentation through the skin or mucous membrane and any other body layers necessary to reach and visualize the site of the procedure
Via Natural or Artificial Opening (7)	**Definition:** Entry of instrumentation through a natural or artificial external opening to reach the site of the procedure
Via Natural or Artificial Opening Endoscopic (8)	**Definition:** Entry of instrumentation through a natural or artificial external opening to reach and visualize the site of the procedure

Section 9 - Chiropractic — Character 5 - Approach

External (X)	**Definition:** Procedures performed directly on the skin or mucous membrane and procedures performed indirectly by the application of external force through the skin or mucous membrane

Section X - New Technology — Character 5 - Approach

External (X)	**Definition:** Procedures performed directly on the skin or mucous membrane and procedures performed indirectly by the application of external force through the skin or mucous membrane
Open (0)	**Definition:** Cutting through the skin or mucous membrane and any other body layers necessary to expose the site of the procedure
Percutaneous (3)	**Definition:** Entry, by puncture or minor incision, of instrumentation through the skin or mucous membrane and any other body layers necessary to reach the site of the procedure
Percutaneous Endoscopic (4)	**Definition:** Entry, by puncture or minor incision, of instrumentation through the skin or mucous membrane and any other body layers necessary to reach and visualize the site of the procedure
Via Natural or Artificial Opening (7)	**Definition:** Entry of instrumentation through a natural or artificial external opening to reach the site of the procedure
Via Natural or Artificial Opening Endoscopic (8)	**Definition:** Entry of instrumentation through a natural or artificial external opening to reach and visualize the site of the procedure

Appendix D: Medical and Surgical Body Parts

Appendices D–F are structured to assist coders with confirming character selections within the Tables. For example, if the coder is considering the body part of Abdomen Muscle, appendix D can be referenced to identify all of the muscles that are included in the body part Abdomen Muscle (see row 2 in the table below). After reviewing the information, the coder can determine if the body part under consideration is correct or if another body part should be reviewed. The same process can be followed for devices which are included in appendix E and substances which are included in appendix F.

Section 0 - Medical and Surgical — Character 4 - Body Part	
1st Toe, Left **1st** Toe, Right	**Includes:** Hallux
Abdomen Muscle, Left **Abdomen** Muscle, Right	**Includes:** External oblique muscle Internal oblique muscle Pyramidalis muscle Rectus abdominis muscle Transversus abdominis muscle
Abdominal Aorta	**Includes:** Inferior phrenic artery Lumbar artery Median sacral artery Middle suprarenal artery Ovarian artery Testicular artery
Abdominal Sympathetic Nerve	**Includes:** Abdominal aortic plexus Auerbach's (myenteric) plexus Celiac (solar) plexus Celiac ganglion Gastric plexus Hepatic plexus Inferior hypogastric plexus Inferior mesenteric ganglion Inferior mesenteric plexus Meissner's (submucous) plexus Myenteric (Auerbach's) plexus Pancreatic plexus Pelvic splanchnic nerve Renal nerve Renal plexus Solar (celiac) plexus Splenic plexus Submucous (Meissner's) plexus Superior hypogastric plexus Superior mesenteric ganglion Superior mesenteric plexus Suprarenal plexus
Abducens Nerve	**Includes:** Sixth cranial nerve
Accessory Nerve	**Includes:** Eleventh cranial nerve
Acoustic Nerve	**Includes:** Cochlear nerve Eighth cranial nerve Scarpa's (vestibular) ganglion Spiral ganglion Vestibular (Scarpa's) ganglion Vestibular nerve Vestibulocochlear nerve
Adenoids	**Includes:** Pharyngeal tonsil

Section 0 - Medical and Surgical — Character 4 - Body Part	
Adrenal Gland **Adrenal** Gland, Left **Adrenal** Gland, Right **Adrenal** Glands, Bilateral	**Includes:** Suprarenal gland
Ampulla of Vater	**Includes:** Duodenal ampulla Hepatopancreatic ampulla
Anal Sphincter	**Includes:** External anal sphincter Internal anal sphincter
Ankle Bursa and Ligament, Left **Ankle** Bursa and Ligament, Right	**Includes:** Calcaneofibular ligament Deltoid ligament Ligament of the lateral malleolus Talofibular ligament
Ankle Joint, Left **Ankle** Joint, Right	**Includes:** Inferior tibiofibular joint Talocrural joint
Anterior Chamber, Left **Anterior** Chamber, Right	**Includes:** Aqueous humour
Anterior Tibial Artery, Left **Anterior** Tibial Artery, Right	**Includes:** Anterior lateral malleolar artery Anterior medial malleolar artery Anterior tibial recurrent artery Dorsalis pedis artery Posterior tibial recurrent artery
Anus	**Includes:** Anal orifice
Aortic Valve	**Includes:** Aortic annulus
Appendix	**Includes:** Vermiform appendix
Atrial Septum	**Includes:** Interatrial septum
Atrium, Left	**Includes:** Atrium pulmonale Left auricular appendix
Atrium, Right	**Includes:** Atrium dextrum cordis Right auricular appendix Sinus venosus
Auditory Ossicle, Left **Auditory** Ossicle, Right	**Includes:** Incus Malleus Stapes

Continued →

Section 0 - Medical and Surgical — Character 4 - Body Part	
Axillary Artery, Left **Axillary** Artery, Right	**Includes:** Anterior circumflex humeral artery Lateral thoracic artery Posterior circumflex humeral artery Subscapular artery Superior thoracic artery Thoracoacromial artery
Azygos Vein	**Includes:** Right ascending lumbar vein Right subcostal vein
Basal Ganglia	**Includes:** Basal nuclei Claustrum Corpus striatum Globus pallidus Substantia nigra Subthalamic nucleus
Basilic Vein, Left **Basilic** Vein, Right	**Includes:** Median antebrachial vein Median cubital vein
Bladder	**Includes:** Trigone of bladder
Brachial Artery, Left **Brachial** Artery, Right	**Includes:** Inferior ulnar collateral artery Profunda brachii Superior ulnar collateral artery
Brachial Plexus	**Includes:** Axillary nerve Dorsal scapular nerve First intercostal nerve Long thoracic nerve Musculocutaneous nerve Subclavius nerve Suprascapular nerve
Brachial Vein, Left **Brachial** Vein, Right	**Includes:** Radial vein Ulnar vein
Brain	**Includes:** Cerebrum Corpus callosum Encephalon
Breast, Bilateral **Breast,** Left **Breast,** Right	**Includes:** Mammary duct Mammary gland
Buccal Mucosa	**Includes:** Buccal gland Molar gland Palatine gland
Carotid Bodies, Bilateral **Carotid** Body, Left **Carotid** Body, Right	**Includes:** Carotid glomus
Carpal Joint, Left **Carpal** Joint, Right	**Includes:** Intercarpal joint Midcarpal joint

Section 0 - Medical and Surgical — Character 4 - Body Part	
Carpal, Left **Carpal,** Right	**Includes:** Capitate bone Hamate bone Lunate bone Pisiform bone Scaphoid bone Trapezium bone Trapezoid bone Triquetral bone
Celiac Artery	**Includes:** Celiac trunk
Cephalic Vein, Left **Cephalic** Vein, Right	**Includes:** Accessory cephalic vein
Cerebellum	**Includes:** Culmen
Cerebral Hemisphere	**Includes:** Frontal lobe Occipital lobe Parietal lobe Temporal lobe
Cerebral Meninges	**Includes:** Arachnoid mater, intracranial Leptomeninges, intracranial Pia mater, intracranial
Cerebral Ventricle	**Includes:** Aqueduct of Sylvius Cerebral aqueduct (Sylvius) Choroid plexus Ependyma Foramen of Monro (intraventricular) Fourth ventricle Interventricular foramen (Monro) Left lateral ventricle Right lateral ventricle Third ventricle
Cervical Nerve	**Includes:** Greater occipital nerve Spinal nerve, cervical Suboccipital nerve Third occipital nerve
Cervical Plexus	**Includes:** Ansa cervicalis Cutaneous (transverse) cervical nerve Great auricular nerve Lesser occipital nerve Supraclavicular nerve Transverse (cutaneous) cervical nerve
Cervical Spinal Cord	Dorsal root ganglion
Cervical Vertebra	**Includes:** Dens Odontoid process Spinous process Transverse foramen Transverse process Vertebral arch Vertebral body Vertebral foramen Vertebral lamina Vertebral pedicle

Continued →

Section 0 - Medical and Surgical — Character 4 - Body Part	
Cervical Vertebral Joint	**Includes:** Atlantoaxial joint Cervical facet joint
Cervical Vertebral Joints, 2 or more	**Includes:** Cervical facet joint
Cervicothoracic Vertebral Joint	**Includes:** Cervicothoracic facet joint
Cisterna Chyli	**Includes:** Intestinal lymphatic trunk Lumbar lymphatic trunk
Coccygeal Glomus	**Includes:** Coccygeal body
Colic Vein	**Includes:** Ileocolic vein Left colic vein Middle colic vein Right colic vein
Conduction Mechanism	**Includes:** Atrioventricular node Bundle of His Bundle of Kent Sinoatrial node
Conjunctiva, Left **Conjunctiva,** Right	**Includes:** Plica semilunaris
Dura Mater	**Includes:** Diaphragma sellae Dura mater, intracranial Falx cerebri Tentorium cerebelli
Elbow Bursa and Ligament, Left **Elbow** Bursa and Ligament, Right	**Includes:** Annular ligament Olecranon bursa Radial collateral ligament Ulnar collateral ligament
Elbow Joint, Left **Elbow** Joint, Right	**Includes:** Distal humerus, involving joint Humeroradial joint Humeroulnar joint Proximal radioulnar joint
Epidural Space, Intracranial	**Includes:** Extradural space, intracranial
Epiglottis	**Includes:** Glossoepiglottic fold
Esophagogastric Junction	**Includes:** Cardia Cardioesophageal junction Gastroesophageal (GE) junction
Esophagus, Lower	**Includes:** Abdominal esophagus
Esophagus, Middle	**Includes:** Thoracic esophagus
Esophagus, Upper	**Includes:** Cervical esophagus
Ethmoid Bone, Left **Ethmoid** Bone, Right	**Includes:** Cribriform plate
Ethmoid Sinus, Left **Ethmoid** Sinus, Right	**Includes:** Ethmoidal air cell

Section 0 - Medical and Surgical — Character 4 - Body Part	
Eustachian Tube, Left **Eustachian** Tube, Right	**Includes:** Auditory tube Pharyngotympanic tube
External Auditory Canal, Left **External** Auditory Canal, Right	**Includes:** External auditory meatus
External Carotid Artery, Left **External** Carotid Artery, Right	**Includes:** Ascending pharyngeal artery Internal maxillary artery Lingual artery Maxillary artery Occipital artery Posterior auricular artery Superior thyroid artery
External Ear, Bilateral **External** Ear, Left **External** Ear, Right	**Includes:** Antihelix Antitragus Auricle Earlobe Helix Pinna Tragus
External Iliac Artery, Left **External** Iliac Artery, Right	**Includes:** Deep circumflex iliac artery Inferior epigastric artery
External Jugular Vein, Left **External** Jugular Vein, Right	**Includes:** Posterior auricular vein
Extraocular Muscle, Left **Extraocular** Muscle, Right	**Includes:** Inferior oblique muscle Inferior rectus muscle Lateral rectus muscle Medial rectus muscle Superior oblique muscle Superior rectus muscle
Eye, Left **Eye,** Right	**Includes:** Ciliary body Posterior chamber
Face Artery	**Includes:** Angular artery Ascending palatine artery External maxillary artery Facial artery Inferior labial artery Submental artery Superior labial artery
Face Vein, Left **Face** Vein, Right	**Includes:** Angular vein Anterior facial vein Common facial vein Deep facial vein Frontal vein Posterior facial (retromandibular) vein Supraorbital vein
Facial Muscle	**Includes:** Buccinator muscle Corrugator supercilii muscle Depressor anguli oris muscle Depressor labii inferioris muscle

Continued →

Section 0 - Medical and Surgical — Character 4 - Body Part	
	Depressor septi nasi muscle Depressor supercilii muscle Levator anguli oris muscle Levator labii superioris alaeque nasi Levator labii superioris alaeque nasi Levator labii superioris alaeque nasi Levator labii superioris muscle Mentalis muscle Nasalis muscle Occipitofrontalis muscle Orbicularis oris muscle Procerus muscle Risorius muscle Zygomaticus muscle
Facial Nerve	**Includes:** Chorda tympani Geniculate ganglion Greater superficial petrosal nerve Nerve to the stapedius Parotid plexus Posterior auricular nerve Seventh cranial nerve Submandibular ganglion
Fallopian Tube, Left **Fallopian** Tube, Right	**Includes:** Oviduct Salpinx Uterine tube
Femoral Artery, Left **Femoral** Artery, Right	**Includes:** Circumflex iliac artery Deep femoral artery Descending genicular artery External pudendal artery Superficial epigastric artery
Femoral Nerve	**Includes:** Anterior crural nerve Saphenous nerve
Femoral Shaft, Left **Femoral** Shaft, Right	**Includes:** Body of femur
Femoral Vein, Left **Femoral** Vein, Right	**Includes:** Deep femoral (profunda femoris) vein Popliteal vein Profunda femoris (deep femoral) vein
Fibula, Left **Fibula,** Right	**Includes:** Body of fibula Head of fibula Lateral malleolus
Finger Nail	**Includes:** Nail bed Nail plate
Finger Phalangeal Joint, Left **Finger** Phalangeal Joint, Right	**Includes:** Interphalangeal (IP) joint
Foot Artery, Left **Foot** Artery, Right	**Includes:** Arcuate artery Dorsal metatarsal artery Lateral plantar artery Lateral tarsal artery Medial plantar artery

Section 0 - Medical and Surgical — Character 4 - Body Part	
Foot Bursa and Ligament, Left **Foot** Bursa and Ligament, Right	**Includes:** Calcaneocuboid ligament Cuneonavicular ligament Intercuneiform ligament Interphalangeal ligament Metatarsal ligament Metatarsophalangeal ligament Subtalar ligament Talocalcaneal ligament Talocalcaneonavicular ligament Tarsometatarsal ligament
Foot Muscle, Left **Foot** Muscle, Right	**Includes:** Abductor hallucis muscle Adductor hallucis muscle Extensor digitorum brevis muscle Extensor hallucis brevis muscle Flexor digitorum brevis muscle Flexor hallucis brevis muscle Quadratus plantae muscle
Foot Vein, Left **Foot** Vein, Right	**Includes:** Common digital vein Dorsal metatarsal vein Dorsal venous arch Plantar digital vein Plantar metatarsal vein Plantar venous arch
Frontal Bone	**Includes:** Zygomatic process of frontal bone
Gastric Artery	**Includes:** Left gastric artery Right gastric artery
Glenoid Cavity, Left **Glenoid** Cavity, Right	**Includes:** Glenoid fossa (of scapula)
Glomus Jugulare	**Includes:** Jugular body
Glossopharyngeal Nerve	**Includes:** Carotid sinus nerve Ninth cranial nerve Tympanic nerve
Hand Artery, Left **Hand** Artery, Right	**Includes:** Deep palmar arch Princeps pollicis artery Radialis indicis Superficial palmar arch
Hand Bursa and Ligament, Left **Hand** Bursa and Ligament, Right	**Includes:** Carpometacarpal ligament Intercarpal ligament Interphalangeal ligament Lunotriquetral ligament Metacarpal ligament Metacarpophalangeal ligament Pisohamate ligament Pisometacarpal ligament Scaphotrapezium ligament
Hand Muscle, Left **Hand** Muscle, Right	**Includes:** Hypothenar muscle Palmar interosseous muscle Thenar muscle

Continued →

Section 0 - Medical and Surgical — Character 4 - Body Part	
Hand Vein, Left **Hand** Vein, Right	**Includes:** Dorsal metacarpal vein Palmar (volar) digital vein Palmar (volar) metacarpal vein Superficial palmar venous arch Volar (palmar) digital vein Volar (palmar) metacarpal vein
Head and Neck Bursa and Ligament	**Includes:** Alar ligament of axis Cervical interspinous ligament Cervical intertransverse ligament Cervical ligamentum flavum Interspinous ligament cervical Intertransverse ligament, cervical Lateral temporomandibular ligament Ligamentum flavum, cervical Sphenomandibular ligament Stylomandibular ligament Transverse ligament of atlas
Head and Neck Sympathetic Nerve	**Includes:** Cavernous plexus Cervical ganglion Ciliary ganglion Internal carotid plexus Otic ganglion Pterygopalatine (sphenopalatine) ganglion Sphenopalatine (pterygopalatine) ganglion Stellate ganglion Submandibular ganglion Submaxillary ganglion
Head Muscle	**Includes:** Auricularis muscle Masseter muscle Pterygoid muscle Splenius capitis muscle Temporalis muscle Temporoparietalis muscle
Heart, Left	**Includes:** Left coronary sulcus Obtuse margin
Heart, Right	**Includes:** Right coronary sulcus
Hemiazygos Vein	**Includes:** Left ascending lumbar vein Left subcostal vein
Hepatic Artery	**Includes:** Common hepatic artery Gastroduodenal artery Hepatic artery proper
Hip Bursa and Ligament, Left **Hip** Bursa and Ligament, Right	**Includes:** Iliofemoral ligament Ischiofemoral ligament Pubofemoral ligament Transverse acetabular ligament Trochanteric bursa
Hip Joint, Left **Hip** Joint, Right	**Includes:** Acetabulofemoral joint

Section 0 - Medical and Surgical — Character 4 - Body Part	
Hip Muscle, Left **Hip** Muscle, Right	**Includes:** Gemellus muscle Gluteus maximus muscle Gluteus medius muscle Gluteus minimus muscle Iliacus muscle Obturator muscle Piriformis muscle Psoas muscle Quadratus femoris muscle Tensor fasciae latae muscle
Humeral Head, Left **Humeral** Head, Right	**Includes:** Greater tuberosity Lesser tuberosity Neck of humerus (anatomical) (surgical)
Humeral Shaft, Left **Humeral** Shaft, Right	**Includes:** Distal humerus Humerus, distal Lateral epicondyle of humerus Medial epicondyle of humerus
Hypogastric Vein, Left **Hypogastric** Vein, Right	**Includes:** Gluteal vein Internal iliac vein Internal pudendal vein Lateral sacral vein Middle hemorrhoidal vein Obturator vein Uterine vein Vaginal vein Vesical vein
Hypoglossal Nerve	**Includes:** Twelfth cranial nerve
Hypothalamus	**Includes:** Mammillary body
Inferior Mesenteric Artery	**Includes:** Sigmoid artery Superior rectal artery
Inferior Mesenteric Vein	**Includes:** Sigmoid vein Superior rectal vein
Inferior Vena Cava	**Includes:** Postcava Right inferior phrenic vein Right ovarian vein Right second lumbar vein Right suprarenal vein Right testicular vein
Inguinal Region, Bilateral **Inguinal** Region, Left **Inguinal** Region, Right	**Includes:** Inguinal canal Inguinal triangle
Inner Ear, Left **Inner** Ear, Right	**Includes:** Bony labyrinth Bony vestibule Cochlea Round window Semicircular canal

Continued →

Section 0 - Medical and Surgical — Character 4 - Body Part

Section 0 - Medical and Surgical — Character 4 - Body Part	
Innominate Artery	**Includes:** Brachiocephalic artery Brachiocephalic trunk
Innominate Vein, Left **Innominate** Vein, Right	**Includes:** Brachiocephalic vein Inferior thyroid vein
Internal Carotid Artery, Left **Internal** Carotid Artery, Right	**Includes:** Caroticotympanic artery Carotid sinus
Internal Iliac Artery, Left **Internal** Iliac Artery, Right	**Includes:** Deferential artery Hypogastric artery Iliolumbar artery Inferior gluteal artery Inferior vesical artery Internal pudendal artery Lateral sacral artery Middle rectal artery Obturator artery Superior gluteal artery Umbilical artery Uterine artery Vaginal artery
Internal Mammary Artery, Left **Internal** Mammary Artery, Right	**Includes:** Anterior intercostal artery Internal thoracic artery Musculophrenic artery Pericardiophrenic artery Superior epigastric artery
Intracranial Artery	**Includes:** Anterior cerebral artery Anterior choroidal artery Anterior communicating artery Basilar artery Circle of Willis Internal carotid artery, intracranial portion Middle cerebral artery Ophthalmic artery Posterior cerebral artery Posterior communicating artery Posterior inferior cerebellar artery (PICA)
Intracranial Vein	**Includes:** Anterior cerebral vein Basal (internal) cerebral vein Dural venous sinus Great cerebral vein Inferior cerebellar vein Inferior cerebral vein Internal (basal) cerebral vein Middle cerebral vein Ophthalmic vein Superior cerebellar vein Superior cerebral vein
Jejunum	**Includes:** Duodenojejunal flexure

Section 0 - Medical and Surgical — Character 4 - Body Part	
Kidney	**Includes:** Renal calyx Renal capsule Renal cortex Renal segment
Kidney Pelvis, Left **Kidney** Pelvis, Right	**Includes:** Ureteropelvic junction (UPJ)
Kidney, Left **Kidney,** Right **Kidneys,** Bilateral	**Includes:** Renal calyx Renal capsule Renal cortex Renal segment
Knee Bursa and Ligament, Left **Knee** Bursa and Ligament, Right	**Includes:** Anterior cruciate ligament (ACL) Lateral collateral ligament (LCL) Ligament of head of fibula Medial collateral ligament (MCL) Patellar ligament Popliteal ligament Posterior cruciate ligament (PCL) Prepatellar bursa
Knee Joint, Femoral Surface, Left **Knee** Joint, Femoral Surface, Right	**Includes:** Femoropatellar joint Patellofemoral joint
Knee Joint, Left **Knee** Joint, Right	**Includes:** Femoropatellar joint Femorotibial joint Lateral meniscus Medial meniscus Patellofemoral joint Tibiofemoral joint
Knee Joint, Tibial Surface, Left **Knee** Joint, Tibial Surface, Right	**Includes:** Femorotibial joint Tibiofemoral joint
Knee Tendon, Left **Knee** Tendon, Right	**Includes:** Patellar tendon
Lacrimal Duct, Left **Lacrimal** Duct, Right	**Includes:** Lacrimal canaliculus Lacrimal punctum Lacrimal sac Nasolacrimal duct
Larynx	**Includes:** Aryepiglottic fold Arytenoid cartilage Corniculate cartilage Cuneiform cartilage False vocal cord Glottis Rima glottidis Thyroid cartilage Ventricular fold
Lens, Left **Lens,** Right	**Includes:** Zonule of Zinn
Liver	**Includes:** Quadrate lobe

Continued →

Section 0 - Medical and Surgical — Character 4 - Body Part	
Lower Arm and Wrist Muscle, Left **Lower** Arm and Wrist Muscle, Right	**Includes:** Anatomical snuffbox Brachioradialis muscle Extensor carpi radialis muscle Extensor carpi ulnaris muscle Flexor carpi radialis muscle Flexor carpi ulnaris muscle Flexor pollicis longus muscle Palmaris longus muscle Pronator quadratus muscle Pronator teres muscle
Lower Artery	Umbilical artery
Lower Eyelid, Left **Lower** Eyelid, Right	**Includes:** Inferior tarsal plate Medial canthus
Lower Femur, Left **Lower** Femur, Right	**Includes:** Lateral condyle of femur Lateral epicondyle of femur Medial condyle of femur Medial epicondyle of femur
Lower Leg Muscle, Left **Lower** Leg Muscle, Right	**Includes:** Extensor digitorum longus muscle Extensor hallucis longus muscle Fibularis brevis muscle Fibularis longus muscle Flexor digitorum longus muscle Flexor hallucis longus muscle Gastrocnemius muscle Peroneus brevis muscle Peroneus longus muscle Popliteus muscle Soleus muscle Tibialis anterior muscle Tibialis posterior muscle
Lower Leg Tendon, Left **Lower** Leg Tendon, Right	**Includes:** Achilles tendon
Lower Lip	**Includes:** Frenulum labii inferioris Labial gland Vermilion border
Lower Spine Bursa and Ligament	Iliolumbar ligament Interspinous ligament, lumbar Intertransverse ligament, lumbar Ligamentum flavum, lumbar Sacrococcygeal ligament Sacroiliac ligament Sacrospinous ligament Sacrotuberous ligament Supraspinous ligament
Lumbar Nerve	**Includes:** Lumbosacral trunk Spinal nerve, lumbar Superior clunic (cluneal) nerve
Lumbar Plexus	**Includes:** Accessory obturator nerve Genitofemoral nerve Iliohypogastric nerve Ilioinguinal nerve Lateral femoral cutaneous nerve Obturator nerve Superior gluteal nerve

Section 0 - Medical and Surgical — Character 4 - Body Part	
Lumbar Spinal Cord	**Includes:** Cauda equina Conus medullaris Dorsal root ganglion
Lumbar Sympathetic Nerve	**Includes:** Lumbar ganglion Lumbar splanchnic nerve
Lumbar Vertebra	**Includes:** Spinous process Transverse process Vertebral arch Vertebral body Vertebral foramen Vertebral lamina Vertebral pedicle
Lumbar Vertebral Joint	**Includes:** Lumbar facet joint
Lumbosacral Joint	**Includes:** Lumbosacral facet joint
Lymphatic, Aortic	**Includes:** Celiac lymph node Gastric lymph node Hepatic lymph node Lumbar lymph node Pancreaticosplenic lymph node Paraaortic lymph node Retroperitoneal lymph node
Lymphatic, Head	**Includes:** Buccinator lymph node Infraauricular lymph node Infraparotid lymph node Parotid lymph node Preauricular lymph node Submandibular lymph node Submaxillary lymph node Submental lymph node Subparotid lymph node Suprahyoid lymph node
Lymphatic, Left Axillary	**Includes:** Anterior (pectoral) lymph node Apical (subclavicular) lymph node Brachial (lateral) lymph node Central axillary lymph node Lateral (brachial) lymph node Pectoral (anterior) lymph node Posterior (subscapular) lymph node Subclavicular (apical) lymph node Subscapular (posterior) lymph node
Lymphatic, Left Lower Extremity	**Includes:** Femoral lymph node Popliteal lymph node
Lymphatic, Left Neck	**Includes:** Cervical lymph node Jugular lymph node Mastoid (postauricular) lymph node Occipital lymph node Postauricular (mastoid) lymph node Retropharyngeal lymph node Supraclavicular (Virchow's) lymph node Virchow's (supraclavicular) lymph node

Continued →

Section 0 - Medical and Surgical — Character 4 - Body Part	
Lymphatic, Left Upper Extremity	**Includes:** Cubital lymph node Deltopectoral (infraclavicular) lymph node Epitrochlear lymph node Infraclavicular (deltopectoral) lymph node Supratrochlear lymph node
Lymphatic, Mesenteric	**Includes:** Inferior mesenteric lymph node Pararectal lymph node Superior mesenteric lymph node
Lymphatic, Pelvis	**Includes:** Common iliac (subaortic) lymph node Gluteal lymph node Iliac lymph node Inferior epigastric lymph node Obturator lymph node Sacral lymph node Subaortic (common iliac) lymph node Suprainguinal lymph node
Lymphatic, Right Axillary	**Includes:** Anterior (pectoral) lymph node Apical (subclavicular) lymph node Brachial (lateral) lymph node Central axillary lymph node Lateral (brachial) lymph node Pectoral (anterior) lymph node Posterior (subscapular) lymph node Subclavicular (apical) lymph node Subscapular (posterior) lymph node
Lymphatic, Right Lower Extremity	**Includes:** Femoral lymph node Popliteal lymph node
Lymphatic, Right Neck	**Includes:** Cervical lymph node Jugular lymph node Mastoid (postauricular) lymph node Occipital lymph node Postauricular (mastoid) lymph node Retropharyngeal lymph node Right jugular trunk Right lymphatic duct Right subclavian trunk Supraclavicular (Virchow's) lymph node Virchow's (supraclavicular) lymph node
Lymphatic, Right Upper Extremity	**Includes:** Cubital lymph node Deltopectoral (infraclavicular) lymph node Epitrochlear lymph node Infraclavicular (deltopectoral) lymph node Supratrochlear lymph node
Lymphatic, Thorax	**Includes:** Intercostal lymph node Mediastinal lymph node Parasternal lymph node Paratracheal lymph node Tracheobronchial lymph node

Section 0 - Medical and Surgical — Character 4 - Body Part	
Main Bronchus, Right	**Includes:** Bronchus Intermedius Intermediate bronchus
Mandible, Left **Mandible,** Right	**Includes:** Alveolar process of mandible Condyloid process Mandibular notch Mental foramen
Mastoid Sinus, Left **Mastoid** Sinus, Right	**Includes:** Mastoid air cells
Maxilla	**Includes:** Alveolar process of maxilla
Maxillary Sinus, Left **Maxillary** Sinus, Right	**Includes:** Antrum of Highmore
Median Nerve	**Includes:** Anterior interosseous nerve Palmar cutaneous nerve
Mediastinum	Mediastinal cavity Mediastinal space
Medulla Oblongata	**Includes:** Myelencephalon
Mesentery	**Includes:** Mesoappendix Mesocolon
Metatarsal, Left **Metatarsal,** Right	Fibular sesamoid Tibial sesamoid
Metatarsal-Phalangeal Joint, Left **Metatarsal-Phalangeal** Joint, Right	**Includes:** Metatarsophalangeal (MTP) joint
Middle Ear, Left **Middle** Ear, Right	**Includes:** Oval window Tympanic cavity
Minor Salivary Gland	**Includes:** Anterior lingual gland
Mitral Valve	**Includes:** Bicuspid valve Left atrioventricular valve Mitral annulus
Nasal Bone	**Includes:** Vomer of nasal septum
Nasal Mucosa and Soft Tissue	Columella External naris Greater alar cartilage Internal naris Lateral nasal cartilage Lesser alar cartilage Nasal cavity Nostril
Nasal Septum	**Includes:** Quadrangular cartilage Septal cartilage Vomer bone
Nasal Turbinate	**Includes:** Inferior turbinate Middle turbinate Nasal concha Superior turbinate

Continued →

Section 0 - Medical and Surgical — Character 4 - Body Part	
Nasopharynx	**Includes:** Choana Fossa of Rosenmuller Pharyngeal recess Rhinopharynx
Neck	Parapharyngeal space Retropharyngeal space
Neck Muscle, Left **Neck** Muscle, Right	**Includes:** Anterior vertebral muscle Arytenoid muscle Cricothyroid muscle Infrahyoid muscle Levator scapulae muscle Platysma muscle Scalene muscle Splenius cervicis muscle Sternocleidomastoid muscle Suprahyoid muscle Thyroarytenoid muscle
Nipple, Left **Nipple,** Right	**Includes:** Areola
Occipital Bone	**Includes:** Foramen magnum
Oculomotor Nerve	**Includes:** Third cranial nerve
Olfactory Nerve	**Includes:** First cranial nerve Olfactory bulb
Omentum	Gastrocolic ligament Gastrocolic omentum Gastrohepatic omentum Gastrophrenic ligament Gastrosplenic ligament Greater Omentum Hepatogastric liagment Lesser Omentum
Optic Nerve	**Includes:** Optic chiasma Second cranial nerve
Orbit, Left **Orbit,** Right	**Includes:** Bony orbit Orbital portion of ethmoid bone Orbital portion of frontal bone Orbital portion of lacrimal bone Orbital portion of maxilla Orbital portion of palatine bone Orbital portion of sphenoid bone Orbital portion of zygomatic bone
Pancreatic Duct	**Includes:** Duct of Wirsung
Pancreatic Duct, Accessory	**Includes:** Duct of Santorini
Parotid Duct, Left **Parotid** Duct, Right	**Includes:** Stensen's duct
Pelvic Bone, Left **Pelvic** Bone, Right	**Includes:** Iliac crest Ilium Ischium Pubis
Pelvic Cavity	**Includes:** Retropubic space

Section 0 - Medical and Surgical — Character 4 - Body Part	
Penis	**Includes:** Corpus cavernosum Corpus spongiosum
Perineum Muscle	**Includes:** Bulbospongiosus muscle Cremaster muscle Deep transverse perineal muscle Ischiocavernosus muscle Levator ani muscle Superficial transverse perineal muscle
Peritoneum	**Includes:** Epiploic foramen
Peroneal Artery, Left **Peroneal** Artery, Right	**Includes:** Fibular artery
Peroneal Nerve	**Includes:** Common fibular nerve Common peroneal nerve External popliteal nerve Lateral sural cutaneous nerve
Pharynx	**Includes:** Base of Tongue Hypopharynx Laryngopharynx Lignual tonsil Oropharynx Piriform recess (sinus) Tongue, base of
Phrenic Nerve	**Includes:** Accessory phrenic nerve
Pituitary Gland	**Includes:** Adenohypophysis Hypophysis Neurohypophysis
Pons	**Includes:** Apneustic center Basis pontis Locus ceruleus Pneumotaxic center Pontine tegmentum Superior olivary nucleus
Popliteal Artery, Left **Popliteal** Artery, Right	**Includes:** Inferior genicular artery Middle genicular artery Superior genicular artery Sural artery Tibioperoneal trunk
Portal Vein	**Includes:** Hepatic portal vein
Prepuce	**Includes:** Foreskin Glans penis
Pudendal Nerve	**Includes:** Posterior labial nerve Posterior scrotal nerve
Pulmonary Artery, Left	**Includes:** Arterial canal (duct) Botallo's duct Pulmoaortic canal
Pulmonary Valve	**Includes:** Pulmonary annulus Pulmonic valve

Continued →

Section 0 - Medical and Surgical — Character 4 - Body Part

Pulmonary Vein, Left	**Includes:** Left inferior pulmonary vein Left superior pulmonary vein
Pulmonary Vein, Right	**Includes:** Right inferior pulmonary vein Right superior pulmonary vein
Radial Artery, Left **Radial** Artery, Right	**Includes:** Radial recurrent artery
Radial Nerve	**Includes:** Dorsal digital nerve Musculospiral nerve Palmar cutaneous nerve Posterior interosseous nerve
Radius, Left **Radius,** Right	**Includes:** Ulnar notch
Rectum	**Includes:** Anorectal junction
Renal Artery, Left **Renal** Artery, Right	**Includes:** Inferior suprarenal artery Renal segmental artery
Renal Vein, Left	**Includes:** Left inferior phrenic vein Left ovarian vein Left second lumbar vein Left suprarenal vein Left testicular vein
Retina, Left **Retina,** Right	**Includes:** Fovea Macula Optic disc
Retroperitoneum	**Includes:** Retroperitoneal cavity Retroperitoneal space
Rib(s) Bursa and Ligament	Costotransverse ligament
Sacral Nerve	**Includes:** Spinal nerve, sacral
Sacral Plexus	**Includes:** Inferior gluteal nerve Posterior femoral cutaneous nerve Pudendal nerve
Sacral Sympathetic Nerve	**Includes:** Ganglion impar (ganglion of Walther) Pelvic splanchnic nerve Sacral ganglion Sacral splanchnic nerve
Sacrococcygeal Joint	**Includes:** Sacrococcygeal symphysis
Saphenous Vein, Left **Saphenous** Vein, Right	External pudendal vein Great(er) saphenous vein Lesser saphenous vein Small saphenous vein Superficial circumflex iliac vein Superficial epigastric vein
Scapula, Left **Scapula,** Right	**Includes:** Acromion (process) Coracoid process
Sciatic Nerve	**Includes:** Ischiatic nerve

Section 0 - Medical and Surgical — Character 4 - Body Part

Shoulder Bursa and Ligament, Left **Shoulder** Bursa and Ligament, Right	**Includes:** Acromioclavicular ligament Coracoacromial ligament Coracoclavicular ligament Coracohumeral ligament
	Costoclavicular ligament Glenohumeral ligament Interclavicular ligament Sternoclavicular ligament Subacromial bursa Transverse humeral ligament Transverse scapular ligament
Shoulder Joint, Left **Shoulder** Joint, Right	**Includes:** Glenohumeral joint Glenoid ligament (labrum)
Shoulder Muscle, Left **Shoulder** Muscle, Right	**Includes:** Deltoid muscle Infraspinatus muscle Subscapularis muscle Supraspinatus muscle Teres major muscle Teres minor muscle
Sigmoid Colon	**Includes:** Rectosigmoid junction Sigmoid flexure
Skin	**Includes:** Dermis Epidermis Sebaceous gland Sweat gland
Skin, Chest	Breast procedures, skin only
Sphenoid Bone	**Includes:** Greater wing Lesser wing Optic foramen Pterygoid process Sella turcica
Spinal Canal	**Includes:** Epidural space, spinal Extradural space, spinal Subarachnoid space, spinal Subdural space, spinal Vertebral canal
Spinal Cord	Dorsal root ganglion
Spinal Meninges	**Includes:** Arachnoid mater, spinal Denticulate (dentate) ligament Dura mater, spinal Filum terminale Leptomeninges, spinal Pia mater, spinal
Spleen	**Includes:** Accessory spleen
Splenic Artery	**Includes:** Left gastroepiploic artery Pancreatic artery Short gastric artery
Splenic Vein	**Includes:** Left gastroepiploic vein Pancreatic vein

Continued →

Section 0 - Medical and Surgical — Character 4 - Body Part	
Sternum	**Includes:** Manubrium Suprasternal notch Xiphoid process
Sternum Bursa and Ligament	Costotransverse ligament Costoxiphoid ligament Sternocostal ligament
Stomach, Pylorus	**Includes:** Pyloric antrum Pyloric canal Pyloric sphincter
Subclavian Artery, Left **Subclavian** Artery, Right	**Includes:** Costocervical trunk Dorsal scapular artery Internal thoracic artery
Subcutaneous Tissue and Fascia, Chest	**Includes:** Pectoral fascia
Subcutaneous Tissue and Fascia, Face	**Includes:** Masseteric fascia Orbital fascia Submandibular space
Subcutaneous Tissue and Fascia, Left Foot	**Includes:** Plantar fascia (aponeurosis)
Subcutaneous Tissue and Fascia, Left Hand	**Includes:** Palmar fascia (aponeurosis)
Subcutaneous Tissue and Fascia, Left Lower Arm	**Includes:** Antebrachial fascia Bicipital aponeurosis
Subcutaneous Tissue and Fascia, Left Neck	Deep cervical fascia Pretracheal fascia Prevertebral fascia
Subcutaneous Tissue and Fascia, Left Upper Arm	**Includes:** Axillary fascia Deltoid fascia Infraspinatus fascia Subscapular aponeurosis Supraspinatus fascia
Subcutaneous Tissue and Fascia, Left Upper Leg	**Includes:** Crural fascia Fascia lata Iliac fascia Iliotibial tract (band)
Subcutaneous Tissue and Fascia, Right Foot	**Includes:** Plantar fascia (aponeurosis)
Subcutaneous Tissue and Fascia, Right Hand	**Includes:** Palmar fascia (aponeurosis)
Subcutaneous Tissue and Fascia, Right Lower Arm	**Includes:** Antebrachial fascia Bicipital aponeurosis
Subcutaneous Tissue and Fascia, Right Neck	Deep cervical fascia Pretracheal fascia Prevertebral fascia
Subcutaneous Tissue and Fascia, Right Upper Arm	**Includes:** Axillary fascia Deltoid fascia Infraspinatus fascia Subscapular aponeurosis Supraspinatus fascia

Section 0 - Medical and Surgical — Character 4 - Body Part	
Subcutaneous Tissue and Fascia, Right Upper Leg	**Includes:** Crural fascia Fascia lata Iliac fascia Iliotibial tract (band)
Subcutaneous Tissue and Fascia, Scalp	**Includes:** Galea aponeurotica
Subcutaneous Tissue and Fascia, Trunk	**Includes:** External oblique aponeurosis Transversalis fascia
Submaxillary Gland, Left **Submaxillary** Gland, Right	**Includes:** Submandibular gland
Superior Mesenteric Artery	**Includes:** Ileal artery Ileocolic artery Inferior pancreaticoduodenal artery Jejunal artery
Superior Mesenteric Vein	**Includes:** Right gastroepiploic vein
Superior Vena Cava	**Includes:** Precava
Tarsal Joint, Left **Tarsal** Joint, Right	**Includes:** Calcaneocuboid joint Cuboideonavicular joint Cuneonavicular joint Intercuneiform joint Subtalar (talocalcaneal) joint Talocalcaneal (subtalar) joint Talocalcaneonavicular joint
Tarsal, Left **Tarsal,** Right	**Includes:** Calcaneus Cuboid bone Intermediate cuneiform bone Lateral cuneiform bone Medial cuneiform bone Navicular bone Talus bone
Temporal Artery, Left **Temporal** Artery, Right	**Includes:** Middle temporal artery Superficial temporal artery Transverse facial artery
Temporal Bone, Left **Temporal** Bone, Right	**Includes:** Mastoid process Petrous part of temoporal bone Tympanic part of temoporal bone Zygomatic process of temporal bone
Thalamus	**Includes:** Epithalamus Geniculate nucleus Metathalamus Pulvinar
Thoracic Aorta Ascending/Arch	**Includes:** Aortic arch Ascending aorta

Continued →

Section 0 - Medical and Surgical — Character 4 - Body Part	
Thoracic Duct	**Includes:** Left jugular trunk Left subclavian trunk
Thoracic Nerve	**Includes:** Intercostal nerve Intercostobrachial nerve Spinal nerve, thoracic Subcostal nerve
Thoracic Spinal Cord	Dorsal root ganglion
Thoracic Sympathetic Nerve	**Includes:** Cardiac plexus Esophageal plexus Greater splanchnic nerve Inferior cardiac nerve Least splanchnic nerve Lesser splanchnic nerve Middle cardiac nerve Pulmonary plexus Superior cardiac nerve Thoracic aortic plexus Thoracic ganglion
Thoracic Vertebra	**Includes:** Spinous process Transverse process Vertebral arch Vertebral body Vertebral foramen Vertebral lamina Vertebral pedicle
Thoracic Vertebral Joint	**Includes:** Costotransverse joint Costovertebral joint Thoracic facet joint
Thoracolumbar Vertebral Joint	**Includes:** Thoracolumbar facet joint
Thorax Muscle, Left **Thorax** Muscle, Right	**Includes:** Intercostal muscle Levatores costarum muscle Pectoralis major muscle Pectoralis minor muscle Serratus anterior muscle Subclavius muscle Subcostal muscle Transverse thoracis muscle
Thymus	**Includes:** Thymus gland
Thyroid Artery, Left **Thyroid** Artery, Right	**Includes:** Cricothyroid artery Hyoid artery Sternocleidomastoid artery Superior laryngeal artery Superior thyroid artery Thyrocervical trunk
Tibia, Left **Tibia,** Right	**Includes:** Lateral condyle of tibia Medial condyle of tibia Medial malleolus
Tibial Nerve	**Includes:** Lateral plantar nerve Medial plantar nerve Medial popliteal nerve Medial sural cutaneous nerve

Section 0 - Medical and Surgical — Character 4 - Body Part	
Toe Nail	**Includes:** Nail bed Nail plate
Toe Phalangeal Joint, Left **Toe** Phalangeal Joint, Right	**Includes:** Interphalangeal (IP) joint
Tongue	**Includes:** Frenulum linguae
Tongue, Palate, Pharynx Muscle	**Includes:** Chondroglossus muscle Genioglossus muscle Hyoglossus muscle Inferior longitudinal muscle Levator veli palatini muscle Palatoglossal muscle Palatopharyngeal muscle Pharyngeal constrictor muscle Salpingopharyngeus muscle Styloglossus muscle Stylopharyngeus muscle Superior longitudinal muscle Tensor veli palatini muscle
Tonsils	**Includes:** Palatine tonsil
Trachea	**Includes:** Cricoid cartilage
Transverse Colon	**Includes:** Hepatic flexure Splenic flexure
Tricuspid Valve	**Includes:** Right atrioventricular valve Tricuspid annulus
Trigeminal Nerve	**Includes:** Fifth cranial nerve Gasserian ganglion Mandibular nerve Maxillary nerve Ophthalmic nerve Trifacial nerve
Trochlear Nerve	**Includes:** Fourth cranial nerve
Trunk Muscle, Left **Trunk** Muscle, Right	**Includes:** Coccygeus muscle Erector spinae muscle Interspinalis muscle Intertransversarius muscle Latissimus dorsi muscle Quadratus lumborum muscle Rhomboid major muscle Rhomboid minor muscle Serratus posterior muscle Transversospinalis muscle Trapezius muscle
Tympanic Membrane, Left **Tympanic** Membrane, Right	**Includes:** Pars flaccida
Ulna, Left **Ulna,** Right	**Includes:** Olecranon process Radial notch

Continued →

Section 0 - Medical and Surgical — Character 4 - Body Part	
Ulnar Artery, Left **Ulnar** Artery, Right	**Includes:** Anterior ulnar recurrent artery Common interosseous artery Posterior ulnar recurrent artery
Ulnar Nerve	**Includes:** Cubital nerve
Upper Arm Muscle, Left **Upper** Arm Muscle, Right	**Includes:** Biceps brachii muscle Brachialis muscle Coracobrachialis muscle Triceps brachii muscle
Upper Artery	**Includes:** Aortic intercostal artery Bronchial artery Esophageal artery Subcostal artery
Upper Eyelid, Left **Upper** Eyelid, Right	**Includes:** Lateral canthus Levator palpebrae superioris muscle Orbicularis oculi muscle Superior tarsal plate
Upper Femur, Left **Upper** Femur, Right	**Includes:** Femoral head Greater trochanter Lesser trochanter Neck of femur
Upper Leg Muscle, Left **Upper** Leg Muscle, Right	**Includes:** Adductor brevis muscle Adductor longus muscle Adductor magnus muscle Biceps femoris muscle Gracilis muscle Pectineus muscle Quadriceps (femoris) Rectus femoris muscle Sartorius muscle Semimembranosus muscle Semitendinosus muscle Vastus intermedius muscle Vastus lateralis muscle Vastus medialis muscle
Upper Lip	**Includes:** Frenulum labii superioris Labial gland Vermilion border
Upper Spine Bursa and Ligament	Interspinous ligament, thoracic Intertransverse ligament, thoracic Ligamentum flavum, thoracic Supraspinous ligament
Ureter **Ureter,** Left **Ureter,** Right **Ureters,** Bilateral	**Includes:** Ureteral orifice Ureterovesical orifice
Urethra	**Includes:** Bulbourethral (Cowper's) gland Cowper's (bulbourethral) gland External urethral sphincter Internal urethral sphincter Membranous urethra Penile urethra Prostatic urethra

Section 0 - Medical and Surgical — Character 4 - Body Part	
Uterine Supporting Structure	**Includes:** Broad ligament Infundibulopelvic ligament Ovarian ligament Round ligament of uterus
Uterus	**Includes:** Fundus uteri Myometrium Perimetrium Uterine cornu
Uvula	**Includes:** Palatine uvula
Vagus Nerve	**Includes:** Anterior vagal trunk Pharyngeal plexus Pneumogastric nerve Posterior vagal trunk Pulmonary plexus Recurrent laryngeal nerve Superior laryngeal nerve Tenth cranial nerve
Vas Deferens **Vas** Deferens, Bilateral **Vas** Deferens, Left **Vas** Deferens, Right	**Includes:** Ductus deferens Ejaculatory duct
Ventricle, Right	**Includes:** Conus arteriosus
Ventricular Septum	**Includes:** Interventricular septum
Vertebral Artery, Left **Vertebral** Artery, Right	**Includes:** Anterior spinal artery Posterior spinal artery
Vertebral Vein, Left **Vertebral** Vein, Right	**Includes:** Deep cervical vein Suboccipital venous plexus
Vestibular Gland	**Includes:** Bartholin's (greater vestibular) gland Greater vestibular (Bartholin's) gland Paraurethral (Skene's) gland Skene's (paraurethral) gland
Vitreous, Left **Vitreous,** Right	**Includes:** Vitreous body
Vocal Cord, Left **Vocal** Cord, Right	**Includes:** Vocal fold
Vulva	**Includes:** Labia majora Labia minora
Wrist Bursa and Ligament, Left **Wrist** Bursa and Ligament, Right	**Includes:** Palmar ulnocarpal ligament Radial collateral carpal ligament Radiocarpal ligament Radioulnar ligament Scapholunate ligament Ulnar collateral carpal ligament
Wrist Joint, Left **Wrist** Joint, Right	**Includes:** Distal radioulnar joint Radiocarpal joint

Appendix E: Medical and Surgical Device Table (Device Key) and Device Aggregation Table

Section 0 - Medical and Surgical — Character 6 - Device	
Articulating Spacer in Lower Joints	**Includes:** Articulating Spacer (Antibiotic) Spacer, Articulating (Antibiotic)
Artificial Sphincter in Gastrointestinal System	**Includes:** Artificial anal sphincter (AAS) Artificial bowel sphincter (neosphincter)
Artificial Sphincter in Urinary System	**Includes:** AMS 800® Urinary Control System Artificial urinary sphincter (AUS)
Autologous Arterial Tissue in Heart and Great Vessels	**Includes:** Autologous artery graft
Autologous Arterial Tissue in Lower Arteries	**Includes:** Autologous artery graft
Autologous Arterial Tissue in Lower Veins	**Includes:** Autologous artery graft
Autologous Arterial Tissue in Upper Arteries	**Includes:** Autologous artery graft
Autologous Arterial Tissue in Upper Veins	**Includes:** Autologous artery graft
Autologous Tissue Substitute	**Includes:** Autograft Cultured epidermal cell autograft Epicel® cultured epidermal autograft
Autologous Venous Tissue in Heart and Great Vessels	**Includes:** Autologous vein graft
Autologous Venous Tissue in Lower Arteries	**Includes:** Autologous vein graft
Autologous Venous Tissue in Lower Veins	**Includes:** Autologous vein graft
Autologous Venous Tissue in Upper Arteries	**Includes:** Autologous vein graft
Autologous Venous Tissue in Upper Veins	**Includes:** Autologous vein graft
Biologic with Synthetic Substitute, Autoregulated Electrohydraulic for Replacement in Heart and Great Vessels	**Includes:** Carmat total artificial heart (TAH)
Bone Growth Stimulator in Head and Facial Bones	**Includes:** Electrical bone growth stimulator (EBGS) Ultrasonic osteogenic stimulator Ultrasound bone healing system
Bone Growth Stimulator in Lower Bones	**Includes:** Electrical bone growth stimulator (EBGS) Ultrasonic osteogenic stimulator Ultrasound bone healing system
Bone Growth Stimulator in Upper Bones	**Includes:** Electrical bone growth stimulator (EBGS) Ultrasonic osteogenic stimulator Ultrasound bone healing system

Section 0 - Medical and Surgical — Character 6 - Device	
Cardiac Lead in Heart and Great Vessels	**Includes:** Cardiac contractility modulation lead
Cardiac Lead, Defibrillator for Insertion in Heart and Great Vessels	**Includes:** ACUITY™ Steerable Lead Attain Ability® lead Attain StarFix® (OTW) lead Cardiac resynchronization therapy (CRT) lead Corox (OTW) Bipolar Lead Durata® Defibrillation Lead ENDOTAK RELIANCE® (G) Defibrillation Lead
Cardiac Lead, Pacemaker for Insertion in Heart and Great Vessels	**Includes:** ACUITY™ Steerable Lead Attain Ability® lead Attain StarFix® (OTW) lead Cardiac resynchronization therapy (CRT) lead Corox (OTW) Bipolar Lead
Cardiac Resynchronization Defibrillator Pulse Generator for Insertion in Subcutaneous Tissue and Fascia	**Includes:** COGNIS® CRT-D Concerto II CRT-D Consulta CRT-D CONTAK RENEWAL® 3 RF (HE) CRT-D LIVIAN™ CRT-D Maximo II DR CRT-D Ovatio™ CRT-D Protecta XT CRT-D Viva (XT)(S)
Cardiac Resynchronization Pacemaker Pulse Generator for Insertion in Subcutaneous Tissue and Fascia	**Includes:** Consulta CRT-P Stratos LV Synchra CRT-P
Contraceptive Device in Female Reproductive System	**Includes:** Intrauterine device (IUD)
Contraceptive Device in Subcutaneous Tissue and Fascia	**Includes:** Subdermal progesterone implant
Contractility Modulation Device for Insertion in Subcutaneous Tissue and Fascia	**Includes:** Optimizer™ III implantable pulse generator
Defibrillator Generator for Insertion in Subcutaneous Tissue and Fascia	**Includes:** Evera (XT)(S)(DR/VR) Implantable cardioverter-defibrillator (ICD) Maximo II DR (VR) Protecta XT DR (XT VR) Secura (DR) (VR) Virtuoso (II) (DR) (VR)
Diaphragmatic Pacemaker Lead in Respiratory System	**Includes:** Phrenic nerve stimulator lead

Continued →

Section 0 - Medical and Surgical — Character 6 - Device	
Drainage Device	**Includes:** Cystostomy tube Foley catheter Percutaneous nephrostomy catheter Thoracostomy tube
External Fixation Device in Head and Facial Bones	**Includes:** External fixator
External Fixation Device in Lower Bones	**Includes:** External fixator
External Fixation Device in Lower Joints	**Includes:** External fixator
External Fixation Device in Upper Bones	**Includes:** External fixator
External Fixation Device in Upper Joints	**Includes:** External fixator
External Fixation Device, Hybrid for Insertion in Upper Bones	**Includes:** Delta frame external fixator Sheffield hybrid external fixator
External Fixation Device, Hybrid for Insertion in Lower Bones	**Includes:** Delta frame external fixator Sheffield hybrid external fixator
External Fixation Device, Hybrid for Reposition in Upper Bones	**Includes:** Delta frame external fixator Sheffield hybrid external fixator
External Fixation Device, Hybrid for Reposition in Lower Bones	**Includes:** Delta frame external fixator Sheffield hybrid external fixator
External Fixation Device, Limb Lengthening for Insertion in Upper Bones	**Includes:** Ilizarov-Vecklich device
External Fixation Device, Limb Lengthening for Insertion in Lower Bones	**Includes:** Ilizarov-Vecklich device
External Fixation Device, Monoplanar for Insertion in Upper Bones	**Includes:** Uniplanar external fixator
External Fixation Device, Monoplanar for Insertion in Lower Bones	**Includes:** Uniplanar external fixator
External Fixation Device, Monoplanar for Reposition in Upper Bones	**Includes:** Uniplanar external fixator
External Fixation Device, Monoplanar for Reposition in Lower Bones	**Includes:** Uniplanar external fixator
External Fixation Device, Ring for Insertion in Upper Bones	**Includes:** Ilizarov external fixator Sheffield ring external fixator
External Fixation Device, Ring for Insertion in Lower Bones	**Includes:** Ilizarov external fixator Sheffield ring external fixator
External Fixation Device, Ring for Reposition in Upper Bones	**Includes:** Ilizarov external fixator Sheffield ring external fixator

Section 0 - Medical and Surgical — Character 6 - Device	
External Fixation Device, Ring for Reposition in Lower Bones	**Includes:** Ilizarov external fixator Sheffield ring external fixator
Extraluminal Device	**Includes:** AtriClip LAA Exclusion System LAP-BAND® adjustable gastric banding system REALIZE® Adjustable Gastric Band
Feeding Device in Gastrointestinal System	**Includes:** Percutaneous endoscopic gastrojejunostomy (PEG/J) tube Percutaneous endoscopic gastrostomy (PEG) tube
Hearing Device in Ear, Nose, Sinus	**Includes:** Esteem® implantable hearing system
Hearing Device in Head and Facial Bones	**Includes:** Bone anchored hearing device
Hearing Device, Bone Conduction for Insertion in Ear, Nose, Sinus	**Includes:** Bone anchored hearing device
Hearing Device, Multiple Channel Cochlear Prosthesis for Insertion in Ear, Nose, Sinus	**Includes:** Cochlear implant (CI), multiple channel (electrode)
Hearing Device, Single Channel Cochlear Prosthesis for Insertion in Ear, Nose, Sinus	**Includes:** Cochlear implant (CI), single channel (electrode)
Implantable Heart Assist System in Heart and Great Vessels	**Includes:** Berlin Heart Ventricular Assist Device DeBakey Left Ventricular Assist Device DuraHeart Left Ventricular Assist System HeartMate II® Left Ventricular Assist Device (LVAD) HeartMate 3® LVAS HeartMate XVE® Left Ventricular Assist Device (LVAD) MicroMed HeartAssist Novacor Left Ventricular Assist Device Thoratec IVAD (Implantable Ventricular Assist Device)
Infusion Device	**Includes:** Ascenda Intrathecal Catheter InDura, intrathecal catheter (1P) (spinal) Non-tunneled central venous catheter Peripherally inserted central catheter (PICC) Tunneled spinal (intrathecal) catheter
Infusion Device, Pump in Subcutaneous Tissue and Fascia	**Includes:** Implantable drug infusion pump (anti-spasmodic)(chemotherapy)(pain) Injection reservoir, pump Pump reservoir Subcutaneous injection reservoir, pump SynchroMed pump

Continued →

Section 0 - Medical and Surgical — Character 6 - Device	
Interbody Fusion Device in Lower Joints	**Includes:** Axial Lumbar Interbody Fusion System AxiaLIF® System CoRoent® XL Direct Lateral Interbody Fusion (DLIF) device EXtreme Lateral Interbody Fusion (XLIF) device Interbody fusion (spine) cage XLIF® System
Interbody Fusion Device in Upper Joints	**Includes:** BAK/C® Interbody Cervical Fusion System Interbody fusion (spine) cage
Internal Fixation Device in Head and Facial Bones	**Includes:** Bone screw (interlocking)(lag)(pedicle)(recessed) Kirschner wire (K-wire) Neutralization plate
Internal Fixation Device in Lower Bones	**Includes:** Bone screw (interlocking)(lag)(pedicle)(recessed) Clamp and rod internal fixation system (CRIF) Kirschner wire (K-wire) Neutralization plate
Internal Fixation Device in Lower Joints	**Includes:** Fusion screw (compression)(lag)(locking) Joint fixation plate Kirschner wire (K-wire)
Internal Fixation Device in Upper Bones	**Includes:** Bone screw (interlocking)(lag)(pedicle)(recessed) Clamp and rod internal fixation system (CRIF) Kirschner wire (K-wire) Neutralization plate
Internal Fixation Device in Upper Joints	**Includes:** Fusion screw (compression)(lag)(locking) Joint fixation plate Kirschner wire (K-wire)
Internal Fixation Device, Intramedullary in Lower Bones	**Includes:** Intramedullary (IM) rod (nail) Intramedullary skeletal kinetic distractor (ISKD) Kuntscher nail
Internal Fixation Device, Intramedullary in Upper Bones	**Includes:** Intramedullary (IM) rod (nail) Intramedullary skeletal kinetic distractor (ISKD) Kuntscher nail
Internal Fixation Device, Intramedullary Limb Lengthening for Insertion in Lower Bones	**Includes:** PRECICE intramedullary limb lengthening system
Internal Fixation Device, Intramedullary Limb Lengthening for Insertion in Upper Bones	**Includes:** PRECICE intramedullary limb lengthening system

Section 0 - Medical and Surgical — Character 6 - Device	
Internal Fixation Device, Rigid Plate for Insertion in Upper Bones	**Includes:** Titanium Sternal Fixation System (TSFS)
Internal Fixation Device, Rigid Plate for Reposition in Upper Bones	**Includes:** Titanium Sternal Fixation System (TSFS)
Internal Fixation Device, Sustained Compression for Fusion in Lower Joints	**Includes:** DynaNail® DynaNail Mini®
Internal Fixation Device, Sustained Compression for Fusion in Upper Joints	**Includes:** DynaNail® DynaNail Mini®
Intraluminal Device	**Includes:** Absolute Pro Vascular (OTW) Self-Expanding Stent System Acculink (RX) Carotid Stent System AFX® Endovascular AAA System AneuRx® AAA Advantage® Assurant (Cobalt) stent Carotid WALLSTENT® Monorail® Endoprosthesis CoAxia NeuroFlo catheter Colonic Z-Stent® Complete (SE) stent Cook Zenith AAA Endovascular Graft Driver stent (RX) (OTW) E-Luminexx™ (Biliary)(Vascular) Stent Embolization coil(s) Endologix AFX® Endovascular AAA System Endurant® II AAA stent graft system Endurant® Endovascular Stent Graft EXCLUDER® AAA Endoprosthesis Express® (LD) Premounted Stent System Express® Biliary SD Monorail® Premounted Stent System Express® SD Renal Monorail® Premounted Stent System FLAIR® Endovascular Stent Graft Formula™ Balloon-Expandable Renal Stent System GORE EXCLUDER® AAA Endoprosthesis GORE TAG® Thoracic Endoprosthesis Herculink (RX) Elite Renal Stent System LifeStent® (Flexstar)(XL) Vascular Stent System Medtronic Endurant® II AAA stent graft system Micro-Driver stent (RX) (OTW) MULTI-LINK (VISION)(MINI-VISION)(ULTRA) Coronary Stent System Omnilink Elite Vascular Balloon Expandable Stent System Protégé® RX Carotid Stent System Stent, intraluminal (cardiovascular)(gastrointestinal)(hepatobiliary)(urinary) Talent® Converter Talent® Occluder

Continued →

Section 0 - Medical and Surgical — Character 6 - Device	
Intraluminal Device (*continued*)	Talent® Stent Graft (abdominal) (thoracic) Therapeutic occlusion coil(s) Ultraflex™ Precision Colonic Stent System Valiant Thoracic Stent Graft WALLSTENT® Endoprosthesis Xact Carotid Stent System Zenith AAA Endovascular Graft Zenith Flex® AAA Endovascular Graft Zenith® Renu™ AAA Ancillary Graft Zenith TX2® TAA Endovascular Graft
Intraluminal Device, Airway in Ear, Nose, Sinus	**Includes:** Nasopharyngeal airway (NPA)
Intraluminal Device, Airway in Gastrointestinal System	**Includes:** Esophageal obturator airway (EOA)
Intraluminal Device, Airway in Mouth and Throat	**Includes:** Guedel airway Oropharyngeal airway (OPA)
Intraluminal Device, Bioactive in Upper Arteries	**Includes:** Bioactive embolization coil(s) Micrus CERECYTE microcoil
Intraluminal Device, Branched or Fenestrated, One or Two Arteries for Restriction in Lower Arteries	**Includes:** Cook Zenith® Fenestrated AAA Endovascular Graft EXCLUDER® AAA Endoprosthesis EXCLUDER® IBE Endoprosthesis GORE EXCLUDER® AAA Endoprosthesis GORE EXCLUDER® IBE Endoprosthesis Zenith® Fenestrated AAA Endovascular Graft
Intraluminal Device, Branched or Fenestrated, Three or More Arteries for Restriction in Lower Arteries	**Includes:** Cook Zenith® Fenestrated AAA Endovascular Graft EXCLUDER® AAA Endoprosthesis GORE EXCLUDER® AAA Endoprosthesis Zenith® Fenestrated AAA Endovascular Graft
Intraluminal Device, Drug-eluting in Heart and Great Vessels	**Includes:** CYPHER® Stent Endeavor® (III)(IV) (Sprint) Zotarolimus-eluting Coronary Stent System Everolimus-eluting coronary stent Paclitaxel-eluting coronary stent Sirolimus-eluting coronary stent TAXUS® Liberté® Paclitaxel-eluting Coronary Stent System XIENCE Everolimus Eluting Coronary Stent System Zotarolimus-eluting coronary stent
Intraluminal Device, Drug-eluting in Lower Arteries	**Includes:** Paclitaxel-eluting peripheral stent Zilver® PTX® (paclitaxel) Drug-Eluting Peripheral Stent
Intraluminal Device, Drug-eluting in Upper Arteries	**Includes:** Paclitaxel-eluting peripheral stent Zilver® PTX® (paclitaxel) Drug-Eluting Peripheral Stent

Section 0 - Medical and Surgical — Character 6 - Device	
Intraluminal Device, Endobronchial Valve in Respiratory System	**Includes:** Spiration IBV™ Valve System
Intraluminal Device, Flow Diverter for Restriction in Upper Arteries	**Includes:** Flow Diverter embolization device Pipeline™ (Flex) embolization device Surpass Streamline™ Flow Diverter
Intraluminal Device, Pessary in Female Reproductive System	**Includes:** Pessary ring Vaginal pessary
Intraluminal Device, Endotracheal Airway in Respiratory System	**Includes:** Endotracheal tube (cuffed)(double-lumen)
Liner in Lower Joints	**Includes:** Acetabular cup Hip (joint) liner Joint liner (insert) Knee (implant) insert Tibial insert
Monitoring Device	**Includes:** Blood glucose monitoring system Cardiac event recorder Continuous Glucose Monitoring (CGM) device Implantable glucose monitoring device Loop recorder, implantable Reveal (LINQ)(DX)(XT)
Monitoring Device, Hemodynamic for Insertion in Subcutaneous Tissue and Fascia	**Includes:** Implantable hemodynamic monitor (IHM) Implantable hemodynamic monitoring system (IHMS)
Monitoring Device, Pressure Sensor for Insertion in Heart and Great Vessels	**Includes:** CardioMEMS® pressure sensor EndoSure® sensor
Neurostimulator Lead in Central Nervous System and Cranial Nerves	**Includes:** Cortical strip neurostimulator lead DBS lead Deep brain neurostimulator lead RNS System lead Spinal cord neurostimulator lead
Neurostimulator Lead in Peripheral Nervous System	**Includes:** InterStim® Therapy lead
Neurostimulator Generator in Head and Facial Bones	**Includes:** RNS system neurostimulator generator
Nonautologous Tissue Substitute	**Includes:** Acellular Hydrated Dermis Bone bank bone graft Cook Biodesign® Fistula Plug(s) Cook Biodesign® Hernia Graft(s) Cook Biodesign® Layered Graft(s) Cook Zenapro™ Layered Grafts(s) Tissue bank graft
Other Device	**Includes:** Alfapump® system

Continued →

Section 0 - Medical and Surgical — Character 6 - Device	
Pacemaker, Dual Chamber for Insertion in Subcutaneous Tissue and Fascia	**Includes:** Advisa (MRI) EnRhythm Kappa Revo MRI™ SureScan® pacemaker Two lead pacemaker Versa
Pacemaker, Single Chamber for Insertion in Subcutaneous Tissue and Fascia	**Includes:** Single lead pacemaker (atrium) (ventricle)
Pacemaker, Single Chamber Rate Responsive for Insertion in Subcutaneous Tissue and Fascia	**Includes:** Single lead rate responsive pacemaker (atrium)(ventricle)
Radioactive Element	**Includes:** Brachytherapy seeds CivaSheet®
Radioactive Element, Cesium-131 Collagen Implant for Insertion in Central Nervous System and Cranial Nerves	Cesium-131 Collagen Implant GammaTile™
Resurfacing Device in Lower Joints	**Includes:** CONSERVE® PLUS Total Resurfacing Hip System Cormet Hip Resurfacing System
Short-term External Heart Assist System in Heart and Great Vessels	Biventricular external heart assist system BVS 5000 Ventricular Assist Device Centrimag® Blood Pump Impella® heart pump TandemHeart® System Thoratec Paracorporeal Ventricular Assist Device
Spacer in Lower Joints	**Includes:** Joint spacer (antibiotic) Spacer, Static (Antibiotic) Static Spacer (Antibiotic)
Spacer in Upper Joints	**Includes:** Joint spacer (antibiotic)
Spinal Stabilization Device, Facet Replacement for Insertion in Upper Joints	**Includes:** Facet replacement spinal stabilization device
Spinal Stabilization Device, Facet Replacement for Insertion in Lower Joints	**Includes:** Facet replacement spinal stabilization device
Spinal Stabilization Device, Interspinous Process for Insertion in Upper Joints	**Includes:** Interspinous process spinal stabilization device X-STOP® Spacer
Spinal Stabilization Device, Interspinous Process for Insertion in Lower Joints	**Includes:** Interspinous process spinal stabilization device X-STOP® Spacer
Spinal Stabilization Device, Pedicle-Based for Insertion in Upper Joints	**Includes:** Dynesys® Dynamic Stabilization System Pedicle-based dynamic stabilization device

Section 0 - Medical and Surgical — Character 6 - Device	
Spinal Stabilization Device, Pedicle-Based for Insertion in Lower Joints	**Includes:** Dynesys® Dynamic Stabilization System Pedicle-based dynamic stabilization device
Stimulator Generator in Subcutaneous Tissue and Fascia	**Includes:** Baroreflex Activation Therapy® (BAT®) Diaphragmatic pacemaker generator Mark IV Breathing Pacemaker System Phrenic nerve stimulator generator Rheos® System device
Stimulator Generator, Multiple Array for Insertion in Subcutaneous Tissue and Fascia	**Includes:** Activa PC neurostimulator Enterra gastric neurostimulator Neurostimulator generator, multiple channel PERCEPT™ PC neurostimulator PrimeAdvanced neurostimulator (SureScan)(MRI Safe)
Stimulator Generator, Multiple Array Rechargeable for Insertion in Subcutaneous Tissue and Fascia	**Includes:** Activa RC neurostimulator Neurostimulator generator, multiple channel rechargeable RestoreAdvanced neurostimulator (SureScan)(MRI Safe) RestoreSensor neurostimulator (SureScan)(MRI Safe) RestoreUltra neurostimulator (SureScan)(MRI Safe)
Stimulator Generator, Single Array for Insertion in Subcutaneous Tissue and Fascia	**Includes:** Activa SC neurostimulator InterStim™ II Therapy neurostimulator Itrel (3)(4) neurostimulator Neurostimulator generator, single channel
Stimulator Generator, Single Array Rechargeable for Insertion in Subcutaneous Tissue and Fascia	**Includes:** InterStim™ Micro Therapy neurostimulator Neurostimulator generator, single channel rechargeable
Stimulator Lead in Gastrointestinal System	**Includes:** Gastric electrical stimulation (GES) lead Gastric pacemaker lead
Stimulator Lead in Muscles	**Includes:** Electrical muscle stimulation (EMS) lead Electronic muscle stimulator lead Neuromuscular electrical stimulation (NEMS) lead
Stimulator Lead in Upper Arteries	**Includes:** Baroreflex Activation Therapy® (BAT®) Carotid (artery) sinus (baroreceptor) lead Rheos® System lead
Stimulator Lead in Urinary System	**Includes:** Sacral nerve modulation (SNM) lead Sacral neuromodulation lead Urinary incontinence stimulator lead
Subcutaneous Defibrillator Lead in Subcutaneous Tissue and Fascia	**Includes:** S-ICD™ lead

Continued →

Section 0 - Medical and Surgical — Character 6 - Device	
Synthetic Substitute	**Includes:** AbioCor® Total Replacement Heart AMPLATZER® Muscular VSD Occluder Annuloplasty ring Bard® Composix® (E/X)(LP) mesh Bard® Composix® Kugel® patch Bard® Dulex™ mesh Bard® Ventralex™ hernia patch Barricaid® Annular Closure Device (ACD) BRYAN® Cervical Disc System Corvia IASD® Ex-PRESS™ mini glaucoma shunt Flexible Composite Mesh GORE® DUALMESH® Holter valve ventricular shunt IASD® (InterAtrial Shunt Device), Corvia InterAtrial Shunt Device IASD®, Corvia MitraClip valve repair system Nitinol framed polymer mesh Open Pivot Aortic Valve Graft (AVG) Open Pivot (mechanical) valve Partially absorbable mesh PHYSIOMESH™ Flexible Composite Mesh Polymethylmethacrylate (PMMA) Polypropylene mesh PRESTIGE® Cervical Disc PROCEED™ Ventral Patch Prodisc-C Prodisc-L PROLENE Polypropylene Hernia System (PHS) Rebound HRD® (Hernia Repair Device) SynCardia Total Artificial Heart Total artificial (replacement) heart ULTRAPRO Hernia System (UHS) ULTRAPRO Partially Absorbable Lightweight Mesh ULTRAPRO Plug V-WAVE Interatrial Shunt System Ventrio™ Hernia Patch Zimmer® NexGen® LPS Mobile Bearing Knee Zimmer® NexGen® LPS-Flex Mobile Knee
Synthetic Substitute, Ceramic for Replacement in Lower Joints	**Includes:** Ceramic on ceramic bearing surface Novation® Ceramic AHS® (Articulation Hip System)
Synthetic Substitute, Intraocular Telescope for Replacement in Eye	**Includes:** Implantable Miniature Telescope™ (IMT)
Synthetic Substitute, Metal for Replacement in Lower Joints	**Includes:** Cobalt/chromium head and socket Metal on metal bearing surface

Section 0 - Medical and Surgical — Character 6 - Device	
Synthetic Substitute, Metal on Polyethylene for Replacement in Lower Joints	**Includes:** Cobalt/chromium head and polyethylene socket
Synthetic Substitute, Oxidized Zirconium on Polyethylene for Replacement in Lower Joints	OXINIUM
Synthetic Substitute, Pneumatic for Replacement in Heart and Great Vessels	**Includes:** SynCardia (temporary) total artificial heart (TAH)
Synthetic Substitute, Polyethylene for Replacement in Lower Joints	**Includes:** Polyethylene socket
Synthetic Substitute, Reverse Ball and Socket for Replacement in Upper Joints	**Includes:** Delta III Reverse shoulder prosthesis Reverse® Shoulder Prosthesis
Tissue Expander in Skin and Breast	**Includes:** Tissue expander (inflatable) (injectable)
Tissue Expander in Subcutaneous Tissue and Fascia	**Includes:** Tissue expander (inflatable) (injectable)
Tracheostomy Device in Respiratory System	**Includes:** Tracheostomy tube
Vascular Access Device, Totally Implantable in Subcutaneous Tissue and Fascia	**Includes:** Implanted (venous)(access) port Injection reservoir, port Subcutaneous injection reservoir, port
Vascular Access Device, Tunneled in Subcutaneous Tissue and Fascia	Tunneled central venous catheter Vectra® Vascular Access Graft
Zooplastic Tissue in Heart and Great Vessels	**Includes:** 3f (Aortic) Bioprosthesis valve Bovine pericardial valve Bovine pericardium graft Contegra Pulmonary Valved Conduit CoreValve transcatheter aortic valve Epic™ Stented Tissue Valve (aortic) Freestyle (Stentless) Aortic Root Bioprosthesis Hancock Bioprosthesis (aortic) (mitral) valve Hancock Bioprosthetic Valved Conduit Melody® transcatheter pulmonary valve Mitroflow® Aortic Pericardial Heart Valve Mosaic Bioprosthesis (aortic) (mitral) valve Porcine (bioprosthetic) valve SAPIEN transcatheter aortic valve SJM Biocor® Stented Valve System Stented tissue valve Trifecta™ Valve (aortic) Xenograft

Device Aggregation Table

Specific Device	for Operation	in Body System	General Device
Autologous Arterial Tissue	All applicable	Heart and Great Vessels Lower Arteries Lower Veins Upper Arteries Upper Veins	**7** Autologous Tissue Substitute
Autologous Venous Tissue	All applicable	Heart and Great Vessels Lower Arteries Lower Veins Upper Arteries Upper Veins	**7** Autologous Tissue Substitute
Cardiac Lead, Defibrillator	Insertion	Heart and Great Vessels	**M** Cardiac Lead
Cardiac Lead, Pacemaker	Insertion	Heart and Great Vessels	**M** Cardiac Lead
Cardiac Resynchronization Defibrillator Pulse Generator	Insertion	Subcutaneous Tissue and Fascia	**P** Cardiac Rhythm Related Device
Cardiac Resynchronization Pacemaker Pulse Generator	Insertion	Subcutaneous Tissue and Fascia	**P** Cardiac Rhythm Related Device
Contractility Modulation Device	Insertion	Subcutaneous Tissue and Fascia	**P** Cardiac Rhythm Related Device
Defibrillator Generator	Insertion	Subcutaneous Tissue and Fascia	**P** Cardiac Rhythm Related Device
Epiretinal Visual Prosthesis	All applicable	Eye	**J** Synthetic Substitute
External Fixation Device, Hybrid	Insertion	Lower Bones Upper Bones	**5** External Fixation Device
External Fixation Device, Hybrid	Reposition	Lower Bones Upper Bones	**5** External Fixation Device
External Fixation Device, Limb Lengthening	Insertion	Lower Bones Upper Bones	**5** External Fixation Device
External Fixation Device, Monoplanar	Insertion	Lower Bones Upper Bones	**5** External Fixation Device
External Fixation Device, Monoplanar	Reposition	Lower Bones Upper Bones	**5** External Fixation Device
External Fixation Device, Ring	Insertion	Lower Bones Upper Bones	**5** External Fixation Device
External Fixation Device, Ring	Reposition	Lower Bones Upper Bones	**5** External Fixation Device
Hearing Device, Bone Conduction	Insertion	Ear, Nose, Sinus	**S** Hearing Device
Hearing Device, Multiple Channel Cochlear Prosthesis	Insertion	Ear, Nose, Sinus	**S** Hearing Device
Hearing Device, Single Channel Cochlear Prosthesis	Insertion	Ear, Nose, Sinus	**S** Hearing Device
Internal Fixation Device, Intramedullary	All applicable	Lower Bones Upper Bones	**4** Internal Fixation Device
Internal Fixation Device, Intramedullary Limb Lengthening	Insertion	Lower Bones Upper Bones	**6** Internal Fixation Device Intramedullary
Internal Fixation Device, Rigid Plate	Insertion	Upper Bones	**4** Internal Fixation Device
Internal Fixation Device, Rigid Plate	Reposition	Upper Bones	**4** Internal Fixation Device

Continued →

Specific Device	for Operation	in Body System	General Device
Intraluminal Device, Airway	All applicable	Ear, Nose, Sinus Gastrointestinal System Mouth and Throat	**D** Intraluminal Device
Intraluminal Device, Bioactive	All applicable	Upper Arteries	**D** Intraluminal Device
Intraluminal Device, Branched or Fenestrated, One or Two Arteries	Restriction	Heart and Great Vessels Lower Arteries	**D** Intraluminal Device
Intraluminal Device, Branched or Fenestrated, Three or More Arteries	Restriction	Heart and Great Vessels Lower Arteries	**D** Intraluminal Device
Intraluminal Device, Drug-eluting	All applicable	Heart and Great Vessels Lower Arteries Upper Arteries	**D** Intraluminal Device
Intraluminal Device, Drug-eluting, Four or More	All applicable	Heart and Great Vessels Lower Arteries Upper Arteries	**D** Intraluminal Device
Intraluminal Device, Drug-eluting, Three	All applicable	Heart and Great Vessels Lower Arteries Upper Arteries	**D** Intraluminal Device
Intraluminal Device, Drug-eluting, Two	All applicable	Heart and Great Vessels Lower Arteries Upper Arteries	**D** Intraluminal Device
Intraluminal Device, Endobronchial Valve	All applicable	Respiratory System	**D** Intraluminal Device
Intraluminal Device, Endotracheal Airway	All applicable	Respiratory System	**D** Intraluminal Device
Intraluminal Device, Flow Diverter	Restriction	Upper Arteries	**D** Intraluminal Device
Intraluminal Device, Four or More	All applicable	Heart and Great Vessels Lower Arteries Upper Arteries	**D** Intraluminal Device
Intraluminal Device, Pessary	All applicable	Female Reproductive System	**D** Intraluminal Device
Intraluminal Device, Radioactive	All applicable	Heart and Great Vessels	**D** Intraluminal Device
Intraluminal Device, Three	All applicable	Heart and Great Vessels Lower Arteries Upper Arteries	**D** Intraluminal Device
Intraluminal Device, Two	All applicable	Heart and Great Vessels Lower Arteries Upper Arteries	**D** Intraluminal Device
Monitoring Device, Hemodynamic	Insertion	Subcutaneous Tissue and Fascia	**2** Monitoring Device
Monitoring Device, Pressure Sensor	Insertion	Heart and Great Vessels	**2** Monitoring Device
Pacemaker, Dual Chamber	Insertion	Subcutaneous Tissue and Fascia	**P** Cardiac Rhythm Related Device
Pacemaker, Single Chamber	Insertion	Subcutaneous Tissue and Fascia	**P** Cardiac Rhythm Related Device
Pacemaker, Single Chamber Rate Responsive	Insertion	Subcutaneous Tissue and Fascia	**P** Cardiac Rhythm Related Device
Spinal Stabilization Device, Facet Replacement	Insertion	Lower Joints Upper Joints	**4** Internal Fixation Device
Spinal Stabilization Device, Interspinous Process	Insertion	Lower Joints Upper Joints	**4** Internal Fixation Device

Continued →

Specific Device	for Operation	in Body System	General Device
Spinal Stabilization Device, Pedicle-Based	Insertion	Lower Joints Upper Joints	**4** Internal Fixation Device
Spinal Stabilization Device, Vertebral Body Tether	Reposition	Lower Bones Upper Bones	**4** Internal Fixation Device
Stimulator Generator, Multiple Array	Insertion	Subcutaneous Tissue and Fascia	**M** Stimulator Generator
Stimulator Generator, Multiple Array Rechargeable	Insertion	Subcutaneous Tissue and Fascia	**M** Stimulator Generator
Stimulator Generator, Single Array	Insertion	Subcutaneous Tissue and Fascia	**M** Stimulator Generator
Stimulator Generator, Single Array Rechargeable	Insertion	Subcutaneous Tissue and Fascia	**M** Stimulator Generator
Synthetic Substitute, Ceramic	Replacement	Lower Joints	**J** Synthetic Substitute
Synthetic Substitute, Ceramic on Polyethylene	Replacement	Lower Joints	**J** Synthetic Substitute
Synthetic Substitute, Intraocular Telescope	Replacement	Eye	**J** Synthetic Substitute
Synthetic Substitute, Metal	Replacement	Lower Joints	**J** Synthetic Substitute
Synthetic Substitute, Metal on Polyethylene	Replacement	Lower Joints	**J** Synthetic Substitute
Synthetic Substitute, Oxidized Zirconium on Polyethylene	Replacement	Lower Joints	**J** Synthetic Substitute
Synthetic Substitute, Polyethylene	Replacement	Lower Joints	**J** Synthetic Substitute
Synthetic Substitute, Reverse Ball and Socket	Replacement	Upper Joints	**J** Synthetic Substitute

Appendix F: Substance Qualifier Table (Key)

Section 3 – Administration Character 6 – Substance	
4-Factor Prothrombin Complex Concentrate	**Includes:** Kcentra
Adhesion Barrier	**Includes:** Seprafilm
Anti-Infective Envelope	**Includes:** AIGISRx Antibacterial Envelope Antibacterial Envelope (TYRX) (AIGISRx) Antimicrobial envelope TYRX Antibacterial Envelope
Clofarabine	**Includes:** Clolar
Globulin	**Includes:** Gammaglobulin Hyperimmune globulin Immunoglobulin Polyclonal hyperimmune globulin
Glucarpidase	**Includes:** Voraxaze
Hematopoietic Stem/ Progenitor Cells, Genetically Modified	**Includes:** OTL-101 OTL-103
Human B-type Natriuretic Peptide	**Includes:** Nesiritide
Other Anti-infective	**Includes:** AVYCAZ® (ceftazidime-avibactam) Ceftazidime-avibactam CRESEMBA® (isavuconazonium sulfate) Isavuconazole (isavuconazonium sulfate)
Other Antineoplastic	**Includes:** Blinatumomab BLINCYTO® (blinatumomab)
Other Therapeutic Substance	**Includes:** Idarucizumab, Pradaxa® (dabigatran) reversal agent Praxbind® (idarucizumab), Pradaxa® (dabigatran) reversal agent
Other Thrombolytic	**Includes:** Tissue Plasinogen Activator (tPA) (r-tPA)
Oxazolidinones	**Includes:** Zyvox
Pathogen Reduced Cryoprecipitated Fibrinogen Complex	**Includes:** INTERCEPT Blood System for Plasma Pathogen Reduced Cryoprecipitated Fibrinogen Complex INTERCEPT Fibrinogen Complex
Recombinant Bone Morphogenetic Protein	**Includes:** Bone morphogenetic protein 2 (BMP 2) rhBMP-2

Section X - New Technology - Character 6 - Device/ Substance/Technology	
Antibiotic-eluting Bone Void Filler	CERAMENT® G
Apalutamide Antineoplastic	ERLEADA™
Atezolizumab Antineoplastic	TECENTRIQ®
Axicabtagene Ciloleucel Immunotherapy	Axicabtagene Ciloleucel Yescarta®
Bezlotoxumab Monoclonal Antibody	ZINPLAVA™
Bioengineered Allogeneic Construct	StrataGraft®
Branched Synthetic Substitute with Intraluminal Device in New Technology	Thoraflex™ Hybrid device
Brexanolone	ZULRESSO™
Brexucabtagene Autoleucel Immunotherapy	Tecartus™
Bromelain-enriched Proteolytic Enzyme	NexoBrid™
Cefiderocol Anti-infective	FETROJA®
Ceftolozane/Tazobactam Anti-infective	ZERBAXA®
Ciltacabtagene Autoleucel	cilta-cel
Coagulation Factor Xa, Inactivated	Andexanet Alfa, Factor Xa Inhibitor Reversal Agent Andexxa Coagulation Factor Xa, (Recombinant) Inactivated Factor Xa Inhibitor Reversal Agent, Andexanet Alfa
Concentrated Bone Marrow Aspirate	CBMA (Concentrated Bone Marrow Aspirate)
Cytarabine and Daunorubicin Liposome Antineoplastic	VYXEOS™
Defibrotide Sodium Anticoagulant	Defitelio
Durvalumab Antineoplastic	IMFINZI®
Eculizumab	Soliris®
Endothelial Damage Inhibitor	DuraGraft® Endothelial Damage Inhibitor
Esketamine Hydrochloride	SPRAVATO™
Fosfomycin Anti-infective	CONTEPO™ Fosfomycin injection
Gilteritinib Antineoplastic	XOSPATA®
High-Dose Intravenous Immune Globulin	GAMUNEX-C, for COVID-19 treatment hdIVIG (high -dose intravenous immunoglobulin), for COVID-19 treatment High-dose intravenous immunoglobulin (hdIVIG), for COVID-19 treatment Octagam 10%, for COVID-19 treatment

Continued →

Section X - New Technology - Character 6 - Device/ Substance/Technology	
Hyperimmune Globulin	Anti-SARS-CoV-2 hyperimmune globulin HIG (hyperimmune intravenous immunoglobulin), for COVID-19 treatment hIVIG (hyperimmune intravenous immunoglobulin), for COVID-19 treatment Hyperimmune intravenous immunoglobulin (hIVIG), for COVID-19 treatment IGIV-C, for COVID-19 treatment
Idecabtagene Vicleucel Immunotherapy	ABECMA® Ide-cel Idecabtagene Vicleucel
Imipenem-cilastatin-relebactam Anti-infective	IMI/REL
Interbody Fusion Device, Customizable in New Technology	aprevo™
Interbody Fusion Device, Nanotextured Surface in New Technology	nanoLOCK™ interbody fusion device
Interbody Fusion Device, Radiolucent Porous in New Technology	COALESCE® radiolucent interbody fusion device COHERE® radiolucent interbody fusion device
Intraluminal Device, Sustained Release Drug-eluting in New Technology	Eluvia™ Drug-Eluting Vascular Stent System SAVAL below-the-knee (BTK) drug-eluting stent system
Intraluminal Device, Sustained Release Drug-eluting, Four or more in New Technology	Eluvia™ Drug-Eluting Vascular Stent System SAVAL below-the-knee (BTK) drug-eluting stent system
Intraluminal Device, Sustained Release Drug-eluting, Three in New Technology	Eluvia™ Drug-Eluting Vascular Stent System SAVAL below-the-knee (BTK) drug-eluting stent system
Intraluminal Device, Sustained Release Drug-eluting, Two in New Technology	Eluvia™ Drug-Eluting Vascular Stent System SAVAL below-the-knee (BTK) drug-eluting stent system
Iobenguane I-131 Antineoplastic	AZEDRA® Iobenguane I-131, High Specific Activity (HSA)
Lefamulin Anti-Infective	XENLETA™
Lifileucel Immunotherapy	Lifileucel
Lisocabtagene Maraleucel Immunotherapy	Lisocabtagene Maraleucel
Lurbinectedin	ZEPZELCA™
Magnetically Controlled Growth Rod(s) in New Technology	MAGEC® Spinal Bracing and Distraction System Spinal growth rods, magnetically controlled

Section X - New Technology - Character 6 - Device/ Substance/Technology	
Meropenem-vaborbactam Anti-infective	Vabomere™
Mineral-based Topical Hemostatic Agent	Hemospray® Endoscopic Hemostat
Nerinitide	NA-1 (Nerinitide)
Nafamostat Anticoagulant	LTX Regional Anticoagulant Niyad™
Omadacycline Anti-infective	NUZYRA™
Other New Technology Therapeutic Substance	STELARA® Ustekinumab
Posterior (Dynamic) Distraction Device in New Technology	ApiFix® Minimally Invasive Deformity Correction (MID-C) System
Reduction Device in New Technology	Neovasc Reducer™ Reducer™ System
REGN-COV2 Monoclonal Antibody	Casirivimab (REGN10933) and Imdevimab (REGN10987) Imdevimab (REGN10987) and Casirivimab (REGN10933)
Remdesivir Anti-infective	GS-5734 Veklury
Ruxolitinib	Jakafi®
Sarilumab	KEVZARA®
Satralizumab-mwge	ENSPRYNG™
Skin Substitute, Porcine Liver Derived in New Technology	MIRODERM™ Biologic Wound Matrix
Synthetic Human Angiotensin II	Angiotensin II GIAPREZA™ Human angiotensin II, synthetic
Synthetic Substitute, Mechanically Expandable (Paired) in New Technology	SpineJack® system
Tagraxofusp-erzs Antineoplastic	ELZONRIS™
Terlipressin	TERLIVAZ®
Tisagenlecleucel Immunotherapy	KYMRIAH® Tisagenlecleucel
Tocilizumab	ACTEMRA®
Trilaciclib	COSELA™
Uridine Triacetate	Vistogard®
Venetoclax Antineoplastic	Venclexta®
Zooplastic Tissue, Rapid Deployment Technique in New Technology	EDWARDS INTUITY Elite valve system INTUITY elite valve system, EDWARDS Perceval sutureless valve Sutureless valve, Perceval

Appendix G: New ICD-10-PCS Codes FY2022

Appendix G is provided online in a format suitable for spreadsheet and/or database use. Go to http://ahimapress.org/casto8482/ click the "Online Resources" link, and enter case sensitive password AHIMAnRn9id2022 to download files.